The Retinal Pigment Epithelium

THE
RETINAL PIGMENT EPITHELIUM
Function and Disease

Edited by

MICHAEL F. MARMOR
Department of Ophthalmology
Stanford University School of Medicine

THOMAS J. WOLFENSBERGER
Hôpital Ophtalmique Jules Gonin
University of Lausanne

New York   Oxford
OXFORD UNIVERSITY PRESS
1998

Oxford University Press

Oxford   New York
Athens   Auckland   Bangkok   Bogota   Buenos Aires   Calcutta
Cape Town   Chennai   Dar es Salaam   Delhi   Florence   Hong Kong   Istanbul
Karachi   Kuala Lumpur   Madras   Melbourne   Mexico City   Mumbai
Nairobi   Paris   Singapore   Taipei   Tokyo   Toronto   Warsaw

and associated companies in
Berlin   Ibadan

Published by Oxford University Press, Inc.
198 Madison Avenue, New York, New York 10016

Oxford is a registered trademark of Oxford University Press

Library of Congress Cataloging-in-Publication Data
The retinal pigment epithelium: function and disease /
[edited by] Michael F. Marmor, Thomas J. Wolfensberger.
p. cm.   Includes bibliographical references and index.
ISBN 0-19-510956-2
1. Retina—Pathophysiology.   2. Retina—Physiology.   3. Epithelium.
I. Marmor, Michael F., 1941– .   II. Wolfensberger, Thomas J.
[DNLM: 1. Retinal Diseases.
2. Pigment Epithelium of Eye.   WW   270 R43853   1998]
RE551.R49   1998   617.47′35—dc21   DNLM/DLC   for Library of Congress   97-18098

987654321

Printed in the United States of America
on acid-free paper

Dedicated to
Roy H. Steinberg, M.D., Ph.D.
1935–1997

Roy Steinberg, who wrote the foreword for this book, died in 1997. He was a friend, mentor and collaborator of the editors and of many others who have worked on the RPE. He recognized early the physiologic importance of the RPE, which he promulgated through superb experimental studies and teaching. Roy is responsible, in no small measure, for current awareness of the roles of the RPE in retinal function and disease, and thus indirectly, for much of the contents of this book.

Foreword

It should be apparent to the reader who approaches the retinal pigment epithelium (RPE) for the first time by reading this volume that the RPE hosts an astonishing collection of functions, both known and hypothesized. The more informed reader will be heartened, I think, by how much the field has grown since the publication 18 years ago of the first version of this book. We now know considerably more about these functions and their roles in disease than we did then. For the expert, those few of us who have studied this tissue for many years, a touch of dissatisfaction may be appropriate. With all of our effort—new researchers enrolled, moneys spent, and knowledge earned—we still have much further to go to reach the understanding of normal and pathological RPE function necessary to prevent and to treat RPE and retinal diseases.

What needs to be done to achieve this end? Until now, we have been held back, I fear, by the overall difficulty in experimenting upon this tissue. It is quite rare, for instance, to find studies of the RPE in its intact condition, sandwiched as it is between the blood supply of the choriocapillaris and a functioning retina. In vitro, it has been nearly impossible to come close to the intact situation. In fact, our preparations are never anatomically complete, and tissue culture of the RPE, perhaps the most straightforward approach, leaves us uncertain about the significance of findings for the intact state. To achieve substantial breakthroughs in knowledge of normal and diseased function we will have to overcome such difficulties.

We must also direct our work to the most genuine problems of normal and diseased RPE function. This should come from defining exactly what the RPE does to support the photoreceptors and retina. We have been given the gift of knowing only two functions for which the needs of the photoreceptor are well documented—the phagocytosis of the tips of their outer segments and the transport of vitamin A and its cohorts to and from the retina. As for the remaining functions, we are much less certain about how significant they are for supporting normal photoreceptor and retinal activity. For instance, we acknowledge that water, salt, and metabolite transport across the RPE must be necessary to feed and cleanse the photoreceptors and retina, as well as to keep it adherent. Yet we must determine which of the myriad aspects of these functions are most vital. We can speculate about possible responses to messengers from retina that modify RPE activity, but what are these messengers and which activities do they modify, and to what end? Conversely, we imagine that trophic factors from RPE act on photoreceptors and cells deeper in the retina, both normally and in the healing of disease. Lastly, we consider it likely that new diseases will be discovered where the RPE is, itself, the source. These clues will lead us directly, I hope, to those areas of research that address the most authentic problems of normal and diseased RPE function.

More than 25 years ago I fell in love with the study of this tissue. The overview of knowledge provided by these chapters convinces me of the rightness of my attraction and more than sustains my current interest. The RPE remains one of a kind rare and beautiful in its complexity, yet so vital for vision. Surely, in the years ahead, we will use what we learn to prevent and cure blinding diseases. We can envision a pharmacology of the RPE, with drugs available to treat RPE disease or to modify RPE function to treat retinal disease. Indeed, the RPE may serve as the pathway through which drugs will enter the retina to protect and preserve its function. No doubt we shall read about all of this in subsequent renditions of this informative volume.

May 3, 1996   Roy H. Steinberg
Tassajara Hot Springs, Cal.

Preface

Nineteen years have passed since the first book devoted to the retinal pigment epithelium (RPE) was published (Zinn and Marmor (Eds.), *The Retinal Pigment Epithelium.* Cambridge, Harvard University Press, 1979). That book covered what was known at the time about the anatomy, physiology and disease of the RPE. These last two decades have seen a wealth of work on the RPE and the emergence of new scientific technology, especially in the area of molecular biology. In almost every major aspect of RPE function and disease, there is not only new knowledge but often a new perspective on the role of this vital tissue in health or disease.

With this explosion of information in mind, we undertook the organization of another book on the RPE. The information in the older book still stood as a foundation of knowledge about the RPE, but so many new topics and new elaborations of knowledge had emerged that it would have been unwieldy to try to cover them within the original framework of chapters. We felt that an entirely new book was needed—one that would build upon the old one, rather than be a second edition of it. Since many chapters now presume some knowledge about the RPE, we have added an Introduction to review the more fundamental properties and clinical science of the RPE and to put the chapters that follow in context.

The subtitle of this book, "Function and Disease," emphasizes our belief that knowledge about both is necessary to understand mechanisms of disease and to recognize the clinical implications of normal physiology. Rather than divide this book into one section on basic science and one on clinical science, as done in Zinn and Marmor (1979), we have organized the material into groups of chapters on major areas of RPE biology or clinical concern, such as "inherited disorders," "de-tachment and adhesion," "cellular growth and transplantation," and "aging and degeneration." In each grouping we include relevant basic and clinical information. For example, the chapter on regulation of immune responses by the RPE is juxtaposed with the chapter on RPE inflammations and infections. We hope this organization will foster and fertilize a bridging of information between basic and clinical scientists.

There are many to whom we owe a great debt of gratitude in making this book possible. Foremost are the contributors whose work is represented here. A number of colleagues contributed illustrations to the book, and they are acknowledged in the text. Jeffrey House, Vice President of Oxford University Press, recognized the scientific and clinical importance of this material. Charles Annis, the Production Editor, expertly shepherded the manuscript through to its published form. Judy Roberts at Stanford University handled, with her usual efficiency and precision, the complex administrative and secretarial work that accompanies a multi-authored work of this scope. We also thank Professors Claude Gailloud and Leonidas Zografos, Chairmen of the Jules Gonin Eye Hospital at the University of Lausanne, for providing TJW with freedom and support to work on the book.

We have dedicated this book to Professor Roy H. Steinberg, M.D., Ph.D., who was a ground-breaking pioneer in the field of RPE research and a contributor to the 1979 RPE book. Sadly, Roy passed away this summer, but the Foreword that he wrote last year remains as both a statement of the importance of what we know about the RPE, and a challenge to learn more.

November, 1997

M.F.M.
T.J.W.

Contents

VI. Cellular Growth and Transplantation

VII. Inflammation and Choroidal Disease

VIII. Exogenous Influences

IX. Aging and Degeneration

Contributors

GUSTAVO D. AGUIRRE, V.M.D., PH.D.
James A. Baker Institute for Animal Health
College of Veterinary Medicine
Cornell University
Ithaca, New York

DON H. ANDERSON, PH.D.
Neuroscience Research Institute
University of California, Santa Barbara
Santa Barbara, California

CAROLINE R. BAUMAL, M.D.
Department of Ophthalmology
Tufts University School of Medicine
Boston, Massachusetts

JOSEPH C. BESHARSE, PH.D.
Department of Cell Biology, Neurobiology, and Anatomy
Medical College of Wisconsin
Milwaukee, Wisconsin

ALAN C. BIRD, M.D.
Institute of Ophthalmology
Moorfields Eye Hospital
London, England

LAURIE BOST-USINGER, PH.D.
Bio-Rad Laboratories
Hercules, California

MICHAEL BOULTON, PH.D.
University Department of Ophthalmology
Manchester Royal Eye Hospital
Manchester, England

NEIL M. BRESSLER, M.D.
Wilmer Ophthalmological Institute
Johns Hopkins University School of Medicine
Baltimore, Maryland

SUSAN B. BRESSLER, M.D.
Wilmer Ophthalmological Institute
Johns Hopkins University School of Medicine
Baltimore, Maryland

JANICE M. BURKE, PH.D.
Department of Ophthalmology
The Eye Institute
Medical College of Wisconsin
Milwaukee, Wisconsin

BETH BURNSIDE, PH.D.
Department of Molecular and Cell Biology
University of California, Berkeley
Berkeley, California

PETER A. CAMPOCHIARO, M.D.
Wilmer Ophthalmological Institute
Johns Hopkins University School of Medicine
Baltimore, Maryland

GERALD J. CHADER, PH.D.
The Foundation Fighting Blindness
Hunt Valley, Maryland

JEFFERY G. COKER, B.S.
New England Eye Center
Tufts University School of Medicine
Boston, Massachusetts

ROSALIE K. CROUCH, PH.D.
Department of Ophthalmology
Medical University of South Carolina
Charleston, South Carolina

DENNIS M. DEFOE, PH.D.
Department of Anatomy and Cell Biology
James H. Quillen College of Medicine
East Tennessee State University
Johnson City, Tennessee

GRAIG E. ELDRED, PH.D.
Pelican Lake, Wisconsin

STEVEN K. FISHER, PH.D.
Neuroscience Research Institute
University of California, Santa Barbara
Santa Barbara, California

FREDERICK W. FITZKE, PH.D.
Institute of Ophthalmology
University College London
London, England

JOHN V. FORRESTER, PH.D.
Department of Ophthalmology
University of Aberdeen Medical School
Aberdeen, Scotland

RON P. GALLEMORE, M.D., PH.D.
Jules Stein Eye Institute
University of California at Los Angeles
Retina-Vitreous Associates
Los Angeles, California

PETER GOURAS, M.D.
Department of Ophthalmology
College of Physicians and Surgeons
Columbia University
New York, New York

DAVID R. GUYER, M.D.
Department of Ophthalmology
Cornell University Medical Center
Manhattan Eye, Ear and Throat Hospital
New York, New York

ROBYN H. GUYMER, M.D., PH.D.
Department of Ophthalmology
University of Melbourne
Royal Victorian Eye and Ear Hospital
East Melbourne, Australia

FARHAD HAFEZI, M.D.
Department of Ophthalmology
University Hospital
Zurich, Switzerland

GREGORY S. HAGEMAN, PH.D.
Department of Ophthalmology and Visual Sciences
University of Iowa Center for Macular Degeneration
University of Iowa Hospitals and Clinics
Iowa City, Iowa

MICHAEL O. HALL, PH.D.
Department of Ophthalmology
Jules Stein Eye Institute
University of California at Los Angeles
Los Angeles, California

PAUL HISCOTT, PH.D.
Unit of Ophthalmology
Department of Medicine
University of Liverpool
Liverpool, England

BRETT A. HUGHES, PH.D.
Departments of Ophthalmology and Physiology
W.K. Kellogg Eye Center
University of Michigan
Ann Arbor, Michigan

ALI A. HUSSAIN, PH.D.
Department of Ophthalmology
United Medical and Dental Schools
University of London
London, England

MARKUS H. KUEHN, M.S.
Department of Ophthalmology and Visual Sciences
University of Iowa Center for Macular Degeneration
University of Iowa Hospitals and Clinics
Iowa City, Iowa

JANET LIVERSIDGE, PH.D.
Department of Ophthalmology
University of Aberdeen Medical School
Aberdeen, Scotland

ANAT LOEWENSTEIN, M.D.
Department of Ophthalmology
Ichilov Hospital
Tel Aviv, Israel

SAM E. MANSOUR, M.D.
Department of Ophthalmology
Stanford University School of Medicine
Stanford, California

MICHAEL F. MARMOR, M.D.
Department of Ophthalmology
Stanford University School of Medicine
Stanford, California

JOHN MARSHALL, PH.D.
Department of Ophthalmology
United Medical and Dental Schools
University of London
London, England

ANDREAS MARTI, M.D.
Department of Ophthalmology
University Hospital
Zurich, Switzerland

FUTOSHI MARUIWA, M.D., PH.D.
Department of Ophthalmology
Miyazaki Medical College
Miyazaki, Japan

SHELDON S. MILLER, PH.D.
Department of Molecular and Cell Biology
    and School of Optometry
University of California, Berkeley
Berkeley, California

DAVID J. MOORE, PH.D.
Department of Ophthalmology
United Medical and Dental Schools
University of London
London, England

KURT MUNZ, M.D.
Laboratory of Retinal Cell Biology
Department of Ophthalmology
University Hospital
Zurich, Switzerland

ANN L. PATMORE, B.SC.
Department of Ophthalmology
United Medical and Dental Schools
University of London
London, England

DAVID R. PEPPERBERG, PH.D.
Department of Ophthalmology and Visual Sciences
College of Medicine
University of Illinois at Chicago
Chicago, Illinois

CARMEN A. PULIAFITO, M.D., M.B.A.
Department of Ophthalmology
Tufts University School of Medicine
Boston, Massachusetts

NARSING A. RAO, M.D.
Departments of Ophthalmology and Pathology
Doheny Eye Institute
University of Southern California School of Medicine
Los Angeles, California

JHARNA RAY, PH.D.
James A. Baker Institute for Animal Health
College of Veterinary Medicine
Cornell University
Ithaca, New York

JÖRG J. REINBOTH, M.D.
Department of Ophthalmology
University Hospital
Zurich, Switzerland

CHARLOTTE E. REMÉ, M.D.
Department of Ophthalmology
Laboratory of Retinal Cell Biology
University Hospital
Zurich, Switzerland

ARTURO SANTOS, M.D.
Centro Universitario de Ciencias de la Salud
University of Guadalajara
Guadalajara, Mexico

STEPHEN G. SCHWARTZ, M.D.
Department of Ophthalmology
New York University Medical Center
New York, New York

CARL M. SHERIDAN, MSC.
Unit of Ophthalmology
Department of Medicine
University of Liverpool
Liverpool, England

KENT W. SMALL, M.D.
Department of Ophthalmology
Jules Stein Eye Institute
University of California at Los Angeles
Los Angeles, California

RICHARD F. SPAIDE, M.D.
Department of Ophthalmology
New York Medical College
Manhattan Eye, Ear and Throat Hospital
New York, New York

CARLA STARITA, M.D.
Department of Ophthalmology
United Medical and Dental Schools
University of London
London, England

LAWRENCE E. STRAMM, PH.D.
Lilly Research Laboratories
Eli Lilly and Co.
Indianapolis, Indiana

ELIAS I. TRABOULSI, M.D.
Pediatric Ophthalmology and Strabismus
The Center for Genetic Eye Disease
Cleveland Clinic Eye Institute
Cleveland, Ohio

ANDREA VON RÜCKMANN, M.D.
Eye Hospital of the University of Giessen
Giessen, Federal Republic of Germany

BARBARA N. WIGGERT, PH.D.
Section on Biochemistry
Laboratory of Retinal Cell and Molecular Biology
National Eye Institute
National Institutes of Health
Bethesda, Maryland

THOMAS J. WOLFENSBERGER, M.D.
Hôpital Ophtalmique Jules Gonin
University of Lausanne
Lausanne, Switzerland

LAWRENCE YANNUZZI, M.D.
Department of Ophthalmology
Columbia University College of Physicians and Surgeons
Manhattan Eye, Ear and Throat Hospital
New York, New York

INTRODUCTION

Structure, function, and disease of the retinal pigment epithelium

MICHAEL F. MARMOR

The retinal pigment epithelium (RPE) is a unique tissue in the eye. It is derived embryologically from the same neural anlage as the sensory retina, but is differentiated into a secretory epithelium. It has no photoreceptive or neural functions, but it is necessary for the support and viability of the photoreceptors (see Chapter 2). It controls the neural environment, synthesizes growth factors, responds to humoral agents, and exhibits regenerative properties that can be helpful or harmful depending on the nature of the insult. Although it was recognized anatomically more than a century ago (see Chapter 1), its vital roles in the eye were largely unappreciated until the past few decades.

In a major compendium called *The Retinal Pigment Epithelium* that appeared in 1979, chapters were devoted to broad topics such as anatomy, biochemistry, and metabolism, as well as dystrophies and degenerations that involve the RPE. Over the past two decades, knowledge of the roles played by the RPE in the eye has become much more sophisticated. Research has focused on specific aspects of RPE function such as the elaboration of growth factors, the mechanisms of pigment migration, and the interaction of RPE with Bruch's membrane in the process of aging. We have organized this new compendium to present the knowledge that has accumulated on these specialized topics, and to integrate clinical information with the relevant basic science.

This introduction gives a brief overview of RPE structure, function, and disease as background for the chapters that follow. More extensive treatment of these fundamentals can be found in Zinn and Marmor (1979) and Soubrane (1995).

STRUCTURE AND FUNCTION OF THE RPE

Tables I-1 and I-2 list some of the major anatomic and functional characteristics of the RPE. The RPE is derived embryologically from the same neural tube tissue that forms the neurosensory retina. The early optic vesicle invaginates to form a cup, the inner layer of which becomes the neurosensory retina and the outer layer of which becomes the RPE. Although the neurosensory retina differentiates into several layers of neurons, the RPE remains a monolayer that takes on the characteristics of a secretory epithelium. The cells (Fig. I-1) are cuboidal in cross-section and hexagonal when viewed from above, and they are all joined near the apical side by tight junctions (zonula occludens) which block the free passage of water and ions. This junctional barrier forms one part of the blood–retinal barrier (the other being formed by the capillary endothelium of the intrinsic retinal vessels).

RPE cells are small (roughly 10–14 μ in diameter) in the macular region, but become flatter and broader (diameter up to 60 μ) toward the periphery. Since the density of photoreceptors also varies across the retina, the number of photoreceptors overlying each RPE cell remains roughly constant, in the range of 45 photoreceptors per RPE cell. This constancy may have physiologic relevance to the extent that each RPE cell is metabolically responsible for a variety of support functions to the overlying retina.

Each RPE cell (see Fig. I-1) is differentiated into an apical portion (facing the photoreceptors) and basal portion (on Bruch's membrane) (see Chapter 5). The apical side has numerous long microvilli which reach up between the outer segments to partially envelop them. The apical cytoplasm contains microfilaments and microtubules (see Chapter 3), and also the greatest concentration of melanin granules. The midportion contains the nucleus and synthetic machinery (golgi apparatus, endoplasmic reticulum, etc.), as well as digestive vesicles (lysosomes). The basal membrane has small convoluted infoldings that increase the surface area for absorption and secretion.

The RPE gets its name from the *melanin pigment* that is present within cytoplasmic granules called *melanosomes* (see Chapter 4). The RPE is the first tissue in the body to become pigmented, and melanogenesis continues to some degree throughout life. With aging, however, these granules begin to fuse with lysosomes and break down, and the elderly fundus typically appears less pigmented. The role of melanin in the eye remains

TABLE I-1. *Anatomic characteristics of the RPE*

Interphotoreceptor matrix—specialized cone and rod domains

Apical microvilli—differential sheathing of rods and cones

Tight junctions—zonula occludens

Cytoskeletal features—microtubules and microfilaments

Lysosomal structures—sometimes merged with other vesicles

Phagosomes and residual bodies

Melanosomes

Lipofuscin

Golgi apparatus and endoplasmic reticulum

Nuclear structures

Basal infoldings

Basement membrane—first layer of Bruch's membrane

Bruch's membrane—collagenous and elastic zones

---

somewhat speculative. The pigment absorbs stray light and minimizes scatter within the eye, which has theoretical optical benefits. However, visual acuity can be excellent even in very blond fundi, so the magnitude of this effect is unclear. Albino eyes lack melanin, but their poor acuity is a result of foveal aplasia rather than optical scatter. Fundus appearance can be misleading with respect to the RPE, since racial differences in fundus appearance are more a result of choroidal pigment than RPE pigment. Melanin serves as a free-radical stabilizer, and it can bind many toxins. However, when melanin binds retinotoxic drugs such as chloroquin and thioridazine, it is unclear whether the effect is beneficial (by removing the toxin) or harmful (by producing a reservoir).

Another RPE pigment, *lipofuscin*, accumulates gradually in RPE cells with age (see Chapter 33). It is an aging pigment throughout the nervous system, and its special significance within the eye remains to be determined. Lipofuscin can be detected even in children, and by old age most RPE cells are severely clogged with the golden autofluorescent pigment. Lipofuscin in the RPE is thought to be derived from outer segment lipids that have been ingested by the RPE, possibly representing membrane fragments that were damaged by light or oxidation and are thus poorly digestible. Because older eyes, which contain large amounts of lipofuscin, can show breakdown of the RPE, as evidenced by drusen formation, atrophy, and choroidal neovascularization (see Chapter 35), the question has been raised whether these degenerative changes are a result of lipofuscin accumulation (or at least whether the lipofuscin is a marker for cellular damage). This remains a hypothesis, however, since many elderly eyes have a considerable quantity of RPE lipofuscin, whereas relatively few have clinically significant macular degeneration. A lipofus-

cin-like substance accumulates in the RPE in several dystrophies, including Stargardt's disease (fundus flavimaculatus) and Best's vitelliform dystrophy.

RPE cells are packed with mitochondria and engage in oxidative metabolism. Enzymes are synthesized for a wide range of functions, including membrane transport, visual pigment metabolism (see Chapter 7), waste product digestion (see Chapter 8), and the elaboration of humoral and growth factors that help respond to and/or regulate the environment of the RPE and photoreceptors (see Chapter 23). The RPE also contributes to the formation and maintenance of the interphotoreceptor matrix (IPM), which is critical for retinal adhesion (see Chapters 18 and 19). Many of these metabolic functions are mediated through the cell membrane, which contains a large variety of receptors and channels for ions and metabolites. These receptors and the elaboration of

TABLE I-2. *Physiologic roles of the RPE*

Pigment functions
  Light adaptation and screening
  Detoxification and binding
  Lipofuscin accumulation
  Antigenic properties

Environment and metabolic control
  Blood–retinal barrier
  Transport of nutrients and ions
  Dehydration of subretinal space
  Synthesis of enzymes, growth factors, pigments
  Interaction with endocrine, vascular and proliferative factors

Visual pigment cycle
  Capture and storage of vitamin A
  Isomerization of all-trans to 11-cis vitamin A

Interphotoreceptor matrix and retinal adhesion
  Specialized matrix ensheathment of rods and cones
  Metabolic control of adhesion

Outer segment phagocytosis and aging
  Phagocytosis of outer segment tips
  Digestion and recycling of membrane material
  Aging effects: lipofuscin, drusen
  Deposits and alterations in Bruch's membrane

Electrical activity
  Responses to light-induced ionic changes: c-wave, fast oscillation
  Response to light-induced chemical signals: EOG
  Nonphotic responses to chemical agents

Repair and reactivity
  Repair and regeneration
  Immunologic interactions
  Scarring and pigment migration
  Modulation of fibrovascular proliferation

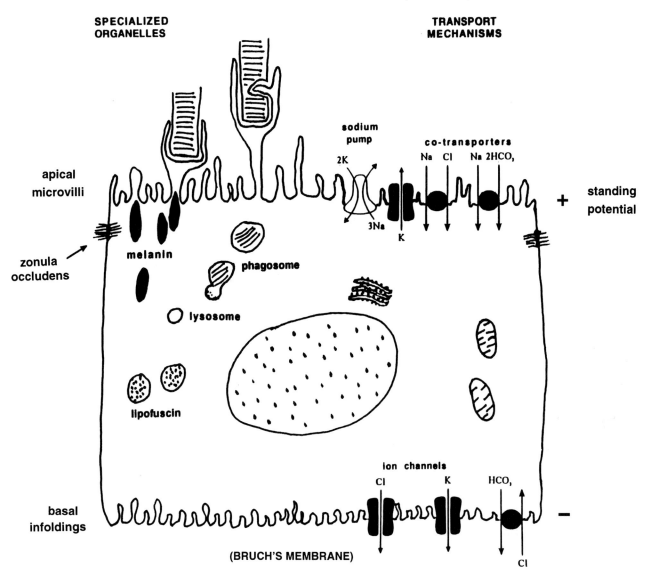

SPECIALIZED ORGANELLES

TRANSPORT MECHANISMS

FIGURE I-1. Idealized RPE cell showing the major anatomic and physiologic features.

humorally active agents are responsible for some of the immunologic properties of the RPE (see Chapter 26) that are relevant to a variety of inflammatory and idiopathic disorders (see Chapters 27 and 28).

The apical and basal membranes of the RPE cells are differentiated with respect to receptoral and ion channel properties (see Chapters 5 and 6). For example, the electrogenic sodium–potassium pump is present on the apical membrane, whereas the chloride–bicarbonate exchange transporter is on the basal membrane (Fig. I-1). The net effect of the pumps, facilitative transport systems, and passive ion channels is a movement of water across the RPE in the apical-to-basal direction, as well as the generation of a voltage difference (the standing potential) across the RPE (see Chapter 6). Stated differ-

ently, several transport systems are moving ions and water in either direction, but the sum of effects is a net movement of water in the retina-to-choroid direction. Thus, water transport could be altered equally well by blocking a transporter that moves ions in the basal direction, or stimulating a transporter that moves ions in the apical direction.

The ability of the RPE to transport water by active transport is very powerful, but passive mechanisms such as hydrostatic and osmotic pressure also work to drive water out of the subretinal space and into the choroid (see Chapter 21). If the RPE barrier is damaged, fluid will actually leave the subretinal space more *quickly* than under normal conditions. In other words, the tight junctions which serve to protect the neural environment of the retina also work, paradoxically, to make the removal of subretinal fluid more difficult—and in a sense it is the presence of these tight junctions that necessitates powerful active transport mechanisms (and the expenditure of metabolic energy to keep the subretinal space dehydrated). These physiologic interactions underlie the mechanisms of clinical serous detachments and central serous chorioretinopathy (see Chapters 21 and 22).

The RPE regulates and/or transports metabolites and nutrients such as glucose and amino acids (see Chapter 6). For example, the RPE absorbs taurine, which is essential to the photoreceptors, and selectively transports D-glucose but not L-glucose. Specialized membrane receptors bind necessary metabolites, required substances such as vitamin A, and many humoral agents such as epinephrine and dopamine. The RPE is being recognized increasingly as a source of growth factors, adhesion molecules, and other substances critical to cellular interaction (see Chapters 5, 18, and 23).

Although the RPE is not a photoreceptive cell, and generates no direct response to light, its membranes will respond electrically to chemical or ionic stimuli (see Chapters 9 and 10). Thus, it responds to local environmental changes that occur as a result of photoreception, and signals such as the light response of the standing potential (the electrooculogram) have been used as clinical diagnostic tests. Chemically induced electrical changes in the RPE have also been studied clinically.

Kühne and Boll demonstrated in 1877 that visual pigments regenerate to maintain the visual process, and that apposition of retina to RPE was required (see Chapter 1). After the initial isomerization of rhodopsin by light, the vitamin A moiety splits off from the opsin, and is carried by a transport protein to the RPE. In the RPE, the vitamin A may be stored in ester form, and is eventually reisomerized to 11-*cis* conformation which can be recombined with opsin (see Chapter 7). This regeneration process is presumed to be the site of pathology in fundus albipunctatus, in which visual pigment regeneration can take several hours instead of thirty minutes.

Another photoreceptor–RPE interaction concerns the process for photoreceptor outer segment renewal (see Chapter 8). Like skin, the photoreceptors are continually exposed to radiant energy (light) and oxygen (from the choroid), both of which facilitate the production of free radicals that can damage membranes over time (see Chapter 29). The outer segments could not last a lifetime without renewal, and every day upwards of 100 discs at the distal end of each photoreceptor are phagocytized by the RPE, while new discs are synthesized. This phagocytosis process follows to some degree a circadian rhythm, with rods shedding discs most vigorously in the morning at the onset of light, and cones

more vigorously at the onset of darkness. The phagocytized disc material becomes encapsulated in vesicles called phagosomes, which merge with lysosomes to facilitate digestion. This is an impressive metabolic task for the RPE, since each cell must ingest and digest more than four thousand discs daily. Normally, critical fatty acids are retained for recycling and waste products are egested across the basal RPE membrane, but some of this membranous material may persist as residual bodies within the RPE cell and contribute to the formation of lipofuscin. Although a strain of rats (RCS) which lacks RPE phagocytosis shows early degeneration of the retina (see Chapter 13), a human disease of phagocytosis has yet to be identified. In retinitis pigmentosa, histologic studies have shown shortened rather than lengthened outer segments.

The RPE is critically involved in the maintenance of retinal adhesion (and thus resistance to retinal detachment). Retinal adhesion is a complex process, which involves several complementary and interactive mechanisms (see Chapter 19). There are passive systems such as the vitreous gel, intraocular fluid pressure, and choroidal osmotic pressure which help keep the retina in place. However, there is also a very strong dependence on metabolic activity, as evidenced by a variety of experiments that show that metabolic blockers or oxygen deprivation lead rapidly to a failure of adhesive strength. The likely basis of these metabolic effects is water transport across the RPE, which controls the hydration and local environment of the subretinal space. The mediator for these effects, and itself a critical element for retinal adhesion, is the interphotoreceptor matrix (IPM).

The IPM was once viewed as merely a viscous filler, composed of proteins, glycosaminoglycans, and other large molecules. However, recent studies have shown that the IPM is a highly structured material with chemically independent domains surrounding the rods and the cones (see Chapter 18). The matrix material bonds firmly to both the outer limiting membrane and the apical membrane of the RPE. The matrix sheaths can be seen to stretch enormously as retina is peeled from the RPE. The bonding properties and viscosity of the IPM depend upon its hydration and its ionic environment, both of which are of course controlled metabolically by the RPE. The matrix also serves as the pathway for nutrients, retinoids, and other substances to cross the subretinal space, and it appears to be an important domain for the elaboration of receptoral and binding proteins that help control the photoreceptor environment.

Although central neural cells do not ordinarily migrate and regenerate, the RPE retains these functions as part of its epithelial character. Small injuries to the

RPE, such as a light laser burn, result in a defect that fills in over 1–2 weeks through migration of cells and through the proliferation of new small RPE cells which fill the cavity. This capacity for growth can have adverse effects, however, when RPE cells migrate into degenerating retina (e.g., in retinitis pigmentosa), or into the vitreous cavity as a component of proliferative vitreoretinopathy (see Chapter 24). The multiplicity of growth and control factors elaborated by the RPE appear under normal conditions to prevent unwanted vascular ingrowth and to promote desirable local healing (see Chapter 23). Under the stress of disease, these same factors may contribute to abnormal vascularization or scarring. As these growth factor interactions become better understood, they offer new avenues of therapy for a variety of serious retinal disorders.

CLINICAL ROLES OF THE RPE

The RPE is involved in many retinal disorders, if for no other reason than that its ability to scar (with hyperpigmentation or depigmentation) is often responsible for the visible manifestations of disease. As the physiologic functions of the RPE become better understood, as outlined above, we are also realizing that the RPE is intimately involved in the pathophysiology of many disorders that were viewed previously as purely choroidal or retinal. Several categories of RPE disease are presented in this book, in part to group together disorders that have similar pathophysiology, but also to allow the juxtaposition of clinical information with relevant basic science.

A number of diagnostic tools exist for evaluation of the RPE. An electrophysiologic test, the electrooculogram (EOG) has been performed clinically for many years, and it is often overinterpreted as a specific test of RPE function (see Chapter 10). That view is too optimistic, since the EOG depends upon the retina (which receives the light) as much as the RPE. The EOG and other electrophysiological responses are now recognized to represent specific voltage changes in the apical or basal RPE membranes (see Chapter 9), but the clinical significance of EOG abnormalities are very poorly understood. The response is severely abnormal only in Best's vitelliform dystrophy, although retinal appearance and function in this disease may be normal throughout most of the eye. It is also possible to stimulate the RPE membranes in the absence of light (i.e., independent from retina), using chemical stimuli such as hyperosmolarity or acetazolamide (see Chapter 10). Unfortunately, these electrical tests, which are all mass responses, have yet to be correlated with specific RPE functions such as retinoid transport or outer segment phagocytosis.

At the other end of the diagnostic spectrum lie imaging techniques which show focal changes. These tests are also hard to correlate with physiological abnormalities, but they can identify local pathologic change. Ophthalmic ultrasound does not discriminate RPE from choroid, but RPE pathology is well demarcated by fluorescein angiography as areas of either hyperfluorescence (depigmentation) or hypofluorescence (hyperpigmentation). Fluorescein angiograms are illustrated in many of the clinical chapters. Optical coherence tomography is a new technique that allows visualization of the RPE layer in the living eye (see Chapter 12), and may show thickening or defects of the RPE under conditions of edema or hemorrhage that make the RPE hard to visualize directly. The scanning laser ophthalmoscope is a powerful tool for in vivo fundus imaging, and can be configured to detect the fluorescence of dyes or natural pigments. For example, autofluorescence from lipofuscin can be visualized (see Chapter 11) to allow correlation with macular degeneration or dystrophic processes (such as fundus flavimaculatus and vitelliform dystrophy).

The RPE is involved in a wide variety of congenital, inherited, and metabolic disorders, although few have been defined in terms of specific cellular dysfunction at the level of the RPE. Congenital abnormalities of the RPE (see Chapter 15) include albinism and congenital hypertrophy of the RPE, which must be distinguished from the pigmentary changes in Gardner's syndrome (intestinal polyposis). Animal models have contributed greatly to our understanding of these hereditary dysfunction syndromes (see Chapters 13 and 14). Retinitis pigmentosa gets its name because of pigment migration from the RPE, but the genes which have been identified so far all represent photoreceptor outer segment proteins (see Chapter 17). One important caveat from new knowledge about the genetics of retinal disease is that the classical attempt to dichotomize disease into retinal or pigment epithelial can be misleading. Retinal degeneration may occur because abnormal proteins lead to death of the outer segments—but it may also occur because abnormal outer segments cause damage to the RPE after they are phagocytized and digested. In this scenario, the subsequent metabolic damage to the RPE may lead to changes that secondarily cause photoreceptor death. These same arguments can apply equally well to diseases thought classically to represent RPE dysfunction (see Chapter 16). Stargardt's disease is characterized histopathologically by an accumulation of lipofuscin-like material throughout the RPE, but the recently isolated gene codes for a lipid transporter in the rod outer segments. In some manner not yet understood, the photoreceptor abnormality indirectly drives the accumulation of abnormal material in the RPE.

The management of retinal detachment has traditionally involved surgical or laser therapy that is designed to tack the retina back in place or seal the conduits that are leaking fluid into the subretinal space. With newer understanding of how the RPE controls fluid movement in and out of the subretinal space, modulates the retinal adhesive process, and responds to retinal separation or reattachment (see Chapter 20), it may be possible to prevent certain types of detachment and to treat others with the therapy that enhances the natural mechanisms of adhesion. This physiologic knowledge has allowed reevaluation of the pathophysiology of some detachment disorders. For example, central serous chorioretinopathy is now recognized to involve broad areas of choroidal and RPE dysfunction that seem to represent the primary pathologic process (see Chapters 21 and 22).

The potential importance of RPE growth factors in retinal scarring and proliferative vitreoretinopathy has already been noted (see Chapter 24). It may eventually be possible to modulate these factors therapeutically (e.g., with antibodies) and thus attack directly the cause of proliferative disorders. Understanding the factors which control RPE growth and proliferation (see Chapter 18) is also central to effective RPE transplantation. It is technically feasible now to transplant RPE cells or sheets of RPE into donor eyes (see Chapter 25), but much work yet remains to make this a safe and reliable enough procedure that it can be done early in age-related or dystrophic disease before permanent retinal dysfunction has taken place.

The RPE is involved in many inflammatory, infectious, and ischemic choroidal diseases, including uveitis and the multifocal chorioretinopathy syndromes (see Chapters 27 and 28). In some of these the RPE may simply be a passive responder to pathology elsewhere. However, its role may also be more direct and critical. Choroidal ischemia or inflammation will have relatively little effect upon the retina unless or until the RPE decompensates above the areas of pathology to allow fluid entry, neovascularization, or metabolic change. The RPE may be antigenically involved in some of the inflammatory syndromes, and it appears clinically to be close to the site of primary disease in many of the multifocal chorioretinopathy syndromes. Understanding how the RPE is affected by and regulates immune responses (see Chapter 26) and responds to local ischemia or metabolic dysfunction will be critical to ultimately understanding and treating these disorders.

The retina is exposed to a lifetime of radiant energy,

and a good portion of this energy is absorbed by the RPE. Light damage to the retina and RPE can be produced very readily in experimental animals, which has raised concern about light as a factor in chronic disorders such as age-related macular degeneration (see Chapter 29). So far, human epidemiologic studies have not given much support to this hypothesis but we may not yet know how to monitor the types of light exposure that are most critical to the human eye. Sunlight effects may be indirect, insofar as the absorption of light creates heat, and even very small changes in retinal temperature can have major metabolic consequences. While low-intensity light is of uncertain pathologic significance in man, high-intensity light (e.g., laser burns) create thermal or other types of tissue damage and play an important role in the therapy of many retinal disorders (see Chapter 30). With new laser techniques it is possible to control the wavelength of incidental light, to limit damage specifically to retinal or RPE tissues, and to choose between thermal or nonthermal tissue-disruptive modes. It remains to be shown how these newer refinements will aid in the management of specific diseases.

The RPE is also affected by many drugs and toxins, which can modulate the various biochemical and physiologic processes outlined above, or damage the tissue metabolically. Studies in the past decade have shown that the RPE contains receptors for a surprising number of humoral agents, including adrenergic receptors, dopaminergic receptors, binding proteins for retinoids and nutrients, hormonal receptors, and binding proteins for adhesion molecules and growth factors (see Chapter 31). Consideration of the toxicology of the RPE similarly involves responses to agents that are toxic generally to all cells, and agents that have a rather specific effect on the RPE, such as thioridazine, chloroquin, and sodium iodate (see Chapter 32). The first two agents are drugs in clinical practice which cause severe visual disability, and it has long been debated whether the propensity of these agents to bind melanin enhances their toxicity or represents a beneficial effect of the RPE in removing the toxins from circulation. Sodium iodate is a general metabolic toxin which nevertheless causes rapid and severe decompensation of the RPE before serious effects on the retina appear. This property has made it a useful drug in the experimental modeling of RPE damage and disease. RPE transport systems can play a role in the management of drugs. For example, fluorescein is actively transported in a retina-to-choroid direction by the RPE, as are other large, acidic molecules such as penicillin. Much remains to be learned about the role of the RPE in maintaining a healthy chemical environment for the photoreceptors.

Finally, the RPE is an integral component of the process of aging within the retina and choroid. Outer segment debris must be metabolically managed by the RPE over a lifetime, and a putative waste product (lipofuscin) accumulates massively in the RPE of older eyes (see Chapter 33). It remains to be determined whether this lipofuscin itself damages the RPE, or whether it is simply a marker for structural or metabolic changes that are taking place in the photoreceptors of the RPE as a part of the aging process (see Chapter 35). In some eyes there is gradual atrophy of the RPE; in others one finds the formation of drusen of various types (that represent in most cases an extrusion of abnormal material from the RPE into different layers of Bruch's membrane). Gradual dysfunction of Bruch's membrane may interfere with the movement of fluid and metabolites to the RPE and retina, and secondarily cause RPE and retinal dysfunction or degeneration (see Chapter 34). Depend-ing on the nature and severity of the RPE and Bruch's membrane damage, the clinical results can range from atrophy, to serous detachment of RPE and/or retina that often involves neovascularization (fibrovascular ingrowth) and threatens a rapid loss of vision (see Chapter 36). Since age-related macular degeneration now represents the major cause of visual disability in the older population of the Western world (see Chapter 37), understanding and preventing these mechanisms represents one of the major public health challenges of our time.

REFERENCES

Soubrane G. (Ed). 1995. Affections acquises de l'épithélium pigmentaire rétinien. Paris: Bull des Sociétés d'Ophtalmologie de France.
Zinn K, Marmor MF. (Eds). 1979. The Retinal Pigment Epithelium. Cambridge (MA): Harvard University Press.

HISTORY AND EVOLUTION OF THE RETINAL PIGMENT EPITHELIUM

1. The historical discovery of the retinal pigment epithelium

THOMAS J. WOLFENSBERGER

During antiquity anatomical knowledge of the retina and its surrounding structures was limited to a few vague ideas. General interest in the transparent vascularised tissue was small and its role was seen as carrying nourishment to the vitreous and the lens, which was considered the visual receptor. This view seemed to satisfy most scholars, and centuries passed with no real attempt to clarify the more fundamental role of the retinal tissues. Even the founders of modern anatomy such as Eustachius, Fallopius, and Vesalius did not consider this an important issue. Although Averroës (1126–1198), the Spanish Moor who wrote extensively on optics, suggested that the retina and not the lens was the visual organ (Münchow 1984), it was not until the early 17th century that Kepler demonstrated with his optical studies the crucial role of the retina in photoreception. Despite these astute observations, characterization of retinal morphology was impossible due to the lack of histological techniques. These became available only at the end of the 17th century when Leeuwenhoek got a first glimpse of "globular bodies" in the frog retina through his improvised microscope. These were presumably cellular elements, probably rods and cones. Since the retinal pigment epithelium is an even thinner layer of cells than the retina and thus cannot be distinguished from the choroid by the naked eye, the discovery of its morphology of necessity was also linked to the advent of the microscope. Thus the earliest known accounts of the histology of the retinal pigment epithelium appeared in the second half of the 18th century. We will start our historical journey, however, with a short account of the discovery of the "netlike structure" since the retinal pigment epithelium is almost inextricably intertwined with the retina—etymologically, morphologically, and functionally speaking. To see the development of anatomical concepts over a period of almost 2000 years will enhance our understanding of the difficulties that arose in the wake of the discovery of the retinal pigment epithelium as a separate entity.

FROM THE RETINA TO THE RETINAL PIGMENT EPITHELIUM: TWO MILLENNIA OF STATUS QUO

Although Aristotle and other Greek scholars were mostly concerned with the outer aspects of the eye, Hippocrates (c.460–c.377 B.C.) described several layers that make up the inner parts of the eye in his treatises "De carnibus" and "De locis in homine." His words were: "There are three coats that protect the eye, a thick outer, a thinner middle and an extremely thin inner coat that protects the fluid." Hippocrates described the innermost coat as thin and transparent, naming it ἀραχνοειδής (arachnoides). This layer lies immediately adjacent to the vitreous, which he called ὑγρόν (to igron) (Fig. 1-1). Knowledge of the inner parts of the globe was rudimentary at that time and stemmed primarily from the observation of eyes that had received severe trauma (Magnus 1878). The hippocratic tradition was expanded by the school of anatomy at Alexandria, where the famous anatomists Erasistratus and Herophilus taught. They provided the first real concept of ocular anatomy; it was not until Zinn (1755) wrote his seminal work that another textbook containing original observations of ocular anatomy was published. Because of the macroscopic resemblance of the ocular tissue to a fishnet, Herophilus (around 300 B.C.) coined the name ἀμφιβληστροειδής (amphiblestroides) (from ἀμφιβαλλειν amphiballein = to throw around), alluding to a net that is thrown around fish. He described its topography as surrounding the vitreous and reaching all the way to the lens with which it finally fuses. Rufus of Ephesus similarly wrote in his treatise "On Naming the Parts of the Human Body": "The third coat of the eye surrounds the glasslike fluid and is compared because of its thinness to a spiderweb. Herophilus, however, compared it to a fishnet and therefore some physicians call it the 'net-like coat'. Others call it the glassy membrane because of the fluid it surrounds." Rufus also mentioned in his Liber 2 that the retina has its own vascular system. Unfortunately, we do

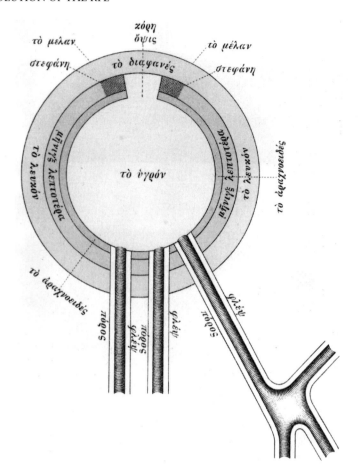

FIGURE 1-1. The eye according to Hippocrates. There are three layers: a thick outer, a thinner middle, and a very thin and transparent inner layer that is immediately adjacent to the vitreous. This innermost layer was termed ἀραχνοειδής, arachnoides. (From Magnus, 1878.)

not have any genuine illustrations of the anatomy of the eye from ancient Greece.

Celsus (25 B.C.–A.D. 50) borrowed the description of a netlike structure from Herophilus, but it was Galen of Pergamum (A.D. 129–c.199), the most important figure after Hippocrates, who summarized the anatomical knowledge gathered to that point and annotated it with his own interpretations. The term *amphiblestroides* was again used by Galen in his manuscript *De usu partium corporis*. He described the retina as part of the brain that merges with the lens and concludes that its function was the registration of changes in the crystalline body and the transmission of these changes to the brain. Here ancient and modern ideas meet for a moment. Galen also suggested a role for the retina in the nourishment of the vitreous and rightly described the abundance of arteries and veins. He called the choroid χοροειδής (*choroides*) and thought it was involved in the nutrition of the retina as well as the reflection of light back to the lens where the image was formed (Fig. 1-2).

As the very strong movement of Islamic ophthalmology emerged in the tenth century, diseases of the retina were discussed by Ibn Muhammad-al-Tabari, who thought they were due to "dyscrasia or to separation of component parts." Similarly, diseases of the choroid were described and interpreted as a wrong mixture of fluids. The anatomy of the eye in the Islamic world, however, was viewed in terms of the concepts laid down by Galen since Islam did not allow the dissection of dead bodies. Avicenna (980–1037) called the retina *rescheth* (netlike), explaining that the retina encloses the vitreous and lens as the fishnet holds the catch. Gerard of Cremona (1114–1187), the medieval scholar who spent most of his life making Latin translations of Islamic texts in Toledo, translated Avicenna's work and used the Latin word *retina*. The term has stayed with us for more than 800 years.

During the Middle Ages in Europe anatomical understanding of the eye followed the tradition of the Arabs or of Galen. Around 1150 Benevenutus Grapheus

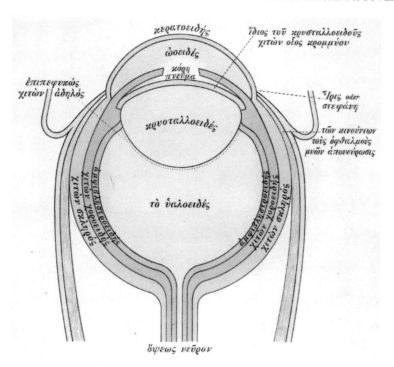

FIGURE 1-2. The eye according to Galen of Pergamum. He describes the retina as part of the brain and calls it ἀμφιβληστροειδής *(amphiblestroides)*. He concluded that the function of the retina was the registration of changes in the crystalline body and the transmission of these changes to the brain. The choroid was called χοροειδής *(choroides)*; it was thought to play a role in the nutrition of the retina and in the reflection of light back to the lens where the image was formed. (From Magnus, 1878.)

of Jerusalem published a book on the treatment of ophthalmic diseases, but without adding anything new to the body of anatomical knowledge. Since little changed until the 16th or 17th century, it has often been assumed that real progress in ophthalmology ceased after Galen. The excellent Belgian anatomist Andreas Vesalius (1514–1564) was the first to dissect humans in almost two millenia (since the School of Alexandria in 300 B.C.), but his contributions to ocular anatomy were small. It wasn't until 1689 that Antoni van Leeuwenhoek (1632–1723) used his newly invented microscope to investigate the eye and discover some of the cellular components of the retina. The introduction of the microscope into the scientific world thus paved the way for fruitful discoveries about the retina (Zinn, 1755) and later the retinal pigment epithelium.

Most observations regarding the pigmented layers in the back of the eye during the next 100 years were made by peeling away different layers of the globe. Naturally, the distinctions between the layers known today were very difficult to make and many reports remained speculative. One of the most prominent scientists of that era was Frederic Ruysch (1638–1731) from Amsterdam (Fig. 1-3). In *Thesaurus Anatomicus,* published in 1702, he described choroidal vessels as seen with the new technique of intravascular injection. From his descriptions the expression *membrana* or *tunica Ruyschiana* was later coined to denote the inner lamella of the choroid, most probably including the RPE and what is known today as Bruch's membrane. This distinction arose since the choroid was peeled off in two layers, *lamina externa* and *lamina interna,* before one could gain access to the retina. This multilayer concept was confirmed a few years later by Jacques Winslow, who wrote in his "Exposito Anatomica Structurae Corporis Humani," of "the choroid having two layers and on the inside a layer of pigment. The choroid is adherent to the retina in this entire area. Usually it is maintained that the retina is the product of the optic nerve substance, the choroid is derived from the arachnoid and the sclera from the dura of the optic nerve." Lorenz Heister subscribed to the same idea in his *Anatomie de Heister* (1735), in which he referred to "the choroid whose internal layer is called the membrane of Ruysch, and one finds a blackish color" (author's translation). Johann Gottfried Zinn (1727–1759) voiced the same concept in his seminal work *Descriptio Anatomica Oculi Humani* (1755). He described the inner surface of the choroid as having a thin layer of black pigment whose thickness decreases in old age. In all these descriptions mention is made of pig-

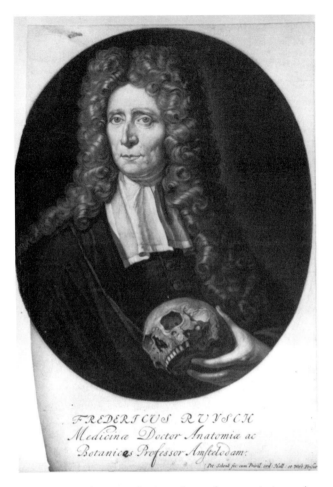

FIGURE 1-3. Frederic Ruysch was professor of anatomy in Amsterdam and distinguished himself with the development of a technique for vascular injection which led to novel insights into vascular distribution and structures. He described the tunica Ruyschiana which comprised at the time the inner lamella of the choroid (presumably with Bruch's membrane and the RPE adherent). (Courtesy Wellcome Institute Library, London.)

ment, although the source of it is assigned to the choroid exclusively. Similarly, the great physiologist and natural scientist Albrecht von Haller (1708–1777) described this pigment as a sort of inorganic mucus: "I see often large black flecks which adhere to the retinal tissue in the human, the bird, and the horse. In the fish these areas form on the surface of the membrane and cover the whole retina" (Haller, 1763—author's translation).

FOCUS ON THE RETINAL PIGMENT EPITHELIUM: THE HISTOLOGY EMERGES

The first real microscopical descriptions of the retinal pigment epithelium date from the end of the 18th century, when the anatomist Carlo Mondini of Bologna de-

scribed the RPE not as a mere mucus or varnish, as was generally believed, but as "a real membrane formed of innumerable globules which make up an excessively delicate network":

If a portion of the membrane composing the pigment be examined with the microscope, it appears composed of small oblong bodies, analogous to globules, which are rendered more or less opaque by the presence of a multitude of small black points, and are more transparent towards the bottom of the eye than on the sides, and still less on the ciliary processes; they are joined together by a very delicate cellular tissue. If a more powerful lens is employed, it is distinctly perceived that each globule is formed of black points, more numerous at its circumference than at the centre. On the posterior surface of the iris they are superposed, one above the other, so as to form two layers—hence the deeper tint of the black colour in this part. With regard to the chemical nature of the black particles, they chiefly consist of carbon and the black oxide of iron. (Mondini, 1790)

Mondini's work was then continued by his son Michele, who elaborated on the findings of his father in 1818 (Mondini, 1818), however, these studies were not pursued any further.

The issue was complicated by the discovery of the Irishman Arthur Jacobs (1790–1874) (Fig. 1-4a) who described the *membrana Jacobi* in human tissue (Jacobs, 1819). By doing so, Jacobs also unknowingly described fragments of the retinal pigment epithelium. This membrane consisted—according to him—of the layer of rods and cones as an individual membrane:

I find that the retina is covered on its external surface by a delicate transparent membrane, united to it by cellular substances and vessels . . . the choroid coat should be gently torn open and turned down, if the exposed surface be now carefully examined, an experienced eye may perceive, that this is not the appearance usually presented by the retina; instead of the blue-white reticulated surface of that membrane, a uniform villous structure, more or less tinged by a black pigment, presents itself. . . . This membrane covers the retina from the optic nerve to the ciliary body. The membrane is also attached to the choroid coat, apparently by fine cellular substance and vessels, but its connection with the retina being stronger, it generally remains attached to that membrane though small portions are sometimes pulled off with the choroid coat." (Jacobs, 1819)

He also adds that "in old eyes this membrane is nearly as dark as the choroid." In a second publication (1822) Jacobs reiterated his observations concerning the membrane and illustrated it as colorless (Fig. 1-4b). These two publications caused widespread discussion in the early 19th century since there also seemed to be some confusion about the exact terminology of the described structures. Ernst Wilhelm von Brücke wrote in 1847 in

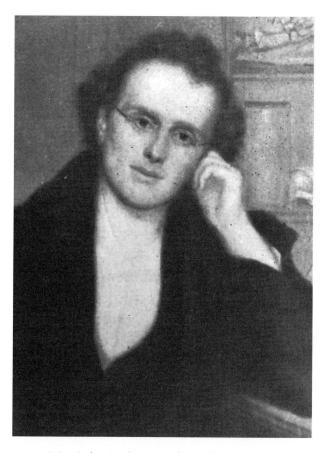

FIGURE 1-4a. Arthur Jacobs was professor of anatomy and physiology to the Royal College of Surgeons in Ireland for 41 years. He was also the first Irish ocular pathologist and described the layer of rods and cones which was named after him.

semitransparent retina; hence we perceive that a part of the functions heretofore assigned by physiologists to the choroid must belong to the membrane of Jacob [or the RPE as we now know]" (Knox, 1826).

The first paper solely devoted to the RPE in its correct morphological sense appeared in 1833 by Thomas Wharton Jones (Fig. 1-5a, 1-5b) in the *Edinburgh Medical and Surgical Journal* (Wharton Jones, 1833). He investigated the tissue of humans, cattle, horse, and sheep and described the epithelium as the "Pigmentum Nigrum, a dark coloured matter that is found . . . on the inner surface of the choroid where it has a very uniform character." In his publication we find an extensive history of the above-mentioned confusion that reigned at that time within the anatomical circles on what really lay between the retina and the choroid. His own description of the RPE then goes as follows: "When . . . the retina is removed, the inner surface of the choroid is found covered by a dark-coloured matter, which may be detached in small pieces. This matter is of a brown colour in the human eye, except over the tapetum in the ox where it is almost transparent. This is what is commonly called the tapetum nigrum." He then added a crucial statement. "But, according to my observations, it is a continuous and curiously organised membrane—

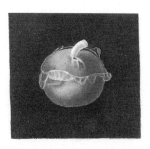

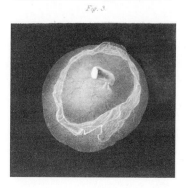

FIGURE 1-4b. Illustration from Arthur Jacobs's second publication in 1822, showing the technique by which he had come to strip the globe from the sclera and the different layers of the choroid arriving at the outer retina in man *(top)* and in sheep *(bottom)*. (Courtesy Wellcome Institute Library, London.)

his anatomical description of the human eyeball: "According to Bidder's proposal [Bidder 1839] we call the layer of the rods and cones usually membrana Jacobi. Hannover [Hannover 1840] objects justifiably against this terminology because 'the name membrana Jacobi has also frequently been used for the pigment epithelium and by some authors even for the ciliary part of the retina. Arthur Jacobs did not know anything about the morphologic elements of this membrane, nor could he at the then state of the arts known anything about them. He apparently had the layer of rods and cones partly with, partly without the pigment epithelium in mind'." Further confusion was created by the Scot Robert Knox, conservator of the Museum of the Royal College of Surgeons in Edinburgh, who seems to have referred to the retinal pigment epithelium as the membrana Jacobi. Although this mixing up of names was unfortunate, Knox's anatomical description was quite astute. He wrote, "The membrane of Jacobi is generally of a brownish colour and sufficiently opaque to arrest the rays of light, supposing them to have passed through the

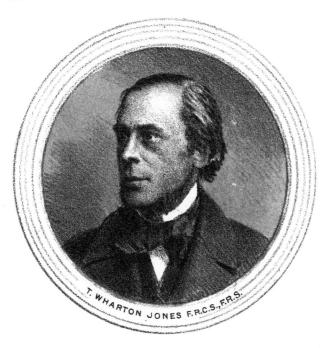

FIGURE 1-5a. Thomas Wharton Jones, fellow of the Royal College of Surgeons and distinguished fellow of the Royal Society, graduated from University College Hospital in London and practiced medicine in London until the second half of the 19th century. (Courtesy Wellcome Institute Library, London.)

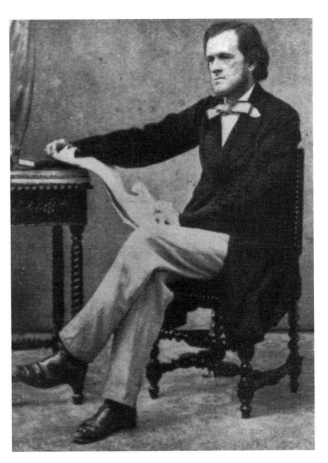

FIGURE 1-6. Carl Ludwig Wilhelm Bruch was born in Mainz and worked at the University of Heidelberg. His seminal work *Untersuchungen zur Kenntniss des körnigen Pigments der Wirbelthiere* was published in Zurich in 1844. He then became professor of anatomy and physiology in Basel and later moved to Giessen in Germany.

the seat of the pigment, but not the pigment itself, which I shall therefore call the membrane of the pigment." (emphasis in original) He then looked at the spread-out and flattened tissue under magnification: "If a portion of this membrane be examined by the aid of the microscope, it is seen to consist of very minute plates, of an hexagonal form, accurately joined together by their edges, in which plates are deposited numerous black particles, which are to be considered as properly constituting the pigment, but not essential to the hexagonal plates composing the membrane; because these may and

ART. IX.—*Notice relative to the* Pigmentum Nigrum *of the Eye.* By Thomas Wharton Jones, Esq. Surgeon.

The *Pigmentum Nigrum* of the eye is that dark-coloured matter which is found on the posterior surface of the *iris,* on the ciliary processes, and on the inner surface of the choroid.

In these different places it does not present the same characters, having on the inner surface of the choroid the appearance of a thin and uniform layer, whilst behind the *iris* and on the ciliary processes, it occurs in greater quantity, particularly in the eyes of the horse, ox, &c. in which it is so loosely contained

FIGURE 1-5b. In 1833 Wharton Jones published the first paper entirely dedicated to the retinal pigment epithelium in the *Edinburgh Medical and Surgical Journal.* He clearly distinguished an epithelial layer of cells, cells filled with small dark pigment granules in normal but not in albino eyes.

do exist without the black particles." He corroborated his hypothesis by examining albino tissue and discovered that "the colouring matter is certainly absent, but. . . . I have found the membrane of the pigment to exist." He further added, "The hexagonal cells appear to be united together by means of mucous or cellular tissue, which is easily torn by a little traction, so that the fragments of the membrane always present a serrated edge, the angles being those of hexagons." He also noted that the pigmented layer ceases to possess the hexagonal structure behind the ciliary processes and the posterior surface of the iris, and that the cells composing the membrane of the pigment are observable in the fetus. These astute observations were later supported by findings of Filipo Pacini in Pisa (Pacini, 1845), who published a new concept of an eight-layered histology of the retina with a correct description of the RPE.

So, after many centuries the interface between retina and choroid had finally been described and characterized. Well, almost. Enter Carl Ludwig Wilhelm Bruch (1819–1884) (Fig. 1-6). In 1844 he published his seminal work *Untersuchungen zur Kenntniss des körnigen Pigments der Wirbelthiere,* in which he described the tapetum of mammals, which had hitherto received little notice, as well as the "structureless membrane" subsequently known by his name. With the techniques available at that time its demonstration was a major achievement, as it involved removing the RPE with a fine brush and then scraping the membrane off horizontally. Further knowledge of Bruch's membrane was later provided by the findings of A.E. Smirnow (1899) who divided it into an outer elastic (mesodermal) layer and an inner cuticular (ectodermal) layer, which represents the basement membrane of the RPE. Thickening of this layer in the form of "colloid" bodies, which were later to be known as drusen, is almost invariable after the age of 30 years as subsequently described by L. Loewenstein (1940).

FROM THE RETINA TO THE RETINAL PIGMENT EPITHELIUM: LESSONS IN EMBRYOLOGY

At around the same time that Wharton Jones published his first extensive work on the morphology of the retinal pigment epithelium, new knowledge on the embryology of the RPE started to become available. The hotly disputed issue then was the fate of the outer layer of the optic vesicle. It was generally agreed that the inner layer developed into the retina, but many scholars believed that the stratum pigmentum of the retina developed from the choroid and was thus of mesodermal origin. This view was chiefly promulgated by Emil Huschke, who published his studies on the development of the chick embryo and the eye in 1835. He saw that the optic vesicle was converted into a two-walled structure by the invagination of its outer wall, resulting in the reduction of the original cavity of the optic vesicle to a narrow cleft lying between the outer and inner walls of the invaginated vesicle. He interpreted the outer layer of the cup as Jacob's membrane, or the layer of rods and cones, and thus failed to ascertain its true fate, the formation of the pigment layer of the retina or the RPE:

There is another question: What becomes of these two layers of the original optic vesicle which have been folded into one another, and, specifically, what becomes of the outer one? That the invaginated layer becomes the retina is easy to trace . . . the outer layer on the other hand has already become thinner in the three-day old chick, and this dwindling increases rapidly . . . on the same day the pigment stratum of the vascular membrane is already visible as a fine membranule lying in close contact with the outer, convex surface of the outer lay-

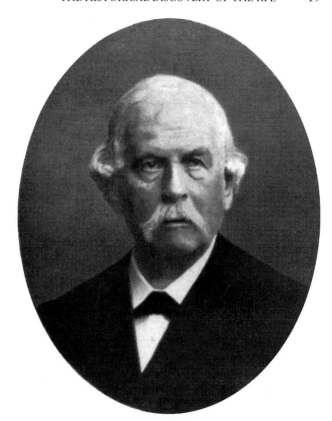

FIGURE 1-7. Rudolf Albert von Kölliker (1817–1905) was born in Zurich. He established that the retinal pigment epithelium developed from the distal lamina of the optic vesicle and was thus neural and not mesodermal in origin. He developed his professional career mostly in Germany, where he was professor of anatomy at the University of Würzburg for many years.

er. After the outer layer has thus become very thin and has come into closer union with the black pigment, it undergoes essentially no further change and finally appears clearly as the membrane of Jacob. . . . [T]he above described transformation of the nervous membrane and origin of Jacob's membrane illuminates completely, as we see, the anatomical significance of the latter.

Of course, Huschke was incorrect in concluding that the outer layer of the optic vesicle gives rise to the photoreceptors. However, nobody challenged this theory for several years. Even the great British anatomist Henry Gray did not shed any new light on the development of the retina, as he again interpreted the outer layer of the optic cup as a part of the choroid (Gray, 1850). This mistake was also partly copied by Robert Remak. He rightly concluded that the outer layer of the optic cup did not become Jacob's membrane; this he said, arose from the inner layer. But he was only partly right in his interpretation of the outer layer of the optic cup, since he went further and derived from it the entire uvea, that is to say, not only the layer now termed the retinal pigment epithelium, but also all the laminae of the choroid which are now known to be of mesodermal origin (Remak, 1855). It was not until 1861 when Albert von Kölliker (Fig. 1-7) published his fundamental work on the embryology of the retina that these misconceptions which had been prevalent for years were put right. He clearly established that the outer layer of the optic cup does not give rise to the layer of rods and cones (as Huschke believed) or to the entire choroid (as Remak thought) but that it is transformed solely into the retinal pigment epithelium. He wrote: "The black eye pigment develops out of the proximal layer of the secondary optic vesicle, and one has proposed to consider it without further ado as part of the retina" (author's translation). Kölliker thus changed once and for all the concept that the RPE was mesodermal or choroidal in origin and convincingly showed that the RPE develops out of the proximal sheath of the secondary eyebulb and is therefore neural in origin. However, it was only later that Babuchin, a student of Kölliker's, attached the embryologically correct term "retinal pigment" to the RPE (Babuchin, 1863; 1865).

FROM THE RETINA TO THE RETINAL PIGMENT EPITHELIUM: THE ADVENT OF THE OPHTHALMOSCOPE

At the same time as these important observations were made on the histology and embryology of the retinal pigment epithelium, the arrival of the ophthalmoscope finally enabled clinicians in the middle of the 19th century to visualize for the first time the retina of patients directly. Although Adolf Kussmaul did not invent the ophthalmoscope, he published in 1845 *Die Farben-Erscheinungen im Grunde des menschlichen Auges* and was the first to describe the optic nerve in an aphakic eye by direct observation with an improvised setup (Kussmaul, 1845). However, it was not until the arrival of Hermann Ludwig Ferdinand von Helmholtz and his popularization of the direct ophthalmoscope in 1851 that the observation of the retina and eventually the retinal pigment epithelium became possible and clinically relevant. In 1855 Eduard Jäger published his seminal atlas of the ocular fundus, "Ergebnisse der Untersuchungen des menschlichen Auges mit dem Augenspiegel" (Jäger, 1855). This was the first time that a wonderful reproduction of the normal fundus with annotations was produced. Jäger described several retinal pathologies in his atlas as well as the retinal pigment epithelium, which he thought was responsible for the yellow-red color of the fundus: "The yellow-red color of the

ocular fundus with its fine granular appearance is mostly produced by the inner continuous layer of the hexagonal pigment cells" (author's translation). He also described pigment atrophy and pigment mottling.

The first photographic documentation of the ocular fundus was reported a few decades later (Howe, 1888; Gerloff, 1891), although the resolution of these cameras did not allow the visualization of many retinal details. With the advent of stereoscopic photography, localization of lesions within and under the retina became possible, and hyperplasia, atrophy, and pigment migration had been demonstrated already by the beginning of this century (Thorner, 1907). Over the next few decades optical systems advanced to the point that Eugene Wolff could claim in 1938 that single normal retinal pigment epithelial cells could be seen by direct ophthalmoscopy in a fair fundus (Wolff, 1938). This would be near the limit of resolution for the optics of the ophthalmoscope, and direct photographic imaging of the normal RPE is still exceedingly difficult.

FOCUS ON THE RETINAL PIGMENT EPITHELIUM: FURTHER STUDIES IN ULTRASTRUCTURE

The second half of the 19th century was characterized by further discoveries of microscopic components of the retinal pigment epithelium. The biggest and most important work to emphasize the histology of the RPE was once more written by Kölliker (1852). He also supplied an exact drawing of the hexagonal cells with the typical basal nucleus (Fig. 1-8) as well as extensive measurements of the diameter and thickness of the cells. In addition, a description of the subretinal space was attached with a discussion of whether this was either a thick cell membrane or an empty space within the cells! Within the same work Kölliker also described Brown's molecular movement of single pigment granules. Kölliker's Würzburg University colleague Heinrich Müller (1820–1864) further expanded the work on the pigment and described pigment migration from the level of the RPE through the retina in patients suffering from retinitis pigmentosa (Müller, 1861). The histology of the RPE was then further elucidated by Willy Kühne (1879) who characterized the pigments in the cells and called them "*Fuscin*," collected preferentially in the apex of the cell, leaving the base with the nucleus next to the choroid relatively pigment free. He also described the enmeshments of the rods and cones by apical RPE processes. His major contribution came, however, with his work on the physiology of what he called *Sehpurpur* (Kühne, 1877; Hubbard, 1977; Marmor and Martin, 1978). After Franz Boll (1876) presented the first findings on the dis-

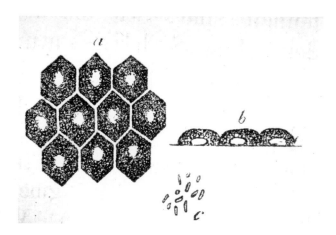

FIGURE 1-8. One of the first original drawings of the hexagonal retinal pigment epithelium cells was done by Kölliker for his *Handbuch der Gewebelehre des Menschen* of 1852. (A) view from above, (b) cross section, (c) single pigment granules.

coloration of the freshly detached frog retina from reddish to transparent, it was Kühne (Fig. 1-9) who finally established the role of the visual purple. He showed that it could be renewed in the dark when the bleached retina was carefully laid back onto the retinal pigment epithelium, and thus he also pointed for the first time to the functional interdependence between retina and RPE in the visual cycle (Kühne, 1877). He also succeeded later in the chemical extraction of rhodopsin from the retina and described the migration of melanin granules in the apical microvilli of the RPE between the photoreceptors during light and dark.

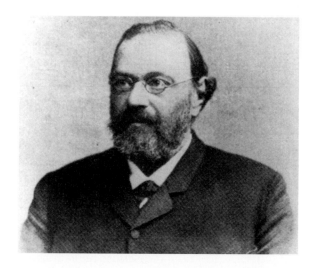

FIGURE 1-9. Willy Kühne (1837–1900) was born in Hamburg and received his doctorate from the University of Göttingen at the age of 19. He trained with several of the greatest scientists of his era, such as Claude Bernard and Rudolf Virchow, and finally succeeded Helmholtz as professor at the University of Heidelberg, a post he held until his death.

At almost the same time Kuhnt (1877) hypothesized on the "cement" that binds the RPE cells together and onto the stratum of the cuticular layer of Bruch's membrane.

FOCUS ON THE RETINAL PIGMENT EPITHELIUM: THE 20TH CENTURY

The term "retinal pigment epithelium" finally entered into the *Nomina Anatomica* of Wilhelm His in 1895 as "stratum pigmenti retinae," and further studies on the RPE continued into the 20th century. Verhoeff (1903) described a layer on the inner surface of the RPE cells which he likened to a condensed cement substance that today we know as the interphotoreceptor matrix. Further detailed measurements of RPE cells were made by Usher in England who found the RPE to become enlarged and multinucleated around the ora serrata (diameter 60 μm) (Usher, 1906). On the continent his contemporary Salzmann described taller cells in the macular region (11–14 μm) as compared to the rest of the fundus (8 μm) as well as the 5 μm–long apical microvilli (Salzmann, 1912). In the next few decades the tissue was mainly studied anatomically; it was not un-til about 1970 that new data became available on the biochemistry, physiology, and electrophysiology of the RPE, which eventually led to the publication of the first complete book on the RPE (Zinn and Marmor, 1979).

What started with the naked eye and the curious scientific amazement over a peeled retina from an isolated globe has in recent years developed into an international multidisciplinary research endeavor supported by hundreds of scientists and clinicians. As new tools of molecular biology have become available, investigations have expanded further and further and a vast body of knowledge on the RPE has thus become available. This has paved the way for the present publication, and the following pages will offer a glimpse of these current concepts.

REFERENCES

Babuchin B. 1863. Beiträge zur Entwicklungsgeschichte des Auges. Würzburger Verhandlungen 4:83.
Babuchin B. 1865. Vergleichend histologische Studien nebst einem Anhange zur Entwicklungsgeschichte der Retina. Würzburger naturwiss Zeitschrift 5.
Bidder F. 1839. Zur Anatomie der Retina. Müllers Archiv.
Boll F. 1876. Zur Anatomie und Physiologie der Retina. Monatsber Akad Wissensch Berlin, 783–787.
Bruch CLW. 1844. Untersuchungen zur Kenntniss des Körnigen Pigments der Wirbelthiere, Zurich.
Galen. De usu Partium Corporis.

Gerloff O. 1891. Ueber die Photographie des Augenhintergrundes. Klin Mbl Augenheilk 29:397–403.

Gray H. 1850. On the development of the retina and optic nerve. Phil Trans Roy Soc Lon 140:189–200.

Haller AV. 1763. Elementa Physiologiae Corporis Humani. Lausanne: Grasset, 365–383.

Hannover R. 1840. Über die Netzhaut. Müllers Archiv.

Heister L. 1735. L'Anatomie de Heister. Paris: Jacques Vincent.

Howe A. 1888. Ueber die photographie des Augenhintergrundes. Klin Mbl Augenheilk 26:381.

Hubbard R. 1977. English translation of Boll's "On the anatomy and physiology of the retina" and of Kühne's "Chemical processes in the retina." Vision Res 17:1245–1316.

Huschke E. 1835. Über einige Streitpunkte aus der Anatomie des Auges. Zeitschrift für die Ophthalmologie 4:272–295.

Jacobs A. 1819. An account of a membrane of the eye, now first described. Philosophical Transactions of the Royal Society of London, 300–307.

Jacobs A. 1822. Inquiries respecting the anatomy of the eye. Med Chir Transactions, 287–519.

Jäger E. 1855. Ergebnisse der Untersuchungen des menschlichen Auges mit dem Augenspiegel. Ber math naturwiss 15(2).

Knox R. 1826. Inquiry into the structure and probably functions of the capsules forming the canal of Petit, and of the marsupium nigrum. Trans Roy Soc Edinburgh 10:249.

Kölliker A. 1852. Handbuch der Gewebelehre des Menschen. Leipzig.

Kölliker A. 1861. Entwicklungsgeschichte des Menschen. Leipzig.

Kühne W. 1877. Zur Photochemie der Netzhaut. Untersuch Physiol Instit Univ Heidelberg 1:1–14.

Kühne W. 1879. Handbuch der Physiologie. Leipzig, 235.

Kuhnt J. 1877. Klin Mbl Augenheilk 15(Beilage 72).

Kussmaul A. 1845. Die Farben-Erscheinungen im Grunde des menschlichen Auges. Heidelberg.

Leeuwenhook A. 1689. Philosophical Transactions of the Royal Society.

Loewenstein L. 1940. Am J Ophthalmol 23:1340.

Magnus H. 1878. Anatomie des Auges bei den Griechen und Römern. Leipzig: von Veit.

Marmor MF, Martin LJ. 1978. 100 years of the visual cycle. Surv Ophthalmol 22:279–285.

Mondini C. 1790. Commentationes Bononienses.

Mondini C. 1818. Opuscoli Scientifici dell' Universita di Bologna.

Müller H. 1861. Quoted in J. Hirschberg (ed), Geschichte der Augenheilkunde. Berlin: Julius Springer, 1918.

Münchow W. 1984. Geschichte der Augenheilkunde. Stuttgart: Enke, 146.

Pacini F. 1845. Nuove ricerche microscopiche sulla tessitura intima della retina nell'uomo, nei vertebrati, nei cefalopodi e negli insetti. Bologna.

Remak R. 1855. Untersuchungen über die Entwicklung der Wirbeltheire. Berlin.

Rufus OE. 1879. The Names of the Parts of the Body [translation]. Paris: Darember & Ruette.

Ruysch F. 1702. Thesaurus Anatomicus. Amsterdam: Wolters.

Salzmann. 1912. Anatomie und Histologie des menschlichen Augapfels. Leipzig.

Smirnow AE. 1899. Graefes Arch Ophthalmol 47:451.

Thorner W. 1907. Die stereoskopische Photographie des Augenhintergrundes. Klin Mbl Augheilk 47:481–490.

Usher. 1906. Trans Ophthalmol Soc UK 26:107.

Verhoeff FH. 1903. Roy Lond Ophthal Hosp Rep 15:309.

Wharton Jones T. 1833. Notice relative to the pigmentum nigrum of the eye. Edin Med Surg J 40:77–83.

Winslow JB. 1753. Expositio Anatomica Structurae Corporis Humani. Frankfurt: Bauer.

Wolff E. 1938. Can the network formed by the retinal pigment epithelium be seen by the ophthalmoscope. Proc Roy Soc Med 31:1104.

Zinn JG. 1755. Descriptio Anatomica Oculi Humani. Göttingen.

Zinn K, Marmor MF. 1979. The Retinal Pigment Epithelium. Cambridge (MA): Harvard University Press.

2. Comparative and evolutionary aspects of the retinal pigment epithelium

MICHAEL F. MARMOR

The retinal pigment epithelium (RPE) serves many functions within the eye, which are the subject of this book and its predecessor (Zinn and Marmor, 1979). To discuss the comparative and evolutionary aspects of the RPE, it is necessary not only to consider the tissue itself but also the way in which functions of the human RPE (Table 2-1) are carried out in other species. All vertebrate RPE is anatomically and embryologically similar (although many variations exist), but invertebrate eyes have different embryologic and anatomic construction. Insects may lack an epithelial pigment layer, but they do have pigment cells that screen light and enhance the optical properties of the photoreceptors. Even in insects, it is necessary to control the ionic environment of the photoreceptors and to recycle visual pigment, although the cells which reform them may not be embryologic analogs of our own RPE. Conversely, functions that we commonly associate with the RPE, such as the absorption of light, may be lacking in some vertebrate eyes, for example, where there is a reflecting tapetum and the overlying RPE is transparent.

This chapter will begin with RPE functions in invertebrates, followed by specializations of the vertebrate RPE. The animal kingdom is vast, and this review is not intended to be comprehensive. However, I hope that selected examples of RPE correlates and diversity will provide perspective on the importance of retinal support functions to the eye, and on the marvelous adaptations of the RPE that serve the different creatures with which we share this planet.

FUNCTIONAL CORRELATES OF THE RPE IN INVERTEBRATES

Screening and Light-Absorptive Pigment

The presence of absorptive or screening pigment is almost universal among eyes, although the location and embryologic origin of this pigment may vary considerably. Even one-celled animals have this optical function. The flagellated protozoan *Euglena* swims toward light through the effects of photoreceptive organelles (con-taining flavoprotein) at the base of the flagellum (Fig. 2-1). This light-receptive region is surrounded by clusters of colored granules (containing carotenoid) that are thought to act as a light filter (Wolken; 1975, 1995; Dodge, 1991).

As organisms evolved, individual cells rather than intracellular organelles became specialized for photoreception—and for optical screening. For example, the isolated light-sensitive cells of sponges, some worms, and even the protochordate *Amphioxus,* are bordered by pigment cells. As visual organs became multicellular, then clusters of visual cells were collectively surrounded by pigmentation (Fig. 2-2). An example is the primitive eyes of the worm, *Planaria,* in which the visual cells lie inside a cup of densely pigmented cells (Duke-Elder, 1958). In some simple eyes (ocelli), in which the photoreceptors directly face the light source, pigment granules appear between the sensory cells rather than behind them. This can be seen in the ocelli of complex worms such as *Nereis* and in many mollusc eyes.

There is a wide range of complexity among mollusc eyes. Many *Planarian* eyes (Fig. 2-2) are primitive cupolas; the chambered nautilus has a "pinhole" eye; the cephalopod eye looks remarkably like our own (although the retina is noninverted). Octopi and squid have pigment granules within their photoreceptors, as well as in supporting cells that send long processes between the outer segments (Fig. 2-3). The pigment within the photoreceptors migrates in response to light: it is distributed throughout the retinal thickness in light adaptation, but retracts to the base of the photoreceptors in the dark (Messenger, 1991). A different strategy for screening and optical support of the photoreceptors is found in the scallop eye. The pigment layers behind the photoreceptors lie outside of a reflecting tapetum, which acts as a focusing mirror to enhance the formation of images upon the retina.

Spiders have simple eyes that are structurally similar to molluscan eyes. The cornea is a major refractive surface in these eyes, and hunting spiders have relatively good acuity. There are many different arrangements of pigment cells, and reflecting tapetal cells, to serve the vi-

TABLE 2-1. *Functions of the RPE*

Optical (pigment)	Structural	Environmental	Visual cycle	Trophic
Light screening	Photoreceptor support	Blood–retinal barrier	Retinoid binding and storage	Ocular development and regeneration
Scatter reduction	Membrane phagocytosis	Ion and water transport	Visual pigment regeneration	Injury/repair
Light reflection (tapetum)	Retinal adhesion	Nutrient control		
		Electrical homeostasis		
		Detoxification		

sual needs and the diurnal or nocturnal habits of the different species.

The most striking ocular adaptation in arthropods is the compound eye, which is built on different optical principles from the vertebrate eye. It is composed of multiple ommatidia, each of which contains a lens and a small number of photoreceptive cells, called retinular cells (Fig. 2-4). These have microvillous extensions, called rhabdomeres, which contain the visual pigment.

There is generally a ring of primary pigment cells surrounding the lens at the apex of each ommatidium, and also a ring of accessory pigment cells around the body of the ommatidium. In species that are adapted for hunting in daylight, like the dragonfly, this pigment prevents light from scattering between adjacent optical elements, and thus improves resolution. Nocturnal insects such as moths lack this screening pigment so that light can cross between the rhabdomeric elements and increase the chance of photon capture (at the expense of acuity). In many arthropod species this screening system is driven by light and dark, and the configuration of the pigment cells, the location of the pigment within cells, or even the shape of the retinular cells, may change with adaptation (Stavenga, 1989). In some compound eyes the pigment cells also contain a reflecting pigment to act like a tapetum near the base of the ommatidial elements. This reflecting layer may be obscured or exposed by the screening pigment as it migrates in response to light or dark (Nilsson, 1989).

A

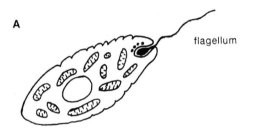

flagellum

B

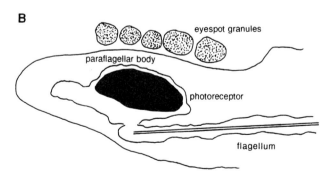

eyespot granules

paraflagellar body

photoreceptor

flagellum

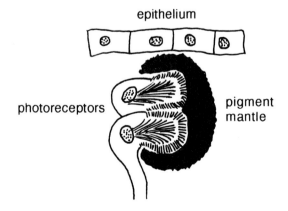

epithelium

photoreceptors

pigment mantle

FIGURE 2-1. Diagram of the *Euglena* eyespot and phototropic mechanism. (A) Dark-grown *Euglena* with eyespot at the base of the flagellum. (B) Enlarged view of eyespot area. (Drawn after Wolken, 1995.)

FIGURE 2-2. Eye of a *Planarian* worm, consisting of two ciliated photoreceptor cells within a pigment mantle. The photoreceptors lie beneath the epithelium. (Drawn after Duke-Elder, 1958.)

A

B

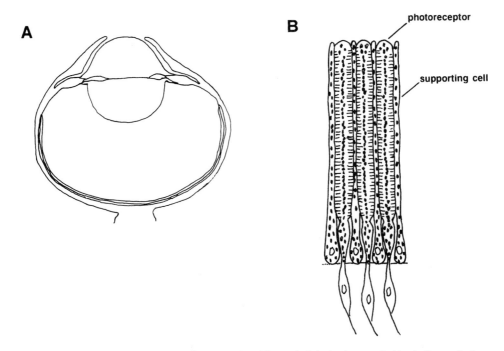

photoreceptor

supporting cell

FIGURE 2-3. Octopus eye. (A) General construction. The optical design is remarkably similar to the human eye, but the retina is not inverted, and there is no pigmented epithelium behind the visual cells. (B) Diagram of retinal elements showing pigment within the photoreceptors as well as in supporting cells that run between them. (Modified from Young, 1962.)

Structural Support and Visual Cell Phagocytosis

In vertebrates, the microvillous extensions of the RPE provide a physical scaffold for the outer segments by reaching between them, and wrapping around them. This scaffolding and the interphotoreceptor matrix help to maintain retinal adherence to the RPE. Ion and water transport across the RPE keep the subretinal space dry and regulate the ionic environment to maximize the adhesive properties of the matrix (see Chapter 19). The RPE also participates intimately in the process of photoreceptor outer segment renewal (see Chapter 8), a necessity in any long-lived animal to remove the membrane material that has been damaged through light absorption, oxidation, or aging. The vertebrate RPE phagocytizes the tips of outer segments on a daily basis, digests the absorbed material, and appropriately recycles or egests the metabolic detritus.

Relatively little has been written about these functions in invertebrates. Some of the physiological issues may not be so critical, insofar as retinal detachment is not an issue for a noninverted retina, and light or oxidative damage may not be serious matters for an animal that lives only a few weeks or months. Furthermore, concepts such as retinal detachment and RPE phagocytosis are truly relevant only for an inverted retina which lies upon an epithelial layer—a configuration essentially limited to vertebrates. The retina cannot detach when it is a direct extension of the optic nerve, and visual cells that directly face the vitreous or that form a rosette within an ommatidial sheath may have no adjacent phagocytic cells.

These comments notwithstanding, studies have shown that photoreceptor membrane renewal is a dy-

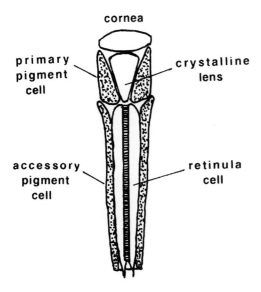

cornea

primary pigment cell

crystalline lens

accessory pigment cell

retinula cell

FIGURE 2-4. Diagram of an arthropod ommatidium.

namic and ongoing process in the compound eyes of many insects (Schwemer, 1989). The need may be less to protect against membrane damage than to facilitate a daily cycle of rhabdomeric expansion and contraction in response to light. In many species, the microvillous rhabdomere shrinks during light, and grows during dark-adaptation. This is accomplished by microvillous shedding and pinocytosis of the membrane material back into the photoreceptor cells where lysozomal enzymes break it down (Schwemer, 1989). In the crane fly, fragments of photoreceptor membrane break off into the extracellular space each dawn, to be engulfed by pseudopods of the retinular cells (Waterman, 1982). In other arthropods, phagocytosis may be accomplished by adjacent glial cells. For example, glial cells are adjacent to the photoreceptors in some spiders, and in the crab *Leptograpsus* there is an almost catastrophic degree of photoreceptor turnover. The photoreceptors extensively dissolve soon after dusk each day, with fresh rhabdomeric microvilli being synthesized via the tubular endoplasmic reticular system during the night. The actual mechanism of new membrane synthesis has not been clearly established. Autoradiographic labeling studies in arthropod eyes have shown a diffuse incorporation of new membrane material into the photoreceptors, somewhat in the fashion of vertebrate cones (Anderson and Andrews, 1982).

Control of Local Environment

One of the most important functions of the vertebrate RPE is to control the local environment of the outer segments. This occurs by ionic and water transport, and also by the regulated transport of glucose, amino acids, and other nutrients. The RPE forms part of the blood-retinal barrier in vertebrates, and thus helps to maintain the optimal extracellular environment for neuronal function. It is hard to define comparable roles in invertebrates, which lack the circulatory distinctions of a somatic and cerebral vasculature. However, the presence of pigment cells and apparent glial cells near the photoreceptors of many invertebrate species suggests that these cells may play some regulatory role, even if the correlation with human RPE function is not very precise. For example, the screening pigments in some compound eyes have been shown also to serve as calcium stores which help maintain homeostasis about the photoreceptive elements (Stavenga, 1989). Willmer (1970) has argued that a prototype of the vertebrate eye is the "cephalic organ" of *Nemertine* worms. This tubular structure contains several neuronal cell types and appears to serve in part as an organ for recognizing and responding to changes in environmental salinity.

Visual Pigment Regeneration

The regeneration of visual pigment that has been altered by the absorption of light is a requirement for all eyes. In vertebrates, the bleached all-*trans* retinal separates from opsin and is transported across the subretinal space to the RPE for reisomerization. The RPE absorbs vitamin A from the circulation, stores it for visual needs, and processes the reformation of 11-*cis* retinal during the visual cycle. Invertebrates that lack an anatomically apposed RPE use other strategies to carry out these functions.

In single-cell organisms, of course, visual pigment regeneration takes place entirely within the cytoplasm of the visual cell. The same strategy in fact serves most of the invertebrate species. Even though many invertebrates utilize vitamin A pigments, the retinal does not separate from the protein opsin after the formation of metarhodopsin as it does in vertebrates. In invertebrates, all-*trans* retinal can be isomerized directly back to 11-*cis* retinal within the structure of metarhodopsin, and this can occur in the photoreceptors and in the presence of light (Wolken, 1995). The absorption of light by the all-*trans* chromophore reisomerizes the retinal to the 11-*cis* form, which then causes the opsin to refold and form rhodopsin. Enzymatic regeneration has also been observed (e.g., in flies and crayfish), but photoregeneration (i.e., driven by light absorption) appears to be the predominant reisomerization mechanism in invertebrates. The exception may be dark-living sea animals (e.g., sea molluscs) that can have a greater proportion of enzymatic pigment regeneration. There are some invertebrate species (e.g., some flies) in which visual pigment appears to regenerate through an associated cellular system analogous to the RPE (Fein and Szuts, 1982; Schwemer, 1989), and invertebrate screening pigments may help the photoregenerative process by concentrating light of the appropriate wavelengths (Stavenga, 1989).

Development and Regeneration

The vertebrate RPE is derived from the same neural *anlage* as the sensory retina, but it is difficult to define homology for the pigment cells in invertebrates. In lower vertebrates (amphibians), isolated RPE cells can regenerate many of the ocular tissues; but this capability is also difficult to compare in invertebrates where the anatomical relationships are so different. Higher mammals lack such regenerative capacity in the RPE, but RPE growth can be triggered by injury so that new cells will spread across a laser burn or other insult.

Invertebrate eyes are generally derived from surface

cells in the developing embryo. Simple ocelli develop from a surface invagination, which becomes a hypodermal pit. The compound eye of insects develops from hypodermal cells that differentiate into pillars that contain the lens, primary pigmented cells, and photoreceptive cells of the ommatidium. Cells left between the pillars develop into the secondary pigment cells that lie along the walls of the ommatidia. To the extent that vertebrate neuroectoderm relates to this primitive ectoderm, the pigment cells of lower animals may bear some distant phylogenetic relationship to the vertebrate RPE. It is perhaps notable that throughout the animal kingdom, pigment cells seem to originate from similar layers as the photoreceptive cells. However, it is hazardous to carry this analogy too far insofar as the vertebrate eye represents a blend of embryologic elements which may have come from a common origin in more primitive organisms (Duke-Elder, 1958).

SPECIALIZATIONS OF THE VERTEBRATE RPE

In all vertebrates, the RPE is a monocellular epithelium of hexagonal cells directly behind the neural retina, containing melanin pigment or the embryological capability of producing it. The epithelial layer is also characterized by tight junctions that form part of the blood–retinal barrier, by apical-to-basal membrane specializations, by cytoplasmic organelles for protein synthesis and storage of metabolites, and by a degree of reparative power and/or polymorphism. Vertebrate RPE carries out all of the functions listed in Table 2.1, but there can be considerable species variation in how this is accomplished. For example, all vertebrates have polarized RPE cells with different apical and basal ionic channels, but the specific nature of these channels and their relative balance varies from species to species (see Chapter 6). All RPE is embryonically equipped to make pigment, but pigment is lacking in some nocturnal species and in fundus regions that have a tapetum lucidum. Lipid droplets have been observed in almost every vertebrate RPE, but they are prominent only in lower vertebrates, and a few mammalian species such as the rabbit.

This section begins with an introduction to features of the RPE that are not found in man, but that are important in lower vertebrate species. This is followed by a review of RPE characteristics in the major categories of vertebrates.

Specializations of Nonhuman RPE

Pigment and cellular movements. In nonmammalian vertebrates, including fish, amphibians and birds, the pig-

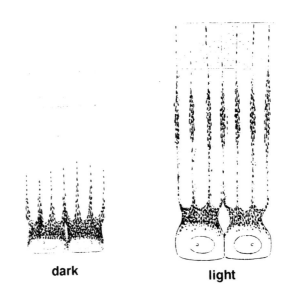

dark   **light**

FIGURE 2-5. Diagram of frog RPE in the light and dark. In the light, pigment granules migrate out into the apical processes. (From Ewald and Kühne, 1878.)

ment granules within the RPE can migrate in response to light or a circadian rhythm. Typically, the granules retract into the cell body during dark-adaptation, to maximize the amount of light reaching the photoreceptors, and move into the apical processes between the photoreceptor cells during light-adaptation (Fig. 2-5). In many species the photoreceptors and/or apical processes of the RPE also contract or elongate in response to light (Fig. 2-6). Neither pigment nor photoreceptor movements have been observed in mammals (Duke-Elder, 1958; Walls, 1942).

The movement of pigment in fish and amphibians involves actin filaments and is modulated by dopamine D2, receptors, and cyclic AMP (Burnside and Dearry, 1986; see Chapter 3). Beside the obvious effect of protecting the photoreceptors from light, the movement of pigment also affects the adhesiveness of the retina. It is very hard to peel retina from the RPE in light-adapted frog eyes without fragmenting the firmly attached microvilli, but in the dark the retina peels off easily and cleanly. Comparable effects in mammals have been suggested in older literature (Duke-Elder, 1958), but have not been observed in more recent experiments (Marmor and Maack, 1982).

Tapetum lucidum. The presence of a tapetum lucidum, or reflective layer behind the retina, is common among vertebrates to facilitate light capture under dim conditions. One function of light-controlled pigment movements, such as were noted above, is to expose or occlude tapetal structures (Walls, 1942; Duke-Elder, 1958; Prince, 1956). The RPE is always modified where it is

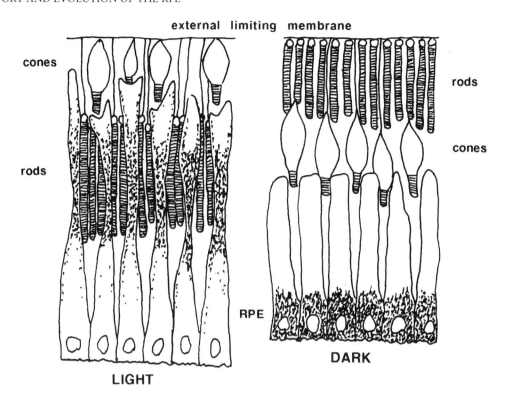

FIGURE 2-6. Diagram of light-induced retinomotor movements in conjunction with RPE pigment migration and apical remodeling in a fish. In the light, the cone outer segments are arrayed along the external limiting membrane, while the rods are screened by pigment in long apical RPE processes. The pigment and processes retract in the dark and the rods switch places with cones to maximize sensitivity. (Modified from Douglas and Djamgoz, 1990, and others.)

associated with a tapetum. In some species the RPE itself becomes a light-reflecting rather than a light-absorptive structure; this is called a *retinal tapetum*. In other species the reflectors are choroidal (*choroidal tapetum*) and the RPE must adapt so that it does not block the path of light. Studies of RPE development in cows have shown that RPE cells over the choroidal tapetum are normally pigmented at embryonic day 40, but by day 65 they are largely unpigmented (Feeney-Burns and Mixon, 1979). The tapetal RPE loses melanin during development by a combination of early termination of melanogenesis, melanin dilution as the eye grows, and autophagy of melanosomes.

Retinal tapeta are found in some teleost fish and crocodilians (Braekevelt, 1977) in whom the RPE contains guanine crystals. In the tapetal areas of the fundus the RPE either lacks pigment, or the pigment granules and/or guanine crystals move in the dark to expose the reflecting crystals (Nicol, 1989). A retinal tapetum is also found in the large fruit-eating bats and in the opossum (Fig. 2-7), both of which have reflecting globules of lipid material (probably cholesterol in the opossum) (Pirie, 1966).

There are several types of choroidal tapetum. In elasmobranch fish such as the sharks and rays, the choroidal tapetum contains plates of guanine crystals, separated by thin processes from adjacent choroidal pigment cells (Fig. 2-8). These pigment cells are distinct from the RPE, which in these animals is a transparent layer between the tapetum and the photoreceptors. The tapetal pigment cell processes fill with melanin during light adaptation, but the melanin retracts behind the tapetum during dark adaptation.

Choroidal tapeta in mammals do not contain guanine and some of their reflectivity is achieved through a dense layering of cells or fibrous tissue. Cats and dogs, other carnivores, and seals have a *tapetum cellulosum*, which consists of a dense array of cells, typically 15 to 30 layers thick, directly behind the RPE (unpigmented) and choriocapillaris (Fig. 2-9). This tapetum usually covers only a portion of the fundus, and the remainder has normally pigmented RPE. The cells of the tapetum in carnivores contain reflective rods or crystals composed most often of a complex of zinc and cysteine (Pirie, 1966). These tapeta can be strikingly effective, as evident to anyone who has spotted the glowing eyes of a

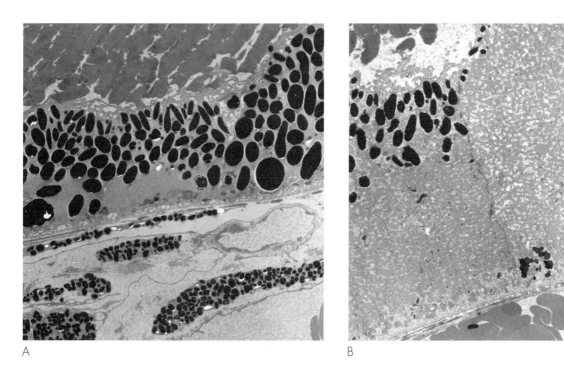

A   B

FIGURE 2-7. Retinal tapetum in the opossum. (A) The nontapetal RPE is normally pigmented. (B) In the tapetal region, the RPE has almost no pigment and is filled with reflective lipid spheres that are thought to contain cholesterol. Electron micrographs, magnification × 3400, courtesy of C. R. Braekevelt.

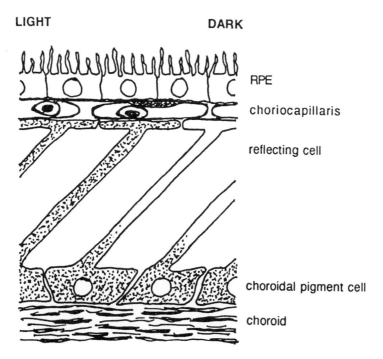

FIGURE 2-8. Diagram of the tapetum of a shark or ray. The tapetum is choroidal, and lies behind a nonpigmented RPE and choriocapillaris. Large reflecting cells are filled with guanine crystals, and processes from special choroidal pigment cells (not RPE) extend be- tween and over the reflecting cells. This diagram artificially combines the light-adapted condition, in which pigment fills the pigment cell processes and occludes the tapetum, with the dark-adapted condition, in which the pigment is retracted behind the reflectors.

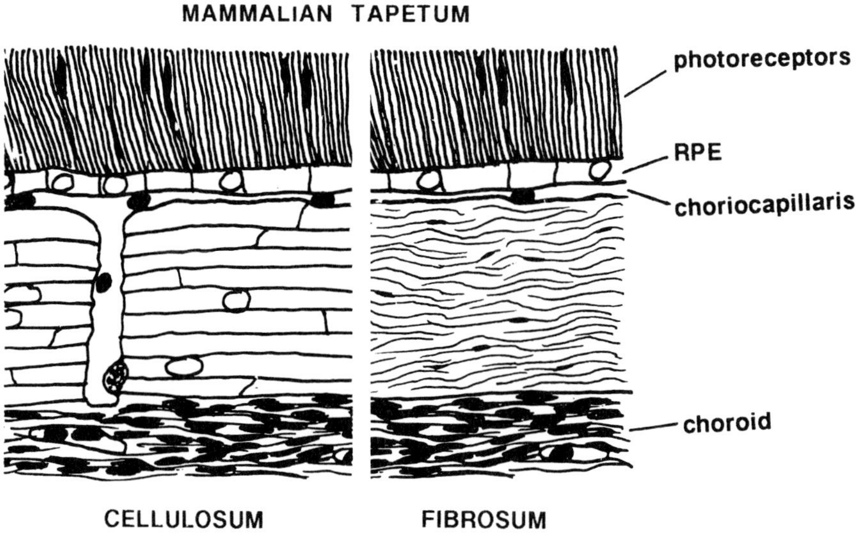

MAMMALIAN TAPETUM

photoreceptors

RPE

choriocapillaris

choroid

CELLULOSUM   FIBROSUM

FIGURE 2-9. Diagram of cellular and fibrous tapeta in mammals. (Drawn after micrographs by Ashton in Duke-Elder, 1958.)

cat (Plate 2-I) or other small carnivore staring back at the light from a flashlight or a campfire. Cellular tapeta are also found in some prosimians such as the lemurs (Duke-Elder, 1958). The tapetal cells in one species of lemur contain riboflavin crystals which, in addition to reflecting light, may actually generate light by fluorescence to UV and deep blue wavelengths (Pirie, 1966).

Virtually all of the ungulates, elephants, whales, some rodents, and some species of marsupial have a *tapetum fibrosum*. This is an acellular choroidal structure consisting of densely packed fibrous tissue directly behind the RPE (Fig. 2-9). The RPE is devoid of pigment over the tapetal region, but in most of these animals only a portion of the fundus is tapetal, and the remainder has pigmented RPE. The array of collagen fibers produces an iridescent reflecting surface. A fibrous tapetum is also found in one primate, the douroucouli (*Aotus*), which is the only known nocturnal monkey and has a striking eye shine.

Species of mammal which lack a tapetum include the rabbit, the pig, and most of the primates (including all of the apes and man).

Myeloid bodies. *Myeloid bodies* are small discrete stacks of membrane material within the RPE cytoplasm (Fig. 2-10). Although once thought to be specialized organelles, they are now believed to represent a condensation or specialization of smooth endoplasmic reticulum within the cytoplasm. They may change in structure within the light and dark cycle, reaching maximum size in the dark (Matthes and Basinger, 1980; Tabor and Fisher, 1983; Yorke and Dickson, 1984). Myeloid bod-

ies are prominent in fish, amphibians, birds, and some reptiles, but are absent in snakes and in most mammals, including man (Nguyen-Legros, 1975). They have been observed in bats, and seen in squirrels early in the dark cycle (Tabor and Fisher, 1983).

Plenipotentiality of the RPE. Classic experiments on salamanders (Stone, 1959; Stroeva and Mitashov, 1983) showed that the RPE in these animals has the capability of giving rise to neural retina, iris, and lens tissue under the right experimental conditions. These studies raise interesting questions concerning the specificity of embryonic tissue origins, relative to the influence of ge-

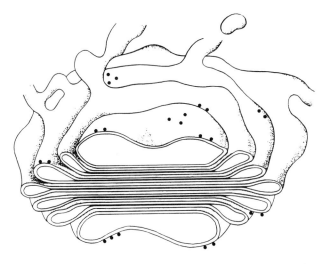

FIGURE 2-10. Diagram of a myeloid body in three-dimensional reconstruction. (From Nguyen-Legros, 1978.)

netic or external trophic factors that modulate tissue differentiation. This plenipotential capacity is lost in higher vertebrates, who also lack the amphibian potential for regenerating limbs. Nevertheless, even the human RPE has the ability to transform, insofar as it can respond to injury with mitosis, repair, and sometimes the acquisition of macrophage or connective-tissue characteristics.

The RPE in Vertebrate Species

Fish. The fish RPE has the basic hexagonal structure common to all vertebrates, but relative to the human RPE it has only sparse basal infoldings, more lipid droplets, and there are myeloid body condensations of the smooth endoplasmic reticulum. Bruch's membrane typically has only three layers in teleost fish, lacking the elastic lamina found in mammals (Nicol, 1989). The apical processes of the RPE are shorter and less complicated than they are in mammals, and may be shortened even further in deep-sea fish that have little use for vision (Nguyen-Legros, 1978; Nicol, 1989). Wandering phagocytic cells are sometimes seen in the subretinal space of bony fish (teleosts) (Braekevelt, 1980c).

One of the most striking features of the fish RPE is the variety of tapetal structures. The more primitive fish like the sharks and rays (elasmobranchs) have a choroidal tapetum containing guanine (see Fig. 2-8). A choroidal tapetum of the fibrosum variety is found in sturgeons, in a few teleosts, and in the coelacanth (Nicol, 1989). Retinal tapeta are found more widely among teleost species (Fig. 2-11) and gars, including fish from all types of habitat (freshwater and deep sea). A number of different reflecting materials have been found in the RPE of these animals, including guanine, lipids, and other substances (Nicol, 1989).

In conjunction with tapetal specialization, fish possess a variety of mechanisms for adjusting to light and dark. In some species the pigment granules migrate up the RPE processes to shield photoreceptors from light (see Fig. 2-6), while in other species melanin shifts location within the cell body to expose the reflecting inclusion bodies of the retinal tapetum (Braekevelt, 1982). The myeloid bodies and even the RPE nucleus can change position or shape in response to the light/dark cycle.

Amphibians and reptiles. The frog RPE is of historical importance, since it was in this species that the regeneration of visual pigment was first demonstrated by Kühne and Boll in 1877 (Marmor and Martin, 1978a). The reddish color of fresh retina had been observed by earlier scientists after the dissection of animal eyes, but

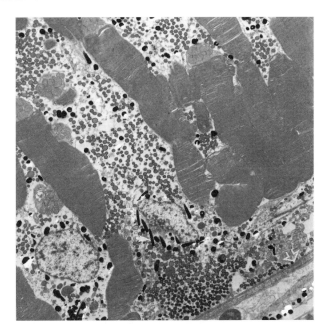

FIGURE 2-11. Retinal tapetum of the scissortail fish. The RPE cells are filled with lipid tapetal spheres, and have only scattered melanosomes (elongate black bodies; *see small white arrow*). Note the long, wide apical RPE processes and trilaminate Bruch's membrane *(open arrow)*. Electron micrograph magnification × 3700, courtesy of C. R. Braekevelt.

it was thought merely to be a vital characteristic that faded with death. It took the insight of Kühne and Boll to recognize that the color itself was the mechanism of light absorption. To prove their hypothesis, they had to show that the pigment could regenerate, which they accomplished by laying frog retina back upon the RPE in the dark (Plate 2-II). This regeneration occurs by way of diffusable substances rather than contact per se, since the color returns even if the retina is replaced upside down (Marmor and Martin, 1978b). These early observers also made careful note of the striking movement of pigment within the frog RPE processes in response to light. This movement of melanin occurs quite rapidly, and affects not only the light sensitivity of the retina but the strength of adhesion between retina and RPE. Frog retina is hard to peel from the RPE in the light, but separates easily in the dark.

Although frogs have not been noted to have tapeta, there are interesting regional variations within the fundus. The bullfrog, for example, has visual pigment based on vitamin A_1 (rhodopsin) and vitamin A_2 (porphyropsin) in the retina at the same time, with the porphyropsin found in the dorsal aspect. No anatomic correlates of this in the RPE have been noted. Curious irregular patches and depigmentation associated with an invasion of macrophages sometimes appear in the inferior fundus of bullfrogs, but this is thought to repre-

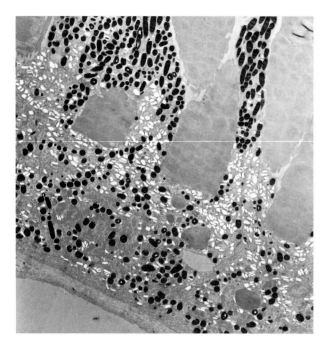

FIGURE 2-12. RPE of the spectacled caiman, at the edge of the retinal tapetum. In this region both melanosomes and guanine-containing tapetal bodies are present. Wide apical processes extend between the photoreceptor outer segments, and Bruch's membrane has five layers. Electron micrograph, magnification × 3600, courtesy of C. R. Braekevelt.

sent damage from ambient light that comes from above (Eckmiller and Steinberg, 1981).

Frogs, like fish, can have large lipid droplets in the RPE. Changes in the frog RPE have been noted during hibernation. There is a generalized decrease in the amount and organization of smooth endoplasmic reticulum and this is associated with a decrease in the size and number of myeloid bodies (Kuwabara, 1975). Bruch's membrane in amphibians is typically pentalaminate, with an elastic lamina present (Braekevelt, 1992). Salamanders that live in dark caves, and are essentially blind, have less-developed RPE in which the cells have little melanin, short apical processes, and less apical-to-basal specialization (Nguyen-Legros, 1978). Crocodilians have retinal tapeta containing guanine (Fig. 2-12).

Birds. The RPE of birds is similar to that of fish and amphibia rather than mammals, insofar as myeloid bodies are observed (Fig. 2-13), lipid droplets are plentiful, and there can be rapid and extensive movements of melanin pigment in response to light and dark (Walls, 1942). Basal RPE infoldings are more prominent than in fish, and Bruch's membrane contains an elastic lamina. Some birds, such as owls and ostriches, have an "eye shine," but tapeta have been only rarely described (Walls, 1942). A few species, such as the nocturnal nighthawk,

have a retinal tapetum in which small reflective spheres are present in the RPE cell bodies (Braekevelt, 1984). In this species and some other birds as well, the myeloid bodies appear continuous with rough rather than smooth endoplasmic reticulum. However, more conventional continuity with smooth endoplasmic reticulum has also been noted in birds, including the barn owl (Dieterich, 1975).

Mammals. Mammals lack the variations of pigmentary and retinomotor movements that characterize lower vertebrates, and the mammalian RPE lacks myeloid bodies. Nevertheless, there is considerable variation among mammals in the nature of tapetal structures, the degree of RPE pigmentation, and the size and abundance of lipid droplets.

Even the more primitive mammals, such as the monotremes and marsupials, have well-developed RPE layers of typical mammalian form. Phagocytes or leukocytes have occasionally been observed in the subretinal space of marsupials (Young and Braekevelt, 1993), similar to their occurrence in fish. The opossum has a striking retinal tapetum (see Fig. 2-7) covering a portion of its superior fundus; the RPE cells in this region contain few or no melanosomes but are full of tiny lipoidal spheres of reflecting material (Braekevelt, 1976). The only other mammals with a retinal tapetum are the larger fruit bats (Megachiroptera) (Duke-Elder, 1958; Walls, 1942).

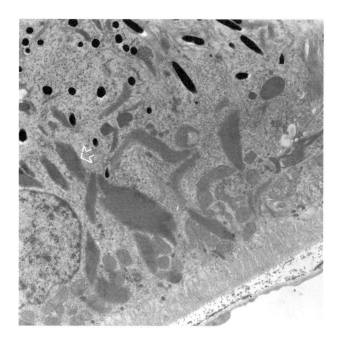

FIGURE 2-13. RPE of the pigeon, showing numerous and prominent myeloid bodies (arrow). Electron micrograph, magnification × 10,000, courtesy of C. R. Braekevelt.

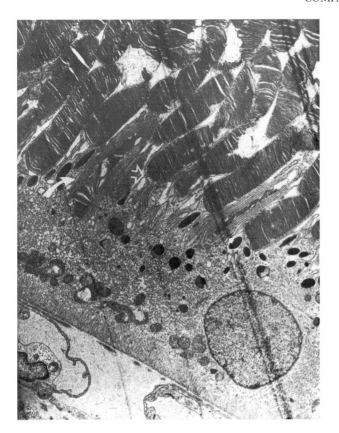

FIGURE 2-14. RPE of the rabbit. The cells are not as thick as in some other mammals. Note the multilayered apical ensheathment of cones *(curved arrow)*, while a simpler sheath envelops the tips of the rods *(open arrow)*. Electron micrograph, original magnification about × 2000.

The RPE of rodents and rabbits (Fig. 2-14) has been studied extensively in conjunction with the use of these animals as experimental models in biomedical research. The RPE is generally similar to other mammals, but a high percentage (70–85%) of the cells are binucleate while such cells are rare (1–3%) in higher species including man (Ts'o and Friedman, 1967). Occasional mitoses are seen in albino rat RPE. Lipid droplets are prominent in the rat and the rabbit; in the rabbit they sometimes span nearly the width of the cytoplasm. The smaller lipid droplets in the rat RPE can form and disappear on a daily cycle correlated with the phagocytosis of outer segment material. At least in the rat, the lipid droplets seem to serve more as a reservoir for fatty acids used in RPE lipid synthesis than as a storage site for retinoids (Baker et al., 1986). In the rabbit one finds cone/rod specialization of the apical RPE processes (Figs. 2-14, 2-15). Leaflike sheaths of microvilli envelop the cones, and are quite distinct from the more fingerlike projections that surround the rods. Similar cone sheaths are present in many mammals (Fig. 2-16) in-

cluding cats and humans (Steinberg and Wood, 1974; Hogan et al., 1971). Tapeta are not common among rodents, but a tapetum fibrosum is found in the cavy and flying squirrel.

During hibernation of bats and ground squirrels, there is a generalized diminution in the amount and organization of the smooth endoplasmic reticulum, similar to the changes that occur in hibernating frogs (Kuwabara, 1975).

A tapetum fibrosum is found in almost all of the ungulates (horses, cows, etc.) (see Fig. 2-17) and in elephants. It is also present in whales and in the only nocturnal simian, the douroucouli, or night monkey. In most of these animals, the tapetum covers only a portion of the fundus, typically the dorsal aspect, and the RPE is devoid of melanin in this region. Elsewhere in the fundus the RPE is heavily pigmented.

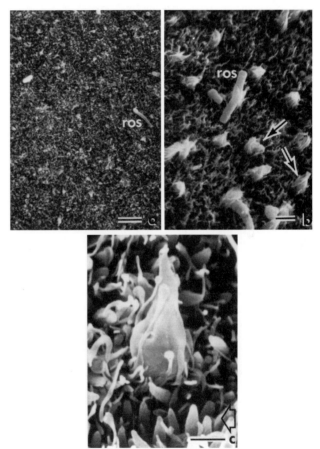

FIGURE 2-15. Scanning electron micrographs of the RPE surface in the rabbit. ros = rod outer segment. (A) At low power (magnification bar = 10 μm) one sees faintly the hexagonal outline of the cells. (B) At medium power (magnification bar = 2 μm), cone sheaths can be seen protruding from the microvillous surface *(arrows)*. (C) Cone sheath structure at high power (magnification bar = 1μm). (From Immel et al., 1968.)

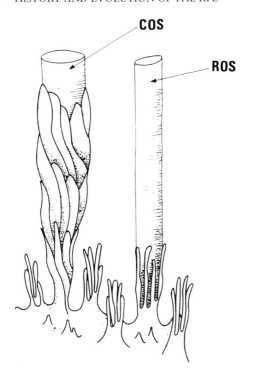

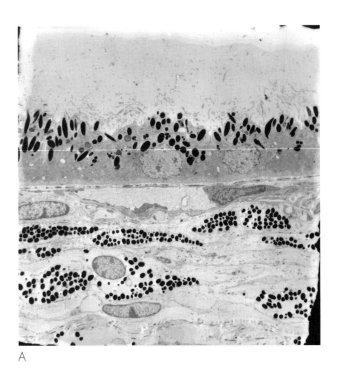

FIGURE 2-16. Diagram of the microvillous ensheathment of cones and rods in mammals. COS and ROS indicate cone and rod outer segments. (From Nguyen-Legros, 1978.)

The most familiar tapeta, of course, are those in carnivores such as the domestic cat (Braekevelt, 1990). These species have a tapetum cellulosum consisting of closely packed cells rather than layers of fibrous tissue (see Fig. 2-18, Plate 2-I and Plates 14-I and 14-V). This cellular tapetum, like the fibrous tapetum, is with rare exception found only in a portion of the upper fundus. The tapetum of the dog and the cat has an extraordinarily high concentration of zinc, associated with cysteine crystals (Pirie, 1966) to enhance the reflective properties of the tissue. Many congenital abnormalities and disease changes of the tapetum have been described in dogs and cats in the veterinary literature. In this species, and others with a cellular tapetum (e.g., seal), the choriocapillaris may indent the RPE cells so that the tapetal surface remains smooth; when this occurs the capillaries split the layers of Bruch's membrane (Nakaizumi, 1964) to lie beneath the first zone (RPE basement membrane) but above the collagenous zone (see Figs. 2-18, 2-19).

The seal has a cellular tapetum (Fig. 2-19) that covers most of the fundus (Braekevelt, 1986). Walls (1942) noted that it is curious to find such an effective tapetum in a diurnal animal which spends considerable time on land during the day. A possible explanation that he proposed relates to the observation that the seal eye has a very high degree of corneal astigmatism. This is neu-

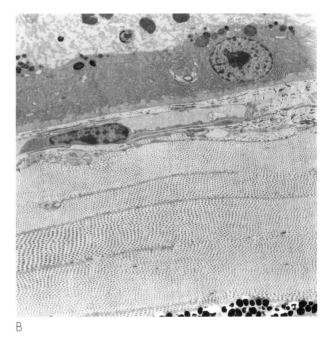

FIGURE 2-17. RPE of the cow. (A) Nontapetal area. There are melanosomes in the apical portion of the RPE cells, and in the choroidal tissue. (B) Tapetal area. The RPE has little or no melanin, and a fibrous (noncellular) tapetum lies immediately behind the choriocapillaris. The tapetal material is a dense array of collagen fibers. Electron micrographs, magnification × 2000 and × 4200, respectively, courtesy of C. R. Braekevelt.

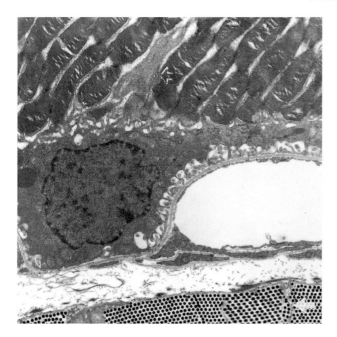

FIGURE 2-18. RPE over the tapetum in the cat. The RPE is amelanotic in this region. A cone sheath of apical RPE processes extends between the rod outer segments *(open arrow)*. The choriocapillaris indents the RPE and overlies the collagenous zones of Bruch's membrane. The tapetum is composed of tightly packed cells *(closed arrow points to a cell junction)*, filled with zinc-cysteine crystals. Electron micrograph, magnification × 9900, courtesy of C. R. Braekevelt.

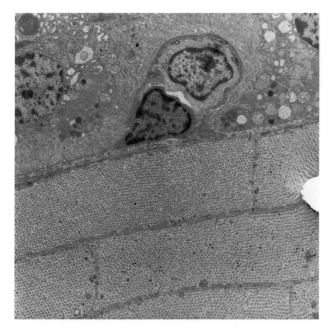

FIGURE 2-19. RPE over the tapetum in the seal. The choriocapillaris indents the RPE and splits Bruch's membrane, as in the cat, and is covered by basal infoldings of the RPE. Note the cellular divisions in the tapetum. Electron micrograph, magnification × 6700, courtesy of C. R. Braekevelt.

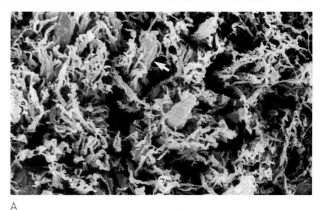

A

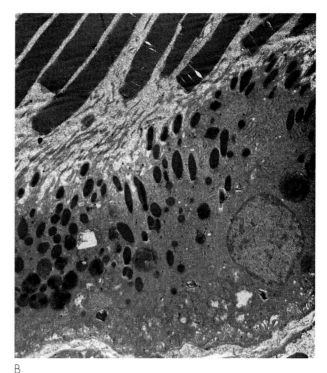

B

FIGURE 2-20. RPE in the rhesus monkey. (A) Scanning electron micrograph of the apical surface, magnification about 2500×. Cone sheaths *(arrow)* are visible among the more fingerlike apical projections that surround the rods. (B) Transmission electron micrograph, magnification about × 3700. (From Marmor et al., 1980.)

tralized under water, of course, but in the air the seal compensates by using a very narrow slit pupil to gain acuity by the principles of a stenopaic slit. The very narrow slit pupil will greatly reduce retinal illumination, however, so that a tapetum becomes useful even during the day.

A cellular tapetum is also found in the nocturnal lemurs and some other prosimians. In the bushbaby (Braekevelt, 1980b), the RPE overlying the tapetum cellulosum is not only depigmented, but the cells are somewhat flattened and squamous in shape (although still joined apically to carry out their epithelial function). The pattern of RPE pigment that interdigitates with receptors at the edge of the tapetum differs among prosimian species, and may relate to their ecological niche (Pariente, 1975). Tapeta are not found in the higher apes or man. The RPE in primates is in general very similar to that in man (Fig. 2-20).

SUMMARY AND CONCLUSIONS

The RPE is remarkably uniform throughout the vertebrate kingdom as a cuboidal hexagonal layer of cells, connected by tight junctions, that serves to isolate and control the environment of the subretinal space. This epithelium phagocytizes the tips of the outer segments on a regular basis and participates in the uptake, storage, and metabolism of the visual pigments. As the name implies, it generally contains melanin pigment which reduces scatter to the photoreceptors, and shields them from excessive light exposure. Many vertebrates have regions of RPE which lack pigment in order to expose a reflecting tapeta which may consist of reflecting material within the RPE itself, or of cellular or fibrous specializations behind the RPE. In submammalian vertebrates, the visual pigment can migrate in and out of the apical RPE processes (or move within the cell body) during light and dark.

Although invertebrates lack a cellular layer directly homologous to the RPE, their eyes still must perform the "RPE functions" of light absorption, neural protection, phagocytosis and visual pigment metabolism. Thus, virtually all invertebrate eyes have pigment cells associated alongside or behind the photoreceptive elements. Some of the other "RPE functions" may be handled by these cells, but are often distributed among nonpigmented cells or the photoreceptors themselves. Visual pigment regeneration in arthropods, for example, is largely photoregenerative within the photoreceptors, while photoreceptor membrane renewal may occur by either pinocytosis into the receptors or phagocytosis by adjacent glial cells.

It is remarkable to look over the animal kingdom and see this homogeneity of RPE structure and function, albeit sometimes achieved in unique and creative ways, to meet the lifestyles of diverse creatures. In this context, human RPE—which has evolved to meet the needs of a particular diurnal primate with high visual acuity and little interest in nocturnal hunting—is a miraculous tissue but does not possess the only or necessarily the best design for all purposes. Through an awareness of the adaptations and correlates of RPE among animals, one may appreciate better the visual role of our own RPE.

ACKNOWLEDGMENT

I am grateful to C.R. Braekevelt, Ph.D., for providing advice and many of the electron micrographs of the vertebrate RPE.

REFERENCES

Anderson RE, Andrews LD. 1982. Biochemistry of retinal photoreceptor membranes in vertebrates and invertebrates. In: Westfall JA, ed, Visual Cells in Evolution. New York: Raven Press, 1–22.

Baker BN, Moriya M, Maude MB, Anderson RE, Williams TP. 1986. Oil droplets of the retinal epithelium of the rat. Exp Eye Res 42:547–557.

Braekevelt CR. 1976. Fine structure of the retinal epithelium and tapetum lucidum of the opossum (Didelphis virginiana). J Morphol 150:213–226.

Braekevelt CR. 1977. Fine structure of the retinal epithelium of the spectacled caiman (Caiman sclerops). Acta Anatomica 97:257–265.

Braekevelt CR. 1980a. The fine structure of the retinal epithelium in the scissortail (Rasbora trileneata) (Teleost). Anat Anz Jena 148:225–235.

Braekevelt CR. 1980b. Fine structure of the retinal epithelium in the bushbaby (Galago senegalensis). Acta Anatomica 107:276–285.

Braekevelt CR. 1980c. Wandering phagocytes at the retinal epithelium–photoreceptor interface in the teleost retina. Vis Res 20:495–499.

Braekevelt CR. 1982. Fine structure of the retinal epithelium and retinal tapetum lucidum of the goldeye Hiodon alosoides. Anat Embryol 164:287–302.

Braekevelt CR. 1984. Retinal pigment epithelial fine structure in the nighthawk (Chordeiles minor). Ophthalmologica Basel 188:222–231.

Braekevelt CR. 1986. Retinal epithelial fine structure in the grey seal (Halichocrus gryphus). Acta Anatomica 127:255–261.

Braekevelt CR. 1990. Retinal epithelial fine structure in the domestic cat (Felis catus). Anat Histol Embryol 19:58–66.

Braekevelt CR. 1992. Retinal pigment epithelial fine structure in the red-backed salamander (Plethodon cinereus). Histol Histopathol 3:471–477.

Burnside B, Dearry A. 1986. Cell motility in the retina. In: Adler R, Farber D, eds, The Retina, part 1, Orlando, FL: Academic Press, 151–206.

Dieterich CE. 1975. On the retinal pigment epithelium of the barn owl (Tyto alba). Albrecht v Graefes Arch Klin Exp Ophthalmol 196:247–254.

Dodge JD. 1991. Photosensory systems in eukaryotic algae. In: Cronly-Dillon JR, Gregory RL, eds, Evolution of the Eye and Visual System, vol 2. Boca Raton: CRC Press, 323–340.

Douglas RH, Djamgoz MBA (eds). 1990. The Visual System of Fish. New York: Chapman and Hall.

Duke-Elder S. 1958. System of Ophthalmology, Vol 1, The Eye in Evolution. London: Henry Kimpton.

Eckmiller MS, Steinberg RH. 1981. Localized depigmentation of the retinal pigment epithelium and macrophage invasion of the retina in the bullfrog. Invest Ophthalmol Vis Sci 21:369–394.

Ewald A, Kühne W. 1978. Untersuchungen über den Sehpurpur III Veränderungen des Sehpurpurs und der Retina im Leben. Untersuch Physiol Inst Univ Heidelberg 1:371–455.

Feeney-Burns L, Mixon RN. 1979. Development of amelanotic retinal pigment epithelium in eyes with a tapetum lucidum: melanosome autophagy and termination of melanogenesis. Develop Biol 72:73–88.

Fein A, Szuts EZ. 1982. Photoreceptors: Their Role in Vision. Cambridge: Cambridge University Press.

Hogan MJ, Alvarado JA, Weddell JE. 1971. Histology of the Human Eye. Philadelphia: Saunders.

Immel J, Negi A, Marmor MF. 1986. Acute changes in RPE apical morphology after retinal detachment in rabbit. Invest Ophthalmol Vis Sci 27:1770–1776.

Kuwabara T. 1975. Cytologic changes of the retina and pigment epithelium during hibernation. Invest Ophthalmol Vis Sci 14:457–467.

Marmor MF, Maack T. 1982. Local environment factors and retinal adhesion in the rabbit. Exp Eye Res 34:727–733.

Marmor MF, Martin LJ. 1978a. 100 years of the visual cycle. Surv Ophthalmol 22:279–285.

Marmor MF, Martin LJ. 1978b. Visual pigment regeneration: occurrence in frog retina upside down upon the pigment epithelium. Experientia 34:374.

Marmor MF, Martin LJ, Tharpe S. 1980. Osmotically induced retinal detachment in the rabbit and primate. Invest Ophthalmol Vis Sci 19:1016–1029.

Matthes MT, Basinger SF. 1980. Myeloid body associations in the frog pigment epithelium. Invest Ophthalmol Vis Sci 19:298–302.

Messenger JB. 1991. Photoreception and vision in molluscs. In: Cronly-Dillon JR, Gregory RL, eds, Evolution of the Eye and Visual System, vol 2. Boca Raton: CRC Press, 364–397.

Nakaizumi Y. 1964. The ultrastructure of Bruch's membrane. Arch Ophthalmol 72:388–394.

Nguyen-Legros J. 1975. Les corps myéloïdes de l'épithélium pigmentaire de la rétine des vertébrés. Arch Ophthalmol 35:759–784.

Nguyen-Legros J. 1978. Fine structure of the pigment epithelium in the vertebrate retina. Intl Rev Cytol 7(Supp):287–328.

Nicol JAC. 1989. The Eyes of Fishes. Oxford: Clarendon Press.

Nilsson D-E. 1989. Optics and evolution of the compound eye. In: Stavenga DG, Hardie RC, eds, Facets of Vision. Berlin, Heidelberg: Springer-Verlag, 30–73.

Pariente GF. 1976. Les differents aspects de la limite du tapetum lucidum chez les prosimiens. Vis Res 16:387–391.

Pirie A. 1966. The chemistry and structure of the tapetum lucidum in animals. In: Graham-Jones O, ed. Aspects of Comparative Ophthalmology. London, Pergamon Press.

Prince JH. 1956. Comparative Anatomy of the Eye. Springfield, IL: Chas C Thomas.

Schwemer J. 1989. Visual pigments of compound eyes—structure, photochemistry, and regeneration. In: Stavenga DG, Hardie RC, eds, Facets of Vision. Berlin, Heidelberg: Springer-Verlag, 112–133.

Stavenga DG. 1989. Pigments in compound eyes. In: Stavenga DG, Hardie RC, eds, Facets of Vision. Berlin, Heidelberg: Springer-Verlag, 152–172.

Steinberg RH, Wood I. 1974. Pigment epithelial cell ensheathment of cone outer segments in the retina of the domestic cat. Proc R Soc Lond B 187:461–478.

Stone LS. 1959. Regeneration of retina, iris and lens. In: Thornton CS, ed, Regeneration in Vertebrates. Chicago: University of Chicago Press, 3–14.

Stroeva OG. 1983. Retinal pigment epithelium: proliferation and differentiation during development and regeneration. Int Rev Cytol 83:221–293.

Tabor GA, Fisher SK. 1983. Myeloid bodies in the mammalian retinal pigment epithelium. Invest Ophthalmol Vis Sci 24:388–391.

Ts'o MOM, Friedman E. 1967. The retinal pigment epithelium. I. Comparative histology. Arch Ophthalmol 78:641–649.

Walls GL. 1942. The Vertebrate Eye and Its Adaptive Radiation (reprinted 1967). New York: Nafner.

Waterman TH. 1982. Fine structure and turnover of photoreceptor membranes. In: Westfall JA, ed, Visual Cells in Evolution. New York: Raven Press, 23–41.

Willmer EN. 1970. Cytology and Evolution. 2nd ed. London: Academic Press, 363–424.

Wolken JJ. 1975. Photoprocesses, Photoreceptors and Evolution. New York: Academic Press.

Wolken JJ. 1995. Light Detectors, Photoreceptors, and Imaging Systems in Nature. New York: Oxford University Press.

Yorke MA, Dickson DH. 1984. Diurnal variations in myeloid bodies of the newt retinal pigment epithelium. Cell Tissue Res 235:177–186.

Young DL, Braekevelt CR. 1993. Fine structure of the retinal epithelial regions of the red kangaroo (Macropus rufus). Anat Anz 175:299–303.

II | FUNDAMENTAL PROPERTIES

3. The retinal pigment epithelial cytoskeleton

BETH BURNSIDE AND LAURIE BOST-USINGER

The last 15 years have seen an explosive increase in our understanding of cytoskeletal composition and function. Genetic and molecular techniques have made it possible to identify and characterize many new cytoskeletal proteins, and powerful in vitro assays for analyzing assembly dynamics and motor function have been developed (see Fuchs and Weber, 1994; Schafer and Cooper, 1995; Maccioni and Cambiazo, 1995; Spudich, 1994). The cytoskeleton has been implicated in mitosis and cytokinesis (see Koshland, 1994; Satterwhite and Pollard, 1992), translocation and localization of messenger RNA (see St Johnston, 1995), directed transport of cytoplasmic components (see Vallee and Bloom, 1991; Fath and Burgess, 1994; Langford, 1995), change and maintenance of cell shape (see Clarke and Spudich, 1977; Kirschner and Mitchison, 1986a), and cell locomotion (see Condeelis, 1993; Lee et al., 1993). Cytoskeletal elements associated with the plasma membrane have been shown to participate in establishment and maintenance of specialized membrane domains (see Bennett and Gilligan, 1993; Hitt and Luna, 1994), regulation of membrane fusion events (see Trifaro and Vitale, 1993), and cell adhesion (see Hynes, 1992; Klymkowsky and Parr, 1995; Huttenlocher et al., 1995). Since the retinal pigment epithelium (RPE) depends on many of these processes for morphogenesis and for carrying out its differentiated functions, and since many RPE functions are critical to photoreceptor survival, the RPE cytoskeleton plays a vital role in maintaining vision (Fig. 3-1). In the review we examine recent studies of the RPE cytoskeleton in relation to the expanding cytoskeleton literature. We emphasize reports published since previous reviews of RPE cytoskeleton appeared (see Burnside, 1976; Burnside and Laties, 1979; Burnside and Nagle, 1983; Burnside and Dearry, 1986; Owaribe, 1988; Hunt, 1994).

COMPONENTS OF THE CYTOSKELETON

The cytoskeleton is composed of three fibrous elements (actin filaments, intermediate filaments, and microtubules) and their associated proteins. Actin filaments and microtubules provide tracks for molecular motors and also provide structural support to the cell. Molecular motors are mechanochemical engines that utilize the energy of ATP hydrolysis to perform mechanical work (see Spudich, 1994). This work is achieved by using the conformational changes generated by ATP hydrolysis to "walk" along an actin filament or microtubule. Intermediate filaments provide mechanical strength and resistance to stretch, but do not appear to serve as tracks for molecular motors (see Fuchs and Weber, 1994).

The membrane cytoskeleton and the cytoplasmic cytoskeleton are structurally and functionally distinct components of the cell. The membrane cytoskeleton coats the cytoplasmic face of the plasma membrane and contributes to membrane contour, stability, and motility (see Hitt and Luna, 1994; Fath and Burgess, 1994; Bennett and Gilligan, 1993). The membrane cytoskeleton is rich in short actin filaments, which may be attached to the membrane either directly by interaction with transmembrane proteins or indirectly by means of actin-binding proteins which themselves interact directly or indirectly with transmembrane proteins (see Luna and Hitt, 1992; Hitt and Luna, 1994; Fath and Burgess, 1994; Bennett and Gilligan, 1993).

The cytoplasmic cytoskeleton is composed of microtubules, actin filaments, and intermediate filaments, and their many associated proteins. The cytoplasmic cytoskeleton is responsible for the structural and tensile properties of the cell, for intracellular transport, and for the contractile and protrusive events which generate cell locomotion and cell shape change (see Cramer et al., 1994; Luby-Phelps, 1994; Heins and Aebi, 1994; Vallee and Bloom, 1991).

The cytoskeleton is highly dynamic. For cells to move and do work, it is crucial that they be able not only to *assemble* cytoskeletal polymers readily, but also to *disassemble* them. To make this possible, the cell utilizes ATP hydrolysis (for actin filaments) or GTP hydrolysis (for microtubules) to maintain the monomer-polymer interaction in a steady state rather than a true equilibrium (see Mitchison, 1992; Heins and Aebi, 1994). Any interference with the dynamics of the cytoskeleton can drastically impair its function.

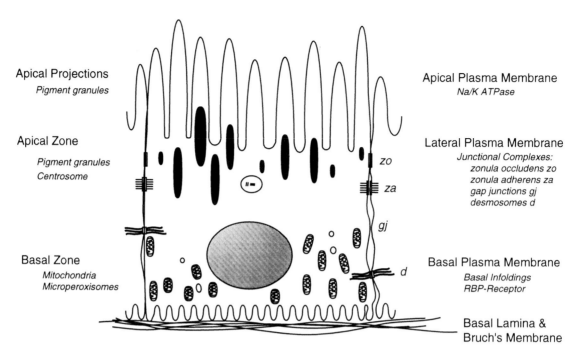

Apical Projections
Pigment granules

Apical Zone

Pigment granules
Centrosome

Basal Zone

Mitochondria
Microperoxisomes

Apical Plasma Membrane
Na/K ATPase

Lateral Plasma Membrane
Junctional Complexes:
zonula occludens zo
zonula adherens za
gap junctions gj
desmosomes d

Basal Plasma Membrane
Basal Infoldings
RBP-Receptor

Basal Lamina &
Bruch's Membrane

zo
za
gj
d

FIGURE 3-1. The polarized phenotype of the differentiated RPE cell. The RPE cell has functionally and biochemically distinct apical and basolateral membrane domains, and asymmetric distributions of cell constituents. The apical plasma membrane is demarcated from the basolat-eral plasma membrane domain by the zonula occludens. The lateral membrane mediates cell contact and adhesion and cell communication via gap junctions. The basal membrane bears the integrins responsible for attachment of the RPE cell to its basal lamina and Bruch's membrane.

The Actin Cytoskeleton

Actin filaments play both structural and motile roles in the cell. They provide anchorage for membrane proteins, influence membrane deformability, and otherwise contribute to the mechanical properties of cytoplasm (see Hitt and Luna, 1994). Actin filaments also interact with myosin motors to produce contraction and intracellular transport of cytoplasmic constituents (see Clarke and Spudich, 1977). When cross-linked into bundles, actin filaments create a stiff scaffolding which can support cell projections or influence cell shape (see Clarke and Spudich, 1977). Enzymes, including those of the glycolytic pathway, and messenger RNAs, including those for cytoskeletal proteins, bind to actin filaments; thus actin filaments mediate localization of enzymes and mRNA in the cell (see Singer, 1992; St Johnston, 1995). Other actin-dependent processes include cell locomotion (see Theriot and Mitchison, 1992; Cramer et al., 1994), cell shape change (see Clarke and Spudich, 1977; Cramer et al., 1994), exocytosis (see Trifaro and Vitale, 1993), organelle transport (see Langford, 1995), the engulfment phase of phagocytosis (see Greenberg, 1995), cytokinesis (see Satterwhite and Pollard, 1992), and cell adhesion (see Huttenlocher et al., 1995).

All known actin functions are performed by actin fil-aments (F-actin). These filaments have inherent polarity (see Mitchison, 1992). One end of the actin filament, designated the plus end, assembles at a lower critical concentration of free subunits and at a faster rate than the minus end. Since myosins can only walk toward the plus ends of actin filaments, the orientation of actin filaments within a cell is a critical aspect of actin-dependent motility.

Cellular motile events depend on dynamic reorganizations of the actin cytoskeleton, as well as on force production by molecular motors (see Mitchinson, 1992; Pollard and Cooper, 1986). The cell regulates the mechanical properties of its cytoplasm by means of numerous actin-binding proteins which variously nucleate, stiffen, stabilize, sever, or cross-link actin filaments in response to intracellular signals (see Pollard and Cooper, 1986). Many actin binding proteins perform more than one of these tasks.

Because of the dynamic nature of the actin cytoskeleton, it has been possible to investigate the roles of actin filaments in cell function by treating cells with drugs that affect actin assembly. The fungal metabolites called cytochalasins readily cross membranes and thus have been particularly useful for identifying actin-mediated processes (Ohmori et al., 1992; Cooper, 1987; Goddette and Frieden, 1986). Cytochalasins bind to and cap the plus ends of actin filaments, thereby preventing further assembly (Ohmori et al., 1992; Cooper, 1987; Goddette and Frieden, 1986). Thus cytochalasins block any on-going net assembly of actin filaments in the cell. If a cell function is blocked by cytochalasin at low concentrations (0.1–0.5 μm range), then it is justified to conclude that the process requires actin assembly. Higher concentrations of cytochalasin produce abnormal clumps of actin filaments, which may nonspecifically obstruct actin-independent motile events. Cytochalasins affect only dynamic actin filaments, they have little or no effect on actin filaments that are stabilized by actin-binding proteins. Thus failure to block a cell process with cytochalasins would not necessarily rule out a role for stable actin filaments, and morphological evaluation of filament disruption is a critical control. Recently, several new drugs have been characterized which sever actin filaments both in vitro and in vivo: tolytoxin (Patterson et al., 1993), latrunculins (Spector et al., 1989), and swinholide A (Bubb et al., 1995). These drugs expand the arsenal of inhibitors for studying the roles of actin filaments in cellular events.

In polarized RPE cells, actin filaments are localized to the basal infoldings, the lateral membrane cytoskeleton, the apical projections, and the dense circumferential microfilament bundles (CMBs) which encircle the cell apex and associate with the zonulae adherens junctions be-

tween adjacent RPE cells (see Nguyen-Legros, 1978; Owaribe, 1988) (Fig. 3-2). Roles for actin filaments in RPE functions have been suggested by numerous reports of cytochalasin effects. High levels of cytochalasin (5–10 μm) induced gaps in well-differentiated cultured RPE cells, suggesting that actin filament disruption impaired the maintenance of epithelial integrity (Crawford et al., 1972; Owaribe et al., 1979; Sakamoto et al., 1994). However, lower levels of cytochalasin blocked similar gap formation induced by thrombin, suggesting a role for actin assembly in producing these gaps (Sakamoto et al., 1994). Cytochalasin has also been reported to inhibit RPE cell migration in vitro (Seldon and Schwartz, 1979; Campochiaro and Glaser, 1986; Gordon and Staley, 1990), wound closure in epithelial monolayers of cultured RPE cells (Verstraeten et al., 1990), migration of pigment granules in fish RPE (Burnside et al., 1983), and engulfment of rod outer segment packets or foreign particles during phagocytosis by RPE cells (Besharse and Dunis, 1982). The possible roles of actin filaments in these processes will be considered in more detail below.

The Myosin Superfamily

To date only one class of motor proteins, the large superfamily of myosins, is known to translocate along

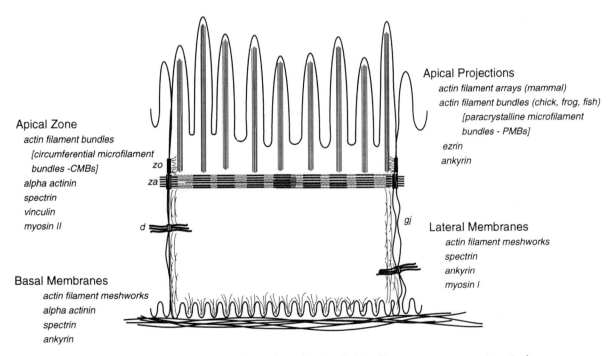

FIGURE 3-2. The actin cytoskeleton of the polarized RPE cell. Actin filaments are most prominent in the apical projections and in the circumferential microfilament bundle (CMB) which encircles the cell apex and attaches to the zonula adherens. The basolateral plasma membranes are lined with a meshwork of short actin filaments. Several actin-binding proteins are asymmetrically distributed.

actin filaments to produce motive force (see Mooseker and Cheney, 1995). Though the myosin superfamily is large and heterogeneous, all myosins have common diagnostic characteristics: all are actin-activated ATPases with conserved ATP- and actin-binding sites in the motor domain (head region). The tail regions of myosins are highly variable and mediate attachment to cargo, dimer formation, or filament formation. Eleven different classes of myosins have been identified to date (Mooseker and Cheney, 1995), and more are likely to come. Many have been identified only by sequence, and their functions are not yet known. Multiple classes of myosins are expressed by individual cells, and most classes have been found in several different species.

Class II myosins are generally called "conventional myosins" because they form the familiar thick filaments of skeletal muscle and other cell types (see Hasson and Mooseker, 1994; Mooseker and Cheney, 1995). Since class II myosins are critical to cytokinesis and other contractile events, they play a role in the lives of all cells. The rest of the myosin classes have been called "unconventional myosins," because they do not form filaments (see Goodson, 1994). The first unconventional myosins identified belonged to the myosin I family. These myosins have the characteristic head region but have very abbreviated tails and do not form dimers or filaments. Functions attributed to myosin I family members include phagocytosis and contractile vacuole formation in *Dictyostelium* and *Acanthamoeba,* cell locomotion and formation and maintenance of microvilli in the brush border of intestinal epithelial cells (see Hasson and Mooseker, 1994; Mooseker and Cheney, 1995).

Class III has only one published member so far: the *Drosophila* ninaC protein. This myosin is localized to the rhabdomeric microvilli of photoreceptors and has a kinase domain in addition to the actin-dependent motor domain found in all myosins (Montell and Rubin, 1988; H. Matsumoto et al., 1987; Porter et al., 1992). Mutations in ninaC produce an altered photoresponse and light-induced retinal degeneration. We have recently identified a vertebrate homologue of ninaC which is expressed in fish and human retina and RPE (Hillman et al., 1998b). Class IV myosin has so far been detected only in *Acanthamoeba;* its function is not known (see Mooseker and Cheney, 1995). Class V myosins, which exhibit some properties of both class I and II myosins, are a particularly interesting group (see Titus, 1993). Chick brain myosin V colocalizes with perinuclear cytoplasmic vesicles and is distributed in a punctate pattern at the tips of neuronal processes (Espreafico et al., 1992). The product of the mouse *dilute* gene is a member of this group (Mercer et al., 1991). Mutations at the *dilute* locus compromise pigment granule transfer by

dermal melanocytes (producing the "dilute" coat color) and also produce nervous system abnormalities. Class VI myosins have been characterized from both *Drosophila* and porcine kidney cells (Hasson and Mooseker, 1994; Kellerman and Miller, 1992). *Drosophila* myosin VI has been shown to mediate particle transport along actin filaments (Mermall and Miller, 1995).

Of particular interest to vision research are the class VII myosins. Defects in the gene for myosin VIIA have recently been shown to be responsible for Usher syndrome type 1B (Weil et al., 1995), which results in both deafness and photoreceptor degeneration (retinitis pigmentosa). Defects in the mouse homologue of this gene produce the shaker-1 phenotype, also associated with deafness but not with photoreceptor degeneration (Gibson et al., 1995). The myosin VIIA gene is expressed in cochlea, RPE, testis, lung, and kidney (Hasson et al., 1995). The functions of class VII myosins are as yet unknown. Class VIII and IX myosins have been identified only in plants and are still being characterized (see Mooseker and Cheney, 1995). Class IX myosins have been cloned and sequenced from rat, human, and pig, and are unique among the known myosins in possessing a domain homologous to GTP-activating proteins (see Mooseker and Cheney, 1995). The functions of class IX myosins and also of class X myosins, which have been partially sequenced from bovine muscle and from bullfrog cochlea, are not yet known.

Immunocytochemical studies have provided information about the subcellular localization of myosins I, II, and VII in RPE cells of a variety of species (Fig. 3-2). An antibody to bovine adrenal myosin I localized primarily to lateral cell membranes and to small vesicles in cultured human RPE cells; little labeling was observed in the apical zone and apical projections (Breckler and Burnside, 1994). Post-Golgi transport vesicles from intestinal epithelial cells have also been shown to bear myosin I on their surfaces, suggesting they may be transported along actin filaments in the cell (Fath and Burgess, 1994). Myosin II is abundant in the apical circumferential bundle of actin filaments in RPE cells, and presumably participates in their contractility (see Owaribe et al., 1988). Myosin VII was immunolocalized to the actin-rich apical region of rat RPE cells, suggesting a possible role for this myosin in phagocytosis (Hasson et al., 1995).

Recently our laboratory has identified several myosin family members that are expressed in teleost RPE (Hillman et al., 1998a). Using degenerate primers for two highly conserved regions which flank the myosin ATP binding site, we have produced PCR products representing eleven distinct myosin isoforms from RPE of the striped bass, *Morone saxatilis.* Although these myosin

TABLE 3-1. *Myosin family members identified in teleost RPE*

Fish sequence	RPE clones (%)	Closest relative	Identity (%)	Family placement	Reference
FM1	7.8	Myosin I (mouse)	93	I	Koslovsky et al., 1993
FM2	6.3	Myosin VIIAA(pig)	96	VIIA	Bement et al., 1994
FM3	7.8	Myosin IB (bovine)	75	IB-like	Reizes et al., 1994
FM4	10.9	Myosin VA (mouse)	93	V	Mercer et al., 1991
FM5	4.7	Myosin VIIBA (pig)	76	X-like	Bement et al., 1994
FM7	15.6	Myosin VIIBA (pig)	69	X-like	Bement et al., 1994
FM12	15.6	Myosin IXBA (human)	92	IXB	Bement et al., 1994
FM16	15.6	NinaC (Drosophila)	*	III	Montell and Rubin, 1988
FM22	4.7	Nonmuscle Myosin II (rat)	94	II	Shohet et al., 1989
FM25	4.7	Myosin IXAA (human)	98	IXA	Bement et al., 1994
FM30	6.3	NinaC (Drosophila)	*	III	Montell and Rubin, 1988

Closest relative for each FM was generated from the UWGCG TFastA search (Devereaux et al., 1984).
*Complete sequences of FM16 and FM30 reveal that they have N-terminal kinase domains and closest homology to *Drosophila* ninaC (Hillman et al., 1997b).

PCR products represent only a part of the motor domain, this region is near the ATP-binding P-loop and appears to contain, in addition to the conserved domains, relatively specific variable domains which are highly diagnostic for myosin classes (see Goodson, 1994). A homology search at the amino acid level identified the most closely related myosin in the GenBank database for each fish myosin PCR product (Table 3-1). Six of the fish myosin PCR products were more than 90% homologous to previously described myosins in the sequenced region and thus represent possible homologues. The remaining five clones were less than 76% homologous to the most closely related myosin in the database. One of these was myosin VIIB-like, and two (FM16A and FM16B) were closely related to one another but only 53% identical to any myosin in the database. These myosins have subsequently been completely sequenced and shown to be members of Class III; thus they are vertebrate homologues of ninaC (Montell and Rubin, 1988). Our myosin screen clearly has not identified all myosins expressed in RPE. An antibody against pig myosin VI (Hasson and Mooseker, 1994) recognizes a protein of the appropriate molecular weight in fish RPE; however we failed to detect a myosin VI in our PCR screen.

Tissue-specific expression patterns of the 11 fish myosin clones were examined by Northern blot analysis against total RNA isolated from RPE, retina, muscle, kidney, brain, and liver of the striped bass. Of the 11 PCR products cloned by RT-PCR from teleost RPE, four were particularly interesting: a class X like myosin appeared to be selectively expressed in RPE; myosin IXB was more highly expressed in RPE than in other tissues;

myosin VIIA was selectively and highly expressed in RPE and retina; and myosin III, the ninaC novel homologue was extremely abundant in retina with lower levels in RPE and brain. Clearly, the RPE expresses many myosin motor isoforms, individual ones of which may be specialized to carry out distinct RPE motile processes.

The Microtubule Cytoskeleton

Microtubules are self-assembling polymers whose soda-straw structure makes them relatively stiff and therefore useful as scaffolding and tracks. The two ends of the microtubule differ structurally, thereby affecting the ease with which new subunits can polymerize onto each end (see Kirschner and Mitchison, 1986b; Mitchison, 1992). Thus, like actin filaments, microtubules have plus and minus ends. Inside the cell, the minus ends of microtubules are usually capped or embedded in microtubule organizing centers (MTOCs—see Mitchison, 1992). Therefore microtubule assembly in the cell is dominated by the dynamics of polymerization at the plus end. Cytoplasmic microtubules and their free subunits coexist in a steady state called *dynamic instability,* in which the microtubule plus end switches spontaneously from slow elongation (assembly) to fast shortening (disassembly) and then back again, with each state persisting for many seconds (see Mitchison and Kirschner, 1984; Mitchison, 1992). Dynamic instability is powered by the hydrolysis of GTP: free microtubule subunits bind GTP, assemble into the polymer, and then hydrolyze the GTP, thereby destabilizing the polymer and permitting disassembly. Because of dynamic instability, the numerous microtubules in a cell are elongating and shortening asynchronously. Newly assembling microtubules can probe all parts of the cell, and selective stabilization of microtubules can lead to altered cytoplasmic organization and/or cell shape change.

Not all microtubules are dynamic. In many cells, microtubules are stabilized by microtubule-associated proteins (MAPs), which bind to their surfaces and inhibit disassembly (see Lee, 1993). These are two distinct types of MAPs: nonmotor MAPs (MAPs 1–5, and tau protein) and microtubule-dependent motor proteins (kinesins and dyneins). Many known MAPs are found only in neurons (Bloom et al., 1984; Sato-Yoshitake et al., 1989); however, MAP3, MAP4, and tau are expressed in a variety of tissues, including epithelial cells (Huber and Matus, 1990; West et al., 1991). Nonmotor MAPs both enhance microtubule assembly and stabilize the polymer (Edson et al., 1993; Hirokawa, 1994). Exogenous tau protein increases the polymerization rate and decreases the depolymerization rate of microtubules in vitro (Drechsel et al., 1992). MAPs can also cross-link microtubules (see Lee, 1993), thereby producing rigid microtubule bundles capable of providing scaffolding for cell projections.

Although MAPs have been studied primarily in neurons, a novel nonneural MAP has recently been characterized. When overexpressed in fibroblasts, this MAP (E-MAP-115) renders the cells' microtubules nocodazole-insensitive, indicating greatly increased stability (Masson and Kreis, 1993). Since E-MAP-115 immunofluorescence increases and microtubules become more stable upon polarization of Caco-2 intestinal epithelial cells in culture, it has been suggested that stabilization of microtubules by E-MAP-115 plays a role in polarization and differentiation of epithelial cells.

Drugs which affect microtubule assembly have been useful for examining the functional roles of microtubules in many cell types. Colchicine binds to free tubulin heterodimer. When the colchicine-dimer binds to the microtubule plus end, it blocks further assembly, leading to catastrophic disassembly of the microtubule. Colchicine is only effective against microtubules that are undergoing dynamic instability; it has no effect on microtubules stabilized by MAPs. Nocodazole binds to a similar site on the tubulin dimer as colchicine and has similar effects on microtubules but has fewer side effects. Taxol binds to and stabilizes the microtubule polymer and prevents microtubule disassembly. Taxol blocks many microtubule-dependent processes, including mitosis, indicating that not only assembly but also disassembly are critical to many microtubule functions (see Mitchison, 1992).

Microtubule-Dependent Motors

Microtubule-dependent motile events are powered by kinesins and dyneins (see Vallee, 1993; Holzbaur et al., 1994). These motors are microtubule-activated ATPases which utilize the energy of ATP hydrolysis to translocate cargo along microtubules. The globular head region of each motor type contains both an ATP-binding site and a microtubule-binding site. Both types of motors also contain α-helical coiled-coil stalk regions which mediate dimerization, and a tail region which interacts with accessory intermediate or light chains and mediates interactions with cargoes. Kinesins and dyneins are constrained in the direction they can move along microtubules; most kinesins walk toward the plus ends of microtubules while dyneins and a small subset of kinesins walk toward the minus ends. Thus, the arrangement of microtubules within a cell is critical to vectorial transport. Motor protein activity in the cell may be regulated either by phosphorylation events or through interactions with accessory proteins (Matthies et al., 1993; Gill et al., 1991).

Because they are smaller and easier to sequence, kinesins have been more thoroughly characterized than dyneins (see Bloom and Endow, 1995; Goldstein, 1993). The first kinesin to be identified was the conventional kinesin heavy chain (KHC) of squid axoplasm. Subsequent studies demonstrated that members of the KHC family were found in most cells and that this family was but one member of a large superfamily of related proteins, termed kinesin family members (KIFs; see Bloom and Endow, 1995). KIFs are defined by the extensive homology they share within the globular motor domain containing the ATP- and microtubule-binding sites. The stalk and tail domains are much more variable and presumably reflect specializations for interaction with different cargoes.

KIFs are classified into seven distinct families based on amino acid sequence and structural similarity (Goldstein, 1993; Sekine et al., 1994). In most cases, members of the same families perform similar functions in vivo. In addition, there are several "orphans" which are not members of the seven conserved families and have no homologues in other organisms. The kinesin heavy chain (KHC) family contains the founding members, about which the most biochemical, structural, and functional information is known (Vale et al., 1985; Bloom et al., 1988). KHC family members have been shown to be involved in fast axonal transport of membranous organelles (Vale et al., 1985), extension of tubular lysosomes in macrophages (Hollenbeck and Swanson, 1990), and pigment granule movement in melanophores

(Rodionov et al., 1991). KIF3 family members have been identified in a variety of species including mouse (Kondo et al., 1994), sea urchin (Cole et al., 1993), and fish (Beech et al., 1996), and in the mouse have been shown to function as anterograde motors in fast axonal transport. KIF1/unc104 family members have been identified in both *Caenorhabditis elegans* (Otsuka et al., 1991) and mouse (Nangaku et al., 1994) and have been shown to be important for synaptic vesicle and mitochondrial transport. The KIF4 family is fairly small with three members; the founding member (KIF4) has been characterized in the mouse, where it functions as an anterograde motor and is developmentally regulated (Sekine et al., 1994). The bimC family of proteins was first identified by their "**b**locked **i**n **m**itosis" phenotype defined in *Aspergillus* (Enos and Morris, 1990), and thus far most of these family members appear to participate in mitotic and meiotic events. The last two families of kinesins (KIF2 and CKIF) are unique in that the motor domains have either a central (KIF2) or C-terminal (CKIF) location, as opposed to the typical N-terminal motor domain. All CKIFs thus far analyzed translocate their cargo toward the minus ends of microtubules, making them the renegades of the KIFs (Bloom and Endow, 1995).

Our laboratory has used a PCR-based cloning strategy to isolate kinesin family members expressed in teleost RPE (King-Smith et al., 1995; Bost-Usinger et al., 1997). We have isolated six different fish kinesin family members (FKIFs1-6) from teleost RPE using degenerate primers which recognize two highly conserved regions in the motor domains of all kinesins (Table 3-2). The partial motor domain of each of the FKIFs was cloned and sequenced, and a predicted amino acid sequence generated for each. A homology search at the amino acid level identified the most closely related kinesin in the GenBank database for each FKIF (Table 3-2). FKIF1 and 5 appear to be members of the KHC family, while FKIF3

appears to be the fish homologue of the mouse KIF1B gene. FKIF4 appears to be a member of the KIF2 family with central motor domains. Because of the low level of identity to their most closely related kinesins, FKIF2 and 6 appear to represent novel kinesin family members.

Of these RPE kinesins, FKIF2 is the most interesting to us. FKIF2 was not only the most prevalent kinesin detected in our PCR screen, but also the most abundantly expressed kinesin in the RPE as assessed by Northern blot analysis. Antibodies to FKIF2 identify an ~80 kDa protein in teleost RPE, and also in cultured human RPE. Complete cDNA sequence analysis has confirmed that FKIF2 is a novel kinesin with a C-terminal motor domain (Bost-Usinger et al., 1997). Both in vitro motility assays and functional studies suggest that most C-terminal KIFs function as minus-end-directed motors (Goldstein, 1993). If FKIF2 is also minus end directed, it would move cargo from base toward apex in the RPE cell. Further analysis and characterization of FKIF2 is needed to clarify the role of FKIF2 in RPE function.

Dyneins comprise a separate superfamily of very large minus-end-directed microtubule motors, including both flagellar and cytoplasmic isoforms (see Vallee, 1993; Collins, 1994). Cytoplasmic dyneins contain two massive heavy chains (~500 kDa), three intermediate chains (~74 kDa), and four associated light chains (~50 kDa). Dynein has been implicated in a number of minus-end-directed microtubule-dependent motile events, including retrograde axonal transport, translocation of secretory vesicles, and poleward migration of chromosomes (see Vallee, 1993; Collins, 1994). Although dynein functions have not been analyzed in RPE cells, dynein has been implicated in vesicle transport in MDCK cells (Lafont et al., 1994). Immunodepletion of cytosolic dynein partially inhibited apical-directed post-Golgi transport in these cells, consistent with a role for dynein in minus-end-directed transport along microtubules.

TABLE 3-2. *Kinesin family members identified in teleost RPE*

Fish sequence	RPE clones (%)	Closest relative	Identity (%)	Family placement	Reference
FKIF1	6.2	KHC (human)	95	KHC	Navone et al., 1992
FKIF2	71.6	KHC (Drosophila)	42	NOVEL	Yang et al., 1989
FKIF3	11.1	KIF1B (mouse)	90	UNC104	Nangaku et al., 1994
FKIF4	3.7	KIF2 (mouse)	64	KIF2	Noda et al., 1995
FKIF5	4.9	KHC (mouse)	87	KHC	Aizawa et al., 1993
FKIF6	2.5	NCD$_1$ (Drosophila)	42	NOVEL	McDonald and Goldstein, 1990

Closest relative for each FKIF was generated from the UWGCG TFastA search (Devereaux et al., 1984).
1 non-claret disjunction

Intermediate Filaments

Intermediate filaments are the third fibrous component of the cytoskeleton (see Fuchs and Weber, 1994). Found in the cytoplasm of most, but not all, animal cells, intermediate filaments are so named because their diameter is between that of thin actin filaments and thick myosin filaments or microtubules. Intermediate filament proteins are classified into five types based upon sequence homology, immunological cross-reactivity, and site of expression. Type I and type II intermediate filaments comprise the acidic and basic cytokeratins, respectively; both are expressed primarily in epithelial cells (see Coulombe, 1993). Type III intermediate filament proteins are expressed in cells of mesenchymal origin and include vimentin, desmin, glial fibrillary acidic protein, and peripherin (see Franke, 1979). Type IV proteins are the low-, medium-, and high-molecular-weight subunits of neurofilaments (see Okabe, 1993). Type V proteins, the lamins, are present in all nucleated cells, where they provide the structural components of the nuclear envelope (Gerace and Burke, 1988).

Intermediate filaments are very heterogeneous in both molecular size and electric charge, but share a common basic molecular arrangement (see Fuchs and Weber, 1994). In contrast to the globular monomeric units of actin filaments and microtubules, intermediate filament protein monomers are elongated fibrous molecules containing variable amino-terminal heads and carboxy-terminal tail regions, and a highly conserved α-helical central rod domain (see Stewart, 1993). The central rod domain mediates the formation of coiled-coil dimers which associate in an antiparallel manner to form a tetrameric subunit. Unlike actin filaments and microtubules, intermediate filaments are nonpolarized.

The functions of intermediate filaments are not nearly as well characterized as those of actin filaments or microtubules (see Fuchs and Weber, 1994). Intermediate filaments are completely lacking in some cells (Hedberg and Chen, 1986) and can be disrupted in others with no deleterious effects (Klymkowsky et al., 1983). Disruption of keratin intermediate filaments by microinjection of antikeratin antibodies had no detectable effect on living cultured fibroblasts. However, intermediate filaments clearly play specialized structural roles in certain tissues. In the human disease epidermolysis bullosa simplex, point mutations in a keratin gene so weaken the mechanical stability of the intermediate filaments in dermal keratinocytes that the epidermis becomes extremely vulnerable to mechanical injury (Coulombe, 1993). Transgenic mice expressing these mutant keratins also exhibit perturbed epidermal architecture (Vassar et al., 1991). Thus, keratin filaments of epithelial cells appear to provide critical structural support for resisting imposed tensile forces and preventing mechanical trauma.

In epithelial cells, intermediate filaments are primarily composed of the acidic type I and basic type II cytokeratins (see Fuchs and Weber, 1994). Cytokeratin intermediate filaments are generally assembled from heterotetramers composed of two type I subunits and two type II subunits. In epithelial cells, cytokeratin intermediate filaments are anchored at desmosomes and hemidesmosomes, where they are optimally situated to reinforce the attachment of cells to adjacent cells or to the basement lamina. Desmosomes and associated intermediate filaments have been observed in RPE of cows (Owaribe et al., 1988), rats (Miki et al., 1975), frogs (Hudspeth and Yee, 1973), and humans (Schlotzer-Schrehardt et al., 1990; Hunt et al., 1989). Surprisingly, chick RPE cells do not contain desmosomes, nor do they express cytokeratins, the intermediate filament type commonly associated with desmosomes (Docherty et al., 1984).

A variety of immunological techniques have been used to identify the intermediate filament expression patterns in RPE cells. These will be only briefly summarized here, since an excellent and detailed review of intermediate filament expression and function in RPE cells has recently appeared (see Hunt, 1994). The expression pattern of intermediate filament proteins in RPE cells varies with species and with culture conditions in vitro. Chick RPE cells are unique in that they express only vimentin intermediate filaments rather than cytokeratins (Doherty et al., 1984; Philp and Nachmias, 1985; Owaribe et al., 1988). In the RPE of amphibia and certain mammals (rats and rabbits), only cytokeratins are expressed (Owaribe et al., 1988; Stroeva et al., 1983). In other mammals (guinea pigs, cows, and humans), RPE cells express both cytokeratins and vimentin (Owaribe et al., 1988; McKechnie et al., 1988; Kasper et al., 1988; Berman et al., 1974). These findings suggest that either vimentin or cytokeratin intermediate filaments can meet the structural needs of RPE cells.

When RPE cells are removed from the eye and put into culture, their cytokeratin expression pattern changes (see Owaribe, 1988; Hunt, 1994). When bovine RPE cells are placed in culture, cytokeratin synthesis decreases and vimentin expression increases. After prolonged culture, all cells seem to express vimentin (Owaribe, 1988). In cat RPE, when cells are subconfluent and dedifferentiated, vimentin filaments are distributed throughout the cytoplasm. When the cells become confluent and display a more differentiated phenotype, vimentin filaments are more concentrated near the cell borders (Matsumoto et al., 1990). Human RPE cells in vivo express cytokeratin 8 and 18 and no vimentin, but when placed in culture express cytokeratins 7, 8, 18, and 19 and vimentin (Hunt and Davis, 1990). Another study reported that cultured human RPE cells express vimentin and a much wider variety of cytokeratins than freshly isolated RPE (McKechnie et al., 1988).

The pattern of intermediate protein expression in vitro is influenced by culture conditions. Exposing cultured RPE cells to vitreous components decreases the proportion of cells coexpressing both cytokeratins and vimentin over time (Vinores et al., 1990). In certain pathological situations RPE cells detach from Bruch's membrane, migrate through the retina, and take up residence on the vitreal surface of the retina in epiretinal membranes (Machemer et al., 1975). The alterations of cytokeratin expression produced by vitreous factors may contribute to dedifferentiated phenotypes in RPE cells.

Intermediate filaments interact with both the actin and microtubule cytoskeletons in RPE cells (Owaribe, 1988). The circumferential bundle of actin filaments is intimately associated with vimentin intermediate filaments to create a central meshwork across the entire apical zone of chick RPE cells. In RPE cells, as in other cell types, microtubules are necessary for maintenance of normal intermediate filament distribution (see Foisner and Wiche, 1991). For example, in cultured chick RPE cells, vimentin filaments are normally dispersed throughout the cytoplasm; however, disruption of the microtubule cytoskeleton with colcemid induces them to collapse into dense bundles which encircle the nucleus (Foisner and Wiche, 1991). Similar clumping of intermediate filaments near the nucleus were seen in teleost RPE cells in vivo after intraocular injections of colchicine (Burnside and Nagle, 1983).

EPITHELIAL POLARITY

The specialized functions of epithelial cells depend upon the establishment of asymmetric membrane domains and polarized distributions of organelles (see Rodriguez-Boulan and Nelson, 1989; Rodriguez-Boulan and Powell, 1992). The apical and basolateral domains of the plasma membrane are segregated by tight junctions and contain distinct compositions of proteins and lipids. This asymmetric distribution is achieved both by targeted delivery of transport vesicles from the Golgi complex to specific domains, and by protein sorting in both the Golgi and in the cell surface membranes (see Rodriguez-Boulan and Nelson, 1989; Rodriguez-Boulan and Powell, 1992; Hitt and Luna, 1994). The cytoskeleton has been shown to participate in targeting and sorting of membrane proteins, in maintenance of

asymmetric distributions of organelles, and in vectorial exocytosis (see Nelson, 1991; Mays et al., 1994; Trifaro and Vitale, 1993; Muallem et al., 1995). Thus cytoskeletal contributions are critical to the establishment and maintenance of epithelial polarity.

Most evidence suggests that the targeted transport of post-Golgi vesicles in epithelial cells depends primarily on microtubules (see Mays et al., 1994). In MDCK (kidney) and Caco-2 (intestinal) epithelial cells in vitro, and in rat and mouse intestinal epithelial cells in vivo, disruption of microtubules resulted in reduced delivery of apical secretory and membrane proteins and the missorting of some apical proteins to the basolateral domain (Achler, 1989; Gilbert et al., 1991; Parczyk et al., 1989; Eilers et al., 1989). The role of microtubules in delivering proteins from the Golgi to the basolateral membrane domain is less clear. Nocodazole failed to inhibit delivery to the basolateral membrane in either MDCK or Caco-2 cells (Gilbert et al., 1991; Parczyk et al., 1989; Eilers et al., 1989); however, complete microtubule disruption may not have been achieved with nocodazole in those studies (Eilers et al., 1989; Van der Sluijs et al., 1990). Both apically directed and basolaterally directed transport vesicles have been shown to bind to microtubules in a specific, cytosol-dependent manner, suggesting that microtubules might in fact participate in basolateral transport (Van der Sluijs et al., 1990). Microtubules also appear to be required for delivery of transport vesicles from the basolateral to the apical plasma membrane domains (transcytosis) but not for transport in the other direction (see Mays et al., 1994). Since cytochalasin disruption of the actin cytoskeleton had no effect on delivery of vesicles from Golgi to either plasma membrane domain, directed transport does not appear to depend on actin filaments (Parczyk et al., 1989; Salas et al., 1986).

Both actin and microtubules have been implicated in mediating some aspects of endocytosis, though these roles appear to differ in different cell types (see Schelling et al., 1992; Gottlieb et al., 1993; Elkjaer et al., 1995). Disruption of microtubules has been reported to inhibit apical endocytosis and maintenance of a polarized distribution of endocytic components and apical membrane proteins (Bomsel et al., 1990; Elkjaer et al., 1995). Actin filament disruption by cytochalasin blocked endocytosis from the apical membrane but not from the basolateral domain, suggesting a role for actin in apical but not basolateral endocytosis (Gottlieb et al., 1993). Since isolated cytoplasmic vesicles from intestinal epithelial cells were found to possess both myosin I and dynein on their surfaces, it seems likely that either actin or microtubule cytoskeletal systems can contribute to intracellular vesicle transport (Fath and Burgess, 1993).

The specific association with particular motors may thus dictate polarity of transport.

RPE cells are said to exhibit "reverse polarity" in comparison to other epithelial cell types because in RPE cells the Na^+/K^+-ATPase is localized to the apical rather than the basolateral plasma membrane (Bok, 1982; Gundersen et al., 1991; Rizzolo, 1990). Nonetheless the RPE does not exhibit reversed polarity in other respects. The distribution of most membrane proteins is more typical, and enveloped viruses bud from the appropriate membranes, suggesting that polarized transport in RPE cells conforms to that of other epithelia (Bok et al., 1992; Gundersen et al., 1991; Philp and Nachmias, 1987; Philp et al., 1990; Rizzolo et al., 1994). As RPE polarity is also discussed in "Determinants of RPE Phenotype and Polarity" by Janice Burke (see Chapter 5), our discussion is specifically directed at the role of the cytoskeleton in maintaining RPE polarity.

The Actin Cytoskeleton in Polarized RPE Cells

The asymmetric distribution of actin filaments and actin-binding proteins in RPE cells resembles that of other polarized epithelia (Rodriguez-Boulan and Nelson, 1989; Mays et al., 1994) (see Fig. 3-2). As cultured epithelial cells reach confluence and assume epithelial polarity, their actin cytoskeletons undergo dramatic rearrangement. Early in culture before confluence, epithelial cells spread and attach to the substratum by focal adhesions, which are associated with bundles of actin filaments called stress fibers (Crawford, 1980; Turksen et al., 1983; Sandig and Kalnins, 1988). These stress fibers contain myosin II, exhibit striations, and extend from one focal adhesion to another, as observed in many other cultured cells, including fibroblasts (see Clarke and Spudich, 1977). As cells assume polarity after confluence, the actin cytoskeleton rearranges. Stress fibers disappear and actin filaments accumulate most abundantly in the apical circumferential microfilament bundle (CMB) associated with the zonula adherens (see Crawford, 1980; Turksen et al., 1983; Sandig and Kalnins, 1988; Owaribe, 1988).

The mature polarized epithelial cell also has an asymmetric distribution of actin-binding proteins (see Pollard and Cooper, 1986) (see Fig. 3-2). Alpha actinin, an actin-binding protein which both cross-links actin filaments and attaches them to membranes in many cell types (see Pollard and Cooper, 1986), is localized to the regions of the zonula adherens and CMB and to the basal infoldings, but is sparse elsewhere in the RPE cell (Nihira et al., 1989; Arikawa and Williams, 1991) (Fig. 3-2). Members of the spectrin superfamily (also called fodrins in nonerythroid cells) cross-link actin filaments into meshworks critical to the stability and flexibility of the plasma membrane (Bennett and Gilligan, 1993; Luna and Hitt, 1992; Hitt and Luna, 1994). In polarized RPE cells, spectrin/fodrin is very abundant in the apical region of the cell in the vicinity of the zonula adherens, and in the basal infoldings and lateral membranes, but sparse or nonexistent in the apical projections (Nihira et al., 1989; Opas and Kalnins, 1985; Opas et al., 1985; Huotari et al., 1995; Rizzolo et al., 1995). It was initially suggested that spectrin localization to apical domains might contribute to the observed localization of Na^+/K^+-ATPase in the apical membranes of rat RPE cells (Gundersen et al., 1991). However, recent studies using chick RPE cells, which have longer apical projections, have been able to show that during development of polarity the Na^+/K^+-ATPase and spectrin pursue different pathways of localization; ultimately the Na^+/K^+-ATPase localizes to the apical membrane but spectrin does not (Rizzolo et al., 1995). Spectrin localizes to the basolateral membranes and to the apical zone containing the zonula adherens and CMB, but not to the apical projections.

Ankyrins are spectrin-binding proteins which link spectrin (and hence actin filaments) to integral membrane proteins in the plasma membrane (see Hitt and Luna, 1994). In several cell types ankyrins serve to anchor the Na^+/K^+-ATPase to spectrin and to the cytoskeleton. Ankyrin is localized to the apical and lateral, but not to the basal membranes of polarized RPE cells (Rizzolo et al., 1995). During polarization of RPE cells ankyrin and spectrin undergo simultaneous changes in localization, appearing in patches on the basal membrane and later moving to lateral and apical membranes. However, the membranes of the developing apical projections contain ankyrin but not spectrin. Thus ankyrin colocalizes with the Na^+/K^+-ATPase in the absence of spectrin in RPE cells. This finding is consistent with the observation that the Na^+/K^+-ATPase could be readily cross-linked to ankyrin but only weakly linked to an ankyrin-spectrin complex in rat RPE (Gundersen et al., 1991). This independent localization of ankyrin in RPE apical projections may contribute to the apical localization of Na^+/K^+-ATPase (Rizzolo and Zhou, 1995).

Members of the ezrin/moesin family of actin-binding proteins have been found in the apical microvilli of a wide variety of polarized epithelial cell types, where they serve to attach microfilaments to the plasma membrane (see Arpin et al., 1994). These proteins undergo tyrosine phosphorylation and are involved in reorganization of the cytoskeleton in response to various stimuli, particularly during induction of microvilli. As in other epithelia, ezrin is localized to the apical plasma membrane in RPE cells (Hofer and Drenckhahn, 1993), where it might be expected to play a role in signal transduction events regulating the actin cytoskeleton of the apical projections.

Microtubules in Polarized RPE Cells

In RPE cells, as in other polarized epithelial cells, the distribution of microtubules is highly ordered (Fig. 3-3). Microtubule distribution has been particularly well characterized in the MDCK cell line, where two distinct microtubule populations have been identified: one population occupies the apical zone between the apical microvilli and the Golgi apparatus and is composed of a dense array of randomly oriented short microtubules; the second population occupies the rest of the cell and is composed of microtubule bundles oriented parallel to the apical-basal axis with minus ends directed toward

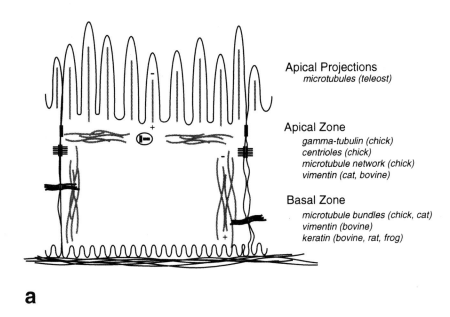

Apical Projections
microtubules (teleost)

Apical Zone
gamma-tubulin (chick)
centrioles (chick)
microtubule network (chick)
vimentin (cat, bovine)

Basal Zone
microtubule bundles (chick, cat)
vimentin (bovine)
keratin (bovine, rat, frog)

a

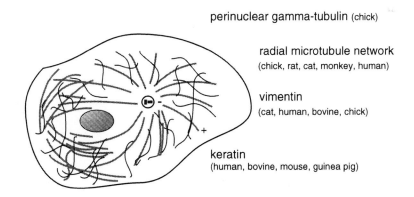

perinuclear gamma-tubulin (chick)

radial microtubule network
(chick, rat, cat, monkey, human)

vimentin
(cat, human, bovine, chick)

keratin
(human, bovine, mouse, guinea pig)

b

FIGURE 3-3. The microtubule and intermediate filament cytoskeletons of (a) a polarized RPE cell and (b) a dedifferentiated RPE cell in culture. (a) The centrosome (containing gamma-tubulin) and a population of horizontally oriented microtubules are located in the apical zone above the nucleus. A population of vertically oriented microtubules occupies the rest of the RPE cell body. Longitudinally oriented microtubules are also found in the apical projections of some species. The entire cell body contains intermediate filaments composed of keratins and/or vimentin, differing with species and whether in situ or in culture. (b) Microtubules radiate from the centrosome-associated gamma-tubulin, extending to the edges of the cell. Intermediate filaments are distributed throughout the cytoplasm. Microtubule polarity indicated by (+) and (−).

the cell apex (Bacallao et al., 1989; Bre et al., 1990). This characteristic microtubule polarity is critical to the vectorial microtubule-dependent targeting of membrane vesicles specifically to the epithelial cell's basolateral membranes (toward microtubule plus ends) or apical membranes (toward microtubule minus ends) (see Mays et al., 1994). As the MDCK cell becomes polarized during development, its centriolar MTOC migrates toward the apical pole. Simultaneously, the previously radially arrayed microtubules lose their perinuclear focus, reorient into bundles, and become aligned parallel to the apical-basal axis (Bacallao et al., 1989; Buendia et al., 1990).

Similar apical localization of the MTOC has been reported in cultured chick RPE cells. Gamma-tubulin (a tubulin family member associated with microtubule nucleation sites, and thus with MTOCs) was shown to be localized in a distinct focus subjacent to the apical membrane, and microtubules emanated from that region (Rizzolo and Joshi, 1993). The authors suggested that microtubules are nucleated at this MTOC at the apical border and extend their plus ends toward the base of the cell parallel to the apical-basal axis, as observed for MDCK cells. Microtubule polarity has been directly ascertained in teleost RPE cells by the hook decoration technique (Troutt and Burnside, 1988). In the long apical projections of these RPE cells, microtubules are uniformly oriented with minus ends toward the apical tips and plus ends toward the cell body. Together these observations suggest that microtubule-dependent transport directed from the tip of the apical projections toward the base of the RPE cell is plus end directed; while movement from base to apex or out into the apical projections is minus end directed.

As epithelial cells become polarized, microtubules may be nucleated at sites other than the centriolar MTOC. At early stages in culture, before confluence and assumption of epithelial morphology, microtubules assume a radial configuration around the perinuclear MTOC in cultured chick and rat RPE cells, as observed in cultured fibroblasts and other epithelial cells (Turksen et al., 1983; Irons and Kalnins, 1984; Bre et al., 1987). Interestingly, in the rat RPE, the greatest concentration of microtubules is actually well separated from the MTOC (Irons and Kalnins, 1984). Thus, all of the microtubules in cultured RPE may not nucleate from a single MTOC, but instead nucleate from several MTOCs scattered throughout the cytoplasm, which is true for other cultured cells (Spiegelman et al., 1979). The microtubules in apical projections of teleost RPE cells appear to be nucleated at the tips of the apical projections, since they are oriented with minus ends distal (Troutt and Burnside, 1988).

ASYMMETRIC DISTRIBUTION OF ORGANELLES AND CYTOPLASMIC COMPONENTS

Maintenance of nonrandom distributions of organelles and other cytoplasmic constituents is likely to be cytoskeletal-dependent in RPE cells (see Nguyen-Legros, 1978). All organelles are excluded from the cytoplasm of the basal infoldings, much as they are from the ruffles and lamellipodia of other cell types by meshworks of actin filaments (see Hogan et al., 1971; Nguyen-Legros, 1978; Cramer et al., 1994). The nucleus, mitochondria, and microperoxisomes are preferentially localized in the basal zone of RPE cells, while pigment granules are primarily localized in the apical zone and in the apical projections. In mammals, pigment granules are often rod- or cigar-shaped and oriented parallel to the path of incoming light (see Burnside and Laties, 1979). The migration of pigment granules that occurs in frog and fish RPE could be considered an extreme case of asymmetric organelle distribution which is modified in response to light (see Burnside and Nagle, 1983).

APICAL PROJECTIONS

Apical projections of RPE cells not only provide the enhanced apical surface area characteristic of polarized epithelia (see Rodriguez-Boulan and Nelson, 1989), but also participate in specialized activities unique to RPE cells, including retinal adhesion (see Hageman et al., 1995), phagocytosis of shed packets of photoreceptor outer-segment disks (see Bok, 1993), and the provision of an oriented, and in some species movable, screen of melanin pigment granules (see Nguyen-Legros, 1978). The size and shape of RPE apical projections are quite variable, ranging from the short (4 μm) fingerlike and leaflike processes of mammalian RPE cells (also classically called *fringes*), to extremely long (up to 100 μm) processes of some fish (see Nguyen-Legros, 1978). In amphibians, reptiles, and birds, the apical projections are also longer than in mammals. In most species of fish, apical projections extend all the way to the tips of the Mueller cell processes, thus enveloping not only the entire photoreceptor outer segment but also much of the inner segment as well. In many species, including monkeys and humans, the apical projections are large enough to contain pigment granules and ER in addition to cytoskeletal components. RPE sheets retain their apical projections when the RPE is detached from the retina, suggesting that the apical projections are supported by their own cytoskeletons and do not require retinal attachment to remain extended (see Burnside and Nagle, 1983; Owaribe, 1988). RPE apical projections have longitudinal bundles or parallel arrays of thin filaments shown to be actin by myosin fragment decoration in mammals (Burnside and Laties, 1976), chicks (Owaribe, 1988), frogs (Murray and Dubin, 1975), and fish (Burnside and Nagle, 1983). Microtubules are abundant in the long apical projections of fish RPE but rare or absent in those of mammals (see Burnside and Laties, 1979).

In mammalian apical projections the usual meshwork of actin filaments associated with the plasma membrane appears to have been modified into parallel arrays which provide much greater mechanical support (Burnside and Laties, 1976; Burnside, 1976). This cytoskeletal arrangement differs from the more familiar central core of bundled actin filaments found in the RPE apical projections of lower vertebrates and in microvilli of many cell types. In the fingerlike and leaflike projections of rat and monkey RPE cells, the plasma membrane is lined on its cytoplasmic face with paraxially aligned, parallel arrays of actin filaments oriented with their plus ends distal and their minus ends toward the cell body, the same orientation seen in intestinal microvilli (Burnside and Laties, 1976) (Fig. 3-4). Similar filaments can be seen in RPE apical projections of other mammalian species, including the very long projections associated with cone outer segments (Steinberg and Wood, 1974).

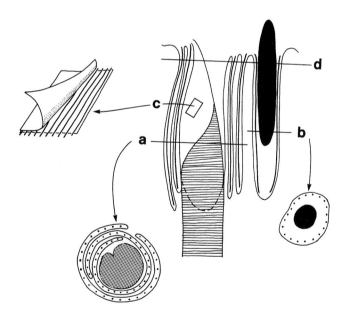

FIGURE 3-4. Actin filaments in apical projections of the mammalian RPE cell (rat). Both leaflike and fingerlike apical projections contain longitudinally oriented, parallel arrays of actin filaments closely associated with the plasma membrane. The tips of outer segments are ensheathed in the leaflike projections, shown in cross-section in (a), and in three dimensions in (c). Pigment granules extend into some fingerlike projections, shown in cross-section in (b). Actin filaments terminate at the base of the projections (d). (From Burnside, 1976, with permission of the publisher, Academic Press.)

These filaments are slightly larger in diameter than typical actin filaments (10 nm as opposed to 6 nm) suggesting that they are associated with actin-binding proteins which perhaps serve to stabilize the filaments. If so, their functions may be difficult to study with cytochalasins.

RPE apical projections play important roles in retinal attachment in mammals (see Marmor, 1993). Ensheathment of the outer segment tips by apical projections may contribute to adhesion by providing frictional or electrostatic resistance to withdrawal (see Marmor, 1993). In human eyes, the insoluble glycoconjugates of the interphotoreceptor matrix, called *cone matrix sheaths* and *rod matrix domains,* are attached firmly to the apical projections of RPE cells and to the retina (see Hageman et al., 1995). In fact, the attachment of the cone matrix sheaths to the surface of the RPE cell appears to be stronger than that between the RPE cell base and Bruch's membrane. If monkey or human retinas are gently peeled back from the eyecup, cone sheaths are stretched but remain attached to the RPE apical surface and actually pull the sheet of RPE off Bruch's membrane. The mechanism of this attachment is extremely sensitive to postmortem changes and is not seen unless the experiment is performed within one minute of death or enucleation. Since the lipid bilayer of the apical projections is unlikely to provide mechanical strength, the actin filament cytoskeleton of the apical projections must play an important role.

The mechanism of retinal attachment in lower vertebrates is less clear. In retinomotor movements, photoreceptors undergo long excursions that create logistical problems for matrix sheaths of the mammalian type. Small junctions with subplasmalemmal densities have been reported between fish RPE apical projections and the cone accessory outer segment (Yacob and Kunz, 1977; Yacob et al., 1977; Burnside et al., 1993). These types of junctions may contribute to retinal adhesion in lower vertebrates.

Actin filaments form paracrystalline bundles in the apical projections of RPE cells in frog (Murray and Dubin, 1975), chick (see Owaribe, 1988) and some fish (Burnside, unpublished observations). These paracrystalline microfilament bundles (PMBs) have been extensively and elegantly studied in chick RPE by Owaribe and coworkers (see Owaribe, 1988). Actin filaments of the PMBs are hexagonally packed with a spacing of approximately 9 nm and oriented in parallel with their plus ends toward the tip of the projection and their minus ends toward the cell body (Owaribe, 1988). Bundling does not appear to be produced by fascin (an actin-binding protein known to produce hexagonally packed actin bundles with similar spacing in other cell types), since no band is present at the appropriate molecular weight in gels of isolated PMBs, and PMBs do not stain with antibodies to fascin (Owaribe, 1988). Immunofluorescence studies to identify actin-binding proteins in PMBs have produced conflicting results: three groups found that PMBs contained little if any myosin II, tropomyosin, alpha-actinin, or vinculin (Drenckhahn and Wagner, 1985; Turksen and Kalnins, 1987; Owaribe, 1988), while another group reported that alpha-actinin, fodrin, myosin II, and vinculin were present in chick PMBs (Philp and Nachmias, 1985). The bundled PMBs are stiff and thus serve as scaffolding and possibly tracks for motor-dependent transport. Particles or membranes transported by myosins along the surface of the PMBs would be moved toward the tip of the apical projection, since all known myosins are plus end directed (see Mooseker and Cheney, 1995).

Before development of the apical projections, the surface of the prospective RPE is attached to the retinal neuroepithelium; RPE apical projections begin to appear as outer segments develop (see Nguyen-Legros, 1978). During development of apical projections in chick RPE the relative actin content dramatically increases (as detected by immunofluorescence, EM, and SDS-PAGE) until actin is approximately 60% of the detergent-insoluble cytoskeleton (Owaribe and Eguchi, 1985). This increase in actin content is accompanied by an increase in actin mRNA but the pool of free actin monomer is not changed, suggesting that increased actin synthesis is directly correlated with increased actin filament assembly (Nachmias et al., 1992). Short PMBs appear at the apical surface and then elongate as the apical projections protrude from the apical surface.

Junctional Complexes

Like all polarized epithelia, RPE cells are held together by junctional complexes composed of tight junctions, or *zonula occludens* (see Citi, 1993), adherens junctions, or *zonula adherens* (see Rodriguez-Boulan and Nelson, 1989), and desmosomes (see Schwarz et al., 1990; Nguyen-Legros, 1978). The tight junctions, located just vitread of the nucleus in the apical zone of the RPE cells (Hudspeth and Yee, 1973), are responsible for maintaining the blood-retinal barrier (Peyman and Bok, 1972). Actin filaments associated with the cytoplasmic face of the tight junction appear to play a functional role in its maintenance, since cytochalasin treatment disrupts tight junctions (see Madara et al., 1992; Stevenson and Begg, 199-4). Tight junction proteins ZO-1, 7H6 antigen, and occludin have all been shown to be present in chicken RPE in vivo but disappear upon plat-

ing the cells into culture (Konari et al., 1995). Chick RPE cells in culture have been shown to form a junctional apparatus in response to a diffusable retinal factor (Rizzolo and Li, 1993). Development of barrier function as measured by transepithelial resistance correlates with the appearance of occludin at the apices of confluent RPE cultures (Konari et al., 1995).

The zonula adherens, a site enriched in actin filaments in all epithelia, is particularly highly developed in RPE cells (see Rodriguez-Boulan and Nelson, 1989; Owaribe, 1988). The actin filaments not only provide mechanical strength to the intercellular attachments but also support contractility. Placoglobin, a protein associated with zonula adherens plaques, has been identified in RPE junctions, along with vinculin and alpha actinin, proteins thought to attach actin filaments to the cytoplasmic face of the plaques (see Owaribe, 1988). The attached actin filaments are oriented with random olarity to form a circumferential microfilament bundle (CMB) encircling the apical ends of the cells. In the particularly large and dense CMBs of RPE cells, actin filaments are associated with the membrane either end-on or laterally, along the membrane-apposed surface of the bundle (see Crawford et al., 1972; Sandig and Kalnins, 1988; Owaribe, 1988; Kodama et al., 1991). Morphological observations suggest that CMBs of the RPE resemble stress fibers in their organization and are contractile: CMBs are striated (Sandig and Kalnins, 1988; Gordon and Essner, 1987) and contain proteins also observed in stress fibers, including myosin II, tropmyosin, filamin, alpha-actinin, and vinculin (Drenckhahn and Wagner, 1985; Gordon and Essner, 1987; Turksen and Kalnins, 1987; Turksen et al., 1983; Kodama et al., 1991). CMBs isolated from chick RPE cells retain their pentagonal or hexagonal shapes and can be induced to contract in vitro (Owaribe et al., 1981; Owaribe and Masuda, 1982). When isolated CMBs were incubated with Mg/ATP, they contracted and still maintained their polygonal shapes. This contraction was blocked by NEM-myosin, which irreversibly binds to actin filaments and obstructs the binding of accessory proteins such as myosins, suggesting a contractile role for myosin II, which is present in the CMBs (Drenkhahn and Wagner, 1985; Owaribe et al., 1988). CMB contraction is ATP dependent but calcium independent (Owaribe et al., 1981), suggesting that myosin II–based contraction of CMBs is not regulated in the conventional manner.

CMBs appear in cultured RPE cells during polarization after confluence (Crawford et al., 1972; Crawford, 1980; Owaribe et al., 1979; Sandig and Kalnins, 1990a), and are reorganized during cytokinesis in dividing RPE cells (see Sandig and Kalnins, 1990b). CMBs appear to be required for maintenance of epithelial organization. Cytochalasin treatment disrupts CMBs and leads to fragmentation of the RPE into islands of cells (Crawford et al., 1972; Owaribe et al., 1979). Cytochalasin appears to induce contraction of the CMBs, thereby pulling the epithelium apart into clumps of twenty to thirty cells which ultimately detach from the substrate. Masses of condensed filamentous material then appear in the subapical region (Owaribe, 1988). Owaribe suggests that CMBs may serve dual roles in RPE cells, acting as mechanical stabilizers of the junctional complexes and also providing a contractile system which can mediate physiologically relevant cell shape changes in the epithelium, for instance in establishment and maintenance of stable hexagonal packing (Crawford, 1980; Honda and Eguchi, 1980). Since cytochalasin treatment leads to rupture of both tight and adherens junctions in cultured RPE (Owaribe et al., 1979; Crawford et al., 1972), it seems likely that dysfunction of the actin cytoskeleton could lead to both disruption of the blood-retinal barrier and detachment of cells from Bruch's membrane in vivo.

Perhaps because the adherens junctions are so well developed, the desmosomes of RPE cells are much less prominent in RPE than in other epithelia. Desmosomes have been identified in bovine RPE both by EM and by the presence of desmosome-specific desmoplakins (Owaribe, 1988; Owaribe et al., 1986). Similar structures have been observed in frog, rat, and human RPE, both in vivo and in vitro (Hudspeth and Yee, 1973; Miki et al., 1975; Hunt et al., 1989), but not in chick RPE (Owaribe, 1988). Desmosomes have been reported to be closely associated with mitochondria in human RPE cells (Schlotzer-Schrehardt et al., 1990). Desmosomes are anchored by intermediate filaments attached to their cytoplasmic faces, as described above.

CYTOSKELETON IN RPE MIGRATION

Under normal conditions RPE cells are stationary and mitotically inactive. In certain pathological situations, including proliferative vitreoretinopathy (PVR) and subretinal neovascularization (SRN), RPE cells detach from the basement membrane and become migratory (see Machemer and Laqua, 1975; Miller et al., 1986). There is evidence to suggest that the migratory behavior results from the loss of receptor-mediated attachments to the underlying matrix, and from chemotactic responses to vitreous components (see Kirchhof et al., 1989) and various growth factors (Hergott et al., 1993; Leschey et al., 1991).

Migrating cells exhibit major differences in their cytoskeletal organization compared to nonmigrating cells. Migrating cells often contain actin filament specializations, including an increased number of stress fibers and short bundles of filaments present at the base of the leading edge (see Rinnerthaler et al., 1988). These actin structures, in association with accessory proteins such as vinculin, are needed to form transient focal contracts and generate tractional forces for cell migration.

The microtubule architecture of RPE cells is also remodeled during migration. The MTOC is reoriented such that it is positioned in front of the nucleus in the direction of cell movement (Gottlieb et al., 1981). New microtubules penetrate into the leading edge and their tips become closely apposed to focal contacts (Rinnerthaler et al., 1988). Moreover, drug disruption of actin filaments or microtubules inhibits cell migration, further suggesting that both microtubules and actin filaments play important roles in migratory activity (see Gordon and Staley, 1990; Seldon and Schwartz, 1979).

The dramatic cytoskeletal reorganization of migrating RPE cells has been studied in "wounded" monolayers of cells in vitro or in special migratory chambers (Robey et al., 1992; Hergott et al., 1993). Nonmigrating cells exhibit a reticular or filamentous actin-staining pattern with few stress fibers (Robey et al., 1992). After migration is initiated, actin filaments reorganize into bundled stress fibers (Robey et al., 1992), and new intermediate filament proteins, cytokeratins 18 and 19, are expressed (Hergott et al., 1993). Cytoskeletal changes have also been studied in RPE cells induced to migrate by wounding in vitro (Hergott et al., 1993). Before wounding, the cuboid RPE cells displayed well-developed CMBs. After wounding, the migrating RPE cells near the wound edge were flat and displayed prominent stress fibers. Vinculin is present at the ends of these stress fibers, indicating that they are associated with focal contacts between the cell and the substratum. Active migration of RPE at the edges of wounds is inhibited by cytochalasin disruption of stress fibers (Verstraeten et al., 1990). These observations suggest that in migrating RPE cells, as in other mobile cells, forces necessary for locomotion over a substrate are generated by interaction of contractile stress fibers with focal contacts (see Cramer et al., 1994). Migration of RPE at wound edges is also inhibited by colchicine, suggesting that microtubules are also important to RPE cell migration in wound healing (Verstraeten et al., 1990).

RPE cells may be induced to migrate by alterations in specific attachments to the underlying basement membrane or by chemotactic factors (see Avery and Glaser, 1986; Chu and Grunwald, 1991a; 1991b; Klymkowsky and Parr, 1995). Cells mediate their attachment to substrates via a family of adhesive integral membrane proteins termed *integrins* (Hynes, 1992). Several integrins have been identified in RPE cells, and antibodies against them inhibit RPE cell adhesion and migration (Chu and Grunwald, 1991a; 1991b). The RGD peptide, which forms part of the cell-binding domain on the fibronectin receptor, also blocks RPE cell attachment to various components of the extracellular matrix (Avery and Glaser, 1986). In a wound-healing organ culture system, antibodies against integrin subunits inhibited RPE cell migration, but not cell spreading and attachment (Hergott et al., 1993). In a different RPE culture system with a less complex substratum, both migration and attachment were blocked by integrin antibody (Chu and Grunwald, 1991b).

There is mounting evidence that association of the cytoskeleton with focal adhesion sites plays a role in signal transduction events (see Lo et al., 1994; Gips et al., 1994). Pharmacological agents which modulate the intracellular calcium and calmodulin signaling systems also affect RPE cell attachment to ECM proteins (Wagner et al., 1995). Both increasing calcium and decreasing calmodulin reduce the adhesion of RPE to matrix components. Modulation of the calcium/calmodulin signal transduction pathway may mediate attachment, and consequently control migration of RPE in pathological conditions such as PVR.

RPE migration is also influenced by both cytokines and growth factors (Leschey et al., 1991; Campochiaro and Glaser, 1986; Kirchhof and Sorgente, 1989). Platelet-derived growth factor (PDGF) is a potent regulator of RPE cell migration (Campochiaro and Glaser, 1985). Agents that inhibit PDGF binding to cell membrane receptors antagonize the migratory response (Leschey et al., 1991). Insulinlike growth factor I (IGF-I), which is present in vitreous, has been shown to have a chemotactic effect on human RPE cells (Grant et al., 1990). Since PVR develops in situations where the vitreous contacts the RPE, it is postulated that RPE contact with vitreous components after trauma may elicit the migratory behavior as seen in PVR. Growth factors elicit a complex signal transduction cascade by binding to and activating their respective receptors (see Bornfeldt et al., 1995). A major signaling pathway for growth factors entails activation of protein kinase C (PKC), and phorbol ester stimulation of PKC also elicits migratory activity in RPE cells (Murphy et al., 1995). In other cells, growth-factor-induced responses include actin-dependent membrane ruffling (Ridley et al., 1992) and stress fiber assembly (Ridley and Hall, 1992), two morphological responses observed in migrating RPE.

Thus, growth factors can induce actin filament reorganization in RPE cells characteristic of cell migration.

ROLES OF THE CYTOSKELETON IN RPE PHAGOCYTOSIS

Phagocytosis is a motile process by which relatively large particles (>0.5 μm) are taken up by the cell into vacuoles by mechanisms that are clathrin independent and usually require actin polymerization (see Rabinovitch, 1995; Swanson and Baer, 1995; Greenberg, 1995). Subsequent phases of phagosome transport and lysosome fusion depend on microtubules (see Swanson and Baer, 1995; Greenberg, 1995). Activation of phagocytosis entails initiation of extensive actin polymerization at the site of attachment, thereby generating pseudopodia which engulf the particle (see Swanson and Baer, 1995; Greenberg, 1995). The binding of a target to receptors on the cell surface produces signals which trigger actin polymerization locally (see Greenberg, 1995). This process is cytochalasin sensitive and thought to entail recruitment of actin-nucleating molecules to the submembranous region underlying ligated phagocytic receptors, and/or the uncapping of the plus ends of preexisting filaments, thereby locally increasing the numbers of elongating actin filaments (see Greenberg, 1995). This stimulated actin polymerization produces an increase in short actin filaments rather than an increase in the length of filaments, so some severing action is likely to accompany uncapping (see Greenberg, 1995).

Two forms of phagocytosis have been described; both depend on actin polymerization, but they differ in several particulars (see Swanson and Baer, 1995). One form entails engulfment by "zippering" the pseudopod around the particle by specific interactions between molecules on the particle surface and receptors on the plasma membrane of the phagocyte, as is observed in Fc-mediated phagocytosis by macrophages. Zippering is highly localized and highly specific. The other form, triggered phagocytosis, entails the activation of highly active ruffling membranes which flop over on the surface and carry out a relatively less specific "macropinocytosis." In this process particles which are sufficiently small are swept in and thus engulfed into macropinosomes. This type of phagocytosis is activated by certain pathogens and also by several growth factors in a variety of cell types (see Swanson and Baer, 1995). The highly specific phagocytosis of outer-segment disks by the RPE appears to be an example of zippering (see Bok, 1982; Besharse, 1982; 1988).

Since they are specialized to phagocytize specific targets (packets of photoreceptor outer segment disks), RPE cells have been classified as "paraprofessional phagocytes" by those who study the "professional phagocytes" like macrophages and neutrophils (see Rabinovitch, 1995). Phagocytosis of photoreceptor outer segments by RPE cells is a daily event critical to survival of photoreceptor cells (Young and Bok, 1969; Bok and Hall, 1971; Besharse, 1982; 1988). Although the tips of the outer segments are in close apposition with lamellar apical projections of RPE cells at all times, phagocytosis occurs in bursts and is triggered by light or circadian signals, depending on the species (see Young and Bok, 1969; LaVail, 1976; Besharse, 1982; 1988). During the phagocytic burst, the frog RPE surface develops phagocytic pseudopods filled with a meshwork of actin filaments which swell to engulf the shedding packet of outer-segment material (B. Matsumoto et al., 1987; Tsukamoto, 1986). These swollen pseudopods differ from the usual apical projections of the frog RPE cells, in that they are filled with an actin meshwork which excludes other cytoplasmic structures. Surprisingly, cytochalasin does not block the early phases of pseudopod formation; however, it does block detachment of the disk packet and engulfment (B. Matsumoto et al., 1987). Similar "actin-rich attachment saucers" appear under attached fragments of outer segments in cultured mammalian RPE cells which have been fed rod outer segments (Chaitin and Hall, 1983a). In monkey and rat RPE in vivo, phagosomes near the apical surface are ensheathed in leaflike projections and thus surrounded by the highly ordered array of parallel actin filaments characteristic of these projections (Burnside, 1976; Burnside and Laties, 1979). These filaments disappear as the phagosome moves into the apical cytoplasm. Subsequent phagosome transport and phagosome-lysosome fusion events in RPE cells are blocked by colchicine disruption of microtubules (Herman and Steinberg, 1982; Beauchemin and Leuenberger, 1977; Keller and Leuenberger, 1977). The requirements for both actin filaments and microtubules in phagocytosis suggests that actin- and microtubule-dependent motor proteins may play critical roles.

In the RCS rat model of retinal degeneration, the ability of the RPE to phagocytize outer-segment material is greatly compromised so that debris accumulates in the subretinal space, eventually leading to photoreceptor degeneration (Bok and Hall, 1971; Herron et al., 1969). Since RPE cells of RCS rats can effectively phagocytize carbon particles and polystyrene microspheres (Custer and Bok, 1975; Reich-D'Almeida and Hockley, 1975a; 1975b), the cytoskeletal mechanisms for phagocytosis appear to be adequate. Thus the defect in RPE phagocytosis appears to lie in the signaling pathway for specific phagocytosis. Recently it has been shown that several different growth factors can produce temporary rescue of the RCS phenotype when injected into the subretinal space before degeneration has become extensive (Faktorovich et al., 1990). Since growth factors have been shown to trigger nonspecific macropinocytosis in a variety of cell types (see Swanson and Baer, 1995), the temporary rescue effect of growth factors in RCS rats may result from growth factor stimulation of nonspecific phagocytic pathways, thereby clearing ROS debris from the subretinal space.

RETINOMOTOR MOVEMENTS IN RPE CELLS

In most lower vertebrates, the distributions of pigment granules in the RPE change in response to change in light condition (see Ali, 1975; Burnside and Nagle, 1983) (Fig. 3-5). Pigment granules are aggregated in the base of the RPE cell in the dark, maximally exposing the rod outer segments. With light onset pigment granules migrate out into the long apical projections of the RPE cells. The dispersed pigment granules shield rod outer segments from complete bleach (Back et al., 1965), and perhaps contribute to acuity by interdigitating between cone outer segments and absorbing scattered light (see Ali, 1975; Burnside and Nagle, 1983). RPE pigment granule migration is most extensive in fish and amphibians, where photoreceptor movements are also dramatic. In birds and mammals, photoreceptor and RPE movements are more modest or lacking (van Genderen Stort, 1887). In mammals, pigment granule migration has been reported only in tree shrews (Immel, 1982) and guinea pigs (Pang et al., 1978).

Regulation of Pigment Migration

The regulation of RPE retinomotor movements by light depends on signals from the retina (see Burnside and Dearry, 1986; Dearry and Burnside, 1989). Though isolated RPE sheets are insensitive to light, they can be induced to disperse their pigment granules by incubation with dopamine or with medium from light-cultured retina (Dearry and Burnside, 1988; 1989). In both cases, induction of dispersion was blocked by antagonists of dopamine D2 family receptors. Intraocular injection of dopamine D2 agonists induced pigment granule dispersion in vivo while light-induced dispersion in vivo was blocked by injecting D2 family antagonists (Dearry and Burnside, 1986). Dopamine and D2 agonists also enhance the dispersion of pigment granules in isolated teleost RPE cells (Bruenner and Burnside, 1986; Garcia

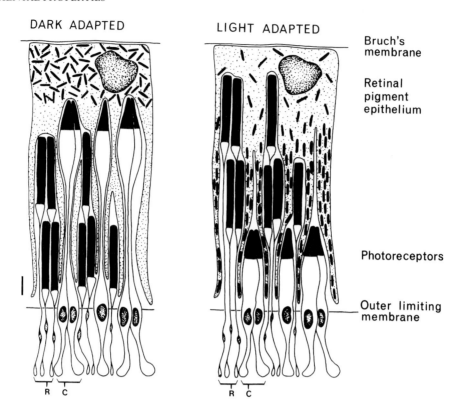

FIGURE 3-5. Retinomotor movements of RPE pigment granules and photoreceptors in the teleost eye. In the dark, cones are long, rods are short, and pigment granules are aggregated into the RPE cell body. In the light, cones are short, rods are long, and pigment granules are dispersed into the long apical projections of the RPE cells. Bar = 10 μm (From Burnside, Nagle, 1983, with permission from the publisher, Pergamon Press.)

and Burnside, 1994). Dopamine also stimulates dispersion of pigment granules in frog RPE, although in this case dopamine appears to act through D1 receptors (Dearry et al., 1990). Other messengers also appear to be capable of conveying a light onset signal from retina to the RPE, since light-induced retinomotor movements reappear in fish RPE two weeks after ablation of retinal dopaminergic cells (Douglas et al., 1992; Ball et al., 1993).

Since D2 family dopamine receptors are usually negatively coupled to adenylate cyclase (see Gingrich and Caron, 1993), these findings implicate cAMP as an intracellular messenger in regulation of RPE retinomotor movements. Furthermore, pigment granule aggregation in teleost RPE is induced by forskolin and cAMP analogs both in vivo and in vitro (Burnside et al., 1982; Burnside and Basinger, 1983; Breunner and Burnside, 1986). Surprisingly, even underivatized cAMP can induce pigment granule aggregation (Bruenner and Burnside, 1986; Garcia and Burnside, 1994). Extracellular cAMP apparently enters the cell through organic ion transporters, since specific inhibitors of organic ion transporters block cAMP-induced but not forskolin-induced aggregation (Garcia

and Burnside, 1994). This finding suggests that cAMP might serve as a first messenger between retina and RPE. Photoreceptors have been shown to have elevated intracellular cAMP levels in the dark (see Cohen, 1982; Denton et al., 1992), and high intracellular cAMP levels produce cAMP efflux in many cell types (Barber and Butcher, 1981; 1983; Nikaido and Takahashi, 1989). Thus dark-induced increases in cAMP levels in photoreceptors could produce extracellular cAMP in the subretinal space, which could in turn signal darkness to the RPE (see Garcia and Burnside, 1994).

Calcium does not appear to play an important role in regulation of RPE pigment granule migration. In isolated teleost RPE cells, elevation of intracellular calcium levels was neither necessary nor sufficient to produce pigment granule aggregation or dispersion (King-Smith et al., 1996). No change in intracellular calcium levels was detected by indicator dyes when pigment granule aggregation or dispersion was induced by cAMP or cAMP washout, respectively. Furthermore, neither aggregation nor dispersion was affected by chelating intra- or extracellular calcium. These observations suggest that cAMP-dependent phosphorylation and dephosphorylation of regulatory proteins may be sufficient to produce aggregation and dispersion, respectively.

Cytoskeletal Roles in RPE Pigment Granule Migration

Kuhne (1887) was the first to suggest that RPE retinomotor movements resulted from pigment granule migration within fixed apical projections, rather than from amoeba-like extension and retraction of the apical projections themselves. Though in some species the lengths of the projections may change slightly (Kunz, 1980), this generalization has held. RPE pigment migration has been extensively studied in fish and frogs in vivo (see Burnside and Nagle, 1983; Douglas et al., 1992; Ball et al., 1993), in isolated fish and frog eyecups (Snyder and Zadunaisky, 1976; Burnside and Basinger, 1983; Dearry et al., 1990), in isolated fish RPE sheets (Dearry and Burnside, 1988; Garcia and Burnside, 1994) and in isolated fish RPE cells (Bruenner and Burnside, 1986; King-Smith et al., 1995; 1996; 1997).

Since aggregation and dispersion can occur in isolated single cells, it is clear that the mechanical basis of pigment granule transport is intrinsic. Isolated fish RPE cells maintain their polarized morphology if prevented from attaching to a substrate in culture (Bruenner and Burnside, 1986); however, when allowed to adhere to coverslips, RPE cells develop a radial array of apical projections (Fig. 3-6 and color plate 3-I). Both attached and unattached isolated RPE cells can aggregate and disperse pigment granules in response to cAMP or forskolin, as observed in vivo. Time-lapse videomicroscopy of isolated attached RPE cells has revealed that pigment granule dispersion is saltatory and bidirectional (King-Smith et al., 1997). Since centrifugal path lengths and average rates are greater, net dispersion is produced. Surprisingly, the dispersed state is highly dynamic. After full dispersion is achieved, bidirectional saltations (shuttling motions) of pigment granules persist in the apical projections. The appearance of pigment granule movement during aggregation is quite different

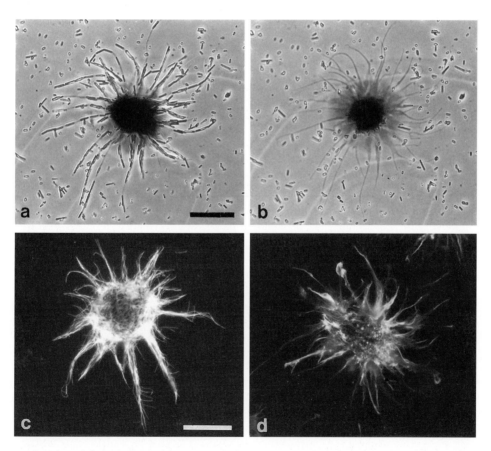

FIGURE 3-6. Dissociated green sunfish RPE cells in culture. Phase contrast micrographs of the same living RPE cell with (a) dispersed and (b) aggregated pigment granules. Apical projections assume a radial arrangement after attachment but still aggregate and disperse pigment effectively. Microtubules in apical projections are shown by antitubulin immunofluorescence of a fixed and permeabilized cell in (c). Actin filaments in apical projections are shown by rhodamine-phalloidin labeling of a fixed and permeabilized cell in (d). Tubulin staining and rhodamine-phalloidin labeling of actin in these cells is shown more clearly in Plate 3-I. Bar = 20 μm (Courtesy of C. King-Smith.)

from that of dispersion. Upon addition of cAMP all centrifugal movement stops, and the entire mass of pigment granules undergoes a smooth, nonsaltatory centripetal migration toward the cell center. The strikingly different appearance of aggregative and dispersive movements suggests they depend on different mechanisms of force production. These characteristic properties of pigment granule movements were also observed in unattached apical projections of isolated cells and of intact RPE sheets, so they are not artifacts of attachment to glass.

In time-lapse videos of isolated RPE cells, it is possible to see other types of motile events taking place in the apical projections, in addition to retinomotor movements of pigment granules. For example, the tips of apical projections undergo repeated cycles of extension and retraction over distances of several micrometers, and cytoplasmic inclusions other than pigment granules also exhibit saltatory excursions. Such constant motile activity may play an important role in turnover of cytoplasm and plasma membrane in the long apical projections. In most epithelia, the equivalent of about 50% of the cell surface is endocytosed per hour; most of that is recycled back into the surface membrane so that only about 5% of the total apical surface per hour is replaced with newly synthesized membrane (see Mostov et al., 1992). For RPE cells with such elaborate apical projections, similar exchange of surface membrane would require a high degree of activity.

The role of microtubules in retinomotor pigment granule migration has been extensively studied in teleost RPE cells (Troutt and Burnside, 1989; King-Smith et al., 1995; 1997). Nocodazole disruption of microtubules in intact RPE/retina cultures inhibited RPE pigment granule aggregation but not dispersion (Troutt and Burnside, 1989). In these preparations the RPE apical projections were in normal association with retinal photoreceptors. A possible role for a plus-end-directed motor protein such as kinesin was implied in pigment granule aggregation, since microtubules in the apical projections are oriented with plus ends toward the cell body (Troutt and Burnside, 1988), and since kinesin heavy chain had been previously shown to mediate pigment migration in teleost melanophores (Rodionov et al., 1991). However, although two forms of kinesin heavy chain were identified in teleost RPE, microinjection of three function-blocking antibodies against kinesin heavy chain failed to block pigment aggregation or dispersion in isolated RPE cells (King-Smith et al., 1995).

Since the antibody microinjection experiments were carried out in isolated cells, microtubule disruption studies were then performed using this preparation (King-Smith et al., 1997). In contrast to the previous re-

sults with RPE/retina preparations, microtubule disruption had no effect on either aggregation or dispersion of pigment granules in isolated RPE cells. The microtubule dependence of pigment aggregation in the RPE/retina preparations perhaps reflects a need for microtubule scaffolding when apical projections are interdigitated with photoreceptors.

The actual force-producing mechanism responsible for pigment granule migration appears to depend on actin filaments rather than microtubules. Disrupting the actin cytoskeleton with cytochalasin D reversibly blocked both aggregation and dispersion in isolated RPE cells (King-Smith et al., 1997). Cytochalasin effects on pigment granule movement were immediate, and recovery occurred within minutes after washout.

Cytochalasin not only blocked pigment granule aggregation and dispersion but also arrested extension and retraction of the tips of apical projections (King-Smith et al., 1996b). Thus the motile machinery responsible for pigment migration and motility of the apical projection tip may be related. Since apical projections of mammalian RPE cells contain actin filaments and also might be expected to be turning over apical membrane components, they too may be more dynamic than might appear from electron micrographs. Perhaps dynamic fluxes of cytoskeletal and membrane components in the apical projections are common to all RPE cells, and the RPE cells of lower vertebrates have harnessed this basic turnover process to translocate their pigment granules.

CONCLUSIONS

In the nearly twenty years that have passed since the last RPE monograph we have vastly increased our understanding of the characteristics and functions of the cytoskeleton in RPE cells. We now have considerably more information about the "parts list" for the machinery, including the struts, cables, and motors that RPE cells use for scaffolding and force production. The next few years should see an enormous proliferation of functional studies. An important realization derived from the recent studies of RPE cytoskeleton is that the cytoskeletal architecture in cultured RPE cells may or may not faithfully reproduce that found in situ. Cytoskeletal organization is particularly sensitive to culture conditions. Since the use of RPE cells in culture is critical to our ability to analyze the roles of the cytoskeleton in RPE functions, we must pay particular attention to the fidelity of cytoskeletal architecture achieved in each culture system. The next review of the RPE cytoskeleton is likely to contain a much more detailed characterization of the specific roles of cytoskeletal components in RPE motile processes critical to normal RPE function, such as morphogenesis of apical projections, development and maintenance of epithelial polarity, and phagocytosis, as well as the role of cytoskeletal dysfunction in pathological conditions such as defective phagocytosis, retinal detachment, failure of the blood–retinal barrier, and detachment and migration of RPE cells.

ACKNOWLEDGMENTS

The authors wish to thank Kris Okumu for preparing Figures 3-1–3-3, Christina King-Smith for Figure 3-6, David Hillman for Table 3-1, and Debbie Tran for help with preparation of the manuscript. We also thank Christina King-Smith for advice and critical feedback on the manuscript.

REFERENCES

Achler C, Filmer D, Merte C, Drenckhahn D. 1989. Role of microtubules in polarized delivery of apical membrane proteins to the brush border of the intestinal epithelium. J Cell Biol 109:179–189.

Aizawa H, Sekine Y, Takemura R, Zhang Z, Nangaku M, Hirokawa N. 1992. Kinesin family in murine central nervous system. J Cell Biol 119:1287–1296.

Ali MA. 1975. Retinomotor responses. In: Ali MA, ed, Vision in Fishes. New York: Plenum Press, 313–355.

Arikawa K, Williams DS. 1991. Alpha-actinin and actin in the outer retina: a double immunoelectron microscopic study. Cell Motil Cytoskeleton 18:15–25.

Arpin M, Algrain M, Louvard D. 1994. Membrane-actin microfilament connections: an increasing diversity of players related to band 4.1. Curr Opin Cell Biol 6:136–141.

Avery RL, Glaser BM. 1986. Inhibition of retinal pigment epithelial cell attachment by a synthetic peptide derived from the cell-binding domain of fibronectin. Arch Ophthalmol 104:1220–1222.

Bacallao R, Antony C, Dotti C, Karsenti E, Stelzer EH, Simons K. 1989. The subcellular organization of Madin-Darby canine kidney cells during the formation of a polarized epithelium. J Cell Biol 109:2817–2832.

Back I, Donner KO, Reuter T. 1965. The screening effect of the pigment epithelium on the retinal rods in the frog. Vision Res 101–111.

Ball AK, Baldridge WH, Fernback TC. 1993. Neuromodulation of pigment movement in the RPE of normal and 6-OHDA-lesioned goldfish retinas. Vis Neurosci 10:529–540.

Barber R, Butcher RW. 1981. The quantitative relationship between intracellular concentration and egress of cyclic AMP from cultured cells. Mol Pharmacol 19:38–43.

Barber R, Butcher RW. 1983. The egress of cyclic AMP from metazoan cells. In: Greengard P, Robison GA, eds, Advances in Cyclic Nucleotide Research, vol 9. New York: Raven Press, 119–138.

Beauchemin ML, Leuenberger PM. 1977. Effects of colchicine on phagosome–lysosome interaction in retinal pigment epithelium. I. In vivo observations in albino rats. Graefes Arch Klin Exp Ophthalmol 203:237–251.

Beech PL, Pagh-Roehl K, Noda Y, Hirokawa N, Burnside B, Rosenbaum JL. 1996. Localization of kinesin superfamily proteins to the connecting cilium of fish photoreceptors. J Cell Sci 109:889–897.

Bement WM, Hasson T, Wirth JA, Cheney RE, Mooseker MS. 1994. Identification and overlapping expression of multiple unconventional myosin genes in vertebrate cell types. Proc Nat Acad Sci USA 91:6549–6553.

Bennett V, Gilligan DM. 1993. The spectrin-based membrane skeleton and micro-scale organization of the plasma membrane. Annu Rev Cell Biol 9:27–66.

Berman ER, Schwell H, Feeney L. 1974. The retinal pigment epithelium: chemical composition and structure. Invest Ophthalmol 13:675–687.

Besharse JC. 1982. The daily light-dark cycle and rhythmic metabolism in the photoreceptor-pigment epithelial complex. In: Osborne NN, Chader GJ, eds, Progress in Retinal Research, vol 1. Oxford: Pergamom Press, 81–124.

Besharse JC, Dunis DA. 1982. Rod photoreceptor shedding in vitro: inhibition by cytochalasin and activation by colchicine. In: Hollyfield JG, ed, The Structure of the Eye. New York: Elsevier, 85–96.

Besharse JC, Iuvone PM, Pierce ME. 1988. Regulation of rhythmic photoreceptor metabolism: a role for postreceptoral neurons. In: Osborne NN, Chader GJ, eds, Progress in Retinal Research. Oxford: Pergamon Press, 21–62.

Bloom GS, Endow S. 1995. Motor proteins I: kinesins. Protein Profile 2:1109–1156.

Bloom GS, Schoenfeld TA, Vallee RB. 1984. Widespread distribution of the major polypeptide component of MAP 1 (microtubule-associated protein 1) in the nervous system. J Cell Biol 98:320–330.

Bloom GS, Wagner MC, Pfister KK, Brady ST. 1988. Native structure and physical properties of bovine brain kinesin and identification of the ATP-binding subunit polypeptide. Biochemistry. 27:3409–3416.

Bok D. 1982. Renewal of photoreceptor cells. Methods Enzymol 81:763–772.

Bok D. 1993. The retinal pigment epithelium: a versatile partner in vision. J Cell Sci Suppl 17:189–195.

Bok D, Hall MO. 1971. The role of the pigment epithelium in the etiology of inherited retinal dystrophy in the rat. J Cell Biol 49:664–682.

Bok D, O'Day W, Rodriguez-Boulan E. 1992. Polarized budding of vesicular stomatitis and influenza virus from cultured human and bovine retinal pigment epithelium. Exp Eye Res 55:853–860.

Bomsel M, Parton R, Kuznetsov SA, Schroer TA, Gruenberg J. 1990. Microtubule- and motor-dependent fusion in vitro between apical and basolateral endocytic vesicles from MDCK cells. Cell 62:719–731.

Bornfeldt KE, Raines EW, Graves LM, Skinner MP, Krebs EG, Ross R. 1995. Platelet-derived growth factor. Distinct signal transduction pathways associated with migration versus proliferation. Ann NY Acad Sci 766:416–430.

Bost-Usinger LM, Chen R, Hillman D, Park H, Burnside M. 1997. Multiple kinesin family members expressed in teleost retina and RPE include a novel c-terminal kinesin. Exp. Eye Res 64:781–794.

Bre MH, Kreis TE, Karsenti E. 1987. Control of microtubule nucleation and stability in Madin-Darby canine kidney cells: the occurrence of noncentrosomal, stable detyrosinated microtubules. J Cell Biol 105:1283–1296.

Bre MH, Pepperkok R, Hill AM, Levilliers N, Ansorge W, Stelzer EHK, Karsenti E. 1990. Regulation of microtubule dynamics and nucleation during polarization in MDCK II cells. J Cell Biol 111:3013–3021.

Breckler J, Burnside B. 1994. Myosin-I in retinal pigment epithelial cells. Invest Ophthalmol Vis Sci 35:2489–2499.

Bruenner U, Burnside B. 1986. Pigment granule migration in isolated cells of the teleost retinal pigment epithelium. Invest Opthalmol Vis Sci 27:1634–1643.

Bubb MR, Spector I, Bershadsky AD, Korn ED. 1995. Swinholide A is a microfilament disrupting marine toxin that stabilizes actin dimers and severs actin filaments. J Biol Chem 270:3463–3466.

Buendia B, Bre MH, Griffiths G, Karsenti E. 1990. Cytoskeletal control of centrioles movement during the establishment of polarity in Madin-Darby canine kidney cells. J Cell Biol 110:1123–1135.

Burnside MB. 1976. Possible roles of microtubules and actin filaments in retinal pigmented epithelium. Exp Eye Res 23:257–275.

Burnside B, Laties AM. 1976. Actin filaments in apical projections of the primate pigmented epithelial cell. Invest Ophthalmol 15:570–575.

Burnside B, Basinger S. 1983. Retinomotor pigment migration in the teleost retinal pigment epithelium. II. Cyclic-3',5'-adenosine monophosphate induction of dark-adaptive movement in vitro. Invest Ophthalmol Vis Sci 24:16–23.

Burnside B, Dearry A. 1986. Cell motility in the retina. In: Adler R, Farber DB, The Retina, vol 12. New York: Academic Press, 151–206.

Burnside B, Laties AM. 1979. Pigment movement and cellular contractility and movement in retinal pigmented epithelium. In: Zinn KM, Marmor MF, eds, The Retinal Pigmented Epithelium. Cambridge, MA: Harvard University Press, 175–191.

Burnside B, Nagle B. 1983. Retinomotor movements of photoreceptors and retinal pigment epithelium: mechanisms and regulation. In: Osborne NN, Chader GJ, eds, Progress in Retinal Research, vol 2. Oxford: Pergamon Press, 67–109.

Burnside B, Evans M, Fletcher RT, Chader GJ. 1982. Induction of dark-adaptive retinomotor movement (cell elongation) in teleost retinal cones by cyclic adenosine 3',5'-monophosphate. J Gen Physiol 79:759–774.

Burnside B, Adler R, O'Connor P. 1983. Retinomotor pigment migration in the teleost retinal pigment epithelium. I. Roles for actin and microtubules in pigment granule transport and cone movement. Invest Ophthalmol Vis Sci 24:1–15.

Burnside B, Wang E, Pagh-Roehl K, Rey H. 1993. Retinomotor movements in isolated teleost retinal cone inner-outer segment preparations (CIS-COS): effects of light, dark and dopamine. Exp Eye Res 57:709–722.

Campochiaro PA, Glaser BM. 1985. Endothelial cells release a chemoattractant for retinal pigment epithelial cells in vitro. Arch Ophthalmol 103:1876–1880.

Campochiaro PA, Glaser BM. 1986. Mechanisms involved in retinal pigment epithelial cell chemotaxis. Arch Ophthalmol 104:277–280.

Chaitin MH, Hall MO. 1983. Defective ingestion of rod outer segments by cultured dystrophic rat pigment epithelial cells. Invest Ophthalmol Vis Sci 24:812–820.

Chu PG, Grunwald GB. 1991a. Identification of the 2A10 antigen of retinal pigment epithelium as a beta 1 subunit of integrin. Invest Ophthalmol Vis Sci 32:1757–1762.

Chu PG, Grunwald GB. 1991b. Functional inhibition of retinal pigment epithelial cell-substrate adhesion with a monoclonal antibody against the beta I subunit of integrin. Invest Ophthalmol Vis Sci 32:1763–1769.

Citi S. 1993. The molecular organization of tight junctions. J Cell Biol 121:485–489.

Clarke M, Spudich JA. 1977. Nonmuscle contractile proteins: the role of actin and myosin in cell motility and shape determination. Annu Rev Biochem 46:797–822.

Cohen AI. 1982. Increased levels of 3',5'-cyclic adenosine monophosphate induced by cobaltous ion or 3-isobutylmethylxanthine in the incubated mouse retina: evidence concerning location and response to ions and light. J Neurochem 38:781–796.

Cole DG, Chinn SW, Wedaman KP, Hall K, Vuong T, Scholey JM. 1993. Novel heterotrimeric kinesin-related protein purified from sea urchin eggs. Nature 366:268–270.

Collins C. 1994. Dynein-based organelle movement. In: Hyams JS, Lloyd CW, eds, Microtubules. New York: Wiley-Liss, 367–380.

Condeelis J. 1993. Life at the leading edge: the formation of cell protrusions. Annu Rev Cell Biol 9:411–444.

Cooper JA. 1987. Effects of cytochalasin and phalloidin on actin. J Cell Biol 105:1473–1478.

Coulombe PA. 1993. The cellular and molecular biology of keratins: beginning a new era. Curr Opin Cell Biol 5:17–29.

Cramer LP, Mitchison TJ, Theriot JA. 1994. Actin-dependent motile forces and cell motility. Curr Opin Cell Biol 6:82–86.

Crawford B, Cloney RA, Cahn RD. 1972. Cloned pigmented retinal cells: the effects of cytochalasin B on ultrastructure and behavior. Z Zellforsch Mikrosk Anat 130:135–151.

Crawford BJ. 1980. Development of the junctional complex during differentiation of chick pigmented epithelial cells in clonal culture. Invest Ophthalmol Vis Sci 19:223–237.

Custer NV, Bok D. 1975. Pigment epithelium–photoreceptor interactions in the normal and dystrophic rat retina. Exp Eye Res 21:153–166.

Dearry A, Burnside B. 1986. Dopaminergic regulation of cone retinomotor movement in isolated teleost retinas: I. Introduction of cone contraction is mediated by D2 receptors. J Neurochem 46:1006–1021.

Dearry A, Burnside B. 1988. Stimulation of distinct D2 dopaminergic and alpha 2-adrenergic receptors induces light-adaptive pigment dispersion in teleost retinal pigment epithelium. J Neurochem 51:1516–1523.

Dearry A, Burnside B. 1989. Light-induced dopamine release from teleost retinas acts as a light-adaptive signal to the retinal pigment epithelium. J Neurochem 53:870–878.

Dearry A, Edelman JL, Miller S, Burnside B. 1990. Dopamine induces light-adaptive retinomotor movements in bullfrog cones via D2 receptors and in retinal pigment epithelium via D1 receptors. J Neurochem 54:1367–1378.

Denton TL, Yamashita CK, Farber DB. 1992. The effects of light on cyclic nucleotide metabolism of isolated cone photoreceptors. Exp Eye Res 54:229–237.

Devereux J, Haeberli P, Smithies O. 1984. A comprehensive set of sequence analysis programs for the VAX. Nucleic Acids Res 12:387–395.

Docherty RJ, Edwards JG, Garrod DR, Mattey DL. 1984. Chick embryonic pigmented retina is one of the group of epithelioid tissues that lack cytokeratins and desmosomes and have intermediate filaments composed of vimentin. J Cell Sci 71:61–74.

Douglas RH, Wagner HJ, Zaunreiter M, Behrens UD, Djamgoz MB. 1992. The effect of dopamine depletion on light-evoked and circadian retinomotor movements in the teleost retina. Vis Neurosci 9:335–343.

Drechsel DN, Hyman AA, Cobb MH, Kirschner MW. 1992. Modulation of the dynamic instability of tubulin assembly by the microtubule-associated protein tau. Mol Biol Cell 3:1141–1154.

Drenckhahn D, Wagner HJ. 1985. Relation of retinomotor responses and contractile proteins in vertebrate retinas. Eur J Cell Biol 37:156–168.

Edson K, Weisshaar B, Matus A. 1993. Actin depolymerisation induces process formation on MAP2-transfected non-neuronal cells. Development 117:689–700.

Eilers U, Klumperman J, Hauri HP. 1989. Nocodazole, a microtubule-active drug, interferes with apical protein delivery in cultured intestinal epithelial cells (Caco-2). J Cell Biol 108:13–22.

Elkjaer ML, Birn H, Agre P, Christensen EI, Nielsen S. 1995. Effects of microtubule disruption on endocytosis, membrane recycling and polarized distribution of Aquaporin-1 and gp330 in proximal tubule cells. Eur J Cell Biol 67:57–72.

Enos AP, Morris NR. 1990. Mutation of a gene that encodes a kinesin-like protein blocks nuclear division in A. nidulans. Cell 60:1019–1027.

Espreafico EM, Cheney RE, Matteoli M, et al. 1992. Primary structure and cellular localization of chicken brain myosin-V (p190), an unconventional myosin with calmodulin light chains. J Cell Biol 119:1541–1557.

Faktorovich EG, Steinberg RH, Yasumura D, Matthes MT, LaVail MM. 1990. Photoreceptor degeneration in inherited retinal dystrophy delayed by basic fibroblast growth factor. Nature 347:83–86.

Fath KR, Burgess DR. 1993. Golgi-derived vesicles from developing epithelial cells bind actin filaments and possess myosin-I as a cytoplasmically oriented peripheral membrane protein. J Cell Biol 120:117–127.

Fath KR, Burgess DR. 1994. Membrane motility mediated by unconventional myosin. Curr Opin Cell Biol 6:131–135.

Fath KR, Trimbur GM, Burgess DR. 1994. Molecular motors are differentially distributed on Golgi membranes from polarized epithelial cells. J Cell Biol 126:661–675.

Foisner R, Wiche G. 1991. Intermediate filament-associated proteins. Curr Opin Cell Biol 3:75–81.

Franke WW, Schmid E, Winter S, Osborn M, Weber K. 1979. Widespread occurrence of intermediate-sized filaments of the vimentin-type in cultured cells from diverse vertebrates. Exp Cell Res 123:25–46.

Fuchs E, Weber K. 1994. Intermediate filaments: structure, dynamics, function, and disease. Annu Rev Biochem 63:345–382.

Garcia DM, Burnside B. 1994. Suppression of cAMP-induced pigment granule aggregation in RPE by organic anion transport inhibitors. Invest Ophthalmol Vis Sci 35:178–188.

Gerace D, Burke G. 1988. Functional organization of the nuclear envelope. Annu Rev Cell Biol 4:355–374.

Gibson F, Walsh J, Mburu P, et al. 1995. A type VII myosin encoded by the mouse deafness gene shaker-1. Nature 374:62–64.

Gilbert T, Le Bivic A, Quaroni A, Rodriguez-Boulan E. 1991. Microtubular organization and its involvement in the biogenetic pathways of plasma membrane proteins in Caco-2 intestinal epithelial cells. J Cell Biol 113:275–288.

Gill SR, Schroer TA, Szilak I, Steuer ER, Sheetz MP, Cleveland DW. 1991. Dynactin, a conserved, ubiquitously expressed component of an activator of vesicle motility mediated by cytoplasmic dynein. J Cell Biol 115:1639–1650.

Gingrich JA, Caron MG. 1993. Recent advances in the molecular biology of dopamine receptors. Annu Rev Neurosci 16:299–321.

Gips SJ, Kandzari DE, Goldschmidt-Clermont PJ. 1994. Growth factor receptors, phospholipases, phospholipid kinases and actin reorganization. Semin Cell Biol 5:201–208.

Goddette DW, Frieden C. 1986. Actin polymerization: the mechanism of action of cytochalasin D. J Biol Chem 261:15974–15980.

Goldstein LS. 1993. With apologies to Scheherazade: tails of 1001 kinesin motors. Annu Rev Genet 27:319–351.

Goodson HV. 1994. Molecular evolution of the myosin superfamily: application of phylogenetic techniques to cell biological questions. In: Fambrought DM, ed, Society of General Physiologists Series, vol 49. New York: Rockefeller University Press, 141–158.

Gordon SR, Essner E. 1987. Investigations on circumferential microfilament bundles in rat retinal pigment epithelium. Eur J Cell Biol 44:97–104.

Gordon SR, Staley CA. 1990. Role of the cytoskeleton during injury-induced cell migration in corneal endothelium. Cell Motil Cytoskeleton 16:47–57.

Gotlieb AI, May LM, Subrahmanyan L, Kalnins VI. 1981. Distribution of microtubule organizing centers in migrating sheets of endothelial cells. J Cell Biol 91:589–594.

Gottlieb TA, Ivanov IE, Adesnik M, Sabatini DD. 1993. Actin microfilaments play a critical role in endocytosis at the apical but not the basolateral surface of polarized epithelial cells. J Cell Biol 120:695–710.

Grant MB, Guay C, Marsh R. 1990. Insulin-like growth factor I stimulates proliferation, migration, and plasminogen activator release by human retinal pigment epithelial cells. Curr Eye Res 9:323–325.

Greenberg S. 1995. Signal transduction of phagocytosis. Trends Cell Biol 5:93–99.

Gundersen D, Orlowski J, Rodriguez-Boulan E. 1991. Apical polarity of Na,K-ATPase in retinal pigment epithelium is linked to a reversal of the ankyrin-fodrin submembrane cytoskeleton. J Cell Biol 112:863–872.

Hageman GS, Marmor MF, Yao XY, Johnson LV. 1995. The interphotoreceptor matrix mediates primate retinal adhesion. Arch Ophthalmol 113:655–660.

Hasson T, Mooseker MS. 1994. Porcine myosin-VI: characterization of a new mammalian unconventional myosin. J Cell Biol 127:425–440.

Hasson T, Heintzelman MB, Santos-Sacchi J, Corey DP, Mooseker MS. 1995. Expression in cochlea and retina of myosin VIIa, the gene product defective in Usher syndrome type 1B. Proc Nat Acad Sci USA 92:9815–9819.

Hedberg KK, Chen LB. 1986. Absence of intermediate filaments in a human adrenal cortex carcinoma-derived cell line. Exp Cell Res 163:509–517.

Heins S, Aebi U. 1994. Making heads and tails of intermediate filament assembly, dynamics and networks. Curr Opin Cell Biol 6:25–33.

Hergott GJ, Nagai H, Kalnins VI. 1993. Inhibition of retinal pigment epithelial cell migration and proliferation with monoclonal antibodies against the beta 1 integrin subunit during wound healing in organ culture. Invest Ophthalmol Vis Sci 34:2761–2768.

Herman KG, Steinberg RH. 1982. Phagosome movement and the diurnal pattern of phagocytosis in the tapetal retinal pigment epithelium of the opossum. Invest Ophthalmol Vis Sci 23:277–290.

Herron WL, Riegel BW, Myers OE, Rubin ML. 1969. Retinal dystrophy in the rat—a pigment epithelial disease. Invest Ophthalmol 8:595–604.

Hillman DW, Cheng J, Bost-Usinger L, and Burnside B. 1998a. Multiple myosins expressed in fish RPE and retina. (submitted)

Hillman DW, Bost-Usinger LM, Lee B, Burnside B. 1998b. A vertebrate class III myosin expressed in fish retina and RPE. (submitted)

Hitt AL, Luna EJ. 1994. Membrane interactions with the actin cytoskeleton. Curr Opin Cell Biol 6:120–130.

Hofer D, Drenckhahn D. 1993. Molecular heterogeneity of the actin filament cytoskeleton associated with microvilli of photoreceptors. Muller's glial cells and pigment epithelial cells of the retina. Histochemistry 99:29–35.

Hogan MJ, Alvarado JA, Esperson-Weddell J. 1971. Histology of the Human Eye. Philadelphia: Saunders.

Hollenbeck PJ, Swanson JA. 1990. Radial extension of macrophage tubular lysosomes supported by kinesin. Nature 346:864–866.

Holzbaur ELF, Mikami A, Paschal BM, Vallee RB. 1994. Molecular characterization of cytoplasmic dynein. In: Hyams JS, Lloyd C, eds, Microtubules. New York: Wiley-Liss, 251–268.

Honda H, Eguchi G. 1980. How much does the cell boundary contract in a monolayered cell sheet? J Theor Biol 84:575–588.

Huber G, Matus A. 1990. Microtubule-associated protein 3 (MAP3) expression in non-neuronal tissues. J Cell Sci 95:237–246.

Hudspeth AJ, Yee AG. 1973. The intercellular junctional complexes of retinal pigment epithelia. Invest Ophthalmol 12:354–365.

Hunt RC. 1994. Intermediate filaments and other cytoskeletal structures in retinal pigment epithelial cells. In: Osborne NN, Chader GJ, eds, Progress in Retinal and Eye Research, vol 13. Oxford: Pergamon Press, 125–145.

Hunt RC, Davis AA. 1990. Altered expression of keratin and vimentin in human retinal pigment epithelial cells in vivo and in vitro. J Cell Physiol 145:187–199.

Hunt RC, Dewey A, Davis AA. 1989. Transferrin receptors on the surfaces of retinal pigment epithelial cells are associated with the cytoskeleton. J Cell Sci 92:655–666.

Huotari V, Sormunen R, Lehto VP, Eskelinen S. 1995. The polarity of the membrane skeleton in retinal pigment epithelial cells of developing chicken embryos and in primary culture. Differentiation 58:205–215.

Huttenlocher A, Sandborg RR, Horwitz AF. 1995. Adhesion in cell migration. Curr Opin Cell Biol 7:697–706.

Hynes RO. 1992. Integrins: versatility, modulation, and signaling in cell adhesion. Cell 69:11–25.

Immel JH. 1982. The Tree Shrew Retina: Photoreceptors and Retinal Pigment Epithelium. Dissertation. University of California, Santa Barbara.

Irons MJ, Kalnins VI. 1984. Distribution of microtubules in cultured RPE cells from normal and dystrophic RCS rats. Invest Ophthalmol Vis Sci 25:434–439.

Kasper M, Moll R, Stosiek P, Karsten U. 1988. Patterns of cytokeratin and vimentin expression in the human eye. Histochemistry 89:369–377.

Keller G, Leuenberger PM. 1977. Effects of colchicine on phagosome-lysosome interaction in retinal pigment epithelium. II. In vitro observations on histio-organotypical retinal pigment epithelial cells of the pig (a preliminary report). Graefes Arch Klin Exp Ophthalmol 203:253–259.

Kellerman KA, Miller KG. 1992. An unconventional myosin heavy chain gene from Drosophila melanogaster. J Cell Biol 119:823–834.

King-Smith C, Bost-Usinger L, Burnside B. 1995. Expression of kinesin heavy chain isoforms in retinal pigment epithelial cells. Cell Motil Cytoskeleton 31:66–81.

King-Smith C, Chen P, Garcia D, Rey H, Burnside B. 1996a. Calcium-independent regulation of pigment granule aggregation and dispersion in teleost retinal pigment epithelial cells. J Cell Sci 109:33–43.

King-Smith C, Paz P, Lee CW, Lam W, Burnside B. 1997. Bidirectional pigment granule migration in isolated retinal pigment epithelial cells requires actin but not microtubules. Cell Motility Cytoskel 38:229–249.

Kinkema M, Schiefelbein J. 1994. A myosin from a higher plant has structural similarities to class V myosins. J Mol Biol 239:591–597.

Kirchhof B, Sorgente N. 1989. Pathogenesis of proliferative vitreoretinopathy: modulation of retinal pigment epithelial cell functions by vitreous and macrophages. Dev Ophthalmol 16:1–53.

Kirchhof B, Kirchhof E, Ryan SJ, Sorgente N. 1989. Vitreous modulation of migration and proliferation of retinal pigment epithelial cells in vitro. Invest Ophthalmol Vis Sci 30:1951–1957.

Kirschner M, Mitchison T. 1986a. Beyond self-assembly: from microtubules to morphogenesis. Cell 45:329–342.

Kirschner NW, Mitchison T. 1986b. Microtubule dynamics [letter]. Nature 324:621.

Klymkowsky MW, Miller RH, Lane EB. 1983. Morphology, behavior, and interaction of cultured epithelial cells after the antibody-induced disruption of keratin filament organization. J Cell Biol 96:494–509.

Klymkowsky MW, Parr B. 1995. The body language of cells: the intimate connection between cell adhesion and behavior. Cell 83:5–8.

Kodama R, Eguchi G, Kelley RO. 1991. Ultrastructural and immunocytochemical analysis of the circumferential microfilament bundle in avian retinal pigmented epithelial cells in vitro. Cell Tissue Res 263:29–40.

Konari K, Sawada N, Zhong Y, Isomura H, Nakagawa T, Mori M. 1995. Development of the blood-retinal barrier in vitro: formation of tight junctions as revealed by occludin and ZO-1 correlates with the barrier function of chick retinal pigment epithelial cells. Exp Eye Res 61:99–108.

Kondo S, Sato-Yoshitake R, Noda Y, et al. 1994. KIF3A is a new microtubule-based anterograde motor in the nerve axon. J Cell Biol 125:1095–1107.

Koshland D. 1994. Mitosis: back to the basics. Cell 77:951–954.

Koslovsky JS, Qian C, Jiang X, Mercer JA. 1993. Molecular cloning of a mouse myosin I expressed in brain. FEBS Lett 320:121–124.

Kuhne W. 1887. Fortgesetzte Untersuchungen uber die Retina und die Pigmente des Auges. Heidelberg: Untersuchungen Physiol Inst Univ, 89–109.

Kunz YW. 1980. Cone mosaics in a teleost retina: changes during light and dark adaptation. Experientia 36:1371–1374.

Lafont F, Burkhardt JK, Simons K. 1994. Involvement of microtubule motors in basolateral and apical transport in kidney cells. Nature 372:801–803.

Langford GM. 1995. Actin- and microtubule-dependent organelle motors: interrelationships between the two motility systems. Curr Opin Cell Biol 7:82–88.

LaVail MM. 1976. Rod outer segment disk shedding in rat retina: relationship to cyclic lighting. Science 194:1071–1074.

Lee G. 1993. Non-motor microtubule-associated proteins. Curr Opin Cell Biol 5:88–94.

Lee J, Ishihara A, Theriot JA, Jacobson K. 1993. Principles of locomotion for simple-shaped cells. 362:167–171.

Leschey KH, Hines J, Singer JH, Hackett SF, Campochiaro PA. 1991. Inhibition of growth factor effects in retinal pigment epithelial cells. Invest Ophthalmol Vis Sci 32:1770–1778.

Lo SH, Weisberg E, Chen LB. 1994. Tensin: a potential link between the cytoskeleton and signal transduction. Bioessays 16:817–823.

Luby-Phelps K. 1994. Physical properties of cytoplasm. Curr Opin Cell Biol 6:3–9.

Luna EJ, Hitt A. 1992. Cytoskeleton–plasma membrane interactions. Science 258:955–964.

Maccioni RB, Cambiazo V. 1995. Role of microtubule-associated proteins in the control of microtubule assembly. Physiol Rev 75:835–864.

Machemer R, Laqua H. 1975. Pigment epithelium proliferation in retinal detachment (massive periretinal proliferation). Am J Ophthalmol 80:1–23.

Madara JL, Parkos C, Colgan S, Nusrat A, Atisook K, Kaoutzani P. 1992. The movement of solutes and cells across tight junctions. Ann NY Acad Sci 664:47–60.

Marmor MF. 1993. Mechanisms of retinal adhesion. In: Osborne N, Chader G, eds, Progress in Retinal Research. New York: Pergamon Press, 179–204.

Masson D, Kreis TE. 1993. Identification and molecular characterization of E-MAP-115, a novel microtubule-associated protein predominantly expressed in epithelial cells. J Cell Biol 123:357–371.

Matsumoto B, Defoe DM, Besharse JC. 1987. Membrane turnover in rod photoreceptors: ensheathment and phagocytosis of outer segment distal tips by pseudopodia of the retinal pigment epithelium. Proc R Soc Lond B Biol Sci 230:339–354.

Matsumoto B, Guerin CJ, Anderson DH. 1990. Cytoskeletal redifferentiation of feline, monkey, and human RPE cells in nature. Invest Ophthalmol Vis Sci 31:879–889.

Matsumoto H, Osono K, Pye Q, Pak WL. 1987. Gene encoding cytoskeletal proteins in Drosophila rhabdomeres. Proc Nat Acad Sci USA 84:985–989.

Matthies HJ, Miller RJ, Palfrey HC. 1993. Calmodulin binding to and cAMP-dependent phosphorylation of kinesin light chains modulate kinesin ATPase activity. J Biol Chem 268:11176–11187.

Mays RW, Beck KA, Nelson WJ. 1994. Organization and function of the cytoskeleton in polarized epithelial cells: a component of the protein sorting machinery. Curr Opin Cell Biol 6:16–24.

McDonald HB, Goldstein LS. 1990. Identification and characterization of a gene encoding a kinesin-like protein in Drosophila. Cell 61:991–1000.

McKechnie NM, Boulton M, Robey HL, Savage FJ, Grierson I. 1988. The cytoskeletal elements of human retinal pigment epithelium: in vitro and in vivo. J Cell Sci 91:303–312.

Mercer JA, Seperack PK, Strobel MC, Copeland NG, Jenkins NA. 1991. Novel myosin heavy chain encoded by murine dilute coat colour locus. Nature 349:709–713; erratum, 352:547.

Mermall V, Miller KG. 1995. The 95F unconventional myosin is required for proper organization of the Drosophila syncytial blastoderm. J Cell Biol 129:1575–1588.

Miki H, Bellhorn MB, Henkind P. 1975. Specializations of the retinochoroidal juncture. Invest Ophthalmol 14:701–707.

Miller H, Miller B, Ryan SJ. 1986. The role of retinal pigment epithelium in the involution of subretinal neovascularization. Invest Ophthalmol Vis Sci 27:1644–1652.

Mitchison T, Kirschner M. 1984. Dynamic instability of microtubule growth. Nature 312:237–242.

Mitchison TJ. 1309–1315. Compare and contrast actin filaments and microtubules. Mol Biol Cell 3:1309–1315.

Montell C, Rubin GM. 1988. The Drosophila ninaC locus encodes two photoreceptor cell specific proteins with domains homologous to protein kinases and the myosin heavy chain head. Cell 52:757–772.

Mooseker MS, Cheney RE. 1995. Unconventional myosins. In: Spudich JA, Gerhart J, McKnight SL, Schekman R, eds, Annual Review of Cell and Developmental Biology, vol 11. Palo Alto: Annual Reviews, 633–676.

Mostov K, Apodaca G, Aroeti B, Okamoto C. 1992. Plasma membrane protein sorting in polarized epithelial cells. J Cell Biol 116:577–583.

Muallem S, Kwiatkowska K, Xu X, Yin HL. 1995. Actin filament disassembly is a sufficient final trigger for exocytosis in nonexcitable cells. J Cell Biol 128:589–598.

Murphy TL, Sakamoto T, Hinton DR, et al. 1995. Migration of retinal pigment epithelium cells in vitro is regulated by protein kinase C. Exp Eye Res 60:683–695.

Murray R, Dubin M. 1975. The occurrence of actinlike filaments in association with migrating pigment granules in frog retinal pigment epithelium. J Cell Biol 64:705–710.

Nachmias VT, Philp N, Momoyama Y, Choi JK. 1992. G-actin pool and actin messenger RNA during development of the apical processes of the retinal pigment epithelial cells of the chick. Dev Biol 149:239–246.

Nangaku M, Sato-Yoshitake R, Okada Y, et al. 1994. KIF1B, a novel microtubule plus end–directed monomeric motor protein for transport of mitochondria. Cell 79:1209–1220.

Navone F, Niclas J, Hom-Booher N, et al. 1992. Cloning and expression of a human kinesin heavy chain gene: interaction of the COOH-terminal domain with cytoplasmic microtubules in transfected CV-1 cells. J Cell Biol 117:1263–1275.

Nelson WJ. 1991. Cytoskeleton functions in membrane traffic in polarized epithelial cells. Semin Cell Biol 2:375–385.

Nguyen-Legros J. 1978. Fine structure of the pigment epithelium in the vertebrate retina. Int Rev Cytol, Suppl 7:287–328.

Nihira M, Fujimoto T, Honda Y, Ogawa K. 1989. Distribution of fodrin and a-actinin in the rat retinal pigment epithelium in vivo. Acta Histochem Cytochem 22:625–637.

Nikaido SS, Takahashi JS. 1989. Twenty-four hour oscillation of cAMP in chick pineal cells: role of cAMP in the acute and circadian regulation of melatonin production. Neuron 3:609–619.

Noda Y, Sato-Yoshitake R, Kondo S, Nangaku M, Hirokawa N. 1995. KIF2 is a new microtubule-based anterograde motor that transports membranous organelles distinct from those carried by kinesin heavy chain or KIF3A/B. J Cell Biol 129:157–167.

Ohmori H, Toyama S, Toyama S. 1992. Direct proof that the primary site of action of cytochalasin on cell motility processes is actin. J Cell Biol 116:933–941.

Okabe S, Miyasaka H, Hirokawa N. 1993. Dynamics of the neuronal intermediate filaments. J Cell Biol 121:375–386.

Opas M, Kalnins VI. 1985. Distribution of spectrin and lectin-binding materials in surface lamina of RPE cells. Invest Ophthalmol Vis Sci 26:621–627.

Opas M, Turksen K, Kalnins VI. 1985. Adhesiveness and distribution of vinculin and spectrin in retinal pigmented epithelial cells during growth and differentiation in vitro. Dev Biol 107:269–280.

Otsuka AJ, Jeyaprakash A, Garcia-Anoveros J, et al. 1991. The C. elegans unc-104 gene encodes a putative kinesin heavy chain-like protein. Neuron 6:113–122.

Owaribe K. 1988. The cytoskeleton of retinal pigment epithelial cells. In: Osborne N, Chader J, eds, Progress in Retinal Research, vol 8. New York: Pergamon Press, 23–49.

Owaribe K, Eguchi G. 1985. Increase in actin contents and elongation of apical projections in retinal pigmented epithelial cells during development of the chicken eye. J Cell Biol 101:590–596.

Owaribe K, Masuda H. 1982. Isolation and characterization of circumferential microfilament bundles from retinal pigmented epithelial cells. J Cell Biol 95:310–315.

Owaribe K, Araki M, Eguchi G. 1979. Cell shape and actin filaments. In: Hatano S, Ishikawa H, Sato H, eds, Cell Motility: Molecules and Organizations. Tokyo: University of Tokyo Press, 491–500.

Owaribe K, Kodama R, Eguchi G. 1981. Demonstration of contractility of circumferential actin bundles and its morphogenetic significance in pigmented epithelium in vitro and in vivo. J Cell Biol 90:507–514.

Owaribe K, Sugino H, Masuda H. 1986. Characterization of intermediate filaments and their structural organization during epithelium formation in pigmented epithelial cells of the retina in vitro. Cell Tissue Res 244:87–93.

Owaribe K, Kartenbeck J, Rungger-Brandle E, Franke WW. 1988. Cytoskeletons of retinal pigment epithelial cells: interspecies differences of expression patterns indicate independence of cell function from the specific complement of cytoskeletal proteins. Cell Tissue Res 254:301–315.

Pang SF, Yew DT, Tsui HW. 1978. Photomechanical changes in the retina and choroid of guinea pigs, Cavia porcellus. Neurosci Lett 10:221–224.

Parczyk K, Haase W, Kondor-Koch C. 1989. Microtubules are involved in the secretion of proteins at the apical cell surface of the polarized epithelial cell, Madin-Darby canine kidney. J Biol Chem 264:16837–16846.

Patterson GM, Smith CD, Kimura LH, Britton BA, Carmeli S. 1993. Action of tolytoxin on cell morphology, cytoskeletal organization, and actin polymerization. Cell Motil Cytoskeleton 24:39–48.

Peyman GA, Bok D. 1972. Peroxidase diffusion in the normal and laser-coagulated primate retina. Invest Ophthalmol 11:35–45.

Philp NJ, Nachmias VT. 1985. Components of the cytoskeleton in the retinal pigmented epithelium of the chick. J Cell Biol 101:358–362.

Philp NJ, Nachmias VT. 1987. Polarized distribution of integrin and fibronectin in retinal pigment epithelium. Invest Ophthalmol Vis Sci 28:1275–1280.

Philp NJ, Yoon MY, Hock RS. 1990. Identification and localization of talin in chick retinal pigment epithelial cells. Exp Eye Res 51:191–198.

Pollard TD, Cooper JA. 1986. Actin and actin-binding proteins: a critical evaluation of mechanisms and functions. Annu Rev Biochem 55:987–1035.

Rabinovitch M. 1995. Professional and non-professional phagocytes: an introduction. Trends Cell Biol 5:85.

Reich-d'Almeida FB, Hockley DJ. 1975a. In situ reactivity of the retinal pigment epithelium. I. Phagocytosis in the normal rat. Exp Eye Res 21:333–345.

Reich-d'Almeida FB, Hockley DJ. 1975b. In situ reactivity of the retinal pigment epithelium. II. Phagocytosis in the dystrophic rat. Exp Eye Res 21:347–357.

Reizes O, Barylko B, Li C, Sudhof TC, Albanesi JP. 1994. Domain structure of a mammalian myosin I beta. Proc Nat Acad Sci USA 91:6349–6353.

Ridley AJ, Hall A. 1992. The small GTP-binding protein rho regulates the assembly of focal adhesions and actin stress fibers in response to growth factors. Cell 70:389–399.

Ridley AJ, Paterson HF, Johnston CL, Diekmann D, Hall A. 1992. The small GTP-binding protein rac regulates growth factor-induced membrane ruffling. Cell 70:401–410.

Rinnerthaler G, Geiger B, Small JV. 1988. Contact formation during fibroblast locomotion: involvement of membrane ruffles and microtubules. J Cell Biol 106:747–760.

Rizzolo LJ. 1990. The distribution of Na+,K(+)-ATPase in the retinal pigmented epithelium from chicken embryo is polarized in vivo but not in primary cell culture. Exp Eye Res 51:435–446.

Rizzolo LJ, Joshi HC. 1993. Apical orientation of the microtubule organizing center and associated gamma-tubulin during the polarization of the retinal pigment epithelium in vivo. Dev Biol 157:147–156.

Rizzolo LJ, Li ZQ. 1993. Diffusible, retinal factors stimulate the barrier properties of junctional complexes in the retinal pigment epithelium. J Cell Sci 106:859–867.

Rizzolo LJ, Zhou S, Li ZQ. 1994. The neural retina maintains integrins in the apical membrane of the RPE early in development. Invest Ophthalmol Vis Sci 35:2567–2576.

Robey HL, Hiscott PS, Grierson I. 1992. Cytokeratins and retinal epithelial cell behaviour. J Cell Sci 102:329–340.

Rodionov VI, Gyoeva FK, Gelfand VI. 1991. Kinesin is responsible for centrifugal movement of pigment granules in melanophores. Proc Nat Acad Sci USA 88:4956–4960.

Rodriguez-Boulan E, Nelson WJ. 1989. Morphogenesis of the polarized epithelial cell phenotype. Science 245:718–725.

Rodriguez-Boulan E, Powell SK. 1992. Polarity of epithelial and neuronal cells. Annu Rev Cell Biol 8:395–427.

Sakamoto T, Sakamoto H, Sheu SJ, Gabrielian K, Ryan SJ, Hinton DR. 1994. Intercellular gap formation induced by thrombin in confluent cultured bovine retinal pigment epithelial cells. Invest Ophthalmol Vis Sci 35:720–729.

Salas PJ, Misek DE, Vega-Salas DE, Gundersen D, Cereijido M, Rodriguez-Boulan E. 1986. Microtubules and actin filaments are not critically involved in the biogenesis of epithelial cell surface polarity. J Cell Biol 102:1853–1867.

Sandig M, Kalnins VI. 1988. Subunits in zonulae adhaerentes and striations in the associated circumferential microfilament bundles in chicken retinal pigment epithelial cells in situ. Exp Cell Res 175:1–14.

Sandig M, Kalnins VI. 1990a. Reorganization of circumferential microfilament bundles in retinal epithelial cells during mitosis. Cell Motil Cytoskeleton 17:133–141.

Sandig M, Kalnins VI. 1990b. Morphological changes in the zonula adhaerens during embryonic development of chick retinal pigment epithelial cells. Cell Tissue Res 259:455–461.

Sato-Yoshitake R, Shiomura Y, Miyasaka H, Hirokawa N. 1989. Microtubule-associated protein 1B: molecular structure, localization, and phosphorylation-dependent expression in developing neurons. Neuron 3:229–238.

Satterwhite LL, Pollard TD. 1992. Cytokinesis. Curr Opin Cell Biol 4:43–52.

Schafer DA, Cooper JA. 1995. Control of actin assembly at filament ends. In: Spudich JA, Gerhart J, McKnight SL, Schekman, R, eds, Annual Review of Cell and Developmental Biology, vol 11. Palo Alto: Annual Reviews, 497–518.

Schelling JR, Hanson AS, Marzec R, Linas SL. 1992. Cytoskeleton-dependent endocytosis is required for apical type 1 angiotensin II receptor-mediated phospholipase C activation in cultured rat proximal tubule cells. J Clin Invest 90:2472–2480.

Schlotzer-Schrehardt U, Muller HG, Wirtz PM, Naumann GO. 1990. Desmosomal-mitochondrial complexes in human nonpigmented ciliary and retinal pigment epithelia. Invest Ophthalmol Vis Sci 31:664–669.

Schwarz MA, Owaribe K, Kartenbeck J, Franke WW. 1990. Desmosomes and hemidesmosomes: constitutive molecular components. Annu Rev Cell Biol 6:461–491.

Sekine Y, Okada Y, Noda Y, et al. 1994. A novel microtubule-based motor protein (KIF4) for organelle transports, whose expression is regulated developmentally. J Cell Biol 127:187–201.

Selden S, Schwartz SM. 1979. Cytochalasin B inhibition of endothelial proliferation at wound edges in vitro. J Cell Biol 81:348–354.

Shohet RV, Conti MA, Kawamoto S, Preston YA, Brill DA, Adelstein RS. 1989. Cloning of the cDNA encoding the myosin heavy chain of a vertebrate cellular myosin. Proc Nat Acad Sci USA 86:7726–7730.

Singer RH. 1992. The cytoskeleton and mRNA localization. Curr Opin Cell Biol 4:15–19.

Snyder WZ, Zadunaisky JA. 1976. A role for calcium in the migration of retinal screening pigment in the frog. Exp Eye Res 22:377–388.

Spector I, Shochet NR, Blasberger D, Kashman Y. 1989. Latrunculins—novel marine macrolides that disrupt microfilament organization and affect cell growth: I. Comparison with cytochalasin D. Cell Motil Cytoskeleton 13:127–144.

Spiegelman BM, Lopata MA, Kirschner MW. 1979. Multiple sites for the initiation of microtubule assembly in mammalian cells. Cell 16:239–252.

Spudich JA. 1994. How molecular motors work. Nature 372:515–518.

St Johnston D. 1995. The intracellular localization of messenger RNAs. Cell 81:161–170.

Steinberg RH, Wood I. 1974. Pigment epithelial cell ensheathment of cone outer segments in the retina of the domestic cat. Proc R Soc Lond B Biol Sci 187:461–478.

Stevenson BR, Begg DA. 1994. Concentration-dependent effects of cytochalasin D on tight junctions and actin filaments in MDCK epithelial cells. J Cell Sci 107:367–375.

Stewart M. 1993. Intermediate filament structure and assembly. Curr Opin Cell Biol 5:3–11.

Stroeva OG, Mitashov VI. 1983. Retinal pigment epithelium: proliferation and differentiation during development and regeneration. Int Rev Cytol 83:221–293.

Swanson JA, Baer SC. 1995. Phagocytosis by zippers and triggers. Trends Cell Biol 5:89–92.

Theriot JA, Mitchison TJ. 1992. Comparison of actin and cell surface dynamics in motile fibroblasts. J Cell Biol 119:367–377.

Titus MA. 1993. Myosins. Curr Opin Cell Biol 5:77–81.

Trifaro JM, Vitale ML. 1993. Cytoskeleton dynamics during neurotransmitter release. Trends Neurosci 16:466–472.

Troutt LL, Burnside B. 1988. The unusual microtubule polarity in teleost retinal pigment epithelial cells. J Cell Biol 107:1461–1464.

Troutt LL, Burnside B. 1989. Role of microtubules in pigment granule migration in teleost retinal pigment epithelial cells. Exp Eye Res 48:433–443.

Tsukamoto Y. 1986. Pigment epithelial ensheathment and phagocytosis of rod tips in the retina of Rana catesbeiana. J Morphol 188:303–313.

Turksen K, Opas M, Aubin JE, Kalnins VI. 1983. Microtubules, microfilaments and adhesion patterns in differentiating chick retinal pigment epithelial (RPE) cells in vitro. Exp Cell Res 147:379–391.

Turksen K, Kalnins VI. 1987. The cytoskeleton of chick retinal pigment epithelial cells in situ. Cell Tissue Res 248:95–101.

Vale RD, Reese TS, Sheetz MP. 1985. Identification of a novel force-generating protein, kinesin, involved in microtubule-based motility. Cell 42:39–50.

Vallee R. 1993. Molecular analysis of the microtubule motor dynein. Proc Nat Acad Sci USA 90:8769–8772.

Vallee RB, Bloom GS. 1991. Mechanisms of fast and slow axonal transport. Annu Rev Neurosci 14:59–92.

Van der Sluijs P, Bennett MK, Antony C, Simons K, Kreis TE. 1990. Binding of exocytic vesicles from MDCK cells to microtubules in vitro. J Cell Sci 95:545–553.

Van Genderen Stort AGH. 1887. Mouvements des elements de la retine sous l'influence de la lumiere. Arch neerlandaises des Sci exact ef Nat 21:316–386.

Vassar R, Coulombe PA, Degenstein L, Albers K, Fuchs E. 1991. Mutant keratin expression in transgenic mice causes marked abnormalities resembling a human genetic skin disease. Cell 64:365–380.

Verstraeten TC, Buzney S, Macdonald S, Neufeld A. 1990. Retinal pigment epithelium wound closure in vitro: pharmacologic inhibition. Invest Ophthalmol Vis Sci 31:481–488.

Vinores SA, Campochiaro PA, McGehee R, Orman W, Hackett SF, Hjelmeland LM. 1990. Ultrastructural and immunocytochemical changes in retinal pigment epithelium, retinal glia, and fibroblasts in vitreous culture. Invest Ophthalmol Vis Sci 31:2529–2545.

Wagner M, Benson MT, Rennie IG, MacNeil S. 1995. Effects of pharmacological modulation of intracellular signalling systems on retinal pigment epithelial cell attachment to extracellular matrix proteins. Curr Eye Res 14:373–384.

Weil D, Blanchard S, Kaplan J, et al. 1995. Defective myosin VIIA gene responsible for Usher syndrome type 1B. Nature 374:60–61.

West RR, Tenbarge KM, Olmsted JB. 1991. A model for microtubule-associated protein 4 structure: domains defined by comparisons of human, mouse, and bovine sequences. J Biol Chem 266:21886–21896.

Yacob A, Kunz YW. 1977. "Disk shedding" in the cone outer segments of the teleost, Poecilia reticulata P. Cell Tissue Res 181:487–492.

Yacob A, Wise C, Kunz YW. 1977. The accessory outer segment of rods and cones in the retina of the guppy, Poecilia reticulata P. (Teleostei): an electron microscopical study. Cell Tissue Res 177:181–193.

Yang JT, Laymon RA, Goldstein LS. 1989. A three-domain structure of kinesin heavy chain revealed by DNA sequence and microtubule binding analyses. Cell 56:879–889.

Young RW, Bok D. 1969. Participation of the retinal pigment epithelium in the rod outer segment renewal process. J Cell Biol 42:392–403.

4. Melanin and the retinal pigment epithelium

MICHAEL BOULTON

Melanin pigments are found in most living organisms, including bacteria, plants, and animals (Nicolaus, 1968; Prota, 1992) and are a common element of a variety of vertebrate tissues, e.g. skin, hair, eye, inner ear, and leptomeninges (Boissy, 1988; Nordlund et al., 1989; Prota, 1992). While melanin is not a vital compound, as mutants lacking it are viable, albinos are at a disadvantage in many ways compared to normal pigmented individuals (Drager and Balkema, 1987). Melanin granules consist of a protein matrix containing polymerized melanin and are often referred to as melanosomes (Seiji et al., 1961; Feeney, 1978; Mishima, 1992; Prota, 1992). It is the presence of melanin, the primary pigment in vertebrates, within these granules that gives them their characteristic color: yellowish to reddish in the case of pheomelanins (e.g. in red hair) or the brown and black of eumelanins (e.g. in black hair) (Gornitz, 1923; Nicolaus, 1968). The melanin granules of the eye mainly contain eumelanin and are present in the pigmented epithelium of the retina (RPE), ciliary body, and iris as well as in the melanocytes of the stroma of the iris and choroid (Hogan et al., 1971; Feeney, 1978; Boissy, 1988; Sarna, 1992). With the exception of the skin, in which melanin is generally accepted to play a photoprotective role (Quevedo et al., 1985; Tosti and Costelli, 1990), the biological role of melanin in ocular tissues is still open to intense debate, as will be discussed in detail later in this chapter.

MELANIN-PRODUCING CELLS

The most common and widely studied melanin-producing cell in vertebrates is the melanocyte. Embryologically, the neural crest generates a stem cell population of mesodermal cells called melanoblasts that migrate and populate various regions of the body (Duncker, 1985; Prota, 1992). Once these melanoblasts reach the appropriate environment, they differentiate into functionally active melanocytes that can be observed readily in the skin, hair, and uvea (Mintz, 1967; Holbrook et al., 1988). By contrast, the RPE, ciliary epithelium, and iris pigment epithelium are neuroectodermal in origin (Mann, 1969; Spitznas, 1971). These neuroepithelia are derived from the outer layer of the optic vesicle and form a single continuous layer of cells within the eye.

Melanin-producing cells either (a) transfer melanin granules into a second cell type, or (b) retain their complement of pigment granules throughout life (see Prota, 1992). Cutaneous melanocytes transfer mature pigment granules into adjacent cells, i.e. from epidermal melanocytes to keratinocytes (Nordlund et al., 1989; Prota, 1992). By contrast, extracutaneous melanin-producing cells, of which ocular cells are no exception, do not normally transfer their melanin granules to other cell types (Feeney, 1978; Sarna, 1992; Prota, 1992). This is true for both the pigmented neuroepithelium of the eye and the uveal stromal melanocytes. Furthermore, while cutaneous melanocytes synthesize melanin throughout life, extracutaneous melanin-producing cells have classically been reported to synthesize melanin only during the early stages of their embryonic development (Mann, 1969; Prota, 1992; Sarna, 1992). More recently, however, de novo synthesis of melanin has been observed in the iris, choroid, and RPE (see Schraermeyer, 1993), a feature which will be discussed in more detail later.

MELANOGENESIS

Melanogenesis, the formation of intracellular pigment granules, has been extensively studied in skin melanocytes (see Nordlund et al., 1989; Mishima, 1992; Prota, 1992; Riley, 1993). However, it is widely accepted that the same enzymes (albeit possibly different isoforms [Varela et al., 1995]) and synthetic pathways are involved in melanogenesis in melanin-containing neuroepithelial cells (Hearing et al., 1973; Mishima et al., 1978; Sarna, 1992; Varela, 1995; Schraermeyer, 1996).

Numerous histological and tracer studies have demonstrated that melanogenesis is initiated via two separate events (Seiji et al., 1961; 1963; Wick et al., 1987); (a) the generation of premelanosomes (containing the structural proteins of melanosomes) and (b) the synthesis of tyrosinase, an enzyme essential for melanogenesis (Fig. 4-1). Premelanosomes appear to be assembled in the smooth endoplasmic reticulum of multivesicular bodies that are connected to the rough endoplasmic

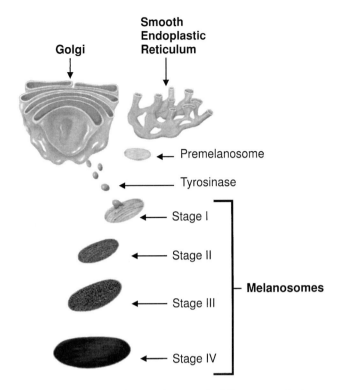

Golgi

**Smooth
Endoplastic
Reticulum**

← Premelanosome

← Tyrosinase

← Stage I

← Stage II

— **Melanosomes**

← Stage III

← Stage IV

FIGURE 4-1. Schematic diagram depicting the different stages in the assembly of melanosomes.

reticulum and are released into the cytoplasm (Toda and Fitzpatrick, 1972; Mishima et al., 1979; Garcia et al., 1979; Stanka et al., 1981; Boissy, 1988). On the other hand, tyrosinase is synthesized by ribosomes on the rough endoplasmic reticulum, and is transported via the smooth endoplasmic reticulum to a particular area of the Golgi apparatus termed the *Golgi-associated endoplasmic reticulum of lysosome,* while undergoing varying stages of post-translational modification (Mishima, 1992). Glycosylation of the enzyme is initiated in the endoplasmic reticulum shortly after synthesis, and further glycosylation and processing is carried out within the Golgi apparatus (Mishima and Imokawa, 1985; Mishima, 1992; Prota, 1992). This glycosylation results in a significant increase in the molecular weight of tyrosinase (Mishima, 1992). The fully glycosylated tyrosinase is then assembled into coated vesicles which bud off from the Golgi and are transferred to the premelanosomes (see Mishima, 1992; Prota, 1992). It appears that glycosylation of the tyrosinase polypeptide is essential for its translocation through the Golgi apparatus to the premelanosome. Glycosylation of tyrosinase can be inhibited by both glucosamine and tunicamycin (Imokawa and Mishima, 1984). Such treatment results in the absence of the higher-molecular-weight form of tyrosinase and prevents the nascent protein from exit-

ing the Golgi apparatus. Glycosylation inhibitors also interfere with the assembly of microfilaments in the premelanosome (Mishima and Imokawa, 1985). Premelanosomes can only melanize after receiving the fully glycosylated form of tyrosinase from such coated vesicles.

In mammals, approximately 160 genes present at nearly 70 loci are estimated to influence melanin pigmentation in melanocytes (Jimbow et al., 1994). Recently identified genes and encoding proteins include (a) TRP-1 (tyrosinase-related protein) (Shibahara, 1993), (b) TRP-2 (dopachrome tautomerase) (Jackson et al., 1992) (c) p-locus protein, which may function as a tyrosine transporter (Spritz, 1993) and (d) lysosomal-associated membrane proteins which are associated with the melanosomal surface (Jimbow et al., 1994). However, it remains to be determined how many of these genes are involved in melanogenesis in the RPE.

The synthesis of melanin depends on translocation of tyrosinase to the premelanosomes, the availability of its substrate L-tyrosine, the fate of the oxidation products generated during the different stages of melanogenesis, and other factors influencing the degree of polymerization (see Mishima, 1992; Prota, 1992; Riley, 1993). Although it is now evident that other enzymes are also involved, it is clear that the most important enzyme in the melanogenic pathway is indeed tyrosinase (Hearing and Jiminez, 1987; Tsukamoto et al., 1992; Riley, 1993), i.e. in the absence of tyrosinase activity no melanin is formed (Giebel and Spritz, 1992). Tyrosinase is a multifunctional copper-containing enzyme which catalyzes the conversion of the amino acid L-tyrosine, through a complex series of intermediates, to the highly polymerized end product melanin (Fig. 4-2) (see Prota, 1992; Riley, 1993). The reaction scheme is further complicated by the highly unstable nature of the intermediates and the extremely insoluble nature of polymerized melanin. Figure 4-2 highlights the main stages in the formation of melanin. In the first step tyrosinase catalyzes two sequential reactions—the hydroxylation of tyrosine to 3,4-dihydroxyphenylalanine (DOPA) and the immediate oxidation of DOPA to dopaquinone. It appears that these two reactions are inseparable and that DOPA, the initial product, also functions as a cofactor of the first reaction (see Riley, 1993). At this point the melanogenesis pathway can take one of two directions, depending on the type of melanin to be generated; eumelanin or pheomelanin. For eumelanin, dopaquinone undergoes spontaneous endocyclic ring formation to give rise to leucodopachrome, which is rapidly oxidized by redox exchange with dopaquinone, generating dopachrome and dopa (see Riley, 1993). Dopachrome is relatively stable whereas DOPA is rapidly reoxidized

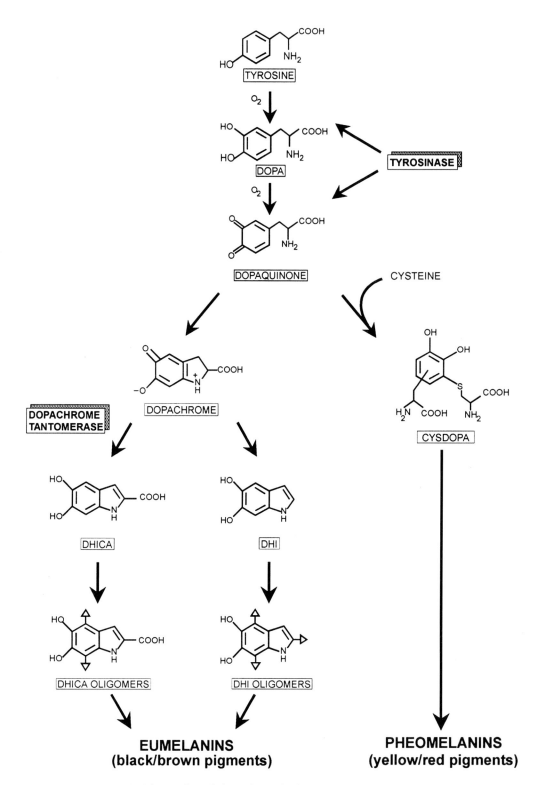

FIGURE 4-2. Scheme of metabolic pathways leading to eumelanin and pheomelanin.

by tyrosinase to form dopaquinone. The dopaquinone/ DOPA cycle thus established is the oxidative dynamo of melanogenesis (Riley, 1993). The next stage of eumelanin generation appears to be mainly under the control of dopachrome tautomerase, which ensures that the major proportion of dopachrome is converted to 5,6-dihydroxyindole-2-carboxylic acid (DHICA) (Bernd et al., 1994; Salinas et al., 1994). An alternative pathway leads to spontaneous decarboxylation and the formation of 5,6-dihydroxyindole (DHI) (Prota, 1988; Riley, 1993; Salinas et al., 1994). Finally, the oxidative polymerization of DHICA and DHI (possibly under the control of TRP-1, DHICA oxidase) results in the melanin polymer, which is strongly attached to the protein matrix of the melanosomes. The details of this process are unclear but give rise to an irregular melanin polymer (Prota, 1980). By contrast, if dopaquinone reacts with cysteine to form cysdopa the result is pheomelanin, which may contain more than 10% sulfur (Prota, 1980; 1992). Any biological melanin is probably a copolymer comprising different proportions of eumelanin and pheomelanin (Sealy et al., 1982; Sarna, 1992), an observation which is supported by the observation that eumelanogenesis and pheomelanogenesis can occur concurrently within the same pigment cell (Inazu and Mishima, 1993). Free-radical intermediates have also been proposed to be involved in the synthesis of melanin, but their precise role requires further investigation (Sealy, 1984; Sarna, 1992).

Why melanin synthesis appears to cease once a melanosome has reached maturity is unclear, particularly since in some cell types tyrosinase is still present. One proposed explanation is that tyrosinase is functionally active in coated vesicles and premelanosomes but that melanization is interrupted, perhaps by an indole-blocking factor, until the enzyme inhibitor complex enters the melanosomes (Pawelek et al., 1980; Chakraborty et al., 1989). Alternatively, melanogenesis may be regulated by the degree of tyrosinase glycosylation (Imokawa and Mishima, 1984); a reduction in tyrosinase activity in mouse hair follicle melanocytes is associated with decreased glycosylation of tyrosinase (Burchill et al., 1989).

While the metabolic pathways leading to melanin have been elucidated from studies on dermal melanocytes, it appears that a similar pathway exists for RPE melanogenesis. The RPE has been shown (a) to exhibit premelanosomes and the varying stages of melanosome maturation (Mann, 1969; Feeney-Burns, 1978; 1980), (b) to have tyrosinase activity (Novikoff et al., 1979; Dryja et al., 1978; Varela et al., 1995), (c) to fail to produce melanin if the tyrosinase gene is defective, as occurs in oculocutaneous albinism (Oetting and King,

1994; Spritz, 1994) and (d) to contain low levels of TRP-1 (Smith-Thomas et al., 1996).

MORPHOLOGY AND TIMING OF OCULAR MELANOGENESIS

Melanogenesis progresses through a number of stages, as identified by electron microscopy (Fig. 4-3) (Garcia et al., 1979; Feeney-Burns, 1980; Sarna, 1992; Mishima, 1992; Prota, 1992). The description of the number of stages and their appearance differ according to author and tissue studied. The following description is based on that of Feeney-Burns (1980) for the RPE (Fig. 4-1). First a nonpigmented, ovoid, poorly defined membrane-bound protein matrix—a premelanosome—is formed. Then tyrosinase, the enzyme responsible for melanogenesis, is delivered either to the premelanosome or to the stage I melanosome, and melanin synthesis begins. The stage I melanosome assumes an ordered protein matrix in which protein filaments extend from pole to pole. Melanin is deposited on the protein matrix and osmophilia becomes apparent. Melanization continues through stages II and III until a fully melanized (stage IV) melanosome is formed, which is often referred to as a *melanin granule*.

In the eye, melanogenesis always occurs first in the RPE, with immature melanosomes visible as early as 7 weeks of gestation in man (Mann, 1969; Hogan et al., 1971; Taylor, 1978). Between the 8th and 14th week melanosomes at all stages of maturation can be ob-

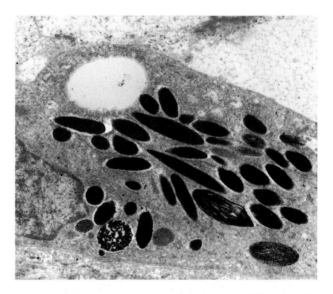

FIGURE 4-3. Electron micrographs of fetal human RPE (15 weeks' gestation) showing melanosomes at different stages of maturation. Magnification ×6500. (Reproduced courtesy of Professor John Marshall, St Thomas's Hospital, London.)

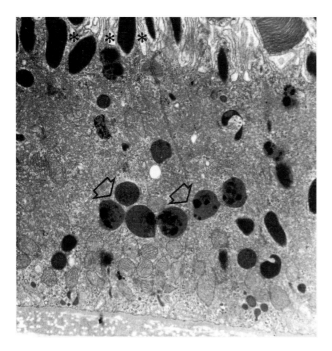

FIGURE 4-4. Electron micrograph of human RPE from a 52-year-old donor. Mature melanin granules can be seen in the apical portion of the cell and are predominantly vertically orientated (*). Lipofuscin granules *(open arrows)* can be observed in the midportion of the cell and are often associated with small melanin deposits. Magnification ×11,500. (Reproduced courtesy of Professor John Marshall, St Thomas's Hospital, London.)

served (Fig. 4-3). Production then ceases within a few weeks, as the cells attain their full complement of melanosomes. However, polymerization of melanin continues to occur in these granules until the RPE acquires a full complement of mature melanin granules (at approximately two years of age in human RPE cells) (Mann, 1969; Feeney-Burns, 1980) (Fig. 4-4).

By contrast, melanogenesis in uveal stromal melanocytes begins during late gestation (20 weeks in man) and by birth the stromal melanocytes have almost completed their quota of melanosomes. However, these are predominantly immature and continue to actively synthesize melanin (Mann, 1969; Hogan et al., 1971; Taylor, 1978). This is apparent in the iris of caucasians, where the iris is usually blue at birth but later becomes darker as more melanin accumulates in the superficial stromal melanocytes. These stages of melanogenesis apply to all species studied through the timing depends on gestation period.

IS MELANIN SYNTHESIZED IN ADULT RPE CELLS?

It has long been the majority view that mammalian RPE cells do not undergo melanogenesis after birth (see Boul-

ton, 1991; Smith-Thomas et al., 1996). However, support for the concept of melanin production in the RPE throughout life (albeit at a slow rate) is now increasing (see Schraermeyer, 1993). Spitznas (1971) presented morphological evidence consistent with active melanin synthesis in adult human RPE, while tyrosinase activity has been identified in the RPE of adult black mice (Novikoff et al., 1979), mature bovine RPE (Dryja et al., 1978), and adult rabbit retina/RPE (Varela et al., 1995). However, the identification of tyrosinase, the principle enzyme in melanogenesis, is not confirmation of melanin formation, since other factors are also involved (Fig. 4-2). There is indirect evidence for melanin synthesis in adult RPE in vivo. Boulton and colleagues (1990) reported that melanin granules isolated from human donors of varying age demonstrated an age-dependent increase in light absorption at the shorter wavelengths and proposed that this reflected a slow increase in the melanin content per granule with age. Electron micrographs of aging human RPE cells clearly demonstrate melanin granules of varying size (Fig. 4-4). While the smaller melanin deposits (often found associated with lipofuscin granules) have been attributed to lysosomal degradation of melanin granules, they could equally reflect the deposition of newly synthesized melanin. Despite evidence for melanin synthesis in adult human RPE, however, premelanosomes have not been identified. This raises two possibilities for melanin synthesis; (a) melanin synthesis is occurring at a slow rate in preexisting melanosomes and/or (b) melanin is being synthesized on an alternative matrix, e.g. phagosomes (Schraermeyer, 1993) or lipofuscin granules.

In addition to in vivo studies, melanin formation has been reported in RPE cells in vitro. Primary cultures of pigmented RPE cells undergo division until a confluent monolayer of poorly pigmented hexanocuboidal cells is formed. Subculturing results in a cell population devoid of pigment granules (Flood and Gouras, 1981; Boulton et al., 1982). This depigmentation is due to the dilution of pigment granules among daughter cells. However, there is evidence of melanogenesis in vitro in depigmented adult human (Campochiaro and Hackett, 1993), porcine (Dorey et al., 1990), bovine (Schraemeyer and Stieve, 1994), and canine (McLellan, personal communication) RPE cells if maintained for sufficient time under the appropriate conditions. Cultured cells synthesize multilamellar bodies, which combine with tyrosinase eventually to form highly pigmented bodies. While it is clear that these multilamellar bodies act in a similar way to that of premelanosomes, their origin is unclear, but they may be derived via the lysosomal system (Dorey et al., 1990; Schraemeyer and Stieve, 1994). Furthermore, it appears that melanogenesis in cultured human RPE cells is regulated by both extracellular matrix and exogenous growth factors (Campochiaro and Hackett, 1993). While melanogenesis in vitro may be an artifact of the tissue culture environment, it does demonstrate that adult RPE cells can, given the right conditions, express the genes necessary for pigment production in vivo, a finding that is supported by the finding that tyrosinase and TRP genes were expressed in RPE cells from patients with proliferative vitreoretinopathy (Abe et al., 1996).

Further studies are required to elucidate (a) the magnitude, and importance (if any), of melanogenesis and (b) the degree of intragranular melanin synthesis and turnover throughout life in adult RPE in vivo.

RPE MELANIN

The color of the RPE is due to its melanin content. Melanin granules are abundant in the cytoplasm of adult RPE cells, predominantly in the apical and midportions of the cell, while virtually absent from the basal cell cytoplasm (Hogan et al., 1971; Feeney, 1978) (Fig. 4-4). Two shapes of granules are apparent; ellipsoid granules (1 μm in diameter and 2–3 μm in length) primarily located toward the apical portion of the cell and spherical granules in the midportion of the cell (Hogan et al., 1971). It is interesting to note that the ellipsoid granules are, for the most part, vertically orientated, lying parallel to one another at the base of, or within, the apical processes (Hogan et al., 1971). However, the distribution of melanin granules within the RPE can vary between species (see Fig. 4-4, 4-5). With the electron microscope the pigment granules are seen to be surrounded by a thin membrane, the internal surface of which is in direct contact with the melanoprotein which fills the space (Hogan et al., 1971; Feeney, 1978). Most of the granules lack any recognizable substructure at the electron microscopic level.

Typical eumelanins such as those of the eye, appear to be polymers or, more precisely, mixtures of polymers consisting mainly of DHI and DHICA units (Sarna, 1992). Unfortunately, the insolubility of eumelanins makes determination of their molecular structure a dif-

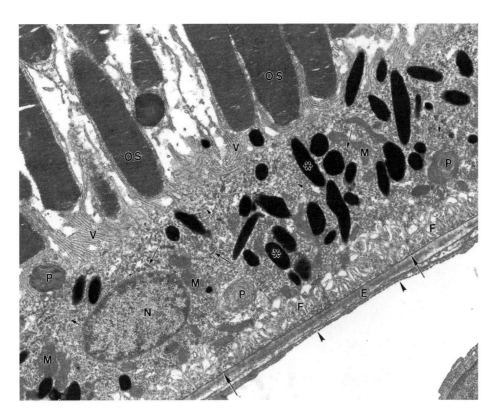

FIGURE 4-5. Electron micrograph of normal adult mouse RPE. (N), nucleus; (F), basal infoldings; (V), microvilli; (M), mitochondria; (P), phagosomes; (OS), outer segments; (E), elastic zone of Bruch's membrane; (*), melanin granules; *large arrows*, basement membrane of RPE: *arrowheads*, fenestration of choriocapillaris; *small long arrows*, rough endoplasmic reticulum; *small short arrows*, smooth endoplasmic reticulum. Magnification ×13,200. (Reproduced courtesy of Lily Zong-Yi Li, M.D., Retinitis Pigmentosa Histopathology Center, University of Washington, Seattle.)

ficult task. The only approach currently available for classifying natural melanins relies on elemental analysis and degradation experiments to define the nature and origin of the main structural units of the pigment polymer. Unlike pheomelanin, which contains more than 10% sulfur, eumelanin should contain no sulfur. However, as already discussed, most biological melanins are a copolymer consisting of different proportions of eumelanin and pheomelanin (Sarna, 1992). While reports are limited for RPE melanin, there is evidence of a significant sulfur content for both bovine and human RPE (Dryja et al., 1979; Ulshafer et al., 1990) indicating that it is a copolymer, albeit with eumelanin predominating. Dryja et al. (1979) compared the sulfur content of melanin from hair, choroid, iris, and RPE from black-haired and red-haired cattle. They found that, in black-haired cattle, sulfur contents of hair and ocular melanins were all between 0.6% and 0.94%, consistent with the predominant eumelanin character of this pigmentation. In red-haired cattle, hair melanin had a sulfur content of 8.66% (similar to pheomelanin) which differed markedly from that of melanin in the choroid (0.94%) or RPE (1.72%). Thus it appears that, in individual animals, ocular melanins can have very different chemical structures from hair melanins. Elemental analysis of melanin pigments isolated from human donor eyes with blue and brown irises revealed that the sulfur content is rather similar in both melanin pigments, in the range 2–2.34% (Menon et al., 1981). In addition to sulfur, RPE melanin also contains detectable amounts of zinc, copper, calcium, and iron (Ulshafer et al., 1990; Samuelson et al., 1993). Melanin granules are generally considered to be relatively insoluble, usually requiring boiling hydroxide solution for solubilisation. However, a recent report suggests that melanin can be degraded by lysosomal enzymes (Schraermeyer and Dohms, 1996).

REGIONAL DISTRIBUTION OF MELANIN GRANULES IN THE RPE

The most obvious regional distribution of melanin granules is seen in the eyes of those animals (e.g. cattle, cats, and dogs) with a tapetal fundus; a brightly colored "iridescent" reflex derives from a semicircular area superior to the optic disc. An important feature of this area is that the RPE cells are devoid of melanosomes, while adjacent regions contain their normal complement of melanin granules (Braekevelt 1989a,b).

In man, the darker pigmentation of the macula has been attributed to the greater distribution of RPE melanin granules in this region (Feeney-Burns et al., 1984; Weiter et al., 1986; Van Norren and Tiemeijer,

1986). Topographically, melanin density shows a slight decrease from the peripheral retina to the posterior pole but with an increase in the macular region (Weiter et al., 1986). However, the peak in melanin density at the macula may be attributed in part to the denser packing of melanin per unit area (RPE cells in the macula are taller and narrower compared to the shorter, wider extra-macular cells) rather than an increased number of melanin granules per cell; the percentage area of the RPE cell occupied by melanin granules is the same for both the macular and equatorial fundus (8%) and highest for the peripheral region (15%) during the first two decades of life (Feeney-Burns et al., 1984). Despite the observation that choroidal melanin concentration in blacks is approximately double that in whites, Weiter and colleagues (1986) were unable to demonstrate a difference in melanin content of the RPE between blacks and whites. These tissue differences may reflect the embryological origin of pigmented cells. Melanocytes, which are neural crest in origin, show marked racial variability (uveal stroma and skin are typical examples) while neuroepithelial pigmentation does not vary significantly with race (Weiter et al., 1986).

AGE-RELATED CHANGES IN RPE MELANIN GRANULES

Apical polarization of the melanosomes within the RPE tends to disappear with senescence (granules are either disoriented or absent from the apex of cells) with the majority of melanin granules distributed throughout the cytoplasm (Hogan et al., 1971; Feeney, 1978). The differential topographical distribution of melanin granules is maintained throughout life, but a significant decline in the total numbers of granules is observed in all regions after the age of 40 (Feeney-Burns et al., 1984; Weiter et al., 1986; Schmidt and Peish, 1986). Comparisons between three age groups (1–20, 21–60, and 61–100 years) demonstrate a decline in melanosome numbers in the macular RPE between the early and late decades of about 25% (Feeney-Burns et al., 1984). Taken as a percentage of cell volume, about 8% of the macular RPE cell is occupied by melanin in the first two decades of life, decreasing to 6% in the subsequent two decades and to 3.5% in later decades. Some compensation for this age-related decrease in melanosome numbers may be achieved through a slow increase in the melanin content per granule with age (Boulton et al., 1990).

The loss in "true" melanin granules correlates with an increase in the numbers of "complex" melanin granules. With increasing age two types of melanin-containing "complex" granules can be identified within the RPE;

melanin with a cortex of lipofuscin (melanolipofuscin) and melanin with a cortex of enzyme-reactive material (melanolysosomes) (Feeney, 1978; Feeney-Burns et al., 1984; 1990). Electron microscopic analysis of RPE from eyes over 90 years old demonstrated that the cells were virtually devoid of unadulterated melanin granules, i.e. they were all "melanin-complexes" (Feeney-Burns et al., 1990). These complexes exhibited a regional distribution similar to that of lipofuscin (Marshall, 1987), with the highest density in the extrafoveal macula and decreasing density toward the periphery and fovea (Feeney-Burns et al., 1984). Expressed as a percentage of the area within the cell, the complex granules range from 3.3% in the first decade of life to 8–10% in the sixth. These complex granules may represent melanin in the process of repair, modification, or degradation.

The loss of RPE melanin with age results in the transition of melanin particles with a high extinction coefficient to weakly absorbing aggregates containing less melanin per unit area and manifest as the fading of eye color with age (Feeney-Burns et al., 1984; Sarna, 1992). The age-related loss of RPE melanin probably results from lysosomal digestion of melanin granules; the lysosomes are postulated to undergo direct fusion with melanin granules (Feeney-Burns et al., 1984). Digestion is slow and the consolidation and reorganization of melanin residues, secondary lysosomes, and lipofuscin that occurs throughout life results in great variation in the morphology of melanin "complexes" in older eyes (Feeney-Burns et al., 1984). Furthermore, such degradation, in tandem with melanin synthesis in adult RPE, may be important in negating damage to melanin caused by light and/or free radicals. It has also been suggested that melanin loss may occur via extrusion of melanin and its incorporation by the lysosomal system of neighboring cells (Burns and Feeney-Burns, 1980). While an interesting concept, this mechanism is unlikely to account for an overall loss of RPE melanin but rather for a redistribution of existing melanin.

In addition to morphological features, the photophysical characteristics of melanin granules also change with age (Boulton et al., 1990). While dissolved human RPE melanin granules from all ages exhibit a typical melanin absorbance profile, which increases as the wavelength decreases from 700 to 250 nm, absorption increases at the shorter wavelengths with increasing age (Fig. 4-6) (Boulton et al., 1990). Dissolved melanosomes from human fetal eyes show an absorbance four times greater at 250 nm than at 700 nm. This ratio increases with increasing age up to a factor of eight in the case of melanin isolated from donor eyes greater than 50 years of age. The fluorescence characteristics of melanosomes also change with age, i.e. a decrease in the blue and a

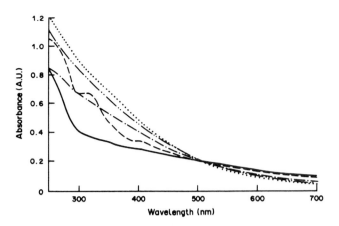

FIGURE 4-6. Absorption spectra of dissolved human RPE melanin fractions from different donor age groups: (——), fetal; (— · —), 5–29 years; (— ·· —), 30–49 years; (·······), greater than 50 years. Bovine melanin from 2-year-old animals is included for comparison (– – –). Absorption (optical density) is expressed in arbitrary units (A.U.) (Reproduced courtesy of Vision Research.)

shift toward the red in the fluorescence spectra with increasing age (Boulton et al., 1990).

PIGMENT MIGRATION

The RPE cells of mammals possess orderly arrangements of melanin granules which normally retain a constant position within the cell. By contrast, dramatic movements of melanin granules in response to light are observed in the RPE cells of fish, amphibians, and some birds (Burnside and Laties, 1979). This intracellular migration of pigment in response to light was identified in the frog RPE as early as 1877 (Boll, 1877; Kuhne, 1878) and has subsequently been purported to reduce the bleaching effect of light on rod outer segments by about one-third (Back et al., 1965; Burnside and Laties, 1979). The absence of melanin migration in mammalian RPE is probably due to ocular adaptations, such as prompt iris sphincter and dilator action affecting pupil size which renders rod-outer-segment protection from light (via pigment migration) superfluous (Ali, 1975; Burnside and Laties, 1979). The apical localization of melanin granules in mammalian RPE cells and their movement in fish and amphibians is thought to be achieved through the complex array of actin filaments (Burnside and Laties, 1979; Grierson et al., 1994).

ROLE OF MELANIN IN THE RPE

It has become clear that cellular melanin is not an inert substance. The role of melanin in cellular metabolism, including the protection it affords against light and other agents, reflects its physical and chemical properties (Pathak and Fitzpatrick, 1974; Kolias et al., 1991; Sarna, 1992; Prota, 1992). Melanin (a) acts as a neutral density filter, (b) attenuates the impinging radiation by light scattering when located in the melanosome, (c) absorbs radiant energy in the UV and visible spectrum and dissipates the absorbed energy as heat, (d) has the capacity to bind many chemicals, (e) utilizes absorbed energy to undergo immediate oxidation through the generation of semiquinoid free radicals in the polymer, and (f) as a stable free radical, has a capacity to act as a biological exchange polymer.

Photophysical Properties of RPE Melanin

While the color of the RPE is due to its melanin content, the color of RPE melanin is probably due to the combined effects of repeated absorption and scattering of light within the pigment granule (Kurtz et al., 1986). Hence the size of the pigment granule is at least as important in determining the melanin color as the molecular structure of the melanin polymer itself. Thus the brown or black colour of melanin in the RPE is the result of its broadband optical absorption spectrum and a low yield of fluorescence and phosphoresence emission (Sarna, 1992).

By acting as a neutral density filter and by scattering light, melanin can protect organisms in a variety of ways. The squid uses melanin as a "smoke screen" against predators; vertebrate skin is protected against UV light by epidermal melanin (Szabo, 1975); and melanin filters light in the eye. It is now well accepted that melanin contributes to vision by preventing light reflection in the fundus that may otherwise give rise to spurious signals and by protecting photoreceptor cells from an excess of dispersed light (Garten, 1907; Walls, 1942). The light passing through the vertebrate retina is almost fully absorbed by melanosomes, and defects in RPE melanin result in increased light sensitivity and susceptibility to light damage (Robison et al., 1975; Van Norren and Tiemeijer, 1986).

Melanin granules present in the RPE and the choroid contribute to the absorption of light in the fundus at almost any wavelength studied (Wolbarsht et al., 1981; Boulton et al., 1990; Sarna, 1992). The increase in absorption by melanin (either whole or solubilized granules) from the visible to the UV end of the spectrum is a general feature of both ocular and nonocular melanin (Fig. 4-6) (Gabel et al., 1979; Kollias and Baqer, 1985; 1986; Menon et al., 1983; Wolbarsht et al., 1981; Boulton et al., 1990). Absorption spectra of intact RPE melanin granules in suspension demonstrate a "mask-ing effect," owing to the high individual optical density of each granule (Boulton et al., 1990). RPE melanosomes are associated with a weak fluorescence (Eldred and Katz, 1988; Boulton et al., 1990; Docchio et al., 1991). In general, adult RPE melanin granules exhibit an excitation maximum at 450 nm and emission peaks at 440 and 560 nm, but the position and intensity of these peaks is age dependent, as discussed above. Weak fluorescence has also been reported for dermal melanin (Arico et al., 1983).

The absorption capabilities of RPE melanin confer some protection from chronic light damage, since melanin is an efficient radiation trap that harmlessly dissipates the energy of high-energy photons. However, this process can result in severe tissue damage from acute light exposures. Thus, three different scenarios can emerge for light absorption by melanin (see Mellerio, 1994); (a) protection from the potential phototoxicity caused by high-energy, short-wavelength light (Dillon, 1991; Sarna, 1992), (b) actinic damage (Ham, 1978; 1980; 1984; Marshall, 1985; Mellerio, 1994), and/or (c) thermal damage (Marshall, 1988; Mellerio, 1994). The potential for melanin to confer photoprotection both for epidermal and ocular cells has received considerable attention. Despite extensive studies, the contribution melanin makes toward photoprotection is still unclear, though intracellular melanin appears to play an important role in vitro by preventing UV-induced cell death by reducing DNA damage (Kobayashi et al., 1993). In vivo data are more difficult to assess, and results are often contradictory. The suggestion that RPE melanosomes are photoprotective for the overlying photoreceptor cells is based on studies in rodent species with variable degrees of pigmentation (Lawill et al., 1973; La Vail, 1980; Rapp and Williams, 1980; Ginsberg and La Vail, 1985; Sanyal and Zeilmaker, 1988), in which light damage was consistently greater in photoreceptors overlying nonpigmented RPE cells than photoreceptors overlying pigmented RPE cells. However, it has been argued that the melanosomes of the RPE provide only minimal protection from light damage, and that this role is achieved only by absorption of light and prevention of light reflection back through the receptors (Noell et al., 1966; Rapp and Williams, 1980; Howell et al., 1982). La Vail and Gorrin (1987) exposed mice strains with alternating pigmented and nonpigmented cells of the RPE to various periods of constant fluorescent light. Photoreceptor degeneration was always more severe in the central retina than in the peripheral retina, and it was independent of the pigmentation phenotype of the immediately underlying RPE.

Free-Radical Scavenging Properties of RPE Melanin

An alternative photoprotective role for melanin could be as a free-radical scavenger (Ostrovsky et al., 1987; Sarna, 1992). The environment (light and high oxygen) and composition (high levels of polyunsaturated fatty acids) of the retina make it an ideal environment for free-radical formation (Boulton, 1991). All melanins exhibit electron exchange properties (Sarna and Swartz, 1993), which probably contributes to melanin's antioxidant activity. Thus, synthetic melanin polymers have been shown to be efficient scavengers of free radicals from water radiolysis and quenchers of singlet oxygen (Sarna et al., 1985; Prota, 1992; Sarna, 1992). However, the level of antioxidant activity differs between synthetic and natural melanin (Sarna, 1992). The electron transfer qualities of melanin have been extensively described (see Sarna, 1992; Prota, 1992; Debing et al., 1988; Gan et al., 1974; 1976). A commonly quoted example is the observation that ferricyanide greatly accelerates the melanin-induced oxidation of NADH, owing to coupled reactions between NADH-melanin and melanin-ferricyanide complexes (Debing et al., 1988; Gan et al., 1988). The efficiency of melanin to scavenge hydroxyl radicals generated uniformly depends strongly on the state of the melanin aggregation; in the case of natural melanin from bovine choroid the apparent rate of the interaction is several orders of magnitude lower than with synthetic melanin (Sarna et al., 1986). It has also been established that the percentage of superoxide anion that is reduced by melanin and that is oxidized depends on the type of melanin polymer. Aggregated dopamelanin and insoluble melanin isolated from the choroid of bovine eyes were significantly less reactive with singlet oxygen, generated homogenously, than either soluble dopamelanin or cysteinyldopamelanin (Sarna et al., 1985). Hence, melanin can be viewed as a pseudodismutase (Sarna, 1992). Furthermore, melanins can inhibit peroxidation of lipids in model systems (Ostrovsky et al., 1987; Korytowski et al., 1995). Thus, while RPE melanin has the potential for electron exchange and free-radical scavenging, its antioxidant activity in vivo is likely to be minimal, bearing in mind that the RPE contains high levels of other antioxidants, including superoxide dismutase, glutathione peroxidase, catalase, and α-tocopherol (Boulton et al., 1991; Friedrichson et al., 1995).

Free Radical Generating Properties of RPE Melanin

Melanins, both in vivo and in vitro, exhibit relatively high concentrations of free-radical centers (Sealy, 1984), which makes the material weakly paramagnetic. The resultant paramagnetic centers probably reflect intrinsic melanin radicals that were generated during polymer formation and trapped within the growing polymer (see Sarna, 1992). Electron paramagnetic resonance spectroscopy allows the nondestructive analysis and differentiation of natural melanins with high sensitivity and accuracy (Sealy et al., 1982; Pilas and Sarna, 1985) by generating characteristic EPR spectra (Sarna et al., 1992). A typical human RPE EPR spectrum is shown in Figure 4-7. The spectrum is characteristic of eumelanin with the X-band showing a single line of width 0.4–0.6 mT with g factor close to 2.004. While melanin free-radical centers are relatively stable, owing to restricted access to extrinsic agents, light is able to induce transient melanin free-radical generation. Irradiation of melanin with either UV or visible light (a) causes an increase in free-radical content, (b) promotes oxygen consumption under aerobic conditions, (c) results in the formation of superoxide anions, hydrogen peroxide, and hydroxyl radicals (Felix et al., 1978; Crippa and Mazzini, 1983), and (d) oxidation of ascorbate (Rozanowska et al., 1997). The action spectrum from oxygen consumption is closely related to that for free-radical production. Thus, the free-radical potential of melanin reflects both intrinsic melanin radicals trapped within the polymer and extrinsic melanin radicals generated via the intramolecular redox potential of the polymer.

The light-induced generation of superoxide and hydrogen peroxide by melanin (Felix et al., 1978; Crippa and Mazzini, 1983) may have a cytotoxic potential, and some authors suggest that this process may intensify the damaging effect of illumination on RPE and retina (Ham et al., 1978; 1980). The light damage first described by Ham and colleagues is held to originate in the RPE and appears to correlate with relatively higher retinal irradiances delivered over short time spans (seconds to minutes) (Marshall, 1987). Ham measured the action spectra of the damage and showed that its sensitivity increased with reducing wavelength of light. Consequently this type of damage became known as "blue-light damage." Melanin has been suggested as the chromophore responsible, with the ensuing cytotoxicity occurring via photochemical or "actinic" responses generated by melanin within the RPE. Histological changes in the melanin of such light-damaged RPE cells include irregular clumping and a decrease in melanin granules (probably via autophagocytosis). However, evidence is now accumulating to refute a direct role for melanin in such photochemical-based retinal light damage. Mellerio (1994) reports that the blue-light-damage action spectrum neither matches the melanin action spectrum

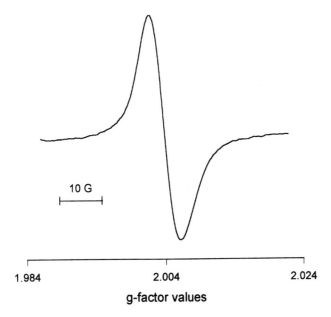

10 G
├───────┤

| 1.984 | 2.004 | 2.024 |

g-factor values

FIGURE 4-7. EPR signal of human RPE melanosomes isolated from donors 60–70 years old. Experimental conditions: temperature, 70 °K; microwave power, 0.063 mW; modulation amplitude, 2.603 G; time constant, 2.62 s; sweep time, 167.77 s; spectrum averaged 5 times. (Figure kindly provided by Professor T. Sarna, Jagiellonian University, Poland.)

for uptake of oxygen nor the absorption spectrum for melanin solution. Furthermore, Putting and colleagues (1993; 1994) reported a significant increase in the permeability of the blood retinal barrier after exposure to light at 418 nm but not at 408 nm (this does not correlate with the increase in light absorption by melanin from the visible to the UV end of the spectrum). Although dispersion and clumping of melanin granules was observed, the action spectra for permeability changes in the blood retinal barrier did not support a melanin-mediated toxicity for the RPE. Alternative chromophores in the RPE that might be responsible for light-induced blood-retinal barrier dysfunction are (a) lipofuscin and/or (b) mitochondrial respiratory enzymes such as cytochrome c oxidase. Recent evidence suggests that lipofuscin is the most potent photosensitizer in human RPE and is more likely to be responsible for the resultant blue-light damage than melanin (Rozanowska et al., 1995). Illumination of human retinal pigment epithelial cells induced both a wavelength- and age-dependent uptake of oxygen, which was primarily due to the presence of lipofuscin. Furthermore, lipofuscin proves (a) to be a photoinducible generator of several oxygen-reactive species, including singlet oxygen, superoxide anion, and H_2O_2 (Boulton et al., 1993; Rozanowska et al., 1995) and (b) to enhance lipid per-

oxidation (Rozanowska et al., 1995). The observation that oxygen uptake by lipofuscin was an order of magnitude greater than RPE melanin implies that lipofuscin is likely to make a far greater contribution to light damage than melanin, at least in older eyes.

RPE Melanin and Thermal Damage

If RPE cells receive relatively short exposures of high-energy light, as is seen with argon and krypton laser treatment of the retina, they will undergo thermal damage or photocoagulation (Marshall, 1988). Thermal effects can occur if incident energy is trapped or absorbed in the substrate molecules (Mellerio, 1994). This absorption is easily measured, and it is generally expected that the absorption value of a substrate will provide an indication of what increase in temperature might result. A sufficient increase in melanin granule temperature (usually quoted as >10 °C) will result in either (a) a zone of denaturation around the granule that would spread with the conduction of heat away from the granule source of (b) the generation of steam at the granule cytoplasm interface if the energy influx is great enough (Hansen and Fine, 1968). The heat would lead first to thermal coagulative damage and then to steam and physical disruptive damage. Hayes and Wolbarsht (1968) pointed out that there would be considerable amplification of lesion size (more than a thousand times) once steam was formed (which could account for the large area of outer retinal damage which occurs following laser photocoagulation), and that further amplification would come from the ensuing biologic effects of inflammatory processes.

Chemical Binding Properties of RPE Melanin

Melanin has the capacity to bind and accumulate many chemicals (Lindquist, 1973; Koneru et al., 1986; Persad et al., 1986; Larsson, 1993). Pigmented cells contain high amounts of calcium, reflecting the enormous calcium-binding capacity of melanin (Drager, 1985; Drager and Balkema, 1987). No tissue in the entire body of the embryo or adult exceeds the calcium binding capacity of pigmented tissues. For instance bone, whose calcium concentration is one thousand times that of pigmented tissues, has a rather low binding capacity; calcium is not bound but is deposited in mineral form (Drager and Balkema, 1987). Binding of chemicals to melanin covers a broad range of affinities; there are relatively fewer high-affinity sites, with a Kd in the low micromolar range (5–10 μM or lower) but many more sites with lower binding affinity. Such binding properties could potentially make melanin an effective calcium buffer over a broad range of concentrations. The binding is pH dependent, and the high-affinity binding sites are relatively selective for calcium over magnesium, but heavy metals compete effectively for the same sites (Drager and Balkema, 1987). The high-affinity binding is not influenced by light or by cyclic compounds like chloroquine. The total calcium concentration is melanosomes is about six times higher than the cytoplasm-free concentration. This binding may have significant implications in development and homeostasis by modulating the coupling/uncoupling of gap junctions.

Melanin-containing cells may be protected from oxidative damage by melanin binding of oxidative catalytic metal ions, which are thus removed from the biochemical arena of the cell. Sarna (1992) concluded that melanin would not normally release free radicals in vivo, notwithstanding such observations having been made in vitro. With aging, the constant exposure of RPE cells to high oxygen levels from the choroid and the decades of daily exposure to light might diminish the antioxidant properties of melanin and allow its pro-oxidative proclivities to gain the upper hand, so inducing the damage we know as age-related macular degeneration. Sarna's conclusion would seem to support the doubts that melanin is the chromophore that initiates "Ham-type" or "blue-light" damage in the retina. However, it is conceivable that the redox activity of melanin could lead to adverse effects. This may happen if melanin reduces, and thus activates, ferric or cupric ions that are present in the melanotic system (Zareba et al., 1995).

If melanin is able to influence, by whatever mechanism, the concentration of rare compounds that are toxic to hair cells (Drager and Balkema, 1987), it may have a similar effect on endogenous compounds which are regularly present and which are of benefit to the sensory receptor cells. Candidates for such endogenous compounds with high melanin affinity are the biogenic amines and calcium.

ROLE OF MELANIN IN OCULAR DISEASE

Ocular disorders associated with melanin can be subdivided into two groups, genetic and oculotoxic.

Genetic

Albinism is a heterogeneous group of genetic disorders characterized by a congenital reduction or absence of melanin synthesis in association with specific ocular changes resulting from hypopigmentation in the developing eye (Oetting and King, 1994; Spritz, 1993; 1994). In oculocutaneous albinism (OCA), pigment is reduced or absent in the skin, hair, and eyes, whereas in ocular albinism (OA), eye involvement is accompanied by relatively normal pigmentation of the skin and hair. If melanin levels are below a critical level there is aberrant neuronal migration in the visual pathways, lack of foveal development, low vision, nystagmus, and strabismus. In general, the severity of the visual defect correlates with the severity of the pigmentation deficit in the eye (Spritz, 1994).

OCA can be subdivided into two types: OCA1 (tyrosinase-deficient OCA) and OCA2 (tyrosinase-positive OCA) (Oetting and King, 1994; Spritz, 1994). OCA1 is an autosomal recessive disorder which results from absence or reduced activity of tyrosinase, an essential enzyme in melanogenesis, as has been discussed in detail above. The human tyrosinase gene is located within chromosome segment 11q14–q21 (Barton et al., 1988) and consists of five exons spanning more than 50 kb of genomic DNA (Giebel et al., 1991). Tyrosinase is initially translated as a 529 amino acid–precursor polypeptide that is cleaved to generate the mature tyrosinase protein. Analysis of the tyrosinase gene in individuals with OCA1 has revealed a large number of mutations; most are single-base substitutions that produce a corresponding amino acid substitution in the protein (Oetting and King, 1994). Missense mutations cluster into four regions of the tyrosinase gene, and it is thought that these clusters represent important functional regions of tyrosinase; two of these regions are the copper-binding sites of this copper-containing enzyme (Oetting and King, 1994). OCA2 is an autosomal recessive disorder with less severe visual defects than those observed in OCA1. The gene responsible for OCA2 has been identified as the human homologue to the mouse pink-eyed dilution (p) gene (Rinchik et al., 1993). The human p gene is located in chromosome segment 15q11–q13 (Ramsay et al., 1992). It has been postulated that the function of the p locus product may be as a tyrosine transporter, but further studies are necessary to confirm the true function of this protein (Oetting and King, 1994).

Described in the literature (Park et al., 1992) have been at least five types of OA, which can be either X-linked recessive (and associated with macromelanosomes) or autosomal recessive (Oetting and King, 1994). The ophthalmic manifestations of OA are similar to but less severe than those in OCA. The gene responsible for OA type 1 is exclusively expressed in pigment cells and encodes a protein of 404 amino acids. This protein appears to be a membrane glycoprotein localized to melanosomes (Schiaffino et al., 1996).

Oculotoxic

Melanin has the capacity to bind and accumulate many chemicals and drugs which can result in chronic lesions affecting pigmented tissues (Lindquist, 1973; Koneru et al., 1986; Persad et al., 1986; Larsson, 1993). Melanins are polyanions with a relatively high content of negatively charged carboxyl groups and o-semiquinones (Prota, 1992). This means that they have an affinity for substances with cationic properties (e.g. amines and metals) which bind by ionic interaction (Larsson and Tjalve, 17778; 1979). The binding of amines can be further enhanced by van der Waal's attractions (Larsson, 1993). Binding can also occur through charge-transfer interactions with electron-donating substances (e.g. chlorpromazine) (Larsson and Tjalve, 1979), as well as through hydrophobic interactions in some instances (Stepien and Wilczok, 1982; Larsson et al., 1988). Thus, melanin-binding is complex and will often involve more than one binding class for an individual substance.

Most studies on melanin binding have been undertaken in vitro and have used either synthetic melanin or solubilized, partially solubilized, or intact melanin granules. While these provide a useful substrate for melanin binding, they often fail to mimic melanin binding in vivo or the potential cellular toxicity (Larsson, 1993). Nevertheless, it is clear that drugs such as chlorpromazine and chloroquine can bind irreversibly to melanin (Larsson and Tjalve, 1979) and that such binding is via multiple binding sites. Incubation of native human RPE melanin granules with varying concentrations of either chlorpromazine or chloroquine reveals at least two classes of binding site (Dayhaw-Barker et al., 1988)—high affinity sites and low affinity sites. At saturation of all binding sites, the total binding capacity was found to be 0.1 mg and 3 mg per gram of melanin granules for higher- and lower-affinity binding sites respectively for chlorpromazine, and 6 mg and 20 mg respectively for chloroquine. Whole-body autoradiographic examinations of mice receiving radio-labeled chlorpromazine (^{35}S) and chloroquine (^{14}C) demonstrated that radioactivity was selectively concentrated in pigmented tissues (Lindquist and Ullberg, 1972). A high concentration of radioactivity from both drugs was observed in the eye for up to 90 days and 1 year for chlorpromazine and chloroquine, respectively. A similar distribution profile was observed following administration of a ^{125}I-labeled chloroquine analogue to a macaca monkey (Denker et al., 1975). Melanin is also able to bind photosensitizers such as 8-methoxypsoralen and protoporphyrin (Persad et al., 1986).

As discussed in the previous section, a variety of metals, including transition metals (e.g. zinc, copper, calcium, manganese, molybdenum, and iron [Ulshafer et al., 1990; Samuelson et al., 1993]) are found in melanin granules and may reflect accumulation from chronic exposure throughout life (Sarna, 1992; Larsson et al., 1993). Metal binding is dependent on the pH and the metal ion concentration (Sarna et al., 1980; Froncisz et al., 1980) with the metal-melanin complexes generated involving different functional groups of the polymer and showing different stabilities. Bound metal ions can be replaced by other cations if they have a greater binding affinity for melanin or are present in sufficiently high concentrations (Sarna et al., 1976). However, some ions (e.g. copper, iron, and magnesium) may not be amenable to displacement either by prolonged acid treatment or by exposure to strong chelators (Sarna et al., 1980).

The importance of melanin binding is unclear; it is considered by some to confer tissue protection and by others to contribute to tissue toxicity. It has been suggested that tissue homeostasis may be augmented by the local regulation of endogenous cations via melanin binding (see Drager and Balkema, 1987). Furthermore, melanin may act to mop up potentially harmful substances; in the RPE melanin is located in close proximity to the photoreceptor cells and may act as a filter for nutrients and toxic compounds emanating from the choriocapillaries (see Sarna, 1992). However, under certain circumstances this "protective mechanism" may be detrimental to RPE cell function and result in cell toxicity. Chronic exposure to toxic substances with an affinity for melanin (e.g. phenothiazine derivatives and chloroquine) can result in histological lesions in pigment cells or in adjacent tissues (photoreceptors) (Larsson and Tjalve, 1979; Ings, 1984; Koneru et al., 1986; Persad et al., 1988). The chorioretinopathy which results from long-term exposure to chloroquine may be the result of either inhibition of protein synthesis (Roskoski and Jaskunas, 1972) or lysosomal enzyme activity (Homewood et al., 1972). Thus, the presence of melanin is not always beneficial; the phenomenon of drug binding to melanin is a case in point, whereby cellular melanin leads to cytotoxicity and visual loss.

ROLE OF MELANIN IN RETINAL DEVELOPMENT

Interestingly, there is evidence from albino mammals to support a role for melanin, or an affiliated agent, in the regulation and maturation of the retina (Stone et al., 1978; Jeffrey et al., 1994a). The central retina is underdeveloped in each of the nuclear layers and the many ganglion cells in the temporal retina, which should not cross in the optic chiasm, instead project contralaterally (Guillery, 1986). Furthermore, in human and other primate albinos the fovea fails to develop (Kinnear et al., 1985), though Jeffrey and colleagues (1994a) reported that the reduction in outer retinal cellularity was exclusive to rod photoreceptors and that the number and distribution of cones was not affected. It has been hypothesized that these abnormalities are related to the paucity of melanin, since introduction of a functional tyrosinase gene into albino mice corrects the abnormal retinal pathways associated with albinism (Jeffrey et al., 1994b). However, the mechanism by which RPE melanin, or the genes involved in its synthesis, regulates the development of the neural retina remains to be elucidated, but may involve modulation of the cell cycle in the developing neural retina (Ilia and Jeffrey, 1996).

SUMMARY

This chapter has attempted to review current knowledge of melanin and its contribution to retinal pathophysiology. The precise role for melanin in the retina is still open to considerable debate. It is currently thought that RPE melanin (a) contributes to visual acuity by preventing light reflection from the fundus that may otherwise give rise to spurious signals, though its role in photoprotection is unclear; (b) may confer little protection against light damage; (c) is a weak free-radical scavenger which probably offers little protection against oxidative damage in vivo; (d) is probably not the principal chromophore in blue-light damage to the retina; (e) is the main point of light absorption and temperature dissipation in the generation of thermal damage; (f) plays a possible cytotoxic role in retinal damage (Sarna, 1992); and (g) may act as a filter or detoxicant for toxic drugs and metals—however, the "filter hypothesis" is difficult to accept given the poor self-purifying capacity of melanin. Furthermore, RPE melanin or components involved in its synthesis (i.e. tyrosinase) may control aspects of retinal development. It is evident that we have made major advances in developing a greater understanding of melanin since the publication of the first edition of *The Retinal Pigment Epithelium* (Zinn and Marmor, 1979). However, it is equally clear that there is still much to learn about the properties of melanin, which will hopefully be covered in the next volume.

REFERENCES

Abe T, Durlu Y, Tamai M. 1996. The properties of retinal pigment epithelial cells in proliferative vitreoretinopathy compared with cultured retinal pigment epithelial cells. Exp Eye Res. 63:201–210.

Ali MA. 1975. Retinomotor responses. In: Ali MA, ed, Vision and Fishes, Series A. NATO Advanced Study Institute, 313–355.

Arico M, Barcellona M, Gianmarinaro MS, Micciancio S. 1983. Time-resolved spectrofluorimetry of melanin in human melanoma. In: Martelluci S, Chester AN, eds, Laser Photobiology and Photomedicine. New York: Plenum Press, 101–106.

Back I, Donner KO, Reuter T. 1965. The screening effect of the retinal pigment epithelium on the retinal rods in the frog. Vision Res 5:101–111.

Barton DE, Kwon BS, Francke U. 1988. Human tyrosinase gene, mapped to chromosome 11(q14–q21), defines second region of homology with mouse chromosome 7. Genomics 3:17–24.

Bernd A, Ramirez-Bosca A, Kippenberger S, Martinez-Liarte JH, Holzmann H, Solano F. 1994. Levels of dopachrome tautomerase in human melanocytes cultured in vitro. Melanoma Res 4:287–291.

Boissy RE. 1988. The melanocyte: its structure, function, and subpopulations in skin, eyes and hair. Dermatologic Clinics 6:161–173.

Boll F. 1877. Zur anatomie und physiologie der retina. Arch Anat Physiol 4:783–787.

Boulton ME. 1991. Ageing of the retinal pigment epithelium. In: Osborne NN, Chader GJ, eds, Progress in Retinal Research, vol 11. Oxford: Pergamon Press, 125–151.

Boulton ME, Marshall J, Mellerio J. 1982. Human retinal pigment epithelial cells in culture: a means of studying inherited retinal disease. In: Cotlier E, Maumanee IH, Berman ER, eds, Genetic Eye Diseases: Retinitis Pigmentosa and Other Inherited Eye Disorders. New York: Liss, 101–118.

Boulton ME, Docchio F, Dayhaw-Barker P, Ramponi R, Cubeddu R. 1990. Age-related changes in the morphology, absorption and fluorescence of melanosomes and lipofuscin granules of the retinal pigment epithelium. Vison Res 30:1291–1303.

Boulton M, Dontsov A, Jarvis-Evans J, Ostrovsky M, Svistunencko D. 1993. Lipofuscin is a photoinducible free radical generator. J Photochem Photobiol B 19:201–204.

Braekevelt CR. 1989a. Fine structure of the retinal pigment epithelium and tapetum lucidum of the ranch mink Mustela vision. Acta Anat 135:296–302.

Braekevelt CR. 1989b. Fine structure of the bovine tapetum fibrosum. Anat Histol Embryol 15:215–222.

Burchill SA, Virden R, Thody AJ. 1984. Regulation of tyrosine synthesis and its processing in the hair follicular melanocytes of the mouse during eumelanogenesis and pheomelanogenesis. J Invest Dermatol 93:235–240.

Burns RP, Feeney-Burns L. 1980. Clinico-morphologic correlations of drusen of Bruch's membrane. Tr Am J Ophthalmol Soc 78: 206–211.

Burnside B, Laties AM. Pigment movement and cellular contractility in the retinal pigment epithelium. In: Zinn K, Marmor MF, eds, The Retinal Pigment Epithelium. Cambridge, MA, and London: Harvard University Press, 175–191.

Campochiaro PA, Hachett SF. 1993. Corneal endothelial cell matrix promotes expression of differentiated features of retinal pigment epithelial cells: implications of laminin and basic fibroblast growth factor as active components. Exp Eye Res 57:539–547.

Chakraborty AK, Mishima Y, Inazu M, Hatta S, Ichihashi M. 1989. Melanogenic regulatory factors in coated vesicles from melanoma cells. J Invest Dermatol 93:616–620.

Crippa PR, Mazzini A. 1983. Involvement of superoxide anions in the oxidation of NADH by melanins. Physiol Chem Phys Med NMR 15:51–56.

Dayhaw-Barker P, Unger W, Bouma E, Boulton ME. 1988. Binding characteristics of drugs to melanin granules from human RPE. Invest Ophthalmol Vis Sci 29(Suppl):285.

Debing AP, Ijzerman AP, Vanguelin G. 1988. Melanosome binding and oxidation-reduction properties of synthetic L-dopa-melanin as in vitro tests for drug toxicity. Mel Pharmacol 33:470–476.

Denker L, Lindquist NG, Ullberg S. 1975. Distribution of ^{125}I-labelled chloroquine analogue in a pregnant macaca monkey. Toxicology 5:255–265.

Dillon J. 1991. Photophysics and photobiology of the eye. J Photochem Photobiol B 10:23–40.

Docchio F, Boulton M, Cubeddu R, Ramponi R, Dayhaw-Barker P. 1991. Age-related changes in the fluorescence of melanin and lipofuscin granules of the retinal pigment epithelium: a time resolved fluorescence spectroscopy study. Photochem Photobiol 54:247–253.

Dorey CK, Torres X, Swart T. 1990. Evidence of melanogenesis in porcine retinal pigment epithelial cells in vitro. Exp Eye Res 50:1–10.

Drager UC. 1985. Calcium binding in pigmented and albino eyes. Proc Nat Acad Sci USA 82:6716–6720.

Drager UC, Balkema GW. 1987. Does melanin do more than protect from light? Neurosci Res Suppl 6:S75–S86.

Dryja PP, O'Neil-Dryja M, Pawelek JM, Albert DM. 1978. Demonstration of tyrosine activity in the adult bovine uveal tract and retinal pigment epithelium. Invest Ophthalmol Vis Sci 17:511–514.

Dryja PP, O'Neil-Dryja M, Albert DM. 1979. Elemental analysis of melanins from bovine hair, iris, choroid and retinal pigment epithelium. Invest Ophthalmol Vis Sci 18:231–236.

Duncker HR. 1985. The neural crest. In: Bagnara JT, Klaus S, Paul E, Schartl M, eds, Pigment Cell 1985: Biological, Molecular and Clinical Aspects, vol 7. Tokyo: University of Tokyo Press, 255–269.

Eldred GE, Katz ML. 1988. Fluorophores of the human retinal pigment epithelium: separation and spectral characteristics. Exp Eye Res 47:71–86.

Feeney L. 1978. Lipofuscin and melanin of human retinal pigment epithelium: fluorescence, enzyme cytochemical and ultrastructural studies. Invest Ophthalmol Vis Sci 17:583–600.

Feeney-Burns L. 1980. The pigments of the RPE. In: Zudanaisky JA, Davson H, eds, Current Topics in Eye Research. New York: Academic Press, 119–178.

Feeney-Burns L, Hilderbrand ES, Eldridge S. 1984. Aging human RPE: morphometric analysis of macular, equatorial and peripheral cells. Invest Ophthalmol Vis Sci 25:195–200.

Feeney-Burns L, Burns RP, Gao CL. 1990. Age-related macular changes in humans over 90 years old. Am J Ophthalmol 109:265–278.

Felik CC, Hyde JS, Sarna T, Sealy RC. 1978. Melanin photoreactions in aerated media: electron spin resonance evidence for production of superoxide and hydrogen peroxide. Biochem Biophys Res Comm 84:335–341.

Flood M, Gouras P. 1981. The organisation of retinal pigment epithelium in vitro. Vision Res 21:119–126.

Friedrichson T, Kalbach H, Buck P, van Kujik F. 1995. Vitamin E in macular and peripheral tissues of the eye. Curr Eye Res 14:693–701.

Froncisz W, Sarna T, Hyde JS. 1980. Cu^{2+} probe of metal-ion binding sites in melanin using electron paramagnetic resonance spectroscopy. I. Synthetic melanins. Arch Biochem Biophys 202:289–303.

Gabel V-P, Birngruber R, Hillenkamp F. 1979. Visible and near infrared light absorption in pigment epithelium and choroid. Excerpta Medica Int Congress Series 450:658–662.

Gan EV, Haberman HF, Menon IA. 1974. Oxidation of NADH by melanin and melanoproteins. Biochem Biophys Acta 370:62–69.

Gan EV, Haberman HF, Menon IA. 1976. Electron transfer properties of melanin. Arch Biochem Biophys 173:666–672.

Garcia RI, Szabo G, Fitzpatrick TB. 1979. Molecular and cell biology of melanin. In: Zinn K, Marmor MF, eds, The Retinal Pigment Epithelium. Cambridge, MA, and London: Harvard University Press, 124–147.

Garten S. Die veranderungen der netzhaut durch licht. Graefe-Saemish Handbuch Gesamten Augenheilkunde (Leipzig). 2:250–280.

Giebel LB, Spritz RA. 1992. The molecular basis of type I (tyrosinase deficient) human oculocutaneous albinism. Pigment Cell Res Suppl 2:101–106.

Ginsberg HM, LaVail MM. 1985. Light-induced retinal degeneration in the mouse: analysis of pigmentation mutants. In: LaVail MM, Hollyfield JG, Anderson RE, eds, Retinal Degeneration: Experimental and Clinical Studies. New York: Liss, 449–469.

Gornitz K. 1923. Versuch einer klassifikation der haufigsten Federfarbuger. Jahrb f Ornithol. 71:127–131.

Grierson I, Hiscott P, Hogg P, Robey H, Mazure A, Larkin G. 1994. Development, repair and regeneration of the retinal pigment epithelium. Eye 8:252–262.

Guillery RW. 1986. Neural abnormalities of albinos. Trends Neurosci 9:364–367.

Ham WT, Ruffolo JJ, Mueller HA, Clarke AM, Moon ME. 1978. Histologic analysis of photochemical lesion produced in rhesus retina by short wavelength light. Invest Ophthalmol Vis Sci 17:1029–1035.

Ham WT, Ruffolo JJ, Mueller HA, Guerry D. 1980. The nature of retina radiation damage as a function of wavelength, power level and exposure time. Vision Res 20:1105–1111.

Ham WT, Mueller HA, Ruffolo JJ, Millen JE, Cleary SF, Guerry RK, Guerry D 3rd. 1984. Basic mechanism underlying production of photochemical lesion in the mammalian retina. Curr Eye Res 3:165–174.

Hansen WP, Fine S. 1968. Melanin granule models for pulsed laser induced retinal injury. Appl Opt 7:155–167.

Hayes JR, Wolbarsht ML. 1968. Thermal model for retinal damage induced by pulsed lasers. Aerospace Med 39:474–480.

Hearing VJ, Jimenez M. 1987. Mammalian tyrosinase—the critical regulatory point in melanocyte pigmentation. Int J Biochem 19:1141–1147.

Hearing VJ, Philips P, Lutzner MA. 1973. The fine structure of melanogenesis in coat colour mutants of the mouse. J Ultrastruct Res 43:88–106.

Hogan MJ, Alvarado JA, Weddell JE. 1971. Histology of the Human Eye. Philadelphia: Saunders.

Holbrook KA, Vogel AM, Underwood RA, Foster CA. 1988. Melanocytes in human embryonic and fetal skin: a review and new finding. Pigment Cell Res 1S:6–17.

Homewood CA, Warhurst DC, Peters W, Baggaley VC. 1972. Lysosomes, pH and the antimalarial action of chloroquine. Nature 235:50–52.

Howell WL, Rapp M, William T. 1982. Distribution of melanosomes across the retinal pigment epithelium of the hooded rat: implications for light damage. Invest Ophthalmol Vis Sci 22:139–144.

Ilia M, Jeffrey G. 1996. Delayed neurogenesis in the albino retina: Evidence for a role for melanin in regulating the pace of cell generation. Brain Res Dev Brain Res 95:176–183.

Imokawa G, Mishima Y. 1984. Functional analysis of tyrosinase isoenzymes of cultured malignant melanoma cells during the recovery period following interrupted melanogenesis induced by glycosylation inhibitors. J Invest Dermatol 83:196–201.

Inazu M, Mishima Y. 1993. Detection of eumelanogenic and pheomelanogenic melanosomes in the same normal human melanocyte. J Invest Dermatol 100:172S–175S.

Ings RM. 1984. The melanin binding of drugs and its implications. Drug Metabol Rev 15:1183–1212.

Jackson IJ, Chambers DM, Tsukamoto K, Copeland NG, Gilbert DJ, Jenkins NA, Hearing VJ. 1992. A second tyrosinase-related protein TRP-2, maps to and is mutated at the mouse slaty locus. EMBO J 11:527–535.

Jeffrey G, Darling K, Whitmore A. 1994a. Melanin and regulation of mammalian photoreceptor topography. Eur J Neurosci 6:657–667.

Jeffrey G, Schutz G, Montoliu L. 1994b. Correction of abnormal retinal pathways found with albinism with the introduction of a functional tyrosinase gene in transgenic mice. Developmental Biol 166:460–464.

Jimbo K, Hara H, Vinayagamoorthy T, Luo D, Dakour J, Yamada K, Dixon W, Che H. 1994. Molecular control of melanogenesis in malignant melanoma: functional assessment of tyrosinase and lamp gene families by UV exposure and gene co-transfection, cloning of a cDNA encoding clanexin, a possible melanogenesis "chaperone." J Dermatol 21:894–906.

Kinnear PE, Jay B, Witkop CJ. 1985. Albinism. Surv Ophthalmol 30:75–101.

Kollias N, Baqer A. 1985. Spectroscopic characteristics of human melanin in vivo. J Invest Dermatol 85:38–42.

Kollias N, Baqer A. 1986. On the assessment of melanin in human skin in vivo. Photochem Photobiol 43:49–54.

Kollias N, Sayre RM, Zeise L, Chedekel MR. 1991. Photoprotection by melanin. J Photochem Photobiol B 9:135–160.

Koneru PB, Lien EJ, Koda RT. 1986. Review: oculotoxicities of systemically administered drugs. J Ocular Pharmacol 2:385–404.

Korytowski W, Pilas B, Sarna T, Kalyanaraman B. 1987. Photoinduced generation of hydrogen peroxide and hydroxyl radicals in melanins. J Photochem Photobiol 45:185–190.

Korytowski W, Sarna T, Zareba M. 1995. Antioxidant action of neuromelanin: the mechanism of inhibitory effect on lipid peroxidation. Arch Biochem Biophys 319:142–148.

Kobayashi N, Muramatsu T, Yamashina Y, Shirai T, Onishi T, Mori T. 1993. Melanin reduces ultraviolet-induced DNA damage formation and killing rate in cultured human melanoma cells. J Invest Dermatol 101:685–689.

Kuhne W. 1878. Fortgesetzte untersuchungen uber die retina und die pigmente des auges. Untersuch Physiol Inst Univ Heidelberg 2:89.

Kurtz SK, Kozikowski SD, Wolfram LJ. 1986. Nonlinear optical and electro-optical properties of biopolymers. In: Gunter P, ed, Proceedings of the International School of Material Science and Technology, Erice. Berlin: Springer, 110–130.

Larsson B, Tjalve H. 1978. Studies on the melanin affinity of metal ions. Physiol Scand 104:479–484.

Larsson B, Tjalve H. 1979. Studies on the mechanism of drug binding to melanin. Biochem Pharmacol 28:1181–1187.

Larsson P, Larsson B, Tjalve H. 1988. Binding of aflatoxinB$_1$ to melanin. Fd Chem Toxicol 26:579–586.

Larsson BS. 1993. Interaction between chemicals and melanin. Pigment Cell Res 6:127–133.

LaVail MM. 1980. Eye pigmentation and constant light damage in the rat retina. In: Williams TP, Baker BN, eds, The Effect of Constant Light on Visual Processes. New York: Plenum Press, 357–387.

LaVail MM, Gorrin GM. 1987. Protection from light damage by ocular pigmentation: analysis using experimental chimeras and translocation mice. Exp Eye Res 44:877–889.

Lawill T. 1973. Effects of prolonged exposure of rabbit retina to low intensity light. Invest Ophthalmol Vis Sci 12:45–51.

Lindquist NG. 1973. Accumulation of drugs in melanin. Acta Radiol (Stockh) 325:1–92.

Lindquist NG, Ullberg S. 1972. The melanin affinity of chloroquine and chlorpromazine studied by whole body autoradiography. Acta Pharmacol Toxicol 32(Suppl 2):1–32.

Mann I. 1969. The Development of the Human Eye. London: BMA.

Marshall J. 1985. Radiation and the ageing eye. Ophthal Physiol Opt 5:241–263.

Marshall J. 1987. The ageing retina: physiology or pathology. Eye 1:282–295.

Marshall J. 1988. Lasers in ophthalmology: the basic principles. 2(suppl):S98–S112.

Mellerio J. 1994. Light effects on the retina. In: Albert DM, Jakobiec FA, eds, Principles and Practice of Ophthalmology: Basic Sciences. Philadelphia: Saunders, 1326–1345.

Menon IA, Persad S, Haberman HF, Kurian CJ, Basu PK. 1981. Do the melanins from blue and brown human eyes differ? In: Seiji M, ed, Proceedings 11th International Pigment Cell Conference, Sendai. Tokyo: University of Tokyo Press, 17–22.

Menon IA, Persad S, Haberman HF, Kurian CJ. 1983. A comparative study of the physical and chemical properties of melanins isolated from human black and red hair. J Invest Dermatol 80:203–206.

Mintz B. 1967. Gene control of mammalian pigmentary differentiation. I. Clonal origin of melanocytes. Proc Nat Acad Sci USA. 58:344–351.

Mishima Y. 1992. A post melanosomal era: control of melanogenesis and melanoma growth. Pigment Cell Res Suppl 2:3–16.

Mishima Y, Imokawa G. 1985. Role of glycosylation in initial melanogenesis: post inhibition dynamics. In: Bagnara J, Klaus SN, Paul E, Scharl M, eds, Pigment Cell 1985: Biological and Molecular Aspects of Pigmentation. Tokyo: University of Tokyo Press, 17–30.

Mishima Y, Imokawa G, Ogura R. 1979. Functional three-dimensional differentiation of smooth membrane structure in melanogenesis. In: Klaus SN, ed, Pigment Cell: Biological Basis of Pigmentation, vol 4. Basel: Karger, 277–290.

Nicolaus RA. Melanins. Paris: Hermann, 1968.

Noell WK, Walker VS, Kang BS, Berman S. 1966. Retinal damage by light in rats. Invest Ophthalmol Vis Sci 5:450–473.

Nordlund JJ, Abel-Malek ZA, Boissy RE, Rheins LA. 1989. Pigment cell biology: an historical review. J Invest Dermatol 92:53S–60S.

Novikoff AB, Neuenberger PM, Novikoff PM, Quintana N. 1979. Retinal pigment epithelium. Interrelationships of endoplasmic reticulum and melanolysosomes in the black mouse and its beige mutant. Lab Invest 40:155–165.

Oetting WS, King RA. 1994. Molecular basis of oculocutaneous albinism. J Invest Dermatol 103:131S–136S.

Ostrovsky M, Sakina NL, Dontsov AE. 1987. An antioxidative role of ocular screening pigments. Vision Res 27:893–899.

Park S, Albert DM, Bolognia JL. 1992. Ocular manifestations of pigmentary disorders. Dermatologic Clinics 10:609–622.

Pathak MA, Fitzpatrick TB. 1974. The role of natural protective agents in human skin. In: Fitzpatrick TB, Pathak MA, Harber LC, Seiji M, Kukita A, eds, Sunlight and Man: Normal and Abnormal Photobiologic Responses. Tokyo: University of Tokyo Press, 725–750.

Pawelek J, Korner A, Bergstrom A, Bologna J. 1980. New regulators of melanin biosynthesis and the autodestruction of melanoma cells. Nature 286:617–619.

Persad S, Menon IA, Basu PK, Haberman HF. 1986. Binding of imipramine, 8-methoxypsoralen, and epinephrine to human blue and brown eye melanins. J Toxicol Cutaneous Toxicol 5:125–132.

Pilas B, Sarna T. 1985. Quantitative determination of melanin in pigmented cells by electron spin resonance. In: Bagnara J, Klaus SN, Paul E, Smartl M, eds, Proceedings 12th International Pigment Cell Conference, Giessen. Tokyo: University of Tokyo Press, 97–103.

Prota G. 1980. Recent advances in the chemistry of melanogenesis in mammals. J Invest Dermatol 75:122–127.

Prota G. 1988. Some new aspects of eumelanin chemistry. In: Advances in Pigment Cell Research. New York: Liss, 101–124.

Prota G. 1992. Melanins and Melanogenesis. San Diego, London: Academic Press.

Putting BJ, van Best JA, Zweypfennig R, Vrensen G, Oosterhuis JA. 1993. Spectral sensitivity of the blood-retinal barrier at the retinal pigment epithelium for blue light in the 400–500nm range. Graefes Arch Clin Exp Ophthalmol 231:600–606.

Putting BJ, van Best JA, Vrensen G, Oosterhuis JA. 1994. Blue light-induced dysfunction of the blood retinal barrier at the pigment epithelium in albino versus pigmented rabbits. Exp Eye Res 58:31–40.

Quevedo WC, Fitzpatrick TB, Jimbow K. 1985. Human skin color: origin, variation and significance. J Human Evolution 14:43–56.

Quevedo WC, Fitzpatrick TB, Szabo G, Jimbow K. 1987. Biology of the melanin pigmentary system. In: Fitzpatrick TB, Eisen HS, Wolff K, Freedberg M, Austen K, eds, Dermatology in General Medicine, vol 1. New York: McGraw-Hill, 224–251.

Ramsay M, Colman MA, Stevens G, Zwane E, Kromberg J, Farrall M, Jenkins T. 1992. The tyrosinase-positive oculocutaneous albinism locus maps to chromosome 15q11.2–q12. Am J Hum Genetics 51:879–884.

Rapp LM, Williams TP. 1980. The role of ocular pigmentation in protecting against retinal light damage. Vision Res 20:1127–1131.

Riley PA. 1993. Mechanistic aspects of the control of tyrosinase activity. Pigment Cell Res 6:182–185.

Rinchik EM, Bultman SJ, Horsthemke B, Lee ST, Strunk K, Spritz RA, Avidano KM, Jong MTC, Nicholls RD. 1993. A gene for the mouse pink-eyed dilution locus and for human type II oculocutaneous albinism. Nature 361:72–76.

Robison WG, Kuwabara T, Cogan DG. 1975. Lysosomes and melanin granules of the retinal pigment epithelium in a mouse model of Chediak-Higashi syndrome. Invest Ophthalmol Vis Sci 14:312–317.

Roskoski R, Jaskunas SR. 1972. Chloroquine and primaquine inhibition of rat liver cell-free polynucleotide-dependent polypeptide synthesis. Biochem Pharmacol 21:391–399.

Rozanowska M, Jarvis-Evans J, Korytowski W, Boulton ME, Burke JM, Sarna T. 1995. Blue light-induced reactivity of retinal age pigment. J Biol Chem 270:18825–18830.

Rozanowska M, Bober A, Burke J, Sarna T. 1997. The role of retinal pigment epithelium melanin in photoinduced oxidation of ascorbate. Photochem Photobiol. 65:472–479.

Salinas C, Garcia-Borron JC, Solano F, Lozano JA. 1994. Dopachrome tautomerase decreases the binding of indolic melanogenesis intermediates to proteins. Biochem Biophys Acta 1204:53–60.

Samuelson DA, Smith P, Ulshafer RJ, Hendricks DG, Whitley RD, Hendricks H, Leone NC. 1993. X-ray microanalysis of ocular melanin in pigs maintained on normal and low zinc diets. Exp Eye Res 56:63–70.

Sanyal S, Zeilmaker GH. 1988. Retinal damage by constant light in chimaeric mice: implications for the protective role of melanin. Exp Eye Res 46:731–743.

Sarna T. 1992. Properties and function of the ocular melanin—a photophysical view. J Photochem Photobiol B: Biol 12:215–258.

Sarna T, Swartz HM. 1993. Interactions of melanin with oxygen (and related species). In: Scott G, ed, Atmospheric Oxygen and Antioxidants, vol 3. Amsterdam: Elsevier Press, 129–169.

Sarna T, Hyde JS, Swartz HM. 1976. Ion exchange in melanin, an electron spin resonance study with lanthanide probes. Science 192: 1132–1134.

Sarna T, Froncisz W, Hyde JS. Cu^{2+} probe of metal-ion binding sites in melanin using electron paramagnetic resonance spectroscopy. II. Natural melanin. Arch Biochem Biophys 202:304–313.

Sarna T, Menon IA, Sealy RC. 1985. Photosensitization of melanins: a comparative study. Photochem Photobiol 42:429–532.

Sarna T, Pilas B, Land EJ, Truscott TG. 1986. Interaction of radicals from water radiolysis with melanin. Biochim Biophys Acta 833:162–167.

Schiaffino M, Baschirotto C, Pellegrini G, Monafti S, Tacchetti C, De Luca M, Ballabio A. 1996. The ocular albinism type 1 gene product is a membrane glycoprotein localized to melanosomes. Proc Natl Acad Sci USA 93:9055–9060.

Schmidt SY, Peisch RD. 1986. Melanin concentration in normal human retinal pigment epithelium. Invest Ophthalmol Vis Sci 27: 1063–1067.

Schraermeyer U. 1993. Does melanin turnover occur in the eyes of adult vertebrates? Pigment Cell Res 6:193–204.

Schraermeyer U, Stieve H. 1994. A newly discovered pathway of melanin formation in cultured retinal pigment epithelium of cattle. Cell Tissue Res 276:273–279.

Schraermeyer U. 1996. The intracellular origin of the melanosome in pigment cells: A review of ultrastructural data. Histol Histopathol. 11:445–462.

Schraermeyer U, Dohms M. 1996. Detection of a fine lamellar gridwork after degradation of ocular melanin granules by cultured peritoneal macrophages. Pigment Cell Res. 9:248–254.

Sealy RC. 1984. Free radicals in melanin formation, structure and reactions. In: Armstrong D, Sohal RS, Cutler RG, Slater TF, eds, Free Radicals in Molecular Biology, Aging and Disease. New York: Raven Press, 67–76.

Sealy RC, Hyde JS, Felix CC, Menon IA, Prota G. 1982. Eumelanins and pheomelanins: characterization by electron spin resonance spectroscopy. Science 217:545–547.

Seiji M, Fitzpatrick TB, Birbeck MS. 1961. The melanosome: a distinctive subcellular particle of mammalian tyrosinase and the site of melanogenesis. J Invest Dermatol 36:243–252.

Seiji M, Shimao K, Birkbeck M, Fitzpatrick T. 1963. Subcellular localisation of melanin biosynthesis. Ann NY Acad Sci 100:497–533.

Shibahara S. 1993. Functional analysis of the tyrosinase gene and brown-locus protein gene promoters. J Invest Dermatol 100:164S–149S.

Smith-Thomas L, Richardson P, Thody A, Graham A, Palmer I, Flemming L, Parsons M, Rennie I, MacNeil S. 1996. Human ocular melanocytes and retinal pigment epithelial cells differ in their melanogenic properties in vivo and in vitro. Curr Eye Res 15: 1079–1091.

Spitznas M. 1971. Morphogenesis and nature of the pigment granules in the adult human retinal pigment epithelium. Zeitschrift fur Zellforschung Mikroskopie und Anatomie. 122:378–388.

Spritz RA. 1993. Molecular genetics of oculocutaneous albinism. Seminars in Dermatology 12:167–172.

Spritz RA. 1994. Molecular genetics of oculocutaneous albinism. Human Molecular Genetics 3:1469–1475.

Stanka P, Rathjen P, Sahlman B. 1981. Evidence of membrane transformation during melanogenesis. An electron microscopic study of the retinal pigment epithelium of chick embryo. Cell Tissue Res 214:343–353.

Stepien K, Wilczok T. 1982. Studies of the mechanism of chloroquine binding to synthetic dopa-melanin. Biochem Pharmacol 31:3359–3365.

Stone J, Rowe MH, Campion JE. 1978. Retinal abnormalities in the Siamese cat. J Comp Neurol 180:773–782.

Szabo G. 1975. Skin is an adaptive organ. In: Damon A, ed, Physiological Anthropology. New York: Oxford University Press, 39–58.

Taylor W. Visual disabilities of oculocutaneous albinism and their alleviation. Trans Ophthalmol Soc UK 98:423–445.

Toda K, Fitzpatrick TB. 1972. Ultrastructural and biochemical studies of the formation of melanosomes in the embryonic chick retinal pigment epithelium. In: Riley V, ed, Pigmentation: Its Genesis and Biological Control. New York: Appleton-Century-Crofts, 125–141.

Tosti A, Costelli E. 1990. The function of melanocytes. In: Cascinelli N, Santinami M, Veronesi U, eds, Cutaneous Melanoma Biology and Management. Milan: Masson, 75–77.

Tsukamoto K, Jimenez M, Hearing VJ. 1992. The nature of tyrosinase isoenzymes. Pigment Cell Res 2(suppl):84–89.

Ulshafer RJ, Allen CB, Rubin ML. 1990. Distributions of elements in the human retinal pigment epithelium. Arch Ophthalmol 108: 113–117.

Van Norren D, Tiemeijer LF. 1986. Spectral reflectance of the human eye. Vision Res 26:313–320.

Varela JM, Stempels NA, Vandenberghe DA, Tassignon MJ. 1995. Isoenzyme patterns of tyrosinase in the rabbit choroid and retina/retinal pigment epithelium. Exp Eye Res 60:621–629.

Walls GL. 1942. The Vertebrate Eye and Its Adaptive Radiation. Cranbrook Institute of Science Bulletin, vol 19. Bloomfield Hills, MI: Cranbrook Institute.

Weiter JJ, Delori FC, Wing GL, Fitch KA. 1986. Retinal pigment epithelial lipofuscin and melanin and choroidal melanin in human eyes. Invest Ophthalmol Vis Sci 27:145–152.

Wick MM, Hearing VJ, Rorsman H. 1987. Biochemistry of melanization. In: Fitzpatrick TB, Eisen AZ, Wolff K, Freedberg M, Austen KF, eds, Dermatology of General Medicine, vol 1. New York: McGraw-Hill, 251–258.

Wolbarsht ML, Walsh AW, George G. 1981. Melanin, a unique biological absorber. Appl Opt 20:2184–2186.

Yokoyama K, Yasumoto K, Suzuki H, Shibahara S. 1994. Cloning of the human DOPAchrome tautomerase/tyrosinase-related protein 2 gene and identification of two regulatory regions required for its pigment cell-specific expression. J Biol Chem 269:27080–27087.

Zareba M, Bober A, Korytowski W, Zecca L, Sarna T. 1995. The effect of synthetic neuromelanin on yield of free hydroxyl radicals generated in model systems. Biochim Biophys Acta 1271:343–348.

Zinn K, Marmor MF, eds. 1979. The Retinal Pigment Epithelium. Cambridge, MA, and London: Harvard University Press.

5. Determinants of retinal pigment epithelial cell phenotype and polarity

JANICE M. BURKE

Cells derived from the retinal pigment epithelium (RPE) of animal and human eyes have been propagated in culture for more than thirty years and used for hundreds of studies of cell structure and function. As with most cultured cells, it is assumed that RPE cells in vitro are similar to cells in situ and that cultures therefore can be used to determine tissue-specific properties of the RPE. This assumption, however, can be questioned on the basis of cell morphology: cultured RPE cells simply do not look like their counterparts within eyes. This criticism can be leveled at cells cultured from most epithelial tissues but it is particularly acute for RPE cells, which have a high degree of epithelial regularity in the normal tissue in situ. In comparison, confluent monolayers of cultured cells are phenotypically variable, lacking a well-ordered epithelial organization. Attempts have been made to manipulate culture conditions for RPE to produce a more epithelioid morphology, but this approach has met with limited success. The problem of variable RPE phenotype in vitro remains, and it is commonly addressed either by electing to study cultures that appear more grossly epithelioid, or by simply ignoring the phenotypic imperfection of the cultured monolayers.

Over the past decade the molecular mechanisms whereby cells develop an epithelial phenotype have begun to be revealed, largely through studies of epithelial cell lines. It is becoming clear that the morphology of cultured epithelial cells is not a chance occurrence that must be accepted as a weakness of culture systems, but rather the result of a complex intrinsic morphogenetic program that is modulated in time and place by extrinsic signals.

BIOGENESIS OF AN EPITHELIAL PHENOTYPE AND THE CENTRAL ROLE OF THE CELL–CELL ADHERENS JUNCTION

The epithelial phenotype is characterized by a compartmentation of the cytoplasm and a molecular asymmetry of the cell surface. Organelles and cytoplasmic filaments are localized to positions along the cell's apico–basal axis. Some cell–cell junctions adopt a zonular pattern, and certain plasma membrane molecules are polarized to apical, lateral, or basal domains. Investigations of epithelial cell lines, primarily from kidney and gut, indicate that this epithelial cell topography is established and maintained by interactions between the actin microfilament and intermediate filament systems and the cell surface at sites of cell–cell and cell–substrate attachment (Hitt and Luna, 1994; Luna and Hitt, 1992; Rodriguez-Boulan and Nelson, 1989).

Fully dissociated cells in suspension lack polarity, and the spatial cues for organizing the cytoplasm and cell surface are provided by both cell–cell and cell–substrate attachment (Nelson, 1991; Wang et al., 1990; Wollner and Nelson, 1992). Substrate attachment induces a different distribution of some membrane molecules on the basal surface relative to the free apical surface in most cells. Additional cues which induce the development of an epithelial phenotype require cell-to-cell contact, which triggers an extensive remodeling of the cytoarchitecture and a further molecular polarization of the cell surface. A central morphoregulatory role in these latter events has been ascribed to the cell–cell adherens junction (Näthke et al., 1993; Takeichi, 1991; 1995).

The cell–cell binding elements of the adherens junction are members of the cadherin family of adhesion molecules (Geiger and Ayalon, 1992; Takeichi, 1995), especially E-cadherin in epithelial cells (Rodriguez-Boulan and Nelson, 1989; Takeichi, 1991). Cell contact initiates the time-dependent formation of cadherin-mediated adhesions, during which the cytoplasmic domain of the cadherin molecule forms a complex with proteins that link it with the actin cytoskeleton (Gumbiner and McCrea, 1993; Hinck et al., 1994b; Näthke et al., 1993). The number of proteins that appear to participate in cadherin-to-actin linkages is growing (Brady-Kalnay et al., 1995; Hurksen et al., 1994; Reynolds et al., 1994; Shibamoto et al., 1995), with the major linkage function currently attributed to members of the catenin family (α-catenin, β-catenin, plakoglobin). When cell contacts first form, E-cadherin is readily solubilized in buffers containing Triton-X-100, but it later becomes resistant to detergent extraction and localized to junctional sites (Hinck et al., 1994b; McNeill et al., 1993). As the formation of cadherin adhesions in epithelial cells progresses, actin filaments organize into circumferential bundles to produce a zonular adherens junction (Yonemura et al., 1995). By mechanisms that are not yet clarified, E-cadherin junctions appear to induce a remodeling of the cell surface membrane cytoskeleton and associated plasma membrane molecules such as Na/K ATPase (McNeill et al., 1990), leading to the development of distinct apical, lateral, and basal membrane domains (Näthke et al., 1993; Rodriguez-Boulan and Nelson, 1989).

Attention has been focused on the sodium pump in studies of epithelial surface polarity, because this ion transporter plays a central role in maintaining the sodium gradient responsible for the transport of virtually all nutrients and metabolites (Kyte, 1981). In epithelial monolayers the sodium pump is restricted to a cell-type-specific domain, so that molecules are transported vectorially as required for normal tissue-level function. Polarization of Na/K ATPase has been studied in epithelial cell lines, especially canine kidney-derived MDCK cells where the pump is lateral. The picture that is emerging is a complicated one, in which multiple mechanisms contribute to the enrichment of Na/K ATPase in the basolateral domain. These mechanisms include a combination of targeting to and selective retention at the appropriate cell surface (Gottardi and Caplan, 1993; Hammerton et al., 1991; McNeill et al., 1990; Nelson, 1991; Nelson and Veshnock, 1987; Siemers et al., 1993; Wollner and Nelson, 1992; Zurzolo and Rodriguez-Boulan, 1993). The relative contribution of these mechanisms may differ among cell types and at different stages of epithelial morphogenesis; differences even exist among clones of MDCK cells (Gottardi and Caplan, 1993; Mays et al., 1995). Selective retention in MDCK cells is hypothesized to result from tethering of sodium pumps to the fodrin-based membrane cytoskeleton (Hammerton et al., 1991; McNeill et al., 1990) via linkage of the α subunit of the sodium pump to ankyrin (Nelson and Veshnock, 1987), which in turn is capable of complexing with the actin-binding protein fodrin (Kennedy et al., 1991). Soluble complexes of ankyrin-fodrin-Na/K ATPase are extracted with detergent buffers from MDCK cells in early confluency. Then, following formation of cadherin-containing cell–cell junctions, the sodium pump accumulates at junctional sites and becomes preferentially retained basal to the junctional complex (Hammerton et al., 1991; Marrs et al., 1993; Wollner et al., 1992).

RPE IN SITU: CELL–CELL ADHERENS JUNCTIONS AND MOLECULAR POLARITY

There is limited information regarding the components of the RPE cell–cell adherens junction and the polarization of surface molecules to discrete domains of the RPE plasma membrane within the normal tissue. Several morphological studies of the zonula adherens junction of RPE cells in situ have focused on the associated actin circumferential microfilament bundles. Using fluorescent compounds tagged to phalloidin to visualize F-actin in RPE monolayers in situ, the striking uniformity in shape of RPE cells is revealed (Gordon and Essner, 1987; Philp and Nachmias, 1985; Turksen and Kalnins, 1987) (Fig. 5-1). In bovine RPE striations can be seen in

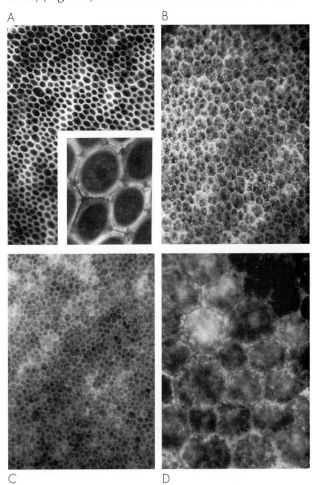

FIGURE 5-1. Fluorescence micrographs of RPE in bovine (A), rabbit (B), and human (C) eyes. Tissues were treated with rhodamine phalloidin to stain circumferential actin microfilament bundles and photographed at the same low magnification to show the regularity, if not uniformity, in cell shape in situ. A higher magnification of bovine actin is provided (inset in [A]) to show the substructure of the thick peripheral actin bundles in this species. A higher magnification of an unstained preparation of human RPE (D) shows variations among cells in pigment and autofluorescent lipofuscin, as well as in cell size and shape. Magnification: (A)–(C), ×28; inset (A) and (D), ×180.

the thick actin bundle (Fig. 5-1) that are similar to those shown by electron microscopy in rat RPE after treatment with phalloidin (Gordon and Essner, 1987). Actin-associated proteins filamen (Kodama et al., 1991), tropomyosin (Turksen and Kalnins, 1987), and myosin (Gordon and Essner, 1987; Philp and Nachmias, 1985) have been shown to colocalize with circumferential actin in RPE cells.

Regarding molecules comprising the cadherin/catenin complex, RPE cells are known to express N-cadherin, and B-cadherin in the chick embryo (Lagunowich and Grunwald, 1989; 1991; Murphy-Erdosh et al., 1994). The RPE has been reported to lack the common epithelial cadherin, E-cadherin (Gundersen et al., 1993), although more recent evidence indicates that E-cadherin is expressed by human RPE *in situ* (Cao et al., 1997). RPE of avian and of several mammalian species (including humans) has been shown to express plakoglobin/γ-catenin (Owaribe et al., 1988), which manifests a zonular distribution consistent with its participation in the adherens junction. Also codistributing with circumferential actin in RPE cells is α-actinin (Arikawa and Williams, 1991; Philp and Nachmias, 1985; Turksen and Kalnins, 1987) and vinculin (Turksen and Kalnins, 1987), a protein related to α-catenin (Herrenknecht et al., 1991; Nagafuchi et al., 1991). Alpha-actinin has been found in complexes with cadherins in some cells (Knudsen et al., 1995).

Other adhesion molecules have also been localized to subcellular domains of RPE cells in situ. An adhesion molecule in the integrin family was shown in the basolateral domain of late-stage chick embryo and adult rat RPE (Philp and Nachmias, 1987). Beta-1 integrin has been demonstrated in the apical or apicolateral domains of chick (Chu and Grunwald, 1991) and primate RPE (Anderson et al., 1990). Although there is some discrepancy in published reports as to N-CAM expression and distribution in RPE cells (Fliesler et al., 1990; Neill and Barnstable, 1990), this cell adhesion molecule has been localized to the apical surface of rat RPE in situ (Gundersen et al., 1993).

Several ion transport molecules have also been localized to discrete plasma membrane domains of RPE cells in situ. Na/K ATPase is found on apical plasma membranes of RPE cells (Bok, 1982; Gundersen et al., 1991), in contrast to the basolateral distribution found in most monolayer epithelia (Rodriguez-Boulan and Nelson, 1989). Electrophysiological studies of RPE-choroid preparations of frog, bovine, and human tissues have localized other transporters to apical (proton-lactate cotransporter, Na/K/Cl cotransporter, $NaHCO_3$ cotransporter, Na-H antiporter) or basolateral (Na-dependent lactate transporter, $Cl-HCO_3$ exchanger) domains of

RPE cells in situ (DiMattio et al., 1983; Joseph and Miller, 1991; Kenyon et al., 1994; la Cour et al., 1994; Lin and Miller, 1991; 1994; Lin et al., 1994; Quinn and Miller, 1992). Other molecules with an enrichment in apical (mannose-6-phosphate receptors, carbonic anhydrase, α1 adrenergic receptors) or basolateral (alkaline phosphatase, retinol-binding protein receptors) RPE membranes have also been described (Bok and Heller, 1976; Edelman and Miller, 1991; Korte et al., 1991; Tarnowski et al., 1988; Wolfensberger et al., 1994).

RPE IN VITRO: PHENOTYPE, ADHERENS JUNCTIONS, AND MOLECULAR POLARITY

The subcellular distribution of relatively few molecules has been determined for RPE cells in vitro, so the extent to which cultured cells develop a topography similar to cells in the normal tissue remains an open question. However, available data indicate that gross cellular phenotype and the subcellular distribution of surface molecules in cultured RPE cells do not fully mimic their in situ counterparts (Zhao et al., 1997).

General Culture Morphology

Phase contrast microscopy is the most common method used to demonstrate the phenotype of cultured cells. Using this criterion, RPE cultures are often described as "epithelioid" or "cobblestone." These descriptors are relative; as compared to fibroblasts the cells are indeed "epithelioid," but relative to RPE cells in situ or to epithelial cell lines derived from other tissues, cultured RPE monolayers appear less epithelioid (Fig. 5-2). Other morphologic methods such as scanning or transmission electron microscopy (TEM) have also been used to examine the epithelial organization of the RPE monolayer. Using these methods, cultured cells have been shown to have well-developed apical microvilli (Ander-

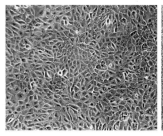

FIGURE 5-2. Phase contrast micrographs of cultures of human RPE *(left)* and MDCK cells *(right)* just at confluency contrasting the phenotypic heterogeneity of RPE cells with the more uniformly epithelioid MDCK cells Both magnified at ×50.

son et al., 1990; Heth et al., 1987), a morphologic feature that provides evidence for some level of epithelial organization, in that microvilli are usually absent from fibroblasts, and their formation requires the polarized distribution of several proteins that bind actin filaments into the tight parallel arrays characteristic of the microvillous core (Mooseker, 1985). Also by TEM, apical intercellular junctions have been identified in cultured cells showing the presence of a morphologic adherens junction with its actin undercoat (Heth et al., 1987; Davis et al., 1995).

It appears therefore that cultured RPE develop some of the structural features of an epithelial tissue. However, phase and electron microscopy are limited in the type of information they provide. The presence of structures like microvilli and apical junctions in discrete domains of the cells shown by EM indicates that cells are at least partially polarized, but the extent of molecular polarity within cells cannot be determined by this method. Variations among individual cells are also difficult to identify in tissue sections. This is a significant issue because nearly all cells must achieve a similar high level of epithelial organization, characterized by complete zonular junctions and an asymmetric distribution of cell surface molecules such as ion transporters, in order for an RPE monolayer to function as a transporting epithelium.

Cell–Cell Adherens Junctions

To examine the epithelial character of broader expanses of the culture monolayer, fluorescence microscopy has been used to visualize the zonular pattern of the actin cytoskeleton. As indicated above, this is an important measure of epithelialization since one of the prominent features that distinguishes an epithelial cell is the organization of its dominant actin network. In epithelial cells actin forms circumferential bundles near the cell apex at sites of cell–cell contact during cell polarization, whereas in fibroblasts the most prominent actin filaments form longitudinal bundles (stress fibers) that associate with the plasma membrane at cell–substrate focal contacts, and cell–cell actin assemblies in fibroblasts fail to develop a beltlike organization (Yonemura et al., 1995). Poorly formed circumferential actin filament bundles therefore are a marker of incomplete epithelial maturation.

Examination of actin distribution in cultured RPE monolayers shows the presence of circumferential bundles, but the development of zonular actin appears to be incomplete in some cells and the overall regularity of the monolayer is visually less than in situ. The actin cytoskeleton was shown to undergo developmental changes after cell–cell contact at confluency in RPE cells

in vitro in cat, monkey, and human RPE cultures. Cytoplasmic actin in subconfluent cells formed stress fibers (Matsumoto et al., 1990) that terminated at presumed sites of cell–substrate contact where the β1 integrin subunit was localized (Anderson et al., 1990). After confluency actin became organized into a prominent circumferential pattern and into apical microvilli (Matsumoto et al., 1990) coincident with the redistribution of the β1 integrin to lateral and apical domains (Anderson et al., 1990). Integrins, including α-β dimers containing the β1 subunit, have been shown to participate in both cell–cell and cell–substrate adhesion in other epithelial cells (Larjava et al., 1990; Schoenenberger et al., 1994). However, even after several weeks in culture the reorganization of actin to a zonular pattern appeared to be incomplete and was not observed in all cells of the RPE monolayer (Matsumoto et al., 1990). The actin in RPE cells rather resembled actin as it has been shown in earlier stages of the polarization of epithelial cell lines when the adherens junction was incompletely developed (Yonemura et al., 1995).

Circumferential actin bundles were also shown in a spontaneously arising human RPE cell line that was recently described (Davis et al., 1995). The actin ring was associated with apical junctional complexes where N-cadherin was localized (Davis et al., 1995). However, immunostaining for junctional N-cadherin was punctate suggesting spot welds around the cell rather than a complete pericellular ring (Davis et al., 1995). A similar observation was made for the cadherin (as well as catenins) in a rat RPE cell line in which the molecules formed an incomplete ring at sites of cell–cell contact (Marrs et al., 1995). These cadherin distributions in cultured RPE cells are similar to the appearance of junctional E-cadherin prior to the development of polarity in an epithelial cell line (Yonemura et al., 1995), again suggesting that the adherens junction in RPE cells is not fully formed. In rat RPE cells (Marrs et al., 1995), the cadherin formed complexes with α-catenin, β-catenin, and plakoglobin in the detergent-soluble fraction of cell lysates as shown by immunoprecipitation, but the immunostaining pattern of cadherin and catenins, as well as other markers of epithelial organization as described below, indicated incomplete junctional development in this RPE cell line.

Embryonic chick RPE cells have notably prominent circumferential actin associated with sites of cell–cell adhesion (Sandig et al., 1990 and references therein) which have been examined during outgrowth from primary explant. This method contrasts with the methods used in the aforementioned studies of mammalian cells in which the tissue is first dissociated, then the RPE monolayer is examined as it re-forms. Examination of outgrowth from chick RPE explants revealed that the adhesion-associated molecule vinculin was localized to cell–cell contact sites in well-developed cells toward the middle of explanted colonies, and to focal cell–substrate contacts in spreading RPE cells at the colony's edge (Opas et al., 1985; Turksen, 1987). This observation indicates a loss of intercellular junctional organization in early culture, but whether vinculin is restored to cell-cell adhesion sites throughout the monolayer after the primary culture becomes confluent is perhaps a different question that is yet unanswered. Nonetheless, it appears that chick RPE cell–cell junctions are not retained when cells are cultured.

Polarity of Nonjunctional Surface Molecules; Lack of Polarity of the Sodium Pump

Because of the key role in determining epithelial polarity attributed to cadherins (Rodriguez-Boulan and Nelson, 1989; Takeichi, 1991), one might suspect that RPE which lack fully formed cadherin-containing junctions would also have an incomplete development of polarity of cell surface molecules. This indeed appears to be the case. Some molecules do attain a polarized distribution in cultured RPE cells: membrane-bound carbonic anhydrase appears to be apically restricted in cultured RPE cells as it apparently is in situ (Wolfensberger et al., 1994), and domain-specific budding of vesicular stomatitis and influenza viruses also occurs in cultured human, bovine, and rat RPE (Bok et al., 1992; Nabi et al., 1993). However, cultured RPE cells with polarized viral budding did not show apical polarization of Na/K ATPase (Bok et al., 1992; Nabi et al., 1993). Studies by electrophysiologic methods of fetal bovine or human RPE also showed little or no enrichment of the sodium pump in the apical domain of cultured cells (Hu et al., 1994; Hernandez et al., 1995). It is also likely that Na/K ATPase was not restricted to the apical domain of the human RPE cell line described by Davis and coworkers (1995) since the fodrin-based membrane cytoskeleton, with which Na/K ATPase is associated in RPE (Gundersen et al., 1991) and other epithelial cells (Nelson and Hammerton, 1989), was not apically polarized. (See comments below on the membrane cytoskeleton and embryonic chick RPE.) One possible exception is the human RPE cell line ARP-19, which may have an apical enrichment of Na/K ATPase (Tugizov et al., 1996).

The absence of polarization of the sodium pump in RPE cells in which other molecules are polarized illustrates that epithelial cell polarity is not an all-or-none phenomenon but rather a relative state. There appears to be a sequence of molecular events following cell–cell

contact that produces an epithelial phenotype. Comparison of the kinetics for polarization of cadherins and Na/K ATPase in MDCK cells showed that after cell contact, a longer period was required for the sodium pump than for cadherins to become restricted to the lateral membrane (Hammerton et al., 1991; Wollner et al., 1992). If the sequence of events leading to epithelial polarity is called a "morphogenetic program," observations on RPE cells suggest that Na/K ATPase is polarized later in the program such that cells may develop a polarized distribution of some proteins but yet fail to polarize the sodium pump. In contrast to epithelial cell lines derived from other tissues, populations of cultured RPE cells appear to be incapable of following the epithelial morphogenetic program to the stage where pump polarization occurs.

What directs the normal apical enrichment of the sodium pump in RPE cells remains to be determined. Although truncated transcripts for the subunits of Na/K ATPase have been found in human RPE cells (Ruiz et al., 1995), the major isoform of Na/K ATPase in RPE ($\alpha 1/\beta 1$) appears to be the same as in kidney epithelial cells (Gundersen et al., 1991; Ruiz et al., 1995). In the latter cells, the pump has a basolateral distribution (Nelson and Hammerton, 1989) suggesting that the cell-type specificity in polarization does not reside in the pump itself. Indeed, the entire ankyrin-fodrin membrane cytoskeletal complex with which the sodium pump is associated is reversed in RPE cells relative to most other monolayer epithelia (Gundersen et al., 1991) except the choroid plexus epithelium (Marrs et al., 1993). The colocalization of ankyrin and fodrin with Na/K ATPase in RPE cells suggests that selective retention via linkages to the membrane cytoskeleton, a mechanism proposed for basolateral polarization of the pump in kidney epithelia (Nelson and Hammerton, 1989; Wollner et al., 1992), contributes to the apical polarization of the RPE pump at least at some stage of the polarization process (Rizzolo and Zhou, 1995). However, domain-specific apical retention of Na/K ATPase appears not to routinely develop in RPE in vitro.

The fundamental role for E-cadherin in determining polarization of Na/K ATPase in other epithelial cells raises the possibility that the apparent absence of this inducer contributes to the lack of pump polarity in cultured RPE cells. Marrs and colleagues (1995) analyzed the ability of a rat RPE cell line to polarize the sodium pump in the presence of this adhesion molecule. Using cells transfected to express E-cadherin, RPE were found to be competent to polarize the sodium pump, but in RPE cells expressing E-cadherin both the pump and the membrane cytoskeleton accumulated at the lateral rather than apical membrane domain. E-cadherin, therefore, appeared to direct (baso)lateral distribution of Na/K ATPase even in cells in which the pump is normally apical. Accompanying the expression of E-cadherin in RPE cells was the induction of a different isoform of ankyrin and the accumulation of the desmosomal cadherin desmoglein. This observation supports a role for E-cadherin in inducing epithelial polarity and further suggests that E-cadherin regulates the formation of an epithelial phenotype by activating the transcription of components that participate in the formation of epithelial junctional complexes. However, whether endogenous RPE cadherins regulate the apical distribution of Na/K ATPase in RPE cells and how that apical polarization develops remain unknown. One might suspect that the major cadherin of cultured RPE cells, N-cadherin, is not sufficient to support epithelialization since fibroblasts can express N-cadherin and form many of the same cadherin-catenin complexes as epithelial cells (Knudsen et al., 1995). Indeed, the expression of N-cadherin in cells of epithelial origin may disrupt rather than potentiate the development of an epithelial phenotype (Islam et al., 1996). With the recent observation of E-cadherin in RPE cells both in situ and in late-stage postconfluent cultures (Cao et al., 1997), the role of E-cadherin in directing basolateral pump polarity in epithelial cells needs to be re-evaluated. This is especially true in the light of data showing that a subset of cells in human RPE cultures is capable of developing an apically polarized sodium pump, but several weeks at confluency are required for polarization to occur (McKay et al., 1997).

WHAT ARE THE IMPEDIMENTS TO FORMING WELL-EPITHELIALIZED RPE MONOLAYERS IN VITRO?

As indicated above, most RPE cultures appear to be incompletely epithelialized by both morphologic and biochemical measures of confluent cultures. However, evaluations of entire RPE populations or of a few RPE cell lines does not exclude the possibility that some RPE cells within the population have the potential to produce an epithelial phenotype in vitro. Perhaps the existence of the ARPE-19 human RPE cell line is an indication that some RPE cells can develop a high level of epithelial organization in culture (Tugizov et al., 1996). Confluent RPE monolayers could appear to be weakly epithelioid if all cells achieved a similar but low level of organization, or, alternatively, if cells of variable phenotype were intermingled. In the latter case, full expression of epithelial development in highly epithelioid cells could be masked by association with adjacent weakly epithelioid cells. Cell-to-cell variation is low in clonal epithelial cell

lines (which makes them an ideal model for studying the mechanisms of epithelial morphogenesis), but phenotypic heterogeneity might be expected among cells propagated from tissues.

Evidence has existed for some time which suggests that RPE cells are morphologically variable with both "squamous" and epithelioid cells identified in RPE cultures (Aronson, 1983). Phenotypic heterogeneity of human RPE was recently confirmed in studies in which RPE cells were plated very sparsely such that cells were widely spaced on the culture substrate and the progeny of individual cells could be identified (McKay and Burke, 1994). Using this protocol, RPE cells formed colonies of cells of distinctly different phenotypes, including both highly epithelioid and markedly fusiform morphologies. The phenotypes were stable and could be demonstrated for many culture passages if sparse plating protocols were used to reveal them. The phenotypic stability of the fusiform subpopulation was further confirmed by separating them from the epithelioid subpopulation to show that fusiform cells did not develop an epithelial phenotype (Fig. 5-3) even when maintained

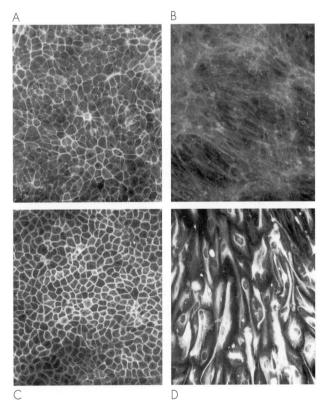

FIGURE 5-3. Fluorescence micrographs of separated subpopulations of epithelioid (A), (C) and fusiform human RPE cells (B), (D). Cells were stained with rhodamine phalloidin for actin (A), (B) or immunostained with antibodies to cytokeratins 8.18.19 (C), (D) to show the markedly different cytoskeletal organizations in these phenotypic variants after two months at confluency. All magnified at ×75. (From McKay and Burke, 1994.)

for extended periods at confluency. The presence of such cells within RPE cultures would be expected to reduce the overall epithelioid appearance of the monolayers in proportion to their representation in the population.

The epithelial character of a cultured monolayer is usually evaluated soon after confluency, on the presumption that epithelial morphology will develop rapidly after cell–cell contact in cells competent to undergo epithelial morphogenesis. However, evidence exists for RPE cells which suggests that final in vitro phenotype is not prominently displayed immediately at confluency. In several studies, RPE cultures from fetal and adult donor eyes were maintained for weeks to months at confluency, prior to analysis of differentiated functions of the monolayer (Hernandez et al., 1995; Hu et al., 1994; Mircheff et al., 1990; Tugizov et al., 1996). Although changes in phenotype during this period were not described, it is presumed that this protocol was used to maximize maturation of the RPE monolayer, and that maturation has a long time course. Matsumoto and colleagues (1990) reported changes in RPE actin organization occurring over weeks in culture, and in the study in which epithelioid and fusiform RPE subpopulations were identified (McKay and Burke, 1994), several weeks at confluency were required for the epithelioid cells to manifest well-formed circumferential actin and intermediate filament bundles. More recently, the epithelioid RPE subpopulation was shown to require several weeks at confluency to develop an adherens junction of zonular and detergent-resistant cadherin (McKay et al., 1997). This time frame of weeks to months for RPE cell morphogenesis differs markedly from epithelial cell lines, which provide the paradigm for epithelialization in vitro, but which require only a few days at confluency to produce an epithelial phenotype (Nelson and Veshnock, 1986; McNeill et al., 1993).

There are therefore at least two gross properties of RPE cultures that differ from epithelial cell lines and which reduce the overall epithelial organization of RPE monolayers at confluency: individual RPE cells differ markedly in phenotype and include some highly fusiform subpopulations, and the development of an epithelial phenotype, even in subpopulations expressing a highly epithelial morphology, is not completed rapidly after confluency but rather has a protracted time course.

EPITHELIALIZATION OF RPE IN VITRO: NATURE VERSUS NURTURE

Why do some cultured RPE cells express a distinctly nonepithelial, fusiform phenotype? One possibility is that conditions of culture are insufficient to support epithelial differentiation. However, standard conditions can support the development of an epithelial phenotype in at least some cells, as shown for the epithelioid subpopulation which coexists in the same cultures as fusiform cells (McKay and Burke, 1994; McKay et al., 1997). It appears, therefore, that all RPE cells from the same donor tissue, even with identical growth conditions, do not respond identically. Stated differently, individual RPE cells appear to vary in the ability to recapitulate the morphogenetic program that produces an epithelial phenotype. This variation raises the question of whether extrinsic signals, perhaps provided by other culture additives, can supplement the intrinsic program of "deficient" cells, increasing the proportion of RPE cells in a population that manifest an epithelial phenotype.

RPE during Embryogenesis

The question of the relative contribution of an intrinsic program and extrinsic signals to the development of an epithelial phenotype in vitro raises yet another question: How do embryonic pigment epithelial cells initially produce their epithelial organization? It is during embryogenesis that the program considered "intrinsic" to adult cells is developed and specific signals in time and place are likely to be provided by the developing eye to induce the formation of the RPE layer. There are relatively little experimental data regarding triggers for RPE morphogenesis during development, although Rizzolo and colleagues have investigated some aspects of the process in the chick embryo. They have observed that the development of an epithelial organization in the RPE in situ in a stepwise process (Rizzolo and Heiges, 1991), with ocular cues provided by adjacent tissues regulating the development of epithelial properties and the polarity of at least some molecules. One of the earliest events in the polarization of the RPE during chick embryogenesis (embryonic day 3) is the development of a distinct apical localization of γ-tubulin, a centrosomal protein which may nucleate microtubule growth (Rizzolo and Joshi, 1993). The signal(s) for this early event have not been determined, although cues have been identified for some later processes. For example, competing cues from interaction with the developing basal substrate and apical sensory retina appear to determine β1 integrin distribution. The β1 integrin subunit is distributed in all domains of the RPE plasma membrane early in development, later becoming basolateral and ultimately basal as development proceeds (Rizzolo and Heiges, 1991). Using RPE from different stages of chick embryo development in a series of tissue reconstitution experiments, Rizzolo (1991) showed that Bruch's membrane and components thereof induce basolateral polarization of the β1 integrin, but association with the immature neurosensory retina or interphotoreceptor matrix could maintain the β1 subunit in the apical membrane at early stages of RPE development (Rizzolo et al., 1994). Diffusible substances from the developing retina provide additional signals for RPE morphogenesis stimulating barrier properties of the developing epithelium (Rizzolo and Li, 1993).

Although basement membrane and factors from retina induced some polarized properties in the developing chick RPE, neither supported the apical polarization of Na/K ATPase (Rizzolo, 1991; Rizzolo and Li, 1993). Perhaps contact between the RPE and the overlying retina induces or maintains the apical localization of Na/K ATPase. As indicated above, the sodium pump is known to complex with proteins of the membrane cytoskeleton which may retain the enzyme in discrete domains of epithelial cells (Hammerton et al., 1991; McNeill et al., 1990; Nelson and Veshnock, 1987). In the chick embryo, during later stages of development the sodium pump no longer codistributes with the spectrin/fodrin membrane cytoskeleton of RPE cells; the latter accumulates at the base of the microvilli and in the basal domain of the cells, whereas the pump is enriched in elongate microvilli (Huotari et al., 1995; Rizzolo and Zhou, 1995). When RPE cells from this stage are removed to cultures there is a rapid loss of polarity of Na/K ATPase, as well as of some cadherin-like molecules (Huotari et al., 1995). This latter observation was interpreted to suggest that the apical distribution of Na/K ATPase may be stabilized by contacts between the RPE and sensory retina, perhaps mediated by cadherin-like molecules.

A Variable Intrinsic Morphogenetic Program in Adult RPE

As investigations of developing systems are extended, it is likely that many additional sequential signals will be identified which induce RPE morphogenesis during development to produce the fully differentiated cells found in the adult monolayer. Considering again RPE cells from adult donors in culture, at least one subpopulation of human RPE cells (epithelioid cells) appears to retain a fairly complete epithelial morphogenetic program. This subpopulation develops the features of a well-organized RPE monolayer under standard conditions of culture (McKay and Burke, 1994), including polarization of the sodium pump (McKay et al., 1997), in the absence of the specific matrix and humoral cues that

were present during development. However, other cells in the RPE population (fusiform cells) do not develop an epithelial phenotype, perhaps because these cells require extrinsic signals to proceed through the stepwise process of morphogenesis. One hypothesis consistent with these observations is that the completeness of the morphogenetic program varies among individual RPE cells. Such a hypothesis would predict that RPE cells might display a spectrum of phenotypes even in the same environment, with morphogenesis proceeding in individual cells until a signal is required that is not provided by the environment, at which point epithelial development ceases and the appearance of the cell at that stage becomes its terminal in vitro phenotype. This hypothesis might explain the multiple phenotypic variants that were recently identified in human RPE cultures (Burke et al., 1996) (Fig. 5-4). Like the epithelioid and fusiform cells previously described (McKay and Burke, 1994), which might be considered the extremes of the phenotypic spectrum, the phenotype of the other RPE variants developed over a long postconfluent time course and then remained unchanged for at least months in vitro. Whether the phenotypes represent a continuum of RPE morphogenetic development, and whether specific culture additives trigger the "next step" in epithelial maturation, remain to be determined.

Modulation of Phenotype by Exogenous Signals

Evidence which suggests that exogenous signals might indeed promote epithelial morphogenesis of adult RPE cells in culture is provided by studies which indicate that humoral substances, substrate association, or tissue interactions can increase (or decrease) the epithelial appearance or molecular polarity of cultured RPE cells. Retinoic acid (Campochiaro et al., 1991) or basic FGF (Campochiaro and Hackett, 1993; Song and Lui, 1990) when added to culture media appear to act as RPE morphogens, increasing the epithelial appearance of cultured cells. In contrast, PDGF, NGF, EGF (Shirikawa et al., 1986), or undefined products of macrophages (Martini et al., 1991) induce a more spindle-shaped morphology. Association with extracellular matrix can, depending on its composition and deformability, increase or decrease the epithelial appearance of cultured RPE cells. Perhaps predictably, RPE cells produced more epithelioid monolayers on basement membrane materials (Campochiaro and Hackett, 1993; Dutt et al., 1991; Opas, 1989; Song and Lui, 1990) and appeared less epithelioid with increasing invasive potential in the presence of fibrillar collagens or when exposed to vitreous (Docherty et al., 1987; Heth et al., 1987; Kirchhof et al.,

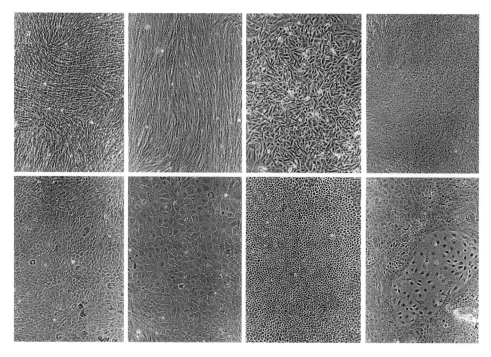

FIGURE 5-4. Phase contrast micrographs of several fields within a single primary human RPE culture illustrating phenotypic variants that were revealed after two months at confluency. Cells with these phenotypes were found in most cultures from 38 donors and could also be identified after passage if cultures were again maintained for extended periods at confluency. All magnified at ×50. (From Burke et al., 1996.)

1988; Martini et al., 1992; Nguyen-Tan and Thompson, 1989; Vidaurri-Leal et al., 1984; Vinores et al., 1990).

The difficulty with studies which have tested the effect of exogenous signals on RPE from adult donors is that gross morphology, shown by phase contrast or transmission electron microscopy, was used to determine outcome. In the absence of additional measures of epithelial organization, such as changes in the distribution of molecules for which the polarized positions are known, it is difficult to dissect the extent to which RPE morphogenesis is modulated by extracellular cues. Two studies, however, suggest that tissue interaction with the sensory retina may be required to maintain a polarized distribution of some RPE surface molecules in the adult tissue. In the rat, NCAM was found on the apical cell surface of RPE cells in situ, but shortly after placing the tissue in culture NCAM redistributed to the basolateral membrane with no accompanying change in the isoform of NCAM expressed by the cells (Gundersen et al., 1993). Similarly, the surface antigen RET-PE2 lost its apical enrichment soon after explantation to primary culture (Marmorstein et al., 1996). These results were considered to result from a loss of interaction with the retina or interphotoreceptor matrix when the tissue was cultured. The factor(s) responsible for maintaining the polarized distribution of these molecules in RPE remain

to be identified, but theoretically such agents could be used as exogenous signals to induce a higher level of molecular polarity in cultured cells.

Identifying the steps in RPE morphogenesis and their controls will require considerable information about the molecular topography of cultured RPE cells. Such investigations would be aided by separated subpopulations of cells expressing different phenotypes, which could then be examined to determine how they differ and whether specific environmental additives convert one phenotype into another. Unfortunately, it is difficult to devise methods to separate cells if it is not known how they differ, and difficult to learn how cells differ if they are not separated. Only for fusiform and epithelioid RPE cells have enriched subcultures been produced (McKay and Burke, 1994), and the molecular basis for their phenotypic differences has not yet been determined. Morphogenesis in cultured RPE cells is likely to be a more complex process than in clonal cell lines selected for their ability to undergo rapid epithelialization in vitro. It is clear, however, that describing RPE cells as "polarized" on the basis of morphology alone is no longer sufficient, since the level of polarity for individual molecules can differ among cells and the factors regulating polarity for each molecule are also likely to differ.

THE RPE MONOLAYER IN SITU: CELL HETEROGENEITY AND PATHOLOGIC IMPLICATIONS OF ALTERED MORPHOLOGY

RPE Heterogeneity In Situ and the Regeneration of the Monolayer

We have questioned the phenotypic variability of cultured RPE cells partly because we perceive that the cells within eyes are homogeneous. But distinctly different RPE phenotypes are revealed in culture almost immediately after cells are isolated from human eyes, as early as the first spreading event (McKay and Burke, 1994), so perhaps despite their grossly similar appearance within the tissue, RPE cells are heterogeneous with regards to the molecular properties that determine phenotype in dissociated cells. Indeed, closer examination reveals that the in situ monolayer is not highly homogeneous even in gross phenotype, but rather consists of a micromosaic of cells varying in size, shape, regularity of cell borders, and amount of melanin and lipofuscin (Fig. 5-1). The extent to which cells differ at the molecular level is largely unknown, although individual RPE cells of bovine eyes have been shown to differ in the expression of the intermediate filament protein vimentin (Burke et al., 1995; Owaribe et al., 1988). Whether differences exist among individual cells in molecules implicated in morphogenesis, such as those comprising the adherens junction and its circumferential actin undercoat, remains to be determined.

Although the extent of molecular heterogeneity of RPE cells is not yet determined, it is clear that when the cells are dissociated and propagated in vitro, they lose epithelial polarity, then repolarize slowly and incompletely in culture. Perhaps this poor morphogenetic potential is to be expected if one considers the properties of the adult tissue. RPE cells originate from neural ectoderm and, as indicated above, there is question as to whether or when RPE cells express the potent epithelial morphogen E-cadherin (Gundersen et al., 1991; Marrs et al., 1993; 1995; Cao et al., 1997), which is found in most other monolayer epithelial cells. RPE cells nonetheless develop a polarized epithelium during embryogenesis, perhaps with the assistance of developmental cues which support epithelialization even in the absence of a potent endogenous morphoregulator. Once epithelialized, however, RPE cells in the adult tissue have little or no cell turnover (Coulombre, 1975), so they may have no ongoing requirement to maintain the machinery to epithelialize. In other words, the RPE monolayer in situ may polarize during a protracted period of embryogenesis, after which it remains essentially undisturbed at "confluency" for most of the organism's life.

Perhaps it is not surprising that cells from this tissue show a limited capacity to reepithelialize in vitro. In this regard the pigment epithelium can be contrasted with tissues like the gut epithelium, which continuously divides in the crypts and polarizes throughout life to form a mature epithelium at the tip of the villus of the intestinal wall.

Although RPE in the normal adult monolayer is quiescent with regards to cell proliferation, the cells are clearly capable of proliferating when they are dissociated and placed in culture. RPE cells in vitro re-form a monolayer that is at least contiguous if not fully epithelialized. It is reasonable to question whether similar events follow damage to the normal RPE monolayer within adult eyes, where after proliferation it is conceivable that the intraocular environment would support a higher level of RPE maturation than culture systems. But it is also possible that the adult eye would fail to support complete RPE reepithelializatin because, like culture systems, it also lacks critical cues that were present during embryogenesis when RPE morphogenesis occurred.

The extent of RPE regeneration within adult eyes has been investigated in animal models in which the RPE is debrided mechanically, photically, or chemically, as summarized in a recent review (Korte et al., 1994). The extent of RPE repair in situ has been shown to correlate with the magnitude of cell loss and with the condition of Bruch's membrane. The monolayer is restored to contiguity relatively rapidly and completely if lesions are small and the underlying matrix is undamaged, but the extent of RPE regeneration declines if large areas of the monolayer are denuded and/or if Bruch's membrane is injured. Monolayer repair is usually assessed by microscopic or clinical measures (e.g., ophthalmoscopy and/or fluorescein angiography) (Heriot and Machemer, 1992; Valentino et al., 1995). Poor repair is characterized by multilayering of the RPE with the persistence of cells with a "fibrocyte-like" appearance (Heriot and Machemer, 1992), whereas more complete regeneration results in RPE cells with a grossly normal appearance, including the presence of morphologically identifiable apicolateral junctional complexes (Valentino et al., 1995). RPE repair, however, in most of these injury models is incomplete if monolayer damage is extensive, and the damaged site remains detectable clinically for extended periods, even in small lesions, at least as a region of variable RPE pigmentation.

In terms of determining the completeness of RPE recovery in situ, these animal model studies suffer from the same limitations as studies of cultured cells in which morphologic measures of cell organization are used: cell–cell heterogeneity throughout and adjacent to the experimental lesion is difficult to appreciate, and the extent of recovery of molecular polarity is not known. The latter question has been addressed in some of the studies conducted by Korte and colleagues using the sodium iodate model of RPE destruction in the rabbit. Intravenous injection of this agent destroys posterior RPE, which is repaired by foci of spared cells in the retinal periphery (see Korte et al., 1994 for review). At least regionally, repaired areas of the RPE monolayer in the rabbit show regeneration of a polarized distribution of alkaline phosphatase (basal) and Na/K ATPase (apical) (Korte et al., 1991; Korte and Wanderman, 1993). The extent of repair throughout the monolayer, however, is unclear.

One rationale for analyzing damaged RPE in animal eyes is to gauge the capacity of the monolayer in human eyes to undergo repair and regeneration in conditions in which cells are lost, as recently discussed (Grierson et al., 1994). Retinal detachment, for example, can damage the RPE monolayer leading to RPE cell proliferation (Anderson et al., 1983; Machemer et al., 1975), which if uncontrolled produces disorders like proliferative vitreoretinopathy (Hiscott et al., 1989; 1991; Marino et al., 1990). Based on animal model studies and investigations of RPE in vitro, one might assume variable and perhaps incomplete regeneration of a normal RPE monolayer at the site of a retinal detachment. We have recently obtained anecdotal evidence that suggests that a well-ordered RPE monolayer may indeed not be restored adjacent to a detached retina. An eye was received from a donor whose history indicated that he had had an idiopathic inferior retinal detachment which was surgically repaired six years prior to his death at the age of 46. The RPE from the detachment site, which was detectable clinically as an area of pigment mottling, was stained with rhodamine-phalloidin to visualize actin circumferential microfilaments as an indicator of RPE cell shape. A few foci of epithelioid cells could be identified, but there were also extensive fields of fusiform cells (Fig. 5-5). This organization contrasted sharply with the regular appearance of the normal RPE monolayer in situ (Fig. 5-1); it rather resembled human RPE cultures which have intermingled fields of the phenotypic variants (Fig. 5-5). The duration of the detachment and the condition of the retina at the time of surgical reattachment for this eye are not known, but this intriguing observation suggests that damage to the RPE monolayer within adult human eyes triggers the development of many RPE phenotypes similar to those seen in vitro. Cultured cells may therefore reliably reflect the shapes that RPE cells will adopt within eyes if the tissue is disrupted. A further implication of the observation of a poorly re-formed monolayer at a detachment site is that

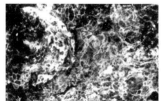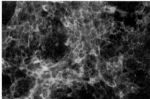

FIGURE 5-5. Fluorescence microscopy of human RPE cells stained with rhodamine phalloidin for actin. The cells shown at the left were in a human eye at the site of a retinal detachment that had been surgically repaired six years previously. A few small foci of epithelioid cells are present *(arrows)*, but the tissue consists primarily of whorls of cells lacking an obvious epithelial appearance. This appearance contrasts markedly with the monolayer in the normal eye (shown in Fig. 5-1C), but rather resembles human RPE cells in culture *(right)*, which after extended periods at confluency also have fields of epithelioid cells among less epithelioid phenotypes. Both magnified at ×75.

the adult eye following detachment may be little better than the culture environment for supporting complete RPE morphogenesis in all cells.

Relationship between Epithelial Function and Phenotype

Because normal epithelial cells have such a high level of cytoplasmic compartmentation, one might expect functional decrements if that compartmentation is disrupted or not fully restored after tissue damage. To what extent might RPE function be impaired if the monolayer is damaged in diseased or injured eyes? Assuming substantial RPE cell loss, markedly diminished barrier and vectorial transport functions might be expected, at least during the period in which the cells are not contiguous before the monolayer is restored. Since these functions of the pigment epithelium regulate the environment of adjacent photoreceptors, one would expect altered photoreceptor activity, although there are no specific data to indicate how well photoreceptors maintain their function when the adjacent RPE layer lacks epithelial organization. Pathogenic consequences have been ascribed to diminished barrier and transport function in epithelial cells (Fish and Molitoris, 1994).

In addition to reduced barrier and transport functions of the RPE when the monolayer is re-forming, these functions might also be affected for an extended period even after contiguity is reestablished. At least in vitro, the process of RPE morphogenesis is protracted, with the cells requiring several weeks after the monolayer is formed before the epithelioid phenotypes are fully developed (Burke et al., 1996), during which time the cells presumably lack polarity. As indicated previously, for other epithelial cell types the morphogenetic process that ensues after cell–cell contact is rapid, so the consequences of reduced function after tissue damage may be greater in the pigment epithelium than in other epithelia in which polarity is reattained more quickly and completely.

In addition to questioning the adequacy of RPE function during tissue repair and subsequent morphogenesis, one might also question the adequacy of function of an RPE monolayer which contains cells that differ in cell size, shape, and regularity. Stated differently, must an RPE monolayer consist of cells in a relatively regular hexagonal array in order to function efficiently? This question may not be merely academic since minor RPE cell loss may produce a monolayer with reduced hexagonality. During normal aging, for example, RPE cell number declines, although there is disagreement as to the extent and topography of the cell loss (Dorey et al., 1989; Feeney-Burns et al., 1990; Gao and Hollyfield, 1992; Watzke et al., 1993). In the fovea a specific diminution in the hexagonality of the RPE has been reported as a consequence of age (Watzke et al., 1993). This portion of the retina is susceptible to age-related degenerative changes and an accompanying reduction in high-acuity vision, so it is clearly of interest to determine whether diminished regularity of RPE cell shape in the aging eye reduces the functional support provided by the RPE for the adjacent retina.

Transport Is Not the Only Function Altered in Epithelial Cells with Disrupted Polarity

As implied above, lack of polarity of transporters like Na/K ATPase is expected to have negative consequences for the function of a transporting epithelium like the RPE, similar to the pathologic consequences described for other monolayer epithelial cells (Fish and Molitoris, 1994). However, lack of cell surface polarity has a much broader impact than a change in transport capabilities. Other molecules are also distributed to specific membrane domains of epithelial cells, notably receptor molecules for growth factors. The distribution of growth factor receptors to specific domains of RPE cells has not been determined, although several have been localized to the basolateral surface of other epithelial cells (Rodrigue-Boulan and Nelson, 1989). Sequestration of receptors to specific domains can limit receptor access to ligand, serving as a mechanism to regulate the cellular response to growth factors. Receptors can then be exposed to their ligands after disruption of epithelial surface polarity, leading to a rapid cellular response in the absence of changes in the levels of either growth factors or their receptors. Whether this mechanism for growth factor regulation occurs in RPE cells is unknown, al-

though there has been considerable interest in growth factors as potential contributors to uncontrolled RPE growth in proliferative ocular disorders. RPE cells in vitro have been shown to express many receptors and to respond by growth or migration to many growth factors (Leschey et al., 1990 and references therein), but the level of epithelial organization of the cultures is usually not reported and the position of receptors on the RPE cell surface has not been determined. However, culture confluency has been known for some time to increase the mitogenic effect of some growth factors (e.g., EGF) and decrease the effect of others (e.g., TNF-α) (Burke, 1989). Culture density also affects bFGF gene expression by RPE cells (Bost et al., 1992; Bost and Hjelmeland, 1993) with higher expression found in cells after disruption of Ca^{2+}-dependent adhesions (Bost et al., 1994). These observations implicate cell contact and adhesion formation, the triggering events for epithelialization (Rodriguez-Boulan and Nelson, 1989; Takeichi, 1991), as modulators of growth factor response and production in RPE cells. Loss of junctional integrity in the RPE monolayer with its concomitant loss of epithelial polarity may therefore profoundly affect the tissue's response to its environment.

Indeed, epithelial junctions have a more direct involvement in regulating the cell's response to its environment than helping to maintain cell surface polarity, since the junction itself is a site of cell-to-cell signaling (Hinck et al., 1994a; Woods and Bryant, 1993). The EGF receptor has been found in a catenin complex in epithelial cell lines (Hoschuetzky et al., 1994), and at least one of the substrates for this receptor tyrosine kinase, pp60[src], has been localized to the adherens junction (Tsukita et al., 1991). Several molecules in cadherin/catenin complexes can be phosphorylated on tyrosine (Hamaguchi et al., 1993; Matsuyoshi et al., 1992), and increased junctional phosphorylation occurs at some stages of junction formation/dissembly in epithelial cells (Volberg et al., 1992) including the RPE (Burke et al., 1996). Further, phosphorylation of adherens junction proteins accompanies exposure of epithelial cells to growth factors like EGF and SF/HGF which regulate cell proliferation, motility, and shape (Hoschuetzky et al., 1994; Shibamoto et al., 1994, 1995). At least for some epithelial cells, therefore, the adherens junction appears to play a key role in growth factor signaling. A junctional distribution has been shown for pp60[src] in RPE cells at some stages of epithelial morphogenesis (Koh, 1992; Moszczynska and Opas, 1994), but little is known about the participation of the RPE adherens junction in the regulation of the cell's response to growth factors. It should be considered, however, that changes in the integrity of RPE junctions, as would occur with damage to the monolayer, will affect not only cellular phenotype but also whether and in what way RPE cells respond to exogenous signaling molecules.

Alteration of RPE phenotype and function by disruption of the monolayer and its limited capacity to re-form a well-epithelialized monolayer also have ramifications for the future success of RPE transplantation therapy. This method is being explored as a technique to replace diseased or damaged RPE cells to restore the support provided by the RPE for the adjacent sensory retina (Bok, 1993; Bok et al., 1993). The focus of the research on RPE transplantation has been on its ability to rescue photoreceptors from degeneration (Gaur et al., 1992; LaVail et al., 1992; Yamamoto et al., 1993), and on developing methods to successfully introduce viable RPE cells into the subretinal space so as to maximize transplant survival while minimizing tissue rejection (Sheng et al., 1995 and references therein). For optimum function of epithelial cells, it is likely that patency of the transplanted tissue will not be enough. The tissue must also be well epithelialized to interact normally with the photoreceptors it is intended to support. The ideal donor tissue would be a polarized RPE monolayer, and the ideal transplantation protocol would cause minimal tissue disruption during insertion. It remains a challenge to identify or produce tissues that would provide good donor material and it is equally challenging to develop strategies to stimulate maturation of the transplanted cells within host eyes. This latter effort is hampered by a lack of information about the morphogenetic program employed by RPE cells to produce an epithelial phenotype, and the triggers required to stimulate a high proportion of cells to complete the program.

SUMMARY

Studies of molecular morphogenesis of epithelial cells from tissues like the RPE lag behind studies of morphogenesis of epithelial cell lines. There is a practical reason for this: cell lines are readily available and easily cloned to produce populations that are homogenous in appearance and synchronous in the events of morphogenesis. Indeed, clones are selected because they express the property slated for investigation, polarization of the cell surface, for example, then the process that is identified in these highly selected cells tends to be generalized to all cells of that type. However, the generalizations may be inaccurate since the level of complexity of tissue-derived epithelial cells such as those propagated from the RPE monolayer may be substantially higher. The discussion here has been focused on the cell–cell ad-

herens junction, which appears to play a pivotal role in the development of epithelial organization in other epithelial cells. The molecular composition of this junction, especially the elements that mediate linkage with the cytoskeleton, and the regulation of junction assembly and dissembly are fruitful areas of future research for all epithelial cells, including the RPE. It has been theorized here that junction formation and cell surface polarization results from a time-dependent series of molecular events partially controlled by an intrinsic morphogenetic program and partially regulated by extrinsic signals. If this is correct, the sequence of events is likely to be complicated, especially in cells of RPE origin in which the program may differ among individual cells, and in which the process may occur over a protracted time course.

It is becoming progressively more obvious as the molecular events of epithelial morphogenesis are dissected that *phenotype* is not merely a descriptive term. The morphology adopted by epithelial cells is both the result of a series of molecular events and a reflection of the functional state of the cell at a given point in time. As the steps in the process of epithelial morphogenesis are identified, the range of functions of the cell will also be revealed. We have considered the phenotypic "imperfection" of RPE cultures undesirable, but such cultures are useful for determining the functional potential of cells from this tissue, and the phenotypes that are displayed in vitro may reflect the phenotypes that are produced in situ when the mature monolayer is damaged. Ultimately, however, as the cues for RPE morphogenesis are revealed, it may be possible to produce the highly ordered RPE monolayers in vitro that we have sought but that have so far eluded us.

ACKNOWLEDGMENTS

Some of the studies described here were conducted with the assistance of Anna Fekete, Christine Brzeski Skumatz, and Pamela Irving, and supported by NEI grants RO1 EY06664, RO1 EY10832, P30 EY01931, and by an unrestricted grant from Research to Prevent Blindness, Inc.

REFERENCES

Anderson DH, Stern WH, Fisher SK, Erickson PA, Borgula GA. 1983. Retinal detachment in the cat: the pigment epithelial-photoreceptor interface. Invest Ophthalmol Vis Sci 24:906–926.

Anderson DH, Guérin CJ, Matsumoto B, Pfeffer BA. 1990. Identification and localization of a beta-1 receptor from the integrin family in mammalian retinal pigment epithelial cells. Invest Ophthalmol Vis Sci 31:81–93.

Arikawa K, Williams FS. 1991. Alpha-actinin and actin in the outer retina: a double immunoelectron microscopic study. Cell Motility and the Cytoskeleton 18:15–25.

Aronson JF. 1983. Human retinal pigment cell culture. In Vitro 19:642–650.

Bok D. 1982. Autoradiographic studies on the polarity of plasma membrane receptors in RPE cells. In: Hollyfield J, ed, The Structure of the Eye. New York: Elsevier North Holland, 247–256.

Bok D. 1993. Retinal transplantation and gene therapy. Invest Ophthalmol Vis Sci 34:473–476.

Bok D, Heller J. 1976. Transport of retinol from the blood to the retina: an autoradiographic study of the pigment epithelial cell surface receptor for plasma retinol-binding protein. Exp Eye Res 22:395.

Bok D, O'Day W, Rodriguez-Boulan E. 1992. Polarized budding of vesicular stomatitis and influenza virus from cultured human and bovine retinal pigment epithelium. Exp Eye Res 55:853–860.

Bok D, Hageman GS, Steinberg RH, for the Photoreceptor/Retinal Pigment Epithelium Panel. 1993. Repair and replacement to restore sight. Arch Ophthalmol 111:463–471.

Bost LM, Hjelmeland LM. 1993. Cell density regulates differential production of bFGF transcripts. Growth Factors 9:195–203.

Bost LM, Aotaki-Keen AE, Hjelmeland LM. 1992. Coexpression of FGF-5 and bFGF by the retinal pigment epithelium in vitro. Exp Eye Res 55:727–734.

Bost LM, Aotaki-Keen AE, Hjelmeland LM. 1994. Cellular adhesion regulates bFGF gene expression in human retinal pigment epithelial cells. Exp Eye Res 58:545–552.

Brady-Kalnay SM, Rimm DL, Tonks NK. 1995. Receptor protein tyrosine phosphatase PTPμ associates with cadherins and catenins in vivo. J Cell Biol 130:977–986.

Burke JM. 1989. Stimulation of DNA synthesis in human and bovine RPE by peptide growth factors: the response to TNF-α and EGF is dependent upon culture density. Curr Eye Res 8:1279–1286.

Burke JM, Skumatz CMB, Irving PE, McKay BS. 1996. Phenotypic heterogeneity of retinal pigment epithelial cells in vitro and in situ. Exp Eye Res 62:63–73.

Campochiaro PA, Hackett SF. 1993. Corneal endothelial cell matrix promotes expression of differentiated features of retinal pigmented epithelial cells: implication of laminin and basic fibroblast growth factor as active components. Exp Eye Res 57:539–547.

Campochiaro PA, Hackett SF, Conway BP. 1991. Retinoic acid promotes density-dependent growth arrest in human retinal pigment epithelial cells. Invest Ophthalmol Vis Sci 32:65–72.

Cao F, Irving PE, Burke JM. 1997. Human retinal pigment epithelium expresses E-cadherin. Mol. Biol. Cell (Suppl.), 8:188a.

Chu P, Grunwald GB. 1991. Identification of the 2A10 antigen of retinal pigment epithelium as a beta-1 subunit of integrin. Invest Ophthalmol Vis Sci 32:1757–1762.

Coulombre AJ. 1979. Roles of the retinal pigment epithelium in the development of ocular tissues. In: Zinn KM, Marmor MF, eds., The Retinal Pigment Epithelium. Cambridge, MA: Harvard University Press, 54.

Davis AA, Bernstein PS, Bok D, Turner J, Nachtigal M, Hunt RC. 1995. A human retinal pigment epithelial cell line that retains epithelial characteristics after prolonged culture. Invest Ophthalmol Vis Sci 36:955–964.

DiMattio J, Degnan KJ, Zadunaisky JA. 1983. A model for transepithelial ion transport across the isolated retinal pigment epithelium of the frog. Exp Eye Res 37:409–420.

Docherty RJ, Forrester JV, Lackie JM. 1987. Type I collagen permits invasive behaviour by retinal pigmented epithelial cells in vitro. J Cell Sci 87:399–409.

Dorey CK, Wu G, Ebenstein D, Garsd A, Weiter JJ. 1989. Cell loss in the aging retina: relationship to lipofuscin accumulation and macular degeneration. Invest Ophthalmol Vis Sci 30:1691–1699.

Dutt K, Scott MM, Del Monte M, Brennan M, Harris-Hooker S, Kaplan HF, Verly G. 1991. Extracellular matrix mediated growth and differentiation in human pigment epithelial cell line 0041. Curr Eye Res 10:1089–1100.

Edelman JL, Miller SS. 1991. Epinephrine stimulates fluid absorption across bovine retinal pigment epithelium. Invest Ophthalmol Vis Sci 32:3033–3040.

Feeney-Burns L, Burns RP, Gao C-L. 1990. Age-related macular changes in humans over 90 years old. Am J Ophthalmol 109: 265–278.

Fish EM, Molitoris BA. 1994. Mechanisms of disease: alterations in epithelial cell polarity and the pathogenesis of disease states. N Engl J Med 330:1580–1588.

Fliesler SJ, Cole GJ, Adler AJ. 1990. Neural cell adhesion molecule (NCAM) in adult vertebrate retinas: tissue localization and evidence against its role in retina-pigment epithelial adhesion. Exp Eye Res 50:475–482.

Gao H, Hollyfield JG. 1992. Aging of the human retina. Differential loss of neurons and retinal pigment epithelial cells. Invest Ophthalmol Vis Sci 33:1–17.

Gaur V, Agarwal N, Li L, Turner JE. 1992. Maintenance of opsin and S-antigen gene expression in RCS dystrophic rats following RPE transplantation. Exp Eye Res 54:91–101.

Geiger B, Ayalon O. 1992. Cadherins. Annu Rev Cell Biol 8:307–332.

Gordon SR, Essner E. 1987. Investigations on circumferential microfilament bundles in rat retinal pigment epithelium. Eur J Cell Biol 44:97–104.

Gottardi CJ, Caplan MJ. 1993. Delivery of Na+,K+-ATPase in polarized epithelial cells. Science 260:552–553.

Grierson I, Hiscott P, Hogg P, Robey H, Mazure A, Larkin G. 1994. Development, repair and regeneration of the retinal pigment epithelium. Eye 8:255–262.

Gumbiner BM, McCrea PD. 1993. Catenins as mediators of the cytoplasmic functions of cadherins. J Cell Sci 17(Suppl):155–158.

Gundersen D, Orlowski J, Rodriguez-Boulan E. 1991. Apical polarity of Na,K-ATPase in retinal pigment epithelium is linked to a reversal of the ankyrin-fodrin submembrane cytoskeleton. J Cell Biol 112:863–872.

Gunderson D, Powell SK, Rodriguez-Boulan E. 1993. Apical polarization of N-CAM in retinal pigment epithelium is dependent on contact with the neural retina. J Cell Biol 121:335–343.

Hamaguchi M, Matsuyoshi N, Ohnishi Y, Gotoh B, Takeichi M, Nagai Y. 1993. p60^v-src causes tyrosine phosphorylation and inactivation of the N-cadherin-catenin cell adhesion system. EMBO J 12:307–314.

Hammerton RW, Krzeminksi KA, Mays RW, Ryan TA, Wollner DA, Nelson WJ. 1991. Mechanism for regulating cell surface distribution of Na+,K+-ATPase in polarized epithelial cells. Science 254:847–850.

Heth CA, Yankauckas MA, Adamian M, Edwards RB. 1987. Characterization of retinal pigment epithelial cells cultured on microporous filters. Curr Eye Res 6:1007–1019.

Heriot WJ, Machemer R. 1992. Pigment epithelial repair. Graefes Arch Clin Exp Ophthalmol 230:91–100.

Hernandez EV, Hu JG, Frambach DA, Gallemore RP. 1995. Potassium conductances in cultured bovine and human retinal pigment epithellium. Invest Ophthalmol Vis Sci 36:113–122.

Herrenknecht K, Ozawa M, Eckerskorn C, Lottspeich F, Lenter M, Kemler R. 1991. The uvomorulin-anchorage protein alpha catenin is a vinculin homologue. Proc Nat Acad Sci USA 88:9156–9160.

Hinck L, Näthke IS, Papkoff J, Nelson WJ. 1994a. β-Catenin: a common target for the regulation of cell adhesion by Wnt-1 and Src signaling pathways. TIBS 19:538–542.

Hinck L, Näthke IS, Papkoff J, Nelson WJ. 1994b. Dynamics of cadherin/catenin complex formation: novel protein interactions and pathways of complex assembly. J Cell Biol 125:1327–1340.

Hiscott P, Grierson I. 1991. Subretinal membranes of proliferative vitreoretinopathy. Br J Ophthalmol 75:53.

Hiscott P, McLeod D, Grierson I, Unger W. 1989. Contractile epiretinal membranes in experimental intraocular inflammation. In: Heimann K, Wiedemann P, eds, Proliferative Vitreoretinopathy. Heidelberg: Kaden Verlag, 58–62.

Hitt AL, Luna EJ. 1994. Membrane interactions with the actin cytoskeleton. Curr Opinion Cell Biol 6:120–130.

Hoschuetzky H, Aberle H, Kemler R. 1994. β-Catenin mediates the interaction of the cadherin-catenin complex with epidermal growth factor receptor. J Cell Biol 127:1375–1380.

Hu JG, Gallemore RP, Bok D, Lee AY, Frambach DA. 1994. Localization of NaK ATPase on cultured human retinal pigment epithelium. Invest Ophthalmol Vis Sci 35:3582–3588.

Hulksen J, Birchmeier W, Behrens J. 1994. E-cadherin and APC compete for the interaction with β-catenin and the cytoskeleton. J Cell Biol 127:2061–2069.

Huotari V, Sormunen R, Veli-Pekka L, Eskelinen S. 1995. The polarity of the membrane skeleton in retinal pigment epithelial cells of developing chicken embryos and in primary culture. Differentiation 58:205–215.

Islam S, Carey TE, Wolf GT, Wheelock MJ, Johnson KR. 1996. Expression of N-cadherin by human squamous carcinoma cells induces a scattered fibroblastic phenotype with disrupted cell-cell adhesion. J Cell Biol 135:1643–1654.

Joseph DP, Miller SS. 1991. Apical and basal membrane ion transport mechanisms in bovine retinal pigment epithelium. J Physiol 435: 439–463.

Kennedy SP, Warren SL, Forget BG, Morrow JS. 1991. Ankyrin binds to the 15th repetitive unit of erythroid and nonerythroid β-spectrin. J Cell Biol 115:267–277.

Kenyon E, Yu K, la Cour M, Miller SS. 1994. Lactate transport mechanisms at the apical and basolateral membranes of bovine retinal pigment epithelium. Am J Physiol 267:C1561–C1573.

Kirchhof B, Kirchhof E, Ryan SJ, Sorgente N. 1988. Human retinal pigment epithelial cell cultures: phenotypic modulation by vitreous and macrophages. Exp Eye Res 47:457–463.

Knudsen KA, Soler AP, Johnson KR, Wheelock MJ. 1995. Interaction of α-actinin with the cadherin/catenin cell-cell adhesion complex via α-catenin. J Cell Biol 130:67–77.

Kodama R, Eguchi G, Kelley RO. 1991. Ultrastructural and immunocytochemical analysis of the circumferential microfilament bundle in avian retinal pigmented epithelial cells in vitro. Cell Tissue Res 263:29–40.

Koh S-WM. 1992. The pp60[c-src] in retinal pigment epithelium and its modulation by vasoactive intestinal peptide. Cell Biol Internatl Rep 16:1003–1014.

Korte GE, Wanderman MC. 1993. Distribution of Na+ K+-ATPase in regenerating retinal pigment epithelium in the rabbit. A study by electron microscopic cytochemistry. Exp Eye Res 56:219–229.

Korte GE, Rappa E, Andracchi S. 1991. Localization of alkaline phosphatase on basolateral plasma membrane of normal and regenerating retinal pigment epithelium. Invest Ophthalmol Vis Sci 32:3187–3197.

Korte GE, Perlman JI, Pollack A. 1994. Regeneration of mammalian retinal pigment epithelium. Int Rev Cytol 152:223–263.

Kyte J. 1981. Molecular mechanisms relevant to the mechanism of active transport. Nature 282:201.

la Cour M, Lin H, Kenyon E, Miller SS. 1994. Lactate transport in freshly isolated human fetal retinal pigment epithelium. Invest Ophthalmol Vis Sci 35:434–442.

Lagunowich LA, Grunwald GB. 1989. Expression of calcium-dependent cell adhesion during ocular development: a biochemical, histochemical and functional analysis. Dev Biol 135:158–171.

Lagunowich LA, Grunwald GB. 1991. Tissue and age-specificity of post-translational modifications of N-cadherin during chick embryo development. Differentiation 47:19–27.

Larjava H, Peltonen J, Akiyama SK, Yamada SS, Gralnick HR, Uitto J, Yamada KM. 1990. Novel function for β1 integrins in keratinocyte cell-cell interactions. J Cell Biol 110:803–815.

LaVail MM, Li L, Turner JE, Yasumura D. 1992. Retinal pigment epithelial cell transplantation in RCS rats: normal metabolism in rescued photoreceptors. Exp Eye Res 55:555–562.

Leschey KH, Hackett SF, Singer SH, Campochiaro PA. 1990. Growth factor responsiveness of human retinal pigment epithelial cells. Invest Ophthalmol Vis Sci 31:839–846.

Lin H, Miller SS. 1991. pH$_i$ regulation in frog retinal pigment epithelium: two apical membrane mechanisms. Am J Physiol 261:C132–C142.

Lin H, Miller SS. 1994. I. pH$_i$ dependent Cl-HCO$_3$ exchange at the basolateral membrane of frog retinal pigment epithelium. Am J Physiol 266:C935–C945.

Lin H, la Cour M, Andersen MVN, Miller SS. 1994. Proton-lactate cotransport in the apical membrane of frog retinal pigment epithelium. Exp Eye Res 59:679–688.

Luna EJ, Hitt AL. 1992. Cytoskeleton-plasma membrane interactions. Science 258:955–963.

Machemer R, Laqua H. 1975. Pigment epithelial proliferation in retinal detachment (massive periretinal proliferation). Am J Ophthalmol 80:1–23.

Marino I, Hiscott P, McKechnie N, Grierson I. 1990. Variation in epiretinal membrane components with clinical derivation of the proliferative tissue. Br J Ophthalmol 74:393–399.

Marmorstein AD, Bonilha VL, Chiflet S, Neill JM, Rodriguez-Boulan F. 1996. The polarity of the plasma membrane protein RET-PE2 in retinal pigment epithelium is developmentally regulated. J. Cell Sci. 109:3025–3034.

Marrs JA, Napolitano EW, Murphy-Erdosh C, Mays RW, Reichardt LF, Nelson WJ. 1993. Distinguishing roles of the membrane-cytoskeleton and cadherin mediated cell-cell adhesion in generating different Na+,K+-ATPase distributions in polarized epithelia. J Cell Biol 123:148–164.

Marrs JA, Andersson-Fisone C, Jeong MC, Cohen-Gould L, Zurzolo C, Nabi IR, Rodriguez-Boulan E, Nelson WJ. 1995. Plasticity in epithelial cell phenotype: modulation by expression of different cadherin cell adhesion molecules. J Cell Biol 129:507–519.

Martini B, Wang H-M, Lee BM, Ogden TE, Ryan SJ, Sorgente N. 1991. Synthesis of extracellular matrix by macrophage-modulated retinal pigment epithelium. Arch Ophthalmol 109:576–580.

Martini B, Pandey R, Ogden TE, Ryan SJ. 1992. Cultures of human retinal pigment epithelium. Invest Ophthalmol Vis Sci 33:516–521.

Matsumoto B, Guérin CJ, Anderson DH. 1990. Cytoskeletal redifferentiation of feline, monkey, and human RPE cells in culture. Invest Ophthalmol Vis Sci 31:879–889.

Matsuyoshi N, Hamaguchi M, Taniguchi S, Nagafuchi A, Tsukita Sh, Takeichi M. 1992. Cadherin-mediated cell-cell adhesion is perturbed by v-src tyrosine phosphorylation in metastatic fibroblasts. J Cell Biol 118:703–714.

Mays RW, Siemers KA, Fritz BA, Lowe AW, van Meer G, Nelson WJ. 1995. Hierarchy of mechanisms involved in generating Na/K-

ATPase polarity in MDCK epithelial cells. J Cell Biol 130:1105–1115.

McKay BS, Burke JM. 1994. Separation of phenotypically distinct subpopulations of cultured human retinal pigment epithelial cells. Exp Cell Res 213:85–92.

McKay BS, Irving PE, Skumatz CMB, Burke JM. 1997. Cell-cell adhesion molecules and the development of an epithelial phenotype in cultured human retinal pigment epithelial cells. Exp. Eye Res., in press.

McNeill H, Ozawa M, Kemler R, Nelson WJ. 1990. Novel function of the cell adhesion molecule uvomorulin as an inducer of cell surface polarity. Cell 62:309–316.

McNeill H, Ryan TA, Smith SJ, Nelson WJ. 1993. Spatial and temporal dissection of immediate and early events following cadherin-mediated epithelial cell adhesion. J Cell Biol 12:1217–1226.

Mircheff AK, Miller SS, Farber DB, Bradley ME, O'Day WT, Bok D. 1990. Isolation and provisional identification of plasma membrane populations from cultured human retinal pigment epithelium. Invest Ophthalmol Vis Sci 31:863–878.

Mooseker MS. 1985. Organization, chemistry, and assembly of the cytoskeletal apparatus of the intestinal brush border. Annu Rev Cell Biol 1:209–242.

Moszczynska A, Opas M. 1994. Regulation of adhesion-related protein tyrosine kinases during in vitro differentiation of retinal pigment epithelial cells: translocation of pp60[c-src] to the nucleus is accompanied by downregulation of pp125[FAK]. Biochem Cell Biol 72:43–47.

Murphy-Erdosh C, Napolitano EW, Reichardt LF. 1994. The expression of B-cadherin during embryonic chick development. Dev Biol 161:107–125.

Nabi IR, Mathews AP, Cohen-Gould L, Gundersen D, Rodriguez-Boulan E. 1993. Immortalization of polarized rat retinal pigment epithelium. J Cell Sci 104:37–49.

Nagafuchi A, Takeichi M, Tsukita S. 1991. The 102 kd cadherin-associated protein: similarity to vinculin and post-transcriptional regulation of expression. Cell 65:849–857.

Näthke IS, Hinck LE, Nelson WJ. Epithelial cell adhesion and development of cell surface polarity: possible mechanisms for modulation of cadherin function, organization and distribution. J Cell Sci 17(Suppl):139–145.

Neill JM, Barnstable CJ. 1990. Expression of the cell surface antigens RET-PE2 and N-CAM by rat retinal pigment epithelial cells during development and in tissue culture. Exp Eye Res 51:573–583.

Nelson WJ. Cytoskeleton functions in membrane traffic in polarized epithelial cells. Cell Biol 2:375–385.

Nelson WJ, Veshnock PJ. 1986. Dynamics of membrane-skeleton (fodrin) organization during development of polarity in Madin-Darby canine kidney epithelial cells. J Cell Biol 103:1751–1766.

Nelson WJ, Veshnock PJ. 1987. Ankyrin binding to Na+,K+-ATPase and implications for the organization of membrane domains in polarized cells. Nature 28:533–536.

Nelson WJ, Hammerton RW. 1989. A membrane-cytoskeletal complex containing Na+,K+-ATPase, ankyrin, and fodrin in Madin-Darby canine kidney (MDCK) cells: implications for the biogenesis of epithelial cell polarity. J Cell Biol 108:893–902.

Nguyen-Tan JQ, Thompson JT. 1989. RPE cell migration into intact vitreous body. Retina 9:203–209.

Opas M. 1989. Expression of the differentiated phenotype by epithelial cells in vitro is regulated by both biochemistry and mechanics of the substratum. Dev Biol 131:281–293.

Opas M, Turksen K, Kalnins VI. 1985. Adhesiveness and distribution of vinculin and spectrin in retinal pigmented epithelial cells during growth and differentiation in vitro. Dev Biol 107:269–280.

Owaribe K, Kartenbeck J, Rungger-Brändle E, Franke WW. 1988. Cytoskeletons of retinal pigment epithelial cells: interspecies differences of expression patterns indicate independence of cell function from the specific complement of cytoskeletal proteins. Cell Tissue Res 254:301–315.

Philp NJ, Nachmias VT. 1985. Components of the cytoskeleton in the retinal pigmented epithelium of the chick. J Cell Biol 101:358–362.

Philp NJ, Nachmias VT. 1987. Polarized distribution of integrin and fibronectin in retinal pigment epithelium. Invest Ophthalmol Vis Sci 28:1275–1280.

Philp NJ, Yoon M-Y, Hock RS. 1990. Identification and localization of talin in chick retinal pigment epithelial cells. Exp Eye Res 51:191–198.

Quinn RH, Miller SS. 1992. Ion transport mechanisms in native human retinal pigment epithelium. Invest Ophthalmol Vis Sci 33:3513–3527.

Reynolds AB, Daniel J, McCrea PD, Wheelock MJ, Wu J, Zhang Z. 1994. Identification of a new catenin: the tyrosine kinase substrate p120[cas] associates with E-cadherin complexes. Mol Cell Biol 14:8333–8342.

Rizzolo LJ. 1990. The distribution of Na+,K+-ATPase in the retinal pigmented epithelium from chicken embryo is polarized in vivo but not in primary cell culture. Exp Eye Res 51:435–446.

Rizzolo LJ. 1991. Basement membrane stimulates the polarized distribution of integrins but not the Na,K-ATPase in the retinal pigment epithelium. Cell Regulation 2:939–949.

Rizzolo LJ, Heiges M. 1991. The polarity of the retinal pigment epithelium is developmentally regulated. Exp Eye Res 53:549–552.

Rizzolo LJ, Joshi HC. 1993. Apical orientation of the microtubule organizing center and associated gamma-tubulin during the polarization of the retinal pigment epithelium in vivo. Dev Biol 157:147–156.

Rizzolo LJ, Li Z-Q. 1993. Diffusible, retinal factors stimulate the barrier properties of junctional complexes in the retinal pigment epithelium. J Cell Sci 106:859–867.

Rizzolo LJ, Zhou S. 1995. The distribution of Na+,K+-ATPase and 5A11 antigen in apical microvilli of the retinal pigment epithelium is unrelated to α-spectrin. J Cell Sci 108:3623–3633.

Rizzolo LJ, Zhou S, Li Z-Q. 1994. The neural retina maintains integrins in the apical membrane of the RPE early in development. Invest Ophthalmol Vis Sci 35:2567–2576.

Rodriguez-Boulan E, Nelson WJ. 1989. Morphogenesis of the polarized epithelial cell phenotype. Science 245:718–725.

Ruiz A, Bhat SP, Bok D. 1995. Characterization and quantification of full-length and truncated Na,K-ATPase α1 and β1 RNA transcripts expressed in human retinal pigment epithelium. Gene 155:179–184.

Sandig M, Hergott GJ, Kalnins VI. 1990. Effects of trypsin and low Ca2+ on zonulae adhaerentes between chick retinal pigment epithelial cells in organ culture. Cell Motility and the Cytoskeleton 17:46–58.

Schoenenberger C-A, Zuk A, Zinkl GM, Kendall D, Matlin KS. 1994. Integrin expression and localization in normal MDCK cells and transformed MDCK cells lacking apical polarity. J Cell Sci 107:527–541.

Sheng Y, Gouras P, Cao H, Berglin L, Kjeldbye H, Lopez R, Rosskothen H. 1995. Patch transplants of human fetal retinal pigment epithelium in rabbit and monkey retina. Invest Ophthalmol Vis Sci 36:381–390.

Shibamoto S, Hayakawa M, Takeuchi K, Hori T, Oku N, Miyazawa K, Kitamura N, Takeichi M, Ito F. 1994. Tyrosine phosphorylation of β-catenin and plakoglobin enhanced by hepatocyte growth factor and epidermal growth factor in human carcinoma cells. Cell Adhesion and Communication 1:295–305.

Shibamoto S, Hayakawa M, Takeuchi K, Hori T, Miyazawa K, Kitamura N, Johnson KR, Wheelock MJ, Matsuyoshi N, Takeichi M, Ito F. 1995. Association of p120, a tyrosine kinase substrate, with E-cadherin/catenin complexes. J Cell Biol 128:949–957.

Shirakawa H, Yoshimura N, Ogino N. 1986. Growth factors induce actin disruption in cultured human retinal pigment epithelial cells. Ophthalmic Res 18:338–342.

Siemers KA, Wilson R, Mays RW, Ryan TA, Wollner DA, Nelson WJ. 1993. Delivery of Na⁺,K⁺-ATPase in polarized epithelial cells. Science 260:554–556.

Song M-K, Lui GM. 1990. Propagation of fetal human RPE cells: preservation of original culture morphology after serial passage. J Cell Physiol 143:196–203.

Takeichi M. 1991. Cadherin cell adhesion receptors as a morphogenetic regulator. Science 251:1451–1455.

Takeichi M. 1995. Morphogenetic roles of classical cadherins. Curr Opinion Cell Biol 7:619–627.

Tarnowski BI, Shepherd VL, McLaughlin BJ. 1988. Mannose 6-phosphate receptors on the plasma membrane of rat retinal pigment epithelial cells. Invest Ophthalmol Vis Sci 29:291–297.

Tsukita Sa, Oishi K, Akiyama T, Yamanashi Y, Yamamoto T, Tsukita Sh. 1991. Specific proto-oncogenic tyrosine kinases of src family are enriched in cell-to-cell adherens junctions where the level of tyrosine phosphorylation is elevated. J Cell Biol 113:867–879.

Tugizov S, Maidji E, Pereira L. 1996. Role of apical and basolateral membranes in replication of human cytomegalovirus in polarized retinal pigment epithelial cells. J Gen Virol 77:61–74.

Turksen K, Kalnins VI. 1987. The cytoskeleton of chick retinal pigment epithelial cells in situ. Cell Tissue Res 248:95–101.

Turksen K, Opas M, Kalnins VI. 1987. Preliminary characterization of cell surface-extracellular matrix linkage complexes in cultured retinal pigmented epithelial cells. Exp Cell Res 171:259–264.

Valentino TL, Kaplan HJ, Del Priore LV, Fang S-R, Berger A, Silverman MS. 1995. Retinal pigment epithelial repopulation in monkeys after submacular surgery. Arch Ophthalmol 113:932–938.

Vidaurri-Leal J, Hohman R, Glaser BM. 1984. Effect of vitreous on morphologic characteristics of retinal pigment epithelial cells. A new approach to the study of proliferative vitreoretinopathy. Arch Ophthalmol 102:1220–1223.

Vinores SA, Campochiaro PA, McGehee R, Orman W, Hackett SF, Hjelmeland LM. 1990. Ultrastructural and immunocytochemical changes in retinal pigment epithelium, retinal glia, and fibroblasts in vitreous culture. Invest Ophthalmol Vis Sci 31:2529–2545.

Volberg T, Zick Y, Dror R, Sabanay I, Gilon C, Levitzki A, Geiger B. 1992. The effect of tyrosine-specific protein phosphorylation on the assembly of adherens-type junctions. EMBO J 11:1733–1742.

Wang AZ, Ojakian GK, Nelson WJ. 1990. Steps in the morphogenesis of a polarized epithelium. I. Uncoupling the roles of cell-cell and cell-substratum contact in establishing plasma membrane polarity in multicellular epithelial (MDCK) cysts. J Cell Sci 95:137–151.

Watzke RC, Soldevilla JD, Trune DR. 1993. Morphometric analysis of human retinal pigment epithelium: correlation with age and location. Curr Eye Res 12:133–142.

Wolfensberger TJ, Mahieu I, Jarvis-Evans J, Boulton M, Carter ND, Nógrádi A, Hollande E, Bird AC. 1994. Membrane-bound carbonic anhydrase in human retinal pigment epithelium. Invest Ophthalmol Vis Sci 35:3401–3407.

Wollner DA, Krzeminski KA, Nelson WJ. 1992. Remodeling the cell surface distribution of membrane proteins during the development of epithelial cell polarity. J Cell Biol 116:889–899.

Wollner DA, Nelson WJ. 1992. Establishing and maintaining epithelial cell polarity: roles of protein sorting, delivery and retention. J Cell Sci 102:185–190.

Woods DF, Bryant PJ. 1993. Apical junctions and cell signalling in epithelia. J Cell Sci 17(Suppl):171–181.

Yamamoto S, Du J, Gouras P, Kjeldbye H. 1993. Retinal pigment epithelial transplants and retinal function in RCS rats. Invest Ophthalmol Vis Sci 34:3068–3075.

Yonemura S, Itoh M, Nagafuchi A, Tsukita Sh. 1995. Cell-to-cell adherens junction formation and actin filament organization: similarities and differences between non-polarized fibroblasts and polarized epithelial cells. J Cell Sci 108:127–142.

Zhao S, Rizzolo LJ, Barnstable CJ. 1997. Differentiation and transdifferentiation of the retinal pigment epithelium. Int. Rev. Cytol. 171:225–266.

Zhou Y, Moszczynska A, Opas M. 1994. Generation and characterization of antibodies to adhesion-related molecules and retinal pigment epithelial cells. Exp Eye Res 58:585–594.

Zurzolo C, Rodriguez-Boulan E. 1993. Delivery of Na⁺,K⁺-ATPase in polarized epithelial cells. Science 260:550–552.

6. Transport mechanisms in the retinal pigment epithelium

BRET A. HUGHES, RON P. GALLEMORE, AND SHELDON S. MILLER

The health and integrity of retinal neurons depends on a well-regulated extracellular environment, and this is achieved by the activities of a variety of accessory cells. One of these cells, the retinal pigment epithelium (RPE), plays a central role in regulating the microenvironment surrounding the photoreceptors in the distal retina, where the events of phototransduction take place. Critical functions of the RPE that contribute to this process include phagocytosis of photoreceptor outer segment tips (Bok, 1994), vitamin A transport and metabolism (Chader et al., 1983; Chader, 1989; Bok, 1990; Saari, 1990; Rando, 1992), and control of the volume and composition of the fluid in the subretinal space through the transport of ions, fluid, and metabolites (Noell et al., 1965; Steinberg and Miller, 1973; Miller and Steinberg, 1977a; Hughes et al., 1984; Steinberg, 1985; Adorante and Miller, 1990; Kenyon et al., 1994b; Bialek and Miller, 1994). This transport is generated by specialized transport proteins present in two distinct RPE membrane domains: the apical membrane, which faces the photoreceptor outer segments across the subretinal space, and the basolateral membrane, which is juxtaposed to the choriocapillaris across Bruch's membrane. A variety of paracrine and endocrine signals originating in the neural retina or choroidal blood supply modulate this transport, enabling the RPE to maintain the specific microenvironment that is required for normal retinal function in the face of changes in retinal activity. The goal of this chapter is to present what is currently known about the physiological mechanisms that help regulate transport across the RPE.

In this chapter, we will summarize a particular set of experimental preparations and methodologies used for the study of RPE transport physiology. Most of the studies we describe were performed on intact layers of RPE (in vivo and in vitro). This information has been incorporated in a model for the transport of ions, fluid, and metabolites across the RPE. In the context of this model, we discuss how the RPE helps regulate the volume and composition of the subretinal space, that is, the extracellular space bounded by the apical membrane of the RPE, the distal portion of Müller cells and the pho-

toreceptor outer segments. Conversely, the RPE can respond to signals from the neural retina, including light-evoked changes in subretinal ion activities, pH, metabolites, and neuromodulators, or from the hormones in the blood. The light-induced modulation of specific RPE transport mechanisms can generate field potentials that are clinically recorded, across the intact eye, as part of the DC ERG (see Chapter 9).

EXPERIMENTAL PREPARATIONS

Characterization of specific transport and regulatory mechanisms of the RPE has been accomplished using several different experimental preparations. The RPE forms a polarized monolayer of cells whose apical and basolateral membranes are morphologically and functionally distinct. The apical membrane often forms villouslike processes that interdigitate with the photoreceptor outer segments in the subretinal space, whereas the basolateral membrane has more limited infoldings apposed to Bruch's membrane. The elaboration of both these membranes increases the surface-to-volume ratio of the cell and is a common feature of transporting epithelia. All of the preparations developed for the study of RPE transport have in common the initial goal of identifying specific types of transport mechanisms at each membrane. With each preparation having specific advantages and disadvantages, the major preparations will be reviewed here.

Isolated RPE-Choroid Preparations

The first in vitro studies of ion transport by the RPE were carried out by Lasansky and De Fisch (1966) on isolated preparations of toad RPE-choroid. The RPE-choroid tissue is isolated from the neural retina and sclera (Fig. 6-1) and then mounted in an Ussing chamber. This chamber mechanically isolates the apical and basolateral membrane surfaces from each other, allowing the ion transport pathways at each surface to be probed by ion substitutions, transport inhibitors, and ion chan-

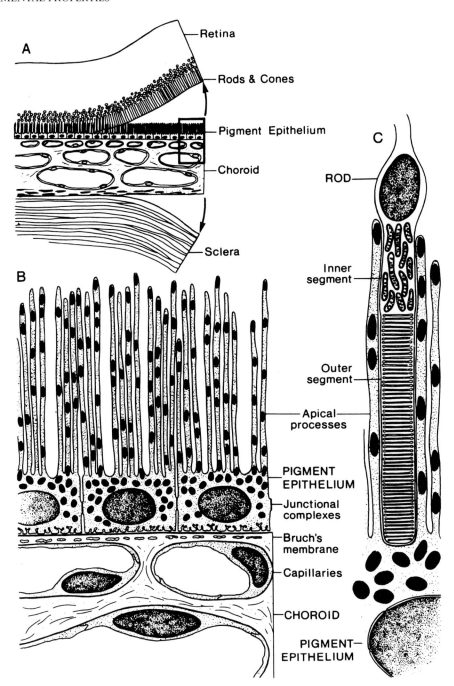

FIGURE 6-1. Experimental preparations. (A) The isolated RPE-choroid tissue is obtained by removal of the neurosensory retina and sclera from the RPE-choroid complex. Removal of the sclera alone creates the retina-RPE-choroid preparation in which light-evoked responses may be studied. (B) Detail of RPE-choroid. (C) Detail of association between RPE apical processes and photoreceptor outer segments in frog. (Reprinted from Miller and Steinberg, 1977b, with permission of the authors and the *Journal of Membrane Biology.*)

nel blockers. For electrophysiological studies, small-volume Ussing chambers allow rapid changes in solution composition.

Isolated RPE-choroid preparations have been developed from toad (Lasansky and De Fisch, 1966), frog

(Miller and Steinberg, 1977a, b), lizard (Griff and Steinberg, 1984), chick (Shirao and Steinberg, 1987; Gallemore et al., 1988), cat (Steinberg et al., 1978; Segawa, 1986), cattle (Crosson and Pautler, 1982; Joseph and Miller, 1991), dog (Tsuboi et al., 1986), monkey (Tsuboi and Pederson, 1988), and man (Quinn and Miller, 1992; la Cour et al., 1994). The bovine isolated RPE-choroid preparation has been a particularly useful mammalian preparation that is available in large quantities for cellular and molecular experiments. It can be easily separated from the neural retina and sclera, and the choroid, although thick, is permeable to ions and pharmacological agents.

Neural Retina-RPE-Choroid Preparations

The isolated neural retina-RPE-choroid preparation was developed to allow in vitro recording of light-evoked responses of the RPE, but it has also been useful in the characterization of transport mechanisms, particularly those present in the RPE basolateral membrane. Like the RPE-choroid, this tissue can be mounted in a small-volume Ussing chamber. Retina-RPE-choroid preparations have been isolated from frog (Oakley et al., 1977), toad (Griff, 1991), lizard (Griff and Steinberg, 1982), and chick (Shirao and Steinberg, 1987; Gallemore et al., 1988). The chick preparation has several advantages, including a thin, permeable choroid, strong adherence between the cone-enriched neural retina and RPE, and, finally, the capacity to generate light-evoked responses typical of warm-blooded vertebrates (Kikawada, 1968). A choroid-free preparation of chick neural retina-RPE also has been developed with the use of enzymatic dissection (Gallemore et al., 1994); this preparation has the added advantage of direct access to the RPE basolateral membrane.

Confluent Monolayers of Cultured RPE

Culture techniques have now been developed that allow the isolation of RPE cells that can be grown to confluence on a semipermeable substrate (Pfeffer et al., 1986; Pfeffer, 1991). Ussing chamber studies have been performed on confluent monolayers of cultured cells derived from frog (Defoe et al., 1994), bovine (Hernandez et al., 1995), and human RPE (Frambach et al., 1990; Hu et al., 1994; Hernandez et al., 1995; Gallemore et al., 1995). The use of cultured cells in place of fresh tissue has several advantages. First, human tissue is in short supply and cell culture can be used to amplify the number of cells needed for the application of molecular and biochemical techniques. Second, in a suitable microenvironment, cultured cells can be maintained for long periods of time (Hu et al., 1994). Third, cultured RPE monolayers allow access to the basolateral membrane in the absence of the choroid. Finally, cultured RPE cells may ultimately be used for RPE transplantation in the treatment of retinal disease (Sheng et al.,

1995), and understanding the physiology of cultured RPE may prove vital to the success of this work.

Cultured RPE preparations, however, have several disadvantages, including phenotypic variability (Burke et al., 1996), loss of polarized expression of the Na/K pump (Rizzolo, 1990; Nabi et al., 1993; Hu et al., 1994; Defoe et al., 1994), and the expression of ion channels that differ from those present in native RPE (Wen et al., 1993; Wen et al., 1994; Botchkin and Matthews, 1994; Hughes and Takahira, 1996). Hence, findings made in cultured RPE must be compared with studies on native tissue to ascertain their physiological relevance. Culture conditions, donor age, and the number of cell passages may be critical factors that affect the cell biology of RPE cells in culture.

EXPERIMENTAL METHODS

A variety of methods have been utilized to study the mechanisms of RPE transport. Each has specific advantages and limitations. By combining several methodologies, however, a more complete and precise understanding of RPE transport can be attained. Specifically, microelectrode recordings, isotope flux measurements, fluid transport measurements, and ion activity measurements can be used to probe the RPE for specific transport pathways. In microelectrode experiments, membrane potential, relative conductances, and properties of electrogenic transport mechanisms can be analyzed. Radioactive isotope flux studies allow one to determine the magnitude and direction of active solute transport across the epithelium and to calculate rates of fluid transport. Measurements with ion-selective microelectrodes or fluorescent dyes allow one to determine the chemical activities of ions and second messengers, as well as calculate driving forces for ion movement across the apical and basolateral membranes.

Microelectrode Recordings

Recording configurations: Isolated RPE-choroid preparation. With an RPE-choroid tissue mounted in a modified Ussing chamber, a number of electrical parameters can be recorded. In vivo and in vitro, the RPE generates a transepithelial potential (TEP) due to the difference between the resting potentials of its apical and basolateral membranes. The different potentials at each membrane result from differences in the types and distribution of ion channels and other transport proteins. Figure 6-2 illustrates the typical recording configuration used in Ussing chamber experiments (in vitro). The TEP is recorded differentially between calomel electrodes con-

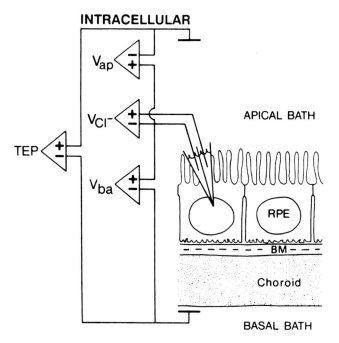

FIGURE 6-2. Recording configuration for the RPE-choroid preparation. The transepithelial potential (TEP) is recorded differentially between the apical and basolateral baths. With a double-barreled Cl⁻-selective microelectrode in the cell, the apical (V_{ap}) and basolateral (V_{ba}) membrane potentials are recorded by referencing the reference barrel to the apical and basolateral baths, respectively. Intracellular activity is determined from the differential signal between the reference and ion selective barrels (V_{Cl}). (Reprinted from Fujii et al., 1992, with the permission of the authors and the *American Journal of Physiology*.)

nected to the apical and basolateral baths by agar salt bridges. With a microelectrode in an RPE cell, the apical membrane potential (V_{ap}) is recorded by referencing to the apical bath electrode and the basolateral membrane potential (V_{ba}) by referencing to the basolateral bath electrode. A double-barreled ion-selective microelectrode may be used to measure simultaneously the two membrane voltages and the intracellular chemical potential of a particular ion, such as Cl (V_{Cl}), which can be readily converted to activity (a_{Cl}^i) (also see "Ion Activity Measurements," below). The double-barreled microelectrode can also be used to measure ion concentrations just outside the RPE basolateral membrane (Immel and Steinberg, 1986; Gallemore et al., 1993).

Equivalent electrical circuits. The analysis of changes in membrane voltage and resistance parameters in epithelia is complicated because the two membranes are electrically coupled by the finite resistance of the paracellular shunt pathway (Frömter, 1972). Potential changes at one membrane are "shunted" across the paracellular resistance by a shunt current, I_S, which causes a passive

voltage change at the other membrane. Quantitative interpretations of experimental results, therefore, are based on equivalent circuit analysis (Miller and Steinberg, 1977a). Figure 6-3 illustrates an equivalent electrical circuit derived for the RPE. The apical membrane is represented by a resistor, R_A, in series with a battery, E_A. Similarly, the basolateral membrane is represented by a resistor, R_B, and a battery, E_B. The apical and basolateral membranes are electrically coupled by the paracellular shunt resistance, R_S, which represents the combined resistance of the tight junctions separating the two membranes (Hudspeth and Yee, 1973) and tissue edge pathways. Since R_S is finite, a battery change at one membrane causes current to flow through R_S. This shunt current reduces the potential change at that membrane and produces a passive voltage change at the opposite membrane. In the steady state, I_S is given by:

$$I_S = \frac{(E_A - E_B)}{(R_A + R_B + R_S)} \qquad (6\text{-}1)$$

Since the TEP is apical-side positive, I_S flows through R_S, into the apical membrane, and out of the basolateral membrane. This current depolarizes the apical membrane and hyperpolarizes the basolateral membrane,

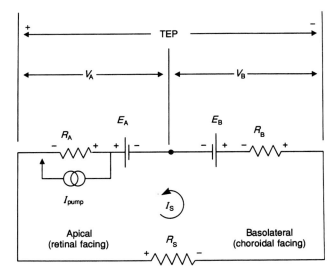

FIGURE 6-3. Equivalent circuit for the retinal pigment epithelium. The apical and basolateral membranes are represented by an EMF (E_A, E_B) in series with a resistor (R_A, R_B). (R_S) is the parallel combination of the junctional complex resistance and the resistance due to tissue edge damage. (I_S) is the loop current which flows through the circuit due to the difference in EMF between (E_A) and (E_B). The electrogenic 3Na/2K pump is modeled as a current source (I_{pump}). (V_A) and (V_B) are the apical and basolateral membrane potentials as recorded by an intracellular microelectrode. (Reprinted from Bialek and Miller, 1994, with permission of the authors and the *Journal of Physiology*.)

and the measured apical and basolateral membrane potentials (V_A and V_B, respectively) are given by:

$$V_A = E_A - I_S R_A \qquad (6\text{-}2)$$

$$V_B = E_B + I_S R_B \qquad (6\text{-}3)$$

Equations 6-1 to 6-3 can be used to derive relationships for the measured changes in V_A and V_B in terms of membrane and shunt resistances. For example, during the c-wave, the apical membrane batter (E_A) changes by ΔE_A as a result of a change in E_K (Steinberg et al., 1985; see Chapter 9). For a change in the apical membrane battery, assuming that E_B, E_S, and the resistance parameters remain constant, V_A, V_B, and I_S would change as follows:

$$\Delta V_A = \Delta E_A - \Delta I_S R_A \qquad (6\text{-}4)$$

$$\Delta V_B = \Delta I_S R_B \qquad (6\text{-}5)$$

$$\Delta I_S = \frac{\Delta E_A}{R_A + R_B + R_S} \qquad (6\text{-}6)$$

Substituting the expression for ΔI_S into Equations 6-4 and 6-5, we arrive at expressions for the polarizations of both membranes in response to the change in the apical battery during the c-wave:

$$\Delta V_A = \Delta E_A \cdot \frac{R_B + R_S}{R_A + R_B + R_S} \qquad (6\text{-}7)$$

$$\Delta V_B = \Delta E_A \cdot \frac{R_B}{R_A + R_B + R_S} \qquad (6\text{-}8)$$

where ΔV_A and ΔV_B are the amplitudes of the c-wave hyperpolarizations of the apical and basolateral membranes, respectively. Thus, ΔV_A is larger than ΔV_B because the potential change originates at the apical membrane, but both ΔV_A and ΔV_B are smaller than the change in the battery, ΔE_A. Since the TEP represents the difference between the apical and basolateral membrane potentials, the amplitude of the transepithelial (RPE) c-wave will be:

$$\Delta TEP = \Delta V_B - \Delta V_A \qquad (6\text{-}9)$$

so that, substituting Equations 6-7 and 6-8, we have:

$$\Delta TEP = -[(R_S)/(R_A + R_B + R_S)] \cdot \Delta E_A \quad (6\text{-}10)$$

(In this example ΔE_A is negative, so ΔTEP is positive.)

Thus, a change in the magnitude of ΔE_A or one or more of the resistive elements of the RPE will change the relative amplitudes of the c-wave membrane hyperpolarizations (ΔV_A and ΔV_B of Equations 6-7 and 6-8, re-

TEP Increase

V_{ap} hyperpolarizes more than V_{ba}

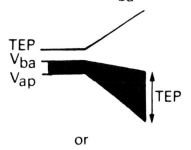

or

V_{ba} depolarizes more than V_{ap}

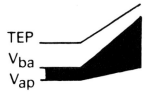

FIGURE 6-4. Schematic representation of membrane voltage changes that may produce an increase in TEP. A TEP increase may result either from a hyperpolarization of V_{ap} relative to V_{ba} *(top)* or from a depolarization of V_{ba} relative to V_{ap} *(bottom)*. (Reprinted from Steinberg and Linsenmeier, 1983, with permission of the authors and *Documentia Ophthalmology Proceedings Series*.)

spectively) and, thus, the amplitude of the RPE c-wave (ΔTEP of Equation 6-9). In addition, Equation 6-9 shows that, in general, the TEP can be decreased (or increased) by a basolateral membrane hyperpolarization (or depolarization), an apical membrane depolarization (or hyperpolarization), or both. This is illustrated schematically in Figure 6-4.

A similar analysis leads to the derivation of the following equations for the measured changes in V_A and V_B that result from a change in basolateral membrane battery (ΔE_B), as occurs, for example, during a step change of $[K]_o$ in the basolateral bath:

$$\Delta V_A = \Delta E_B \cdot \frac{R_A}{R_A + R_B + R_S} \qquad (6\text{-}11)$$

$$\Delta V_B = \Delta E_B \cdot \frac{R_A + R_S}{R_A + R_B + R_S} \qquad (6\text{-}12)$$

In addition to the apical and basolateral membrane batteries, the electrogenic Na/K pump at the apical membrane also contributes to V_A and V_B. The pump generates a source of steady current, part of which flows through R_A and part through R_S and then R_B. The pump current (i_{pump}) hyperpolarizes V_A and V_B by:

$$\Delta V_A = i_{pump} \cdot \frac{R_A(R_B + R_S)}{R_A + R_B + R_S} \qquad (6\text{-}13)$$

$$\Delta V_B = i_{pump} \cdot \frac{R_B + R_S}{R_A + R_B + R_S} \qquad (6\text{-}14)$$

Two resistance parameters can be recorded that allow inferences to be made about the membrane origin of a resistance (or conductance) change. In the RPE, the transepithelial resistance, R_t, and the membrane resistance ratio, R_A/R_B or *a* value, can be measured by passing current (Δi) across the epithelium and measuring the current-induced potential changes across the RPE ($R_t = \Delta TEP/\Delta i$) and across each membrane ($R_A/R_B = \Delta V_A/\Delta V_B$). The relationship between R_t and the membrane and shunt resistances is given by:
    Calculation of the individual membrane and shunt re-

$$R_t = \frac{R_S(R_A + R_B)}{R_A + R_B + R_S} \qquad (6\text{-}15)$$

sistances requires a third, independent measurement in addition to R_t and R_A/R_B (Frömter, 1972). However, the membrane location of a resistance change often can be postulated by comparing changes in R_t and R_A/R_B. In many cases, the simplest explanation for a simultaneous decrease in R_t and increase in R_A/R_B, as occurs during the light peak, is a decrease in R_B (Gallemore and Steinberg, 1993). Table 6-1 summarizes the mean values for TEP, V_A, V_B, R_t, and R_A/R_B for a variety of species and preparations.
    One important measure of the transport properties of a given membrane is the relative conductance of that membrane for a given ion. Although direct measurements of ionic conductances cannot be made in the intact epithelial sheet using conventional recording techniques, experimental approaches are available that allow one to estimate these parameters. The relative conductance of a membrane for a given ion (T_{ion}) is defined as: $T_{ion} = g_{ion}/g_{total}$. T_{ion} can be determined by measuring the change in membrane battery (ΔE_m) produced by a change in the equilibrium potential for that ion (ΔE_{ion}). For example, the relative Cl^- conductance of the basolateral membrane is given by: $T_{Cl} = \Delta E_B/\Delta E_{Cl}$. The change in E_{Cl} can be produced by making a rapid step change in $[Cl]_o$ outside the basolateral membrane. The value for ΔE_{Cl} can be calculated by us-

TABLE 6-1. *RPE electrical parameters*

Species	TEP (mV)	V_A(mV)	R_t(ohm·cm²)	R_A/R_B
RPE-choroid				
Frog[1]	10	−88mV	273	0.42
Toad[2]	14.9	−63	175	0.79
Bovine[3]	6	−61	138	0.22
Cat[4]	9	−67	133–259	0.2–0.5
Fetal human[5]	2.2	−56	206	0.70
Rabbit[6]	12.5		350	
Adult human[5]	1.9	−49	79	0.29
Retina-RPE-choroid				
Frog[7]	6.8	−83	329	0.2
Chick[8]	4.7	−67	115	0.25
Cultured RPE				
Fetal bovine[9]	0.6	−61	70	2.26
Fetal human[9]	1.3	−57	329	1.14
Fetal human[10,*]	1.3	−36	225	2.6
Adult human[10,*]	2.1	−41	215	1.5

   Mean values for electrical parameters in RPE for various species in different preparations. The variability in measurements may be found, when provided, in the original references. TEP, transepithelial potential; R_t, transepithelial resistance; V_A, apical membrane potential; R_A/R_B, apical to basolateral membrane resistance ratio (a-value). All measurements are in HCO_3 Ringer solutions, except for those marked by *, which were obtained in culture medium. References: [1]Miller and Steinberg, 1977; [2]Fujii et al., 1992; [3]Steinberg et al., 1978; [4]Joseph and Miller, 1991; [5]Quinn and Miller, 1992; [6]Frambach et al., 1988; [7]Oakley, 1977 ([+], Griff et al., 1985); [8]Gallemore et al., 1993; [9]Hernandez et al., 1995; [10]Hu et al., 1994.

ing the Nernst equation (assuming a_{Cl}^i remains constant):

$$\Delta E_{Cl} = -61mV \cdot \log\left(\frac{a_{Cl}^o {}^2}{a_{Cl}^o {}^1}\right) \qquad (6\text{-}16)$$

where $a_{Cl}^o {}^1$ and $a_{Cl}^o {}^2$ are the initial and final extracellular Cl activities at 37°C, $\Delta E_{Cl} = E_{Cl}^2 - E_{Cl}^1$, and $E_{Cl} = -61$ mV·$\log(a_{Cl}^o/a_{Cl}^i)$.
    The change in basolateral membrane battery, ΔE_B, is calculated from the measured change in V_B using the following relationship, obtained by rearranging Equation 6-12:

$$\Delta E_B = \Delta V_B \cdot \frac{R_A + R_B + R_S}{R_A + R_S} \qquad (6\text{-}17)$$

Thus, to estimate ΔE_B, the individual resistance parameters must first be estimated. Given R_t and R_A/R_B, one can determine R_A and R_B if R_S is known (Eq. 6-15). The shunt resistance (R_S) has been estimated in the isolated bovine RPE-choroid preparation by inhibiting the apical Na/K pump with ouabain and measuring the resulting changes in apical and basolateral membrane potentials in the first few seconds during which R_t, R_A, and R_B were constant (Joseph and Miller, 1991). In the chick retina-RPE-choroid preparation, this was accomplished by briefly illuminating the tissue and measuring the first few seconds of the apical and basolateral membrane hyperpolarizations of the c-wave (Gallemore et al., 1993); these responses are generated by a rapid light-evoked $[K]_o$ decrease outside the apical membrane (Oakley and Green, 1976; Steinberg et al., 1980; see Chapter 9). In either case, the following relationship can then be used to calculate R_S (Gallemore et al., 1993):

$$R_S = [R_t/(a + 1)] \cdot [(\Delta V_A / \Delta V_B) + a] \quad (6\text{-}18)$$

where R_t and a are as defined above, and $\Delta V_A / \Delta V_B$ is the ratio of the apical to basolateral membrane hyperpolarizations measured during the first 500–1500 msec of the voltage change. During this time period, R_t and a appear constant. Given R_S, R_t, and a, R_A and R_B can then be calculated as follows:

$$R_A = [R_S \cdot R_t \cdot a]/[(a + 1)(R_S - R_t)] \quad (6\text{-}19)$$

$$R_B = R_A/a \quad (6\text{-}20)$$

It also can be shown that, for the equivalent electrical circuit of the RPE, the electromotive forces (batteries) for the apical and basolateral membranes (E_A and E_B, respectively) are given by:

$$E_A = V_A - TEP(R_A/R_S) \quad (6\text{-}21)$$

$$E_B = V_B + TEP(R_B/R_S) \quad (6\text{-}22)$$

Table 6-2 summarizes mean values for E_B, E_A, R_A, R_B, and R_S, as calculated for the frog (Miller and Steinberg, 1977a), toad (R.P. Gallemore, S. Fujii, and R.H. Steinberg, unpublished), and bovine (Joseph and Miller, 1991) RPE-choroid preparations, cultured human RPE

monolayers (F. Maruiwa, R.P. Gallemore, J. Hu and D. Bok, unpublished), and the chick neural retina-RPE-choroid preparation (Gallemore et al., 1993).

Isotope Flux Measurements

An important method for determining the magnitude and direction of ionic fluxes across an epithelium involves the use of radioactive isotope flux measurements. These measurements typically are performed in in vitro preparations mounted in an Ussing chamber with separate apical and basolateral baths. Tracer amounts of radioactive isotopes are introduced into the bath on one side of the tissue and samples are collected periodically from the bath on the opposite side to determine the unidirectional flux (e.g., apical-to-basolateral or retina-to-choroid flux). The unidirectional flux in the opposite direction (basolateral-to-apical or choroid-to-retina flux) is generally measured in a paired tissue from the same animal. The magnitude and direction of the net ionic flux is equal to the difference between the two unidirectional fluxes. In the absence of a transepithelial electrochemical gradient for a particular ion (i.e., the short-circuit condition), the net flux provides a measure of active transport for that ion (Ginzberg and Hogg, 1967; Dawson, 1991).

There are two routes for the transepithelial movement of ions and other solutes: transcellular and paracellular. Active transport across each epithelial cell membrane is the algebraic sum of ion and solute movements through pumps, channels, exchangers, and cotransporters. For each of these transport steps, ATP hydrolysis is the primary source of energy. In vivo (or in vitro, open circuit), there is a transepithelial potential (TEP) and chemical gradient that could drive net ion flux across the epithelium via both the paracellular and transcellular routes. The rate of active cellular transport can be determined

TABLE 6-2. *Calculated electrical parameters of RPE*

Species	E_A (mV)	E_B (mV)	R_A (ohm·cm²)	R_B (ohm·cm²)	R_S (ohm·cm²)
Frog RPE-choroid[1]	−97	−69mV	224	472	426
Toad RPE-choroid[2]	−85	−23	324	373	224
Bovine RPE-choroid[3]	−69	−24	223	1254	179
Chick retina[4]	−77	−45	152	615	138
Cultured fetal human RPE[5]	−77	−38	5006	4660	358

Mean values for the following electrical parameters: apical membrane battery (E_A), basolateral membrane battery (E_B), apical membrane resistance (R_A), basolateral membrane resistance (R_B), and paracellular shunt resistance (R_S). References: [1]Miller and Steinberg, 1977; [2]R. P. Gallemore, S. Fujii and R. H. Steinberg, unpublished; [3]Joseph and Miller, 1991; [4]Gallemore et al., 1993; [5]F. Maruiwa, R. B. Gallemore and D. Bok, unpublished. The reader is directed to these original references for measures of parameter variability.

by measuring the net flux under the short-circuit condition, where the transepithelial potential is clamped to zero and the chemical composition of the solutions on both sides of the tissue are identical (i.e., transepithelial electrochemical gradient is zero). The magnitude of current required to clamp the TEP to zero is termed the short-circuit current (I_{sc}), and is equal to the sum of all net ionic fluxes across the epithelium, that is, $I_{sc} = I_{Cl} + I_{Na} + I_K + I_{HCO_3}$.

Under the open-circuit condition, which more closely resembles the situation in situ, the direction and magnitude of the net flux of an ion can differ from that measured in the short circuit because of passive movement driven by the TEP through the paracellular pathway. For example, under the short-circuit condition, Na is actively *secreted* across the frog RPE-choroid in the choroid-to-retinal direction. In contrast, under the *open-circuit* condition Na is *absorbed* in the retina-to-choroid direction, mainly due to a large passive flux driven through the paracellular pathway by the TEP. Flux measurements in the open-circuit condition allow one to calculate net solute flux and thereby estimate the magnitude and direction of fluid transport (Hughes et al., 1984; Miller and Farber, 1984).

Fluid Transport Measurements

Several techniques have been developed to measure the rate of fluid transport (J_v) and hydraulic conductivity (L_p) across the RPE in vitro. A common feature of all these methods is that they utilize a modified Ussing chamber, which exposes the apical and basolateral surfaces of the RPE-choroid preparation to separate fluid compartments and allows the measurement of electrical parameters as well as J_v. Miller and colleagues (Miller et al., 1982; Hughes et al., 1984) employed a capacitance probe technique to monitor fluid transport across the isolated bullfrog RPE-choroid mounted in a modified Ussing chamber constructed of Kel-F, a water-impermeable plastic. In this apparatus, the hemichambers were closed except for a small cannula that connected the bathing solution to a vertical fluid column. A capacitance probe measured the capacitance of the air gap separating the tip of the probe and the meniscus of the fluid in the column. When the tissue transported fluid, the height of the fluid dropped over time on one side and then rose on the other side of the tissue. This change in fluid height produced a change in capacitance that could be readily converted into a volume change. In principle, a unilateral volumetric measurement might suffice, but the inability to test for leaks and for evaporative artifacts make the unilateral measure-

ments difficult or impossible to interpret (Welsh et al., 1980; Nathanson et al., 1983).

A variation of this technique using glass capillary tubes was originally devised by Reid in 1892 for studies on frog skin (Reid, 1892; Huf, 1979). An adaptation of this capillary technique was used by Tsuboi and colleagues to measure fluid transport across the isolated RPE-choroid of dog (Tsuboi, 1987) and monkey (Tsuboi and Pederson, 1988). Instead of relying on capacitance probes, they monitored J_v by measuring the movement of fluid in capillary tubes connected to apical and basolateral hemichambers. It should be emphasized that these volumetric techniques are valid only for the measurement of steady-state fluid transport, because substantial volume changes can occur simply as a result of the tissue bowing due to the tissue responding to hydrostatic pressure differences or contraction of smooth muscle in the choroid (Hughes et al., 1988).

Frambach and colleagues (1985) measured fluid transport across the isolated RPE-choroid of the bullfrog using a photogrammetric method. The RPE-choroid was mounted in an Ussing chamber modified so that the basolateral surface faced a sealed compartment. Fluid transport into the sealed hemichamber caused bowing of the tissue, which was monitored by analyzing the displacement of a laser image projected onto the apical surface of the RPE.

The rate of fluid reabsorption across the RPE following the injection of fluid into the subretinal space of living rabbits also has been estimated (Frambach and Marmor, 1982). The reader is directed to a review by Marmor (1990) for more details on this topic.

Ion Activity Measurements

Two methods are used for measurement of ion activities: ion-selective microelectrodes and ion-sensitive fluorescent dyes. Double-barreled ion-selective microelectrodes have been used to record intracellularly from RPE cells. As shown in Figure 6-2, these electrodes consist of two barrels lying in parallel, a reference barrel and an ion-selective barrel. The ion-selective barrel is made by first silanizing the inner surface of its glass wall to make it hydrophobic and then filling the electrode tip with an ion-selective resin. For intracellular recordings, the reference barrel is used to sense the membrane voltage (V_m). The voltage sensed by the ion-selective barrel has contributions from both ion activity and membrane voltage, but the chemical potential (V_{ion}) can be readily isolated by taking the difference between the signals from ion-selective and reference barrels. Ion activity (a_{ion}) can then be calculated using the Nicolsky equation (Armstrong and Garcia-Diaz, 1980). For example, the relationship between intracellular Cl activity (a_{Cl}^i) and Cl chemical potential (V_{Cl}) is given by:

$$a_{Cl}^i = (a_{Cl}^o + S_{HCO_3/Cl} \cdot a_{HCO_3}) \cdot 10^{V_{Cl}/M} \quad (6\text{-}23)$$

where $S_{HCO_3/Cl}$ is the selectivity of the electrode for HCO_3 over Cl (ΔV_{ion} for a tenfold change in $[HCO_3]_o$ divided by ΔV_{ion} for a tenfold change in $[Cl]_o$), a_{Cl}^o and $a_{HCO_3}^o$ are the Cl and HCO_3 activities in the extracellular bathing solution, V_{Cl} is the difference in voltages measured by the Cl-sensing barrel and the reference barrel, and M is the slope of the electrode voltage response to $\Delta[Cl]_o$ measured during electrode calibration. Double-barreled ion-selective microelectrodes have been used to record the intracellular ion activities of Cl (Fong et al., 1988; Gallemore and Steinberg, 1989; 1993; Joseph and Miller, 1991; Bialek and Miller, 1994), K (Oakley et al., 1978; la Cour et al., 1986; Bialek and Miller, 1994), H (la Cour, 1989; 1991a; 1991b), and Na (la Cour, 1991a) in the RPE. They also have been used to measure K and Cl activities in the extracellular space outside the basolateral membrane (Immel and Steinberg, 1986; Gallemore et al., 1993), as well as dark-adapted and light-evoked changes in the activities of K, Cl, Na, H, and Ca^{2+} in the subretinal space separating photoreceptor outer segments and apical processes of the RPE (Oakley and Green, 1976; Yamamoto et al., 1992; Gallemore and Steinberg, 1988; Dimitriev et al., 1996).

Intracellular pH and Ca^{2+} measurements also have been made using the pH-sensitive and Ca^{2+}-sensitive fluorescent dyes 2'-7'-bis(carboxyethyl)-5(6)-carboxy-fluorescein (BCECF) and fura-2, respectively. The method was pioneered by Tsien and colleagues (Rink et al., 1982). Cells are loaded with the ester form of an ion-sensitive dye, which easily passes across the cell membrane. Once in the intracellular compartment, the ester is cleaved by endogenous esterases and the dye becomes trapped within the cell. A ratioing technique is then used to measure the intracellular activity of the ion. Miller and colleagues (Lin and Miller, 1991a) have performed these experiments in a modified Ussing chamber mounted on an inverted microscope equipped for epifluorescence, which allows the simultaneous recording of intracellular ion activity, TEP, and R_t.

To estimate intracellular ion activity, the background fluorescence of the tissue must be subtracted from all measurements and the ion-sensitive dye must be calibrated. Calibration can be performed at the end of an experiment using the method of Thomas and colleagues (1979), in which calibration solutions contain a molecule that permeabilizes the cell membrane to the ion of interest, such that changes in the extracellular ion activity lead to linear changes in intracellular ion activity.

TRANSPORT MECHANISMS

Epithelia have the ability to vectorially transport metabolites, ions, and fluid from one extracellular space to another. In this section we summarize what is known about the RPE plasma membrane transport proteins and the intra- or extracellular regulatory signals that help mediate the "traffic" of these molecules across the RPF, either in the retina-to-choroid direction (absorption), or in the opposite direction, from choroid to retina (secretion). The model in Figure 6-5 illustrates many of the ion transport proteins that have been identified in the bovine RPE and provides a framework for the discussion in this section. The distribution of transport proteins that reside in the apical and basolateral membrane domains of the cell is clearly asymmetric, and this difference is what allows the epithelium to carry out vectorial transport. The migration of membrane proteins between the apical and basolateral membrane surfaces is prevented by tight junction proteins, which are part of the junctional complex that surrounds each cell. Intracellularly, the asymmetry or polarity of the cell is maintained because the intracellular molecular machinery is continually synthesizing new proteins and delivering them preferentially to the apical or basolateral cell membranes (Nelson, 1991; Rothman, 1996). The cytoskeleton also plays a fundamental role in determining cell polarity and in regulating transport (Mays et al., 1994; Mills and Mandel, 1994).

Transport across the RPE is regulated by a set of extracellular signals—paracrine, autocrine or hormonal—that arise from the retina, the RPE itself, or from the blood. In the light and dark, these signals differentially activate a whole panoply of cell surface receptors that are coupled via the appropriate G proteins and other mechanisms to a variety of intracellular second-messenger systems. It is the stimulus-induced alterations in second-messenger activity (e.g., IP_3, Ca^{2+}, cAMP, H) that directly alter epithelial transport and function.

Transport across the RPE can be also regulated by "recycling" mechanisms that are located either at the apical or basolateral membranes. For example, Cl recycling at the basolateral membrane involves the efflux of Cl through a Cl channel and its influx through a Cl/HCO_3 exchanger (see Fig. 6-5). Net vectorial transport of Cl is determined by the relative rates of these oppositely directed and separately regulated transport proteins. Several groups of transport proteins at the both

Subretinal Space

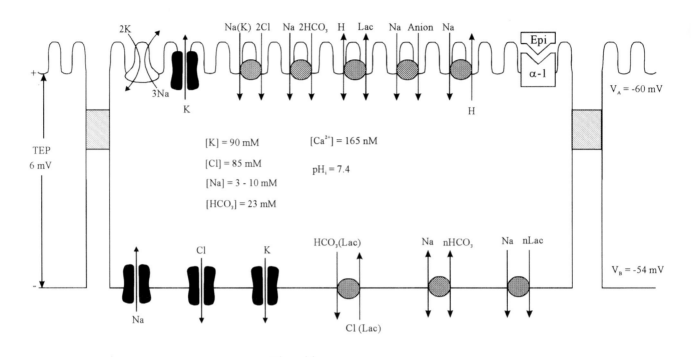

Choroid

FIGURE 6-5. Model of RPE ion transport mechanisms from bovine RPE. Apical membrane; Na/K ATPase, K channel, Na,K,2Cl cotransporter, NaHCO$_3$ cotransporter, H-Lactate cotransporter, Na-anion cotransporter, Na/H exchanger, alpha-1 adrenergic receptor, Epi (epinephrine). Basolateral membrane: Na uptake mechanism (Na channel?), Cl and K channels, Cl/HCO$_3$ exchanger, NaHCO$_3$ cotransporter, and Na-Lactate cotransporter. Average intracellular ion activities, membrane potentials (V_A, V_B) and TEP (transepithelial potential) values are shown.

the apical and basolateral membranes are organized into recycling pathways that can be experimentally manipulated to significantly alter net transepithelial ion and fluid transport. In some cases the RPE can be transformed from an absorbing to a secreting epithelium.

As discussed below (under "Potassium Transport" and "Bicarbonate Transport") recycling pathways at both membranes are affected by physiologically relevant alterations in extracellular (apical) K concentration ($[K]_o$). Similar changes in $[K]_o$ occur in the subretinal space of the vertebrate eye following transitions between light and dark (see Chapter 9). The in vitro results suggest that in the intact eye, these $[K]_o$ changes would alter the transport rates of several apical and basolateral membrane transporters, change RPE cell volume, and alter the chemical composition and hydration of the subretinal space.

We begin with a review of net transport measured under short- and open-circuit conditions. The transport

pathways for K, Na, Cl, HCO$_3$, H, and Ca^{2+} are reviewed. Known transport mechanisms for other substances, including taurine, GABA, lactate, and glucose also are presented. The section ends with a review of fluid transport.

Ion Transport in the Short-Circuit Condition

Radioisotope flux measurements in isolated RPE-choroid preparations have demonstrated that the RPE is capable of actively transporting a variety of ions between the subretinal space and the choroidal blood. Under experimental conditions where the transepithelial potential is short-circuited (TEP set to zero) and the two surfaces of the RPE-choroid are bathed with identical bathing solutions, any net flux (measured as the difference between two unidirectional fluxes) is indicative of *active transport* across the apical and basolateral membranes in series.

TABLE 6-3. *Ion transport in the short circuit*

Species	R_t (ohm·cm²)	I_{sc} (μEq·cm⁻²·h⁻¹)	J_{Cl} (net A→B) (μEq·cm⁻²·h⁻¹)	J_{Na} (net B→A) (μEq·cm⁻²·h⁻¹)	J_K (net A→B) (μEq·cm⁻²·h⁻¹)
Frog[1,2]	364	1.34	0.34	0.32	0.05
Toad[3]	450–600	—	—	0.13	—
Bovine[4]	152	1.28	0.69	0.52	0.0
Dog[5]	129	1.0	0.67	0.76	—

Mean values from the following references: [1]Edelman, Lin, and Miller, 1994a; [2]Miller and Farber, 1984; [3]Lasansky and DeFisch, 1966; [4]Miller and Edelman, 1990; [5]Tsuboi et al., 1986.

The isolated bovine RPE-choroid actively transports Cl and HCO_3 in the retina-to-choroid direction (absorption), and actively transports Na in the opposite direction (secretion) (Miller and Edelman, 1990). Under resting conditions, net K absorption is practically zero, except when K recycling at the apical membrane is reduced (as is produced by adding barium or epinephrine to the apical bath) (Miller and Edelman, 1990; Joseph and Miller, 1992; Edelman and Miller, 1991; 1996). These results are qualitatively similar to those obtained in isolated dog (Tsuboi et al., 1986) and amphibian RPE-choroid (Lasansky and De Fisch, 1966; Miller and Steinberg, 1977b; Miller and Farber, 1984). Measurements in bullfrog RPE-choroid demonstrated active Ca^{2+} secretion (Miller and Steinberg, 1977b), but presently nothing is known about active Ca^{2+} transport in mammalian RPE. Average values for short-circuit ionic fluxes in several species are shown in Table 6-3. The net direction and relative magnitudes of fluxes across bovine RPE are illustrated schematically in the top panel of Figure 6-6.

Ion Transport in the Open-Circuit Condition

In the open-circuit condition, which more closely resembles the situation for the RPE in the eye, there is a spontaneous transepithelial potential on the order of 5 to 15 mV, apical side positive (see Table 6-1). This TEP provides an electrical driving force causing the movement of Na in the retina-to-choroid direction through the paracellular pathway, which presumably is Na selective. In the open circuit this passive absorptive flux of Na through the paracellular pathway exceeds the active secretory Na flux through the transcellular route, leading to net Na absorption. Thus, the net flux under the open-circuit condition includes both active transcellular transport as well as a paracellular flux driven by the TEP. Average values for net transepithelial ionic fluxes measured under the open-circuit condition are shown in

Table 6-4. The direction and relative magnitude of net fluxes in bovine RPE are illustrated schematically in the bottom panel of Figure 6-6.

Potassium Transport

Mechanisms. Active transport of K across the RPE is a complex process involving several different transport proteins that mediate K entry and exit across the apical and basolateral membranes. Potassium movement across the apical membrane is governed by at least three separate transport pathways: (1) an electrogenic Na/K pump (Miller et al., 1978; Joseph and Miller, 1991); (2) an electroneutral Na,K,2Cl cotransporter (Adorante and Miller, 1990; Kennedy, 1990; la Cour, 1992; Kennedy, 1992; Hu

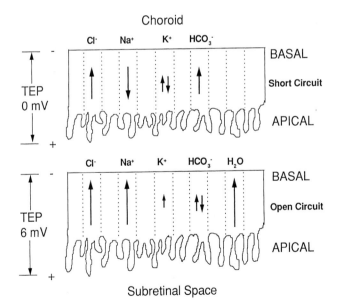

FIGURE 6-6. Schematic diagram of net transepithelial transport in bovine RPE-choroid. Under (A) short-circuit conditions and (B) open-circuit conditions. Numerical values for net transport of specific ions are shown in Tables 6-3 and 6-4. Value for fluid transport measured under open circuit conditions are shown in Table 6-7.

TABLE 6-4. *Ion transport in the open circuit*

Species	TEP (mV)	R_t (ohm·cm²)	J_{Cl} (net A→B) (μEq·cm⁻²·h⁻¹)	J_{Na} (net A→B) (μEq·cm⁻²·h⁻¹)	J_K (net A→B) (μEq·cm⁻²·h⁻¹)
Frog[1]	11	250	0.32	0.43	0.11
Bovine[2]	8.0	160	0.67	0.68	0.05
Dog[3]	1.56	280	0.27	0.32	0.05
Chick[4]	5.1	144	1.62	1.48	—
Cultured human[5]	3.6	385	0.3	—	—

Mean values from the following references: [1]Edelman, Lin, and Miller, 1994a; [2]Miller and Edelman, 1996, unpublished; [3]Tsuboi et al., 1986; [4]Frambach and Misfeldt, 1983; [5]Hu et al., 1996a.

et al., 1996b); and (3) a Ba^{2+}-sensitive and Cs^+-sensitive K conductance (Miller and Steinberg, 1977a; Griff et al., 1985; la Cour et al., 1986; Joseph and Miller, 1991; Hughes et all, 1995b; Takahira and Hughes, 1997). The basolateral membrane contains a K conductance that is relatively large (see Table 6-6) and Ba^{2+} sensitive, although the Ba^{2+} concentration required to produce a block is higher than it is for the apical membrane K conductance (Miller and Steinberg, 1977b; Immel and Steinberg, 1986; Griff et al., 1985; Gallemore et al., 1993; Hernandez et al., 1995). In addition, there is evidence for KCl uptake across the basolateral membrane (Oakley et al., 1978), but the mechanism is not known.

The specific types of K channels that make up the apical and basolateral membrane K conductances have been investigated in patch-clamp studies on freshly amphibian and mammalian RPE cells. Thus far, two voltage-dependent K channels have been identified whose functional properties are compatible with those of the apical and basolateral membrane K conductances: a mildly voltage dependent inward rectifier, which is blocked by Cs^+ and Ba^{2+} (Hughes and Steinberg, 1990; Segawa and Hughes, 1994; Wen et al., 1993; Hughes and Takahira, 1996) and a sustained outward rectifier, which is blocked by millimolar concentrations of Ba^{2+} (Hughes et al., 1995a; Takahira and Hughes, 1997). Recent studies in the intact toad RPE-choroid (Hughes et al., 1995b) and in cultured human RPE monolayers (Maruiwa et al., 1996) indicate that the apical K conductance is largely composed of inward rectifier K channels, but the channels underlying the basolateral membrane K conductance have not yet been determined.

Recycling. In the steady state, the net movement of K between the subretinal space and choroid is equal to the *net* influx of K across the apical membrane, which also must equal the *net* efflux of K across the basolateral membrane. In bovine RPE, the apical K conductance is so large that practically all of the K transported into the

cell by the Na/K pump and Na,K,2Cl cotransporter diffuses back into the apical bath. Therefore, very little K exits the cell across the basolateral membrane and net K absorption is approximately zero (Miller and Edelman, 1990). There are, however, at least two experimental ways in which K recycling at the apical membrane can be blocked or reduced and net K absorption across the epithelium increased. One method is shown in Figure 6-7 (Miller and Edelman, 1990), which plots the unidirectional fluxes of ^{86}Rb (a radioactively labeled tracer for K—Miller and Steinberg, 1982) in the retina-to-choroid (open circles) and choroid-to-retina direction (closed circles), before and after the addition of apical barium. Net active transport across the epithelium is equal to the difference between these two unidirectional fluxes (see "Isotope Flux Measurements," above), which in the absence of barium, is equal to zero. At the time indicated by the arrow, 1 mM barium was added to the apical bath to block recycling of K. This caused a large increase in net active K absorption across the epithelium, which was mediated at the apical membrane by the Na/K pump and the Na,K,2Cl cotransporter, and at the basolateral membrane by K channels. This net flux can be inhibited, almost entirely, by apical ouabain (Miller and Edelman, 1990).

K recycling across the apical membrane is also reduced following the addition of epinephrine to the apical bath (Edelman and Miller, 1992). This leads to a dramatic increase in active K absorption. Epinephrine activates α_1 adrenergic receptors, which presumably are coupled to G-proteins and a secondary rise in intracellular free Ca^{2+} (Lin and Miller, 1991a; Chapter 9).

Spatial buffering. There is good experimental evidence that in the presence of a K concentration gradient across the RPE, a net *passive* K flux can occur through the cellular pathway. In a study on the frog RPE-choroid, Immel and Steinberg (1986) used K-sensitive microelectrodes positioned just outside the basolateral membrane

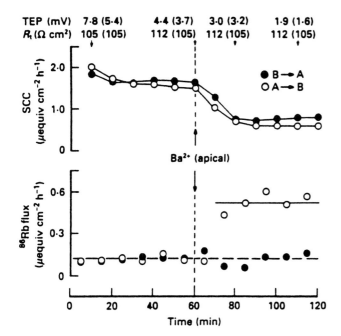

FIGURE 6-7. Effect of apical barium (1 mM) on potassium absorption across the bovine RPE. Unidirectional ^{86}Rb (K) fluxes in the retina-to-choroid (O) and choroid-to-retina (●) directions were measured in paired tissues from the same eye. Apical barium, added at t = 60 min, increased net ^{86}Rb (K) absorption from zero to ≈0.4 μequiv cm^{-2} h^{-1}. Barium also caused the TEP and short-circuit current (SCC) to decrease. (Reprinted from Miller and Edelman, 1990, with permission from the authors and the *Journal of Physiology.*)

to show that $\Delta[K]_o$-induced depolarization of the apical membrane increased the efflux of K through the Ba^{2+}-sensitive K channels in the basolateral membrane. A stimulation of K efflux also was produced by depolarizing the apical membrane by other means, such as blocking the apical K channels with Ba^{2+}, indicating that the mechanism involved electrical coupling of the apical and basolateral membranes. On the basis of these findings, they proposed a "spatial buffering" model that explained how an increase in $[K]_o$ in the apical bath could transfer K to the basolateral side. In other studies on the frog RPE-choroid, la Cour and colleagues (1986; 1993) proposed on the basis of apical $[K]_o$-induced changes in membrane voltage and resistance and intracellular K activity that an increase in apical membrane K permeability could contribute to the buffering of the light-evoked decrease in subretinal [K] by the RPE. Recent patch-clamp studies on isolated RPE cells have shown that the inward rectifier K conductance, which is located on the RPE apical membrane of toad (Hughes et al., 1995b) and cultured human RPE (Maruiwa et al., 1996), *increases* when subretinal [K] is decreased from 5 to 2 mM (Segawa and Hughes, 1994; Hughes and Takahira, 1996; Takahira and Hughes, 1997). This con-

ductance increase may conspire with K-induced changes in driving forces to generate K secretion (see below).

In a recent study on bovine RPE-choroid, Bialek and Miller (1994) measured changes in the apical and basolateral membrane potentials and intracellular K activity caused by decreasing apical $[K]_o$ from 5 to 2 mM. Figure 6-8A shows that the decrease in apical $[K]_o$ hyperpolarized the apical and basolateral membrane potentials and caused the intracellular K$^+$ activity to fall by 19 mM. In the presence of apical barium, the $\Delta[K]_o$-induced changes in membrane potentials and intracellular K activity were significantly smaller (Fig. 6-8B), indicating that the decrease in K activity observed in the absence of barium mainly resulted from the net movement of K through the apical K conductance. Other experiments revealed that much of the $\Delta[K]_o$-induced change in intracellular K activity also could be inhibited by blocking the basolateral membrane Cl$^-$ conductance with DIDS, indicating that the apical membrane K$^+$ conductance and the basolateral membrane Cl$^-$ conductance are electrically coupled. Analysis of the electrochemical driving forces on K movement across the apical and basolateral membranes predicted that a decrease in apical $[K]_o$ from 5 to 2 mM would generate the net secretion of K into the subretinal space, and this prediction was confirmed by ^{86}Rb flux measurements. The results of these experiments helped identify several apical and basolateral membrane mechanisms that work in concert to buffer extracellular K and that, in the intact eye, also might help regulate the hydration and chemical composition of the subretinal space following transitions between light and dark (see Chapter 9).

Sodium Transport

Mechanisms. Active Na secretion across the RPE is generated by the electrogenic Na/K pump, located in the apical membrane (Miller and Steinberg, 1977a, b; Miller et al., 1978). Evidence for the existence and location of this electrogenic pump first came from electrophysiological studies which showed that ouabain depolarized the apical membrane (Miller and Steinberg, 1977a, b; Joseph and Miller, 1991; Quinn and Miller, 1992) and that this depolarization began as soon as the first ouabain molecules reached the apical membrane surface (Miller et al., 1978; Oakley et al., 1978). In contrast, basolateral ouabain had no effect on any of the RPE electrical properties. In addition, ion flux measurements showed that active ^{22}Na secretion is inhibited by apical ouabain (Miller and Steinberg, 1977b; Hughes et al., 1984; Tsuboi et al., 1986; Hughes et al., 1988; Miller and Edelman, 1990). Further evidence for polarization of Na/K pump sites to the apical membrane

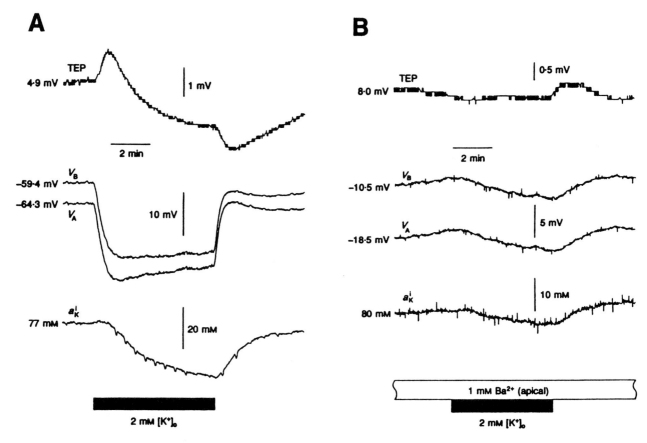

FIGURE 6-8. $\Delta[K]_o$-induced changes in membrane potential and intracellular K activity (a_K^i) in bovine RPE. (A) The effect of changing apical bath $[K]_o$ from 5 to 2 mM on TEP, V_A, V_B, and a_K^i. (B) The effect of changing apical bath $[K]_o$ from 5 to 2 mM on TEP, V_A, V_B, and

a_K^i in the presence of 1 mM apical Ba^{2+}. Ba^{2+} blocked most of the $[K]_o$-induced TEP, V_A, and V_B responses and inhibited the $[K]_o$-induced a_K^i response by 67%. (Reprinted from Bialek and Miller, 1994, with permission from the authors and the *Journal of Physiology*.)

has been provided by autoradiographic studies with tritiated ouabain (Bok, 1982), biochemical studies of purified membrane fractions (Ostwald and Steinberg, 1980; Mircheff et al., 1990) and immunocytochemical studies (Defoe et al., 1994).

Although active Na secretion requires that Na enters the cell across the basolateral membrane, the exact mechanism of entry has not been identified. The presence of a Na conductance is suggested by the finding that Na removal from the basolateral side of the frog RPE-choroid preparation increases the apparent basolateral membrane resistance (Hughes et al., 1988). However, it has not been possible to determine the relative Na conductance of the basolateral membrane from voltage responses to Na concentration changes in the bath (Miller and Steinberg, 1977a), perhaps because of diffusion limitations in the choroid or because they are masked by voltage changes generated across the paracellular pathway and the choroid (Hughes et al., 1989).

No Na-selective ion channels have yet been identified in freshly isolated RPE cells, although nonselective cation conductances have been observed (Hughes and Segawa, 1992). In culture, however, cells derived from human (Wen et al., 1994) and rat (Botchkin and Matthews, 1994) RPE exhibit tetrodotoxin-sensitive Na channels, consistent with a change in phenotype.

Regulation. It has been shown that the elevation of intracellular cAMP in the frog RPE-choroid stimulates the Na/K pump (Hughes et al., 1988), leading to increases in active Na secretion and K absorption (Miller and Farber, 1984; Hughes et al., 1984). Na/K pump activity is directly stimulated by increases in apical bath potassium concentration in the physiological range between 0.2 and 5 mM (Miller and Steinberg, 1982; Griff et al., 1985; see Chapter 9), and by decreases in intracellular K activity (Oakley et al., 1978). The pump is *indirectly* stimulated by apical taurine or GABA (Miller and Steinberg, 1979; Scharschmidt et al., 1988; Peterson and Miller, 1995a; see "Modulation of RPE Transport by Changes in Apical $[K]_o$," below).

Chloride Transport

Mechanisms. A large fraction of active Cl absorption across the RPE is determined by two transport proteins, one located at the apical membrane and the other at the basolateral membrane. The apical membrane protein is a furosemide- and bumetanide-sensitive Na,K,2Cl cotransport mechanism (Frambach et al., 1989; Adorante and Miller, 1990; Kennedy, 1992; Hu et al., 1996a), which mediates the net influx of Cl. Cl influx via this electroneutral cotransporter is tightly coupled to the inward movements of K and Na (Adorante and Miller, 1990; Kennedy, 1990; la Cour, 1992). Normally, the inward Na gradient maintained by the Na/K pump is sufficiently large to drive the "uphill" transport of K and Cl, but the direction of cotransport is predicted to reverse under certain circumstances, such as immediately following reductions in apical $[K]_o$ (Bialek and Miller, 1994).

Evidence strongly suggests that Cl exits across the basolateral membrane via a Cl conductance, comprising Ca^{2+}-activated and cAMP-activated Cl channels (Fong et al., 1988; Gallemore and Steinberg, 1989a; Joseph and Miller, 1991; la Cour, 1992; Fujii et al., 1992; Gallemore et al., 1993; Hughes and Segawa, 1993; Ueda and Steinberg, 1994; Strauss et al., 1996). For example, treatment of the basolateral side of frog, chick, or bovine RPE with DIDS, a stilbene derivative capable of blocking some types of Cl channels (Hanrahan et al., 1985; Anderson and Welsh, 1991), including cAMP-activated and Ca^{2+}-activated Cl channels in isolated RPE cells (Hughes and Segawa, 1993; Ueda and Steinberg, 1994), causes the inhibition of active ^{36}Cl absorption, a rise in intracellular Cl activity, a hyperpolarization of V_B, and an increase in the apparent basolateral membrane resistance (Fong et al., 1988; Miller and Edelman, 1990; Bialek and Miller, 1994; Joseph and Miller, 1991; Gallemore and Steinberg, 1989a; Fujii et al., 1992; Gallemore et al., 1993). Under control conditions, the Cl conductance is estimated to account for 20%–45% of the total basolateral membrane conductance (Joseph and Miller, 1991; Fujii et al., 1992; Gallemore et al., 1993). Average values for basolateral membrane T_{Cl} are shown in Table 6-5.

There also is evidence from patch-clamp studies on single cells for a swelling-activated Cl channel (Botchkin and Matthews, 1993; Ueda and Steinberg, 1994; Gallemore et al., 1996). Studies in cultured monolayers indicate that the channel resides in the basolateral mem-

TABLE 6-5. *Relative K and Cl conductances of RPE membranes*

Species	Apical T_K	Basolateral T_K	Basolateral T_{Cl}
Frog[1,2]	0.7	0.9	~0–0.27
Toad[3,4]	—	0.3–0.4	0.45
Bovine[5,6]	0.7–0.9	0.34	0.6–0.7
Chick[7,8]	0.9	0.61 (dark)	0.23 (dark)

Mean values from the following references: [1]Miller and Steinberg, 1977b; [2]la Cour, 1992; [3]Fujii et al., 1992; [4]Gallemore, Fujii and Steinberg, unpublished (basolateral T_K); [5]Joseph and Miller, 1991; [6]Bialek and Miller, 1994; [7]Gallemore et al., 1993; [8]Gallemore and Steinberg, unpublished (apical T_K estimated from light-evoked $\Delta[K]_o$ and ΔV_{ap}).

brane (Gallemore et al., 1996). Its contribution to the resting Cl conductance remains to be determined.

Recycling. The net movement of Cl out of the cell across the basolateral membrane is determined by the balance between its efflux through the Cl conductance and the activity of a Cl/HCO_3 exchanger. Under control conditions, the exchanger transports Cl into the cell in exchange for intracellular HCO_3 (Lin and Miller, 1994). Thus, Cl is recycled at the basolateral membrane. The rate of exchange is increased by cell alkalinization and decreased by cell acidification. In frog RPE, inhibition of the exchanger by cell acidification leads to a doubling in the rate of Cl and fluid absorption (Edelman and Miller, 1994a).

cAMP. In many epithelia, Cl transport is regulated by cAMP modulation of Cl channel activity (Peterson and Reuss, 1983; Fuller and Benos, 1992; Frizzell, 1995). Several studies on the frog RPE-choroid preparation showed that cAMP increases the basolateral membrane conductance (Miller and Farber, 1984; Hughes et al., 1987; 1988) and decreases intracellular Cl activity (B. Hughes and S. Miller, unpublished), consistent with the activation of Cl channels. Indeed, whole-cell patch-clamp recordings in isolated frog and toad RPE cells have confirmed the presence of cAMP-activated Cl channels (Hughes and Segawa, 1993). Steady-state Cl and fluid absorption, however, is inhibited by cAMP due to an increase in NaCl secretion (Miller and Farber, 1984; Hughes et al., 1984; 1987; 1988). Studies on frog and cultured monkey RPE indicate that elevation of cAMP also inhibits Na,K,2Cl cotransport rate (la Cour, 1992; Kennedy, 1992), which could account for the cAMP-induced decrease in net Cl absorption.

For reasons that are not yet understood, the electrophysiological effects of cAMP in the chick retina-RPE-choroid preparation (Nao-i et al., 1990; Kuntz et al., 1994) and the bovine RPE-choroid preparation (Peterson and Miller, 1995b) are exactly opposite to those of frog and are consistent with a decrease in basolateral membrane Cl conductance. In cultured and native human RPE, however, there is evidence that the elevation of intracellular cAMP activates a Cl channel in the basolateral membrane (Frambach et al., 1990; Hu et al., 1995; Quinn and Miller, 1993). Recent molecular studies suggests that bovine and human RPE express messenger RNA for the cystic fibrosis membrane regulator (CFTR) (Miller et al., 1992), which encodes a cAMP-regulated Cl channel in a number of secretory epithelia (Fuller and Benos, 1992). Interestingly, the fast oscillation component of the electrooculogram, which is mediated by the basolateral membrane Cl conductance (Gallemore and Steinberg, 1993; Bialek et al., 1995), is significantly slower in cystic fibrosis patients than in normal individuals (Miller et al., 1992).

Calcium. Recent studies of bovine RPE-choroid suggest that the basolateral membrane Cl conductance also may be modulated by intracellular Ca^{2+}. Alpha-adrenergic agonists produce electrophysiological changes consistent with an increase in basolateral membrane Cl conductance (Joseph and Miller, 1992), and they stimulate Cl absorption (Edelman and Miller, 1992). Other experiments suggest that this Cl conductance change may be mediated by an increase in $[Ca^{2+}]_i$ (Joseph and Miller, 1992; Lin and Miller, 1991a). Patch-clamp studies on isolated rat RPE cells have shown that conditions expected to increase intracellular Ca^{2+} cause the activation of Cl channels (Ueda and Steinberg, 1994). Thus, the basolateral membrane Cl conductance may comprise cAMP- and Ca^{2+}-modulated Cl channels.

pH_i. In flux studies on frog RPE-choroid, several experimental conditions have been identified that cause a reversal in the direction of active Cl^- transport from absorption to secretion. Miller and colleagues (1994b) found that elevating apical $[K]_o$, $[Ba^{2+}]_o$, or $[HCO_3]_o$, or lowering bath pCO_2 all stimulated active Cl secretion. In each case, the mechanism for the reversal of Cl transport from absorption to secretion is stimulation of the basolateral membrane Cl/HCO_3 exchanger by intracellular alkalinization. Intracellular alkalinization is produced by increases in the inward electrical driving force (membrane depolarization by K or Ba^{2+}) or inward chemical driving force (HCO_3) on the apical $NaHCO_3$ cotransporter, which increases the rate of HCO_3 entry (see "$\Delta[K^+]_o$ (Light)-Induced Changes in pH_i," below). Stimulation of the Cl/HCO_3 exchanger leads to a net influx of Cl across the basolateral membrane; concomitantly, net Cl efflux across the apical

membrane also must occur. The transport mechanism(s) in the apical membrane that mediate Cl exit have not yet been identified.

$\Delta[K]_o$-induced changes. In a study on bovine RPE-choroid, Bialek and Miller (1994) measured changes in the apical and basolateral membrane potentials and intracellular Cl activity that are caused by decreasing apical $[K]_o$ from 5 to 2 mM. Figure 6-9A shows that the decrease in apical $[K]_o$ hyperpolarized V_A and V_B and caused intracellular Cl activity to decrease by 25 mM. This K-induced decrease was significantly inhibited by basolateral DIDS (Fig. 6-9B), implicating electrodiffusion of Cl through the basolateral membrane Cl conductance. Much of the $\Delta[K]_o$-induced change in intracellular Cl activity could also be inhibited by blocking the apical membrane K conductance with barium, indicating electrical coupling between the apical membrane K^+ conductance and the basolateral membrane Cl^- conductance. Considerations of osmotic balance led to the prediction that there would be a loss of cell water associated with the $\Delta[K]_o$-induced decreases in intracellular Cl and K activities (see "RPE regulation of subretinal space volume" below).

Bicarbonate Transport

Mechanisms. The first hint that the RPE may absorb HCO_3 came from the manometric measurements carried out by Lasansky and De Fisch (1966) in toad RPE. Electrophysiological and intracellular pH imaging studies in frog RPE have shown that the first step in active bicarbonate transport is the linked movement of Na *and* HCO_3 into the cell across the apical membrane via an electrogenic $NaHCO_3$ cotransporter (Hughes et al., 1989; la Cour, 1989; 1991a; Lin and Miller, 1991b). Note that this cotransporter also is responsible for driving fluid *across* the frog RPE from retina to choroid (Hughes et al., 1984). This process is initiated at the apical membrane by the linked movement of three ions, two HCO_3 and one Na, into the cell during each transport cycle; the net inward movement of one negative charge per transport cycle is sufficient to hyperpolarize the apical membrane by several millivolts (Hughes et al., 1989). The process of active HCO_3 absorption is completed by the exit of HCO_3 across the basolateral membrane. In frog, bovine, and human RPE the principle mechanism that mediates HCO_3 efflux is a Cl/HCO_3 exchanger (Fong et al., 1988; Lin and Miller, 1991b; Lin and Miller, 1994; Edelman et al., 1994a; 1994b). In fresh bovine and cultured human RPE, an electrogenic $NaHCO_3$ cotransporter in the basolateral membrane

A

B

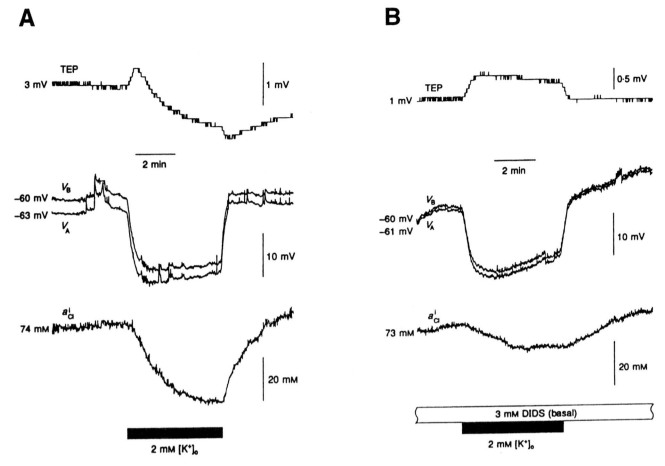

FIGURE 6-9 $\Delta[K]_o$-induced changes in membrane potential and intracellular Cl activity (a_{Cl}^i) in bovine RPE. (A) The effect of changing apical bath $[K]_o$ from 5 to 2 mM on TEP, V_A, V_B, and a_{Cl}^i. (B) The effect of changing apical bath $[K]_o$ from 5 to 2 mM on TEP, V_A, V_B, and a_{Cl}^i in the presence of 3 mM basolateral DIDS. DIDS did not significant-

ly affect the amplitude of the $[K]_o$-induced hyperpolarizations of V_A and V_B but it inhibited the $[K]_o$-induced a_{Cl}^i response by 50%. (Reprinted from Bialek and Miller, 1994, with permission of the authors and the *Journal of Physiology*.)

also may contribute to this process (Kenyon et al., 1997; R.P. Gallemore, F. Maruiwa, and D. Bok, unpublished observations).

$\Delta[K^+]_o$ (light)-induced changes in pH$_i$. The rate of the $NaHCO_3$ cotransporter is determined not only by the intracellular and extracellular activities of Na and HCO_3, but also by the apical membrane potential. Consequently, in the intact eye, intracellular activities of Na and HCO_3 (pH$_i$) would be significantly altered by the apical membrane hyperpolarization that occurs as a result of light-induced $[K]_o$ decreases outside the RPE apical membrane (la Cour, 1991a; Lin and Miller, 1991b; also see Chapter 9). This light-evoked decrease in $[K]_o$ can be mimicked in vitro in the isolated RPE-choroid preparation by decreasing apical $[K]_o$ from 5 to 2 mM.

Figure 6-10 shows that reducing apical $[K]_o$ from 5 to 2 mM acidifies the frog RPE cytoplasm by nearly 0.2 units (Lin and Miller, 1991b). Similar results have been observed in bovine RPE (Kenyon et al., 1997) and human RPE (Lin et al., 1992). The apical hyperpolarization produced by lowering subretinal $[K]_o$ moves V_A toward the reversal potential of the $NaHCO_3$ cotransporter (-114 mV in frog), reducing the driving force for $NaHCO_3$ influx across the apical membrane. This reduction in driving force slows the transporter, causing a depolarization of the apical membrane and acidification of the cell interior.

In frog RPE, it has been shown that the rate of the basolateral membrane exchanger is pH$_i$ sensitive and that it is regulated, in vitro, by changes in apical $[K]_o$ that closely approximate the changes observed in the sub-

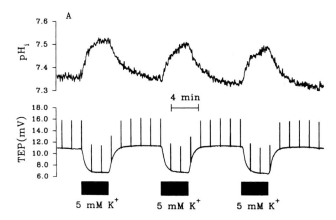

FIGURE 6-10. Changes in pH_i and TEP during step changes in apical $[K]_o$ from 2 to 5 mM in frog RPE. The transition to 5 mM $[K^+]_o$ mimics the light/dark transition while the transition from 5 mM to 2 mM $[K^+]_o$ mimics the transition from dark to light ("light onset"). (Reprinted from Lin and Miller, 1991, with permission of the authors and the *American Journal of Physiology*.)

retinal space following transitions between light and dark. The rate of this exchanger is reduced by cell acidification and increased by cell alkalinization (Lin and Miller, 1994). Any alteration in the rate of HCO_3 entry via the apical membrane cotransporter—for example, that produced by a $\Delta[K]_o$-induced change in apical membrane potential—would alter cell pH with a time course determined by the rate of the apical membrane potential change (Lin and Miller, 1991b).

At the basolateral membrane, Cl exits the cell through a Cl channel, driven by a favorable electrochemical gradient. In HCO_3 Ringer with 2 mM K in the apical bath, a fraction of this outgoing Cl is recycled back into the cell through the Cl/HCO_3 exchanger. When apical [K] is elevated from 2 to 5 mM, approximating the light-dark transition in the intact eye, the apical membrane depolarizes and the cell alkalinizes because the driving force on the apical membrane cotransporter is increased, which brings more HCO_3 into the cell per unit time. This alkalinization activates the basolateral membrane Cl/HCO_3 exchanger, which brings more Cl into the cell per unit time. In this situation (5 mM K in the apical bath), the rate of Cl entry through the Cl/HCO_3 exchanger exceeds the rate of Cl efflux through the basolateral membrane Cl channel. This $\Delta[K]_o$-induced reversal from active transepithelial Cl absorption to active secretion and the subsequent reduction of net fluid absorption from retina to choroid directly stems from the exquisite pH_i sensitivity of the basolateral membrane Cl/HCO_3 exchanger (Lin and Miller, 1994; Edelman et al., 1994b).

Regulation of pH_i. The apical membrane contains two separate pH_i regulatory mechanisms, the $NaHCO_3$ co-

transporter and an amiloride-sensitive Na/H exchanger, which utilizes the inward chemical gradient for Na to drive H out of the cell (Lin and Miller, 1991b). Following a decrease in cell pH both of these mechanisms respond by extruding acid from the cell. The relative contributions of these two mechanisms to pH regulation are species dependent. In frog, the cotransporter accounts for 80%–90% of the acid extruded following an acid load and is therefore the dominant mechanism in physiological Ringer (HCO_3/CO_2 buffered). In fresh bovine RPE (Kenyon et al., 1997), both of the apical membrane mechanisms contribute approximately equally to acid extrusion. In native human RPE, from adult donor and fetal eyes, the results lead to a different conclusion; here, the apical membrane Na/H exchanger is the dominant acid extrusion mechanism (Lin et al., 1992).

A more complete analysis of pH_i regulatory mechanisms has been carried out using fresh explants of bovine RPE (Kenyon et al., 1997). In bovine RPE there are three apical and two basolateral membrane mechanisms that all contribute to the regulation of pH_i. The important functional feature of these mechanisms is that they are very tightly coupled; sufficiently so, that changes in pH_i can only occur after two or more of them are inhibited. Four mechanisms contribute to acid extrusion; apical Na/H exchange, H-Lac cotransport (Kenyon et al., 1994b), and $NaHCO_3$ cotransport, and basolateral membrane $NaHCO_3$ cotransport. In addition two mechanisms have been identified that contribute to alkali (base) extrusion: apical $NaHCO_3$ cotransport and basolateral membrane Cl/HCO_3 exchange. These two transporters, located on opposite sides of the cell, are functionally important because they act in concert to tightly regulate cell pH and because they provide the pathways for the transepithelial transport of both Na and HCO_3, and thereby help regulate the hydration and pH of the subretinal space.

In sum, the in vitro mechanisms that regulate pH_i in frog, bovine, and human RPE probably serve multiple functions in vivo. By also controlling net ion and fluid transport across the RPE, they serve to spatially buffer the chemical composition (pH_i, lactate, Cl, Na, K) of the extracellular spaces on both sides of the epithelium; in particular, these mechanisms help determine the light-induced changes in the chemical composition of the subretinal space and thus regulate retinal metabolism and photoreceptor activity (Kenyon et al., 1994b; Peterson and Miller, 1995a).

Calcium Transport

Mechanisms. Calcium transport by the RPE is of particular interest because of the important roles Ca^{2+} plays in phototransduction and light adaptation in photoreceptors, and because of its action as an intracellular messenger in general. Ion flux measurements in frog revealed an active transepithelial Ca^{2+} flux in the choroid-to-retina direction of 5.9 nM/cm^2h (Miller and Steinberg, 1977b). This net secretory flux was approximately doubled by apical ouabain. Net Ca^{2+} secretion requires mechanisms for Ca^{2+} uptake at the basolateral membrane and Ca^{2+} efflux at the apical membrane. Studies on apical membrane vesicles from shark and bovine RPE have provided evidence for a Na/Ca^{2+} exchanger that could mediate Ca^{2+} efflux from the cell (Fijisawa et al., 1993). More recent studies indicate that both a Na/Ca^{2+} exchanger (Mangini et al., 1997) and plasma membrane Ca^{2+}-ATPase (Kennedy and Mangini, 1996) are present in cultured human RPE. A mechanism for Ca^{2+} uptake at the basolateral membrane remains to be identified. Patch-clamp experiments in freshly isolated and cultured rat RPE cells (Ueda and Steinberg, 1993) and freshly isolated human (fetal and adult) and monkey RPE (Ueda and Steinberg, 1995) have identified dihydroperidine-sensitive Ca^{2+} channels that appear to be similar to L-type Ca^{2+} channels. These voltage-sensitive channels are inactive at the resting membrane potential, but could be activated by physiological membrane depolarizations produced by light/dark changes in subretinal $[K]_o$. The mechanisms for Ca^{2+} transport under resting conditions require further elucidation.

Transport of Taurine, GABA, and Other Organic Molecules

Mechanism of taurine/GABA transport. Taurine, an uncharged beta-aminosulfonic acid, is important for normal retinal function. Taurine deficiency causes photoreceptor degeneration in cats (Schmidt et al., 1976) and is associated with ERG abnormalities in humans (Geggel et al., 1985). Taurine is concentrated in the outer nuclear layer of the vertebrate retina by a Na-dependent mechanism, reaching intracellular concentrations of 60–80 mM (Pasante-Morales et al., 1972; Lake et al, 1975; 1977; Voaden et al., 1977; Schmidt, 1980). It appears to be released into the subretinal space following light onset (Salceda et al., 1977; Schmidt, 1978), and thus the RPE might be expected to transport taurine out of the subretinal space, buffering the light-evoked concentration change.

Experiments on isolated frog RPE-choroid showed that taurine is actively transported in the retina-to-choroid direction (Miller and Steinberg, 1976; Ostwald and Steinberg, 1981) and that this active absorption involves a Na-dependent mechanism at the apical membrane (Miller and Steinberg, 1979). This mechanism appears to cotransport Na, taurine, and net positive charge into the cell, which depolarizes the apical membrane. With prolonged exposure to taurine, the accompanying load of intracellular Na appears to stimulate the apical membrane electrogenic Na/K pump, and this effect is evident in electrophysiological recordings (Scharschmidt et al., 1988). A similar mechanism may be present in mammalian RPE (Sivakami et al., 1992; Hussain et al., 1995).

In addition to taurine, this Na-dependent uptake mechanism transports β-alanine (Miller and Steinberg, 1976; 1979) and γ-amino butyric acid (GABA) (Miyamoto et al., 1991; Peterson and Miller, 1995a). GABA is the major inhibitory neurotransmitter in the retina (Barnstable, 1993), and in the amphibian retina it is released tonically in the dark by both horizontal and amacrine cells (O'Malley et al., 1992), but it is not taken up by the nearby Müller cells (Neal et al., 1979). Using an electrophysiological assay, Peterson and Miller (1995a) determined that this transporter has a significantly higher affinity for GABA as compared with taurine (GABA: K_m = 160 μM; alanine: K_m = 250 μM; taurine: K_m = 850 μM.

$\Delta[K]_o$ (light)-induced modulation of taurine/GABA transport. The rate of the Na-dependent taurine/GABA cotransporter is determined by the intracellular and extracellular activities of Na, GABA, and taurine, as well as by the apical membrane potential. Decreasing apical $[K]_o$ from 5 to 2 mM, which mimics the transition from dark to light, hyperpolarizes the apical membrane and lowers intracellular Na activity, and both these changes significantly increase the driving force for GABA (or taurine) uptake (Peterson and Miller, 1996). In the intact eye, then, light onset would increase the rate of the Na-dependent transporter, facilitating the removal of GABA and taurine from the subretinal space. Conversely, increasing taurine or GABA concentration increases K absorption across the RPE by stimulating K influx through the apical membrane Na/K pump and K efflux through the basolateral membrane K channels (Miller and Steinberg, 1979; Peterson and Miller, 1995a). Thus, light-induced changes in taurine or GABA concentration may be one of several mechanisms that help regulate $[K]_o$ in the subretinal space.

Since the transporter can carry both GABA and taurine, it is likely that these two amino acids compete for uptake via this carrier in vivo, and that the transport rate of both substrates is regulated by light/dark transitions. Coordinated uptake and release by this carrier in the RPE apical membrane could help determine the activities of GABA and taurine in the subretinal space.

Transport of other amino acids, glucose, and organic molecules

Amino acids. There is evidence for the transport of a number of other amino acids by the RPE. In addition to taurine, GABA, and alanine, leucine (Sellner, 1986a; 1986b; Pautler et al., 1989) and the excitatory neurotransmitter glutamate (Pautler and Tengerdy, 1986; Pautler et al., 1989; Miyamoto and Del Monte, 1994) also are actively absorbed across the RPE. Glutamate is the transmitter of photoreceptor cells and mediates the transmission of signals between the photoreceptors and second-order retinal neurons. Absorption by the RPE may reduce background levels of glutamate in distal retina and enhance the signal-to-noise ratio of photoreceptor transmission.

Glucose. Radioactive tracer flux studies on isolated RPE-choroid preparations have shown that glucose is not actively transported (Miller and Steinberg, 1976; Sellner, 1986b; DiMattio and Streitman, 1986; 1991) but instead is passively transported by facilitated diffusion (Pascuzzo et al., 1980; Masterson and Chader, 1981; Crosson and Pautler, 1982; Stramm and Pautler, 1982; To and Hodson, 1995). Recent molecular studies have demonstrated that the RPE contains the glucose transporter GLUT1 in its apical and basolateral membranes (Harik et al., 1990; Takata et al., 1992; Kumagai et al., 1994), which would provide a pathway for passive glucose transport across the epithelium. In the dark-adapted eye, it is likely that the high rate of glycolysis in photoreceptor cells establishes a significant gradient favoring the movement of glucose from the choroid to the subretinal space.

Changes in choroidal glucose levels affect the standing potential in the isolated, perfused cat eye (Macaluso et al., 1992), but the specific transport mechanisms underlying this response remains to be determined.

Myo-inositol. Myo-inositol transport has been demonstrated in cultured RPE (Khatami, 1990; Khatami et al., 1990; Yokoyama et al., 1993), but has yet to be examined in native tissue.

Ascorbic acid. Uptake studies have identified Na-dependent, active ascorbic acid transport in cultured cat and bovine RPE cells (Khatami, 1987; Khatami et al., 1986). Active ascorbic acid transport also has been demonstrated in the isolated frog RPE-choroid preparation, where it occurs in the retina-to-choroid direction (DiMattio and Streitman, 1991). As in cultured cat and bovine RPE cells, active ascorbic acid transport in frog RPE was inhibited by apical ouabain and by the removal of Na from the bathing solutions, indicating that this transport mechanism is ultimately tied to the activity of the Na/K pump.

Probenicid-sensitive organic anion transport. The movement of fluorescein across the RPE is of particular interest because fluorescein angiography is utilized in identifying abnormalities of the blood-retinal barrier. Surprisingly, the RPE appears to actively transport fluorescein in the retina-to-choroid direction (Tsuboi et al., 1984; Koyano et al., 1993). The active transport of fluorescein appears to be mediated by a probenicid-inhibitable organic anion transporter present in the apical membrane that also carries cAMP (Garcia and Burnside, 1994); the ion-sensitive dyes FURA 2, BCECF, calcium green, and sodium green; and lactate (Kenyon et al., 1994b).

Modulation of RPE Transport by Changes in Apical $[K]_o$: A Summary

The RPE c-wave response is due solely to the light-induced decrease in subretinal space $[K]_o$ (Oakley, 1977; see Chapter 9). In the frog eyecup and in the intact eye of the cat, subretinal space $[K]_o$ is approximately 5 mM in the dark and, depending on stimulus intensity and duration, as low as 1 mM in the light (Oakley and Green, 1976; Steinberg et al., 1983). Clearly, the light-induced change in subretinal space $[K]_o$ is a paracrine signal that helps inform the RPE when the light is on ($[K]_o \approx 2$ mM) or off ($[K]_o \approx 5$ mM). As discussed in Chapter 9, these $\Delta[K]_o$ changes can be used in vitro to approximate the transition between light and dark. The range of changes in RPE physiology produced by this particular signal, presumably one of many retinal paracrine signals, has been elaborated using a variety of in vitro RPE-choroid preparations from frog, chick, bovine, and human eyes. The work on frog and bovine preparations will be summarized here; it is representative of the others and the most complete.

In frog RPE, it has been shown that $[K]_o$ changes in the range between 2 and 5 mM alter the rate of the Na/K pump (Miller and Steinberg, 1982), the Na,K,2Cl cotransporter (Adorante and Miller, 1990) and the $NaHCO_3$ cotransporter (Hughes et al., 1989; Lin and Miller, 1991a). As $[K]_o$ is elevated from 2 to 5 mM, the Na/K pump rate is increased toward saturation and the Na,K,2Cl cotransport rate is increased, while the $NaHCO_3$ cotransporter is stimulated by an increase in the electrical driving force that moves Na and HCO_3 into the cell with a stoichiometry of approximately 1:2 (Hughes et al., 1989). These rate changes alter the hydration and chemical composition of the extracellular spaces on both sides of the epithelium (see "RPE regulation of subretinal space volume," below and Chapter 9) as well as the intracellular milieu (see "RPE cell volume regulation," below). For example, the $\Delta[K]_o$-induced increase in HCO_3 uptake increases cell pH, which in turn increases the rate of the basolateral membrane Cl/HCO_3 exchanger, bringing more Cl into the cell per unit time (Lin and Miller, 1994). This $\Delta[K]_o$-induced, pH_i-dependent change in Cl recycling at the basolateral membrane (see "Recycling," above) determines whether Cl is actively absorbed ($[K]_o = 2$ mM) or secreted ($[K]_o = 5$ mM) across the epithelium; the rate of transepithelial fluid absorption also is reduced as $[K]_o$ is elevated (Edelman et al., 1994a; 1994b). Elevating $[K]_o$ from 2 to 5 mM also decreases the rate of taurine and GABA uptake into the RPE, a finding that has potentially important implications for the regulation of photoreceptor activity following light/dark transitions (Miller and Steinberg, 1979; Peterson and Miller, 1995a). Finally, elevating $[K]_o$ from 2 to 5 mM increases RPE cell volume (Adorante and Miller, 1990) and decreases subretinal space volume (Huang and Karwoski, 1989; 1992).

A major difference between bovine and frog RPE is that the intracellular Cl concentration is approximately three times higher in bovine RPE than in frog (≈ 60 versus 20 mM—Joseph and Miller, 1991; Fong et al., 1988). Part of this difference occurs because bovine control Ringer contains 5 mM K, whereas frog Ringer contains 2 mM K. In bovine RPE, a reduction of apical $[K]_o$, to mimic the transition from dark to light, slows down the apical membrane cotransporter and stimulates the efflux of KCl through apical membrane K and basolateral membrane Cl channels (Bialek and Miller, 1994; Bialek et al., 1995). The mean $\Delta[K]_o$-induced decrease in Cl activity is approximately 25 mM (see Fig. 6-9). Because the intracellular Cl concentration is high in bovine RPE bathed in control Ringer, the basolateral membrane Cl/HCO_3 exchanger is close to equilibrium and is not significantly altered by $\Delta[K]_o$-induced changes in pH_i (approximately 0.3 pH units).

In addition, there is evidence that this decrease in $[K]_o$ also causes K, HCO_3, and fluid to be secreted into the apical bath (Bialek and Miller, 1994; Kenyon et al., 1997). The comparison of the light-induced changes in subretinal space volume (Li et al., 1994a) with the in vitro analysis of the mechanisms that regulate RPE volume strongly suggests that the $\Delta[K]_o$-induced changes in RPE physiology generate feedback signals, which in turn modulate the relative hydration and chemical composition of the subretinal space (see Chapter 9).

In addition to K, the transition between light and dark induces changes in the subretinal concentration of other ions, such as H (Yamamoto et al., 1992) and Ca^{2+} (Gallemore and Steinberg, 1988; Livsey et al., 1990; Gallemore et al., 1994). The extent to which changes in apical concentration of these ions modulates RPE transport, however, remains to be determined.

Lactate Transport

Mechanisms. Under dark-adapted conditions, oxygen tension in the distal mammalian retina approaches 0 mm Hg and the RPE and photoreceptors exist in a relative state of anoxia (Linsenmeier and Braun, 1992). Anaerobic glycolysis is therefore required for energy production, and lactic acid is a byproduct of this pathway (Winkler, 1981; 1989; Miceli et al., 1990). Evidence for lactic acid generation in vivo comes from studies on pig. Lactate levels in choroidal venous blood were found to exceed levels in arterial blood (Tornquist and Alm, 1979; Alm and Tornquist, 1985), and a lactate gradient has been measured in the subretinal space, which increases from the outer limiting membrane to the RPE (Adler and Southwick, 1990). Lactate accumulation in the distal retina would impose an osmotic load and cause a marked reduction in extracellular pH. As part of the blood-retinal barrier, then, the RPE might be expected to participate in the removal of lactate and protons from the subretinal space.

Tracer flux studies in bovine RPE-choroid preparation revealed active transcellular absorption of lactate (Kenyon et al., 1994b). Intracellular pH measurements during perturbations of apical and basolateral bath lactate levels revealed two mechanisms for lactate transport: H-lactate cotransport for lactate uptake at the apical membrane and electrogenic Na-lactate cotransport for lactate efflux across the basolateral membrane. While basolateral lactate transport is mediated predominantly by Na-dependent lactate transport, there is also a minor contribution of the DIDS-sensitive Cl/HCO_3 exchanger, which can carry lactate in place of Cl. Recently, Philp and colleagues (Philp et al., 1995; Yoon et al., 1997) identified an RPE-specific monocarboxylate transporter and localized it immunohistochemically to the basolateral membrane of chick RPE. The relationship between this transporter and the Na-dependent lactate transporter in bovine RPE unclear, but it seems likely that it provides an important mechanism for lactate transport across the basolateral membrane. Apical membrane H-lactate cotransport also has been characterized in frog RPE (Lin et al., 1994) and lactate transport has been characterized in native fetal human RPE as well (la Cour et al., 1994).

Light-induced changes. Thermodynamic considerations suggest the possibility of light/dark differences in lactate transport across the RPE and a brief summary from the recent work of Miller and colleagues (1994b) is presented here. In the dark-adapted retina, where photoreceptor metabolism is highest, lactate and hydrogen ion production would be highest, favoring lactate absorption across the RPE. At light onset, the light-evoked hyperpolarization of the RPE cell membranes (see Chapter 9) would increase the driving force for electrogenic lactate exit across the basolateral membrane, transiently stimulating lactate absorption across the RPE. With maintained illumination, however, lactate and proton production would fall as a result of a decrease in photoreceptor metabolism, and the electrochemical gradient for lactate would now favor its transport from choroid to retina. This postulated secretion of lactate may provide an alternative fuel to the photoreceptors when the oxygen supply is no longer limited (in the light). The hypothesis that Müller cells also provide energy substrates (lactate, pyruvate) that support photoreceptor activity has recently been reviewed by Tsacopoulos and Magistretti (1996) in the more general context of metabolic coupling between glia and neurons.

Contributions to fluid transport. Another possible physiological role for lactate transport is the generation of fluid absorption across the RPE. When the RPE is bathed with solutions containing putative dark-adapted levels of retinal and choroidal lactate, there is net lactate absorption across the RPE (Kenyon et al., 1994b). Assuming isotonic coupling between fluid and net solute fluxes, this lactate transport (coupled to Na absorption) is calculated to drive fluid absorption at a rate of 4.6 μl/cm^2·hr. In situ, this lactate-induced flux would add significantly to the transepithelial fluid transport coupled to net salt movement (1.4–4 μl/cm^2·hr). Thus, water flow coupled to Na lactate transport may represent a significant portion of the total transport rate and could have clinical significance.

Fluid Transport

Fluid absorption by the RPE is thought to play a role in normal retinal adhesion and recovery from retinal detachment, and as a pathway for fluid outflow from the eye under normal conditions (Marmor, 1994; Pederson, 1994). Fluid transport rates across the RPE have now been estimated by a variety of methods, both in vivo and in vitro. In vivo, a number of factors may conspire to determine the rate of net fluid transport across the RPE. These include osmotic and oncotic pressures, hydrostatic pressure, and solute-linked fluid transport. Estimates of each of these contributions have been made and, overall, solute-linked fluid absorption appears to be the predominant factor, with only minor contributions from the others (Pederson, 1994). The average fluid transport rates estimated in various species are shown in Table 6-6, along with the technique of measurement

TABLE 6-6. *RPE fluid transport rates measured in vitro and in vivo*

Species/preparation	$J_V (\mu l \cdot cm^{-2} \cdot h^{-1})$	Method
Frog, RPE-choroid[1]	4.8	Capacitance probe
Bovine, RPE-choroid[2]	1.4	Capacitance probe
Dog, RPE-choroid[3]	6.4	Capillary
Monkey, RPE-choroid[4]	7.2	Capillary
Human (cultured fetal)[5]	2.7	Capacitance probe
Human (native fetal)[5]	4	Capacitance probe
Rabbit[6]	4	Subretinal bleb, photometric
Human, in vivo[7]	11.0	B-scan ultrasonography

Mean values from the following references: [1]Hughes et al., 1984; [2]Edelman and Miller, 1991; [3]Tsuboi, 1987; [4]Tsuboi and Pederson, 1987; [5]Miller, unpublished; [6]Wolfensberger et al., 1996; [7]Chihara and Nao-i, 1984.

and the preparation used. The values range from 1.42 to 11 μl/cm^2·h.

The rates measured in the in vitro preparations are remarkably similar to those measured in vivo, even though the in vitro preparations are undoubtedly missing at least some of the normal paracrine and hormonal input signals from the retina and blood that would normally help regulate fluid transport out of the subretinal space. It has been shown that many of the apical and basolateral membrane transport proteins that mediate fluid transport across the epithelium also serve to regulate the volume of the RPE following osmotic perturbations that shrink or swell the cells (Adorante and Miller, 1990; Kennedy, 1994; Bialek and Miller, 1994; Adorante, 1995). These proteins include the apical membrane Na,K,2Cl cotransporter, basolateral membrane Cl channels and the apical and basolateral membrane K channels. In the intact eye, measurements of light-induced changes in subretinal space volume (Huang and Karwoski, 1992; Li et al., 1994a; 1994b) show that these same mechanisms play an important role in controlling the hydration and chemical composition of the subretinal space (for more details, see "RPE Regulation of Subretinal Space Volume," below, and Chapter 9). The remarkable similarity of fluid transport rates in vitro and in vivo, and the realization that proteins that mediate RPE volume regulation also determine subretinal space volume suggests that our understanding of in situ physiology will continue to benefit from a close comparison of cellular and in situ preparations.

Mechanism of solute-linked fluid flow. The ion transport proteins and pathways that generate transepithelial fluid absorption across the RPE have been studied in a variety of in vitro preparations, including frog (Miller et al., 1982; Hughes et al., 1984; 1987; 1989; Adorante and Miller, 1990; Edelman et al., 1994a; 1994b), dog (Tsuboi, 1987), cattle (Miller and Edelman, 1990; Edelman and Miller, 1991; Bialek and Miller, 1994), monkey (Tsuboi and Pederson, 1986), and human (Quinn and Miller, 1992; Quong et al., 1996; K. Yu and S.S. Miller, unpublished observations). In each of these studies, there is evidence for a fluid-entry step at the apical (retina-facing) membrane that is mediated in part by the apical membrane Na,K,2Cl cotransporter. The molecular mechanisms that might link ion and fluid transport in other epithelia have been recently reviewed (Fischbarg et al., 1993; Zeuthen, 1995). In the frog, bovine, and human preparations it also has been shown that in steady-state, fluid exit across the basolateral membrane is coupled to Cl exit through a basolateral membrane Cl channel. Taken together, these studies show that fluid absorption across the RPE is coupled to the Cl transport pathway, which consists of an apical membrane Na,K,2Cl cotransporter and a basolateral membrane Cl channel.

In frog RPE, it has been shown that a significant portion of the absorbed fluid is driven across the RPE via the HCO_3 transport pathway, which consists of the apical membrane $NaHCO_3$ cotransporter (Hughes et al., 1984; 1987) and the basolateral membrane Cl/HCO_3 exchanger (Lin and Miller, 1994; Edelman et al., 1994a; 1994b; see "Bicarbonate Transport," above). There is good evidence to suggest that this fluid transport is isotonic, as expected for "leaky" epithelia (Zeuthen, 1995). The comparison of flux and fluid transport measurements in control and cAMP-stimulated tissues (Hughes et al., 1984; 1987) show that net "solute" flux is linearly related to the separately measured fluid transport rate, and that the constant of proportionality is the osmolarity of the bathing solution, as expected for isotonic transport (House, 1974). In this case, the net solute flux is defined as the vectorial sum of all steady-state net ion tracer fluxes (Na, Cl, K) measured in the open circuit plus a net HCO_3 flux inferred from the constraint that the net current must be equal to zero (Ginsburg and Hogg, 1967). In bovine RPE, a similar kind of comparison also showed that the sum of measured solute fluxes and the fluid transport rate are linearly related. Again, the constant of proportionality is the osmolarity of the bathing solution, as predicted for isotonic transport (Edelman and Miller, 1991; 1996). However, in this case, the possibility of contributions from other solutes such as lactate remain to be evaluated (Kenyon et al., 1994b).

Ion and fluid secretion by the RPE. As in other epithelia, net fluid transport across the RPE is determined by ion

transport pathways that allow the absorption or the secretion of ions. The vector sum of separate absorptive and secretory ion transport pathways determines the direction and magnitude of net fluid transport (Jiang et al., 1993). It has been shown in frog RPE that active Cl transport across the epithelium can be reversed from absorption to secretion by a small, physiologically relevant increase in apical bath [K] (from 2 to 5 mM), and that this reversal in the direction of Cl transport significantly reduces net fluid absorption (Edelman et al., 1994b). There is accumulating evidence that bovine and human RPE can spontaneously secrete fluid in physiologically relevant bathing media (Edelman and Miller, 1991; K. Yu and S.S. Miller, unpublished observations). Although the exact mechanisms that mediate this process have not yet been identified, there is evidence for the involvement of HCO_3 and K secretory pathways (Tsuboi et al., 1986; Bialek and Miller, 1994). Recent studies in bovine RPE identified a specific HCO_3-dependent-secretory pathway that could mediate the secretory component of net fluid transport (Kenyon et al., 1994a; Kenyon et al., 1997).

The observations that some unstimulated tissues secrete while others absorb fluid in the steady state is perhaps not surprising, given the reversibility of active Cl transport across frog RPE (Edelman et al., 1994b) and a similar observation in bovine RPE (J. Edelman and S. Miller, unpublished observations). The recent demonstration of pH_i-dependent changes in fluid transport and Cl/HCO_3 exchange at the basolateral membrane of frog and bovine RPE (Lin and Miller, 1994; Edelman et al., 1994a; Kenyon et al., 1997) indicates that significant amounts of Cl are recycled at the basolateral membrane. It has been shown that the Cl exit pathway in the basolateral membrane is a Ca^{2+}-sensitive Cl channel (Joseph and Miller, 1992). Hence, any drug or intracellular messenger that decreases Cl conductance, such as flufenamic acid, pH_i, or low $[Ca^{2+}]_i$, would tend to decrease net Cl and fluid absorption and therefore increase the likelihood of net Cl secretion via the Cl/HCO_3 exchanger. For example, in bovine RPE the flufenamic-acid-induced decrease in basolateral membrane Cl conductance can cause net fluid secretion (basolateral to apical or choroid to retina). The counterion that must accompany Cl in this secretory process is probably Na or K (Bialek et al., 1996; Kenyon et al., 1997).

Basolateral membrane Cl conductance regulates fluid transport. There is undoubtedly a wide range of paracrine, autocrine, and hormonal signals that differentially affect RPE fluid transport in light or dark. The size and time course of these signals in light and dark, their activation of specific apical or basolateral membrane receptors, and their intracellular signal transduction pathways are all co-ordinated to determine whether fluid is absorbed (retina to choroid) or secreted (choroid to retina). For example, in control HCO_3-buffered Ringer, fluid absorption across the bovine RPE is driven by the absorption of Na and Cl (Edelman and Miller, 1992). Solute (KCl)-coupled fluid absorption (J_v) is significantly increased by the presence of nanomolar amounts of epinephrine, which activate alpha-1 adrenergic receptors at the apical membrane. Epinephrine-induced receptor activation leads to an elevation of cell free Ca^{2+} levels, which causes a increase in basolateral membrane Cl conductance followed by a decrease in apical membrane K conductance (Joseph and Miller, 1992; Lin and Miller, 1991a; Edelman and Miller, 1992). These epinephrine-induced changes in conductances lead to an increase in fluid absorption across the RPE (Joseph and Miller, 1991; 1992), mediated in part by the Cl transport pathway. Other catecholamines, such as dopamine, have similar effects and form a class of putative paracrine signals that would allow the retinal to "tell" the RPE when the light is on or off. Nonsteroidal anti-inflammatory drugs (NSAIDs), such as indomethacin and niflumic acid, also increase fluid absorption by increasing basolateral membrane Cl conductance (Bialek et al., 1996). In striking contrast, other members of the fenamate family, such as flufenamic acid, have the opposite effect: they decrease basolateral membrane Cl conductance and block fluid absorption. Because these compounds decrease $[Ca^{2+}]_i$ and have no effect on K conductance, the mechanism by which they modulate fluid absorption most likely involves direct effects on basolateral membrane Cl channels (Bialek et al., 1996).

Acetazolamide. Evidence from several animal studies indicates that the systemic administration of high doses of acetazolamide (Diamox) can enhance fluid absorption across the RPE (Marmor and Maack, 1982; Tsuboi and Pederson, 1987; Wolfensberger et al., in press). The mechanism underlying this stimulation of fluid absorption is unknown, but it could involve a number of effects, including the inhibition of membrane-bound or cytosolic carbonic anhydrase, leading to changes in intracellular pH and HCO_3^-, or the direct inhibition of transporters. Several in vitro and in vivo studies have shown that acetazolamide causes changes in TEP or standing potential, but the polarity of these voltage changes is not consistent, even among mammalian species (Miller and Steinberg, 1977b; Kawasaki et al., 1986; Yonemura et al., 1978; Yamamoto and Steinberg, 1992). Although these TEP changes may reflect alterations in ion transport, their origin remains obscure. Because fluid transport across the RPE is isotonically cou-pled to solute transport, acetazolamide would be expected to cause an increase in net solute absorption. In a study on the isolated frog RPE-choroid preparation, however, Miller and Steinberg (1977b) found that acetazolamide inhibited Cl absorption, which would tend to reduce, not enhance, fluid absorption. Because Cl transport and pH_i are regulated somewhat differently in bovine RPE than they are in frog (see "Regulation of pH_i" and "Modulation of RPE Transport by Changes in Apical $[K]_o$," above), it is possible that acetazolamide affects Cl transport differently in mammalian RPE. Future experiments should determine the effect of acetazolamide on pH_i and Cl transport in mammalian RPE and ascertain whether the transport of other osmotically active solutes are modulated.

RPE cell volume regulation. As in other cell types, the RPE responds to changes in cell volume by activation of solute transport mechanisms that move osmotically obliged water into or out of the cell, returning cell volume toward normal. In the intact eye, osmotic perturbations are likely to occur in the subretinal space as a result of changes in photoreceptor activity or fluid and solute transport by the RPE itself. Studies in frog RPE have shown that following hyperosmotic shrinkage, cells reswell as a result of stimulation of the apical Na,K,2Cl cotransporter (Adorante and Miller, 1990). This regulatory volume increase (RVI) was found to depend on apical $[K]_o$ and took place when the apical bath contained 5 mM K but not when it contained 2 mM K. Consistent with the view that the Na,K,2Cl cotransporter mediates the RVI, Kennedy (1990; 1992; 1994) has shown in cultured human and monkey RPE cells that hyperosmotic conditions produce a 2.5-fold increase in the rate of the bumetanide-sensitive ^{86}Rb influx. Other investigators working on cultured human RPE cells, however, found evidence suggesting that regulatory volume increase was likely mediated by Na/H and Cl/HCO_3 exchangers in parallel, rather than the Na,K,2Cl cotransporter (Civan et al., 1994).

The regulatory volume decrease of RPE cells following hypotonic cell swelling has been found to be mediated by basolateral membrane K channels in the frog RPE-choroid preparation (Adorante, 1995). In cultured human RPE cells, K channels appear to be involved in the regulatory volume decrease, but Cl channels (Civan et al., 1994) and KCl symport (Kennedy, 1994) also have been implicated. In patch-clamp studies, the activation of Cl channels by cell swelling has been observed in freshly isolated rat (Botchkin and Matthews, 1993; Ueda and Steinberg, 1994) and bovine RPE cells (M. Takahira and B.A. Hughes, unpublished observations) and in cultured human RPE cells (Gallemore et al., 1996), but the activation of K channels has not been reported.

RPE regulation of subretinal space volume.

In vitro studies have demonstrated that the RPE apical membrane Na,K,2Cl cotransporter, apical membrane K channel, and basolateral membrane K and Cl channels are all important determinants of RPE cell volume (Adorante and Miller, 1990; Bialek and Miller, 1994; Kennedy, 1994; Adorante, 1995). It has been shown that decreasing apical $[K]_o$ from 5 to 2 mM produces a decrease in RPE cell volume (Adorante and Miller, 1990) and a decrease or reversal in Na,K,2Cl cotransport (Bialek and Miller, 1994). These findings suggested the possibility that illumination of the retina in situ could result in a significant increase in the volume of the subretinal space, which has subsequently been observed (Huang and Karwoski, 1989; Huang and Karwoski, 1992; Li et al., 1994a; 1994b). Changes in subretinal volume will not only affect the concentration of ions and metabolites outside the photoreceptor outer segments, but may also alter the state of hydration of the interphotoreceptor matrix (IPM), affecting retinal adhesion (Marmor, 1994) and other photoreceptor–RPE interactions.

Alterations in net ion and fluid transport across the RPE could cause the light-evoked changes in subretinal-space volume. This possibility was investigated in the in vitro frog and chick preparations. In their studies on the frog eyecup preparation, Huang and Karwoski (1989; 1992) found that retinal furosemide had no effect on the light-evoked decrease in subretinal $[TMA]_o$, and that retinal bumetanide either had no effect or it depressed all retinal functions. In chick, it was found that inhibiting Cl uptake across the apical membrane by the Na,K,2Cl cotransporter with bumetanide or furosemide reduced the size of the light-evoked decrease in $[TMA]_o$ by more than 50%. These results in chick support the notion that the Na,K,2Cl cotransporter not only regulates the volume of the RPE cell but also the volume of the subretinal space. The negative result in frog may reflect the perfusion limitations of the eyecup preparation.

The involvement of the apical membrane K conductance and the basolateral membrane Cl conductance in retinal hydration was proposed by Huang and Karwoski (1992) on the basis of their observation that the light-evoked decrease in subretinal $[TMA]_o$ was partially inhibited by retinal Ba^{2+}. In bovine RPE, decreases in apical $[K]_o$ produced large increases in the electrochemical driving forces for conductive K and Cl exit across the apical and basolateral membranes, respectively (Bialek and Miller, 1994). Because the K and Cl conductances are electrically coupled, blocking either the apical K conductance with Ba^{2+} or the basolateral membrane Cl conductance with DIDS significantly reduced the apical $[K]_o$-induced efflux of KCl. These in vitro data led to the prediction that RPE cell volume would be decreased in situ by an amount comparable to the light-induced increase in subretinal space volume, and that these changes in RPE and subretinal volume would be decreased by blockade of either of the conductances. This prediction is supported by in situ data obtained from the chick retina-RPE-choroid preparation. It was shown that either retinal Ba^{2+} or basolateral DIDS inhibited the light-evoked decrease in subretinal $[TMA]_o$ (Li et al., 1994a), indicating that a portion of the cell water lost from the RPE contributes to subretinal hydration.

It is possible that other RPE transport mechanisms are involved. For example, Huang and Karwoski (1992) showed in frog retina that the light-evoked decrease in subretinal $[TMA]_o$ was partially inhibited by retinal amiloride (2 mM), suggesting that the Na/H exchanger in the RPE apical membrane might play a role in the light-evoked hydration of subretinal space. Interestingly, superfusing the retina with DIDS (1 mM) had no effect on the TMA response, suggesting that the $NaHCO_3$ cotransporter in the RPE apical membrane does not participate in the light-evoked decrease in subretinal volume. This result is not definitive, however, since DIDS may not have reached the RPE apical membrane in sufficient concentration to block the cotransporter.

In summary, two RPE transport mechanisms that contribute to the light-evoked hydration of the subretinal space have been identified. First, the light-evoked decrease in subretinal $[K]_o$ causes a slowing of the Na,K,2Cl contransporter in the RPE apical membrane, resulting in a decrease in the solute-linked movement of water from the subretinal space into the RPE cell. Second, the decrease in subretinal $[K]_o$ also stimulates a massive efflux of KCl from the RPE cell, causing a reduction in RPE cell volume; evidently, some of the lost cell water moves out across the apical membrane and into the subretinal space. Future experiments should ascertain whether the transport of other osmotically active solutes, such as lactate, may be involved in this process (Kenyon et al., 1994b).

Clinical implications.

Abnormalities in fluid *absorption* across the RPE may contribute to the etiology of certain diseases of the photoreceptor-RPE complex. These abnormalities could stem from disease-induced (1) alterations in active ion and solute-linked fluid transport; (2) alterations in oncotic or hydrostatic pressure gradients, which are normally directed in the retina to choroid direction (Fould, 1976; Negi and Marmor, 1983; 1984; Pederson, 1994); (3) alterations in fluid (or hydraulic) conductivity of the RPE cell membranes or adjacent tissues; (4) changes in the interphotoreceptor matrix, which normally forms a "glue" between the neural retina and RPE (Fischer and Anderson, 1994). In retinal pigment epithelial detachments, for example, fluid accumulates between the RPE and Bruch's membrane, leading to localized detachment of the RPE (Bird, 1994). This detachment may occur as a result of an age-related decrease in the hydraulic conductivity of Bruch's membrane (Starita et al., 1995) leading to the accumulation of subepithelial fluid (Bird, 1995).

The formation of serous retinal detachments in a variety of conditions may be related to impaired fluid absorption by the RPE secondary to factors released in these disease states (Bird, 1994; Marmor, 1994). Increased fluid absorption, driven by active ion or solute transport across the RPE, could significantly contribute to recovery from rhegmatogenous retinal detachments and facilitate adherence between the neural retina and RPE (Chihara and Nao-i, 1984; Kirchhof and Ryan, 1993; Marmor, 1994; Steinberg, 1986). Serous detachments of the retina could also occur from a reversal of active ion- (or solute-) linked fluid transport from absorption to secretion. This in vitro observation seems particularly relevant in the case of central serous retinopathy, where focal serous detachments of the sensory retina can occur. While a "hole" in the RPE allowing fluid to pass from the choroid to subretinal space has been proposed as the mechanism for this disease (Judson and Yannuzzi, 1994), a defect in the barrier function of the RPE alone would not necessarily detach the retina. The discovery of experimental conditions that can slow or reverse the direction of fluid transport across the RPE may thus have particular clinical relevance.

Some pharmacological agents that can alter fluid absorption across the RPE have been identified and hopefully some of them will be important in treating diseases where accumulation of subretinal and intraretinal fluid occur. For example, stimulation of fluid absorption by epinephrine in isolated RPE-choroid preparations has been well characterized, and involves stimulation of KCl absorption across the RPE (Edelman and Miller, 1991; 1992). In vivo, however, adrenergic agents may impair fluid absorption across the RPE and lead to retinal edema (Swartz, 1994). Since a number of paracrine- and endocrine-activated membrane receptors are positively and negatively coupled to adenylate cyclase (Dearry et al., 1990; Nash and Osborne, 1995), and since cAMP is known to alter fluid transport across the RPE (Hughes et al., 1984), cAMP may be a crucial second messenger

regulating fluid transport across the RPE in vivo. The efficacy of Diamox in treating certain forms of macular edema is another such example (Cox et al., 1988; Fishman et al., 1989; Marmor, 1994), although the cellular mechanisms by which carbonic anhydrase inhibitors may alter fluid transport across the RPE remain elusive. Steroids and nonsteroidal anti-inflammatory agents have also been used in the treatment of macular edema (Flach, 1992). The recent observation that certain NSAIDs increase the Cl conductance of the basolateral membrane of the RPE may be relevant to the clinical utility of these agents (Bialek et al., 1996).

SUMMARY

Fluid absorption across the RPE from retina to choroid is mediated mainly by two transport proteins, an apical membrane Na,K,2Cl cotransporter and a basolateral membrane Cl channel. Chloride and fluid absorption can be modulated by small extracellular changes in $[K]_o$, by catecholamines such as epinephrine or dopamine, and by nonsteroidal anti-inflammatory drugs such as indomethecin and flufenamic acid, but relatively little is known about the intracellular messengers that regulate these functionally important transport proteins. The intracellular messengers or plasma membrane mechanisms that mediate the reversal of fluid transport, from absorption to secretion have not yet been determined. The role of water channels and the molecular basis of RPE fluid transport are also not understood. CFTR mRNA, which encodes a cAMP-activated Cl channel, has been localized in the RPE and it would be interesting to explore further the role this channel plays in normal RPE transport and in disease. In general, it will be important to learn which transport proteins are targets for disease and which proteins can be modulated for therapeutic benefit.

ACKNOWLEDGMENTS

The writing of this chapter was supported by NIH grants EY-02205 (SSM), EY-08850 (BAH), a Stein/Oppenheimer Research Grant (RPG), the Stella-Joseph Research Endowment (RPG), and the Patricia Morrison Fund (RPG). It is our pleasure to thank Roy Steinberg, Rob Linsenmeier, and Victor Govardovsky for their thoughtful comments on various portions of the manuscript. The authors are also indebted to Ms. Jane Hu for her assistance.

REFERENCES

Adorante JS. 1995. Regulatory volume decrease in frog retinal pigment epithelium. Am J Physiol 268:C89–100 (with erratum following table of contents).
Adorante J, Miller S. 1990. Potassium-dependent volume regulation

in retinal pigment epithelium is mediated by Na,K,Cl cotransport. J Gen Physiol 96:1153–1176.

Alm A, Tornquist P. 1985. Lactate transport through the blood-retinal and the blood-brain barrier in rats. Ophthalmic Res 17:181–184.

Anderson M, Welsh M. 1991. Calcium and cAMP activate different chloride channels in the apical membrane of normal and cystic fibrosis epithelia. Proc Nat Acad Sci USA 88:6003–6007.

Armstrong WM, Garcia-Diaz JF. 1980. Ion-selective microelectrodes: theory and technique. Fed Proc 39:2851–2859.

Barnstable C. 1993. Glutamate and GABA in retinal circuitry. Curr Opin Neurobiol 3:520–525.

Bialek S, Joseph D, Miller S. 1995. The delayed basolateral membrane hyperpolarization of the bovine retinal pigment epithelium: mechanism of generation. J Physiol (Lond) 484:53–67.

Bialek S, Miller S. 1994. K+ and Cl+ transport mechanisms in bovine pigment epithelium that could modulate subretinal space volume and composition. J Physiol (Lond) 475:401–417.

Bialek S, Quong J, Yu K, Miller SS. 1996. Non-steroidal anti-inflammatory drugs modulated Cl conductance and fluid transport in bovine pigment epithelium. Am J Physiol 270:C1175–C1189.

Bird A. 1994. Pathogenesis of serous detachment of the retina and pigment epithelium. In: Ryan SJ, ed, Retina. Vol 2. St. Louis: Mosby, 1019–1026.

Bird AC. 1995. Retinal photoreceptor dystrophies. LI. Edward Jackson Memorial Lecture. Am J Ophthalmol 119:543–562.

Bok D. 1982. Autoradiographic studies on the polarity of plasma membrane receptors in retinal pigment epithelial cells. In: Hollyfield J, ed, The Structure of the Eye. New York: Elsevier, 247–256.

Bok D. 1990. Processing and transport of retinoids by the retinal pigment epithelium. Eye 4:326–332.

Bok D. 1994. Retinal photoreceptor disc shedding and pigment epithelium phagocytosis. In: Ryan SJ, ed, Retina. Vol. 1. St. Louis: Mosby, 81–94.

Botchkin LM, Matthews G. 1993. Chloride current activated by swelling in retinal pigment epithelium cells. Am J Physiol 265:C1037–C1045.

Botchkin LM, Matthews G. 1994. Voltage-dependent sodium channels develop in rat retinal pigment epithelium cells in culture. Proc Natl Acad Sci USA 91:4564–4568.

Bretag A. 1987. Muscle chloride channels. Physiol Rev 67:618–720.

Burke JM, Skumatz CMB, Irving PE, McKay BS. 1996. Phenotypic heterogeneity of retinal pigment epithelial cells in vitro and in situ. Exp Eye Res 62:63–73.

Chader G. 1989. Interphotoreceptor retinol-binding protein (IRBP): a model protein for molecular biological and clinically relevant studies. Invest Ophthalmol Vis Sci 30:7–22.

Chader G, Wiggert B, Lai Y, Lee L, Fletcher R. 1983. Interphotoreceptor retinol-binding protein: a possible role in retinoid transport to the retina. In: Osborne N, Chader G, eds, Progress in Retinal Research. Oxford: Pergamon Press, 163–189.

Chihara E, Nao-i N. 1984. Transport of subretinal fluid by the retinal pigment epithelium: studies on rhegmatogenous retinal detachment surgery without drainage of the subretinal fluid. Nippon Ganka Gakkai Zasshi 88:1318–1323.

Civan MM, Marano CW, Matschinsky FW, Peterson-Yantorno K. 1994. Prolonged incubation with elevated glucose inhibits the regulatory response to shrinkage of cultured human retinal pigment epithelial cells. J Membr Biol 139:1–13.

Collins FS. 1992. Cystic fibrosis: molecular biology and therapeutic implications. Science 256:774–779.

Cox SN, Hay E, Bird AC. 1988. Treatment of chronic macular edema with acetazolamide. Arch Ophthalmol 106:1190–1195.

Crosson CE, Pautler EL. 1982. Glucose transport across isolated bovine pigment epithelium. Exp Eye Res 35:371–377.

Dawson DC. 1991. Principles of membrane transport. In: Handbook of Physiology. The Gastrointestinal System, SG Schultz, section ed, M Field, RA Frizzell, vol. eds.), Bethesda: American Physiological Society, sect 6, vol 4, pp 1–44.

Dearry A, Edelman JL, Miller SS, Burnside B. 1990. Dopamine induces light-adaptive retinomotor movements in bullfrog cones via D2 receptors and in retinal pigment epithelium via D1 receptors. J Neurochem 54:1367–1378.

Defoe DM, Ahmad A, Chen W, Hughes BA. 1994. Membrane polarity of the Na+-K+ pump in primary cultures of Xenopus retinal pigment epithelium. Exp Eye Res 59:587–596.

DiMattio J, Streitman J. 1986. Facilitated glucose transport across the retinal pigment epithelium of the bullfrog (Rana catesbeiana). Exp Eye Res 43:15–28.

DiMattio J, Streitman J. 1991. Active transport of ascorbic acid across the retinal pigment epithelium of the bullfrog. Curr Eye Res 10:959–965.

Dimitriev AV, Govardovskii VI, Steinberg RH. 1996. Light-induced changes of principal extracellular ions and extracellular space volume in the chick retina. Invest Ophthal Vis Sci 37:S140.

Dowling JE. 1960. The chemistry of visual adaptation in the rat. Nature 188:114–118.

Edelman J, Miller S. 1991. Epinephrine stimulates fluid absorption across bovine retinal pigment epithelium. Invest Ophthalmol Vis Sci 32:3033–3040.

Edelman J, Miller S. 1992. Epinephrine (EP) stimulates KCl and fluid absorption across the bovine retinal pigment epithelium (RPE). Invest Ophthalmol Vis Sci 33:1111 (abstract).

Edelman J, Lin H, Miller S. 1994a. Acidification stimulates chloride and fluid absorption across frog retinal pigment epithelium. Am J Physiol 266:C946–956.

Edelman J, Lin H, Miller S. 1994b. Potassium-induced chloride secretion across the frog retinal pigment epithelium. Am J Physiol 266:C957–966.

Faber DS. 1969. Analysis of the slow transretinal potentials in response to light. Ph.D. dissertation. State University of New York, Buffalo.

Fijisawa K, Ye J, Zadunaisky J. 1993. A Na+/Ca2+ exchange mechanism in apical membrane vesicles of the retinal pigment epithelium. Curr Eye Res 12:261–70.

Fischer SK, Anderson DH. 1994. Cellular effects of detachment on the neural retina and the retinal pigment epithelium. In: Ryan SJ, ed, Retina. vol 3. St. Louis: Mosby, 2035–2062.

Fischbarg J, Kuang K, Li J, Arant-Hickman S, Vera J, Silverstein S, Loike J. 1993. Facilitative and sodium-dependent glucose transporters behave as water channel. In: Ussing H, Fischbarg J, Sten-Knudsen O, Larsen E, Willumsen N, eds, Isotonic Transport in Leaky Epithelia. Copenhagen: Munksgaard.

Fishman GA, Gilbert LD, Fiscella RG, Kimura AE, Jampol LM. 1989. Acetazolamide for treatment of chronic macular edema in retinitis pigmentosa. Arch Ophthalmol 107:1445–1452.

Flach AJ. 1992. Cyclooxygenase inhibitors in ophthalmology. Survey of Ophthalmol 36:259–284.

Fong C, Bialek S, Hughes B, Miller S. 1988. Modulation of intracellular chloride in bullfrog retinal pigment epithelium (RPE). FASEB J (Abstract) 2:A1722.

Fould W. 1976. Clinical significance of transscleral fluid transfer. Doyne memorial lecture. Trans Ophthalmol Soc UK 96:290–308.

Frambach DA, Marmor MF. 1982. The rate and route of fluid resorption from the subretinal space of the rabbit. Invest Ophthalmol Vis Sci 22:292–302.

Frambach D, Misfeldt D. 1983. Furosemide-sensitive Cl transport in embryonic chicken retinal pigment epithelium. Am J Physiol 244:F679–F685.

Frambach D, Weiter J, Adler A. 1985. A photogrammetric method to measure fluid movement across isolated frog retinal pigment epithelium. Biophys J 47:547–552.

Frambach DA, Valentine JL, Weiter JJ. 1988. Initial observations of rabbit retinal pigment epithelium-choroid-sclera preparation. Invest Ophthalmol Vis Sci 29:814–817.

Frambach DA, Valentine JL, Weiter JJ. 1989. Furosemide-sensitive Cl transport in bovine retinal pigment epithelium. Invest Ophthalmol Vis Sci 30:2271–2274.

Frambach D, Fain G, Farber D, Bok D. 1990. Beta adrenergic receptors on cultured human retinal pigment epithelium. Invest Ophthalmol Vis Sci 31:1767–1772.

Frizzell RA. 1995. Functions of the cystic fibrosis transmembrane conductance regulator protein. Am J Respir Crit Care Med 151:S54–S58.

Frömter E. 1972. The route of passive ion movement through the epithelium of Necturus gallbladder. J Membr Biol 8:259–301.

Fujii S, Gallemore RP, Hughes BH, Steinberg R. 1992. Direct evidence for a basal membrane Cl$^-$ conductance in toad retinal pigment epithelium. Am J Physiol 262:C374–C383.

Fuller C, Benos D. 1992. CFTR! Am J Physiol 263:C267–C286.

Gallemore RP, Steinberg RH. 1988. Light-evoked changes in [Ca^{2+}]$_o$ in chick retina. Invest Ophthalmol Vis Sci 29:103 (abstract).

Gallemore R, Steinberg R. 1989. Effects of DIDS on the chick retinal pigment epithelium. I. Membrane potentials, apparent resistances and mechanisms. J Neurosci 9:1968–1976.

Gallemore R, Steinberg R. 1993. Light-evoked modulation of basolateral membrane Cl$^-$ conductance in chick retinal pigment epithelium: the light peak and fast oscillation. J Neurophysiol 70:1669–1680.

Gallemore R, Hernandez E, Tayyanipour R, Fujii S, Steinberg R. 1993. Basolateral membrane Cl$^-$ and K$^+$ conductances of the dark-adapted chick retinal pigment epithelium. J Neurophysiol 70:1656–1668.

Gallemore R, Hernandez E, Steinberg R. 1994. Choroid-free preparation of explant retinal pigment epithelium. Invest Ophthalmol Vis Sci 35:2348 (ARVO Abstract).

Gallemore RP, Hu J, Frambach DA, Bok D. 1995. Ion transport in cultured fetal human retinal pigment epithelium. Invest Ophthalmol Vis Sci 36:S216 (abstract).

Garcia DM, Burnside B. 1994. Suppression of cAMP-induced pigment granule aggregation in RPE by organic anion transport inhibitors. Invest Ophthalmol Vis Sci 35:178–188.

Geggel H, Ament M, Heckenlively J, Martin D, Kopple J. 1985. Nutritional requirement for taurine in patients receiving long-term paraenteral nutrition. N Engl J Med 312:142–146.

Ginzburg B, Hogg J. 1967. What does a short circuit current measure in biological systems? J Theoretical Biol 14:316–322.

Griff E. 1991. Potassium-evoked responses from the retinal pigment epithelium of the toad Bufo marinus. Exp Eye Res 53:219–228.

Griff E, Steinberg R. 1982. Origin of the light peak: in vitro study of Gekko gekko. J Physiol (Lond) 331:637–652.

Griff E, Steinberg R. 1984. Changes in apical [K$^+$]$_o$ produce delayed basal membrane responses of the retinal pigment epithelium in the gekko. J Gen Physiol 83:193–211.

Griff E, Shirao Y, Steinberg R. 1985. Ba^{2+} unmasks K$^+$ modulation of the Na$^+$-K$^+$ pump in the frog pigment epithelium. J Gen Physiol 86:853–876.

Hanrahan J, Alles W, Lewis S. 1985. Single anion-selective channels in basolateral membrane of a mammalian tight epithelium. Proc Nat Acad Sci USA 82:7791–7795.

Harik SI, Kalaria RN, Whitney PM, Andersson L, Lundahl P, Ledbetter SR, Perry G. 1990. Glucose transporters are abundant in cells with "occluding" junctions at the blood-eye barriers. Proc Natl Acad Sci USA 87:4261–4264.

He S, Wang HM, Ye J, Ogden TE, Ryan SJ, Hinton DR. 1994. Dexamethasone-induced proliferation of cultured retinal pigment epithelial cells. Curr Eye Res 13:257–261.

Hernandez E, Hu J, Frambach D, Gallemore R. 1995. Potassium conductances in cultured bovine and human retinal pigment epithelium. Invest Ophthalmol Vis Sci 36:113–122.

House CR. 1974. *Water Transport in Cells and Tissues.* London: Edward Arnold, 390–470.

Hille B. 1992. *Ionic Channels of Excitable Membranes.* 2nd ed. Sunderland, MA: Sinauer, 341–347.

Hu J, Gallemore R, Bok D, Lee Y, Frambach D. 1994. Localization of Na,K ATPase on cultured human retinal pigment epithelium. Invest Ophthalmol Vis Sci 35:3582–3588.

Hu J, Bok D, Frambach D, Gallemore R. 1995. Beta-2 adrenergic receptors activate basal membrane ion channels in cultured fetal human retinal pigment epithelium. Invest Opthalmol Vis Sci 36:2726 (Abstract).

Hu J, Gallemore R, Bok D, Frambach D. 1996a. Chloride transport in cultured fetal human retinal pigment epithelium. Exp Eye Res 62:443–448.

Hu J, Gallemore R, Maruiwa F, Bok D. 1996b. Retinal potassium modulates multiple ion transport mechanisms in cultured human retinal pigment epithelium. Invest Ophthalmol Vis Sci (ARVO Abstract).

Huang B, Karwoski C. 1989. Change in extracellular space in the frog retina. Invest Ophthalmol Vis Sci 30:64 (Abstract).

Huang B, Karwoski C. 1992. Light-evoked expansion of subretinal space volume in the retina of the frog. J Neurosci 12:4243–4252.

Hudspeth A, Yee A. 1973. The intercellular junctional complexes of the retinal pigment epithelia. Invest Ophthalmol Vis Sci 12:354–365.

Huf EG. 1979. Echos of the past: reflections on the early history of the concept of active transport. Physiologist 22:18–24.

Hughes BA, Segawa Y. 1992. Cation currents in isolated retinal pigment epithelial cells of toad. Exp Eye Res 55(suppl 1):s11 (abstract).

Hughes B, Segawa Y. 1993. cAMP-activated chloride currents in amphibian retinal pigment epithelial cells. J Physiol (Lond) 466:749–766.

Hughes BA, Steinberg RH. 1990. Voltage-dependent currents in isolated cells of the frog retinal pigment epithelium. J Physiol (Lond) 428:273–297.

Hughes BA, Takahira M. 1996. Inwardly rectifying K$^+$ currents in isolated human retinal pigment epithelial cells. Invest Ophthalmol Vis Sci 37:1125–1139.

Hughes B, Miller S, Machen TE. 1984. Effects of cyclic AMP on fluid absorption and ion transport across frog retinal pigment epithelium: measurements in the open-circuit state. J Gen Physiol 83:875–899.

Hughes B, Miller S, Farber DB. 1987. Adenylate cyclase alters transport in frog retinal pigment epithelium. Am J Physiol 252:C385–C395.

Hughes B, Miller S, Joseph D, Edelman J. 1988. cAMP stimulates the Na$^+$-K$^+$ pump in frog retinal pigment epithelium. Am J Physiol 254:C84–98.

Hughes B, Adorante J, Miller S, Lin H. 1989. Apical electrogenic NaHCO$_3$ cotransport: a mechanism for HCO$_3$ absorption across the retinal pigment epithelium. J Gen Physiol 94:125–150.

Hughes BA, Takahira M, Segawa Y. 1995a. An outwardly rectifying K$^+$ current active near resting potential in human retinal pigment epithelial cells. Am J Physiol 269:C179–C187.

Hughes BA, Shaikh A, Ahmad A. 1995b. Effects of Ba^{2+} and Cs$^+$ on apical membrane K⁺ conductance in toad retinal pigment epithelium. Am J Physiol 268:C1164–1172.

Hussain A, Kundaiker S, Marshall J. 1995. Regulatory vectorial transport of taurine across bovine RPE. Invest Ophthalmol Vis Sci 36:2730 (Abstract).

Immel J, Steinberg R. 1986. Spatial buffering of K⁺ by the retinal pigment epithelium in frog. J Neurosci 6:3197–3204.

Jiang C, Finkbeiner W, Widdicombe J, McCray P Jr, Miller S. 1993. Altered fluid transport across airway epithelium in cystic fibrosis. Science 263:424–427.

Joseph D, Miller S. 1991. Apical and basal membrane ion transport mechanisms in bovine retinal pigment epithelium. J Physiol 435:439–463.

Joseph D, Miller S. 1992. Alpha-1-adrenergic modulation of K and Cl transport in bovine retinal pigment epithelium. J Gen Physiol 99:263–290.

Judson PH, Yannuzzi LA. 1994. Macular hole. In: Ryan SJ, ed, Retina vol. 2. St. Louis: Mosby, 1165–1185.

Kawasaki K, Mukoh S, Yonemura D, Fujii S, Segawa Y. 1986. Acetazolamide-induced changes of the membrane potentials of the retinal pigment epithelial cell. Doc Ophthalmol 63:375–381.

Kikawada N. 1968. Variations in the corneo-retinal standing potential of the vertebrate eye during light and dark adaptation. Jap J Physiol 18:687–702.

Karwoski CJ, Lu HK, Newman EA. 1989. Spatial buffering of light-evoked potassium increases by retinal Müller (glial) cells. Science 244:578–580.

Kennedy B. 1990. Na⁺-K⁺-Cl⁻ cotransport in cultured cells derived from human retinal pigment epithelium. Am J Physiol 28:C29–C34.

Kennedy BG. 1992. Rubidium transport in cultured monkey retinal pigment epithelium. Exp Eye Res 55:289–296.

Kennedy BG. 1994. Volume regulation in cultured cells derived from human retinal pigment epithelium. Am J Physiol 266:C676–683.

Kennedy BG, Mangini NJ. 1996. Plasma membrane calcium-ATPase in cultured human retinal pigment epithelium. Exp Eye Res 63:547–556.

Kenyon E, Joseph D, Miller S. 1994a. Evidence for electrogenic Cl-dependent Na-HCO₃ cotransport at the apical membrane of bovine RPE. Invest Ophthalmol Vis Sci (abstract) 35:1759.

Kenyon E, Yu K, la Cour M, Miller S. 1994b. Lactate transport mechanism at the apical and basolateral membranes of bovine retinal pigment epithelium. Am J Physiol 267:C1561–C1573.

Kenyon E, Joseph DP, Miller SS. 1997. Apical and basolateral membrane mechanisms that regulate pHᵢ in bovine retinal pigment epithelium. Am J Physiol 273:C456–C472.

Khatami M. 1987. Na⁺-linked active transport of ascorbate into cultured bovine retinal pigment epithelial cells: heterologous inhibition by glucose. Membr Biochem 7:115–130.

Khatami M. 1990. Regulation of MI transport in retinal pigment epithelium by sugars, amiloride, and pH gradients: potential impairment of pump-leak balance in diabetic maculopathy. Membr Biochem 9:279–292.

Khatami M, Stramm LE, Rockey JH. 1986. Ascorbate transport in cultured cat retinal pigment epithelial cells. Exp Eye Res 43:607–615.

Khatami M, Cernadas M, Geroff A, Chandra P, Cohen F. 1990. Direct regulation of Na⁺-dependent myo-inositol transport by sugars in retinal pigment epithelium: role of phorbol ester and staurosporin. Membr Biochem 9:263–277.

Kirchof B, Ryan SJ. 1993. Differential permeance of retina and retinal pigment epithelium to water: implications for retinal adhesion. Int Ophthalmol 17:19–22.

Koyano S, Araie M, Eguchi S. 1993. Movement of fluorescein and its glucuronide across retinal pigment epithelium-choroid. Invest Ophthalmol Vis Sci 34:531–538.

Kumagai AK, Glasgow BJ, Pardridge WM. 1994. GLUT1 glucose transporter expression in the diabetic and nondiabetic human eye. Invest Ophthalmol Vis Sci 35:2887–2894.

Kuntz C, Crook R, Dmitriev A, Steinberg R. 1994. Modification by cyclic adenosine monophosphate of basolateral membrane chloride conductance in chick retinal pigment epithelium. Invest Ophthalmol Vis Sci 35:422–433.

la Cour M. 1989. Rheogenic sodium-bicarbonate co-transport across the retinal membrane of the frog retinal pigment epithelium. J Physiol (Lond) 419:539–553; erratum, 445:779.

la Cour M. 1991a. Kinetic properties and Na⁺ dependence of rheogenic Na⁺-HCO₃⁻ co-transport in frog retinal pigment epithelium. J Physiol (Lond) 439:59–72.

la Cour M. 1991b. pH homeostasis in the frog retina: the role of Na⁺:HCO₃⁻ co-transport in the retinal pigment epithelium. Acta Ophthalmol (Copenh) 69(4):496–504.

la Cour M. 1992. Cl⁻ transport in frog retinal pigment epithelium. Exp Eye Res 54(6):921–931.

la Cour M. 1993. Ion transport in the retinal pigment epithelium: a study with ion-selective microelectrodes. Acta Ophthalmol 209(suppl):1–32.

la Cour M, Lund-Andersen H, Zeuthen T. 1986. Potassium transport of the frog retinal pigment epithelium: autoregulation of potassium activity in the subretinal space. J Physiol (Lond) 375:461–479.

la Cour M, Lin H, Kenyon E, Miller SS. 1994. Lactate transport in freshly isolated human fetal retinal pigment epithelium. Invest Ophthalmol Vis Sci 35:434–42; erratum 36(5):757.

Lake N, Marshall J, Voaden MJ. 1975. Studies on the uptake of taurine by the isolated neural retina and pigment epithelium of the frog. Biochem Soc Trans 3:524–525.

Lake N, Marshall J, Voaden MJ. 1977. The entry of taurine into the neural retina and pigment epithelium of the frog. Brain Res. 128:497–503.

Lasansky A, De Fisch F. 1966. Potential, current and ionic fluxes across isolated retinal pigment epithelium and choroid. J Gen Physiol 49:913–924.

Li JD, Gallemore RP, Dmitriev A, Steinberg RH. 1994a. Light-dependent hydration of the space surrounding photoreceptors in chick retina. Invest Ophthalmol Vis Sci 35:2700–2711.

Li JD, Govardovskii VI, Steinberg RH. 1994b. Light-dependent hydration of the space surrounding photoreceptors in the cat retina. Vis Neurosci 11:743–752.

Lin H, Miller S. 1994. pHᵢ-dependent Cl-HCO₃ exchange at the basolateral membrane of frog retinal pigment epithelium. Am J Physiol 266:C935–945.

Lin H, Kenyon E, Miller SS. 1992. Sodium dependent pHᵢ regulatory mechanisms in native human retinal pigment epithelium. Invest Ophthalmol Vis Sci 33:3528–3538.

Lin H, Miller S. 1991a. Apical epinephrine modulates [Ca²⁺]ᵢ in bovine retinal pigment epithelium. Invest Ophthalmol Vis Sci 32:671 (Abstract).

Lin H, Miller S. 1991b. pHᵢ regulation in frog retinal pigment epithelium: two apical membrane mechanisms. Am J Physiol 261:C132–C142.

Lin H, la Cour M, Anderson M, Miller S. 1994. Proton-lactate cotransport in the apical membrane of frog retinal pigment epithelium. Exp Eye Res 59:679–688.

Linsenmeier R, Braun R. 1992. Oxygen distribution and consumption in the cat retina during normoxia and hypoxemia. J Gen Physiol 99:177–197.

Macaluso C, Onoe S, Niemeyer G. 1992. Changes in glucose level affect rod function more than cone function in the isolated, perfused cat eye. Invest Ophthalmol Vis Sci 33:2798–2808.

Mangini NJ, Valle J, Haugh-Scheidt L, Kennedy BG. 1997. Characterization of Na$^+$/Ca^{2+} exchange protein and cDNA in cultured human retinal pigment epithelial cells. Invest Ophthal Vis Sci 35:S467 (abstract).

Marmor M. 1979. Dystrophies of the retinal pigment epithelium. In: Zinn K, Marmor, eds, The Retinal Pigment Epithelium. Cambridge, MA: Harvard University Press, 424–453.

Marmor MF. 1990. Control of subretinal fluid: experimental and clinical studies. Eye 4:340–344.

Marmor MF. 1994. Mechanisms of normal retinal adhesion. In: Ryan SJ, ed, Retina. St. Louis: Mosby, 1931–1953.

Marmor M, Lurie M. 1979. Light-induced electrical responses of the retinal pigment epithelium. In: Zinn K, Marmor M, eds, The Retinal Pigment Epithelium. Cambridge, MA: Harvard University Press, 226–244.

Marmor MF, Maack T. 1982. Enhancement of retinal adhesion and subretinal fluid resorption by acetazolamide. Invest Ophthalmol Vis Sci 23:121–124.s.

Maruiwa F, Gallemore RP, Takahira M, Hughes B, Hu J, Bok D. 1996. Membrane polarization of potassium conductances in cultured retinal pigment epithelium. Invest Ophthal Vis Sci 37:S229 (abstract).

Masterson E, Chader GJ. 1981. Characterization of glucose transport by cultured chick pigmented epithelium. Exp Eye Res 32:279–289.

Mays RW, Beck KA, Nelson JW. 1994. Organization and function of the cytoskeleton in polarized epithelial cells: a component of the protein sorting machinery. Curr Opin Cell Biol 6:16–24.

Miceli M, Newsome D, Schriver G. 1990. Glucose uptake, hexose monophosphate shunt activity, and oxygen consumption in cultured human retinal pigment epithelial cell. Invest Ophthalmol Vis Sci 31:277–283.

Miller RF, Dowling JE. 1970. Intracellular responses of the Müller (glial) cells of mudpuppy retina: their relation to b-wave of the electroretinogram. J Neurophysiol 33:323–341.

Miller S, Edelman J. 1990. Active ion transport pathways in the bovine retinal pigment epithelium. J Physiol (Lond) 424:283–300.

Miller S, Farber D. 1984. Cyclic AMP modulation of ion transport across frog retinal pigment epithelium: Measurements in the short-circuit state. J Gen Physiol 83:853–874.

Miller S, Steinberg R. 1976. Transport of taurine, L-methionine and 3-o-methyl-D-glucose across frog retinal pigment epithelium. Exp Eye Res 23(2):177–189.

Miller S, Steinberg R. 1977a. Passive ionic properties of frog retinal pigment epithelium. J Membr Biol 36:337–372.

Miller S, Steinberg R. 1977b. Active transport of ions across the frog retinal pigment epithelium. Exp Eye Res 25:235–248.

Miller S, Steinberg R. 1979. Potassium modulation of taurine transport across the frog retinal pigment epithelium. J Gen Physiol 74:237–259.

Miller S, Steinberg R. 1982. Potassium transport across the frog retinal pigment epithelium. J Membr Biol 67:199–209.

Miller S, Steinberg R, Oakley B II. 1978. The electrogenic sodium pump of the frog retinal pigment epithelium. J Membr Biol 44:259–279.

Miller SS, Hughes BA, Machen TE. 1982. Fluid transport across retinal pigment epithelium is inhibited by cyclic AMP. Proc Nat Acad Sci USA 79:2111–2115.

Miller SS, Rabin J, Strong T, Iannuzzi M, Adams AJ, Collins F, Reenstra W, McCray P Jr. 1992. Cystic fibrosis (CF) gene product is expressed in retina and retinal pigment epithelium. Invest Ophthamol Vis Sci 33:1009 (abstract).

Mills JW, Mandel LJ. 1994. Cytoskeletal regulation of membrane transport events. FASEB J 8:1161–1165.

Mircheff AK, Miller SS, Farber DB, Bradley ME, O'Day WT, Bok D. 1990. Isolation and provisional identification of plasma membrane populations from cultured human retinal pigment epithelium. Invest Ophthalmol Vis Sci 31:863–878.

Miyamoto Y, Del Monte MA. 1994. Na(+)-dependent glutamate transporter in human retinal pigment epithelial cells. Invest Ophthalmol Vis Sci 35:3589–3598.

Miyamoto Y, Kulanthaivel P, Leibach FH, Ganapathy V. 1991. Taurine uptake in apical membrane vesicles from the bovine retinal pigment epithelium. Invest Ophthalmol Vis Sci 32:2542–2551.

Nabi IR, Mathews AP, Cohen-Gould L, Gundersen D, Rodriguez-Boulan E. 1993. Immortalization of polarized rat retinal pigment epithelium. J Cell Sci 104:37–49.

Nao-i N, Gallemore R, Steinberg R. 1990. Effects of cAMP and IBMX on the chick retinal pigment epithelium: membrane potentials and light-evoked responses. Invest Ophthalmol Vis Sci 31:54–66.

Nash MS, Osborne NN. 1995. Pertussis toxin-sensitive melatonin receptors negatively coupled to adenylate cyclase associated with cultured human and rat retinal pigment epithelial cells. Invest Ophthalmol Vis Sci 36:95–102.

Nathanson L, Widdicombe JH, Nadel JA. 1983. Effect of amphotericin B on ion and fluid transport across dog tracheal epithelium. J Appl Physiol 55:1257–1261.

Neal M, Cunningham J, Marshall J. 1979. The uptake and radioautographical localization in the frog retina of [^{3}H] (+/−) aminocyclohexane carboxylic acid, a selective inhibitor of neuronal GABA transport. Brain Res 176:285–296.

Negi A, Marmor MF. 1983. The resorption of subretinal fluid after diffuse damage to the retinal pigment epithelium. Invest Ophthalmol Vis Sci 24:1475–1459.

Negi A, Marmor MF. 1984. Effects of subretinal and systemic osmolality on the rate of subretinal fluid resorption. Invest Ophthalmol Vis Sci 25:616–620.

Nelson WJ. 1991. Mechanisms for regulating cell surface distribution of Na$^+$,K$^+$-ATPase in polarized epithelial cells. Science 254:847–850.

Noell WK, Crapper DR, Paganelli CV. 1965. Transretinal currents and ion fluxes. In: Snell F, Noell WK, eds, Transcellular Membrane Potentials and Ion Fluxes. New York: Gordon and Breach, 92–130.

Oakley B II. 1977. Potassium and the photoreceptor dependent pigment epithelial hyperpolarization. J Gen Physiol 70:405–425.

Oakley B II, Green DG. 1976. Correlation of light-induced changes in retinal extracellular potassium concentration with the c-wave of the electroretinogram. J Neurophysiol 39:1117–1133.

Oakley B II, Steinberg R, Miller S, Nilsson S. 1977. The in vitro frog pigment epithelial cell hyperpolarization in response to light. Invest Ophthalmol Vis Sci 16(8):771–774.

Oakley B II, Miller S, Steinberg R. 1978. Intracellular K$^+$ modulates the Na$^+$/K$^+$ pump in frog retinal pigment epithelium. J Membr Biol 44:281–307.

O'Malley D, Sandell J, Masland R. 1992. Co-release of acetylcholine and GABA by starburst amacrine cell. J Neurosci 12:1394–1408.

Ostwald T, Steinberg R. 1980. Localization of frog retinal pigment epithelium Na$^+$-K$^+$ ATPase. Exp Eye Res 31:351–360.

Ostwald T, Steinberg R. 1981. Transmembrane components of taurine flux across frog retinal pigment epithelium. Curr Eye Res 1:437–443.

Pasante-Morales H, Klethi J, Ledig M, Mandel P. 1972. Free amino acids of chicken and rat retina. Brain Res 41:494–497.

Pascuzzo GJ, Johnson JE, Pautler EL. 1980. Glucose transport in isolated mammalian pigment epithelium. Exp Eye Res 30:53–58.

Pautler EL, Tengerdy C. 1986. Transport of acidic amino acids by the bovine pigment epithelium. Exp Eye Res 43:207–214; erratum, 44:following 329.

Pautler EL, Tengerdy C, Beyer J, Beezley D. 1989. Modification of leucine transport across bovine pigment epithelium by metabolic stress. Am J Physiol 257:C940–C947.

Pederson JE. 1994. Fluid physiology of the subretinal space. In: Ryan SJ, ed, Retina, vol 3. St. Louis: Mosby, 1955–1968.

Peterson R-U, Reuss L. 1983. Cyclic-AMP induced chloride permeability in the apical membrane of Necturus gallbladder epithelium. J Gen Physiol 81:705–729.

Peterson WM, Miller SS. 1995a. Identification and functional characterization of a dual GABA/taurine transporter in the bullfrog retinal pigment epithelium. J Gen Physiol 106:1089–1122.

Peterson W, Miller S. 1995b. Elevation of cyclic AMP levels in the bovine retinal pigment epithelium (RPE) closes basolateral membrane Cl channels. Invest Ophthalmol Vis Sci 36:S216 (Abstract).

Pfeffer BA. 1991. Improved methodology for cell culture of human and monkey retinal pigment epithelium. In: Osborne N, Chader G, eds, Progress in Retinal Research. Oxford: Pergamon Press, 251–291.

Philp N, Chu P, Pan TC, Zhang RZ, Chu ML, Stank K, Boettiger D, Yoon A, Kieber-Emmons T. 1995. Developmental expression and molecular cloning of REMP, a novel retinal epithelial membrane protein. Exp Cell Res 219:64–73.

Quinn R, Miller S. 1992. Ion transport mechanisms in native human retinal pigment epithelium. Invest Ophthalmol Vis Sci 33:3513–3527.

Quinn RH, Miller SS. 1993. Apical epinephrine or cyclic AMP modulates K and Cl transport in native human fetal retinal pigment epithelium. Invest Ophthalmol Vis Sci 34:872 (abstract).

Quong JN, Quinn RH, Miller SS. 1996. Evidence for two types of chloride channels in native fetal human retinal pigment epithelium. Invest Ophthalmol Vis Sci 37:51109 (Abstract).

Rando R. 1992. Molecular mechanisms in visual pigment regeneration. Photochem Photobiol 56(6):1145–1156.

Reid WW. 1892. Experiments upon "absorption without osmosis." Brit Med J 1:323–326.

Rink T, Tsien R, Pozzan T. 1982. Cytoplasmic pH and free Mg in lymphocytes. J Cell Biol 96:189–196.

Rizzolo LJ. 1990. The distribution of Na$^+$,K$^+$-ATPase in the retinal pigmented epithelium from chicken embryo is polarized in vivo but not in primary cell culture. Exp Eye Res 51:435–446.

Roos A, Boron W. 1981. Intracellular pH. Physiol Rev 61:296–434.

Rothman JE. 1996. Protein sorting by transport vesicles. Science 272:227–234.

Saari J. 1990. Enzymes and proteins of the mammalian visual cycle. In: Osborne N, Chader G, eds, Progress in Retinal Research. New York: Pergamon Press, 363–381.

Salceda R, Lopez-Colome A, Pasante-Morales H. 1977. Light-stimulated release of [^{35}S]-taurine from frog retinal rod outer segments. Brain Res 135:186–191.

Scharschmidt B, Griff E, Steinberg R. 1988. Effect of taurine on the isolated retinal pigment epithelium of the frog: electrophysiologic evidence for stimulation of an apical, electrogenic Na$^+$-K$^+$ pump. J Membr Biol 106:71–81.

Schmidt SY. 1978. Taurine fluxes in isolated cat and rat retinas: effects of illumination. Exp Eye Res 26:529–535.

Schmidt S. 1980. High-affinity uptake of [^{3}H] taurine in isolated cat retinas: effects of Na$^+$ and K$^+$. Exp Eye Res 31:373–379.

Schmidt SY, Berson EL, Hayes KC. 1976. Retinal degeneration in cats fed casein. I. Taurine deficiency. Invest Ophthalmol 15:47–52.

Segawa Y. 1987. Electrical responses of the retinal pigment epithelium to sodium bicarbonate (I). Experimental studies in animals. J Juzen Med Soc 96:1008–1021.

Segawa Y, Hughes BA. 1994. Properties of the inwardly rectifying K$^+$ conductance in the toad retinal pigment epithelium. J Physiol (Lond) 476:41–53.

Sellner P. 1986a. The blood-retinal barrier: leucine transport by the retinal pigment epithelium. J Neurosci 6:2823–2828.

Sellner PA. 1986b. The movement of organic solutes between the retina and pigment epithelium. Exp Eye Res 43:631–639.

Sheng Y, Gouras P, Cao H, Berglin L, Kjeldbye H, Lopez R, Rosskothen H. 1995. Patch transplants of human fetal retinal pigment epithelium in rabbit and monkey retina. Invest Ophthalmol Vis Sci 36:381–390.

Shirao Y, Steinberg R. 1987. Mechanisms of effects of small hyperosmotic gradients on the chick RPE. Invest Ophthalmol Vis Sci 280:2015–2025.

Sivakami S, Ganapathy V, Leibach F, Miyamoto Y. 1992. The γ-aminobutyric acid transporter and its interaction with taurine in the apical membrane of the bovine retinal pigment epithelium. Biochem J 283:391–397.

Starita C, Hussain AA, Marshall J. 1995. Decreasing hydraulic conductivity of Bruch's membrane: relevance to photoreceptor survival and lipofuscinoses. Am J Med Genet 57:235–237.

Steinberg R. 1985. Interaction between the retinal pigment epithelium and the neural retina. Doc Ophthalmol 60:327–346.

Steinberg R. 1986. Research update: report from workshop on cell biology of retinal detachment. Exp Eye Res 43:695–706.

Steinberg R. 1987. Monitoring communications between photoreceptors and pigment epithelial cells: effects of "mild" systemic hypoxia. Friedenwald lecture. Invest Ophthalmol Vis Sci 28:1888–1904.

Steinberg R, Miller S. 1973. Aspects of electrolyte transport in frog pigment epithelium. Exp Eye Res 16:365–372.

Steinberg R, Miller S, Stern W. 1978. Initial observations on the isolated retinal pigment epithelium-choroid of the cat. Invest Ophthalmol Vis Sci 17:675–678.

Steinberg R, Linsenmeier R, Griff E. 1983. Three light-evoked responses of the retinal pigment epithelium. Vision Res 23:1315–1323.

Steinberg R, Linsenmeier R, Griff E. 1985. Retinal pigment epithelial cell contributions to the electrooculogram. In: Osborne N, Chader G, eds, Progress in Retinal Research, vol 4. New York: Pergamon Press, 33–36.

Stoddard J, Reuss L. 1989. pH effects on basolateral membrane ion conductances in gallbladder epithelium. Am J Physiol 256:C1184–C1195.

Stramm LE, Pautler EL. 1982. Transport of 3-O-methylglucose in isolated rat retinal pigment epithelial cells. Exp Eye Res 35:91–97.

Strauss O, Wiederholt M, Wienrich M. 1996. Activation of Cl$^-$ currents in cultured rat retinal pigment epithelial cells by intracellular applications of ionositol-1,4,5-triphosphate: differences between rats with retinal dystrophy (RCS) and normal rats. J Membr Biol 151:189–200.

Swartz M. 1994. Other diseases: drug toxicity and metabolic and nutritional conditions. In: Ryan SJ, ed, Retina, vol 2. St. Louis: Mosby, 1755–1766.

Takahira M, Hughes BA. 1997. Isolated bovine retinal pigment epithelial cells express delayed rectifier type and M-type K$^+$ currents. Am J Physiol 273:C790–C803.

Takata K, Kasahara T, Kasahara M, Ezaki O, Hirano H. 1992. Ultracytochemical localization of the erythrocyte/HepG2-type glucose transporter (GLUT1) in cells of the blood-retinal barrier in the rat. Invest Ophthalmol Vis Sci 33:377–383.

Tarnowski BI, Shepherd VL, McLaughlin BJ. 1988. Mannose 6-phosphate receptors on the plasma membrane on rat retinal pigment epithelial cells. Invest Ophthalmol Vis Sci 29:291–297.

Thomas J, Buchsbaum R, Ximniak A, Racker E. 1979. Intracellular pH measurements in Ehrlich ascites tumor cells utilizing spectroscopic probes generated in situ. Biochem 18:2210–2218.

To C, Hodson S. 1995. Glucose supply to the photoreceptor cells by retinal pigment epithelium. Invest Ophthalmol Vis Sci 36:S216 (ARVO Abstract).

Tornquist P, Alm A. 1979. Retinal and choroidal contribution to retinal metabolism in vivo: a study in pigs. Acta Physiol Scand 106:351–357.

Tsacopoulos M, Magistretti PJ. 1996. Metabolic coupling between glia and neurons. J Neurosci 16(3):877–885.

Tsuboi S. 1987. Measurement of the volume flow and hydraulic conductivity across the isolated dog retinal pigment epithelium. Invest Ophthalmol Vis Sci 28:1776–1782.

Tsuboi S, Pederson JE. 1988. Volume flow across the isolated retinal pigment epithelium of cynomolgus monkey eyes. Invest Ophthalmol Vis Sci 29:1652–1655.

Tsuboi S, Fujimoto T, Uchihori Y, Emi K, Iizuka S, Kishida K, Manage R. 1984. Measurement of retinal permeability to sodium fluorescein in vitro. Invest Ophthalmol Vis Sci 25:1146–1150.

Tsuboi S, Manabe R, Iizuka S. 1986. Aspects of electrolyte transport across isolated dog retinal pigment epithelium. Am J Physiol 250:F781–F784.

Tsuboi S, Pederson JE. 1987. Acetazolamide effect on the inward permeability of the blood-retinal barrier to carboxyfluorescein. Invest Ophthalmol Vis Sci 28:92–95.

Ueda Y, Steinberg R. 1993. Voltage-operated calcium channels in fresh and cultured rat retinal pigment epithelial cells. Invest Ophthalmol Vis Sci 34:3408–3418.

Ueda Y, Steinberg R. 1994. Chloride currents in freshly isolated rat retinal pigment epithelial cells. Exp Eye Res 58:331–342.

Ueda Y, Steinberg RH. 1995. Dihydropyridine-sensitive calcium currents in freshly isolated human and monkey retinal pigment epithelial cells. Invest Ophthalmol Vis Sci 36:373–380.

Voaden MJ, Lake N, Marshall J, Morjaria B. 1977. Studies on the distribution of taurine and other neuroactive amino acids in the retina. Exp Eye Res 25:249–257.

Welsh MJ, Widdicombe JE, Nadel JN. 1980. Fluid transport across the canine tracheal epithelium. J Applied Physiol 49:905–909.

Wen R, Lui G, Steinberg R. 1993. Whole-cell K+ currents in fresh and cultured cells of the human and monkey retinal pigment epithelium. J Physiol (Lond) 465:121–147.

Wen R, Lui GM, Steinberg RH. 1994. Expression of a tetrodotoxin-sensitive Na+ current in cultured human retinal pigment epithelial cells. J Physiol (Lond) 476:187–196.

Winkler BS. 1981. Glycolytic and oxidative metabolism in relation to retinal function. J Gen Physiol 77:667–692.

Winkler BS. 1989. Retinal aerobic glycolysis revisited [editorial]. Invest Ophthalmol Vis Sci 30:1023.

Wolfensberger TJ, Chiang RK, Takeuchi A, Marmor MF. In press. Inhibition of membrane bound carbonic anhydrase enhances subretinal fluid absorption and retinal adhesiveness. Invest Ophthalmol Vis Sci.

Yamamoto F, Borgula G, Steinberg R. 1992. Effects of light and darkness on pH outside rod photoreceptors in the cat retina. Exp Eye Res 54:685–697.

Yamamoto F, Steinberg RH. 1992. Effects of intravenous acetazolamide on retinal pH in the cat. Exp Eye Res 54:711–718.

Yonemura D, Kawasaki K, Tanabe J, Yamamoto S. 1978. Susceptibility of the standing potential of the eye to acetazolamide and its clinical application. Folia Ophthalmol Jpn 29:408–416.

Yokoyama T, Lin L-R, Chakrapani B, Reddy VN. 1993. Hypertonic stress increases NaK ATPase, taurine, myoinositol in human lens and retinal pigment epithelial cultures. Invest Ophthalmol Vis Sci 34:2512–2517.

Yoon H, Fanelli A, Grollman EF, Philp NJ. 1997. Identification of a unique monocarboxylate transporter (MCT3) in retinal pigment epithelium. Biochem Biophys Res Comm 234:90–94.

Zeuthen T. 1995. Molecular mechanisms for passive and active transport of water. Int Rev Cytol 160:99–161.

7. Retinoids and the retinal pigment epithelium

GERALD J. CHADER, DAVID R. PEPPERBERG, ROSALIE CROUCH, AND BARBARA WIGGERT

The retinal pigment epithelium (RPE) is now recognized as a true partner of the neurosensory retina in the visual cycle. The last few years in particular have seen the solving of one of the central problems in vision, namely, discovering the site of formation and the probable mechanism involved in the generation of 11-*cis*-retinoids for subsequent use in the synthesis of rhodopsin. There is also mounting evidence that the interphotoreceptor matrix (IPM), juxtaposed between the RPE cell layer and the photoreceptor outer segments of the neural retina, is also of importance in the cycle. It is through this extracellular matrix that potentially large amounts of retinoids travel in a vectorial manner back and forth between storage in the RPE and use in photoreceptor outer segments for rhodopsin synthesis. Thus, in considering the role of the RPE in vision, it is best to consider the reactions taking place in the entire retina-IPM-RPE complex, as proper processing of retinoids in all three compartments is necessary for normal visual functioning. The present chapter updates progress in this area, focusing on new information on retinoid reactions in the RPE and on retinoid transport through the IPM as it relates to the RPE. Since this book was last published, excellent "minireviews" have been written on retinoid transformations in the visual cycle by Rando (1991; 1992) and Rando and colleagues (1991), on enzymes and binding proteins involved in the visual cycle by Saari (1989; 1994), on general RPE cell functioning by Bok (1990; 1993), and on retinoid movement in the IPM by Pepperberg and colleagues (1993).

VITAMIN A AND THE RPE: EARLY WORK

Although it has been known for many years that the RPE is somehow involved in vision, retinoid processing in this cell layer has been little understood until quite recently. It is only within the last decade that the RPE has been pinpointed as the actual site of retinoid isomerization as well as uptake and storage. Dr. George Wald was the first to describe the presence of vitamin A in the retina (Wald, 1934), finding that, with a strong light bleach, the bulk of the "retinene" (i.e., retinaldehyde) is converted to "Vitamin A" (i.e., retinol) (Wald, 1935–6). Interestingly, he found that most of this Vitamin A then disappeared from the neural retina (Wald, 1935–6). Even then, the prime suspect in vitamin A uptake was the RPE, since vitamin A fluorescence was observed in the rat RPE shortly after exposure to light but not after a longer period of dark adaptation (Jancso and Jancso, 1936). This notion was strengthened when it was found that the total ocular content of retinoids was not changed in cycles of light and dark (Hubbard and Coleman, 1959). The cycling of retinoid between neural retina and RPE (i.e., the visual cycle) only became clear, however, with the pioneering work of Dowling (1960; 1963) who examined the relative distribution of retinol and retinaldehyde in the retina and RPE of the rat eye under conditions of light and dark adaptation (Fig. 7-1). It was found that, in dark-adapted retinas, >95% of the "potential vitamin A" was present as retinaldehyde in the rhodopsin of the outer segments, with little if any in the RPE-choroid. Rhodopsin bleaching led to a release of retinaldehyde from the opsin protein moiety, as was well known, followed by conversion to retinol (vitamin A) and a sharp rise in vitamin A in the RPE. With an increasing period of illumination (light adaptation), total retinoid was found to decrease in the neural retina and to increase in the RPE cells. Little retinaldehyde was detected in the RPE during this time, and it was concluded that "it is only vitamin A that migrates from the retina into the pigmented layers" (Dowling, 1960). Upon dark adaptation, a marked fall in the vitamin A content of the RPE was noted, with a concomitant rise in "retinene" within the rhodopsin moiety of the photoreceptor outer segments, as noted above. Other investigators, notably Zimmerman and colleagues (1974; 1975), also did much to establish this cycle and begin to describe the enzyme activities needed to perform the isomeric conversions intrinsic to the visual process. Figure 7-2 summarizes the knowledge of the visual cycle until the mid-1980s. Due to the work of Wald, Hubbard,

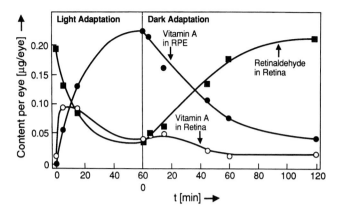

FIGURE 7-1. Distribution of retinoids in the retina and pigment epithelium during light- and dark-adaptation in the rat. (Adapted from Dowling, 1960.)

Dowling, and many others, it was established that 11-cis-retinaldehyde is the form of retinoid that is covalently bound to rhodopsin and that serves as the chromophore in the visual pigment. Furthermore, it was recognized that illumination initiates a process that results in both isomerization of the retinoid to the *trans* configuration and retinoid release from the opsin protein. In this scheme, however, many unanswered questions remained: How is retinoid taken up and stored in the RPE? What is the mechanism of transit of retinoids between RPE and photoreceptor? Where is retinoid isomerized back to the 11-*cis* conformation and is this an active, enzyme-mediated process? Helpful in answering many of these questions in the last few years is the realization not only that several enzymes are involved but that a number of specific retinoid-binding proteins are present in the RPE cell and IPM that seem to facilitate retinoid processing.

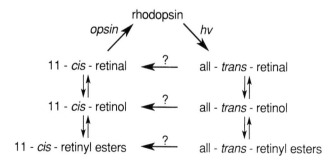

FIGURE 7-2. Classical scheme of retinoid movement between the neural retina and retinal pigment epithelium (RPE). With bleaching, retinoid (vitamin A) moves from retina to RPE and, with dark adaptation, the process is reversed. Question marks indicate pathways in doubt. (Taken from Rando, 1991.)

RETINOID UPTAKE FROM SERUM INTO THE RPE CELL

The visual cycle is truly a tightly regulated "cycle," in which retinoid moves back and forth from RPE cell to photoreceptor outer segment through the IPM and is strongly retained in this loop (Dowling, 1964). Since retinoid is not synthesized in the eye, however, retinol must first be taken up into the RPE from the blood, where it is bound in a 1:1 ratio to the serum retinol-binding protein (RBP). RBP is a 21 kDa protein synthesized in the liver; with its bound retinol, it is released into the bloodstream in response to tissue demands for retinoid (Goodman, 1984). RBP is also complexed with another protein, transthyretin (TTR, prealbumin), which is important in the plasma transport of thyroxine (van Jaarsveld et al., 1973). Such a double complex (approximately 75 kDa) probably protects the RBP from clearance by glomerular filtration. In the mid-1970s, Bok and Heller (1976) demonstrated that plasma RBP does not cross the blood-retina barrier into RPE cells, and thus a mechanism must be present to remove the retinol from its RBP binding site and to translocate it through the plasma membrane into the RPE cell. Using detached sheets of RPE cells and radiolabeled RBP with and without bound retinol, Bok and Heller (1976) autoradiographically demonstrated specific membrane binding sites for RBP on the basal and lateral surfaces of the RPE cell. Since retinol is concentrated only by RPE and a limited number of other cell types, a receptor-mediated mechanism of uptake was thus suggested (Heller, 1975). At this time, Maraini and colleagues (1977) reported that they were able to extract a 14.5 kDa retinol-binding protein from RPE cell plasma membranes, although our current knowledge of RPE cell retinoid-binding proteins indicates that this could be the soluble cellular retinol-binding protein (CRBP) which binds retinol within the RPE cell (see below). More recently, Båvik and colleagues (1992) have proposed that a particular 63 kDa protein (p63) within a high molecular weight complex could function as the basal-surface "receptor" in RPE cells. Biochemical characterization of this protein demonstrates that p63 has a high affinity for RBP (K_d of 30–75 nM) but that it is not an ordinary integral membrane protein since it exists in multiple extractable forms and in complex with other proteins. It is also reported to be found only in RPE cells and to be expressed highest on basolateral surfaces of the RPE. Båvik and colleagues (1993) have recently reported the isolation of the p63 protein and its cDNA. This protein is unusual in that, based on the cDNA-deduced amino acid sequence, it does not have an N-terminal signal sequence or transmembrane regions, nor does the in vitro translated protein become membrane inserted in the presence of heterologous microsomes.

An identical protein has been purified and cloned by Hamel and colleagues (1993a; 1993b). Called RPE65, this protein was originally isolated using an RPE-cell-specific monoclonal antibody. Their analyses have demonstrated two areas having an ampipathic α-helical structure in the protein which can interact with membranes. Questions remain as to the localization of this protein, however, since Hamel and colleagues (1993b) have detected RPE65 mainly in association with microsomal membranes. A second point in need of resolution is that Hamel and colleagues (1993b) have reported that cultured RPE cells soon lose their ability to synthesize RPE65. If p63/RPE65 functions as an obligatory receptor, this would seem to be incompatible with the fact that cultured cells in general appear to have the ability to take up retinol in a normal manner, that is, bound to RBP—as demonstrated by Carlson and Bok (1992). Despite these questions, much evidence yet remains indicating that RPE cells uptake of retinol from the choroid is both specific and receptor mediated. In such a scheme, plasma retinol, bound to RBP (probably also complexed to TTR) passes out of the choroidal vessels in a manner yet to be determined and is recognized by specific receptors (putatively p63/RPE65) on the basolateral side of RPE cells. Also in an unknown manner, the retinol is then translocated across the membrane into the RPE cell where it can be bound by an "acceptor" protein such as CRBP. Because of its strong affinity for plasma RPB in an in vitro binding assay (Båvik et al., 1993), p63 is the current candidate for consideration as a basolateral membrane receptor that functions in retinol uptake into the RPE cell. Supporting the general idea that there is a specific interaction between serum RBP and an RPE cell receptor, Melhus and colleagues (1995) have demonstrated that a monoclonal antibody to RBP effectively blocks binding of RBP to the its receptor on RPE cell membranes.

RETINOID-BINDING PROTEINS OF THE RPE-IPM-RETINA COMPLEX

The occurrence of retinoids in three oxidative states (alcohol, aldehyde, and acid) and in *cis/trans* isomeric forms, as well as the capacity of the alcohol to be esterified, presents several challenges to understanding retinoid metabolism in the RPE. Once within the RPE cell, for example, retinol is subject to several metabolic paths. As in blood, soluble intracellular retinoid-binding proteins have been identified that are fairly specific for many of the different types of retinoids and seem to be involved in retinoid transfer within the RPE cell and across the interphotoreceptor matrix (IPM) to the neural retina. Such proteins could be useful in several regards. First, retinoids are, to varying degrees, intrinsically insoluble and unstable in aqueous media. Furthermore, at higher concentrations, retinol can be toxic to cell membranes and organelles (Meeks and colleagues, 1981). Protein binding can "solubilize" retinoids and protect them from oxidative or enzymatic attack as well as protect the RPE cell from membranolysis induced by retinoid. Finally, these proteins also may actively specify pathways of retinoid processing and participate in the chemical transformations within the cell. Following is a description of the retinoid-binding proteins found in the RPE-IPM-retina complex (Table 7-1). As seen in Figure 7-3, these have been depicted by Bok (1983) as carrying their endogenous ligands within the scheme of the visual cycle.

Over twenty years ago, Bashor and colleagues (1973) reported the presence in a number of tissues of a novel,

TABLE 7-1. *Retinoid-binding proteins*

Binding protein	Mol. size (approx kDa)	Retinoid specificity	Tissue localization
Retinol-binding protein (RBP)	21	Retinol	Serum and eye
Cellular retinol-binding protein (CRBP)	15	Retinol	Many tissues; RPE and Müller cells
Cellular retinoic acid-binding protein (CRABP)	15	Retinoic acid	Many tissues; amacrine and Müller cells
Cellular retinaldehyde-binding protein (CRALBP)	36	*cis* conformation of retinoids	RPE, Müller cells, pineal
Interphotoreceptor retinoid-binding protein (IRBP)	135–140	Binds most retinoids and fatty acids	Interphotoreceptor matrix and pineal

small (16 kDa) protein, the cellular retinol-binding protein (CRBP), which bound retinol with relatively high affinity and specificity. Wiggert and Chader (1975) were the first to use this information to explore ocular tissues for the occurrence of soluble retinol-binding proteins, establishing the presence of such proteins in eye tissues including retina, pigment epithelium, and cornea (Wiggert and colleagues, 1976; 1977). Saari and Futterman (1976) established the separate nature of retinol and retinoic acid binding in retina; only all-*trans*-retinol has been found to bind to CRBP in vitro (Wiggert et al., 1977) and to be present on the purified protein (Saari et al., 1982). Marked cell specificity also exists, in that, within the retina-RPE complex, CRBP is found exclusively in RPE cells and Müller glia of the neural retina (Bok et al., 1984; de Leeuw et al., 1990). It is now known that CRBP belongs to a large supergene family whose protein products bind ligands such as retinoic acid and fatty acids. The cellular retinoic acid-binding protein (CRABP) is a member of this family. In general, CRBP probably functions to facilitate intracellular transport of the retinol as well as to protect it during transit. In the eye, all-*trans*-retinol bound to CRBP has been found to be a good substrate for esterification by retinyl ester synthase (LRAT) in RPE cell microsomes (Berman et al., 1980; Saari et al., 1984). Ottonello and colleagues (1987) also have presented evidence that CRBP is probably an important factor in general retinol binding within the RPE cell and, specifically, in the regulation of retinyl ester hydrolase.

Although not involved in the visual process per se, retinoic acid is thought to be an important mediator of cellular development (Gudas, 1994) and, within many cell types, is bound to a specific cellular retinoic acid-binding protein (CRABP). In the adult eye, CRABP is mainly found in the retina (Saari and Futterman, 1976; Wiggert et al., 1978), specifically within Müller glia and GABAergic amacrine cells (Milam et al., 1990). Cullum and colleagues (1984) have reported the presence of CRABP in fetal but not adult RPE. Doyle and colleagues (1995) have demonstrated, however, that cultured RPE cells can readily metabolize retinoic acid and therefore could be an ocular site of retinoic acid "deactivation." De Leeuw and colleagues (1990) have detected CRABP in rat retina during the early embryonic period and have suggested that it plays a role in neuronal differentiation in the inner retina.

In comparison to the relatively ubiquitous CRBP and CRABP, cellular retinaldehyde protein (CRALBP) appears to be mainly restricted to retina/RPE and pineal gland although Saari and colleagues (1996) have reported its presence in glia of optic nerve and brain. With retina/RPE, however, it is found in relatively high amounts. Bunt-Milam and Saari (1983) have immunocytochemically localized CRALBP to RPE and to Müller cells within the neural retina. The protein was first described by Futterman et al. (1977). It is now known to be about 36 kDa in size (Stubbs et al., 1979) and to have no sequence similarities to other proteins (Crabb et al., 1988). It binds both retinol and retinaldehyde but only in the *cis* conformation (Stubbs et al., 1979). Within this specificity, however, Saari and colleagues (1982) have found that this protein binds different ligands in retina versus RPE. CRALBP purified from RPE only has endogenous 11-*cis*-retinaldehyde bound to it, whereas CRALBP purified from retina contains 11-*cis*-retinol as well as 11-*cis*-retinaldehyde. Importantly, Saari and colleagues (1994) have presented evidence that CRALBP can determine which metabolic pathway 11-*cis*-retinol takes in the RPE cell. It is known that 11-*cis*-retinol is a pivotal substrate that can be either oxidized to 11-*cis*-retinaldehyde for use in the visual process in the outer segments or be esterified for storage within the RPE cell. Saari and colleagues (1994) have demonstrated that 11-*cis*-retinol is oxidized more readily to retinaldehyde (a two- to threefold increase) and is esterified more slowly to its ester form (about a tenfold decrease) when bound to CRALBP. CRALBP may thus act as a "substrate-routing protein" in vivo and, as such, could be an important factor in supplying 11-*cis*-retinaldehyde for rhodopsin formation.

Along with these cellular retinoid-binding proteins, both the plasma RBP and TTR have been shown to be synthesized in the eye. Martone and colleagues (1988) and Herbert and colleagues (1991) have reported that, although RPB mRNA is only detected in RPE cells, the RBP protein is found in several ocular areas, including retinal ganglion cells and corneal epithelium. Dwork and colleagues (1988) and Cavallaro and colleagues (1990) have pinpointed TTR synthesis also to the retinal RPE layer. As with RPB, the TTR protein is immunocytochemically detectable in many eye areas including RPE, iris, ciliary body, cornea, retina, and lens capsule. Ong and colleagues (1994) have demonstrated the apical secretion of both RBP and TTR in cultured RPE cells although the secretion does not have the 1:1 stoichiometry that seems to be obligatory in the secretion of the RBP-TTR complex by liver. Although direct functional evidence is yet not available, it is postulated that these proteins could take part in retinoid translocation within the eye.

The exchange of retinoid between the RPE and retina in the visual cycle seems to be strongly dependent on an extracellular retinoid-binding protein, the interphotoreceptor retinoid-binding protein (IRBP). IRBP was first seen as a large, ^{3}H-retinol-binding protein in sucrose gradients of retinal supernatant fractions now known to contain adherent interphotoreceptor matrix (Wiggert et al., 1976; 1977). Early studies also demonstrated the association of this binding protein with the photoreceptor outer segment layer (Bergsma et al., 1977) and with an apparent differential light-dark binding of retinoid (Wiggert et al., 1979). The extracellular nature of IRBP and its occurrence as a major component of the IPM were subsequently established in several laboratories and led to the hypothesis that IRBP is involved in the transport of retinoid between RPE and neural retina (Adler and Martin, 1982; Liou et al., 1982; Lai et al., 1982; Bunt-Milam and Saari, 1983). IRBP is now known to be a large (approximately 135 kDa) lipoglycoprotein (Fong et al., 1984; Adler et al., 1985; Saari et al., 1985) that is synthesized by retinal photoreceptors (van Veen et al., 1986). The bovine (Borst et al., 1989), frog (Gonzalez-Fernandez et al., 1993), and human (Liou et al., 1989; Fong et al., 1990) genes have been cloned and characterized; they all demonstrate an interesting fourfold repeat structure and do not seem to belong to a large gene family, as do CRBP and CRABP.

IRBP readily binds fatty acids as well as retinoids (Bazan et al., 1985; Chen et al., 1993; Putilina et al., 1993) and thus could be involved in the transport of fatty acids as well as retinoids in the interphotoreceptor matrix. Chen and Noy (1996) have recently found that docosahexaenoic acid (DHA) comprises a large fraction of the fatty acids bound to IRBP to "target 11-*cis*-retinal to its site of action in photoreceptor cells." Chen and Anderson (1993) have provided evidence that triglycerides within the RPE cell are the source within the interphotoreceptor space of free fatty acids that can be recycled back to the photoreceptors on IRBP and/or other proteins. Originally, IRBP was reported to bind 2 M retinoid/M protein by Fong and colleagues (1984) and Saari and colleagues (1985) or 1 M retinoid/M protein by Adler and colleagues (1985) and Okajima and colleagues (1989). This apparent discrepancy is most probably due to differences in isolation, loading, and assay conditions since IRBP has a relatively low binding affinity (~1 μM) for retinol (Adler et al., 1985; Okajima et al., 1989) and binds a number of retinoids in both *trans* and *cis* conformations with a sharp increase in the amount of all-*trans*-retinol endogenously carried by the protein observed after bleaching (Adler and Martin, 1982; Saari et al., 1985). More recently, Chen and colleagues (1993) have reported two binding sites on IRBP for all-*trans*-retinol, one high-affinity site (dissociation constant of 0.1 μM) and one of lower affinity. Importantly, fatty acids such as docosahexaenoic acid were found to compete for the higher-affinity retinoid-binding site on IRBP, indicating that "in vivo, retinoid bind-

ing by this protein will be affected by the amount and identity of the fatty acids associated with it" (Chen et al., 1993).

The high concentration of IRBP in the IPM as well as its relatively low affinity and specificity for retinoids and fatty acids are properties consistent with the need for rapid shuttling of bulk amounts of different retinoids (specifically all-*trans*-retinol and 11-*cis*-retinaldehyde) back and forth between photoreceptors and RPE and the return of important fatty acids to the neural retina from the RPE. Importantly, IRBP has been shown to protect retinol from chemical oxidation and isomerization in vitro (Crouch et al., 1992); it thus may also act as a protective "buffer" for retinoids traversing the heavily oxygenated IPM.

RETINOID REACTIONS WITHIN THE RPE CELL

The basic function of the RPE cell in the visual process is to generate the 11-*cis*-retinaldehyde that is used in the formation of rhodopsin. Important but ancillary to this are its functions in retinoid uptake and storage. Retinol uptake appears to occur in three ways (Fig. 7-3). As described above, there is putative receptor-mediated uptake from blood through the basal surface of the RPE cell. Less well understood is the return of retinol from the retinal photoreceptors. This latter process begins in the outer segment with the reduction of *trans*-retinaldehyde (generated by the bleaching of rhodopsin) to all-*trans*-retinol by retinol dehydrogenase (Futterman, 1963; Zimmerman et al., 1975). Recent studies indicate that the reduction of retinaldehyde to retinol is relatively slow, requiring minutes for completion, and that its progress influences the quenching kinetics of activated photoproducts in the visual process (Palczewski et al., 1994). Importantly, Hofmann and colleagues (1992) have found that all-*trans*-retinaldehyde can form complexes with opsin and that these complexes are capable of activity in the phototransduction cascade. Thus, the reductase, by controlling the level of all-*trans*-retinaldehyde, may regulate the level of the active opsin-all-*trans*-retinaldehyde complex as well as the amount of opsin available for interaction with 11-*cis*-retinaldehyde to regenerate rhodopsin (Jin et al., 1993; Palczewski et al., 1994).

Retinoid is then moved to the RPE through the IPM (probably bound to IRBP) and by phagocytosis of shed tips of photoreceptor outer segments. In most animals, a significant fraction of the outer segment and its complement of proteins, fatty acids, and retinoids is shed each day and phagocytized by RPE cells. In the rat, for example, there is turnover of the complete length of the

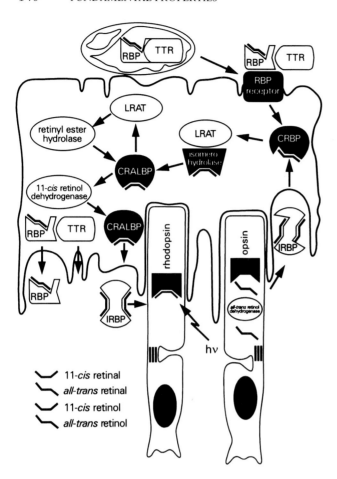

11-*cis* retinal

all-trans retinal

11-*cis* retinol

all-trans retinol

FIGURE 7-3. Schematic depiction of proteins and enzymes involved in the movement of retinoids in and around the RPE cell during the visual cycle. (TTR): transthyretin; (IRBP): interphotoreceptor retinoid-binding protein; (LRAT): lecithin:retinol acetyltransferase. Other retinoid-binding proteins are defined in Table 7-1. (Modified from Bok, 1993.)

rod outer segment in only about nine days (Young, 1967), making this a potentially important route for entry of retinol and fatty acids into the RPE cell. Once the shed disc packet is engulfed within the cell as a phagosome, there is fusion with the lysosomes, protein digestion, and release of retinoid, where it is free to bind to an appropriate binding protein and reenter into the visual cycle. Similarly, it is assumed that retinol, recycled apically by IRBP to the RPE or delivered basally by plasma RBP, is bound to CRBP upon entry into the cell. The bound retinol can then be esterified by an ester synthase activity present in RPE cell microsomes. Krinsky (1958) first showed that RPE cell homogenates readily convert all-*trans*-retinol to an ester even without the addition of an exogenous acyl donor. Berman et al. (1980) subsequently demonstrated the localization of the synthase activity to the RPE microsomal fraction. In an important series of experiments, Saari and Bredberg (1988)

demonstrated that endogenous fatty acyl-CoAs in RPE microsomes are not present at sufficiently high concentrations to support synthase activity and that a yet unknown lipid functions as the endogenous donor. Saari and colleagues (Saari and Bredberg, 1989; Saari et al., 1993) then identified the enzymatic transfer of an acyl group from the 1-position of phosphatidylcholine to all-*trans*-retinol and, as with a similar activity described by MacDonald and Ong (1988) in intestine, referred to this esterifying activity as "lecithin:retinol acetyltransferase (LRAT)." In the RPE cell, there is positional selectivity in transfer of the acyl group from lecithin to retinoid, in that transfer occurs almost exclusively from the 1-position of the phospholipid (Barry et al., 1989). Several kinetic parameters, including the mechanism by which LRAT from RPE cells catalyzes acyl group transfer, have more recently been established (Shi et al., 1993); for example, the reaction proceeds as an ordered, "ping-pong bi-bi" mechanism.

Esterification of retinol has now been identified as a key reaction in the visual cycle, since not only does it produce a stable, nontoxic form of retinoid that can be easily stored but the ester actually serves as the substrate in the isomerization reaction that converts the all-*trans*-retinoid to the 11-*cis*-conformation. Until the mid-1980s, the retinoid isomerizing system of the eye remained elusive. Not only were investigators unable to establish whether the *trans-cis* isomerization process was enzymatically driven, but the site of the isomerization (i.e., retina *vs.* RPE) was controversial. In groundbreaking work soon thereafter, though, Bernstein and colleagues (1987a) firmly established both the enzymatic nature of the isomerizing reactions and the fact that the "isomerase" resides in the RPE. Moreover, it was established that the isomerization reaction is an energy-transducing process that uses endogenous membrane lipid as a thermodynamic energy source (Deigner et al., 1989). Of particular interest was the finding of a close connection between the action of the isomerase and the energetics of formation of all-*trans* retinyl ester, the immediate substrate of the reaction.

The enzymatic nature and the site of the isomerase reaction in the RPE cell were unequivocally established by Bernstein and colleagues (1987a), who showed that retina/RPE membranes catalyze the conversion of exogenously added ^{3}H-all-*trans*-retinol to a mixture of 11-*cis*-retinaldehyde, 11-*cis*-retinol, and 11-*cis*-retinyl palmitate. This apparent enzymatic activity was primarily found in the RPE, (Fulton and Rando, 1987). At about this same time, Trehan and colleagues (1990) also made the important observation that a large number of diverse reagents have parallel inhibitory effects on retinyl isomerization and retinyl synthetase activity. For example, treatment of RPE membranes with all-*trans*-retinyl-α-bromoacetate (a potent inhibitor of retinyl ester synthase) not only inhibited the synthase activity as expected but markedly reduced the production of 11-*cis*-retinoids. These results demonstrated that it is the ester, rather than the free alcohol or aldehyde forms of the retinoid, that serves as the substrate in the isomerase reaction. The enzyme catalyzing this combined isomerization and hydrolysis of all-*trans*-retinyl ester is thus best referred to as an "isomerohydrolase." Gueil and colleagues (1991) reported the presence of retinal ester hydrolase in the RPE. In parallel studies, Mata and colleagues (1992) partially characterized a retinyl ester hydrolase activity (REH) in bovine RPE cell microsomes that catalyzes the hydrolysis of both *cis* and *trans* retinyl esters; they concluded that esters of the two isomers are hydrolyzed at distinct catalytic sites.

Also of importance is that retinyl esters contain high-energy bonds which, upon hydrolysis, release up to 5 kcal/M. Coupling of the free energy of hydrolysis to the "thermodynamically uphill" isomerization process was shown to supply the energy that drives the isomerization reaction (Deigner et al., 1989; Rando, 1991). As depicted in Figure 7-4, a coupled, energy-producing reaction can drive the isomerization process. First, it is assumed that all-*trans*-retinol is converted to an all-*trans*-retinyl ester using a phospholipid-OX donor. Second, the ester is isomerized in a reaction that utilizes the free energy of ester hydrolysis to produce the *trans* to *cis* conversion. This overall reaction, i.e., all-*trans*-ester to 11-*cis* retinol, is energetically favorable since the net Gibbs free energy is −1 kcal/M. This pathway was tested by Deigner et al. (1989) by following the fate of

[18]oxygen in the C-O bond of all-*trans*-retinol during the isomerohydrolysase reaction. Theoretically, if C-O cleavage occurs during the process as predicted in the pathway, then the [18]O should be lost and the 11-*cis*-retinol initially formed should not contain the label. Using a field desorption mass-spectrometry technique, label was indeed found to be lost and, on this basis, the overall process was thought to be consistent with the two-step pathway. Bernstein and colleagues (1987b) also used a double-label experiment to demonstrate that retinoid isomerization occurs at the alcohol level of oxidation. When 15-[3]H- and 15-^{14}C-all-*trans*-retinol were used as substrates with RPE cell membranes, the ^{3}H-label was retained in the resultant 11-*cis*-retinol product. Although several kinetic parameters of the isomerase system have been reported (Bernstein et al., 1987b; Livrea et al., 1991), the enzyme has remained elusive and difficult to purify. In spite of such difficulties, the pattern of the flow of retinoids in the RPE cell proposed by Rando and his colleagues seems well established; a similar scheme for retinoid transformation and movement has been proposed by Timmers and colleagues (1991).

What is the source of the energy needed for the *trans* to *cis* conversion? As depicted in Figure 7-5, Rando and his collaborators envisioned that lecithin and retinyl esters in conjunction with an ester synthetase and an isomerohydrolase enzyme (exhibiting both hydrolase and isomerase activities as shown) play pivotal roles in the biosynthesis of 11-*cis*-retinoids. Here, lecithin works in a group transfer reaction as would ATP, supplying the energy to drive the endergonic isomerization reaction. In this scheme, the ester synthetase (LRAT) and the iso-

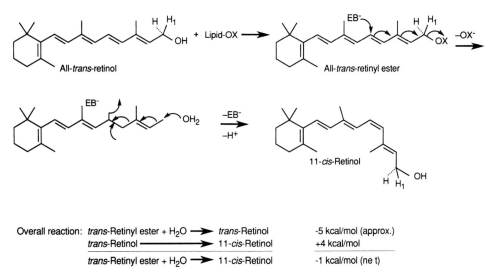

FIGURE 7-4. Proposed reactions leading to retinoid isomerization in the RPE cell. (Lipid-OX): phospholipid acyl donor; (EB⁻): enzyme active-site nucleophile. (Taken from Deigner et al. 1989.)

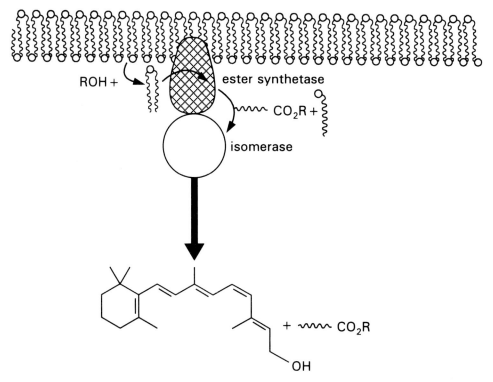

FIGURE 7-5. Schematic depiction of the involvement of membrane phospholipids in the formation of 11-*cis*-retinol. The ester synthetase, LRAT (lecithin:retinol acyltransferase), converts free retinol (ROH) to an all-*trans*-retinyl ester form (⌇⌇⌇CO$_2$R) using lecithin (⌇⌇⌇O) from the general membrane phospholipids as the acyl donor. The isomerase (isomerohydrolase reaction) then converts the ester into 11-*cis*-retinol. (Taken from Rando, 1991.)

merase (isomerohydrolase) are depicted as membrane-associated proteins although their physical relationship to RPE cell membranes has yet to be elucidated. It is also likely that CRBP and CRALBP could be at least transiently associated with the complex as carrier proteins for retinol and 11-*cis*-retinoid, respectively. Once the isomerization reaction produces the 11-*cis*-conformation, the retinoid can be oxidized and the 11-*cis*-retinaldehyde moved to the outer segment for rhodopsin regeneration. Suzuki and colleagues (1993) have reported the partial purification of the *cis*-specific retinoid dehydrogenase involved in retinoid chromophore regeneration and, with an anti-33 kDa monoclonal antibody, determined the protein to be present only in RPE cells. Simon and colleagues (1995) and Driessen and colleagues (1995) have recently described the cloning of a protein specific to the RPE that appears to be the 11-*cis*-retinol dehydrogenase. This 32 kDa protein (p32) is stereospecific for 11-*cis*-retinol and belongs to a gene family of short-chain alcohol dehydrogenases. The closest homolog is the human D-β-hydroxybutyrate precursor protein. Interestingly, p32 interacts with p63, the putative RPB membrane receptor, leading Simon and

colleagues (1995) to hypothesize that "cellular uptake and metabolism are coupled events in the RPE."

RETINOID TRANSPORT BETWEEN RPE CELLS AND PHOTORECEPTORS

As with our understanding of retinoid reactions within the RPE cell, the last ten years have seen marked advances in elucidating the possible mechanism by which retinoid moves between RPE and neural retina in the interphotoreceptor matrix (IPM). This mechanism must satisfy the requirements for both ligand protection and vectorial bulk transport. Concerning the protective effect, it has been mentioned above that Crouch and colleagues (1992) have provided evidence that binding of retinol to IRBP markedly protects the retinoid from chemical degradation. Along with this, IRBP could provide physiological protection of the delicate ROS/RPE cell membranes and normal retinoid pathways from disruptive effects of retinoid buildup. In this regard, Jones and colleagues (1989) have demonstrated that 11-*cis*-retinol is actually "toxic" to rod outer segments, in that the ROS lose electrophysiological sensitivity in its presence, but that IRBP reverses the effect by exerting a protective or "buffering" action.

The mechanism responsible for the movement of retinoids must also account for the vectorial transfer of all-*trans*-retinol from outer segment membranes to RPE cells under bleaching conditions and the movement of 11-*cis*-retinaldehyde back to the photoreceptors in the dark. All this must be done for bulk amounts of retinoid and within the electrophysiologically established time frames of the reactions. Ho and colleagues (1989) have argued that IRBP is an unlikely candidate for actual participation in retinoid transport within the IPM, since they found that all-*trans*-retinol was rapidly transferred between liposome reservoirs and ROS membranes in vitro and that IRBP addition retarded rather than facilitated the transfer process. The visual cycle is not a particularly speedy process, however, and Jones et al. (1989) have provided evidence that electrophysiological recovery of sensitivity of bleached, isolated rods after addition of 11-*cis*-retinaldehyde bound to IRBP "occurs in times that are not markedly different than those within the intact eye."

With light adaptation, Okajima and colleagues (1989) have demonstrated that IRBP not only increases the delivery of retinol to the RPE but promotes an increase in ester formation within the RPE cell as well. These studies employed the "RPE-eyecup" preparation from the posterior hemisphere of the eye of the toad

(*Bufo marinus)*, which is devoid of the vitreous and neural retina. ^{3}H-all-*trans*-retinol can then be added to the exposed apical surface of the RPE in the presence of IRBP or other test agents. They found that IRBP was more efficient than phosphatidyl choline vesicles, serum RBP, or albumin in effecting the synthesis of ^{3}H-retinyl ester within the RPE. Figure 7-6 demonstrates that the time course of ester formation is markedly faster in RPE eyecups receiving ^{3}H-retinol with 3 μM IRBP than in those receiving the retinoid with 90 μM albumin.

During dark adaptation in vivo, retinoid moves out of the RPE cell, across the IPM and into the photoreceptor cell, where it interacts with opsin to form the visual pigment rhodopsin. Okajima and colleagues (1990) used the toad RPE-eyecup preparation and obtained evidence that IRBP affects both the amount and type of retinoid released by the RPE as well as the formation of rhodopsin in ROS. They observed that when a buffer solution containing IRBP was incubated in the vitreal cavity of the RPE-eyecup, retinoid was released by the RPE (Fig. 7-7A). In contrast, no retinoid was released when the eyecup contained buffer alone or buffer containing albumin. Furthermore, virtually all of the released retinoid was found to be 11-*cis*-retinaldehyde (Fig. 7-7A insert and Fig. 7-7B), the isomer needed to combine with opsin and the isomer previously found to be the major endogenous retinoid bound to IRBP isolated from dark-adapted eyes (Saari et al., 1985). Adler and Spencer (1991) also found that the major endogenous ligand of IRBP is 11-*cis*-retinaldehyde in the dark and all-*trans*-retinol in the light. Finally, experiments also demonstrated a direct involvement of IRBP in the regeneration of rhodopsin (Okajima et al., 1990). Bleached rod outer segments (ROS) were incubated with or without retinoid-free IRBP in the RPE-eyecup (where the RPE supplies an endogenous source of retinoids) or in a test tube (where there is no retinoid source). Only in the case where both IRBP and RPE were present was substantial rhodopsin formation seen. Together, these studies provide strong evidence that IRBP promotes (1) the selective release of only 11-*cis*-retinaldehyde from the RPE cell and (2) the efficient transfer of this retinoid from RPE to photoreceptor ROS, thereby facilitating the formation of visual pigment.

IRBP-induced release of 11-*cis*-retinaldehyde from apical RPE cell membranes has also been demonstrated by Carlson and Bok (1992). They used a sophisticated RPE cell tissue culture system in which medium at the basal and apical surfaces of the cell could be independently varied and sampled. It was found that, when ^{3}H-all-*trans*-retinol bound to RBP is presented basally to the cultured cells, only IRBP successfully induces the apical release of ^{3}H-*cis*-retinaldehyde. More recent

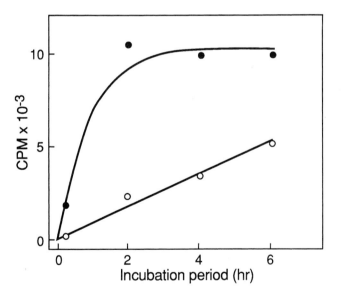

FIGURE 7-6. Time course of formation of ^{3}H-retinyl ester in toad RPE eyecups. The vitreal cavity contained 0.05 μM ^{3}H-all-*trans*-retinol with either 3 μM IRBP (●) or 90 μM bovine serum albumin (○). Subsequent HPLC testing demonstrated a much more rapid formation of retinyl ester in RPE samples incubated with IRBP. (Taken from Okajima et al., 1989.)

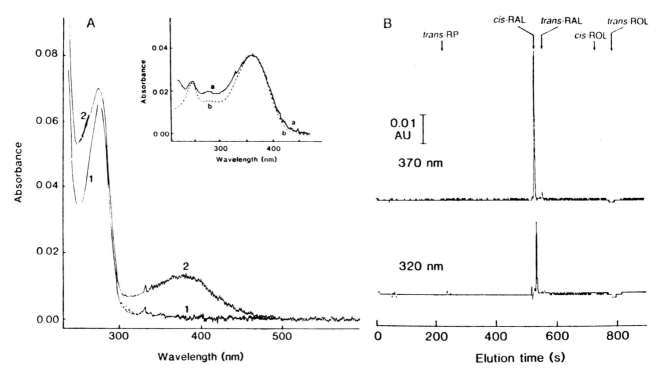

FIGURE 7-7. (A) Absorbance spectra demonstrating the influence of IRBP on retinoid release into the vitreal cavity of toad RPE eyecups. (Sample 1): 250 μl buffer sample containing 2.8 nmol IRBP placed in vitreal cavity and immediately withdrawn. (Sample 2): Identical sample incubated for 3 hrs. showing extraction of 380 nm–absorbing material. No retinoid was withdrawn in the absence of IRBP. (Insert; curve a): Absorbance spectrum of material extracted from sample 2. (Curve b): Absorbance spectrum of 11-*cis*-retinaldehyde in hexane. (B) HPLC profiles of the 380 nm–absorbing material extracted from the vitreal cavity of the eyecup. The retinoid is identified as 11-*cis*-retinaldehyde. (Taken from Okajima et al., 1990.)

studies by Duffy and colleagues (1993) confirm and extend these results. They used a skate eyecup preparation in which the neural retina could be experimentally detached and then reapplied to the underlying RPE. After detachment, the concentration of IRBP in the subretinal space could be decreased (by fluid lavage) or increased (by addition of exogenous IRBP). With lavage, a marked deficit was seen in both the rate and total amount of rhodopsin regenerated after bleaching. Specifically, it was found by fundus reflectometry that instillation of IRBP into the subretinal space before replacement of the neural retina on the RPE markedly increased both the rate of regeneration and the amount of rhodopsin formed during a subsequent period of dark adaptation.

Okajima and colleagues (1994) used the toad RPE-eyecup system to track the fate of radiolabeled retinoids in the RPE cell and to investigate the effects of IRBP on the formation and release of 11-*cis*-retinaldehyde (Fig. 7-8). Eyecups were first incubated with ³H-all-*trans*-retinol (loading phase) and then fresh medium (with or without IRBP) was added to the vitreal cavities (test phase). It was found that the presence of RBP increased

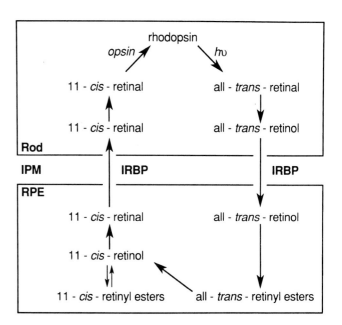

FIGURE 7-8. Current scheme depicting retinoid movement in the visual cycle. (Adapted from Rando, 1991.)

both the amount and specific radioactivity of 11-*cis*-retinaldehyde released by RPE cells. Interestingly, the specific radioactivity of the released 11-*cis*-retinaldehyde exceeded that of the all-*trans*-retinyl ester within the RPE. These data demonstrate that IRBP promotes the formation of 11-*cis*-retinaldehyde from all-*trans*-precursors within the RPE as well as its release from RPE cells. Moreover, it appears that recently incorporated and esterified all-*trans*-retinol is utilized in the synthesis and release of 11-*cis*-retinaldehyde in a "last in/first out" manner. The possibility of retinoid compartmentalization and specific routing pathways within the RPE cell, as perhaps defined by intracellular retinoid-binding proteins, should be an interesting area for future investigation.

CURRENT MODELS OF RETINOID PROCESSING IN THE RPE CELL

Rando (1991) and Okajima and colleagues (1994) have proposed composite schemes, outlining the known features of retinoid movement in the visual cycle and of retinoid processing in the RPE. Figure 7-9 outlines the current concept of retinoid transformations and flow within and between the compartments of the RPE-IPM-retina complex as compared with the classical view given in Figure 7-2. Of greatest importance is that we now know that it is the all-*trans*-ester that plays a central role

in formation of the 11-*cis*-retinaldehyde chromophore and that the process takes place within the RPE cell. In concert, the energy needed to drive the endergonic isomerization reaction is known to be derived from RPE cell membrane phospholipids.

It also now seems clear that retinoid reactions within and outside of the RPE cell are markedly affected and probably mediated by a number of retinoid-binding proteins such as CRBP, CRALBP, and IRBP. As mentioned earlier, IRBP facilitates the delivery of retinol to the RPE and enhances subsequent ester synthesis (Okajima et al., 1989). IRBP also promotes the formation of 11-*cis*-retinaldehyde in the RPE and its release for use in photoreceptor outer segments (Okajima et al., 1990; 1994; Carlson and Bok, 1992). As depicted in the model shown in Figures 7-8 and 7-9, retinoid movement is initiated in this pathway by bleaching of rhodopsin, the loss of retinoid from opsin, and the appearance of all-*trans*-retinol in the IPM. Either actively or by simple mass action, IRBP appears to facilitate the movement of retinol to the RPE cell. Although the transmembrane uptake process for retinol remains to be determined, Edwards and Adler (1994) have studied the kinetics of retinol exchange between IRBP and CRBP and have found CRBP to efficiently remove retinol from IRBP, a finding consistent with the almost 100-fold higher affinity for the retinoid of CRBP than IRBP. They suggest that this difference in affinity could contribute "to the flow of retinol to the RPE during a bleach *in vivo*."

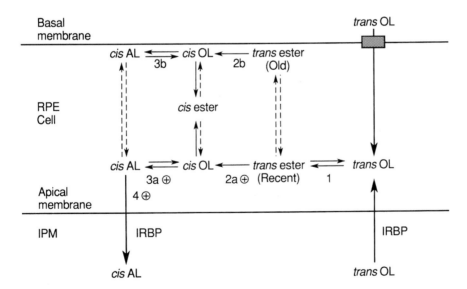

FIGURE 7-9. Current scheme of retinoid processing in the RPE cell. (OL): retinol; (AL): retinaldehyde; (IPM): interphotoreceptor matrix. Dual symbols for the same retinoid signify dual pools for the same retinoid. *Plus signs:* IRBP-stimulated reactions. *Dashed arrows:* unstimulated, sluggish reactions. Numbered reactions are catalyzed as follows: (1): all-*trans*-retinyl ester synthase; (2a) and (2b): retinyl isomerohydrolase; (3a) and (3b): 11-*cis*-retinol oxidoreductase. Box on basal membrane indicates uptake receptor for retinol. (Adapted from Okajima et al., 1994.)

Within the RPE cell, Okajima and colleagues (1994) have postulated that there is an "IRBP-stimulated pathway" that preferentially uses recently synthesized all-*trans*-retinyl ester for generation of 11-*cis*-retinaldehyde on a last in/first out basis. Central to this postulated pathway is the notion that, through a direct or indirect action of IRBP, recently arrived and esterified *trans*-retinol is processed to 11-*cis*-retinaldehyde without first entering the bulk ester pool. It will be interesting to determine in future work if the critical *trans*-to-*cis* isomerization step is mediated by a subpopulation of the isomerohydrolase enzyme that is preferentially stimulated by IRBP. Specifically, extracellular binding of 11-*cis*-retinaldehyde by IRBP (Fig. 7-9, Reaction 4) could significantly decrease the concentration of free 11-*cis*-retinaldehyde in the RPE and, by mass action or by a more active process, promote increased oxidoreductase (Reaction 3a) and/or isomerohydrolase (Reaction 2a) activities.

Within the RPE cell, elegant work by Saari and colleagues has demonstrated that both CRBP and CRALBP also function in an active manner to control the flow of substrate in the retinoid reactions within the RPE cell. By binding retinol, CRBP could control processes such as retinyl ester synthesis (Saari et al., 1984). As described above, CRALBP stimulates the oxidation of 11-*cis*-retinol and thus is probably a critical factor in production of 11-*cis*-retinaldehyde (Saari et al., 1994). Thus, a concerted effect of both extracellular and intracellular binding proteins could work with the appropriate enzyme activities to ensure proper movement of retinoids back and forth between retinal photoreceptors and RPE cells. Significantly, a new retinaldehyde-binding protein has been described in RPE that preferentially binds all-*trans*-retinaldehyde (Jiang et al., 1993; Shen et al., 1994). This 32 kDa RPE-retinal G-protein-coupled receptor (RGR) is related to the visual pigment genes (e.g. opsin and retinochrome) and, as with CRALBP, is found in the cytoplasm of both RPE and Müller glial cells. As with CRBP, CRALBP, and IRBP, RGR could participate in the visual process by passive binding of the *trans* isomer or by directing the flow of retinoids in a more active manner.

FUTURE DIRECTIONS

Although the major pathways of retinoid routing in the RPE-IPM-retina complex are now known, more work is needed to fully understand the complex reactions and regulatory mechanisms within the visual cycle. For example, the process of retinoid uptake from blood, through phagocytosis of shed ROS disc membranes and by direct uptake from the IPM, remain to be clarified.

Although it is clear that the eye forms a "closed" system of retinoid recycling, both quantitative and qualitative aspects of these three separate modes of retinoid entry into the RPE cell need to be determined. One of the most pressing problems concerns the actual translocation of retinoid across the RPE cell membrane. This includes (1) the search for IRBP "receptors" on the apical surface of the RPE (and retina as well) that might mediate the extracellular transfer of retinoid across the IPM and (2) the need for a better definition of RBP receptors on the basolateral surface of the RPE. In preliminary work, a putative cell surface receptor for IRBP has been identified on cultured RPE cells using photoaffinity-labeled IRBP and chemical cross-linking techniques (Duncan et al., 1995). Concerning the RPB receptor, it is as yet unclear why, if it is a specific basolateral membrane receptor and if it is identical to RPE65, it is present in such large amounts in the RPE and why it is mainly present in the microsomal membrane fraction of the cell, as reported by Hamel and colleagues (1993b). In spite of this, Båvik and colleagues (1995) have recently demonstrated that the binding of retinol to RPB markedly increases the biological effects of retinol on terminal differentiation of cultured human keratinocytes. In contrast, experiments on retinoid uptake into human keratinocytes by Hodam and colleagues (1991) concluded that RBP mediation is not necessary for retinol uptake into the cells nor for its biological actions and that no specific or saturable binding of RPB could be identified on the cell surface membranes. In fact, the necessity of either membrane receptors or soluble binding proteins has been questioned from several quarters. As with the experiments of Ho and colleagues (1989) cited above, Rando and Bangerter (1982) demonstrated rapid transfer between liposomes and between liposomes and erythrocyte membranes in the absence of carrier proteins. Supporting this notion is the finding of Szuts and Harosi (1991) that the solubility of retinol and retinaldehyde in aqueous medium is 0.06 μM and 0.11 μM respectively, levels that could allow for low but physiologically significant movement of the retinoids through aqueous solutions unaided by solubilizing binding proteins. Studies by Noy and Xu (1990) on dissociation of retinol from RBP also conclude that at least retinol can move freely between lipophilic compartments without the need for membrane receptors or binding proteins. Bulk quantities, as are possibly moved in the visual cycle, would be difficult to handle in this manner, however. Thus, although it is obvious that more work has to be done, the available evidence implies that both the membrane receptors and soluble retinoid-binding proteins lend directional specificity to the movement of retinoids into and within the RPE cell. Support for this hypothesis comes from the finding that 11-*cis*-retinaldehyde and all-*trans*-retinol are the retinoids with the highest affinity for IRBP, corresponding to the "physiological need to shuttle these particular retinoids between RPE and photoreceptor cells across the IPM in the visual cycle" (Chen and Noy, 1994). Moreover, it is evident that IRBP can perform the critical physiological function of protecting retinoid from degradation during passage through the IPM (Crouch et al., 1992).

The natures of the various enzymes involved in retinoid transformations within the RPE cell will also need to be further explored. In particular, it will be necessary to purify and clone the enzymes involved in isomerization, particularly the LRAT and isomerohydrolase protein moieties, and to determine the factors that regulate their activities. In this regard, Edwards and colleagues (1991) have provided evidence that retinyl ester synthetase activity is retained in cultured RPE cells when insulin or IGF-1 are added to the medium at physiological levels, implicating growth factors in at least the maintenance of ester synthesis. The possibly tight coupling of multiple enzyme activities (e.g. the isomerohydrolase with the ester synthase) is intriguing and should be further investigated. Similarly, interactions of these enzyme complexes with CRBP, CRALBP, and RGR may constitute major checkpoints for controlling substrate flow in the visual process and/or facilitating vectorial retinoid transport within the RPE cell.

The large amount of new information revealing the critical role of the RPE cell in retinoid processing emphasizes the possibility that abnormalities in RPE cell function most probably lead to visual impairment and blindness. For example, the unique character of many of the retinoid-processing enzymes and proteins being uncovered in the RPE cell makes them immediate candidates for involvement in hereditary diseases of the visual system. Smith and colleagues (1994), for example, have presented evidence that perturbations in ocular retinoid levels occur in the vitiligo mouse model of hereditary retinal degeneration. Specifically, they found that the concentrations of retinol and retinyl palmitate were markedly increased in RPE and liver of vitiligo mice. IRBP levels in eyes of young adult animals were also elevated. A hereditary perturbation in retinoid metabolism thus seems to be present in the mutant mouse that, even though systemic, particularly affects the RPE, causing or at least contributing to blindness. Pinpointing the site of the metabolic lesion in the vitiligo mutant may allow for a better understanding of enzymes or pathways in the human RPE cell at greatest risk to mutation and subsequent dysfunction.

More specifically, there is now evidence that mutations in RPE-specific genes thought to be involved in retinoid processing directly lead to inherited degenerations of the neural retina. Maw and colleagues (1997) have demonstrated that mutations in the CRALBP gene lead to a form of autosomal recessive retinitis pigmentosa. Gu and colleagues (1997) have shown that mutations in the RPE65 gene cause an early-onset, severe form of autosomal recessive retinal degeneration. Similarly, Marlhens and coworkers (1997) have reported mutations in the RPE65 gene specifically in patients with Leber's congenital amaurosis.

Problems of aging and environmental stress (e.g. phototoxicity) can also disrupt the delicately balanced flow of retinoids within the RPE cell and lead to retinal degeneration. An area ripe for investigation is that of macular degeneration, the leading cause of irreversible blindness in the United States and other developed countries, as cited in the *NEI Report of the Retinal and Choroidal Disease Panel* (1983–1987; NIH publication 83-2471). Although the cause(s) of macular degeneration are unknown except in a few special cases, the RPE cell is thought to play a central role in the etiology of this family of diseases. In particular, the accumulation of lipofuscin granules ("aging pigment"), as is seen in the RPE cells of older animals, is thought to lead to progressive loss of visual function. Robison and colleagues (1980) were the first to document the involvement of vitamin A as well as other lipophilic substances in lipofuscin formation. In animals, vitamin A–deficient diets have been shown to markedly lower the number of lipofuscin inclusion bodies in the RPE, demonstrating the direct involvement of retinoids in lipofuscin fluorophore formation (Katz and Norberg, 1992). Eldred and Lasky (1993) reported that the major orange-emitting fluorophore of the aging pigments of the RPE cell is a Schiff base product formed by the reaction of retinaldehyde and ethanolamine, an abundant substance in the RPE cell. They suggested that this product should display "lysosomotrophic detergent behavior" and could account for many of the degenerative changes seen in the aging process. More recent evidence suggests that the structure of the orange ocular aging pigment (A2-E) is that of a pyridinium *bis*-retinoid (Sakai et al., 1996). Importantly, lipofuscin photolysis can lead to superoxide formation, further contributing to age-related problems of the RPE-retina complex (Reszka et al., 1995). Thus, both hereditary retinal degenerations and those that are age related and environmentally induced need to be carefully examined as to primary or secondary problems in retinoid metabolism within the RPE cell.

CONCLUSION

In the last ten years, great progress has been made in understanding the processing of retinoids in the RPE cell, as well as the movement of retinoids between and within RPE, IPM, and neural retinal compartments. Most importantly, the RPE cell has been recognized as a full partner with the photoreceptor cell in retinoid processing, containing the unique isomerizing system that is critical in formation of the 11-*cis*-retinoid conformation. Although the broad outlines of retinoid movement and transformation are now known, much work yet remains to be done in understanding the molecular mechanisms underlying these pathways. Progress in this area should also greatly aid in our studies of the causes of inherited retinal degeneration such as retinitis pigmentosa and macular degeneration.

ACKNOWLEDGMENT

The authors are grateful to Drs. Dean Bok and Alice Adler for very helpful suggestions in modifying the text of the chapter and to Drs. Bok and A. Carlson for allowing us to use their updated version of Figure 7-3. Dr. Pepperberg was supported by NIH grant EY-05494 and Dr. Crouch by EY-04939.

REFERENCES

Adler A, Martin K. 1982. Retinol-binding proteins in bovine interphotoreceptor matrix. Biochem Biophys Res Commun 108:1601–1608.

Adler A, Evans C, Stafford W. 1985. Molecular properties of bovine interphotoreceptor retinol-binding protein. J Biol Chem 260:4850–4855.

Adler A, Spencer S. 1991. Effect of light on endogenous ligands carried by interphotoreceptor retinoid-binding protein. Exp Eye Res 53:337–346.

Barry R, Cañada F, Rando R. 1989. Solubilization and partial purification of retinyl ester synthase and retinoid isomerase from bovine ocular pigment epithelium. J Biol Chem 264:9231–9238.

Bashor M, Thoft D, Chytil F. 1973. In vitro binding of retinol to rat-tissue components. Proc Nat Acad Sci USA 70:3483–3487.

Båvik C-O, Busch C, Eriksson U. 1992. Characterization of a plasma retinol-binding protein membrane receptor expressed in the retinal pigment epithelium. J Biol Chem 267:23035–23042.

Båvik C-O, Levy F, Hellman L, Wernsted C, Eriksson U. 1993. The retinal pigment epithelium membrane receptor for plasma retinol-binding protein: isolation and cloning of the 63 kDa protein. J Biol Chem 268:20540–20546.

Båvik C-O, Peterson P, Eriksson U. 1995. Retinol-binding protein mediates uptake of retinol to cultured human keratinocytes. Exp Cell Res 216:358–362.

Bazan N, Reddy T, Redmond T, Wiggert B, Chader G. 1985. Endogenous fatty acids are covalently and noncovalently bound to interphotoreceptor retinoid-binding protein in the monkey retina. J Biol Chem 260:13677–13680.

Bergsma D, Wiggert B, Funahashi M, Kuwabara T, Chader G. 1977. Vitamin A receptors in normal and dystrophic human retina. Nature 265:66–67.

Berman E, Horowitz J, Segal N, Fisher S, Feeny-Burns L. 1980. Enzymatic esterification of vitamin A in the pigment epithelium of bovine retina. Biochim Biophys Acta 630:36–46.

Bernstein P, Law W, Rando R. 1987a. Isomerization of all-*trans*-retinoids to 11-*cis*-retinoids in vitro. Proc Nat Acad Sci USA 84:1849–1853.

Bernstein P, Law W, Rando R. 1987b. Biochemical characteriza-

tion of the retinoid isomerase system of the eye. J Biol Chem 262:16848–16857.

Bok D. 1990. Processing and transport of retinoids by retinal pigment epithelium. Eye 4:326–332.

Bok D. 1993. The retinal pigment epithelium: a versatile partner in vision. J Cell Sci 17(suppl):189–195.

Bok D, Heller J. 1976. Transport of retinol from the blood to the retina: an autoradiographic study of the pigment epithelial cell surface receptor for plasma retinol-binding protein. Exp Eye Res 22:395–402.

Bok D, Ong DE, Chytil F. 1984. Immunocytochemical localization of cellular retinol-binding protein in the rat retina. Invest Ophthalmol Vis Sci 25:877–883.

Borst D, Redmond T, Elser J, Gonda M, Wiggert B, Chader G, Nickerson J. 1989. Interphotoreceptor retinoid-binding protein: gene characterization, protein repeat structure and its evolution. J Biol Chem 264:1115–1123.

Bridges C, Alvarez R, Fong S-L, Gonzalez-Fernandez F, Lam D, Liou G. 1984. Visual cycle in the mammalian eye: retinoid binding proteins and the distribution of 11-*cis*-retinoids. Vision Res 24:1581–1594.

Bunt-Milam A, Saari J. 1983. Immunocytochemical localization of two retinoid-binding proteins in vertebrate retina. J Cell Biol 97:703–712.

Carlson A, Bok D. 1992. Promotion of the release of 11-*cis*-retinal from cultured retinal pigment epithelium by interphotoreceptor retinoid-binding protein. Biochemistry 31:9056–9062.

Cavallaro T, Martone R, Dwork A, Schon E, Herbert J. 1990. The retinal pigment epithelium is the unique site of transthyretin synthesis in the rat eye. Invest Ophthalmol Vis Sci 31:497–501.

Chen H, Anderson E. 1993. Metabolism in frog retinal pigment epithelium of docosahexaenoic and arachadonic acids derived from rod outer segment membranes. Exp Eye Res 57:369–377.

Chen Y, Noy N. 1994. Retinoid specificity of interphotoreceptor retinoid-binding protein. Biochemistry 33:10658–10665.

Chen Y, Noy N. 1996. Interrelationships between the interactions of bovine interphotoreceptor retinoid-binding protein with long-chain fatty acids and with retinoids. Invest Ophthalmol Vis Sci 37:S801.

Chen Y, Saari J, Noy N. 1993. Interactions of all-*trans* retinol and long-chain fatty acids with interphotoreceptor retinoid-binding protein. Biochemistry 32:11311–11317.

Crabb J, Johnson C, Carr S, Armes L, Saari J. 1988. The complete primary structure of the cellular retinaldehyde-binding protein from bovine retina. J Biol Chem 263:18678–18687.

Crouch R, Hazard E, Lind T, Wiggert B, Chader G, Corson D. 1992. Interphotoreceptor retinoid-binding protein and α-tocopherol preserve the isomeric and oxidative state of retinol. Photochem Photobiol 56:251–255.

Cullum M, Johnson B, Zile M. 1984. Comparison of fetal and adult retinol and retinoic acid-binding proteins in bovine serum and pigment epithelium. Int J Vit Nutr Res 54:297–305.

Deigner P, Law W, Cañada F, Rando R. 1989. Membranes as the energy source in the endergonic transformation of vitamin A to 11-*cis*-retinol. Science 244:968–971.

de Leeuw AM, Gaur VP, Saari J, Milam AH. 1990. Immunolocalization of cellular retinol-, retinaldehyde- and retinoic acid-binding proteins in rat retina during postnatal development. J Neurocytol 19:253–264.

Dowling J. 1960. Chemistry of visual adaptation in the rat. Nature 168:114–118.

Dowling J. 1963. Neural and photochemical mechanisms of visual adaptation in the rat. J Gen Physiol 46:1287–1301.

Dowling J. 1964. Nutrition and inherited blindness in the rat. Exp Eye Res 3:348–356.

Doyle J, Dowgiert R, Buzney S. 1995. Retinoic acid metabolism in cultured retinal pigment epithelial cells. Invest Ophthalmol Vis Sci 36:708–717.

Driessen C, Janssen B, Winkens H, van Vugt A, de Leeuw T, Jansses J. 1995. Cloning and expression of a cDNA encoding bovine retinal pigment epithelial 11-*cis* retinol dehydrogenase. Invest Ophthalmol Vis Sci 36:1988–1996.

Duffy M, Sun Y, Wiggert B, Duncan T, Chader G, Ripps H. 1993. Interphotoreceptor retinoid-binding protein (IRBP) enhances rhodopsin regeneration in the experimentally-detached retina. Exp Eye Res 57:771–782.

Duncan T, Palmer K, Chader G, Wiggert B. 1995. A putative retinal pigment epithelial cell surface receptor for interphotoreceptor retinoid-binding protein. Invest Ophthalmol Vis Sci 36(suppl):S122.

Dwork A, Cavallaro T, Martone R, Goodman D, Schon E, Herbert J. 1990. Distribution of transthyretin in the rat eye. Invest Ophthalmol Vis Sci 31:489–496.

Edwards R, Adler A. 1994. Exchange of retinol between IRBP and CRBP. Exp Eye Res 59:161–170.

Edwards R, Adler A, Claycomb R. 1991. Requirement of insulin or IGF-I for the maintenance of retinyl ester synthetase activity by cultured retinal pigment epithelial cells. Exp Eye Res 52:51–57.

Eldred G, Lasky M. 1993. Retinal age pigments generated by self-assemblying lysosomotrophic detergents. Nature 361:724–726.

Fong S-L, Liou G, Landers R, Alvarez R, Bridges CD. 1984. Purification and characterization of a retinol-binding glycoprotein synthesized and secreted by bovine neural retina. J Biol Chem 259:6534–6542.

Fong S-L, Fong W-B, Morris T, Kedzie K, Bridges C. 1990. Characterization and comparative features of the gene for human interstitial retinol-binding protein. J Biol Chem 265:3648–3653.

Fulton B, Rando R. 1987. Retinyl ester formation in the biosynthesis of 11-*cis*-retinoids by bovine pigment epithelium membranes. Biochemistry 26:7938–7945.

Futterman S, Saari JC, Blair S. 1977. Occurrence of a binding protein for 11-*cis*-retinal in retina. J Biol Chem 252:3267–3271.

Futterman S. 1963. Metabolism of the retina. III. The role of reduced triphosphopyridine nucleotides in the visual cycle. J Biol Chem 238:1145–1150.

Goodman DS. 1984. Retinal transport in human plasma. In: Sporn MB, Roberts AB, Goodman DS, eds, The Retinoids, vol. 2. Orlando, FL: Academic Press, 42–82.

Gonzalez-Fernandez F, Kitteridge K, Rayborn M, Hollyfield J, Landers R, Saha M, Granger R. 1993. Interphotoreceptor retinoid-binding protein (IRBP), a major 124 kDa glycoprotein in the interphotoreceptor matrix of X. laevis. J Cell Sci 105:7–21.

Gu SM, Thompson D, Srikumari C, Lorenz B, Finckh L, Nicolette A, Murthy K, Rathmann M, Kumaramanickavel G, Denton M, Gal A. 1997. Mutations in RPE65 cause autosomal recessive childhood-onset severe retinal dystrophy. Nature Genetics 17:194–197.

Gudas L. 1994. Retinoids and vertebrate development. J Biol Chem 269:15399–15402.

Gueli M, Nicotra C, Pintaudi A, Paganini A, Pandolfo L, DeLeo G, Di Bella M. 1991. Retinyl ester hydrolase in retinal pigment epithelium. Arch Biochem Biophys 228:572–577.

Hamel C, Tsilou E, Pfeffer B, Hooks J, Detrick B, Redmond TM. 1993a. Molecular cloning and expression of RPE65, a novel retinal pigment epithelium-specific microsomal protein that is post-translationally regulated in vitro. J Biol Chem 268:15751–15757.

Hamel C, Tsilou E, Harris E, Pfeffer B, Hooks J, Detrick B, Redmond TM. 1993b. A developmentally regulated microsomal protein specific for the pigment epithelium of the vertebrate retina. J Neurosci Res 34:414–425.

Heller J. 1975. Interactions of plasma retinol-binding protein with its receptor. J Biol Chem 250:3613–3620.

Herbert J, Cavallero T, Martone R. 1991. The distribution of retinol-binding protein and its mRNA in the mammalian eye. Invest Ophthalmol Vis Sci 32:302–309.

Ho M-T, Massey J, Pownall H, Anderson R, Hollyfield J. 1989. Mechanism of vitamin A movement between rod outer segments, interphotoreceptor retinoid-binding protein and liposomes. J Biol Chem 264:928–935.

Hodam J, Hilaire P, Creek K. 1991. Comparison of the rate of uptake and biologic effects of retinol added to human keratinocytes either directly to the culture medium or bound to serum retinol-binding protein. J Invest Dermatol 97:298–304.

Hofmann K, Pulvermüller A, Buczylko J, Van Hooser P, Palczewski K. 1992. The role of arrestin and retinoids in the regulation pathway of rhodopsin. J Biol Chem 267:15701–15706.

Hubbard R, Colman A. 1959. Vitamin A content of the frog eye during light and dark adaptation. Science 130:997–998.

Hubbard R, Dowling J. 1962. Formation and utilization of 11-*cis* vitamin A by the eye tissues during light and dark adaptation. Nature 193:341–343.

Jancso N, Jancso H. 1936. Fluoreszenzmikroscopische biobachtungen der reversiblen vitamin A bildung in der netzhaut wahrend des sehatkes. Biochem Z 287:289–290.

Jiang M, Pandey S, Fong H. 1993. An opsin homologue in the retina and pigment epithelium. Invest Ophthalmol Vis Sci 34:3669–3678.

Jin J, Crouch R, Corson D, Katz B, MacNichol E, Cornwall M. 1993. Non-covalent occupancy of the chromophore binding pocket of opsin mediates bleaching and adaptation of retinal cones. Neuron 11:513–522.

Jones G, Crouch R, Wiggert B, Cornwall MC, Chader G. 1989. Retinoid requirements for recovery of sensitivity after visual-pigment bleaching in isolated photoreceptors. Proc Nat Acad Sci USA 86:9606–9610.

Katz M, Norberg M. 1992. Influence of dietary vitamin A on autofluorescence of leupeptin-induced inclusions in the retinal pigment epithelium. Exp Eye Res 54:239–246.

Krinsky N. 1958. The enzymatic esterification of vitamin A. J Biol Chem 232:881–894.

Lai Y-L, Wiggert B, Liu Y-P, Chader GJ. 1982. Interphotoreceptor retinol-binding proteins: possible transport vehicles between compartments of the retina. Nature 298:848–849.

Liou G, Bridges C, Fong S-L, Alvarez R, Gonzalez-Fernandez F. 1982. Vitamin A transport between retina and pigment epithelium—an interstitial protein carrying endogenous retinol (interstitial retinol-binding protein). Vision Res 22:1457–1467.

Liou G, Ma DP, Yang Y-W, Geng L, Zhu C, Baehr W. 1989. Human interstitial retinoid-binding protein. Gene structure and primary sequence. J Biol Chem 264:8200–8206.

Livrea M, Tesoriere L, Bongiorno A. 1991. All-*trans*-to 11-*cis*-retinol isomerization in nuclear membrane fraction from bovine retinal pigment epithelium. Exp Eye Res 52:451–459.

Mariani G, Ottonello S, Gozzoli F, Merli A. 1977. Identification of a membrane protein binding the retinol in retinal pigment epithelium. Nature 265:68–69.

Marlhens F, Bariel C, Griffoin J-M, Zrenner E, Amalric P, Eliaou C, Liu S-Y, Harris E, Redmond T, Arnaud B, Claustres M, Hamel C. 1997. Mutations in RPE65 cause Leber's congenital amaurosis. Nature Genetics 17:139–141.

Martone R, Schon E, Goodman D, Soprano D, Herbert J. 1988.

Retinol-binding protein is synthesized in the mammalian eye. Biochem Biophys Res Commun 157:1078–1084.

Mata N, Tsin A, Chambers J. 1992. Hydrolysis of 11-*cis* and all-*trans*-retinyl palmitate by retinal pigment epithelium microsomes. J Biol Chem 267:9794–9799.

Maw M, Kennedy B, Knight A, Bridges R, Roth K, Mani E, Mukkadan D, Crabb J, Denton M. 1997. Mutation of the gene encoding cellular retinaldehyde-protein in autosomal recessive retinitis pigmentosa. Nature Genetics 17:198–200.

McDonald P, Ong D. 1988. Evidence for a lecithin-retinol acyltransferase activity in the rat small intestine. J Bio Chem 263:12478–12482.

Meeks R, Zaharevitz D, Chen R. 1981. Membrane effects of retinoids: possible correlation with toxicity. Arch Biochem Biophys 207:141–147.

Melhus H, Båvik CO, Rask L, Peterson P, Eriksson U. 1995. Epitope mapping of a monoclonal antibody that blocks the binding of retinol-binding protein to its receptor. Biochem Biophys Res Commun 210:105–112.

Milam A, deLeeuw A, Gaur V, Saari J. 1990. Immunolocalization of cellular retinoic acid-binding protein to Müller cells and/or a subpopulation of GABA-positive amacrine cells in retinas of different species. J Comp Neurol 296:123–129.

Noy N, Xu Z-J. 1990. Interactions of retinol with binding proteins: implications for the mechanism of uptake by cells. Biochemistry 29:3878–3883.

Okajima T-I, Pepperberg D, Ripps H, Wiggert B, Chader G. 1989. Interphotoreceptor retinoid-binding protein: role in delivery of retinol to the pigment epithelium. Exp Eye Res 49:629–644.

Okajima T-I, Pepperberg D, Ripps H, Wiggert B, Chader G. 1990. Interphotoreceptor retinoid-binding proteins promotes rhodopsin regeneration in toad photoreceptors. Proc Nat Acad Sci USA 87:6907–6911.

Okajima T-I, Wiggert B, Chader G, Pepperberg D. 1994. Retinoid processing in retinal pigment epithelium of toad. J Biol Chem 269:21983–21989.

Ong D, Davis J, O'Day W, Bok D. 1994. Synthesis and secretion of retinol-binding protein and transthyretin by cultured retinal pigment epithelium. Biochemistry 33:1835–1842.

Ottonello S, Petrucci S, Maraini G. 1987. Vitamin A uptake from retinol-binding protein in a cell-free system from pigment epithelial cells. J Biol Chem 262:3975–3981.

Palczewski K, Jager S, Buczylko J, Crouch R, Bredberg L, Hofmann KP, Asson-Batres M, Saari J. 1994. Rod outer segment retinol dehydrogenase: substrate specificity and role in phototransduction. Biochemistry 33:13741–13750.

Pepperberg D, Okajima T-I, Wiggert B, Ripps H, Crouch R, Chader G. 1993. Interphotoreceptor retinoid-binding protein: molecular biology and physiological role in the visual cycle of rhodopsin. Mol Neurobiol 7:61–84.

Putilina T, Sittenfeld D, Chader G, Wiggert B. 1993. Study of a fatty acid-binding site of interphotoreceptor retinoid-binding protein using fluorescent fatty acids. Biochemistry 32:3793–3803.

Rando R. 1991. Membrane phospholipids as an energy source in the operation of the visual cycle. Biochemistry 30:595–602.

Rando R. 1992. Molecular mechanism in visual pigment regeneration. Photochem Photobiol 56:1145–1156.

Rando R, Bangerter F. 1982. The rapid intermembraneous transfer of retinoids. Biochem Biophys Res Commun 104:430–436.

Rando R, Bernstein P, Barry R. 1991. New insights into the visual cycle. In: Osborne N, Chader G, eds, Progress in Retinal Research. Oxford: Pergamon Press, 161–178.

Reszka K, Eldred G, Wang R-H, Chignell C, Dillon J. 1995. The pho-

tochemistry of human retinal lipofuscin as studied by ERP. Photochem Photobiol 62:1005–1008.

Robison W, Kuwabara T, Bieri J. 1980. Deficiencies of vitamin E and A in the rat: retinal damage and lipofiscin accumulation. Invest Ophthalmol Vis Sci 19:1030–1037.

Saari J. 1989. Enzymes and proteins of the visual cycle. In: Osborn NN, Chader GJ, eds, Progress in Retinal Research. Oxford: Pergamon Press, 363–381.

Saari J. 1994. Retinoids in photosensitive systems. In: Sporn M, Roberts A, Goodman D, eds, The Retinoids. New York: Raven Press, 351–385.

Saari J, Bredberg L. 1988. CoA- and non-CoA-dependent retinol esterification in retinal pigment epithelium. J Biol Chem 263:8084–8090.

Saari J, Bredberg L. 1989. Lecithin: retinol acetyltransferase in retinal pigment epithelium. J Biol Chem 264:8636–8640.

Saari J, Futterman S. 1976. Separable binding proteins for retinoic acid and retinol in bovine retina. Biochim Biophys Acta 444:789–793.

Saari J, Bredberg L, Garwin G. 1982. Identification of the endogenous retinoids associated with three retinoid-binding proteins from bovine retina. Vision Res 24:1595–1603.

Saari J, Bunt-Milan A, Bredberg D, Garwin G. 1984. Properties and immunocytochemical localization of three retinoid-binding proteins from bovine retina. Vision Res 24:11595–11603.

Saari J, Teller D, Crabb J, Bredberg L. 1985. Properties of an interphotoreceptor retinoid-binding protein from bovine retina. J Biol Chem 260:195–201.

Saari J, Bredberg L, Farrell D. 1993. Retinol esterification in bovine pigment epithelium: reversibility of lecithin:retinol acyltransferase. Biochem J 291:697–700.

Saari J, Bredberg L, Noy N. 1994. Control of substrate flow at a branch point in the visual cycle. Biochemistry 33:3106–3112.

Saari J, Huang J, Possin D, Fariss R, Charurat M, Busby D, Milam A. 1996. CRALBP is present in glia of optic nerve and brain. Invest Ophthalmol Vis Sci 37:S1042.

Sakai N, Decatur J. Nakanishi K, Eldred G. Ocular age pigment "A2-E": an unprecedented pyridinium bisretinoid. J Am Chem Soc 118:1559–1560.

Shen D, Jiang M, Hao W, Tao L, Salazar M, Fong H. 1994. A human opsin-related gene that encodes a retinaldehyde-binding protein. Biochemistry 33:13117–13125.

Shi Y-Q, Hubacek I, Rando RR. 1993. Kinetic mechanism of lecithin retinol acyl transferase. Biochemistry 32:1257–1263.

Simon A, Hellman U, Wernstedt C, Eriksson U. 1995. The retinal pigment epithelial-specific 11-*cis*-retinol dehydrogenase belongs to the family of short chain alcohol dehydrogenases. J Biol Chem 270:1107–1112.

Smith S, Duncan T, Kutty G, Kutty R, Wiggert B. 1994. Increase in retinyl palmitate concentration in eyes and livers and the concentration of interphotoreceptor retinoid-binding protein in eyes of vitiligo mutant mice. Biochem J 300:63–68.

Stubbs G, Saari J, Futterman S. 1979. 11-*cis*- retinal-binding protein from bovine retina. J Biol Chem 254:8529–8533.

Suzuki Y, Ishiguru S, Tamai M. 1993. Identification and immunohistochemistry of retinol dehydrogenase from bovine pigment epithelium. Biochim Biophys Acta 1163:201–208.

Szuts E, Harosi F. 1991. Solubility of retinoids in water. Arch Biochem Biophys 287:297–304.

Timmers A, van Groningen-Luyben D, DeGrip W. 1991. Uptake and isomerization of all-*trans*-retinol by isolated bovine retinal pigment epithelial cells: further clues to the visual cycle. Exp Eye Res 52:129–138.

Trehan A, Cañada F, Rando RR. 1990. Inhibitors of retinyl ester formation also prevent the biosynthesis of 11-*cis*-retinol. Biochemistry 29:309–312.

Van Jaarsfeld P, Edelhoch H, Goodman D, Robbins J. 1973. The interaction of human plasma retinol-binding protein with prealbumin. J Biol Chem 248:4698–4704.

van Veen T, Katial A, Shinohara T, Barrett D, Wiggert B, Chader G, Nickerson J. 1986. Retinal photoreceptor neurons and pinealocytes accumulate mRNA for interphotoreceptor retinoid-binding protein (IRBP). FEBS Lett. 208:133–137.

Wald G. 1934. Carotenoids and the vitamin A cycle in vision. Nature 134:65–75.

Wald G. 1935–6. Carotenoids and the visual cycle. J Gen Physiol 19:351–371.

Wiggert B, Chader GJ. 1975. A receptor for retinol in the developing retina and pigment epithelium. Exp Eye Res 21:143–149.

Wiggert B, Bergsma D, Chader G. 1976. Retinol receptors of the retina and pigment epithelium: further characterization and species variation. Exp Eye Res 22:411–419.

Wiggert B, Bergsma D, Lewis M, Chader G. 1977. Vitamin A receptors: retinol binding in neural retina and pigment epithelium. J Neurochem 29:947–953.

Wiggert B, Bergsma D, Helmsen D, Chader G. 1978. Vitamin A receptors: retinoic acid binding in ocular tissues. Biochem J 169:87–94.

Wiggert B, Derr J, Fitzpatrick M, Chader G. 1979. Vitamin A receptors of the retina: differential binding in light and dark. Biochim Biophys Acta 582:115–121.

Young RW. 1967. The renewal of photoreceptor outer segments. J Cell Biol 33:61–72.

Zimmerman W, Yost M, Daemen F. 1974. Dynamics and function of vitamin A compounds in rat retina after a small bleach of rhodopsin. Nature 250:66.

Zimmerman W, Lion F, Daemen F, Bonting S. 1975. Biochemical aspects of the visual process. XXX. Distribution of steriospecific retinol dehydrogenase activities in subcellular fractions of bovine retina and pigment epithelium. Exp Eye Res 21:325–332.

8. Role of the retinal pigment epithelium in photoreceptor membrane turnover

JOSEPH C. BESHARSE AND DENNIS M. DEFOE

The retinal pigment epithelium (RPE) plays a crucial role in turnover of the photosensitive membrane of both rod and cone photoreceptors. There are two major aspects of this role. First, pigment epithelial cells phagocytize and degrade protein and lipid components of the shed photoreceptor discs. Second, during degradation of disc macromolecules, some of the building blocks are recycled to photoreceptors for use in the synthesis and assembly of new discs. Although foreshadowed in early studies of the ultrastructure of pigment epithelium (Bairati and Orzalesi, 1963), these findings emerged from early work defining both the mechanism and the quantitative aspects of photoreceptor outer segment turnover (Droz, 1963; Young, 1967; 1971a; Young and Droz, 1968; Young and Bok, 1969) . They are of major significance in understanding RPE function because photosensitive membrane turnover is prodigious in magnitude and thus a major factor in pigment epithelium metabolism. It is now recognized that lipofuscin in RPE is derived from photosensitive membrane and that age-related accumulation of lipofuscin reflects the turnover of photosensitive membrane over the lifetime of the cell. In addition, disruption of photosensitive membrane turnover can lead to disruption in the balance between photosensitive membrane assembly with the consequence of impaired photoreceptor function and blindness. For example, a mutation impairing phagocytosis in the RCS rat RPE leads ultimately to photoreceptor degeneration (see Chapter 13). This chapter describes the role of RPE in photosensitive disc turnover with particular emphasis on cellular mechanisms and regulation of disc shedding. Related work on the role of the RPE cytoskeleton in phagocytosis and on lysosomes and lipofuscin accumulation is covered in Chapters 3 and 33.

EARLY EVIDENCE OF PHOTOSENSITIVE MEMBRANE TURNOVER

Early electron microscopic investigation of pigment epithelium (Porter and Yamada, 1960) illustrated an abundance of lamellar membranes in RPE that were called *myeloid bodies*. These pleiomorphic structures were clearly identified as an elaboration of smooth endoplasmic reticulum (Porter and Yamada, 1960—see Fig. 8-1). It is now recognized that such myeloid bodies take on a variety of structural forms and that they are best studied in RPE of lower vertebrates (Nguyen-Legros, 1978). Initially, the term was used to describe a variety of membranous structures. However, myeloid bodies comparable to those seen in frog were not observed in mouse or human RPE (Cohen, 1960; 1961). In their now classic study on vitamin A deficiency and retinal ultrastructure, Dowling and Gibbons (1961) recognized that structures called "myeloid bodies" in rat were actually inclusion bodies surrounded by a membrane; they were not continuous with smooth endoplasmic reticulum as in frog and other lower vertebrates. Insight into the origin of the inclusion bodies came from studies of human RPE (Bairati and Orzalesi, 1963) in which it was proposed that membrane-bound lamellar bodies were derived from ingested fragments of adjacent photoreceptors. Bairati and Orzalesi (1963) correctly predicted (1) that photoreceptor discs are detached, phagocytized, and degraded in RPE and (2) that detachment of discs would require a compensatory process of disc renewal.

Bairati and Orzalesi had at their disposal contemporaneous autoradiographic data (Droz, 1963) showing that the protein component of rod outer segments was continuously renewed. This data indicated that new proteins were synthesized in the inner segment and then incorporated into the outer segment. Other studies of the ultrastructure of photoreceptors indicated that they might continue to assemble new discs at their base after differentiation was completed (Cohen, 1963; Nilsson, 1964). Furthermore, Feeney and colleagues (1965) provided additional structural evidence that the so-called myeloid bodies in human RPE were actually detached discs engulfed by the pigment epithelial cell. Today we reserve the term *myeloid body* for those lamellar organelles in RPE that are derived from and associated with smooth endoplasmic reticulum (Fig. 8-1A) and refer to inclusion bodies derived from phagocytosis of outer segment membranes as *phagosomes* (Fig. 8-1B).

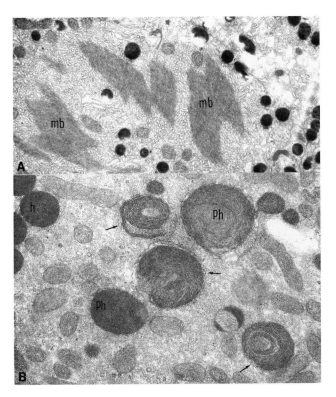

FIGURE 8-1. Electron micrographs illustrating myeloid bodies and phagosomes in RPE. (A) Myeloid bodies (mb) in the RPE of the desert night lizard, *Xantusia vigilis* (×22,790). These organelles are pleiomorphic and represent differentiated portions of the smooth endoplasmic reticulum. (B) Phagosomes (ph) derived from rod outer segments in various stages of degradation within the RPE of the rhesus monkey (×22,790). Phagosomes contain discs that are surrounded by a limiting membrane *(arrows)* derived from the RPE plasma membrane during internalization. Those on the left are highly compacted. As discs are degraded phagosomes take on a more granular appearance *(center)*. (Reproduced from K. M. Zinn and M. F. Marmor (eds), *The Retinal Pigment Epithelium,* with permission of Harvard University Press. Original micrographs courtesy of Dr. Dean Bok of the Jules Stein Eye Institute, Los Angeles, California.)

THE CONCEPT OF OUTER SEGMENT MEMBRANE RENEWAL

The now classic studies of Young (1967), Young and Droz (1968), and Young and Bok (1969) thoroughly established the concept of renewal of rod outer segments. A sequence of events was established in which radioactive protein is initially synthesized in the inner segment, transported to the outer segment and incorporated into new discs formed at the base of the outer segment in association with the connecting cilium (Fig. 8-2). Radioactive protein was concentrated into forming discs, resulting in a band of radioactivity that was displaced distally, eventually disappearing from the distal tip of the outer segment. The vital role of RPE in phagocyto-

sis of rod discs was directly demonstrated in autoradiographic experiments in which tissue was prepared after radioactive "reaction bands" had arrived at the outer segment distal tip (Young and Bok, 1969). In such preparations radioactive phagosomes were observed in RPE, directly demonstrating their origin from outer segment distal tips (Fig. 8-3). Furthermore, gradual transformation of the morphology and disappearance of radioactive phagosomes demonstrated that they were degraded within RPE. The "reaction band" in these experiments reflected the fact that radioactivity was delivered essentially as a pulse and that newly synthesized, nonradioactive discs formed to displace the radioactive discs distally. Because the radioactivity within the band remained relatively constant throughout its sojourn in the outer segment (Hall et al., 1969) it was recognized that the disc protein turned over through the process of disc shedding. These classic studies as well as subsequent work in a variety of species have established that turnover of rod discs is typical among vertebrates and has provided insight into interspecies variability in the magnitude of the process (Table 8-1).

Cone photoreceptors renew their disc membranes through a process similar to that in rods. However, the early finding in autoradiographic experiments, that radioactivity becomes diffusely distributed in cones and that distinct "reaction bands" are not readily seen, led to the hypothesis that cones differed from rods in that they cease to assemble new discs after they differentiate (Young, 1971b; 1971c). However, this hypothesis was inconsistent with subsequent structural studies that indicated cone disc shedding in human retina (Hogan et al., 1974) and demonstrated cone disc shedding (Fig. 8-4) in the cone-dominated retinas of diurnal squirrels (Anderson and Fisher, 1975; 1976; Anderson et al., 1978). In addition, "reaction bands" were found to be lacking in developing chicken and salamander cones during the time that the outer segment was still growing (Ditto, 1975). Finally, autoradiographic studies at early time points after incorporation of radioactive fucose showed transient reaction bands at the base of cone outer segments in diurnal squirrels indicative of basal disc assembly in cones (Anderson et al., 1986).

The general lack or transient nature of "reaction bands" at the base of cone outer segments distinguishes them from rods, but there is still controversy about the meaning of this finding. Cone discs are continuous with the outer segment plasma membrane and with each other. Therefore, it has been widely proposed that radio-labeled membrane proteins would be free to diffuse laterally through cone outer segment membranes, leading to a global distribution of radioactivity (Poo and Cone, 1974; Liebman and Entine, 1974). However, the edge

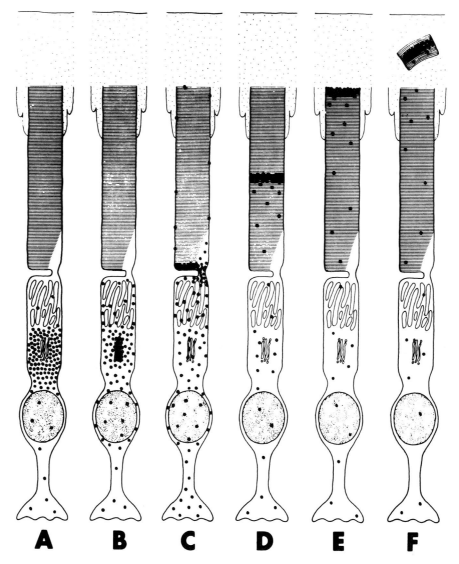

FIGURE 8-2. Diagram illustrating rod outer segment membrane renewal based on the autoradiographic studies of Young (1967) and Young and Bok (1969). (A–C) Radioactive protein *(black dots)* is synthesized in the inner segment and transported to the outer segment where it is incorporated into forming discs. (D–E) Discs containing a band of radiolabeled protein are transported distally to the distal tip of the outer segment. (F) Distal discs are shed and phagocytized by the RPE. (From Young, 1976, with permission of the Association for Research in Vision and Ophthalmology.)

region of both rod and cone discs is a distinct membrane domain and potential barrier to free lateral diffusion (Fetter and Corless, 1987). In addition, disc assembly mechanisms unique to cones may exist. Recent models of cone disc assembly designed to account for their conical shape have proposed either basal disc assembly with recycling of distal disc membranes into forming discs (Corless et al., 1989) or formation of new discs throughout the length of the cone outer segment (Eckmiller, 1987; 1993). Although it is currently difficult to choose between these models, either would be expected to result in a more random distribution of recently synthesized disc components within the cone outer segment.

THE MAGNITUDE OF DISC TURNOVER IS PRODIGIOUS

Since photoreceptors maintain relatively constant outer segment length in normal mature retinas and are constantly renewing their outer segment membranes, it follows that disposal of disc membranes through RPE

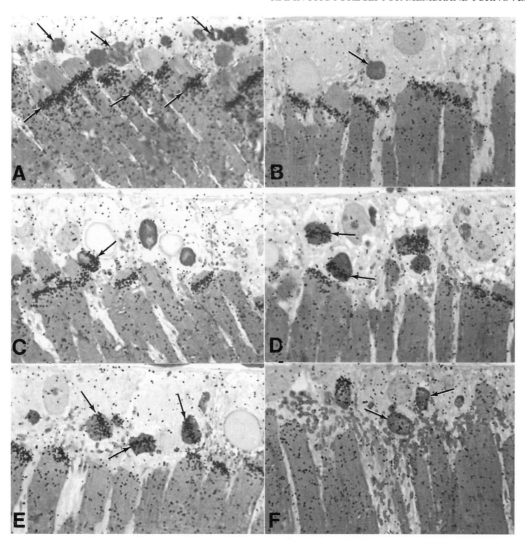

FIGURE 8-3. Light microscopic autoradiograms illustrating the origin of phagosomes through disc shedding in the frog retina. Frogs were injected with a mixture of ^{3}H-leucine and ^{3}H-phenylalanine and sacrificed at times at which the radioactive "reaction bands" were near the outer segment distal tip (47 to 68 days). (A, B) Initially radioactive discs are found in the outer segment distal tip and phagosomes in RPE are not radioactive. (C–E) Disc shedding results in production of phagosomes containing "reaction bands." (F) Eventually radioactive bands are lost from the outer segment distal tips. (Reproduced from K. M. Zinn and M. F. Marmor (eds), *The Retinal Pigment Epithelium,* with permission of Harvard University Press. Original micrograph courtesy of Dr. Dean Bok of the Jules Stein Eye Institute, Los Angeles, California.)

phagocytosis and degradation is a major preoccupation of RPE cells. The rate of disc assembly has been measured in several species and ranges from approximately 36 to 100 discs per day (Table 8-1). For example, each principal rod of adult *Xenopus laevis* assembles about 6004 μm^2 of membrane containing some 1.2×10^8 opsins per day. The phagocytic load per RPE cell is determined by the number of rod cells serviced by each RPE cell. For amphibian species this number is small and the estimate of photosensitive membrane internalized per cell is relatively low. In contrast, for the large binucleate RPE cells of rats this number is large and leads to the estimate that as many as 30,000 discs containing approximately 3.8×10^9 opsin molecules are phagocytized each day (Table 8-1; Bok and Young, 1979). In the case of rhesus monkey the number of rods per RPE cell varies according to retinal location. In the periphery it has been estimated that 4000 discs per RPE cell are degraded daily (Young, 1971a). Finally, in cold blooded amphibians, renewal rate is strongly dependent on temperature with a Q_{10} (rise in rate for each 10°C rise in temperature) exceeding 3.0 (Hollyfield et al.,

TABLE 8-1. *Quantitative aspects of rod disc assembly and disc phagocytosis by RPE on a daily basis*

Species	Photoreceptor disc assembly				Phagocytosis of discs by RPE			
	Discs/ day	Disc diameter (μm)	Disc area/ day[1] (μm sq)	# of opsins/ day	Rods/ RPE Cell[2]	Discs/ RPE Cell	Area/ RPE Cell	Opsins/ RPE Cell
Rhesus monkey[3] periphery	90	1.7	409	8.17×10^6	45	4050	18385	3.68×10^8
rat[4]	100	2.0	628	1.26×10^7	300	30000	188496	3.77×10^9
Rana pipiens[5] adult, 22.5° C.	36	7.0	2771	5.54×10^7	5	180	13854	2.77×10^8
Rana pipiens[6] tadpole, 23° C.	60	7.0	4618	9.24×10^7	5	300	23091	4.62×10^8
Xenopus laevis[7] adult, 22° C.	78	7.0	6004	1.20×10^8	5	390	30018	6.00×10^8
Xenopus laevis[8] tadpole, 28° C.	100	7.0	7697	1.54×10^8	5	500	38485	7.70×10^8

Estimates derived from renewal data in Bok and Young (1979), Young (1971c), Hollyfield, et al. (1977), Besharse, et al. (1977), and Kinney and Fisher (1978).

[1] Based on the assumption of 20,000 opsins per sq μm of disc membrane.
[2] Based on estimates by Bok and Young (1979).
[3] Data from Young (1971c) and Bok and Young (1979).
[4] and [5] Data from Bok and Young (1979).
[6] Data from Hollyfield, et al. (1977).
[7] Data from Kinney and Fisher (1978).
[8] Data from Besharse, et al. (1977).

1977). Thus, at higher temperatures the phagocytic load for each RPE cell increases dramatically. Although the variation in these estimates is broad and highly species dependent, such estimates indicate that phagocytosis and phagosome degradation is a major daily activity of RPE cells.

MECHANISM OF DISC DETACHMENT AND PHAGOCYTOSIS IN SITU

A central question related to disc shedding is the extent to which disc detachment and phagocytosis represent separate and distinct events. Most investigators have favored the view that disc detachment and phagocytosis are separate processes. Young (1971b), using rhesus monkey, observed that discs were often curled toward RPE or were separated from adjacent discs by enfoldings of the outer segment plasma membrane (Fig. 8-5). Similar observations including the finding of distal disc vesiculation have been made in numerous ultrastructural studies in other species for both rods and cones (Anderson and Fisher, 1976; Steinberg et al., 1977; Anderson et al., 1978; Besharse, 1982; Matsumoto et al., 1987; Currie et al., 1978). However, this interpretation

is made ambiguous by the lack of fully formed, incipient phagosomes in the interphotoreceptor space prior to phagocytosis and the frequent observation of RPE processes intruding into distal regions of the outer segment prior to complete disc detachment. Furthermore, disc detachment fails to occur in retinal regions separated from RPE even when adjacent "attached" photoreceptors undergo normal disc shedding (Williams and Fisher, 1987). These findings suggest that the RPE is required for normal disc detachment.

A more active role of RPE in disc detachment was suggested by Spitznas and Hogan (1970) who interpreted their electron microscopic images to mean that distal disc membranes were actively removed from the photoreceptor by apical processes of the RPE which intruded into the outer segment. Partial support for this idea has come from analysis of disc detachment in *Xenopus* and *Rana* eye cups (Besharse et al., 1986; Matsumoto et al., 1987), in which large pseudopodia devoid of membranous organelles and enriched in a cross-linked array of actin filaments intrude around and into the outer segment (Fig. 8-6). It has been suggested that the typical ultrastructural images of disc shedding would be expected if the initiation of disc detachment in photoreceptors were followed by a rapid phagocytic response by the

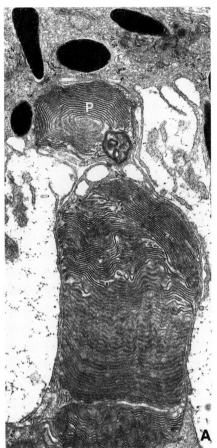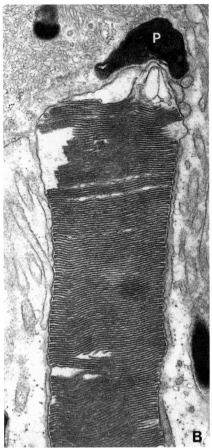

FIGURE 8-4. Cone disc shedding in squirrel retinas. (A) Cone outer segment with detaching disc packet (p) in the retina of the Western gray squirrel. (B) Cone outer segment and cone phagosome (p) in the retina of the California ground squirrel. Note that the phagosome is more electron dense and compressed than the adjacent outer segment. (From Anderson et al., 1978, with permission of the Association for Research in Vision and Ophthalmology.)

RPE (Steinberg et al., 1977). However, an alternative view equally consistent with the data is that RPE plays an active role in both initiation and completion of disc detachment.

The view that disc detachment may be initiated and/or assisted by RPE does not mean that the photoreceptor is completely passive. There is some evidence for an active process localized in distal domains of the rod cell. Generally, disc detachment results in loss of discs with retention of membrane continuity and it has been proposed that this is accomplished through fusion of disc and plasma membrane. This model was proposed by Matsumoto and Besharse (1985) to account for light-modulated labeling of distal rod discs using the water-soluble fluorescent dye Lucifer Yellow (Fig. 8-7). When isolated eye cups with intact RPE are incubated under conditions conducive for disc shedding and the retina isolated and incubated with Lucifer Yellow, discrete fluorescent bands form in distal regions of the rod cell corresponding to regions of expected disc detachment (Fig. 8-7). These bands reflect sequestration of the dye into a compartment associated with discs. The idea that this uptake is associated with membrane fusion events was strengthened by subsequent studies showing a similar distal banding pattern in rod outer segments incubated with fluorescent lipid probes that partition initially into the outer segment plasma membrane (Besharse and Hageman, 1990—see Figs. 8-7C and 8-7D). Distal tip labeling was also shown to be characteristic of both amphibian and mammalian rod photoreceptors. EM evaluation of distal domains indicates that discs break down locally to form small vesicles and micelles.

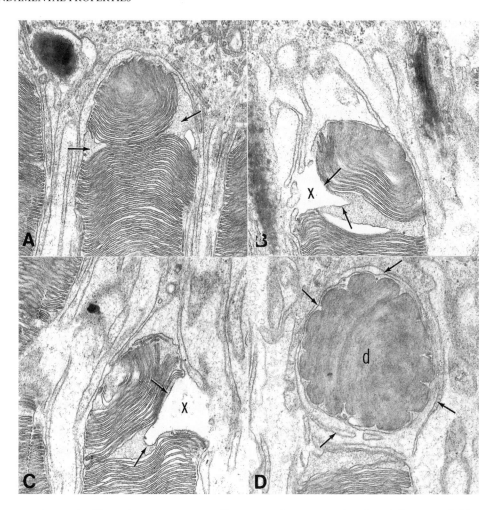

FIGURE 8-5. Electron micrographs illustrating outer segment disc shedding in the rhesus monkey. (A–C) illustrate curled discs partially separated from the outer segment and the appearance of granular cytoplasm within the ROS at the site of detachment. Arrows indicate site of apparent detachment and (X) indicates the extracellular space. (D) Completely detached packet of discs with plasma membrane intact *(upper arrows)* and partially surrounded by processes from the RPE *(lower arrows)*. Magnification: ×32,570. (Reproduced from K. M. Zinn and M. F. Marmor (eds), *The Retinal Pigment Epithelium,* with permission of Harvard University Press. Original micrograph courtesy of Dr. Dean Bok of the Jules Stein Eye Institute, Los Angeles, California.)

These experiments suggest that disc shedding is initiated through a process involving interaction of RPE and outer segment distal tip (Fig. 8-8). Subsequently, membrane fusion events continue within the outer segment separated from RPE but disc detachment is not completed. These events occurring at the distal tip of the outer segment may identify the location of Ca^{2+}-dependent membrane fusion studied biochemically in isolated outer segments (Boesze-Battaglia et al., 1992).

A further ultrastructural feature of distal photoreceptor domains in mammalian photoreceptors is the distal "cap" (Hageman and Besharse, 1990). "Caps" are part of the outer segment and are frequently seen to be contiguous with the outer segment region that contains the connecting cilium (Fig. 8-9). They lack discs or other membranes and contain a granular, homogenous cytoplasm. The cap extends between the distal discs and the adjacent RPE. Cytoplasmic caps on rod photoreceptors are visible in published EM images from prior ultrastructural investigations (see for example Young, 1971c), but their temporal relationship to disc shedding was overlooked. One reason may be that they are dynamic structures that form principally during the night. For example, quantitative analysis using hamsters in constant darkness indicates that 95% of the rod cells have distal caps at subjective midnight, and that this number is reduced to 15% during the middle of expected daytime. The circadian rhythm in distal caps peaks

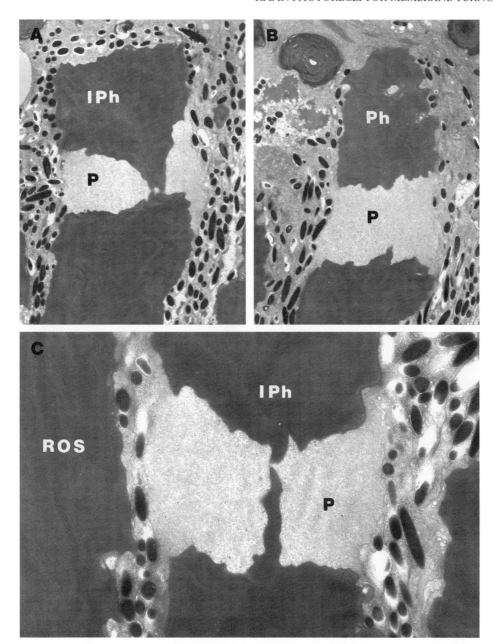

FIGURE 8-6. Electron micrographs illustrating stages of rod disc shedding in frog retina captured at early times after light onset (15 minutes). (A) and (B) illustrate an incipient (IPh) and complete (Ph) phagosome while (C) illustrates an incipient phagosome at higher magnification. In each case pseudopodia (P) from the RPE intrude into the site of disc detachment. The cytoplasm of the pseudopods has a fine granular appearance with exclusion of other organelles characteristic of the RPE. Pseudopods form transiently and are distinct from villous processes that contain melanin granules. Magnifications: (A) and (B) ×6375; (C) ×12,750. (From Besharse et al., 1986, with permission of Alan R. Liss, Inc., New York.)

during nighttime (Hageman and Besharse, 1990), while the peak of disc shedding is near the time of expected light onset (LaVail, 1976). These findings suggest that cap formation is an active, photoreceptor-based process that prepares the distal rod outer segment for subsequent to disc detachment and phagocytosis.

OUTER SEGMENT LIPID TURNOVER AND RECYCLING OF DOCOSAHEXANOIC ACID

Our view of disc turnover in rod cells is based on the protein component, which exhibits little or no turnover until it is lost into the RPE through disc shedding at the

FIGURE 8-7. Fluorescent microscopic images showing specific staining of rod outer segment distal tips with the fluorescent dye, Lucifer Yellow CH (A and B) or the fluorescent lipid probe, 1,1′-dihexadecyloxacarbocyanine (DIOC$_{16}$) (C and D). (A) Fluorescent image of a piece of whole mounted retina from a constant light treated animal that had been isolated, incubated in medium containing Lucifer Yellow for 5 minutes. Fluorescent bands *(top)* are in the distal region of rod tips. Large arrowhead indicates an outer segment tip in which one of the bands is incomplete. (B) Same view as in (A) but with white light background illumination to reveal the outer segments and fluorescent tips. (C) and (D) illustrate outer segments shaken from freshly isolated retinas onto glass slides and incubated for 5 minutes with DIOC$_{16}$. Proximal ends of outer segments are indicated by arrowheads. In (C) part of the inner segment is present. In (D) proximal disc labeling *(arrowhead)* as well as distal disc labeling is seen. Approximate magnification: (A) and (B) ×775; (C) and (D) ×700.

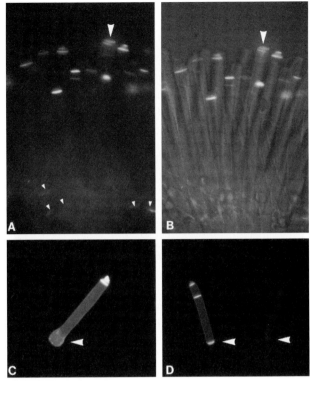

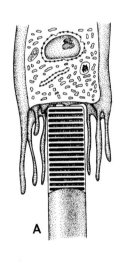
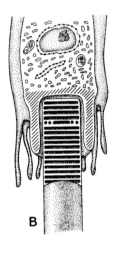
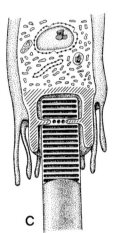

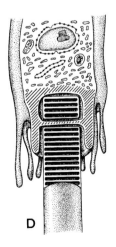
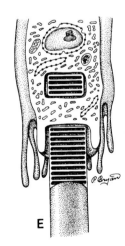

FIGURE 8-8. Diagram illustrating mechanism of disc detachment and phagocytosis inferred from studies on amphibian retina. The basic model is similar to that described by Steinberg et al., 1977 based on mammalian retina. (A–D) The rod outer segment distal tip is ensheathed by pseudopodial processes of the RPE which disappear only after engulfment of the disc packet (E). Pseudopods *(cross-hatched area)* are transient in nature, distinct from villous processes of RPE, and enriched in actin containing filaments. Concurrent with pseudopod formation, an active process in the outer segment distal tip involving membrane fusion results in detachment of the disc packet (B–D). (From Matsumoto et al., 1987, with permission of the Royal Society.)

160

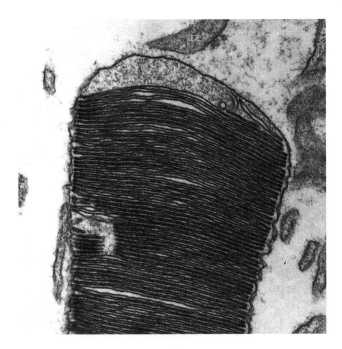

FIGURE 8-9. Electron microscopic image showing a distal cap on a rod photoreceptor in the rat retina. (Original electron micrograph provided by Gregory Hageman).

outer segment distal tip (Young and Bok, 1969; Hall et al., 1969). In contrast, turnover of most lipid components of discs appears to be an exponential process related to the random distribution of newly synthesized membrane lipids throughout the outer segment. Bibb and Young (1974a; 1974b) first showed that membrane lipid precursors are incorporated in the inner segment and transferred to the outer segment, where they quickly attain a random distribution. The lack of a "reaction band" at the outer segment base of rod outer segments indicates that mechanisms exist for exchange of membrane lipids throughout the outer segment. The subject of outer segment membrane lipid metabolism is complex and is beyond the scope of this chapter. Nonetheless, there are two aspects of photoreceptor lipid metabolism that have a direct bearing on our understanding of mechanisms of photoreceptor-RPE interaction. First, it appears that mechanisms other than disc shedding account for a significant component of disc phospholipid turnover. Second, docosahexanoic acid, which is highly enriched within phospholipids of photoreceptor discs, is at least in part removed from the outer segment through disc shedding and then recycled from RPE to photoreceptors for new phospholipid synthesis.

The random distribution of newly synthesized phospholipid throughout the outer segment first described by Bibb and Young (1974a; 1974b) has been observed in several subsequent studies using phospholipid precursors such as choline, glycerol, and inositol (Mercu-

rio and Holtzman, 1982; Matheke and Holtzman, 1984; Wetzel et al., 1993; Wetzel and Besharse, 1995). Using the model of disc turnover by shedding in rods, Anderson and colleagues (1980a) estimated the half-life of randomly distributed radioactive phospholipids based on the assumption that disc shedding was the exclusive mechanism for turnover. They then determined the actual half-lives of rod outer segment phosphatidylcholine, phosphatidylethanolamine, and phosphatidylinositol (Anderson et al., 1980a–1980c). The half-lives were different for the three phospholipids. In addition, all three were shorter than expected from the disc-shedding model. Subsequent work showed that even specific docosahexanoic-acid-containing species within a phospholipid class exhibited different turnover rates (Louie et al., 1988). These data indicate that phospholipid turnover proceeds at rates exceeding that expected if disc shedding were the sole mechanism for turnover, and that different phospholipids have different rates of turnover. This suggests phospholipids may be either transported back to the inner segment for degradation and/or degraded by outer segment lipases. The observation that outer segments contain high levels of diacylglycerol (Anderson et al., 1980d) and specific phospholipases (Zimmerman, 1984; Ghalayini and Anderson, 1984; 1992; Hayashi and Amakawa, 1985) indicates that local breakdown within the outer segment may be significant. Interestingly, breakdown products such as diacylglycerol are known to be membrane fusogenic agents. This leads directly to the idea that phospholipid turnover within the outer segment may be related to distal membrane changes that occur during disc detachment at the outer segment distal tip (see Fig. 8-8).

Although most radio-labeled lipid precursors are randomly distributed when incorporated into the outer segment, a different pattern is seen when tritiated docosahexanoic acid is used as a precursor for phospholipids. Docosahexanoic acid containing phospholipids appear to associate at least in part with newly formed discs and to retain that association throughout their sojourn through the outer segment (Gordon and Bazan, 1993; Gordon et al., 1992). Recent experiments have demonstrated the appearance of radiolabeled phagosomes within the RPE by autoradiography after incorporation of ^{3}H-docosahexanoic acid into outer segments (Gordon et al., 1992) and biochemical incorporation of docosahexanoic acid in RPE after disc shedding (Chen et al., 1992). In addition, docosahexaenoic acid appears to be conserved in photoreceptors by recycling from RPE back to photoreceptors (Gordon et al., 1992; Chen and Anderson, 1993). It is released from outer segment membranes and incorporated into a metabolically active pool of triglycerides, from which it can be hydrolyzed and released (Chen and Anderson, 1993). Do-

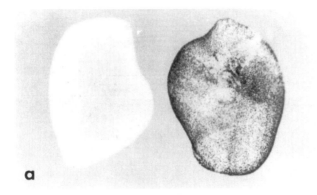

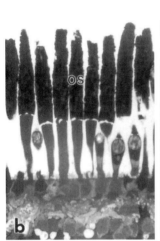
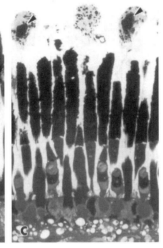

FIGURE 8-10. (A) Photomicrograph of two isolated *Xenopus laevis* retinas (photoreceptor side up) isolated from eyecups incubated for 1 hour in darkness in standard medium *(left)* or medium containing 12 mM L-glutamate. The one on the left separated cleanly from adjacent RPE, while the one on the right has adherent melanin pigment distributed over its surface. (B) and (C) are light micrographs from sections incubated, as in (A), in normal medium (B) or in medium containing 12 mM L-glutamate (C). (C) illustrates apical domains containing melanin pigment and phagocytized disc membranes that partitioned with photoreceptors in the presence of glutamate. These organelles lack nuclei and basal cytoplasmic organelles such as mitochondria. Magnifications: (a) ×24; (b) and (c) ×819. (From Figure 1 in Defoe et al., 1989, with permission of Academic Press, New York.)

cosahexanoic acid is highly enriched in photoreceptors and critical for outer segment function. Although the precise RPE mechanism for lipid recycling remains undefined, this process may be important for maintaining the high degree of enrichment of docosahexaenoic acid in outer segments.

RELATIONSHIP OF RETINAL ADHESIVENESS TO SHEDDING AND PHAGOCYTOSIS

Disc membrane phagocytosis has been most extensively studied using cultured RPE cells (Edwards and Sza-

mier, 1977; Chaitin and Hall, 1983; Hall and Abrams, 1987; Reid et al., 1992—see also Chapter 13). Such studies have generally been modeled after comparable work in macrophages and polymorphonuclear granulocytes in which phagocytosis can be broken down into the separate events of attachment, internalization, intracellular transport, and degradation (Greenberg and Silverstein, 1993). Generally, it is thought that receptor-ligand interaction leads to activation of the machinery for internalization. Similar concepts apply to RPE cells in culture and recent work has identified several putative RPE receptor candidates that mediate attachment and internalization (see below). However, phagocytosis of outer segment tips in the intact retina differs in one important respect from the constitutive uptake of particles by cultured epithelia or phagocytic leukocytes. In cultured cells, engulfment is initiated by particle binding to the phagocyte surface, whereas the photoreceptor distal tip remains in close apposition to the RPE surface during both quiescent and active periods of disc shedding and phagocytosis. Such considerations prompt the question of whether these two adhesive interactions, retinal attachment and phagocytosis, are mediated through the same or distinct receptor-ligand mechanisms (Besharse, 1982).

Evidence obtained using *Xenopus laevis* eyecup tissues in vitro is suggestive of a difference in these adhesive systems. Adherence of neural retinas to the RPE, which is normally relatively weak in *Xenopus* eyecups, is enhanced during L-aspartate- and L-glutamate-induced shedding (Matsumoto et al., 1987; Defoe et al., 1989). This can easily be monitored through measurement of increased partitioning of apical RPE domains containing melanin pigment with photoreceptors (Fig. 8-10) when retinas are "peeled" from RPE (Matsumoto et al., 1987; Defoe et al., 1989). The apical RPE domains that partition with photoreceptors have been shown (Matsumoto et al., 1987) to include pseudopodia, highly enriched in actin filaments (see Plate 8-I). It has also been found that cytochalasin D, a disrupter of actin filaments, blocks disc shedding and pseudopod formation (Besharse and Dunis, 1982; Matsumoto et al., 1987). These observations suggest that the increased adhesiveness observed during glutamate-induced disc shedding is due to the pseudopods adhering to distal tips of outer segments. However, glutamate-induced adhesive changes have been shown to take place when pseudopod extension and disc ingestion are blocked by cytochalasin D (Defoe et al., 1989), indicating that pseudopods *per se* may not be responsible for the adhesive changes. Thus, there may be qualitative or quantitative differences in the interaction of photoreceptors and epithelium during periods of active shedding, versus relatively quiescent periods.

Similarly, in cultured cell systems, there is evidence that ROS binding is not always sufficient to initiate phagocytic uptake. For example, while epithelial cultures from RCS rats are able to bind ROS as well as their normal counterparts, these same cells are unable to phagocytize ROS (Chaitin and Hall, 1983). This has been interpreted to indicate that cells from mutant animals are defective in a phagocytosis-specific signaling pathway. However, the data can also be accommodated by a hypothesis proposing that binding and internalization are two distinctive parts of the phagocytic process (McLaughlin et al., 1994).

Recently, these questions have also been addressed by studies using immunological reagents to block ROS phagocytosis. Gregory and Hall (1992) have obtained an antiserum that inhibits binding of ROS to the RPE and also significantly reduces the ingestion phase, lending support to a model of phagocytosis in which attachment and internalization can be viewed as two phases of a sequential process. Somewhat different results have been reported by McLaughlin and colleagues (1994), using antisera directed against an apical membrane-enriched fraction of RPE (Guo et al., 1991). While two of the reagents were effective in blocking both binding and ingestion of ROS, a third produced inhibitory effects only upon internalization. Based on these data, it has been suggested that binding and internalization may be subserved by different molecules (McLaughlin et al., 1994).

Recent investigations into the role of cell–cell adhesiveness in epithelial phagocytosis have begun to focus on specific surface receptors, particularly those which have been demonstrated to promote ingestion in phagocytic leukocytes. For example, it has been known for some time that monkey RPE cells, like macrophages, have receptors for the Fc portion of antibodies, as well as the C3 component of complement, and can phagocytize erythrocytes coated (opsonized) with both of these proteins (Elner et al., 1981). Immunoglobulins have been detected in the space between photoreceptors and epithelium (Hageman and Johnson, 1986). However, since antibody-coated ROS are bound and ingested to the same extent as unopsonized ROS (Mayerson and Hall, 1986; Laird and Molday, 1988), the significance of these receptors for outer segment phagocytosis is unclear.

A mannose recognition system, similar to that used by macrophages to ingest unopsonized bacteria and yeast particles (Sung et al., 1983; Ezekowitz et al., 1991) may be involved in ROS phagocytosis by RPE. Mannose receptors have been shown to be present on apical membranes and microvilli by immunoelectron microscopy (Boyle et al., 1991; Shepherd et al., 1991). Furthermore, these receptors participate in the uptake by the epithelium of both soluble and particulate mannose-containing ligands (Tarnowski et al., 1991; Boyle et al., 1991; Shepherd et al., 1991). However, the exclusive use of mannan-coated latex beads as target particles in these initial studies has led others to doubt the role that such a mannose recognition system might play in ROS phagocytosis (Hall and Abrams, 1991). Such concerns have subsequently been addressed by Boyle and colleagues (1991), who reported that phagocytosis of ROS can be inhibited by 80% in the presence of an antibody to the mannose receptor. Furthermore, when ROS themselves are preabsorbed with the purified mannose-receptor protein, there is a dramatic inhibition (93%) of ROS phagocytosis (Boyle et al., 1991). Nevertheless, unlike macrophage phagocytosis of yeast zymosan, which is inhibitable by soluble mannose-containing ligands, binding and uptake of ROS by the RPE is unaffected by high concentrations of mannose (Lentrichia et al., 1987; Hall and Abrams, 1991) or mannan (Philp et al., 1988; Hall and Abrams, 1991). Thus, definitive evidence for involvement of a mannose receptor must await identification of the specific ligand on the surface of ROS, as well as verification that such a system operates in the intact retina. In this regard, there is compelling evidence that rhodopsin, the major mannose-containing plasma membrane protein of outer segments, is not involved in binding or phagocytosis (Shirakawa et al., 1987; Laird and Molday, 1988; Philp et al., 1988).

Recently, Ryeom and colleagues (1996) have reported that CD36, a multifunctional cell surface receptor found in RPE, is capable of mediating the phagocytosis of isolated outer segments when expressed by exogenous cells. In macrophages, as well as a number of other cell types, CD36 has been shown to serve as a "scavenger receptor" for oxidized LDL (Endemann et al., 1993) and as a receptor mediating the internalization of oxidatively damaged red blood cells and apoptotic neutrophils (Sambrano et al., 1994; Ren et al., 1995). Bowes melanoma cells transfected with CD36 cDNA show increased binding of ^{125}I-ROS, and this binding is reduced by 61% when the cells are preincubated with monoclonal antibody to CD36. In phagocytosis assays, greater numbers of ROS/cell (more than 15-fold) were detected in transfected cells than nontransfected cells. Evidence obtained in other systems indicates that CD36 cooperates with an integrin, the vitronectin receptor ($\alpha_v\beta_3$), in macrophage phagocytosis of apoptotic neutrophils (Savill et al., 1990; 1992). Interestingly, expression of this receptor has been demonstrated in epithelial tissues from chick embryo eyes and adult primate retinas, where α_v subunits have been localized immunocytochemically to the apical RPE surface (Rizzolo et al., 1994; Anderson et al., 1995). While this integrin could potentially play a role in several adhesive phenomena within the retina, there is no data to indicate that these receptors promote disc phagocytosis.

Although the in vitro evidence supporting a role for the mannose receptor and CD36 is substantial, their precise role remains to be determined. Although expression of CD36 and mannose receptors by the RPE has been demonstrated immunocytochemically and by Western blotting, there is as yet no direct evidence for involvement of these proteins in ROS uptake by intact systems under conditions in which disc shedding is physiologically controlled. In addition, CD36 function in ROS phagocytosis has not been demonstrated in RPE cells. Furthermore, there is evidence that other as yet unidentified factors may be involved. For example, an antiserum known to block binding and phagocytosis of ROS (Gregory and Hall, 1992), has recently been used to affinity-purify membrane proteins as candidate receptors. Neither CD36 nor mannose receptors were among the purified proteins (Hall et al., 1996). These data suggest that factors in addition to CD36 and mannose receptors may play a role in ROS recognition and phagocytosis.

In all studies examining phagocytosis by cultured RPE cells, serum in the culture medium is required for significant ingestion of isolated ROS (Edwards and Flaherty, 1986; Mayerson and Hall, 1986), specifically when present at the RPE apical surface (Edwards, 1991). Experiments using red blood cells or outer segments pretreated with serum or antibodies make it unlikely that this effect is due to particle opsonization (Mayerson and Hall, 1986; Reid et al., 1992). Nevertheless, the necessity for serum stimulation remains unexplained, and contrasts with studies using frog RPE cultures for tissue reconstitution in vitro. In the latter experiments, reattachment of isolated neural retinas to epithelial monolayers was achieved with cultures previously maintained for 1–2 weeks in a serum-free defined medium (Defoe and Easterling, 1994). While shedding and phagocytosis, as well as retinal adhesiveness, were low under basal conditions, these processes could be greatly enhanced by L-glutamate treatment. Such data indicate that additional regulatory mechanisms are likely to be operating in intact retinal tissues, and that there may be significant differences in the behavior of intact versus isolated cell systems. They also point to the need for testing potential candidates for receptor-ligand interactions in phagocytosis in intact systems.

THE LIGHT-DARK CYCLE AND RHYTHMIC DISC SHEDDING

A major advance in our understanding of disc shedding was the finding by LaVail (1976) of a burst of rod disc shedding and phagocytosis in rats during a period immediately after light onset each day. This report led immediately to similar findings for rod disc shedding in amphibian retinas (Basinger et al., 1976; Hollyfield et al., 1976; Besharse et al., 1977) and to an explosive growth in literature describing the phenomenon of rhythmic disc shedding (reviewed in Besharse, 1982). It quickly became clear that rhythmic disc shedding involved interaction of the daily light/dark cycle and a circadian clock mechanism. For example, in rats (LaVail, 1976; 1980) and hamsters (Grace et al., 1996) the rod disc shedding rhythm persists for many days in constant darkness without substantial damping of amplitude. This indicates a primary role for a circadian oscillator (or clock) in control of the rhythm. Circadian clocks are timing systems that provide endogenous timing signals. In circadian systems light serves to synchronize the internal clock to the external cyclic environment. In contrast to the rat, rod disc shedding in the frog, Rana pipiens, was found to be driven by light onset each day (Basinger et al., 1976), while in the African clawed frog, Xenopus laevis, both light onset and a circadian clock were found to influence the disc shedding rhythm (Besharse et al., 1977; Besharse, 1982).

The concept of rhythmic disc shedding was extended to cones in goldfish, chicken, and lizard retinas with the novel twist that it occurred primarily after light offset (O'Day and Young, 1978; Young, 1977; 1978). However, unlike rods, which shed discs after light onset in all species examined to date, subsequent studies of the timing of the burst in cone disc shedding in mammalian retinas showed that it occurred primarily after light onset in the tree shrew (Immel and Fisher, 1985), while in tree squirrels cone disc shedding predominates in the middle of the dark period (Tabor et al., 1980). In addition, a detailed analysis of rhesus monkey (Anderson et al., 1980e) has provided clear evidence of both rod and cone disc shedding both after light onset and offset. Although rhythmic disc shedding appears to be the rule for both rod and cone photoreceptors, there is substantial variability among species in the shedding patterns observed. To date, the possible persistence of cone disc shedding in constant darkness has not been studied.

Constant light blocks rhythmic rod disc shedding and subsequent initiation of shedding requires exposure to darkness (Currie et al., 1978; Goldman et al., 1980). This has led to the concept that light initiates rod disc shedding in the morning but is subsequently inhibitory until after a subsequent "dark-priming" period. This period in darkness may require as little as 30 minutes in the frog (Currie et al., 1978). In rats constant light appears to block disc shedding without disruption of the underlying circadian mechanism (Goldman et al., 1980). Thus, two-hour periods of dark exposure followed by light are sufficient to reinitiate disc shedding but the magnitude of the response is optimal only if it occurs at the time of normal expected disc shedding in the circadian cycle. Although constant light blocks disc shedding, it does not block disc assembly (Besharse et al., 1977) which in *Xenopus laevis* continues at a maximal rate. Consequently, constant light treatment in amphibians leads to dramatic increases in outer segment length; when disc shedding is reinitiated by dark treatment followed by light, a larger than normal burst of disc shedding occurs (Currie et al., 1978; Besharse et al., 1980; Besharse et al., 1986). Perhaps related, at least in part, to these mechanisms is the finding that constant light eventually results in damage to photoreceptors in the rat (Organisciak and Winkler, 1994).

Quantitative analysis indicates that rhythmic disc shedding does not account for all of the disc shedding expected during the day. In a steady state in which average rod outer segment length remains relatively constant, the total number of discs removed from a photoreceptor should equal the number of new discs assembled. In his earliest analysis, LaVail (1976) indicated that the number and size of phagosomes after light onset were not sufficient to account for daily turnover expected from data on disc assembly and suggested that disc shedding might be occurring at other times of day. Similar observations were reported in pigmented mice (Besharse and Hollyfield, 1979), and Anderson and colleagues (1980) reported significant levels of nighttime rod disc shedding in rhesus monkeys. In a detailed analysis of disc assembly and disc shedding in relationship to temperature in the frog, *Rana pipiens*, Hollyfield and colleagues (1977) found that the number of discs in individual phagosomes were remarkably uniform in size, containing 130 to 140 discs. This would account for about 80% of the expected disc disposal (Table 8-2). They went on to show evidence for an additional mechanism of disc shedding involving small fragments

TABLE 8-2. *Quantitative aspects of light-evoked disc shedding in the frog* Rana pipiens

Measurement	23C	28C	33C
Mean number of rods shedding per day (%)	18	33	42
Mean number of days between shedding events per rod	5.6	3.0	2.4
Mean number of discs shed per phagosome	139.5	129.4	129.9
Mean number of discs added per day per rod	32.4	55.9	65.5
Mean number of discs added between successive shedding events	181.4	167.7	157.2

Data compiled from work on effects of temperature on both disc shedding and phagocytosis of discs (Hollyfield et al., 1977).

of the outer segment that occurred around the clock and suggested that this process might account for the remainder of the expected disc disposal. The general conclusion is that disc shedding may occur at any time during the light/dark cycle. Nonetheless, endogenous timing signals from a circadian oscillator and/or direct exposure to the light/dark cycle provides a mechanism for temporal regulation of disc turnover.

FACTORS REGULATING RHYTHMIC DISC SHEDDING ARE INTRINSIC TO THE EYE

Rhythmic rod disc shedding is controlled locally within the eye. For example, rhythmic disc shedding in the rat persists after removal of the pineal gland, the superior cervical ganglia, the hypophysis, and the thyroid/parathyroid glands (Tamai et al., 1978; LaVail and Ward, 1978). In addition, lesions of the suprachiasmatic nucleus abolish most circadian rhythms in the rat while leaving that of rod disc shedding intact (Terman et al., 1993). Furthermore, eye occlusion experiments (Fig. 8-11) indicate that circadian shedding in the rat (Tierstein et al., 1980) and light-evoked shedding in the frog (Hollyfield and Basinger, 1978) can be regulated independently in the two eyes. This, along with the finding that light-regulated disc shedding persists in both *Xenopus laevis* (Besharse et al., 1980; Besharse and Dunis, 1983; Flannery and Fisher, 1984) and *Rana pipiens* (Basinger and Hoffman, 1982; Besharse et al., 1986) eye cups in culture, indicates that disc shedding is controlled through mechanisms intrinsic to the eye.

Recently, it has been possible to localize a circadian clock mechanism controlling melatonin synthesis to photoreceptors (Besharse and Iuvone, 1983; Cahill and Besharse, 1993). Early evidence for this came from the in vitro demonstration of persistent oscillation of a melatonin synthetic enzyme, serotonin N-acetyltransferase, in *Xenopus laevis* eye cups kept for three days in culture (Besharse and Iuvone, 1983). Subsequently, measurement of circadian release of melatonin for up to five days from single eye cups maintained in flow-through culture showed that single eye cups have a circadian oscillator that persists in constant darkness and that the phase of the oscillation can be altered by exposure to brief treatments of light or dopamine (Cahill and Besharse, 1991). With development of a lesioning system that permitted analysis of living photoreceptor layers, either in association with RPE or in isolation, it was shown that melatonin is released from photoreceptors and that the clock and entrainment mechanism regulating its release is an intrinsic property of photoreceptors (Cahill and Besharse, 1992; 1993).

The identification of a photoreceptor circadian clock

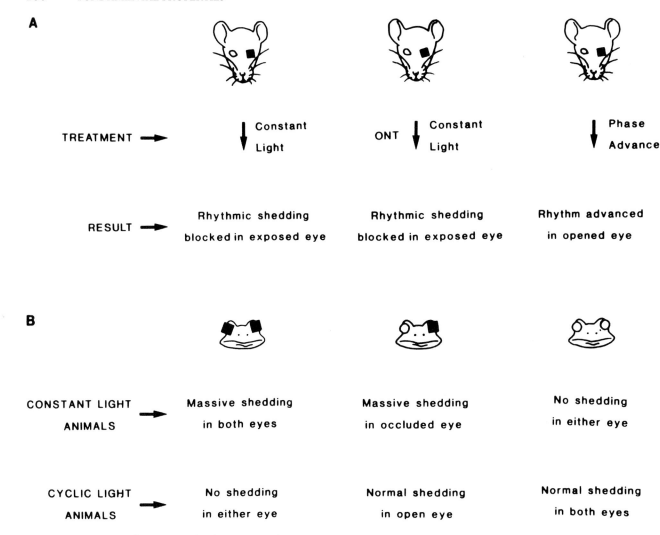

FIGURE 8-11. Diagram illustrating early observations indicating that factors controlling rhythmic disc shedding are intrinsic to the eye. (A) Eyepatch experiments in the rat (Tierstein et al., 1980) indicate that constant light blockade and phase shifting can occur in a single unpatched eye independently of the other patched eye; constant light effects are also seen after optic nerve transection (ONT). (B) Eyepatch experiments in *Rana pipiens* (Hollyfield and Basinger, 1978) indicate that in constant-light-treated animals disc shedding occurred only in eyes that were patched, indicating that a dark-dependent process necessary for disc shedding occurs monocularly. Shedding in cyclic light was blocked by the patches indicating monocular control of "light-triggered" disc shedding. (Modified from Besharse, 1982, with permission of Pergamon Press, New York.)

(Cahill and Besharse, 1993) suggests that this system may be responsible for circadian control of disc shedding and RPE phagocytosis known to occur in *Xenopus laevis* (Besharse et al., 1977; Flannery and Fisher, 1984). It seems likely that a similar circadian clock may be a general phenomenon in vertebrate photoreceptors. Iodopsin gene expression is rhythmic in dissociated cultures of chicken embryonic retina (Pierce et al., 1993) and melatonin is released rhythmically in hamster and rat retinas maintained in flow-through culture (Tosini and Menaker, 1996). The latter findings directly support earlier conclusions from in vivo experiments for intrinsic oscillators controlling retinal melatonin synthe-sis in Japanese quail (Underwood et al., 1990) and disc shedding in the rat (Tierstein et al., 1980; Remé et al., 1991; Terman et al., 1993). A point of potential interest is that, with the exception of experiments on rat (Tierstein et al., 1980), all such studies suggest that a light-entrainment pathway responsible for maintaining synchrony with the external light/dark cycle (see Cahill and Besharse, 1995) is also intrinsic to the eye. In the experiments on rat, however, it was reported that lesioning of the optic nerve permitted continuation of a disc-shedding rhythm that could not be reentrained to a different light cycle. Although this experiment needs to be replicated, it implies that interaction with a central mechanism is required for phase shifting the retinal oscillator.

RHYTHMIC REGULATION OF DISC SHEDDING BY MELATONIN AND DOPAMINE

Development of an eye cup culture system that supports light-evoked disc shedding (Besharse et al., 1980) has permitted pharmacological investigation of some of the factors involved in regulation. This work has lead to a model in which rhythmic physiology is regulated through neuromodulators such as melatonin and dopamine. Because of its relationship to circadian phenomena, melatonin was among the first agents studied (Besharse and Dunis, 1983; Pierce and Besharse, 1986). Melatonin and a related methoxyindole, 5 methoxy-tryptophol, activate light-evoked disc shedding when applied in darkness prior to light onset. In addition, using constant-light-treated eye cups that require darkness (i.e., dark priming) before disc shedding can be initiated, melatonin was found to mimic darkness by causing disc shedding. Because melatonin was most effective as a mimic for darkness and is normally synthesized by photoreceptors at night (Cahill and Besharse, 1992; 1993), it has been suggested that it or a related methoxyindole may be a primary signal regulating circadian phenomena including disc shedding (Besharse et al., 1988). Melatonin has been shown to inhibit retinal dopamine release (Dubocovich, 1983; Boatright et al., 1994), and dopamine is known to inhibit disc shedding (Pierce and Besharse, 1986; Besharse et al., 1988).

Dopamine and agonists selective for the D_2 family of dopamine receptors have no effect on light-evoked disc shedding. However, they block the dark-dependent process required for disc shedding (Pierce and Besharse, 1986; Besharse et al., 1988). Since dopamine receptors are found on both photoreceptors and RPE (Brann and Young, 1986; Dearry and Burnside, 1986; Dearry et al., 1990; Muresan and Besharse, 1993; Cahill and Besharse, 1993; Cohen et al., 1992; Vuvan et al., 1993; Wagner et al., 1993), it has been suggested that dopamine is a direct effector, at least in part responsible for the inhibitory effect of constant light on disc shedding. The current model for melatonin-dopamine interaction in control of rhythmic physiology suggests that dopamine acts within the photoreceptor-pigment epithelial complex to control disc shedding and other rhythmic phenomena while melatonin, synthesized in photoreceptors (Cahill and Besharse, 1992), regulates dopamine release from retinal interplexiform and amacrine cells in a rhythmic pattern. This is consistent with both dopaminergic regulation of disc shedding and

rhythmic regulation of dopamine metabolism in mammalian retinas (Remé and Wirz-Justice, 1984; Wirz-Justice et al., 1984).

Current data suggest that melatonin and dopamine act, respectively, at receptors in the inner retina and photoreceptor-RPE complex to influence disc shedding and other rhythms (reviewed in Besharse et al., 1988). However, direct effects of both agents on RPE are likely. Melatonin receptors have been cloned from melanin containing pigment cells in Xenopus skin (Ebisawa et al., 1994). In addition, melatonin has been reported to alter phagocytosis of polystyrene spheres in cultured chicken epithelial cells (Ogino et al., 1983). This, along with reports of melatonin effects on melanin pigment migration in RPE (Kraus-Ruppert and Lembeck, 1965), raises the possibility that melatonin may have direct functions in addition to control of retinal dopamine release. The same can be said of dopamine as well. In frog, movement of melanin pigment occurs in isolated RPE cells and can be regulated pharmacologically with dopamine agonists selective for D_1 receptors in a process that involves increases in cellular cAMP levels (Dearry et al., 1990). Increased cAMP levels inhibit ROS phagocytosis in cultured RPE and disc shedding in amphibian eye cups (Edwards and Bakshian, 1982; Besharse et al., 1982). Thus, in addition to its direct effects on photoreceptors, it is possible that dopamine directly affects RPE to control disc shedding and phagocytosis.

REGULATION OF DISC DETACHMENT AND PHAGOCYTOSIS

A major unanswered question in the biology of the RPE is the exact mechanism by which light/dark cycles and a circadian clock regulate disc detachment and phagocytosis. From the foregoing it is clear that a circadian clock resides in photoreceptors and that the mechanism of the effect of both light and the clock must be initiated at this level. It is tempting to conclude that RPE is capable of phagocytizing outer segments whenever disc detachment is initiated within retina. This is consistent with the finding that disc shedding can be observed throughout the day and that phagocytosis of damaged outer segments occurs whenever they are available (Custer and Bok, 1975). It is also clear that detachment and phagocytosis normally involves controlled interaction between the apical surface of RPE and the outer segment tip. We have modeled disc detachment and phagocytosis as involving intrinsic changes in the outer segment tip that occur synchronously with extension of pseudopodial processes from the RPE (Fig. 8-9). This is necessary because experimental separation of disc detachment from phagocytosis has not been possible in situ. In partially detached retinas it has been shown that ROS with normal interdigitation with RPE undergo disc shedding while adjacent separated ROS do not (Williams and Fisher, 1987). Furthermore, isolated retinas do not detach discs but disc detachment and phagocytosis can be reinitiated when retinas are reattached in eye cup cultures or to monolayer RPE cultures (Defoe et al., 1992; Defoe and Easterling, 1994; 1995). The dependence of disc detachment on the presence of RPE suggests that the normal signalling mechanism requires the presence of RPE, and that the process is controlled through RPE-photoreceptor interaction.

It is likely that this signaling mechanism normally involves local interaction between a single outer segment and RPE. In amphibian retina only a subset of photoreceptors shed their tip at light onset each day (Basinger et al., 1976; Besharse et al., 1977; Hollyfield et al., 1977). This has been studied quantitatively in *Rana pipiens* in relationship to increases in temperature (Hollyfield et al., 1977). Among the basic findings is that each rod does not undergo light-evoked shedding each day; for example, at 28°C only about one-third of the rods undergo disc shedding (Table 8-2). This means that individual rods undergo light-evoked disc shedding on average every third day. From the morphology it is clear that disc shedding is randomly distributed across the retina. Since five or more rod cells are serviced by a single RPE cell (Table 8-1), it follows that in association with a single RPE cell some rods are undergoing disc detachment while others are not. This is consistent with the frequent observation of adjacent rod tips in a single RPE cell, one shedding and the other quiescent. This is similar to the local regulation known to occur in macrophage phagocytosis (Griffin and Silverstein, 1974).These observations imply local signaling between single photoreceptors and RPE. Several mechanisms could account for this. For example, local changes in the ROS distal tip or surrounding interphotoreceptor matrix, or highly localized release of a factor in this region could locally activate the apical domain of RPE and/or distal domain of the outer segment. Alternatively, signaling could involve an inhibitory process or factor that is removed locally.

Several factors have been identified that result in global disc shedding across the entire photoreceptor-RPE complex. Since light-evoked disc shedding in frogs normally involves a controlled response of a subset of cells, such factors may be assumed to disrupt one or more normal regulatory systems. When eye cups are incubated with glutamate, aspartate, kainic acid, taurine or several other nonmetabolizable amino acids, uncontrolled disc shedding involving most of the rods in the retina is induced (Greenberger and Besharse, 1985). Similar effects are seen when medium sodium is replaced with choline, when eye cups are incubated with ouabain (Williams et al., 1984), or when potassium concentration is increased (Greenberger and Besharse, 1985). These effects involve a direct response to culture conditions and occur in either light or darkness. The site of action of these effectors of disc shedding has not been identified. They could act within either the retina or the RPE or both. For example, ouabain would be expected to block the Na+/K+ ATPase of both photoreceptors and RPE, high K+ would cause depolarization-dependent release of neuronal transmitters in retina and alter RPE membrane polarization. Excitatory amino acids could affect retinal glutamate receptors and/or alter RPE transport.

It seems likely that at least the excitatory amino acids are active in retina. For example, analysis using excitatory amino acid receptor agonists and antagonists indicates that glutamate receptors selectively responsive to kainic acid may be involved (Besharse and Spratt, 1988). Kainic acid among several excitatory amino acid receptor agonists is a highly potent effector of disc shedding. Furthermore, some excitatory amino acid antagonists block both kainic acid induced disc shedding and light evoked disc shedding (Besharse et al., 1988b). Such data have led to the suggestion that an excitatory amino acid receptor system in retina is involved in the acute regulation of disc shedding by light and that activation of this system by agonists results in uncontrolled disc shedding. It has also been suggested that effects of substances like ouabain and high potassium could act through the same mechanism because they cause release of retinal transmitters such as glutamate (Besharse et al., 1988b). Although the mode of action of factors that disregulate disc shedding remains poorly resolved, such factors have profound effects on RPE (Fig. 8-10). This includes the global elaboration of pseudopods that ensheath photoreceptor tips (Matsumoto et al., 1987) and dramatic increases in retinal adhesivity to the RPE (Defoe et al., 1989). In addition to serving as useful tools for studies of photoreceptor RPE interaction, eventual understanding of their mode of action is likely to yield insight into local mechanisms controlling disc shedding.

SUMMARY

Although membrane turnover is a general attribute of cells, it is accomplished in most cells through intrinsic synthetic and degradative mechanisms. The unique feature of photoreceptor outer segment turnover is the involvement of supporting cells of the retinal pigment epithelium in the degradation of membrane components synthesized and assembled in the photoreceptor. At least in the case of docosahexaenoic acid, this mechanism also provides a means for recycling back to photoreceptors. Although RPE involvement provides a mechanism for disposal of large quantities of photosensitive membrane, this mechanism requires a high degree of coordination between synthetic pathways in the photoreceptor and degradative pathways in the RPE. As elegantly summarized by Young (1976), photoreceptor function ultimately depends on maintenance of a balance between synthetic and degradative processes. The importance of this balance is seen in constant light, in which rod disc shedding is inhibited at the same time that assembly of new discs is maximized. The result is abnormal elongation of rod outer segments. Ultimately, failure of the turnover mechanism can lead to photoreceptor death, as is true in the RCS rat that carries a mutation that impairs the phagocytic ability of the RPE (see Chapter 13). Recent advances in our understanding of outer segment turnover indicate that it is highly regulated both temporally and spatially. The finding that the light/dark cycle and a circadian clock control photoreceptor disc shedding has led to development of models for temporal regulation that involve the action of a photoreceptor circadian clock and neurochemical agents from retina. At the same time, cell biological studies of the photoreceptor-RPE interface have led to a general understanding of the spatial organization of disc shedding in which pseudopods from RPE interact with distal domains of individual photoreceptor outer segments. Furthermore, studies using phagocytic assays in cell culture have begun to yield insight into the receptor mechanisms that mediate phagocytosis. Ultimately, a merger of these lines of analysis will be necessary to fully understand the cellular-molecular mechanisms involved in disc shedding.

REFERENCES

Anderson DH, Fisher SK. 1975. Disc shedding in the rod-like and cone-like photoreceptors of tree squirrels. Science 187:953–955.

Anderson DH, Fisher SK. 1976. The photoreceptors of diurnal squirrels: outer segment structure, disc shedding and protein renewal. J Ultrastruct Res 55:119–141.

Anderson DH, Fisher SK, Breding DJ. 1986. A concentration of fucosylated glycoconjugates at the base of cone outer segments: quantitative electron microscope autoradiography. Exp Eye Res 42:267–283.

Anderson DH, Fisher SK, Steinberg RH. 1978. Mammalian cones: disc shedding, phagocytosis and renewal. Invest Ophthalmol Vis Sci 17:117–133.

Anderson RE, Maude MB, Kelleher PA, Maida TM, Basinger SF. 1980a. Metabolism of phosphatidylcholine in the frog retina. Biochim Biophys Acta 620:212–226.

Anderson RE, Kelleher PA, Maude MB. 1980b. Metabolism of phosphatidylserine in the frog retina. Biochim Biophys Acta 620:227–235.

Anderson RE, Maude MB, Kelleher PA. 1980c. Metabolism of phosphatidylinositol in the frog retina. Biochim Biophys Acta 620:236–246.

Anderson RE, Kelleher PA, Maude MB, Maida TM. 1980d. Synthesis and turnover of lipid and protein components of frog retinal rod outer segments. In: Bazan NG, Lolley RN, (eds), Neurochemistry of the Retina. New York: Pergamon, 29–42.

Anderson DH, Fisher SK, Erickson PA, Tabor GA. 1980e. Rod and cone disc shedding in the rhesus monkey retina: a quantitative study. Exp Eye Res 30:559–574.

Anderson DH, Johnson LV, Hageman GS. 1995. Vitronectin receptor expression and distribution at the photoreceptor-retinal pigment epithelial interface. J Comp Neurol 360:1–16.

Bairati A, Orzalesi N. 1963. The ultrastructure of the pigment epithelium and of the photoreceptor-pigment epithelium junction in the human retina. J Ultrastruct Res 9:484–496.

Basinger SF, Hoffman RT. 1982. Regulation of rod shedding in the frog retina. In: Hollyfield JG, ed The Structure of the Eye. Amsterdam: Elsevier, 75–83.

Basinger S, Hoffman R, Matthes M. 1976. Photoreceptor shedding is initiated by light in the frog retina. Science. 194:1074–1076.

Besharse JC. 1982. The daily light-dark cycle and rhythmic metabolism in the photoreceptor-pigment epithelial complex. Prog Retinal Res 1:81–124.

Besharse JC, Dunis DA. 1982. Rod photoreceptor disc shedding in vitro: inhibition by cytochalasins and activation by colchicine. In: Hollyfield JG, ed, The Structure of the Eye. Amsterdam: Elsevier, 85–96.

Besharse JC, Dunis DA. 1983. Methoxyindoles and photoreceptor metabolism: activation of rod shedding. Science 219:1341–1343.

Besharse JC, Hageman GS. 1990. Incorporation of lipid probes into rod photoreceptor distal tips suggests formation of transient disc-plasma membrane continuities associated with disc shedding. Invest Ophthalmol Vis Sci 31(Abstract Suppl):5.

Besharse JC, Hollyfield JG. 1979. Turnover of mouse photoreceptor outer segments in constant light and darkness. Invest Ophthalmol Vis Sci 18:1019–1024.

Besharse JC, Iuvone PM. 1983. Circadian clock in Xenopus eye controlling retinal serotonin N-acetyltransferase. Nature 305:133–135.

Besharse JC, Spratt G. 1988. Excitatory amino acids and rod photoreceptor disc shedding: analysis using specific agonists. Exp Eye Res 47:609–620.

Besharse JC, Hollyfield JG, Rayborn ME. 1977. Turnover of rod photoreceptor outer segments II. Membrane addition and loss in relationship to light. J Cell Biol 75:507–527.

Besharse JC, Terrill RO, Dunis DA. 1980. Light-evoked disc shedding by rod photoreceptors in vitro: relationship to medium bicarbonate concentration. Invest Ophthalmol Vis Sci 19:1512–1517.

Besharse JC, Dunis DA, Burnside B. 1982. Effects of adenosine 3′, 5′ cyclic monophosphate on photoreceptor disc shedding and retinomotor movement: inhibition of rod shedding and stimulation of cone elongation. J Gen Physiol 79:775–790.

Besharse JC, Spratt G, Forestner DM. 1986. Light-evoked and kainic acid-induced disc shedding by rod photoreceptors: differential sensitivity to extracellular calcium. J Comp Neurol 251:185–197.

Besharse JC, Iuvone PM, Pierce ME. 1988a. Regulation of rhythmic photoreceptor metabolism: a role for post-receptoral neurons. Prog Retinal Res 7:21–61.

Besharse JC, Spratt G, Reif-Lehrer L. 1988b. Effects of kynurenate and other excitatory amino acid antagonists as blockers of light-

and kainate-induced retinal rod photoreceptor disc shedding. J Comp Neurol 274:295–303.

Bibb C, Young RW. 1974a. Renewal of fatty acids in the membranes of visual cell outer segments. J Cell Biol 61:327–343.

Bibb C, Young RW. 1974b. Renewal of glycerol in the visual cells and pigment epithelium of the frog retina. J Cell Biol 62:378–389.

Boatright JH, Rubim NM, Iuvone PM. 1994. Regulation of endogenous dopamine release in amphibian retina by melatonin: the role of GABA. Vis Neurosci 11:1013–1018.

Boesze-Battaglia K, Albert AD, Yeagle PL. 1992. Fusion between disc membranes and plasma membrane of bovine photoreceptor cells is calcium dependent. Biochemistry 31:3733–3737.

Bok D, Young RW. 1979. Phagocytic properties of the retinal pigment epithelium. In Marmor, MF and Zinn, KM eds. The Retinal Pigment Epithelium. Cambridge, MA: Harvard University Press, 148–174.

Boyle DL, Tien L, Cooper NGF, Shepherd V, McLaughlin BJ. 1991. A mannose receptor is involved in retinal phagocytosis. Invest Ophthalmol Vis Sci 32:1464–1470.

Brann MR, III, and Young WS. 1986. Dopamine receptors are located on rods in bovine retina. Neurosci Lett 69:221–226.

Cahill GM, Besharse JC. 1991. Resetting the circadian clock in cultured Xenopus eyecups: regulation of retinal melatonin rhythms by light and D2 dopamine receptors. J Neurosci 11:2959–2971.

Cahill GM, Besharse JC. 1992. Light-sensitive melatonin synthesis by Xenopus photoreceptors after destruction of the inner retina. Vis Neurosci 8:487–490.

Cahill GM, Besharse JC. 1993. Circadian clock functions localized in Xenopus retinal photoreceptors. Neuron 10:573–577.

Cahill GM, Besharse JC. 1995. Circadian rhythmicity in vertebrate retinas: regulation by a photoreceptor oscillator. Prog Ret Eye Res 14:267–291.

Chaitin MH, Hall MO. 1983. Defective ingestion of rod outer segments by cultured dystrophic rat pigment epithelial cells. Invest Ophthalmol Vis Sci 24:812–820.

Chen H, Anderson RE. 1993. Metabolism in frog retinal pigment epithelium of docosahexaenoic and arachidonic acids derived from rod outer segment membranes. Exp Eye Res 57:369–377.

Chen H, Wiegand RD, Koutz CA, Anderson RE. 1992. Docosahexaenoic acid increases in frog retinal pigment epithelium following rod photoreceptor shedding. Exp Eye Res 55:93–100.

Cohen AI. 1960. The ultrastructure of the rods of the mouse retina. Am J Anat 107:23–48.

Cohen AI. 1961. The fine structure of the extrafoveal receptors of the rhesus monkey. Exp Eye Res 1:128–136.

Cohen AI. 1963. Vertebrate retinal cells and their organization. Biol Rev 38:427–459.

Cohen AI, Todd RD, Harmon S, O'Malley KL. 1992. Photoreceptors of mouse retinas possess D4 receptors coupled to adenylate cyclase. Proc Nat Acad Sci USA 89:12093–12097.

Corless JM, Worniallo E, Fetter RD. 1989. Modulation of disk margin structure during renewal of cone outer segments in the vertebrate retina. J Comp Neurol 287:531–544.

Currie JR, Hollyfield JG, Rayborn ME. 1978. Rod outer segments elongate in constant light: darkness is required for normal shedding. Vision Res 18:995–1003.

Custer NV, Bok D. 1975. Pigment epithelium-photoreceptor interactions in the normal and dystrophic rat retina. Exp Eye Res 21:153–166.

Dearry A, Burnside B. 1986. Dopaminergic regulation of cone retinomotor movement in isolated teleost retinas: I. Induction of cone contraction is mediated by D2 receptors. J Neurochem 46:1006–1021.

Dearry A, Edelman JL, Miller S, Burnside B. 1990. Dopamine induces

light-adaptive retinomotor movements in bullfrog cones via D2 receptors and in retinal pigment epithelium via D1 receptors. J Neurochem 54:1367–1378.

Defoe DM, Easterling KC. 1994. Reattachment of retinas to cultured pigment epithelial monolayers from Xenopus laevis. Invest Ophthalmol Vis Sci 35:2466–2476.

Defoe DM, Easterling KC. 1995. Light-evoked shedding in recombined eyecups from Xenopus laevis. Exp Eye Res 60:107–109.

Defoe DM, Matsumoto B, Besharse JC. 1989. Cytochalasin D inhibits L-glutamate-induced disc shedding without altering L-glutamate-induced increase in adhesiveness. Exp Eye Res 48:641–652.

Defoe DM, Matsumoto B, Besharse JC. 1992. Reconstitution of the photoreceptor-pigment epithelium interface: L-glutamate stimulation of adhesive interactions and rod disc shedding after recombination of dissociated Xenopus laevis eyecups. Exp Eye Res 54:903–911.

Ditto M. 1975. A difference between developing rods and cones in the formation of outer segment membranes. Vision Res 15:535–536.

Dowling JE, Gibbons IR. 1961. The effect of vitamin A deficiency on the fine structure of the retina. In: Smelser GK, ed, The Structure of the Eye. New York: Academic Press, 85–99.

Droz B. 1963. Dynamic condition of proteins in the visual cells of rats and mice as shown by radioautography with labeled amino acids. Anat Rec 145:157–168.

Dubocovich ML. 1983. Melatonin is a potent modulator of dopamine release in the retina. Nature 204:183–184.

Ebisawa T, Karne S, Lerner MR, Reppert SM. 1994. Expression cloning of a high-affinity melatonin receptor from Xenopus dermal melanophores. Proc Nat Acad Sci USA 91:6133–6137.

Eckmiller MS. 1987. Cone outer segment morphogenesis: taper change and distal invaginations. J Cell Biol 105:2267–2277.

Eckmiller MS. 1993. Shifting distribution of autoradiographic label in cone outer segments and its implications for renewal. J Hirnforsch 34:179–191.

Edwards RB. 1991. Stimulation of rod outer segment phagocytosis by serum occurs only at the RPE apical surface. Exp Eye Res 53:229–232.

Edwards RB, Bakshian S. 1982. Phagocytosis of outer segments by cultured rat pigment epithelium: reduction by cAMP and phosphodiesterase inhibitors. Invest Ophthalmol Vis Sci 19:1184–1188.

Edwards RB, Flaherty PM. 1986. Increased phagocytosis of outer segments in the presence of serum by cultured normal, but not dystrophic, rat retinal pigment epithelium. J Cell Physiol 127:293–296.

Edwards RB, Szamier RB. 1977. Defective phagocytosis of isolated rod outer segments by RCS rat retinal pigment epithelium in culture. Science 197:1001–1003.

Elner VM, Schaffner T, Taylor K, Glagov S. 1981. Immunophagocytic properties of retinal pigment epithelial cells. Science 211:74–76.

Endemann G, Stanton LW, Madden KS, Bryant CM, White RT, Protter AA. 1993. CD36 is a receptor for oxidized low density lipoprotein. J Biol Chem 268:11811–11816.

Ezekowitz RAB, Sastry K, Bailly P, Warner A. 1990. Molecular characterization of the human macrophage mannose receptor: demonstration of multiple carbohydrate recognition domains and phagocytosis of yeast in COS-I cells. J Exp Med 172:1785–1794.

Feeney L, Grieshaber JA, Hogan MJ. 1965. Studies on human ocular pigment. In Rohen JW ed, The Structure of the Eye. Stuttgart: FK Schattauer-Verlag, 535–548.

Fetter RD, Corless JM. 1987. Morphological components associated with frog cone outer segment disc margins. Invest Ophthalmol Vis Sci 28:646–657.

Flannery JG, Fisher SK. 1984. Circadian disc shedding in Xenopus retina in vitro. Invest Ophthalmol Vis Sci 25:229–232.

Ghalayini A, Anderson RE. 1984. Phosphatidylinositol 4,5-bisphosphate: light-mediated breakdown in the vertebrate retina. Biochem Biophys Res Commun 124:503–506.

Ghalayini A, Anderson RE. 1992. Activation of bovine rod outer segment phospholipase C by arrestin. J Biol Chem 267:17977–17982.

Goldman AI, Tierstein PS, O'Brien P. 1980. The role of ambient lighting in circadian disc shedding in the rod outer segment of the rat retina. Invest Ophthalmol Vis Sci 19:1257–1267.

Gordon WC, Bazan NG. 1993. Visualization of [³H]docosahexaenoic acid trafficking through photoreceptors and retinal pigment epithelium by electron microscopic autoradiography. Invest Ophthalmol Vis Sci 34:2402–2411.

Gordon WC, Rodriguez de Turco EB, Bazan NG. 1992. Retinal pigment epithelial cells play a central role in the conservation of docosahexaenoic acid by photoreceptor cells after shedding and phagocytosis. Curr Eye Res 11:73–83.

Grace MS, Wang LA, Pickard, GE, Besharse JC, Menaker M. 1996. The tau mutation shortens the period of rhythmic photoreceptor outer segment disk shedding in the hamster. Brain Res 735:93–100.

Gregory CY, Hall MO. 1992. The phagocytosis of ROS by RPE is inhibited by an antiserum to rat RPE cell plasma membranes. Exp Eye Res 54:843–851.

Greenberg S, Silverstein SC. 1993. Phagocytosis. In: Paul WE, ed, Fundamental Immunology. New York: Raven Press, 941–964.

Greenberger LM, Besharse JC. 1985. Stimulation of photoreceptor disc shedding and pigment epithelial phagocytosis by glutamate, aspartate and other amino acids. J Comp Neurol 239:361–372.

Griffin FM, Silverstein SC. 1974. Segmental response of the macrophage plasma membrane to a phagocytic stimulus. J Exp Med 139:323–336.

Guo Y, Boyle DL, Tien L, Cooper NGF, McLaughlin BJ. 1991. Inhibition of rod outer segment phagocytosis with antibodies to retinal pigment epithelium membrane-associated protein. Invest Ophthalmol Vis Sci 32(suppl):890.

Hageman GS, Besharse JC. 1990. "Cytoplasmic Caps" at the apices of mammalian photoreceptors exhibit a circadian rhythm that peaks at night. Invest Ophthalmol Vis Sci 31(suppl):5.

Hageman GS, Johnson LV. 1986. Distribution of IgA and IgG within the interphotoreceptor matrix: selective association with cone photoreceptors. Invest Ophthalmol Vis Sci 27(suppl):239.

Hall MO, Abrams T. 1987. Kinetic studies of rod outer segment binding and ingestion by cultured rat RPE cells. Exp Eye Res 45:907–922.

Hall MO, Abrams T. 1991. The phagocytosis of ROS by RPE cells is not inhibited by mannose-containing ligands. Exp Eye Res 53:167–170.

Hall MO, Bok D, Bacharach ADE. 1969. Biosynthesis and assembly of the rod outer segment membrane system. J Mol Biol 45:397–406.

Hall MO, Burgess BL, Abrams TA, Ershov AV, Gregory CY. 1996. Further studies on the identification of the phagocytosis receptor of rat pigment epithelial cells. Exp Eye Res 63:255–264.

Hayashi F, Amakawa T. 1985. Light-mediated breakdown of phosphatidylinositol-4,5-bisphosphate in isolated rod outer segments of frog photoreceptor. Biochem Biophys Res Commun 128:954–959.

Hogan MJ, Wood I, Steinberg RH. 1974. Phagocytosis by pigment epithelium of human retinal cones. Nature. 252:305–307.

Hollyfield JG, Basinger S. 1978. Photoreceptor shedding can be initiated within the eye. Nature 274:794–796.

Hollyfield JG, Besharse JC, Rayborn ME. 1976. The effect of light on the quantity of phagosomes in the pigment epithelium. Exp Eye Res 23:623–635.

Hollyfield JG, Besharse JC, Rayborn ME. 1977. Turnover of rod photoreceptor outer segments: I. Membrane addition and loss in relationship to temperature. J Cell Biol 75:490–506.

Immel JH, Fisher SK. 1985. Cone photoreceptor shedding in the tree shrew (Tupaia belangerii). Cell Tissue Res 239:667–675.

Kraus-Ruppert R, Lembeck F. 1965. Die wirkung von melatonin auf die pigmentzellen der retina von fröschen. Pflügers Arch Eur J Physiol 284:160–168.

Kinney MS, Fisher SK. 1978. The photoreceptors and pigment epithelium of the adult Xenopus retina: morphology and outer segment renewal. Proc Royal Soc Lond B 201:131–147.

Laird DW, Molday RS. 1988. Evidence against the role of rhodopsin in rod outer segment binding to RPE cells. Invest Ophthalmol Vis Sci 29:419–428.

LaVail MM. 1976. Rod outer segment disc shedding in rat retina: relationship to cyclic lighting. Science 194:1071–1074.

LaVail MM. 1980. Circadian nature of rod outer segment disc shedding in the rat. Invest Ophthalmol Vis Sci 19:407–411.

LaVail MM, Ward PA. 1978. Studies on the hormonal control of circadian outer segment disc shedding in the rat retina. Invest Ophthalmol Vis Sci 17:1189–1193.

Lentrichia BB, Itoh Y, Plantner JJ, Kean EL. 1987. The influence of Carbohydrates on the binding of rod outer-segment (ROS) disc membranes and intact ROS by the cells of the retinal pigment epithelium of the embryonic chick. Exp Eye Res 44:127–142.

Liebman PA, Entine G. 1974. Lateral diffusion of visual pigment in photoreceptor disk membranes. Science 185:457–459.

Louie K, Wiegand RD, Anderson RE. 1988. Docosahexaenoic acid-containing molecular species of glycerophospholipids from frog retinal rod outer segments show different rates of biosynthesis and turnover. Biochemistry 27:9014–9020.

Matheke ML, Holtzman E. 1984. The effects of monensin and of puromycin on transport of membrane components in the frog retinal photoreceptor. II. Electron microscopic autoradiography of proteins and glycerolipids. J Neurosci 4:1093–1103.

Matsumoto B, Besharse JC. 1985. Light and temperature modulated staining of the rod outer segment distal tips with lucifer yellow. Invest Ophthalmol Vis Sci 26:628–635.

Matsumoto B, Defoe DM, Besharse JC. 1987. Membrane turnover in rod photoreceptors: ensheathment and phagocytosis of outer segment distal tips by pseudopodia of the retinal pigment epithelium. Proc Royal Soc Lond B 230:339–354.

Mayerson PL, Hall MO. 1986. Rat retinal pigment epithelial cells show specificity of phagocytosis in vitro. J Cell Biol 103:299–308.

McLaughlin BJ, Cooper NGF, Shepherd VL. 1994. How good is the evidence to suggest that phagocytosis of ROS by RPE is receptor mediated? Prog Ret Eye Res 13:147–164.

Mercurio AM, Holtzman E. 1982. Ultrastructural localization of glycerolipid synthesis in rod cells of the isolated frog retina. J Neurocytol 11:295–322.

Muresan Z, Besharse JC. 1993. D2-like dopamine receptors in amphibian retina: localization with fluorescent ligands. J Comp Neurol 331:149–160.

Nguyen-Legros J. 1978. Fine structure of the pigment epithelium in the vertebrate retina. Int Rev Cytol Supp 7:287–328.

Nilsson SEG. 1964. Receptor cell outer segment development and ultrastructure of the disk membranes in the retina of the tadpole Rana pipiens. J Ultrastruct Res 11:581–620.

O'Day WT, Young RW. 1978. Rhythmic daily shedding of outer segment membranes by visual cells in the goldfish. J Cell Biol 76:593–604.

Ogino N, Matsumura M, Shirakawa H, Tsukahara I. 1983. Phagocytic activity of cultured retinal pigment epithelial cells from chick embryo: inhibition by melatonin and cyclic AMP, and its reversal by taurine and cyclic GMP. Ophthalmic Res 15:72–89.

Organisciak DT, Winkler BS. 1994. Retinal light damage: practical and theoretical considerations. Prog Ret Eye Res 13:1–29.

Philp NJ, Nachmias VT, Lee D, Stramm L, Buzdygon B. 1988. Is rhodopsin the ligand for receptor-mediated phagocytosis of rod outer segments by retinal pigment epithelium? Exp Eye Res 46:21–28.

Pierce ME, Besharse JC. 1986. Melatonin and dopamine interactions in the regulation of rhythmic photoreceptor metabolism. In O'Brien PJ, Klein DC Pineal and Retinal Relationships. New York: Academic Press, 219–237.

Pierce ME, Sheshberadaran H, Zhang Z, Fox LE, Applebury ML, Takahashi JS. 1993. Circadian regulation of iodopsin gene expression in embryonic photoreceptors in retinal cell cultures. Neuron 10:579–584.

Poo M, Cone RA. 1974. Lateral diffusion of rhodopsin in the photoreceptor membrane. Nature 247:438–441.

Porter KR, Yamada E. 1960. Studies on the endoplasmic reticulum. V. Its form and differentiation in pigment epithelial cells of the frog retina. Biophys Biochem Cytol 8:181–205.

Reid DM, Laird DW, Molday RS. 1992. Characterization and application of an in vitro detection system for studying the binding and phagocytosis of rod outer segments by retinal pigment epithelial cells. Exp Eye Res 54:775–783.

Remé C, Wirz-Justice A, Aberhard B, Rhyner A. 1984. Chronic clorgyline dampens rat retinal rhythms. Brain Res 298:99–106.

Remé C, Wirz-Justice A, Terman M. 1991. The visual input stage of the mammalian circadian pacemaking system. I. Is there a clock in the mammalian eye? J Biol Rhythms 6:5–29.

Ren Y, Silverstein RL, Allen J, Savill J. 1995. CD36 gene transfer confers capacity for phagocytosis of cells undergoing apoptosis. J Exp Med 181:1857–1862.

Rizzolo LJ, Zhou S, Li Z-Q. 1994. Neural retina maintains integrins in the apical membrane of the RPE early in development. Invest Ophthalmol Vis Sci 35:2567–2576.

Ryeom SW, Sparrow JR, Silverstein RL. 1996. CD36 participates in the phagocytosis of rod outer segments by retinal pigment epithelium. J Cell Sci 109:387–395.

Sambrano GR, Parthasarathy S, Steinberg D. 1994. Recognition of oxidatively damaged erythrocytes by a macrophage receptor with specificity for oxidized low density lipoprotein. Proc Natl Acad Sci USA 91:3265–3269.

Savill J, Dransfield I, Hogg N, Haslett C. 1990. Vitronectin receptor-mediated phagocytosis of cells undergoing apoptosis. Nature 343:170–173.

Savill J, Hogg N, Ren Y, Haslett C. 1992. Thrombospondin cooperates with CD36 and the vitronectin receptor in macrophage recognition of neutrophils undergoing apoptosis. J Clin Invest 90:1513–1522.

Shepherd VL, Tarnowski BI, McLaughlin BJ. 1991. Isolation and characterization of a mannose receptor from human pigment epithelium. Invest Ophthalmol Vis Sci 32:1779–1784.

Shirakawa H, Ishiguro SI, Itoh Y, Plantner JJ, Kean EL. 1987. Are sugars involved in the binding of rhodopsin-membranes by the retinal pigment epithelium? Invest Ophthalmol Vis Sci 28:628–632.

Spitznas M, Hogan MJ. 1970. Outer segments of photoreceptors and the retinal pigment epithelium. Arch Ophthalmol 84:810–819.

Steinberg RH, Wood I, Hogan MJ. 1977. Pigment epithelial ensheathment and phagocytosis of extrafoveal cones in human retina. Phil Trans Royal Soc Lond 277:459–474.

Sung S-SJ, Nelson RS, Silverstein SC. 1983. Yeast mannans inhibit binding and phagocytosis of zymosan by mouse peritoneal macrophages. J Cell Biol 96:160–166.

Tabor GA, Fisher SK, Anderson DH. 1980. Rod and cone disc shedding in light-entrained tree squirrels. Exp Eye Res 30:545–557.

Tamai M, Tierstein P, Goldman A, O'Brien P. 1978. The pineal gland does not control rod outer segment disc shedding and phagocytosis in the rat retina and pigment epithelium. Invest Ophthalmol Vis Sci 17:558–562.

Tarnowski BI, Shepherd VL, McLaughlin BJ. 1991. Expression of mannose receptors for pinocytosis and phagocytosis on rat retinal pigment epithelium. Invest Ophthalmol Vis Sci 29:742–748.

Terman JS, Remé CE, Terman M. 1993. Rod outer segment disk shedding in rats with lesions of the suprachiasmatic nucleus. Brain Res 605:256–264.

Tierstein PS, Goldman AI, O'Brien PJ. 1980. Evidence for both local and central regulation of rat rod outer segment disc shedding. Invest Ophthalmol Vis Sci 19:1268–1273.

Tosini G, Menaker M. 1996. Circadian rhythms in cultured mammalian retina. Science 272:419–421.

Underwood H, Barrett RK, Siopes T. 1990. The quail's eye: a biological clock. J Biol Rhythms 5:257–265.

Vuvan T, Geffard M, Denis P, Simon A, Nguyen-Legros J. 1993. Radioimmunoligand characterization and immunohistochemical localization of dopamine D_2 receptors on rods in the rat retina. Brain Res 614:57–64.

Wagner H-J, Luo B-G, Ariano MA, Sibley DR, Stell W. 1993. Localization of D_2 dopamine receptors in vertebrate retina with antipeptide antibodies. J Comp Neurol 331:469–481.

Wetzel MG, Bendala-Tufanisco E, Besharse JC. 1993. Tunicamycin does not inhibit transport of phosphatidylinositol to Xenopus rod outer segments. J Neurocytol 22:397–412.

Wetzel MG, Besharse JC. 1994. Transport of phosphatidylcholine to Xenopus photoreceptor rod outer segments in the presence of tunicamycin. J Neurocytol 23:333–342.

Williams DS, Fisher SK. 1987. Prevention of rod disk shedding by detachment from the retinal pigment epithelium. Invest Ophthalmol Vis Sci 28:184–187.

Williams DS, Wilson C, Linberg K, Fisher S. 1984. Effects of low sodium, ouabain, and strophanthidin on the shedding of rod outer segment discs. J Comp Physiol A 155:763–770.

Wirz-Justice A, DaPrada M, Remé C. 1984. Circadian rhythm in rat retinal dopamine. Neurosci Lett 45:21–25.

Young RW. 1967. The renewal of photoreceptor cell outer segments. J Cell Biol 33:61–72.

Young RW. 1971a. The renewal of rod and cone outer segments in the rhesus monkey. J Cell Biol 49:303–318.

Young RW. 1971b. Shedding of discs from rod outer segments in the rhesus monkey. J Ultrastruct Res 34:190–203.

Young RW. 1971c. An hypothesis to account for a basic distinction between rods and cones. Vision Res 11:1–5.

Young RW. 1976. Visual cells and the concept of renewal. Invest Ophthalmol Vis Sci 15:700–725.

Young RW. 1977. The daily rhythm of shedding and degradation of cone outer segment membranes in the lizard retina. J Ultrastruct Res 61:172–185.

Young RW. 1978. The daily rhythm of shedding of rod and cone outer segment membranes in the chick retina. Invest Ophthalmol Vis Sci 17:105–116.

Young RW, Bok D. 1969. Participation of the retinal pigment epithelium in the rod outer segment renewal process. J Cell Biol 42:392–403.

Young RW, Droz B. 1968. The renewal of protein in retinal rods and cones. J Cell Biol 39:169–184.

Zimmerman WF. 1984. Enzymes of phospholipid metabolism in bovine rod outer segments. Invest Ophthalmol Vis Sci 25:(suppl):113.

III | DIAGNOSTIC EVALUATION

9. Light-induced responses of the retinal pigment epithelium

RON P. GALLEMORE, BRET A. HUGHES, AND SHELDON S. MILLER

Nearly 150 years ago du Bois-Reymond (1849) reported that the dark-adapted eye generates a standing potential, with the cornea positive to the posterior pole. In the ensuing years, Holmgren (1865; 1879) and, independently, Dewar and M'Kendrick (1873a–1873c; Dewar, 1877) discovered that illumination of the eye produced a series of changes in this standing potential. These potential changes were further characterized and defined as distinct components of the electroretinogram (Einthoven and Jolly, 1908; Piper, 1911; Granit, 1933). Figure 9-1 illustrates a typical electroretinogram recorded with direct current (DC) amplification in a higher vertebrate with its components identified by contemporary terminology. The response begins with the fast a- and b-waves, which are followed by three slower potential changes: the c-wave, the fast-oscillation trough, and the light peak. At light offset, responses of opposite polarity are recorded.

While a number of investigators realized that the neural retina must contribute to these electrical responses of the eye (Armington, 1974), it was Noell in the 1950s who proposed and demonstrated that the retinal pigment epithelium (RPE) could contribute to both the standing potential and the ERG. Using a variety of pharmacological agents, Noell was able to selectively damage either the neural retina or the RPE. He demonstrated that the RPE is the primary source of the standing potential of the eye and that both the neural retina and the RPE contribute to components of the electroretinogram (Noell, 1952; 1953; 1954). In the course of analyzing the retinal origins of the fast a- and b-waves, he provided the first demonstration that the RPE contributes to the slower c-wave (Noell, 1954). Based on his analysis of RPE transport (Noell et al., 1965), Noell went on to propose that the c-wave originates from a light-induced change in ion concentration originating from the photoreceptors, which somehow affects the retinal (apical) side of the RPE (Noell, 1954).

In the ensuing years, the cellular mechanism of the c-wave was defined. Steinberg, Schmidt, and Brown (1970) discovered a light-evoked hyperpolarization of the RPE apical membrane that followed the time course of the c-wave and had identical stimulus-response characteristics. Miller and Steinberg (1977; Steinberg and Miller, 1973) demonstrated that the RPE apical membrane had a very large K conductance, suggesting that a decrease in K concentration (or other ion activity change) could contribute to the c-wave. Using K-selective microelectrodes, Oakley and Green (1976) and Oakley (1977) measured the light-evoked decrease in subretinal K concentration that generates the c-wave.

In recent years, the ionic mechanisms of other light-induced responses of the RPE have been elucidated, in part, by considering the fundamental transport properties of the RPE. In Chapter 6 we reviewed the basic transport mechanisms involved in fluid, ion, and metabolite transport. These studies were conducted on in vitro RPE preparations in the absence of the neural retina, and the transport mechanisms at both the retinal (apical) and choroidal (basolateral) facing membranes were identified. This work led to the discovery that both the fast-oscillation and light-peak voltages originate from modulation of the Cl transport pathways of the RPE. The same K concentration decrease underlying the c-wave also generates the fast oscillation. The retinal paracrine signal that generates the light peak remains unknown. In addition to these ERG components, the effects of K and other signaling molecules whose concentration may change during illumination have also been elucidated.

In this chapter we focus on the ionic mechanisms underlying the light-induced electrical responses of the RPE. In addition to the origins of the DC ERG, we review the effects of signaling molecules on the transport and electrical properties of the RPE. Finally, the origin of light-evoked changes in subretinal space volume are covered as well. The clinical applications of RPE electrophysiology are considered in Chapter 10.

EXPERIMENTAL PREPARATIONS

A number of preparations have been used to study the light-induced responses of the RPE. In vitro preparations

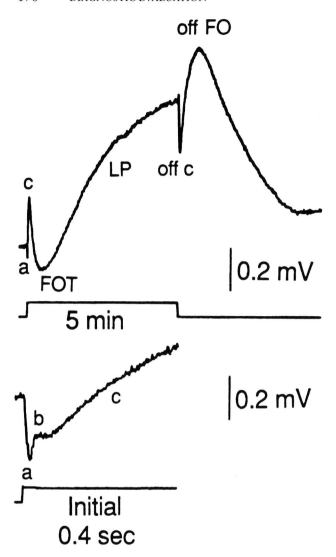

FIGURE 9-1. Direct-current electroretinogram (DC-ERG). Recorded in vitro in the chick neural retina-RPE-choroid preparation. Responses in temporal order are: onset of illumination—a-wave, fast-oscillation trough (FOT), and light peak (LP); offset of illumination—off c-wave and the "off" of the fast oscillation (off FO). The stimulus diffusely illuminated in the retina with 6.0×10^{-5} W/cm²; stimulus duration was 5 min, indicated by an upward deflection of the trace below the response. The initial components of the ERG are shown below on an expanded time scale. The apparent reduction in a-wave amplitude in the complete response is an artifact of digitization. The small b-wave is due to the addition of extra magnesium (3 mM total) to the perfusate to suppress spreading depression (Martins-Ferreira and Oliveira Castro, 1971). (From Gallemore and Steinberg, 1989).

include the eye cup (Karwoski and Proenza, 1977; Miller et al., 1986), isolated perfused mammalian eye (Niemeyer, 1981; Dawis and Niemeyer, 1986), and RPE-choroid tissues with and without the neural retina (Lasansky and De Fisch, 1966; Miller and Steinberg, 1977; Joseph and Miller, 1991; Oakley et al., 1977; Shirao and Steinberg,

1987; Gallemore et al., 1988). The predominant in vivo preparation has been the intact cat (Steinberg et al., 1970; Linsenmeier and Steinberg, 1982; Steinberg et al., 1985; Steinberg, 1987). Each preparation has particular advantages and disadvantages. Of these preparations, the RPE-choroid and retina-RPE choroid tissues have provided the most information regarding the ionic mechanisms of the light-induced RPE responses. Here, we briefly review these two preparations.

The RPE-choroid and neural retina-RPE-choroid preparations are studied in a similar fashion. Both tissues are mounted in an Üssing chamber in which the apical and basolateral sides of the RPE can be separately perfused. Chemical changes in the basal bath reach the basolateral membrane after diffusion through the choroid. In the RPE-choroid preparation, changes in the apical bath chemical composition reach the apical membrane rapidly after diffusion through a thin unstirred layer, but in the retina-RPE-choroid preparation, changes are slower, due to diffusion through the relatively thick neural retina. The transport mechanisms at each membrane can then be characterized by using ion substitutions, transport inhibitors, and ion channel blockers.

The RPE-choroid preparation has been used primarily to characterize the specific transport mechanisms that are present in the apical and basolateral membranes of the RPE (see Chapter 6). It has also been utilized, however, to study the origin of light-evoked RPE responses. This is possible because two of these light-evoked responses, the c-wave and the fast-oscillation trough, are generated by the photoreceptor-dependent decrease in subretinal K concentration ($[K]_0$). Decreasing the K concentration outside the apical membrane from 5 to 2 mM mimics the transition from dark to light and the $\Delta[K]_0$-induced responses of the RPE, in the absence of the neural retina, can then be studied.

The isolated neural retina-RPE-choroid preparation was developed to allow in vitro recording of light-evoked responses of the RPE. Isolated retina-RPE-choroid preparations have been developed from frog (Oakley et al., 1977), toad (Griff, 1991), lizard (Griff and Steinberg, 1982), and chick (Shirao and Steinberg, 1987; Gallemore et al., 1988). The chick preparation has several advantages, including a thin, permeable choroid, strong adherence between the cone-enriched neural retina and RPE, and, finally, the capacity to generate light-evoked responses typical of warm-blooded vertebrates. A choroid-free preparation of chick neural retina-RPE has also been developed with the use of enzymatic dissection (Gallemore et al., 1994b); this preparation has the added benefit of direct access to the RPE basal membrane.

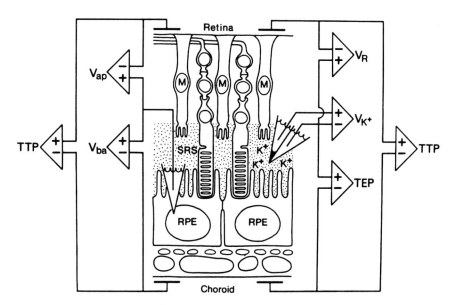

FIGURE 9-2. Recording configurations for the neural retina-RPE-choroid preparation. The transtissue potential (TTP) is recorded differentially between the retinal and choroidal baths and the change in TTP in response to light is the DC electroretinogram. With a microelectrode positioned in an RPE cell *(left)*, the apical (V_{ap}) and basal (V_{ba}) membrane potentials are recorded differentially by referencing to the retinal and choroidal baths, respectively. With a double-barreled K$^+$-specific electrode positioned in the subretinal space *(right)*, the transretinal potential (V_R) and transepithelial potential (TEP) are recorded differentially by referencing the nonselective (reference) barrel to the retinal and choroidal baths, respectively. (V_{K+}) represents the differential signal between the reference barrel and K$^+$-selective barrel (note liquid ion exchange resin in the tip), and is a measure of the local K$^+$ concentration in the subretinal space (SRS). (From Gallemore and Steinberg, 1991).

EXPERIMENTAL METHODS

Electrophysiological techniques have been used to study the light-induced responses of the RPE. Here we use the neural retina-RPE-choroid preparation as an example. The same principles can be applied to the other preparations. Figure 9-2 illustrates the signals recorded in the preparation. The transtissue potential (TTP) is recorded between extracellular agar-salt bridge electrodes placed in the apical (retinal) and basal (choroidal) baths. The TTP is the in vitro equivalent of the standing potential of the eye and originates primarily from the RPE (Steinberg et al., 1985). The light-evoked changes in TTP recorded with direct-current (DC) amplification represent the DC electroretinogram (DC ERG). The transtissue potential is the sum of two separate potentials generated by the neural retina and RPE, respectively. With a microelectrode positioned extracellularly within the subretinal space (Fig. 9-2, right side), the transretinal potential (V_R) is recorded by referencing to the apical (retinal) bath and the transepithelial potential (TEP) is recorded by referencing to the choroidal (basal) bath. The subretinal recording is used to localize an ERG potential to the RPE or neural retina. In addition,

with a double-barreled microelectrode, as shown here, changes in the extracellular chemical potential of an ion (V_K) outside the photoreceptors (subretinal space) can be recorded as well.

Once a potential change has been localized to the RPE, a microelectrode is placed within the RPE cell to localize the potential change to the apical or basolateral membrane (Fig. 9-2, left side). The apical membrane potential (V_{ap}) is recorded by referencing to the retinal bath; this signal actually includes the transretinal potential (V_R), but its contribution is generally small. Referencing the microelectrode to the basal bath gives the basolateral membrane potential (V_{ba}), assuming no potential difference across the choroid. Double-barreled ion-selective microelectrodes also can be placed intracellularly within the RPE to record, for example, light-evoked changes in intracellular ion activity.

The membrane events underlying voltage changes recorded extracellularly within the retina and intracellularly from the RPE often can be elucidated by equivalent electrical circuit analysis. This type of analysis is particularly important for the RPE, since the interpretation of changes in membrane voltage and conductance in an epithelium is complicated by electrical coupling

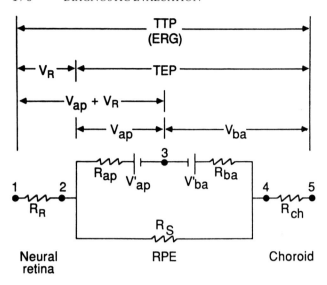

FIGURE 9-3. Equivalent circuit for the neural retina-RPE-choroid preparation. The neural retina and choroid are represented by resistors, (R_r) and (R_{ch}), respectively. The RPE apical and basal membranes are represented by an EMF (V'_{ap}, V'_{ba}) in series with a resistor (R_{ap}, R_{ba}). (R_s) is the parallel combination of the junctional complex resistance (shunt) and the resistance due to tissue edge damage. (From Gallemore and Steinberg, 1989a).

between the two membranes of the cell (Miller and Steinberg, 1977). The apical and basolateral membranes of the RPE are not electrically isolated, since the tight junctions that separate them have a finite resistance. As a result, potential changes at one membrane are shunted passively to the other membrane (Miller and Steinberg, 1977). A more detailed analysis of this problem is presented in Chapter 6. In much the same way, the neural retina and the RPE are also electrically coupled and potential changes in one may be shunted to the other. However, this coupling is generally of negligible significance due to the relatively small resistance of the neural retina in comparison to the RPE (Steinberg et al., 1985).

Figure 9-3 illustrates the equivalent electrical circuit for the neural retina-RPE-choroid preparation. The neural retina is represented by the resistance R_r and the choroid is represented by the resistance R_{ch}. In this simplified circuit, the retina and choroid do not generate any potential. The RPE is represented by three components. The apical membrane is represented by a battery, V_{ap}, and resistance, R_{ap}; the basolateral membrane is represented by a resistance, R_{ba}, and a battery, V_{ba}; and the paracellular shunt is represented by the resistance R_s. Equations derived from this equivalent electrical circuit can be used to interpret potential changes recorded during the DC ERG (see Chapter 6).

LIGHT-EVOKED ELECTRICAL RESPONSES: THE DC ERG AND EOG

The transepithelial potential (TEP) of the RPE is the primary source of the corneal-positive standing potential of the vertebrate eye. In response to illumination, a complex series of changes in the standing potential can be recorded with DC amplification as components of the DC ERG. Figure 9-1 illustrates the normal DC ERG of an in vitro preparation of chick retina-RPE-choroid in response to 5 minutes of diffuse illumination; the DC ERG of chick, a warm-blooded higher vertebrate, is remarkably similar to that of mammals, including human (Kikawada, 1968; Marmor and Lurie, 1979). The response begins with the fast a- and b-waves, shown on an expanded time scale in the lower portion of the figure, which are followed by three slower changes in potential, the c-wave, the fast-oscillation trough (FOT), and the light peak (LP). Each of these slower components has its counterpart at the offset of illumination. While the a- and b-waves are manifestations of voltage changes within the neural retina itself (Miller and Dowling, 1970; Rodiek, 1972), all three slower components of the DC ERG result largely from light-evoked changes in RPE cell membrane potentials (Steinberg et al., 1983; 1985; van Norren and Heyman, 1986; Valeton and van Norren, 1982). Figure 9-4 illustrates the relationship between the DC ERG and the intracellularly recorded changes in RPE membrane potentials and resistance parameters. The underlying changes in RPE ion transport associated with each component of the ERG are discussed in the following sections.

C-Wave

The c-wave is the first component of the DC ERG having contributions from the RPE (Noell, 1954). Intraretinal depth profiles and intracellular recordings from cat RPE cells demonstrated that the positive-going c-wave originates from a hyperpolarization of the RPE apical membrane (Steinberg et al., 1970). Noell (1954) suggested that the c-wave could be generated by a light-induced change in the activity of an ion (K) in the subretinal space. Miller and Steinberg (1977) observed that the apical membrane of the isolated frog RPE had a large K conductance and proposed that a light-evoked decrease in subretinal K might underlie the c-wave hyperpolarization. Experiments with K-selective electrodes in frog (Oakley and Green, 1976; Oakley, 1977; Oakley et al., 1977; Oakley and Steinberg, 1982), turtle (Matsura et al., 1978), and cat (Steinberg et al., 1980) bore out this hypothesis: a light-evoked decrease in subretinal $[K]_o$ was observed with the same stimulus-

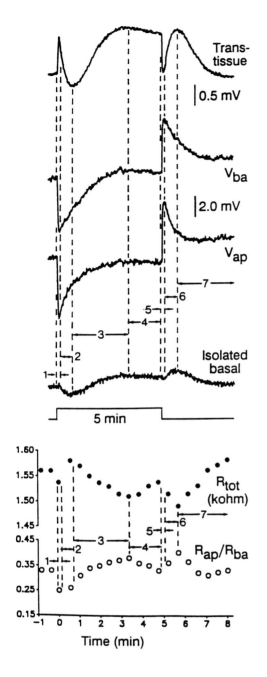

FIGURE 9-4. Changes in transtissue potential (TTP), the intracellular responses of the retinal pigment epithelium (RPE; V_{ba} and V_{ap}) and in resistance parameters (R_{tot} and R_{ap}/R_{ba}) in response to 5 min of illumination. The isolated basolateral membrane voltage response is generated by subtraction of the shunted portion of the apical membrane voltage (see Steinberg et al., 1985 and Linsenmeier and Steinberg, 1984b). The transtissue resistance (R_{tot}), reflects changes in R_t (RPE resistance) because R_{ret} (retinal resistance) is small and constant. Intracellular responses began with the large membrane hyperpolarizations of the c-wave (phase 1). After the c-wave there was a "delayed" hyperpolarization of the basal membrane (phase 2), seen clearly in the isolated basal response (generated by computer subtraction). This is the RPE contribution to the fast oscillation trough (FOT). During phase 2, R_{ap}/R_{ba} remained below its dark-adapted value, whereas R_{tot} increased. The basal membrane then depolarized with the same time course as the light peak (phase 3), during which R_{ap}/R_{ba} increased and R_{tot} decreased. At the offset of illumination, the former sequence of events was reversed (phases 5, 6, 7). The stimulus diffusely illuminated the retinal with 6.0×10^{-5} W/cm²; stimulus duration is indicated by an upward deflection of the trace below the response. (From Gallemore and Steinberg, 1993).

response characteristics as the c-wave and could account for the time course and amplitude of the c-wave hyperpolarization of the RPE apical membrane.

The light-evoked $[K]_o$ decrease is generated by the photoreceptors when they hyperpolarize in response to light due to the closure of cGMP-gated channels in the outer segment (Oakley et al., 1979; Steinberg, 1987). The light-evoked $[K]_o$ decrease in the subretinal space of the cat is shown in Figure 9-5 (Steinberg, 1987). This light-induced hyperpolarization of the photoreceptor cell membrane causes a reduction in the passive efflux of K through inner segment K channels, and since K up-

take via the Na/K pump persists, there is a fall in $[K]_o$ (Fig. 9-5A). In response to this light-induced $[K]_o$ decrease, the apical membrane of the RPE and the distal ends of Müller cells hyperpolarize (Fig. 9-5B). The RPE hyperpolarization produces one component of the c-wave and the Müller cell hyperpolarization produces another, a negative-going potential across the neural retina, termed *slowPIII*, which has approximately the same time course as the c-wave (Faber, 1969; Witkovsky et al., 1975; Karwoski and Proenza, 1977). Examples of these components are shown in Figure 9-6, which depicts a recording from the intact cat eye. Thus, the DC

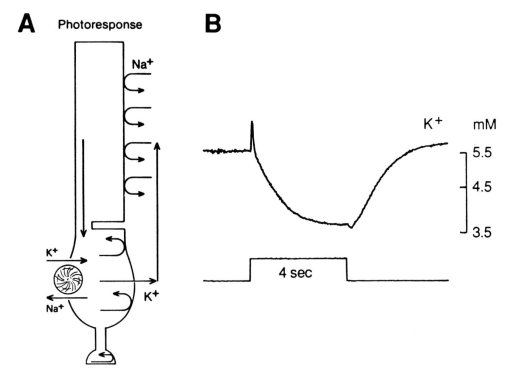

FIGURE 9-5. The light-induced shutdown of photocurrent and the decrease in subretinal $[K^+]_o$. (A) Diagram depicting membrane events underlying the shutdown of the photocurrent. Light closes channels in the outer segment, reducing the inward movement of Na at the outer segment and reducing the leakage of K^+ from the inner segment. Na/K pump rate is maintained at the dark level in the first moments after stimulus onset. (B) Subretinal $[K^+]_o$ in response to 4.0 sec of illumination in cat. Illumination causes a decrease in subretinal $[K^+]_o$ that reaches a minimum about 4.0 sec after stimulus onset. Illumination at 8.3 log quanta $deg^{-2} sec^{-1}$. (From Steinberg, 1987).

ERG c-wave has contributions from both the neural retina and RPE; these responses are of opposite polarity, but the RPE component is generally larger, resulting in a positive potential at the cornea.

Figure 9-7 illustrates the c-wave hyperpolarization of the RPE apical membrane in cat, along with the light-evoked decrease in subretinal $[K]_o$. The decrease in $[K]_o$ causes the K equilibrium potential across the apical membrane to become more negative; because the apical membrane has a large K conductance, it hyperpolarizes. The changes in transepithelial, transretinal, and apical membrane potentials closely reflect the decrease in $[K]_o$ (Steinberg et al., 1985). It is important to note that the basolateral membrane also hyperpolarizes during the c-wave (Fig. 9-4). This is the result of electrical coupling between the two membranes so that a fraction of the apical membrane voltage response is shunted to the basolateral side.

Recent work indicates that the membrane voltage changes in the RPE during the c-wave also include a minor contribution from the apical membrane Na/K pump. Griff and colleagues (1985) showed in the isolated frog RPE-choroid preparation that the light-evoked $[K]_o$ decrease slows the electrogenic Na/K pump, producing a membrane depolarization that re-duces the amplitude of the c-wave hyperpolarization of the apical membrane. This modulation of the Na/K pump by $\Delta[K]_o$ was "unmasked" by using barium to block the apical K conductance (Fig. 9-8). Similar results have been obtained in toad, bovine, and human RPE (Griff, 1991; Joseph and Miller, 1991; Hernandez et al., 1995).

The membrane hyperpolarization also changes the driving force on any electrogenic transport mechanism in the RPE. These effects are considered further in Chapter 6 and include slowing of the apical membrane $NaHCO_3$ cotransporter (Hughes et al., 1989; La Cour, 1989; 1991a; 1991b), which alkalinizes the cell; stimulation of the NaGABA (taurine) cotransporter (Scharshmidt et al., 1988; Peterson and Miller, 1995a), which increases the removal of amino acids from the subretinal space; and increasing K and Cl efflux, which drives water out of the cell, decreasing RPE cell volume and hydrating the subretinal space (Bialek and Miller, 1995; Li et al., 1994a; Huang and Karwoski, 1992—see also "Light-Evoked Modulation of Subretinal Volume," below).

In summary, the c-wave voltage of the DC ERG, recorded at the cornea, reflects the modulation of at least two ion transport mechanisms at the apical mem-

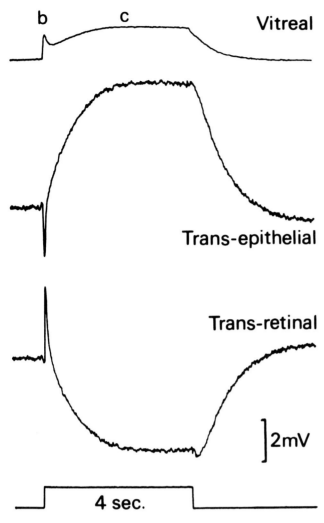

FIGURE 9-6. The ERG c-wave along with its transepithelial and trans-retinal components. With a microelectrode in the subretinal space, the RPE c-wave (transepithelial) is recorded across the RPE while the transretinal component (slow PIII) is recorded across the neural retinal. (From Steinberg et al., 1985).

brane of the RPE. The light-evoked decrease in subretinal $[K]_o$ underlying the c-wave produces (1) a diffusion potential across Ba^{2+}-sensitive K channels, which hyperpolarizes the apical membrane, and (2) a slowing of the ouabain-sensitive Na/K pump, which produces a smaller apical membrane depolarization. The net result is a hyperpolarization of both membranes, which modulates a variety of transporters and leads to significant changes in intracellular K, Cl, HCO_3, pH, and cell volume (see Chapter 6).

Fast Oscillation

The second slow component of the DC ERG, the fast-oscillation trough (FOT), represents the recovery of potential following the c-wave to a level at or below the

dark-adapted baseline (Fig. 9-4, Phase 2). Studies in lizard (Griff and Steinberg, 1984) and cat (Linsenmeier and Steinberg, 1984a) have shown that the trough originates from a hyperpolarization of the RPE basolateral membrane that is "delayed" with respect to the c-wave hyperpolarization of the apical membrane (see also Steinberg, 1985). A similar delayed basal hyperpolarization can be produced by decreasing $[K]_o$ outside the apical membrane of the isolated RPE-choroid, implicating the light-evoked decrease in subretinal $[K]_o$ in the generation of the fast-oscillation trough (Griff and Steinberg, 1984).

Mechanism: isolated RPE preparation. Experiments in the isolated bovine RPE-choroid preparation have clarified the sequence of events that probably generate the delayed basolateral hyperpolarization in the intact eye (Joseph and Miller, 1991; Bialek et al., 1995): (1) the light-evoked decrease in subretinal $[K]_o$ slows Cl uptake by the apical membrane Na,K,2Cl cotransporter,; (2) this leads to a reduction in intracellular Cl activity (a^i_{Cl}); (3) this decrease in a^i_{Cl} changes the Cl equilibrium potential across the basolateral membrane Cl channel, producing a hyperpolarization. A delayed basal membrane depolarization can be produced in the isolated RPE-choroid by decreasing apical $[K]_o$ from 5 to 2 mM. This mimics the light-evoked change in subretinal $[K]_o$ but does not evoke a light peak, which simplifies analy-

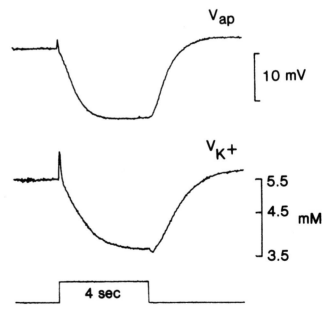

FIGURE 9-7. RPE apical membrane and subretinal $[K^+]_o$ in response to 4.0 sec of illumination in cat. These responses were obtained in separate experiments at an illumination of 8.3 log quanta $deg^{-2} sec^{-1}$. The apical membrane potential V_{ap}, was derived by subtracting an intracellular recording of basal membrane potential from the transepithelial recording. (From Steinberg et al., 1985).

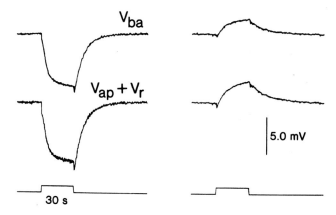

FIGURE 9-8. Barium unmasks light-evoked (ΔK) modulation of the Na/K pump. Under control conditions (left), a 30-second flash evokes hyperpolarizations of the apical and basal membranes. In the presence of the K-channel blocker, barium (right), a light-evoked depolarization of both membranes is seen. See text for additional details. (From Griff, Shirao, and Steinberg, 1985).

sis of the resultant electrophysiological changes (Steinberg and Niemeyer, 1981). Figure 9-9 illustrates the changes in TEP, membrane voltage, and a^i_{Cl} that accompany the decrease in apical $[K]_o$ from 5 to 2 mM. The important feature of this recording is the large decrease in intracellular Cl activity that accompanies the delayed basal membrane hyperpolarization. Miller and colleagues (Joseph and Miller, 1991; Bialek et al., 1995) showed that this Cl activity decrease was sufficient to cause the delayed basolateral membrane hyperpolarization. They also corroborated the observation, made previously in lizard (Griff and Steinberg, 1984), that the delayed basal membrane hyperpolarization is associated with an apparent decrease in basolateral membrane conductance.

The decrease in a^i_{Cl} could cause a delayed hyperpolarization of the basal membrane by two mechanisms: (1) shifting the equilibrium potential for Cl (E_{Cl}) in the negative direction, and (2) decreasing the basolateral membrane Cl conductance (g_{Cl}) by reducing the number of charge carriers for the Cl channel, as predicted by the Goldman-Hodgkin-Katz current equation (Hille, 1992). The following equation for steady-state membrane potential shows how changes in E_{Cl} and g_{Cl} would effect the basal membrane battery, E_B (V'_{ba} in Fig. 9-3).

$$E_B = (g_K E_K + g_{Cl} E_{Cl})/(g_K + g_{Cl}) \qquad (9\text{-}1)$$

where g_K and g_{Cl} are the resting K and Cl conductances of the basolateral membrane and E_K and E_{Cl} are the equilibrium (Nernst) potentials for K and Cl across the membrane. This relationship assumes that the total basal membrane conductance comprises only Cl and K conductances, which appears to be largely the case (Joseph and Miller, 1991; Gallemore et al., 1993). From this equation it can readily be seen that either a hyper-

polarization of E_{Cl} or a reduction of g_{Cl} could hyperpolarize E_B. E_B would also be hyperpolarized by an increase in E_K or an increase in g_K, but an increase in g_K would increase the basolateral membrane conductance, opposite to what is observed. A detailed analysis of the changes in E_{Cl}, g_{Cl}, E_K, and g_K during the delayed basal membrane hyperpolarization in bovine RPE indicates that the response is mainly due to the a^i_{Cl}-induced changes in E_{Cl} (Bialek et al., 1995).

Experiments with transport blockers indicate that the decrease in intracellular Cl activity is generated by modulation of the Cl transport pathway. The delayed basolateral membrane hyperpolarization is severely reduced by apical bumetanide, a blocker of Na,K,2Cl cotransport, or by basal DIDS, a blocker of the Cl channels (Bialek et al., 1995). Similar results with these blockers were observed in cultured human RPE monolayers (Hu et al., 1996).

In situ studies. While the delayed basal hyperpolarization studied in isolated RPE-choroid tissues has similarities to the fast-oscillation trough of the DC ERG, there are important differences. For example, the step decrease in apical $[K]_o$ is not identical in time course to the light-evoked changes in subretinal $[K]_o$, where $[K]_o$ falls to a minimum in 3–5 sec and then slowly recovers (Steinberg et al., 1980). Furthermore, while the light-evoked $[K]_o$ decrease appears to be sufficient to generate the fast oscillation, this light-evoked response involves the interaction between the neural retina and RPE, and other factors may modify or contribute to its generation in situ.

Nevertheless, studies in the chick retina-RPE-choroid preparation support the model of Miller and colleagues for the generation of the fast oscillation in situ (Gallemore and Steinberg, 1993). As illustrated in Figure 9-10, a light-evoked decrease in intracellular Cl activity was measured during the delayed basal membrane hyperpolarization of the fast oscillation. Analysis showed that the time course and magnitude of the light-evoked decrease in a^i_{Cl} can account for the time course and magnitude of the delayed basolateral membrane hyperpolarization. In addition, blockade of the Cl transport pathway also suppressed the delayed basal membrane hyperpolarization and the fast-oscillation trough. An example of suppression with blockade of basolateral membrane Cl channels with DIDS is shown in Figure 9-11.

Light Peak

The light peak is the increase in potential following the fast-oscillation trough and forms the slowest and largest component of the DC ERG (Kris, 1958; Kolder, 1959; Kikawada, 1968; Griff and Steinberg, 1982; Linsen-

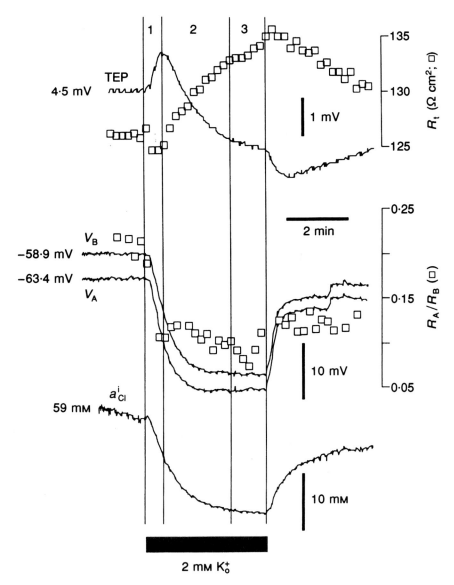

FIGURE 9-9. Changes in TEP, V_{ap}, V_{ba}, and a^i_{Cl} accompanying a step decrease in apical $[K^+]_o$ from 5 to 2 mM in bovine RPE. The response is divided into three phases. Phases 1 and 2 resemble the c-wave hyperpolarization and the delayed basal membrane hyperpolarization respectively, recorded in situ. See text for additional details. (From Joseph and Miller, 1991).

meier and Steinberg, 1982; Valeton and van Norren, 1982; Steinberg et al., 1985). Like the fast oscillation, the light peak also originates from a potential change at the RPE basolateral membrane (Fig. 9-4, Phase 3), but in this case a depolarization is accompanied by an apparent increase in basolateral membrane conductance (Griff and Steinberg, 1982; Linsenmeier and Steinberg, 1982). The light peak does not appear to depend on changes in subretinal $[K]_o$ (Steinberg and Niemeyer, 1981) and cannot be produced in the isolated RPE-choroid by decreasing apical $[K]_o$ from 5 to 2 mM (e.g., Griff and Steinberg, 1984). The signal between the neu-

ral retina and RPE mediating this response remains unknown. Blockage of transmission in the neural retina proximal to the photoreceptors with a number of agents does not suppress the light peak, which supports a photoreceptoral origin for the "light-peak substance" (Gallemore et al., 1988). Possible candidates for the light-peak substance are discussed below, in "Paracrine and Endocrine Signals."

The light-peak voltage is now understood to originate from an increase in basolateral membrane Cl conductance. This conclusion is based on several experimental results obtained in the chick retina-RPE-choroid prepa-

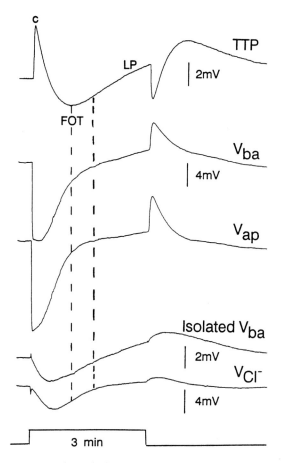

FIGURE 9-10. Light-evoked changes in intracellular Cl activity during the DC-ERG in the isolated chick retina-RPE-choroid preparation. Changes in TTP, V_{ba}, V_{ap}, and V_{Cl^-} were recorded with a double-barrel Cl-selective microelectrode positioned in an RPE cell. The isolated V_{ba} trace was obtained by computer subtraction (Linsenmeier and Steinberg, 1984b). After the onset of illumination, V_{Cl} rapidly fell with the same time course as the delayed hyperpolarization of the basal membrane (see isolated V_{ba} trace), the RPE generator of the FOT. While V_{ba} began to depolarize during the light peak (between the vertical interrupted lines), V_{Cl} was recovering, and after the second vertical line, V_{Cl} began to plateau and no longer followed the time course of the depolarizing isolated V_{ba} trace. In this illustration, the time course of the fast oscillation (TTP) is clearly different than the time course of the delayed basal hyperpolarization seen in the isolated response. This difference is due to other potentials that also modify the time course of the response, namely the transretinal potential (slow PIII) and the changes in apical membrane voltage related to recovery from the c-wave. These contributions are reviewed in detail elsewhere (Steinberg et al., 1985). (From Gallemore and Steinberg, 1993).

ration (Gallemore, 1992; Gallemore and Steinberg, 1989a; 1989b; 1991b; 1993). First, as shown in Figure 9-10, changes in intracellular Cl activity during the light peak were small and could not account for the response. Second, the relative Cl conductance of the basal membrane (T_{Cl}) was found to increase in the light. This was determined by making a rapid decrease in Cl concentration outside the basal membrane to produce Cl diffusion

potentials before and during the light peak. As shown in Figure 9-12, the Cl diffusion potential increased in amplitude during the light peak, providing direct evidence for an increase in the relative Cl conductance of the basal membrane. The relative Cl conductance of the basal membrane (T_{Cl}) was estimated to increase an average of 55% during the light peak (Gallemore and Steinberg, 1993), and the light peak was suppressed by the Cl channel blocker DIDS (Fig. 9-11). Finally, the reversal potential of the conductance that increases during the light peak was found to equal the chloride equilibrium potential (E_{Cl}), and shifting E_{Cl} shifted the reversal potential of the "light peak conductance" in the same direction (Gallemore and Steinberg, 1993).

The data indicate that an increase in basolateral membrane Cl conductance generates the light-peak voltage. The slow time course of the light peak suggests that the increase in Cl conductance is probably mediated by a second messenger. In RPE cells from several species, the Cl conductance of the basal membrane may be modulated by changes in the intracellular activity of Ca^{2+} or cyclic AMP (Hughes et al., 1988; Joseph and Miller, 1989; 1992; Lin and Miller, 1991; Nao-i et al., 1990a; Gallemore and Steinberg, 1990; Hughes and Segawa, 1993; Ueda and Steinberg, 1994; Gallemore et al., 1995). In frog RPE-choroid tissues (Hughes et al., 1988), cultured human RPE (Hu et al., 1995; Gallemore et al., 1995), and native human RPE (Quinn and Miller, 1993), elevating cAMP depolarizes the basolateral membrane by increasing the Cl conductance of that membrane. In contrast, in fresh chick and bovine preparations, cAMP hyperpolarizes the basal membrane and decreases its conductance by closing basal membrane Cl channels (Nao-i et al., 1990a; Kuntz et al., 1994; Peterson and Miller, 1995b). These opposite effects of cAMP on RPE voltage and resistance in species that have similar light peaks, argue against cAMP as the intracellular messenger for the light peak. Intracellular pH is also known to modify the conductance of some ion channels (Roos and Boron, 1981; Stoddard and Reuss, 1989), and given the evidence for pH-sensitive Cl channels in other cells (e.g., Bretag, 1987), pH could also regulate the Cl conductance of the RPE (Edelman et al., 1994). Thus, changes in intracellular Ca^{2+} or pH could lead to activation of the light peak conductance and future research will focus on determining the role of these two messengers in the "light-peak cascade."

Summary of DC ERG Mechanisms

Figure 9-13 presents a diagrammatic summary of current knowledge regarding the generation of each component of the DC ERG. Each response is summarized below.

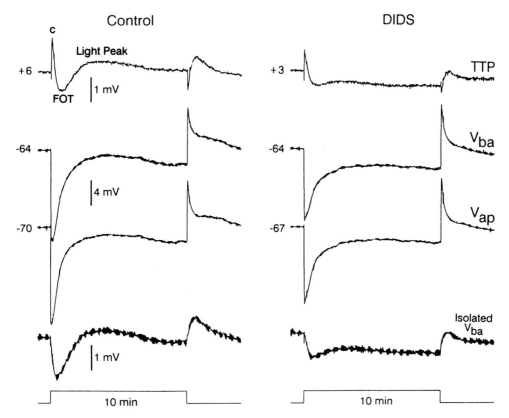

FIGURE 9-11. Intracellular recording of the DC-ERG in response to 10 min. steps of diffuse illumination before and 20 min. after perfusion of the basal membrane with 500 μM 4,4'-diisothiocyanostilbene-2,2'-disulfonate (DIDS). The intracellular DC-ERG consists of the c-wave hyperpolarization of V_{ap} (V_{ba} also hyperpolarizes, probably due to the presence of intercellular junctional complexes that electrically couple the apical and basolateral membranes), the delayed basal membrane hyperpolarization of the FOT, and, last, the slow basal depolarization of the light peak. Basal membrane voltage changes are seen most clearly in the isolated V_{ba} responses obtained by scaling and subtracting the apical response from the basal response. In DIDS, the delayed basal hyperpolarization and the light-peak depolarization were suppressed. (From Gallemore and Steinberg, 1993).

C-wave. The c-wave is generated directly by a light-evoked decrease in subretinal $[K]_o$ resulting from changes in photoreceptor activity. This $[K]_o$ change hyperpolarizes the apical membrane of the RPE and distal processes of Müller cells, generating the RPE c-wave and slow PIII, respectively. The decrease in apical $[K]_o$ also slows the apical Na/K pump, which contributes an underlying membrane depolarization. As a result of the apical and basolateral membrane hyperpolarizations and Na/K pump inhibition, the transmembrane fluxes of ions, metabolites, and fluid are altered (see Chapter 6).

Fast-oscillation trough. The light-evoked $[K]_o$ decrease underlying the c-wave also generates the fast-oscillation of the DC ERG. This is caused by a $\Delta[K]_o$-induced slowing of the apical Na,K,2Cl cotransporter, which decreases net Cl uptake and reduces intracellular Cl activity. This changes the Cl equilibrium potential across the basolateral membrane Cl channel, causing a hyperpolarization of the basolateral membrane.

Light peak. The light-peak voltage originates as a depolarization of the basolateral membrane accompanied by an increase in its conductance. The mechanism is an increase in basolateral membrane Cl conductance. This response may be triggered by a neuromodulator released by the photoreceptors or possibly other retinal cells. The intracellular messenger leading to activation of the Cl channel remains unknown. Cyclic AMP does not appear to mediate the response. Likely candidates include Ca^{2+} and pH, but other second messengers need to be considered as well.

Species Differences

It was noted from the earliest investigations of the DC ERG that significant differences were present between species (Kikawada, 1968). The greatest difference is in the apparent absence of the fast oscillation and light peak in amphibians. Lower vertebrates appeared to exhibit only the c-wave component, while reptiles, birds,

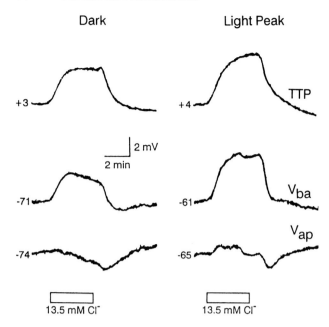

FIGURE 9-12. Intracellular recording of TTP, V_{ba}, and V_{ap} in chick RPE during decreases in $[Cl]_o$ in the basal bath from 134.6 to 13.5 mM in the dark and at the light peak. All records were obtained from the same cell. The tissue was exposed to the low Cl solution (gluconate substitution) for 3.5 min. (From Gallemore and Steinberg, 1993).

and mammals exhibited all three components. More recent studies suggest that these differences may only reflect the relative magnitude of the responses, not their complete absence. Griff (Griff and Bossano, 1990; Griff, 1991) was able to record a fast oscillation and light peak in an in vitro toad preparation (*Bufo marinus*). The difficulty of recording the basolateral membrane contributions in lower vertebrates may reflect a smaller resting Cl conductance at the basolateral membrane (Fujii et al., 1992; Gallemore et al., 1993).

Clinical Significance

In humans, the fast oscillation and light peak are recorded in the electrooculogram (EOG). In combination with the "clinical ERG" (recording of the a- and b-waves), which can be used to assess specific aspects of neural retinal function, the EOG is used in the diagnosis and follow-up of a number of specific diseases known to affect the RPE and of other diseases whose pathogeneses are not known but which may involve the photoreceptors, RPE, or their interactions (see Chapter 10 and Marmor, 1979; Marmor and Lurie, 1979; Weleber, 1989). Both the fast oscillation and light peak are now

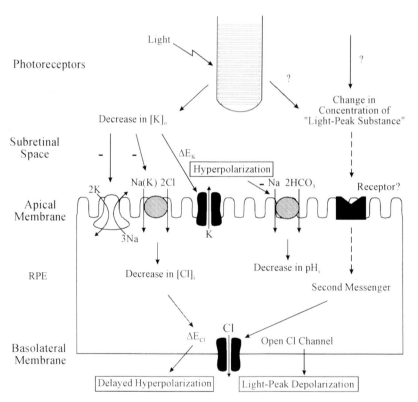

FIGURE 9-13. Summary of mechanisms of light-evoked electrical responses of the RPE. The sequence of steps leading to each response is shown.

considered to reflect changes in RPE Cl transport pathways. This knowledge can now be applied to disease mechanisms. In fact, Miller et al. (1992) recently studied these responses in patients with cystic fibrosis, a disease that results from mutations in the gene that codes for cAMP-activated Cl channels in many epithelia—the cystic fibrosis transmembrane conductance regulator (CFTR) (Collins, 1992; Fuller and Benos, 1992; Frizzell, 1995). EOG measurements in these patients revealed a suppressed fast oscillation with a normal light peak, raising the possibility that the two EOG responses involve different types of Cl channels or regulatory pathways and that the light peak is not mediated by CFTR. In airway epithelia, for example, cAMP and Ca^{2+} activate different Cl channels (Anderson and Welsh, 1991). The possible role of Cl transport defects in other diseases where the EOG is altered remains to be determined. Chapter 10 provides a more detailed review of the clinical application of the ERG responses of the RPE.

PARACRINE AND ENDOCRINE SIGNALS

Receptors and Second Messengers

Light-induced modulation of RPE transport must be mediated by a variety of paracrine and endocrine signals that continuously impinge upon the RPE apical and basolateral membranes. These signals are thought to regulate the transport of metabolites into and out of the distal retina, by activating apical or basolateral membrane receptors that modulate transport mechanisms in the RPE via second messengers such as calcium, cAMP, and phosphatydylinositol metabolites. Recently, extensive reviews of RPE receptors have been published by Nash and Osborne (1996) and by Campachioro and colleagues (1996 and see Chapter 23), but most of this information comes from cultured cells, whose phenotype may differ from native, intact epithelia (see Burke, Chapter 5) and in most cases the apical or basolateral membrane location of these receptors is not known. Moreover, relatively little is known about how these receptors work individually or in concert to modulate RPE function.

Several neuromodulators have been found to affect RPE transport physiology in the intact, native tissue. Neurotransmitters have been found that are stored and released by retinal neurons or hormones present in the circulation and that modulate RPE membrane voltage and resistance, fluid and ion transport and, in lower vertebrates, pigment granule migration. In some cases, effects have been localized to specific membrane receptors on the apical or basolateral membranes and the second messenger systems coupled to these receptors have been defined. Here we review several of the major agents found to affect RPE physiology in intact preparations.

Dopamine

Dopamine is the predominant catecholamine in the vertebrate retina (Ehinger, 1983). It is principally stored and released by neurons, particularly those in the interplexiform layer, and in lower vertebrates it is thought to function in modulating center-surround balance under conditions of light and dark adaptation (Piccolino et al., 1984; Witkovsky et al., 1987; Dacey, 1988). Dopamine receptors in the distal retina may be best known for mediating retinomotor movements in lower vertebrates (Dearry and Burnside, 1988a; 1988b). In the green sunfish, D2 receptors mediate light-adaptive RPE pigment dispersion, rod elongation and cone contraction. D2 receptors are negatively coupled to adenylate cyclase, and a reduction in intracellular cAMP appears to mediate these effects. In frog RPE, D1 receptors mediate RPE pigment migration via elevation of cAMP (Dearry et al., 1990).

In higher vertebrates, the effects of exogenous dopamine on RPE transport appear to result from cross reaction with adrenergic receptors. In bovine RPE, for example, dopamine can activate apical membrane alpha-1 adrenergic receptors and produce electrical effects similar to epinephrine (Joseph and Miller, 1992). Additional effects presumably include reduction of apical membrane K conductance and stimulation of fluid transport. At physiologic concentrations, however, epinephrine is the more active agonist (Joseph and Miller, 1992).

In the isolated perfused cat eye, dopamine produces an increase in the standing potential, presumably by depolarizing the RPE basolateral membrane and increasing the TEP (Dawis and Niemeyer, 1986). The specific receptors mediating these effects were not identified, but are likely adrenergic, since physiologic concentrations of norepinephrine had similar effects (Dawis and Niemeyer, 1988). In chick RPE, the effects of dopamine are more complex (Gallemore and Steinberg, 1990). In most chick retina-RPE-choroid preparations, dopamine added to the retinal or choroidal side produced a transient hyperpolarization of the basal membrane associated with a conductance decrease; this response was inhibited by DIDS, suggesting that it arose from a reduction in basal membrane Cl conductance. In other tissues, however, a basal membrane depolarization accompanied by a conductance increase was observed. This was also blocked by DIDS, suggesting an increase in Cl conductance. Chick RPE cells appear to express both beta-2 and alpha-1 adrenergic receptors, and the complexity of dopamine's effects may relate to variable expression and activity of these receptors (Gallemore and Steinberg, 1990).

An important observation, first made in the isolated perfused cat eye, is that dopamine can suppress the light peak of the DC ERG (Dawis and Niemeyer, 1986). This observation led to the proposal that dopamine may be the light peak substance. Dopamine also suppressed the light peak in chick, but interestingly, this suppression was dependent on the net change in TEP it produced (Gallemore and Steinberg, 1990). Even with large, transient changes in TEP, if dopamine produced little net change in standing potential, the light peak amplitude was not affected significantly. The light peak also survived conditions found to block dopamine release in other preparations (low Ca^{2+}, cobalt), also arguing against this role (Gallemore et al., 1988; Gallemore and Steinberg, 1991a). Because the effects of dopamine appear to be species dependent, but the light peak response is similar in all preparations, it seems unlikely that dopamine is the light peak substance (Gallemore and Steinberg, 1990).

Epinephrine

Epinephrine may function as a neurotransmitter in the vertebrate retina. It is localized to specific retinal neurons and released following light onset (Haggendal and Malmfors, 1965; Hadjiconstantinou et al., 1983; 1984; Dacey, 1988; Dearry and Burnside, 1989). Interest in the effect of epinephrine on the RPE (Frambach et al., 1988a; 1988b; Joseph and Miller, 1988) was sparked by the observation that a variety of catecholamines increased the standing potential and c-wave, and suppressed the light peak in the isolated perfused cat eye (Dawis and Niemeyer, 1986; 1988).

In the bovine RPE-choroid preparation, epinephrine was found to be the most potent of catecholamines in effecting RPE voltage and resistance (epinephrine > norepinephrine > dopamine). Epinephrine activates apical membrane alpha-1 adrenergic receptors, which appear to be coupled to an increase in intracellular [Ca^{2+}] and the opening of basolateral membrane Cl channels (Joseph and Miller, 1992; Lin and Miller, 1991a). Figure 9-14 illustrates the effects of 10^{-8} M epinephrine on electrical parameters (A) under control conditions, (B) in the presence of an alpha-1-selective adrenergic receptor antagonist, prazosin (10^{-7} M), and (C) following recovery. Epinephrine also was found to stimulate fluid absorption across the isolated bovine RPE-choroid (Edelman and Miller, 1991; 1992; Edelman and Miller, 1996). This increase in fluid absorption was found to be coupled to the stimulation of KCl absorption.

Joseph and Miller (1992) proposed epinephrine as a candidate molecule for the light peak substance. There is some evidence that this catecholamine is released by retinal neurons at light onset (Dacey, 1988). It could then diffuse to the RPE, bind to apical membrane alpha-1 adrenergic receptors, elevate intracellular Ca^{2+}, and activate basal membrane Cl channels. Evidence against this hypothesis is that the effects of alpha-1 receptor stimulation are species dependent. In rabbit and chick, epinephrine decreases the TEP, in contrast to the increase observed in bovine (Frambach et al., 1988a; 1988b; Gallemore and Steinberg, 1990). In addition, conditions that block catecholamine release and synaptic transmission in the inner retina do not suppress the light peak (Gallemore et al., 1988). There is currently no in vivo evidence to support the idea that epinephrine

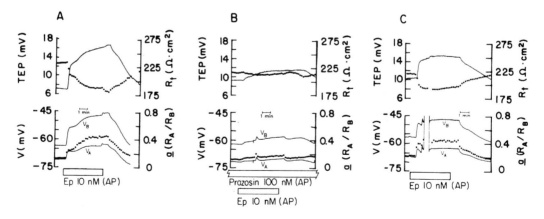

FIGURE 9-14. Effects of epinephrine and prazosin on membrane voltage and resistance in bovine RPE. (A) Control response. (B) Epinephrine response after pretreatment of tissue with 100 nM prazosin. (C) Following control. (From Joseph and Miller, 1992).

is the paracrine signal that mediates the light peak response.

Activation of adrenergic receptors by epinephrine also has been observed in freshly isolated fetal human RPE (Quinn and Miller, 1992). Adrenergic agents, including epinephrine, have been implicated in clinical conditions where defects in RPE transport may be a contributing factor. These include cystoid macular edema (CME) and central serous retinopathy (CSR) (Kolker and Becker, 1968; Bird, 1994). The alpha-1 adrenergic receptors described may play a functional role in these disease states. There is a discrepancy, however, since CME and CSR are associated with an increase in subretinal fluid, but epinephrine stimulates fluid absorption. Long-term treatment with epinephrine, however, may cause the down regulation of receptors, leading to the inhibition of tonic fluid absorption. Alternatively, epinephrine may act by altering choroidal perfusion. Further work is required to elucidate the contribution of adrenergic receptors to these clinical entities.

In addition to alpha-1 adrenergic receptors, beta or beta-2 adrenergic receptors have been identified in several preparations of RPE. These include embryonic chick RPE, postnatal (1–4 weeks) chick RPE, cultured fetal human RPE, and native fetal human RPE (Koh and Chader, 1984; Friedman et al., 1987; Tran, 1992). In cultured and native fetal human RPE, beta adrenergic receptor activation increases the basal membrane Cl conductance, depolarizing the basal membrane and decreasing its resistance (Frambach et al., 1990; Quinn and Miller, 1993; Hu et al., 1995; Gallemore et al., 1995). Studies in single cells using the whole-cell recording configuration of the patch-clamp technique revealed that cAMP and beta-adrenergic receptor activation with isoproterenol activate an outwardly rectifying Cl conductance (M. Takahira and B. Hughes, unpublished observations). While molecular studies have provided evidence for alpha-1 adrenergic receptors in cultured human RPE (Moroi-Fetters et al., 1995), the predominant electrophysiologic effects in cultured fetal human RPE were mediated by the beta-2 adrenergic receptor. As discussed earlier, there may be developmental regulation of adrenergic receptor expression and activity in the RPE. Receptor expression may be modulated by other factors as well. Adrenergic receptors may contribute to physiologic and pathophysiologic mechanisms of RPE function, but their precise roles in human disease remain unclear.

Melatonin

Melatonin is an indolamine hormone synthesized by retinal neurons, and photoreceptor cells may be one source (Pang et al., 1980; Wiechman et al., 1985; 1986; Besharse et al., 1988). In some species, melatonin is thought to participate in circadian changes in retinal function; in frog, for example, it induces cone elongation and RPE pigment aggregation in darkness (for reviews see Besharse et al., 1988; Wiechmann, 1986). Melatonin may also be essential for a process of "dark priming" that precedes photoreceptor disc shedding and RPE phagocytosis (Besharse et al., 1988).

The likely presence of metatonin receptors on the RPE raises the possibility that melatonin may modulate RPE transport as well. In the isolated perfused cat eye, melatonin was found to increase the standing potential, increase the c-wave, and suppress the light peak (Dawis and Niemeyer, 1988). These effects of melatonin were qualitatively similar to those of norepinephrine and seratonin, but smaller in magnitude. To identify the origin of these effects, melatonin was studied in the chick retinal-RPE-choroid preparation (Nao-i et al., 1990b). Melatonin was found to have effects dissimilar to those in cat. Choroidal melatonin hyperpolarized the basal membrane, increased its apparent resistance and decreased the ERG c-wave, consistent with the inhibition of basal membrane Cl channels. Retinal melatonin first depolarized the apical membrane and increased its apparent resistance and this gave way to a basal membrane hyperpolarization and apparent increase in basal membrane resistance. Experiments on isolated RPE-choroid preparations suggested that the effects of choroidal melatonin were independent of the neural retina, while the retinal effect was more complex and probably included a neural retinal component. Effects of melatonin on the light peak were small, arguing against a role in generating the light-evoked response.

Adenosine

In the central nervous system, adenosine is involved in synaptic transmission, regulation of vascular tone, and recovery from ischemic injury (Phillis and Wu, 1981; Dragunow and Faull, 1988). Anatomical studies have been used to localize adenosine receptors in the retina. Adenosine A1 receptors were found in the inner plexiform layer and A2 receptors were localized to the RPE and photoreceptors (Blazynski and Perez, 1991). While the functional roles of adenosine in the retina have not been fully characterized, some of the effects of adenosine on RPE physiology have been studied. In the isolated perfused cat eye, adenosine increases the standing potential, increases the c-wave amplitude, and suppresses the light peak (Blazynski et al., 1989). These observations were corroborated and extended in the in vitro chick retina preparation, where retinal adenosine was found to depolarize the basal membrane and in- crease its apparent conductance (Maruiwa et al., 1995). The Cl$^-$ channel blocker DIDS suppressed the effects of adenosine. Taken together, these studies suggest that adenosine release from the inner retina may bind to A2 receptors on the RPE and activate basal membrane Cl$^-$ channels. Adenosine could play a role in light/dark in- teractions between the retina and RPE. Further studies will be needed to understand the role of adenosine in regulating RPE physiology.

Other Signals

In addition to the neuromodulators described above, other ions and molecules may also modulate RPE trans- port in light and darkness. In addition to K, the sub- retinal concentrations of a number of other ions also change during the transition between light and dark. A light-evoked alkalinization of the subretinal space has been measured in the frog retina (Borgula et al., 1989) as well as in the intact cat eye (Yamamoto et al., 1992). This response was maximal outside the outer nuclear layer, where photoreceptor cells are most densely packed. An example of the light-evoked alkalinization measured in the subretinal space is shown in Figure 9- 15. The light-evoked alkalinization of the distal retina likely reflects a light-evoked inhibition of aerobic gly- colysis by the photoreceptors (Yamamoto et al., 1992). There might also be contributions from a $\Delta[K]_o$-induced decrease in RPE NaHCO$_3$ cotransport (Lin and Miller, 1991b), but this is likely to be small since the alkalin- ization falls off significantly as the RPE is approached.

The light-evoked alkalinization may have functional significance. For example, the photoreceptors and RPE interact across the subretinal space where they are sepa- rated by the interphotoreceptor matrix (IPM). The IPM consists of polyanionic molecules such as glycosamino- glycans that may undergo pH-induced conformational changes. Thus, the discovery of light/dark changes in the distribution of IPM constituents (Uehara et al., 1990) may be related to light/dark changes in extracellular pH (Yamamoto et al., 1992).

Several light-evoked changes in subretinal space Ca^{2+} have been recorded as well. The best known is the Ca^{2+} increase that results from light/dark changes in Ca^{2+} fluxes across the outer segment. This was origi- nally recorded in isolated retinas and single photore- ceptor cells (Gold and Korenbrot, 1980; Yoshikami et al., 1980; Gobradovski et al., 1987; Miller and Koren- brot, 1987). In the intact cat eye, frog eyecup, and chick retina-RPE preparation, an increase in subretinal calci- um content was accompanied by a slow, sustained de- crease in calcium concentration (Gallemore and Stein- berg, 1988; Livsey et al., 1990; Gallemore et al., 1994a;

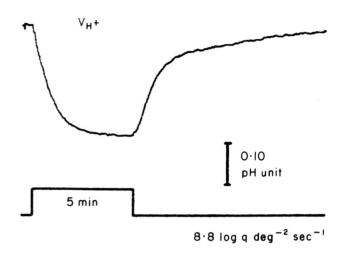

FIGURE 9-15. Light-evoked alkalization in response to 5 min of illu- mination at 8.8 log quanta. This response was obtained with a low resistance microelectrode, so that differencing artifacts at stimulus onset and offset were essentially eliminated by cross-capacitance com- pensation. (From Yamamoto et al., 1992).

Li et al., 1994a, 1994b). In cat, this decrease could be 1 mM or larger (Fig. 9-16) and was maximal near the RPE. One factor contributing to this response is the light-evoked hydration of the subretinal space (Huang and Karwoski, 1989; 1992; Li et al., 1994a; 1994b). Other mechanisms include Ca^{2+} uptake by the RPE and Ca^{2+} binding by components of the IPM (see Gallemore et al., 1994 for further discussion).

Irrespective of the mechanisms, the light-evoked $[Ca^{2+}]_o$ decrease in the distal retina may have signifi- cance for photoreceptor function. Phototransduction is mediated by an enzymatic cascade that leads to the hy- drolysis of cGMP and closure of cGMP-sensitive cation channels in the outer segment membrane (for reviews see Yau, 1994; Koutalos and Yau, 1993). Variations in extracellular and intracellular Ca^{2+} are known to affect the mechanisms of phototransduction and light adapta- tion, as well as synaptic transmission between photore- ceptors and second-order neurons (for reviews see Fain and Matthews, 1990; Koch, 1992). Thus, the RPE may help regulate the adaptive state of the retina by modu- lating subretinal Ca^{2+} in light and darkness. Further work on the cellular mechanisms of Ca^{2+} transport in the RPE will help clarify the mechanisms regulating sub- retinal $[Ca^{2+}]_o$.

Light-induced changes in the subretinal space con- centrations of Na and Cl have also been recorded (Dimi- triev et al., 1996). The Na increase presumably reflects, in part, the cessation of Na influx through light-sensitive channels. The Cl decrease reflects, in part, the light- evoked hydration of subretinal space volume. The effect of these ion concentration changes on RPE transport re- main to be investigated.

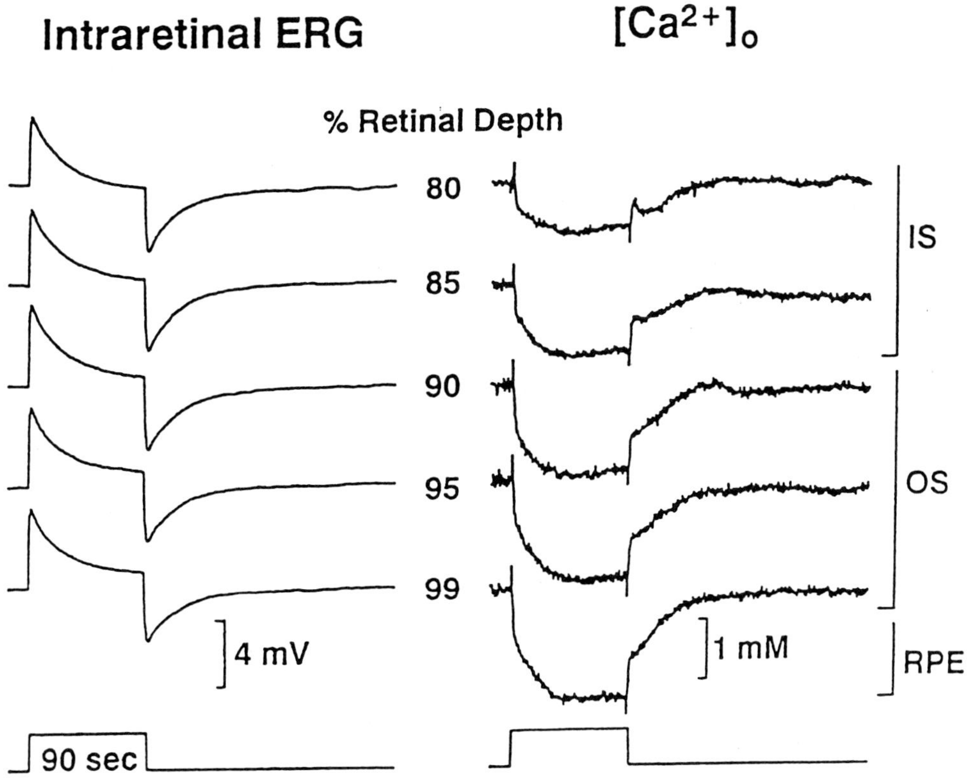

Intraretinal ERG

$[Ca^{2+}]_o$

% Retinal Depth

FIGURE 9-16. Light-evoked changes in $[Ca^{2+}]_o$ and intraretinal ERGs as a function of depth in the subretinal space. Responses are to 90-second steps of diffuse white light delivered at rod saturation (8.2 log quanta/deg^2/s), as indicated by the stimulus marker. The electrode was advanced to 80% retinal depth, and the first response was recorded near the outer limiting membrane which forms the proximal border of the subretinal space. Other responses were recorded at successively more distal retinal depths as the electrode was advanced through the retina in 3 μm steps. The maximal response was recorded in the most distal portion of the subretinal space, at a depth of 99%. The electrode penetrated the RPE at 100% retinal depth. The dark-adapted Ca^{2+} concentration gradient was measured in this retina, allowing conversion of the V_{Ca}^{2+} signals to concentration. The intraretinal ERG is dominated by slow PIII, the retinal ERG c-wave, the amplitude of which remained constant, confirming the subretinal location of the Ca^{2+}-sensitive microelectrode. (From Gallemore et al., 1994).

Transport mechanisms for GABA, taurine, and other organic molecules whose concentration may change in light and darkness have also been localized to the RPE (e.g., Scharschmidt et al., 1988; Peterson and Miller, 1995a). These mechanisms are typically present in the apical membrane and they may help regulate the levels of these signaling molecules in the subretinal space. The RPE may act as both a reservoir and source for these agents. The transport of these molecules and the relative effects of light and darkness are reviewed in Chapter 6.

LIGHT-EVOKED MODULATION OF SUBRETINAL VOLUME

In vitro studies have demonstrated that the apical membrane Na,K,2Cl cotransporter, apical membrane K channel, and basolateral membrane K and Cl channels are all important determinants of RPE cell volume (Adorante and Miller, 1990; Bialek and Miller, 1994; Kennedy, 1994; Adorante, 1995). It has been shown that decreasing apical $[K]_o$ from 5 to 2 mM produces an increase in KCl efflux, a decrease or reversal in Na,K,2CL cotransport (Bialek and Miller, 1994), and a decrease in RPE cell volume (Adorante and Miller, 1990). These findings suggested the possibility that illumination of the retina in situ could result in a significant increase in the volume of the subretinal space, which has subsequently been observed (Huang and Karwoski, 1989; 1992; Li et al., 1994a; 1994b). Changes in subretinal volume will not only affect the concentration of ions and metabolites outside the photoreceptor outer segments, but may also alter the state of hydration of the interphotoreceptor matrix (IPM), affecting retinal adhesion (Marmor, 1994) and other photoreceptor-RPE interactions.

In Vitro Measurements

Light-evoked changes in subretinal volume have been demonstrated using ion-selective microelectrodes (ISMs) to monitor changes in the extracellular concentration of ionic probes that serve as extracellular space markers. In a study on the frog retina-in-eyecup preparation, Huang and Karwoski (1989; 1992) superfused the retina with the relatively cell-impermeant cation tetramethylammonium (TMA, 10 mM) and then used K-selective microelectrodes to measure light-evoked changes in the concentration of this ion after it had equilibrated in the subretinal space. K-sensitive electrodes can be used to accurately measure the concentration of TMA without interference from K, because their selectivity for TMA is nearly two hundred times greater than for K. Figure 9-17 shows that illumination of the frog retina produced a decrease in subretinal $[TMA]_o$ (left panel), which became larger with increasing light intensity. These $[TMA]_o$ changes are converted into changes in extracellular volume in the panel on the right, which indicates a light-evoked expansion of subretinal space with a saturating response of approximately 7% at 8 log units. An underlying assumption of this conversion is that the decreases in $[TMA]_o$ are due to expansion of the subretinal space and not to light-evoked uptake of TMA by retinal cells. In fact, TMA has been shown to be taken up by RPE cells (Adorante and Miller, 1990). However, when other probe cations and anions were used,

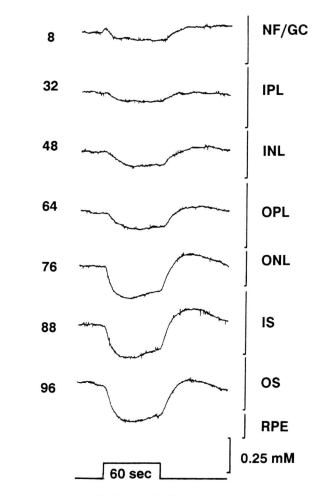

FIGURE 9-18. Depth distribution of light-evoked changes of $[TMA^+]_o$ in chick retina in response to 60 seconds of illumination. Depth profiles were obtained by moving the microelectrode from retina to RPE and stopping at selected depths to record $[TMA^+]_o$ changes. Calculated percentage changes in the extracellular concentration of TMA^+ are shown on the right. Illumination is 6×10^{-5} W/cm² in this and all other figures in this chapter unless indicated. Relationship of retinal depth to position of retinal layers as obtained in previous histological studies (Gallemore and Steinberg, unpublished observation). (NF/GC), nerve fiber–ganglion cell layer; (OPL), outer plexiform layer; (ONL), outer nuclear layer; (IS), inner segments of photoreceptors; (OS), outer segments; (RPE), retinal pigment epithelium. (From Li et al., 1994a).

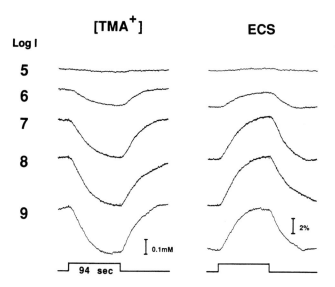

FIGURE 9-17. Light-evoked changes in subretinal space (SRS), $[TMA^+]$, and extracellular space (ECS) as a function of light intensity ($\log_{10}I = 3.2 \times 10^6$ lux). In the ECS plots, an upward shift corresponds to an expansion of ECS volume. Superfusate $[TMA^+]$ was 10.0 mM. Baseline $[TMA^+]$ in SRS was 5.3 mM; baseline ESC = 100%. See text for additional details. (From Huang and Karwoski, 1992).

light-evoked concentration changes were of similar polarity and magnitude, strongly suggesting that the $[TMA]_o$ response indeed reflects changes in extracellular volume.

Figure 9-18 illustrates a depth profile of light-evoked changes in $[TMA]_o$ in the chick neural retina-RPE-choroid preparation (Li et al., 1994a). The response is dominated by a light-evoked decrease in $[TMA]_o$, which increases in amplitude from more proximal to distal retina and is maximal in the subretinal space near the RPE. The response in chick is similar in magnitude and waveform to that in frog, although the time course is significantly faster, as might be expected for a preparation from a warm-blooded animal.

With maintained illumination of the chick retina, the $[TMA]_o$ decrease was transient and returned to the dark-adapted baseline in about 3 minutes (not shown). The transient nature of the $[TMA]_o$ decrease seems to be due to TMA diffusion, which tends to equilibrate the concentration gradient across the retina. When a mathematical model of TMA diffusion (Govardovskii et al., 1994) was used to estimate the light-evoked changes in subretinal hydration from changes in $[TMA]_o$, the inferred volume changes were 2.2 to 3.8 times larger and more prolonged than the responses derived directly from $[TMA]_o$ changes, with a peak subretinal volume expansion of about 20%.

In Vivo Measurements

Light-evoked changes in subretinal $[TMA]_o$ have also been measured in the intact cat retina, where TMA loading of the retina was achieved by intravitreal injection (Li et al., 1994b). Retinal illumination produced a decrease in $[TMA]_o$, which was maximal near the RPE. The TMA response in cat also was transient and resembled the light-evoked $[TMA]_o$ decreases recorded in frog and chick, but it was considerably larger in amplitude—about 22% compared with 7%. Analysis of these $[TMA]_o$ changes with the diffusion model predicted that the subretinal volume in cat increases by an average of 63%, compared with the volume increase of 20% calculated for frog and chick. In the intact cat eye, this volume expansion can last for minutes.

Contributions of RPE Transport Mechanisms

The possibility that alterations in net ion and fluid transport across the RPE could cause the light-evoked changes in subretinal space volume was investigated in both in vitro frog and chick preparations. In their studies on the frog eyecup preparation, Huang and Karwoski (1989; 1992) found that retinal furosemide had no effect on the light-evoked decrease in subretinal $[TMA]_o$ and that retinal bumetanide either had no effect or it depressed all retinal functions. In chick, it was found that inhibiting Cl uptake across the apical membrane by the Na,K,2Cl cotransporter with bumetanide or furosemide reduced the size of the light-evoked de-

crease in $[TMA]_o$ by more than 50%. These results in chick support the notion that the Na,K,2Cl cotransporter not only regulates the volume of the RPE cell, but also the volume of the subretinal space. The negative result in frog may reflect the perfusion limitations of the eyecup preparation.

The involvement of the apical membrane K conductance and the basolateral membrane Cl conductance in retinal hydration was proposed by Huang and Karwoski (1992) on the basis of their observation that the light-evoked decrease in subretinal $[TMA]_o$ was partially inhibited by retinal Ba^{2+}. In bovine RPE, decreases in apical $[K]_o$ produced large increases in the electrochemical driving forces for conductive K and Cl exit across the apical and basolateral membranes, respectively (Bialek and Miller, 1994). Because the K and Cl conductances are electrically coupled, blocking either the apical K conductance with Ba^{2+} or the basolateral membrane Cl conductance with DIDS significantly reduced the apical $\Delta[K]_o$-induced efflux of KCl. These in vitro data led to the prediction that RPE cell volume would be decreased in situ by an amount comparable to the light-induced increase in subretinal space volume, and that these changes in RPE and subretinal volume would be decreased by blockade of either of the conductances. This prediction is supported by in situ data obtained from the chick retina-RPE-choroid preparation. It was shown that either retinal Ba^{2+} or basal DIDS inhibited the light-evoked decrease in subretinal $[TMA]_o$ (Li et al., 1994a), indicating that a portion of the cell water lost from the RPE contributes to subretinal hydration.

It is possible that other RPE transport mechanisms are involved. For example, Huang and Karwoski (1992) showed in frog retina that the light-evoked decrease in subretinal $[TMA]_o$ was partially inhibited by retinal amiloride (2 mM), suggesting that the Na/H exchanger in the RPE apical membrane might play a role in the light-evoked hydration of subretinal space. Interestingly, superfusing the retina with DIDS (1 mM) had no effect on the TMA response, suggesting that the $NaHCO_3$ cotransporter in the RPE apical membrane does not participate in the light-evoked decrease in subretinal volume. This result is not definitive, however, since DIDS may not have reached the RPE apical membrane in sufficient concentration to block the cotransporter.

In summary, two mechanisms for the light-evoked hydration of the subretinal space have been identified. First, the light-evoked decrease in subretinal $[K]_o$ causes a slowing of the Na,K,2Cl cotransporter in the RPE apical membrane, resulting in a decrease in the solute-linked movement of water from the subretinal space into the RPE cell. Second, the decrease in subretinal $[K]_o$ also stimulates a massive efflux of KCl from the RPE cell, causing a reduction in RPE cell volume; evidently, some of the lost cell water moves out across the apical membrane and into the subretinal space. Future experiments should ascertain whether the transport of other osmotically active solutes, such as lactate, may be involved in this process (Kenyon et al., 1994).

SUMMARY

We now have a relatively detailed understanding of some of the cellular mechanisms that underlie the RPE-dependent electrical responses recorded in the DC ERG. The c-wave, fast oscillation, and light peak all originate from a light-induced interaction between the RPE and the photoreceptors and involve the modulation of specific ion-transport mechanisms at the apical and/or basolateral membranes of the RPE cell. The c-wave involves apical membrane K channels, whereas the fast oscillation and light peak are generated by the Cl transport pathway, which mainly consists of two transport proteins, the apical membrane Na,K,Cl cotransporter and the basolateral membrane Cl channel. The Cl transport pathway has several distinct functions, including the regulation of RPE and subretinal volume and the absorption of fluid and ions out of the subretinal space. Both the c-wave and the fast oscillation are produced by the light-evoked decrease in subretinal K concentration. However, the specific events that initiate the light-peak response remain to be determined, but most likely involve a paracrine signal or signals from the retina, the activation of RPE apical membrane receptors, and the generation of intracellular messengers. There are undoubtedly a host of neurotransmitters and neuromodulators that are released by retinal neurons during the light and dark, which, along with hormones present in the choroidal blood, could help regulate RPE function. The presence of receptors for an array of neuromodulators provides support for the idea that RPE function is modulated by paracrine and hormonal molecules. Although the effects of select signaling molecules on RPE transport have been investigated, in most cases it remains to be shown if these putative paracrine or hormonal signals are released in sufficient quantities to reach the RPE apical or basolateral membranes by diffusion through the extracellular spaces on either side of the epithelium. It is of particular interest to identify the specific intercellular signals that mediate communication among the cells that border the subretinal space: the RPE, the photoreceptors and the Müller cells. These signaling molecules presumably coordinate the transport activity of all three cell types and thereby determine the chemical composition and hydration of the subretinal space, in addition to allowing the RPE to help modulate its phagocytic activity.

ACKNOWLEDGMENTS

The writing of this review was supported by NIH grants EY-02205 (SSM), EY-08850 (BAH), the RP Foundation Fighting Blindness (BAH), a Stein/Oppenheimer Research Grant (RPG), the Jules Stein Eye Institute (JSEI) Stella-Joseph Research Endowment (RPG), and the JSEI Patricia Morrison Fund (RPG). It is our pleasure to thank Roy Steinberg, Rob Linsenmeier, and Victor Govardovsky for their thoughtful comments on various portions of the manuscript.

REFERENCES

Adorante JS. 1995. Regulatory volume decrease in frog retinal pigment epithelium. Am J Physiol 268:C89–100 (with erratum following table of contents).

Adorante J, Miller S. 1990. Potassium-dependent volume regulation in retinal pigment epithelium is mediated by Na,K,Cl cotransport. J Gen Physiol 96:1153–1176.

Anderson M, Welsh M. 1991. Calcium and cAMP activate different chloride channels in the apical membrane of normal and cystic fibrosis epithelia. Proc Nat Acad Sci USA 88:6003–6007.

Armington JC. 1974. The Electroretinogram. New York: Academic Press.

Besharse J, Iuvone P, Pierce M. 1988. Regulation of rhythmic photoreceptor metabolism: a role for post-receptoral neurons. In: Osborne N, Chader G (eds), Progress in Retinal Research, vol. 7. Oxford: Pergamon Press, 21–61.

Bialek S, Miller S. 1994. K^+ and Cl^- transport mechanisms in bovine pigment epithelium that could modulate subretinal space volume and composition. J Physiol (Lond) 475:40–17.

Bialek S, Joseph D, Miller S. 1995. The delayed basolateral membrane hyperpolarization of the bovine retinal pigment epithelium: mechanism of generation. J Physiol (Lond) 484:53–67.

Bird A. 1994. Pathogenesis of serous detachment of the retina and pigment epithelium. In: Ryan SJ, ed, Retina, vol. 2. St. Louis: Mosby, 1019–1026.

Blazynski C, Perez MT. 1991. Adenosine in the vertebrate retina: localization, receptor characterization, and function. Cell Mol Neurobiol 11:463–484.

Blazynski C, Cohen A, Fruh B, Niemeyer G. 1989. Adenosine: autoradiographic localization and electrophysiologic effects in the cat retina. Invest Ophthalmol Vis Sci 30:2533–2536.

Borgula GA, Karwoski CJ, Steinberg RH. 1989. Light-evoked changes in extracellular pH in frog retina. Vision Res 29:1069–1077.

Bretag A. 1987. Muscle chloride channels. Physiol Rev 67:618–720.

Campochiaro PA, Hackett SF, Vinores SA. 1996. Growth factors in the retina and retinal pigmented epithelium. Prog Ret Eye Res 15(2):547–565.

Collins, FS. 1992. Cystic fibrosis: molecular biology and therapeutic implications. Science 256:774–779.

Dacey DD. 1988. Dopamine-accumulating retinal neurons revealed by in vitro fluorescence display a unique morphology. Science 240:1196–1198.

Dawis S, Niemeyer G. 1986. Dopamine influences the light peak in the perfused mammalian eye. Invest Ophthalmol Vis Sci 27:330.

Dawis SM, Niemeyer G. 1988. Similarity and diversity of monoamines in their effects on the standing potential, light peak and electroretinogram of the perfused cat eye. Clin Vis Sci 3:108–119.

Dearry A, Burnside B. 1988a. Stimulation of distinct D2 dopaminergic and alpha 2-adrenergic receptors induces light-adaptive pigment dispersion in teleost retinal pigment epithelium. J Neurochem 51:1516–1523.

Dearry A, Burnside B. 1988b. Dopamine induces light-adaptive retino-motor movements in teleost photoreceptors and retinal pigment epithelium. In: Bodis-Wollner I, ed, Dopaminergic Mechanisms in Vision. New York: Liss, 109–135.

Dearry A, Burnside B. 1989. Light-induced dopamine release from teleost retinas acts as a light-adaptive signal to the retinal pigment epithelium. J Neurochem 53:870–878.

Dearry A, Edelman JL, Miller SS, Burnside B. 1990. Dopamine induces light-adaptive retinomotor movements in bullfrog cones via D2 receptors and in retinal pigment epithelium via D1 receptors. J Neurochem 54:1367–1378.

Dewar J. 1877. On the physiological action of light. Parts 1 and 2. Nature, 1555:433–435; 452–454.

Dewar J, M'Kendrick JG. 1873a. On the physiological action of light. Proc Royal Soc Edinb 8:100–104.

Dewar J, M'Kendrick JG. 1873b. On the physiological action of light. Proc Royal Soc Edinb 8:110–114.

Dewar J, M'Kendrick JG. 1873c. On the physiological action of light. Proc Royal Soc Edinb 8:179–182.

Dimitriev AV, Govardovskii VI, Steinberg RH. 1996. Light-induced changes of principal extracellular ions and extracellular space volume in the chick retina. Invest Ophthal Vis Sci 37:S140.

Dragunow M, Faull R. 1988. Neuroprotective effects of adenosine. Trends Pharmacol Sci USA 9:193.

de Bois-Reymond E. 1849. Untersuchungen über thierische Elektricität. vol. 2, Berlin: Reimer, 256–257.

Edelman J, Miller S. 1991. Epinephrine stimulates fluid absorption across bovine retinal pigment epithelium. Invest Ophthalmol Vis Sci 32:3033–3040.

Edelman J, Miller S. 1992. Epinephrine (EP) stimulates KCl and fluid absorption across the bovine retinal pigment epithelium (RPE). Invest Ophthalmol Vis Sci 33:1111 (Abstract).

Edelman J, Miller S. 1996. Isotonic fluid transport in bovine RPE (in preparation).

Edelman J, Lin H, Miller S. 1994. Acidification stimulates chloride and fluid absorption across frog retinal pigment epithelium. Am J Physiol 266:C946–956.

Ehinger B. 1983. Functional role of dopamine in the retina. In: Osborne N, Chader G, eds, Progress in Retinal Research, vol 2. Oxford: Pergamon Press, 213–232.

Einthoven W, Jolly WA. 1908. The form and magnitude of the electrical response of the eye to stimulation by light at various intensities. Quart J Exp Physiol 1:373–416.

Fain GL, Matthews HR. 1990. Calcium and the mechanism of light adaptation in vertebrate photoreceptors. Trends Neurosci 13:378–384.

Farber DS. 1969. Analysis of the slow transretinal potentials in response to light. Ph.D. dissertation. State University of New York, Buffalo.

Frambach DA, Valentine JL, Weiter JJ. 1988a. Alpha-1 adrenergic receptors on rabbit retinal pigment epithelium. Invest Ophthalmol Vis Sci 29:737–741.

Frambach DA, Valentine JL, Weiter JJ. 1988b. Modulation of rabbit retinal pigment epithelium electrogenic transport by alpha-1 adrenergic stimulation. Invest Ophthalmol Vis Sci 29:814–817.

Frambach D, Fain G, Farber D, Bok D. 1990. Beta adrenergic receptors on cultured human retinal pigment epithelium. Invest Ophthalmol Vis Sci 31:1767–1772.

Friedman Z, Hackett SF, Campochiaro PA. 1987. Characterization of adenylate cyclase in human retinal pigment epithelial cells in vitro. Exp Eye Res 44:471–479.

Frizzel RA. 1995. Functions of the cystic fibrosis transmembrane conductance regulator protein. Am J Respir Crit Care Med 151: S54–S58.

Fujii S, Gallemore RP, Hughes BH, Steinberg R. 1992. Direct evidence for a basal membrane Cl^- conductance in toad retinal pigment epithelium. Am J Physiol 262:C374–C383.

Fuller C, Benos D. 1992. CFTR! Am J Physiol 263:C267–C286.

Gallemore RP. 1992. Ionic mechanism of the light-peak voltage of the DC electroretinogram. Ph.D. dissertation. University of California, San Francisco.

Gallemore R, Griff E, Steinberg R. 1988. Evidence in support of a photoreceptoral origin for the "light-peak substance." Invest Ophthalmol Vis Sci 29:566–571.

Gallemore RP, Steinberg RH. 1988. Light-evoked changes in $[Ca^{2+}]_o$ in chick retina. Invest Ophthalmol Vis Sci 29:103 (abstract).

Gallemore R, Steinberg R. 1989a. Effects of DIDS on the chick retinal pigment epithelium. I. membrane potentials, apparent resistances and mechanisms. J Neurosci 9:1968–1976.

Gallemore R, Steinberg R. 1989b. Effects of DIDS on the chick retinal pigment epithelium. II. mechanism of the light peak and other responses originating at the basal membrane. J Neurosci 9:1977–1984.

Gallemore R, Steinberg R. 1990. Effects of dopamine on the chick retinal pigment epithelium: membrane potentials and light-evoked responses. Invest Ophthalmol Vis Sci 31:67–80.

Gallemore RP, Steinberg RH. 1991a. Cobalt increases photoreceptor-dependent responses of the chick retinal pigment epithelium. Invest Ophthalmol Vis Sci 32:3041–3052.

Gallemore RP, Steinberg RH. 1991b. The light peak of the DC ERG is associated with an increase in Cl^- conductance in chick RPE. Invest Ophthalmol Vis Sci (ARVO abstr) 32:837.

Gallemore R, Steinberg R. 1993. Light-evoked modulation of basolateral membrane Cl^- conductance in chick retinal pigment epithelium: the light peak and fast oscillation. J Neurophysiol 70:1669–1680.

Gallemore R, Hernandez E, Tayyanipour R, Fujii S, Steinberg R. 1993. Basolateral membrane Cl^- and K^+ conductances of the dark-adapted chick retinal pigment epithelium. J Neurophysiol 70:1656–1668.

Gallemore R, Li J, Govardovskii V, Steinberg R. 1994a. Calcium gradients and light-evoked calcium changes outside rods in the intact cat retina. Vis Neurosci 11:753–761.

Gallemore R, Hernandez E, Steinberg R. 1994b. Choroid-free preparation of explant retinal pigment epithelium. Invest Ophthalmol Vis Sci (ARVO Abstract) 35:2348.

Gallemore RP, Hu J, Frambach DA, Bok D. 1995. Ion transport in cultured fetal human retinal pigment epithelium. Invest Ophthalmol Vis Sci 36:S216 (abstract).

Gold GH, Korenbrot JI. 1980. Light-induced calcium release by intact retinal rods. Proc Nat Acad Sci USA 77:5557–5561.

Govardovskii V, Berman A, Bykov K, Skachkov S. 1987. The role of Ca^{++} and cyclic GMP in excitation and adaptation of vertebrate photoreceptors. In: Ovchinnikov Y, ed, Retinal Proteins: Proceedings of an International Conference. Utrecht: VNU Science Press, 15–31.

Govardovskii V, Li J, Dmitriev A, Steinberg R. 1994. Mathematical model of TMA^+ diffusion and prediction of light-dependent subretinal hydration in chick retina. Invest Ophthalmol Vis Sci 35(6):2712–2724.

Granit R. 1933. The components of the retinal action potential in mammals and their relation to the discharge in the optic nerve. J Physiol 77:207–239.

Griff E. 1991. Potassium-evoked responses from the retinal pigment epithelium of the toad Bufo marinus. Exp Eye Res 53:219–228.

Griff E, Steinberg R. 1982. Origin of the light peak: in vitro study of Gekko gekko. J Physiol (Lond) 331:637–652.

Griff E, Steinberg R. 1984. Changes in apical [K$^+$]$_o$ produce delayed basal membrane responses of the retinal pigment epithelium in the gekko. J Gen Physiol 83:193–211.

Griff E, Bonasso C. 1990. A light peak in the toad, Bufo marinus. Invest Ophthalmol Vis Sci 31:391 (Abstract).

Griff E, Shirao Y, Steinberg R. 1985. Ba^{2+} unmasks K$^+$ modulation of the Na$^+$-K$^+$ pump in the frog pigment epithelium. J Gen Physiol 86:853–876.

Hadjiconstantinou M, Cohen J, Neff N. 1983. Epinephrine: a potential neurotransmitter in retina. J Neurochem 41:1440–1444.

Hadjiconstantinou M, Mariani A, Panula P, Joh T, Neff H. 1984. Immunohistochemical evidence for epinephrine-containing retinal amacrine cell. Neurosci 13:547–551.

Haggendal J, Malmfors T. 1965. Evidence of dopamine-containing neurons in the retina of rabbit. Acta Physiol Scand 59:295–296.

Hernandez E, Hu J, Frambach D, Gallemore R. 1995. Potassium conductances in cultured bovine and human retinal pigment epithelium. Invest Ophthalmol Vis Sci 36:113–122.

Hille B. 1992. Ionic Channels of Excitable Membranes. 2nd ed. Sunderland, MA: Sinanuer, 341–347.

Homgren F. 1865–66. En method att objektivera effecten af ljusintryck pä retina. Upsala Läkareförenings Förehandlingar 1:177–191.

Homgren F. 1879–80. Über die Retinaströme. Untersuchung Physiolisches Institüt der Universität Heidelberg 3:278–326.

Hu J, Bok D, Frambach D, Gallemore R. 1995. Beta-2 adrenergic receptors activate basal membrane ion channels in cultured fetal human retinal pigment epithelium. Invest Ophthalmol Vis Sci 36:2726 (Abstract).

Hu J, Gallemore R, Maruiwa F, Bok D. 1996. Retinal potassium modulates multiple ion transport mechanisms in cultured human retinal pigment epithelium. Invest Ophthalmol Vis Sci 37:5229. (ARVO Abstract).

Huang B, Karwoski C. 1989. Change in extracellular space in the frog retina. Invest Ophthalmol Vis Sci 30:64 (Abstract).

Huang B, Karwoski C. 1992. Light-evoked expansion of subretinal space volume in the retina of the frog. J Neurosci 12:4243–4252.

Hughes B, Segawa Y. 1993. cAMP-activated chloride currents in amphibian retinal pigment epithelial cells. J Physiol (Lond) 466:749–766.

Hughes B, Miller S, Joseph D, Edelman J. 1988. cAMP stimulates the Na$^+$-K$^+$ pump in frog retinal pigment epithelium. Am J Physiol 254:C84–98.

Joseph D, Miller SS. 1988. Alpha adrenergic receptors mediate membrane voltage and resistance changes in bovine retinal pigment epithelium. Invest Ophthalmol Vis Sci 29:20 (Abstract).

Joseph D, Miller S. 1989. Alpha-adrenergic receptor activation at bovine RPE apical membrane affects basolateral membrane Cl channels. Invest Ophthalmol Vis Sci 30:413 (Abstract).

Joseph D, Miller S. 1991. Apical and basal membrane ion transport mechanisms in bovine retinal pigment epithelium. J Physiol 435:439–463.

Joseph D, Miller S. 1992. Alpha-1-adrenergic modulation of K and Cl transport in bovine retinal pigment epithelium. J Gen Physiol 99:263–290.

Karwoski C, Proenza L. 1977. Relationship between Müller cell responses, a local transretinal potential, and potassium flux. J Neurophysiol 40:244–259.

Kennedy BG. 1994. Volume regulation in cultured cells derived from human retinal pigment epithelium. Am J Physiol 266:C676–683.

Kenyon E, Yu K, La Cour M, Miller S. 1994. Lactate transport mechanism at the apical and basolateral membranes of bovine retinal pigment epithelium. Am J Physiol 267:C1561–C1573.

Kikawada N. 1968. Variations in the corneo-retinal standing potential of the vertebrate eye during light and dark adaptation. Jap J Physiol 18:687–702.

Koch K-W. 1992. Biochemical mechanism of light adaptation in vertebrate photoreceptors. Trends Bicohem Sci 17:307–311.

Koh SW, Chader GJ. 1984. Retinal pigment epithelium in culture demonstrates a distinct beta-adrenergic receptor. Exp Eye Res 38:7–13.

Kolder H. 1959. Spontane und experimentelle Angerungen des Bestandpotentials des menschlichen Auges. Pflugers Arch 268:258–272.

Kolker A, Becker B. 1968. Epinephrine maculopathy. Arch Ophthal 79:552–562.

Koutalos Y, Yau KW. 1993. A rich complexity emerges in photo-transduction. Curr Opin Neurobiol 3(4):5513–5519.

Kris C. 1958. Corneofundal potential variations during light and dark adaptation. Nature 182:1027–1028.

Kuntz C, Crook R, Dmitriev A, Steinberg R. 1994. Modification by cyclic adenosine monophosphate of basolateral membrane chloride conductance in chick retinal pigment epithelium. Invest Ophthalmol Vis Sci 35:422–433.

la Cour M. 1989. Rheogenic sodium-bicarbonate co-transport across the retinal membrane of the frog retinal pigment epithelium. J Physiol (Lond) 419:539–553; erratum, 445:779.

la Cour M. 1991a. Kinetic properties and Na$^+$ dependence of rheogenic Na$^+$-HCO$_3$$^-$ co-transport in frog retinal pigment epithelium. J Physiol (Lond) 439:59–72.

la Cour M. 1991b. pH homeostasis in the frog retina: the role of Na$^+$:HCO$_3^-$ co-transport in the retinal pigment epithelium. Acta Ophthalmol (Copenh) 69(4):496–504.

Lasansky A, De Fisch F. 1966. Potential, current and ionic fluxes across isolated retinal pigment epithelium and choroid. J Gen Physiol 49:913–924.

Li JD, Gallemore RP, Dmitriev A, Steinberg RH. 1994a. Light-dependent hydration of the space surrounding photoreceptors in chick retina. Invest Ophthalmol Vis Sci 35:2700–2711.

Li JD, Govardovskii VI, Steinberg RH. 1994b. Light-dependent hydration of the space surrounding photoreceptors in the cat retina. Vis Neurosci 11:743–752.

Lin H, Miller S. 1991a. Apical epinephrine modulates [Ca^{2+}]i in bovine retinal pigment epithelium. Invest Ophthalmol Vis Sci 32:671 (Abstract).

Lin H, Miller S. 1991b. pH$_i$ regulation in frog retinal pigment epithelium: two apical membrane mechanisms. Am J Physiol 261:C132–C142.

Linsenmeier R, Steinberg R. 1982. Origin and sensitivity of the light peak in the intact cat eye. J Physiol (Lond) 331:653–673.

Linsenmeier R, Steinberg R. 1984a. Delayed basal hyperpolarization of the cat retinal pigment epithelium, and its relation to the fast-oscillation of the DC ERG. J Gen Physiol 83:213–232.

Linsenmeier R, Steinberg R. 1984b. Effects of hypoxia on potassium homeostasis and pigment epithelial cells in the cat retina. J Gen Physiol 84:945–970.

Livsey C, Huang B, Xu J, Karwoski C. 1990. Light-evoked changes in extracellular calcium concentration in frog retina. Vision Res 30:853–861.

Marmor M. 1979. Dystrophies of the retinal pigment epithelium. In: Zinn K, Marmor M, eds, The Retinal Pigment Epithelium. Cambridge, MA: Harvard University press, 424–453.

Marmor MF. 1994. Mechanisms of normal retinal adhesion: In: Ryan SJ, ed, Retina, vol 3. St Louis: Mosby, 1931–1953.

Marmor M, Lurie M. 1979. Light-induced electrical responses of the retinal pigment epithelium. In: Zinn K, Marmor M, eds, The Retinal Pigment Epithelium. Cambridge, MA: Harvard University Press, 226–244.

Martins-Ferreira H, Oliveira Castro G. 1971. Spreading depression in isolated chick retina. Vision Res 3(Suppl):171–174.

Maruiwa F, Nao-i N, Nakazaki S, Sawada A. 1995. Effects of adenosine on chick RPE membrane potentials. Curr Eye Res 14:685–691.

Matsura T, Miller W, Tomita T. 1978. Cone-specific c-wave in the turtle retina. Vision Res 18:767–775.

Miller DL, Korenbrot JI. 1987. Kinetics of light-dependent Ca fluxes across the plasma membrane of rod outer segments: a dynamic model of the regulation of the cytoplasmic Ca concentration. J Gen Physiol 90:397–425.

Miller RF, Dowling JE. 1970. Intracellular responses of the Müller (glial) cells of mudpuppy retina: their relation to b-wave of the electroretinogram. J Neurophysiol 33:323–341.

Miller R, Zalutsky R, Massey S. 1986. A perfused rabbit retina preparation suitable for pharmacological studies. J Neurosci Methods 16:309–322.

Miller S, Steinberg R. 1977. Passive ionic properties of frog retinal pigment epithelium. J Membr Biol 36:337–372.

Miller SS, Rabin J, Strong T, Iannuzzi M, Adams AJ, Collins F, Reenstra W, McCray P Jr. 1992. Cystic fibrosis (CF) gene product is expressed in retina and retina pigment epithelium. Invest Ophthalmol Vis Sci 33:1009 (abstract).

Moroi-Fetters SE, Earley O, Hirakata A, Caron MG, Jaffe GJ. 1995. Binding, coupling, and mRNA subtype heterogeneity of alpha 1-adrenergic receptors in cultured human RPE. Exp Eye Res 60:527–532.

Nao-i N, Gallemore R, Steinberg R. 1990a. Effects of cAMP and IBMX on the chick retinal pigment epithelium: membrane potentials and light-evoked responses. Invest Ophthalmol Vis Sci 31:54–66.

Nao-i N, Nilsson S, Gallemore R, Steinberg R. 1990b. Effects of melatonin on the chick retinal pigment epithelium: membrane potentials and light-evoked responses. Exp Eye Res 49:573–589.

Nash MS, Osborne NN. 1996. Cell surface receptors associated with the retinal pigment epithelium: the adenylate cyclase and phospholipase C signal transduction pathways. Prog Ret Eye Res 15(2):501–546.

Niemeyer G. 1981. Neurobiology of mammalian eyes. Neurosci Methods 3:317–337.

Noell W. 1952. Azide sensitive potential difference across the eye bulb. Am J Physiol 170:217–238.

Noell W. 1953. Studies on the electrophysiology and metabolism of the retina. U.S.A.F. School of Aviation Medicine, Project No. 21-1201-0004. Randolf Field, Texas.

Noell W. 1954. The origin of the electroretinogram. Am J Ophthalmol 38:78–90.

Noell WK, Crapper DR, Paganelli CV. 1965. Transretinal currents and ion fluxes. In: Snell F, Noell WK, eds, Transcellular Membrane Potentials and Ion Fluxes. New York: Gordon and Breach, 92–130.

Oakley B II. 1977. Potassium and the photoreceptor dependent pigment epithelial hyperpolarization. J Gen Physiol 70:405–425.

Oakley B II, Green DG (1976). Correlation of light-induced changes in retinal extracellular potassium concentration with the c-wave of the electroretinogram. J Neurophysiol 39:1117–1133.

Oakley B II, Steinberg R. 1982. Effects of maintained illumination upon [K+]O in the subretinal space of the frog retina. Vision Res 22:767–737.

Oakley B II, Steinberg R, Miller S, Nilsson S. 1977. The in vitro frog pigment epithelial cell hyperpolarization in response to light. Invest Ophthalmol Vis Sci 16(8):771–774.

Oakley B II, Flaming D, Brown K. 1979. Effects of the rod receptor potential upon retinal extracellular potassium concentration. J Gen Physiol 74:713–737.

Pang S, Yu H, Suen H, Brown G. 1980. Melatonin in the retina of rats a diurnal rhythm. J Endocrinol 87:89–93.

Peterson WM, Miller SS. 1995a. Identification and functional characterization of a dual GABA/taurine transporter in the bullfrog retinal pigment epithelium. J Gen Physiol 106:1089–1122.

Peterson W, Miller S. 1995b. Elevation of cyclic AMP levels in the bovine retinal pigment epithelium (RPE) closes basolateral membrane Cl channels. Invest Ophthalmol Vis Sci 36:S216 (Abstract).

Phillis J, Wu P. 1981. The role of adenosine and its nucleotides in central synaptic transmission. Prog Neurobiol 16:187.

Piccolino M, Neyton J, Gerschenfeld H. 1984. Decrease of the gap-junction permeability induced by dopamine and cyclic 3′,5′-adenosine monophosphate in horizontal cells of the turtle retina. J Neurosci 4:2477.

Piper H. 1911. Über die Netzhauströme. Arch für Anatomie und Physiologie, Physiologische Abteilung (Leipzig), 85–132.

Quinn R, Miller S. 1992. Ion transport mechanisms in native human retinal pigment epithelium. Invest Ophthalmol Vis Sci 33:3513–3527.

Quinn RH, Miller SS. 1993. Apical epinephrine or cyclic AMP modulates K and Cl transport in native human fetal retinal pigment epithelium. Invest Ophthalmol Vis Sci 34:872 (abstract).

Rodieck R. 1972. Components of the electroretinogram—a reappraisal. Vision Res 12:773–780.

Romano C, Price M, Bai HY, Olney JW. 1993. Neuroprotectants in Honghua: glucose attenuates retinal ischemic damage. Invest Ophthal Vis Sci 34:72–80.

Roos A, Boron W. 1981. Intracellular pH. Physiol Rev 61:296–434.

Scharschmidt B, Griff E, Steinberg R. 1988. Effect of taurine on the isolated retinal pigment epithelium of the frog: electrophysiologic evidence for stimulation of an apical, electrogenic Na$^+$-K$^+$ pump. J Membr Biol 106:71–81.

Shirao Y, Steinberg R. 1987. Mechanisms of effects of small hyperosmotic gradients on the chick RPE. Invest Ophthalmol Vis Sci 280:2015–2025.

Steinberg R. 1985. Interaction between the retinal pigment epithelium and the neural retina. Doc Ophthalmol 60:327–346.

Steinberg R. 1987. Monitoring communications between photoreceptors and pigment epithelial cells: effects of "mild" systemic hypoxia. Friedenwald lecture. Invest Ophthalmol Vis Sci 28:1888–1904.

Steinberg R, Miller S. 1973. Aspects of electrolyte transport in frog pigment epithelium. Exp Eye Res 16:365–372.

Steinberg R, Niemeyer G. 1981. Light peak of cat DC electroretinogram: not generated by a change in [K+]o. Invest Ophthalmol Vis Sci 20:414–418.

Steinberg R, Schmidt R, Brown K. 1970. Intracellular responses to light from cat pigment epithelium: origin of the electroretinogram c-wave. Nature 227:728–730.

Steinberg R, Oakley B II, Niemeyer G. 1980. Light-evoked changes in [K$^+$]$_o$ in retina of intact cat eye. J Neurophysiol 44:897–921.

Steinberg R, Linsenmeier R, Griff E. 1983. Three light-evoked responses of the retinal pigment epithelium. Vision Res 23:1315–1323.

Steinberg R, Linsenmeier R, Griff E. 1985. Retinal pigment epithelial cell contributions to the electrooculogram. In: Osborne N, Chader G, eds, Progress in Retinal Research, vol 4. New York: Pergamon Press, 33–36.

Stoddard J, Reuss L. 1989. pH effects on basolateral membrane ion conductances in gallbladder epithelium. Am J Physiol 256:C1184–C1195.

Tran VT. 1992. Human retinal pigment epithelial cells possess beta 2-adrenergic receptors. Exp Eye Res 55:413–417.

Ueda Y, Steinberg R. 1994. Chloride currents in freshly isolated rat retinal pigment epithelial cells. Exp Eye Res 58:331–342.

Uehara F, Mathes M, Yasumura D, LaVail M. 1990. Light-evoked changes in the interphotoreceptor matrix. Science 248:1633–1636.

Valeton J, van Norren D. 1982. Intraretinal recordings of slow electrical responses to steady illumination in monkey: isolation of receptor responses and the origin of the light peak. Vision Res 22:393–399.

van Norren D, Heynen H. 1986. Origin of the fast oscillation in the electroretinogram of the macaque. Vision Res 26:569–575.

Weleber R. 1989. Fast and slow oscillations of the electro-oculogram in Best's macular degeneration and retinitis pigmentosa. Arch Ophthalmol 107:530–537.

Wiechmann A. 1986. Melatonin: parallels in pineal gland and retina. Exp Eye Res 42:507–527.

Wiechmann A, Bok D, Horowitz J. 1985. Localization of hydroxyindole-O-methyltransferase in mammalian pineal gland and retina. Invest Ophthalmol Vis Sci 26:253–265.

Wiechmann A, Bok D, Horowitz J. 1986. Melatonin-binding in the frog retina. Autoradiographic and biochemical analysis. Invest Ophthalmol Vis Sci 27:153–163.

Witkovsky P, Dudek F, Ripps H. 1975. Slow PIII component of the carp electroretinogram. J Gen Physiol 65:119–135.

Witkovsky P, Stone S, Besharse J. 1987. Dopamine mimics light-adaptation in horizontal cells of the Xenopus retina. Soc Neurosci Abstr 13:24.

Yamamoto F, Borgula G, Steinberg R. 1992. Effects of light and darkness on pH outside rod photoreceptors in the cat retina. Exp Eye Res 54:685–697.

Yau K-W. 1994. Phototransduction mechanism in retinal rods and cones. Friedenwald lecture. Invest Ophthalmol Vis Sci 35:9–32.

Yoshikami S, George JS, Hagins WA. 1980. Light-induced calcium-fluxes from outer segment layer of vertebrate retinas. Nature 286:395–398.

10. Clinical electrophysiology of the retinal pigment epithelium

RON P. GALLEMORE, FUTOSHI MARUIWA, AND MICHAEL F. MARMOR

The retinal pigment epithelium (RPE) forms the blood retinal barrier for the distal retina, where it maintains the health and integrity of the photoreceptors and choriocapillaris. It is not surprising, then, that defects in retinal pigment epithelial function have been implicated in a number of ocular diseases. Clinical tests of RPE function could be useful in the diagnosis of such diseases and for their differentiation from other conditions. In this chapter, we will review the electrophysiologic tests of RPE function and their clinical applications.

Clinical tests include both photic and nonphotic responses of the RPE. Photic responses are usually recorded by electrooculography and include the fast oscillation, light peak, and dark trough. The well-known Arden ratio (light peak–to–dark trough ratio) of the electrooculogram (EOG) is the most commonly used electrophysiologic test of RPE function. Each photic response reflects specific light-evoked changes in RPE membrane potentials and resistance, and depends both on the RPE and photoreceptors for its generation.

The nonphotic responses include the hyperosmolarity, acetazolamide (Diamox), and bicarbonate responses. These responses also reflect changes in RPE membrane potentials and resistance. These tests assess RPE integrity more selectively, but could be affected by disease in other retinal cells as well. Hypoxia and ethanol also affect the electrophysiology of the RPE, but their effects have not been used in clinical tests.

In recent years we have gained a greater understanding of the origin and mechanisms of these electrophysiologic tests. Each response reflects changes in the activity of specific ion transport mechanisms in the RPE, many of which have been characterized in physiologic studies (see Chapter 6). The clinical utility of these tests remains, however, limited. As we learn more about these tests, their value will increase for determining mechanisms of disease, distinguishing between diseases, staging diseases, and assessing response to treatment.

PHOTIC MEASURES OF RPE FUNCTION

Standing Potential and DC ERG

In the dark, a potential difference (standing potential) is recorded across the vertebrate eye with the cornea positive to the posterior pole. Illumination produces a series of changes in the standing potential that can be recorded with direct current (DC) amplification as components of the electroretinogram (DC ERG). Figure 10-1 summarizes the major light-evoked responses of the human eye. The response begins with the early receptor potential (ERP), which occurs within 1–2 msec and represents physiological changes in the visual pigment molecules of the photoreceptors. This is followed within 10–20 msec by the a- and b-waves of the ERG, which primarily reflect the receptor potential and activity of neurons in the inner retina, respectively. After a few seconds, the "slow" potentials begin, the c-wave, fast oscillation, light peak, and slow oscillations. Each of these slow responses have significant contributions from the RPE (Steinberg et al., 1985), and their clinical utility will be considered in this review.

Physiology

We now have a much better understanding of the cellular events underlying the standing potential and RPE-dependent photic responses. While this material is covered in detail in Chapter 9, we provide a brief review here as a context for clinical discussion. To discuss the physiology involved, we must consider the transport mechanisms in the RPE since they generate the voltages we record. Figure 10-2 illustrates a current model for ion transport in human RPE (Quinn and Miller, 1992; Gallemore et al., 1995). A diagrammatic representation of the photic response mechanisms is shown in Figure 10-3.

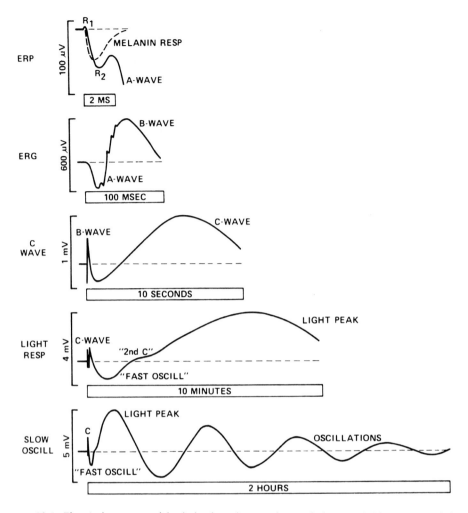

FIGURE 10-1. Electrical responses of the dark-adapted eye, as they might be recorded from a corneal electrode after exposure to a bright light. Note that the time frame changes between each tracing, and each tracing incorporates the responses of the preceding one. (From Marmor and Lurie, 1979.)

Standing potential. The standing potential (SP) of the eye was first described by Du Bois-Reymond in 1849. The SP is essentially a measure of the transepithelial potential (TEP) of the RPE (Noell, 1952; 1953; Faber, 1969; Steinberg et al., 1985; Marmor and Lurie, 1979). The TEP results from different values for the apical and basolateral membrane potentials of the RPE. The apical membrane potential (V_{ap}) is more hyperpolarized than the basolateral membrane (V_{ba}), resulting in a positive value for the TEP (Figure 10-2). This difference in membrane potentials results from differences in the types and distribution of transport mechanisms between the two RPE membranes (see Chapter 6). The major transport mechanisms are illustrated in Figure 10-2: The electrogenic transport mechanisms, which transport net charge across the plasma membrane, are shaded in black. The apical membrane potential is generated primarily by K

channels with smaller contributions from the electrogenic Na/K pump and $NaHCO_3$ cotransporter. The basolateral membrane potential is generated primarily by a balance between Cl and K channels. The basolateral membrane is relatively more depolarized than the apical membrane because of its relatively large Cl conductance. This difference in membranes potentials gives a positive value for the TEP (TEP = $V_{ba} - V_{ap}$).

C-wave. The c-wave is the first slow potential in the DC ERG. This response is the sum of two potentials, a positive potential generated at the RPE (the RPE c-wave) and a negative potential generated by the Müller cells across the neural retina (slow PIII) (Farber, 1969; Witkovsky et al., 1975). Both responses result from membrane hyperpolarizations in response to the photoreceptor-dependent $[K^+]_o$ decrease (Oakley and

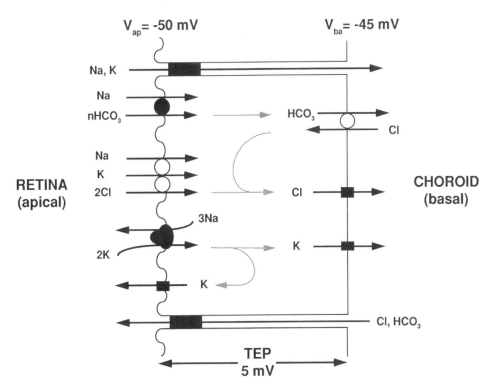

FIGURE 10-2. Model of human RPE ion transport mechanisms.

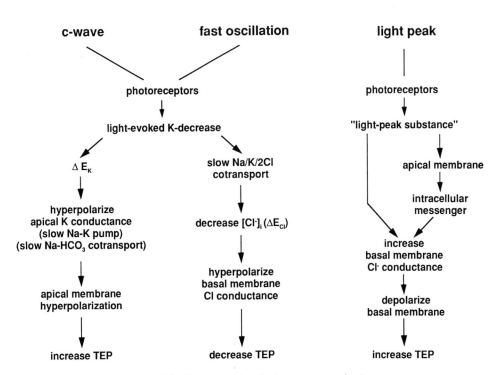

FIGURE 10-3. Diagram of the photic response mechanisms.

Green, 1976; Matsura et al., 1978; Steinberg et al., 1980). These waves add to give the final response, measured at the cornea. The K$^+$ decrease and RPE c-wave voltage are associated with the modulation of a variety of transport mechanisms (see Chapters 6 and 9).

Fast oscillation. The fast oscillation follows the c-wave and is the first negative-going slow potential in the DC ERG (Kris, 1958; Kolder and Brecker, 1966; Kolder and North, 1966). It represents the fall in potential toward or below the dark-adapted baseline. The mechanism underlying this voltage response has been clarified in the past several years (Joseph and Miller, 1991; Gallemore and Steinberg, 1993; Bialek et al., 1995). The response involves modulation of the Cl transport pathway by changes in subretinal [K$^+$]$_o$ (Fig. 10-2). The light-evoked decrease in subretinal [K$^+$]$_o$, which originates at the photoreceptors, slows the activity of the apical membrane Na/K/2Cl cotransporter. This reduces the influx of Cl across the RPE apical membrane. The fall in intracellular Cl, in the presence of the basolateral membrane Cl channel (Fig. 10-2), hyperpolarizes the basolateral membrane. The fast oscillation response is also termed the *delayed basolateral membrane hyperpolarization* (DBMH) since it follows in time the c-wave hyperpolarization of the apical membrane (Griff and Steinberg, 1984; Linsenmeier and Steinberg, 1984a).

The term *fast oscillation* refers to the speed of this response relative to the slower light peak. The initial trough after illumination occurs in about 1 min, whereas the light peak does not reach a maximum for 6–9 min. The fast oscillation is optimally driven by light/dark cycles that alternate every 60–80 sec, whereas the slow oscillation ("light response of the RPE") is best driven by alternations every 12–15 min. The trough of the fast oscillation is the response to illumination; the peak represents an off-response involving the same mechanisms of K concentration and Cl conductance changes (Linsenmeier and Steinberg, 1984a; Gallemore and Steinberg, 1993; Bialek et al., 1995).

Light peak. The light peak is the third slow component of the DC ERG and represents the rise in standing potential following the fast-oscillation trough. In humans and other higher vertebrates, it is actually the first of a series of slow oscillations that may be recorded during continuous illumination or following a bright step of light (Fig. 10-1; Kris, 1958; Kolder, 1959; Arden and Kelsey, 1962). The light peak voltage originates in the chloride transport pathway of the RPE like the fast-oscillation trough (Gallemore, 1992; Gallemore and Steinberg, 1989b; 1991a; 1993). The light peak is gen-

erated by an increase in basolateral membrane Cl conductance, which depolarizes the basal membrane and increases the transepithelial potential (Linsenmeier and Steinberg, 1982; Griff and Steinberg, 1982; Gallemore and Steinberg, 1992; 1993). The steps preceding activation of the Cl channel have not been clearly delineated, although there is strong evidence that a messenger, released by the photoreceptors (Gallemore et al., 1988; Linsenmeier and Steinberg, 1982), activates a cascade of events that leads to Cl channel activation (Fig. 10-3). The light-evoked K decrease does not generate the light peak voltage (Steinberg and Niemeyer, 1981). Candidates for the "light-peak substance" include catecholamines, indolamines, purines, and others (Blazynski et al., 1989; Dawis and Niemeyer, 1985; 1987; Joseph and Miller, 1992; Gallemore and Steinberg, 1990; Nao-i et al., 1989; 1990; Miller et al., 1996). In various species, agents from each of these classes can activate the basolateral membrane Cl channel and increase the TEP. A second messenger such as Ca^{2+} could couple the receptor to the Cl channel.

The Clinical EOG

The RPE-dependent components of the ERG must be recorded with DC amplification due to their slow time course. This contrasts with the a- and b-waves of the clinical ERG, which can be recorded with AC amplification due to their rapid time course (Fig. 10-4). Recording the DC ERG is difficult and unreliable in awake human subjects, however, due to the drifting baseline inherent to DC recording. Thus, an alternative method for recording the slower light-evoked responses of the RPE was developed (Miles, 1940; Kolder, 1959; Arden and Kelsey, 1962; Arden et al., 1962a). This recording method is based on the technique of electrooculography and recordings of the light response are commonly called the electrooculogram (EOG). The same technique can be used to record fast oscillations.

Recording technique. As illustrated in Figure 10-5, electrooculography is a method for measuring the movement of the eyes and, indirectly, the standing potential of the eye. The technique utilizes alternating eye movements. With electrodes at each canthus, the patient rotates the eye between each electrode, moving the cornea-positive ocular dipole. As the eye rotates back and forth, the polarities reverse and the voltage changes are recorded with DC amplification. By maintaining a constant amplitude and frequency of eye movements, an indirect measurement of the standing potential of the eye is obtained. Changes in the standing potential occur

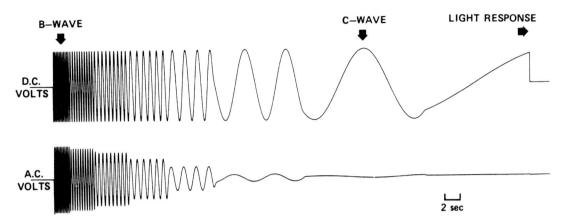

FIGURE 10-4. Comparison of DC and AC amplification. Sine waves at different frequencies were passed through a DC *(above)* and an AC *(below)* amplifier. The AC record was filtered at 2–1000 Hz, typical settings for conventional ERG recording. The arrows show the dominant frequencies of some ocular responses. Note that AC amplification is adequate only for recording a- and b-waves, not for slower components. (From Marmor and Lurie, 1979.)

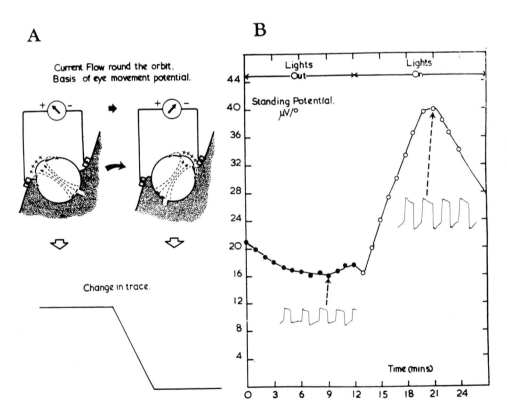

FIGURE 10-5. Diagram illustrating the electrooculographic method of recording the standing potential. (A) Electrode placement at either canthus. The cornea is positive relative to the back of the eye, and as the eye rotates toward and away from a canthal electrode, a voltage shift is recorded. The amplitude of this shift is proportional to the corneofundal potential. (B) Plot of the standing potential (recorded by the EOG) during dark and light adaptation. There is a dark trough *(first arrow)* and light peak *(second arrow)*. The slight drop in potential in the first minute of light adaptation represents the fast oscillation. (From Arden and Fojas, 1962.)

with changes in illumination, but only relative changes in the standing potential are recorded accurately with electrooculography, not absolute values.

The light peak, dark trough, and Arden ratio. The clinical electrooculogram begins with a 15 min period of dark adaptation, which initiates a fall in the standing potential to a dark trough (Fig. 10-5); if darkness is maintained, the standing potential rises somewhat and eventually stabilizes to a steady baseline. At light onset, the signal increases to a maximum after 6–9 min. which represents the light peak. The absolute amplitude of the dark trough represents a base value for the standing potential and is relevant to the health of the RPE. However, the magnitude of the light response is hard to interpret except in context of the baseline from which it arose, and Arden proposed use of the ratio light peak/dark trough as a clinical index (Fig. 10-5). This light-to-dark ratio, or Arden ratio, is the most widely used value for the clinical EOG (although some laboratories measure it as the ratio of the light peak to the dark-adapted baseline rather than the trough). In general, the clinical EOG is less reproducible than the clinical electroretinogram, but variability can be reduced by careful attention to standard recording protocols (see below). The optimal stimulus intensity, balancing response and comfort, is 3–3.5 log trolands (whether pupils are dilated or undilated—see Fig. 10-6). Measuring the light peak against a dark trough gives ratios of higher amplitude but more variability than measurement against a dark adapted baseline value; the overall reproducibility is similar with the two techniques (Lessel et al., 1993; Timmins and Marmor, 1992).

Fast oscillation. The fast oscillation may also be recorded by electrooculography. In conventional EOG recordings the response is seen as a brief fall in potential following the onset of illumination and before the light rise occurs (Fig. 10-5). Optimal recording of this response is achieved by alternating light and dark every 60–80 sec (Fig. 10-7). Clinical measurements include the ratio of peak to trough and the phase shift. The fast oscillation is not often used clinically, but research studies have shown differences in various diseases, as discussed in later sections of this chapter.

Standardization. To facilitate comparisons of EOG measurements throughout the world, the International Society for Clinical Electrophysiology and Vision (ISCEV) has defined standards for two alternative methods for recording the EOG (Marmor et al., 1993): (1) a light peak after a dark trough (Arden ratio) or (2) a light peak after establishing a dark-adapted baseline. Gener-

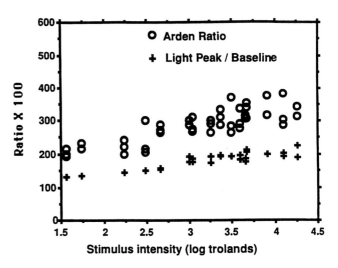

FIGURE 10-6. Relationship of the Arden ratio and the light peak/baseline ratio to stimulus intensity. The ratios increase with stimulus intensity but show a leveling off toward 3.5 log trolands. (From Timmons and Marmor, 1992.)

al guidelines include the use of diffuse (Ganzfeld) illumination, nonpolarizable recording electrodes, fixed saccadic amplitudes (targets subtend 30° visual angle), specific dark and light adaptation protocols and specific stimulus intensities (depending on whether the pupils are dilated). Clinical reporting should include the dark-trough amplitude as well as the light-to-dark ratio. Recommendations were also made for a protocol to record the fast oscillation, using alternating light and dark periods of 60 to 80 sec each, although this response has not been officially standardized. The reader is referred to the original publication for further details.

Clinical Applications

Clinical EOG. The clinical EOG has only limited practical applications at present (Niemeyer, 1989; Nilsson, 1985; and Marmor, 1991). While the physiology of this response has been better explained in the past decade, we have also realized many of its clinical limitations. In particular, since the EOG depends on the photoreceptors for its initiation, it is indiscriminately diminished in any condition where photoreceptor function is diffusely impaired. Since the clinical ERG can inform more precisely about diffuse retinal damage, the EOG adds little to clinical management in most cases. The clinical EOG is most useful when testing for conditions where the clinical ERG and other measures of diffuse retinal function are likely to be normal (Ponte et al., 1986).

As discussed earlier and in Chapter 9, the voltage changes associated with the fast and slow oscillations of the EOG are now understood to reflect modulation of

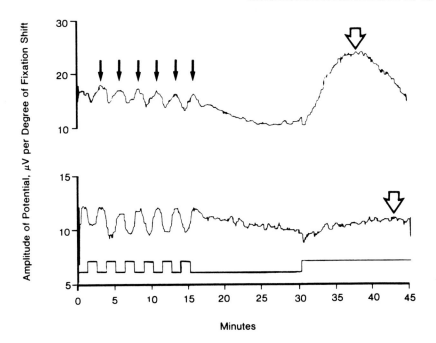

FIGURE 10-7. Electrooculogram (EOG) from *(top)* a normal subject and *(bottom)* a patient with Best's macular dystrophy. Ordinate is amplitude of potential in microvolts per degree of fixation shift. Event marker line below indicates "on" or "off" of the 20 foot-lambert background illumination. Fast oscillation peaks are indicated by closed arrows; the slow light response by open arrows. There is loss and prolongation of the light peak, but preservation of the fast oscillation, in the patient with Best's disease. (After Weleber, 1989.)

the Cl transport pathway in the RPE. Since Cl transport plays a central role in fluid transport, cell volume regulation, and the hydration of the subretinal space (Chapter 6), any of these functions may be abnormal in clinical diseases where the EOG is suppressed. However, interpretation of EOG abnormalities is limited by the lack of correlation with visual functions or even with any RPE function that is measured clinically. Nonexpressing carriers of the Best's dystrophy gene, for example, may be clinically normal but have virtually no EOG light response (Marmor, 1991). Here we review some of the primary conditions where the EOG is altered and its clinical utility in each setting.

Best's vitelliform macular dystrophy. Perhaps the best-known use of the clinical EOG is in the diagnosis of Best's disease. The hallmark of this disease is a markedly reduced EOG with a normal clinical ERG. Visual function is typically normal in the early stages of the disease. At that time, the clinical features are so characteristic that the diagnosis is often made before the EOG is obtained (see Chapter 16). In advanced disease, however, where the condition may mimic other macular degenerative states and visual acuity may be impaired, the EOG may help clinch the diagnosis. The EOG is severely depressed without correlation with patient age or severity of vision loss (Wajima et al., 1993). Since the dystrophy shows variable expression, the EOG will also

identify individuals who have the dominant gene but do not express it (Cross, 1974; Walter et al., 1994). Occasionally adults will present with vitelliform lesions that bear a resemblance to those in Best's disease. Most of these patients do not have Best's disease but one of several conditions that have been termed adult-onset *vitelliform degeneration* (see chapter 16; Fishman et al., 1977; Marmor, 1979a). The EOG can be very helpful in this differential diagnosis, since patients with adult vitelliform degenerations have normal or only slightly reduced EOGs, rather than the severe depression characteristic of Best's disease.

The basis for the abnormal EOG in Best's disease remains unknown. A reduction in EOG amplitude is not associated with any known visual disturbance. Histological studies in Best's disease revealed an accumulation of lipofuscin-like material between the RPE and Bruch's membrane (Frangieh et al., 1982; Weingeist et al., 1982). Since the light-induced change in EOG potential is generated by the basolateral membrane Cl channels, the abnormal EOG potential may relate to an effect on the basolateral membrane of the lipofuscin material. The normal fast oscillation in Best's disease (Fig. 10-7) suggests that the effect may be on a selective type of Cl channel. The relationship between RPE Cl channels and Best's disease may become better defined once the genes for each have been identified.

Retinitis pigmentosa. The clinical electroretinogram is the primary test for following the retinitis pigmentosas, facilitating subclassification of patients in terms of rod and cone involvement and offering a screening tool for early detection in the absence of signs and symptoms (Heckenlively, 1988; Berson, 1993). As the genes for the retinitis pigmentosas have been cloned, molecular diagnostic techniques have begun to play a greater role in the evaluation of these patients. The EOG is usually profoundly suppressed in patients with advanced RP, and is not typically used to follow the course of this disease (Heckenlively, 1988). Weleber (1989) found, however, that some patients with retinitis pigmentosa exhibited suppressed fast oscillations and normal light peaks early in the disease (Fig. 10-8). Thus, while the EOG is not particularly useful in the clinical management of patients with RP, it may provide another means of phenotypic differentiation. This may be of interest, since there can be remarkable phenotypic variation among patients with the same genetic defect (for review see Berson, 1993; Bird, 1995). Thus, phenotypic markers may have some prognostic if not diagnostic utility.

Another potential clinical use of the EOG is in the detection of carriers for some forms of retinitis pigmentosa (van Aarem et al., 1995; Pinckers et al., 1994). Further work will be required before the utility of such screening is established.

An exciting possible use for the EOG in managing RP patients may come when we devise effective treatments for the disease. The EOG may provide some information regarding the stage of disease, patient selection for therapy, and the efficacy of treatment. To this end, it is interesting to note that a patient with vitamin A deficiency and cystic fibrosis exhibited a suppressed light peak–to–dark trough ratio but normal ERG. The Arden ratio normalized after vitamin A supplementation (Leguire et al., 1992).

Retinal vascular occlusions. While the light peak and dark trough appear to originate exclusively from an interaction between the photoreceptors and RPE (Linsenmeier and Steinberg, 1982; Gallemore et al., 1988), retinal vascular occlusions have been found to affect EOG amplitude (Taumer et al., 1982). This is surprising since the choriocapillaris is largely responsible for maintaining the oxygen supply for the cells in the distal retina. Suppression of light peak amplitude, measured with the DC ERG in experimentally induced central retinal artery occlusion was reported by Gouras and Carr (1965). Yonemura and colleagues (1977) reported a decrease of the light peak/dark trough ratio of the EOG in central retinal artery occlusion in humans. Both central retinal vein occlusions (CRVO) and branch retinal vein occlusions (BRVO) have been associated with a decrease in EOG amplitude (Papakostopoulos et al., 1992; Hara

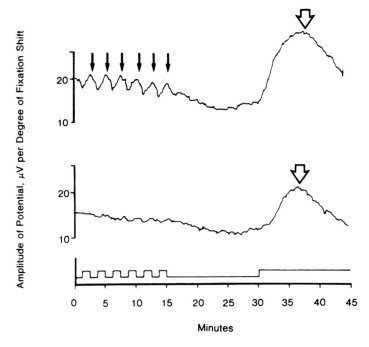

FIGURE 10-8. Electrooculogram (EOG) in a normal subject *(top)* and a patient with autosomal recessive retinitis pigmentosa *(bottom)*. Event marker and arrows as in Figure 10-7. In this patient the light response (slow oscillation) is more preserved than the fast oscillation. (After Weleber, 1989.)

and Miura, 1994; Hara and Nagamoto, 1995). In CRVO, a suppression of greater than 50% in comparison with the EOG light peak of the patient's normal eye was associated with the development of rubeosis; no eyes with EOG light peak amplitudes greater than 48% of normal developed rubeosis (Papakostopoulos et al., 1992). Presumably the extent of retinal damage and ischemia is related to the degree of EOG suppression. A similar differentiation can be made on the basis of ERG criteria (Johnson and McPhee, 1993), although its clinical specificity is uncertain (and presently under investigation by the Central Retinal Vein Occlusion study). In BRVO, normal clinical ERG measurements were found while the EOG was depressed (Hara and Miura, 1994).

The depressed EOG amplitude observed in vascular occlusions likely relates to several factors. One possibility is that the light peak substance is released by inner retinal neurons which are damaged by the ischemic insult (Gouras and Carr, 1965). There is growing evidence, however, that inner retinal neurons are not the source for the light peak substance. Rather, it appears to originate from the photoreceptors (Linsenmeier and Steinberg, 1982; Gallemore et al., 1988). A more likely explanation, then, would involve a direct hypoxic insult to the photoreceptors. Braun and Linsenmeier (1995) found evidence for photoreceptor hypoxia in the setting of vascular occlusion. Central retinal artery occlusion in the cat was associated with a 25% decrease in photoreceptor oxygen consumption. Since the light peak is the most sensitive ERG potential to hypoxia, this degree of hypoxia might account for its suppression (Linsenmeier and Steinberg, 1986; Braun and Linsenmeier, 1995). In addition, factors released from hypoxic retinal cells may have a global effect on RPE function. This could help explain, for example, how a more localized injury such as a BRVO could effect the EOG. The relative contribution of these factors has not been experimentally explored.

Chloroquine and hydroxychloroquine toxicity. These antimalarial agents have been used in the treatment of collagen-vascular disease. With prolonged use they may cause a cumulative dose-related pigmentary retinopathy (see Chapter 32). The safe-dose maximum has been estimated at 3 to 4 mg/kg/day for chloroquine and 5 to 6 mg/kg/day for hydroxychloroquine (Plaquenil) (Brinkley et al., 1979; Mackenzie and Scherbel, 1968; Bernstein, 1992; Easterbrook, 1993), but cumulative dosage may be equally or more important in predisposing to toxicity. These agents have an affinity for melanin, and thus may accumulate in the RPE (Rubin and Slonicki; 1966), although it is unclear whether this binding adds to toxicity or is protective. Suppression of the EOG has been reported (Arden et al., 1962b; Kolb, 1965) but is not necessarily the earliest or most reliable sign of toxicity by these agents. Visual disturbances sometimes occur first and, histologically, degenerative changes in the photoreceptor outer segments and ganglion cell layers may precede effects on the RPE. The mechanism of cell damage appears to involve abnormal cell membrane turnover and this may be related to the cationic amphiphilic nature of these drugs, which could interfere with phospholipid breakdown (Bernstein and Ginsberg, 1964; Abraham and Hendy, 1970; Drenckhan and Lullman-Rauch, 1978; Rosenthal et al., 1978).

Given that other retinal regions may be preferentially affected, tests other than the EOG may be more sensitive screens for toxicity. These include contrast sensitivity (Bishara and Matamoros, 1989), visual fields (MacKenzie, 1983; Hart et al., 1984), Amsler grid testing (Easterbrook, 1984), color vision and quantitative red desaturation testing (Lim et al., 1996), and threshold automated perimetry. Nevertheless ERG and EOG tests should be obtained whenever the question of toxicity has been raised by other tests or fundus appearance, or as a baseline for patients at particularly high risk because of high dose levels or many years of intake.

An important consideration regarding the utility of EOG testing as a screening test for chloroquine and hydroxychloroquine toxicity is the fact that chloroquine is now less commonly used and hydroxychloroquine is much less toxic (Finbloom et al., 1985; Cox and Patterson, 1994), although well-documented cases have been reported (Raines et al., 1989). A recent limited survey of patients in a rheumatology clinic on Plaquinil failed to find evidence of toxicity in any patient (Spalton et al., 1993), which suggests that the risks are low at standard doses. Based on these results, the authors suggested that ancillary tests such as EOG and visual fields may be overused and recommended a reassessment of screening guidelines. Since toxicity can occur and is generally not reversible, some level of screening is warranted and further studies will be required to determine the optimal guidelines.

Other diseases affecting the RPE. The EOG may be mildly reduced, without ERG abnormalities, in pattern dystrophies of the RPE (Marmor and Byers, 1977; Hsieh et al., 1977; Marmor, 1979b), widespread dominant drusen (Deutoman, 1994), and some cases of fundus flavimaculatus and Stargardt's disease (Itabashi et al., 1993). The EOG does not typically add to the diagnosis of any of these conditions, which is based on fundoscopic findings, but an EOG abnormality associated with a normal ERG does suggest a degree of diffuse RPE dysfunction. The EOG was found to be normal in congenital hypertrophy of the retinal pigment epithelium

(CHRPE) associated with familial adenomatous polyposis (Santos et al., 1994). This indicates that while CHRPE has been related to generalized expression of an abnormal gene in the RPE (Olschwang et al., 1993; Wallis et al., 1994), its phenotypic and functional abnormalities tend to be localized. Age-related macular degeneration is not associated with an EOG abnormality, presumably due in part to the focal nature of the RPE disturbance (Sunness et al., 1985; Sunness and Massof, 1986).

The EOG may be of ancillary use in the differential diagnosis of uveal melanoma from choroidal naevi and choroidal metastasis (Brink et al., 1989). In birdshot chorioretinopathy the light peak/dark trough ratio was depressed while the fast oscillation was preserved (Priem et al., 1988).

C-wave. The c-wave has not found a practical clinical application. First, as noted earlier, it has contributions from both the RPE and neural retina. Second, its amplitude can vary widely even in the same patient (Fig. 10-9) perhaps as a result of the dual origin of the c-wave (Hock and Marmor, 1983). The c-wave is also difficult to record in awake human subjects, since the response is too slow to be recorded with AC amplification and too fast for accurate measurement by electrooculography. Experimental studies of the c-wave, however, have provided important insights into RPE physiology (Steinberg et al., 1985; Linsenmeier and Steinberg, 1984b; Dawis and Niemeyer, 1985; Gallemore and Steinberg, 1990). When a condition produces an acute change in the standing potential (e.g., light), there is often an accompanying change in c-wave amplitude which reflects underlying changes in RPE membrane conductance. These conductance changes can be inferred with the corneal recording. For example, increases in standing potential are often accompanied by an increase in c-wave amplitude, which typically reflects an increase in RPE basolateral membrane Cl conductance (Gallemore and Steinberg, 1990).

Fast oscillation. Studies of the fast oscillation have been limited due in part to the difficult methodology required for optimal recording. The fast oscillation and light peak are differentially affected in several diseases. In a few cases where the response has been recorded with the light peak, some interesting differences have been found. The fast oscillation was preferentially suppressed

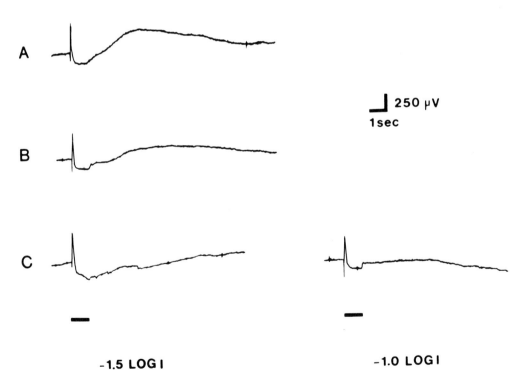

FIGURE 10-9. Human c-wave showing variable appearance from one subject. These responses were obtained during a single recording session. (From Hock and Marmor, 1983.)

over the light peak (and/or Arden ratio) in some cases of retinitis pigmentosa early in the disease (see Fig. 10-8) (Weleber, 1989) and in cystic fibrosis (Miller et al., 1992). The light peak may be affected preferentially over the fast oscillation in Best's macular dystrophy (see Fig. 10-7), chloroquine and hydroxychloroquine maculopathy (De Rouck and Kayembe, 1981), and dominantly inherited drusen (Hess and Niemeyer, 1983).

While the light peak and fast-oscillation voltages both involve the Cl conductance at the basolateral membrane of the RPE, the differential effects of diseases on these two responses suggest that the responses (and diseases) may involve different Cl channel subtypes. There is now evidence to suggest, in fact, that the basolateral membrane Cl conductance may include several different Cl channels or, perhaps, a single channel coupled to different regulatory pathways (see Chapter 6). Calcium-activated, swelling-activated, and cAMP-dependent Cl conductances have all been described (Ueda and Steinberg, 1994; Botchkin and Matthews, 1993; Hughes and Segawa, 1993; Gallemore et al., 1996). In addition, there is a resting Cl conductance at the basal membrane (Fig. 10-2) which may be a distinct channel type as well (Joseph and Miller, 1991; Fujii et al., 1992; Gallemore and Steinberg, 1989a; Gallemore et al., 1993). In the case of cystic fibrosis, the genetic defect is now understood to involve a Cl channel termed CFTR, for cystic fibrosis transmembrane regulator (Anderson et al., 1992; Fuller and Benos, 1992). This was the impetus for studying the fast-oscillation and light peak responses in cystic fibrosis patients (Miller et al., 1992). The CFTR gene product has been identified in the RPE (Miller et al., 1992), but its function as a Cl channel has not yet been explored. It will be interesting to learn how the RPE Cl channels may be directly or indirectly involved in disease mechanisms. Ion transport is involved in a variety of functions in vision, and defects in specific ion transport mechanisms in the RPE and photoreceptors may underlie specific blinding diseases.

Melanin response. The melanin response is largely of historical interest. In the early 1960s it was discovered that intense, nonphysiologic light stimuli applied to the RPE generate potential changes across the epithelium (Brown 1965; Brown and Gage 1966; Brown and Crawford, 1967). This *melanin response* reflects a physicochemical response to light absorption by melanin, analogous in some respects to the early receptor potential of the ERG generated by opsin molecules. Investigators have yet to find a clinical use for the melanin response. Theoretically, it could aid in the assessment of RPE cell membrane properties or melanin distribution, which could be altered by drugs or disease (Arden, 1968). It

does serve as a model for a widespread biological phenomenon, the absorption of light by pigment to initiate an ionic event (Arden et al., 1967; Ebrey and Cone, 1967).

NONPHOTIC RESPONSES OF THE RPE

A major clinical limitation of the EOG and other photic responses of the RPE is their dependence on the photoreceptors for their initiation. Since diseases may affect the RPE alone, photoreceptors alone, or both, clinical tests which assess the integrity of the RPE separately could help localize sites of disease. To this end, several non-photic electrophysiologic responses have been developed which are thought to depend solely on the integrity of the RPE (Yonemura and Kawasaki, 1979; Yonemura et al., 1984; Shirao and Segawa, 1989; Marmor, 1991). These include the hyperosmolarity response, the acetazolamide response, and the bicarbonate response. These responses can be recorded in the intact human and their mechanisms have been studied in in vitro preparations of RPE. The clinical response is typically produced by intravenous infusion of the agent, while the change in standing potential is recorded by electrooculography.

Another nonphotic test of RPE function is the response to hypoxia (Fenn et al., 1949; Kolder, 1959; Marmor et al., 1985). However, this response develops through effects upon the photoreceptors, and may not allow localization of abnormalities to the RPE. It may have other applications, however, which will be considered below. Other nonphotic stimuli that alter the EOG potential are reviewed briefly as well.

The Hyperosmolarity Response

The hyperosmolarity response in humans is elicited by the slow intravenous infusion of a hyperosmolar solution that produces a 15 to 20 mOsm increase in blood osmolarity (e.g. 10% fructose plus 15% mannitol or 25% mannitol alone) (Marmor, 1989; Madachi-Yamamoto et al., 1984a). The response to this infusion is usually recorded with electrooculography and consists of a slow decrease in the standing potential, which reaches a minimum in about 20 min (Fig. 10-10). From a clinical standpoint, examination and use of the hyperosmotic response (and other nonphotic responses) has been limited by the need for drugs and the length of time required to test a patient (especially if photic responses are also desired). To make these nonphotic responses somewhat more palatable as a clinical test and facilitate their use for both routine and investigative purpose, Mori et

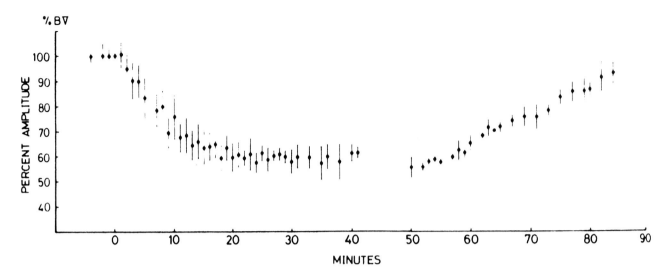

FIGURE 10-10. The clinical hyperosmolarity response and its recovery recorded with electrooculography in normal human subjects. A solution of 1400 mOsm was injected intravenously for 15–30 min beginning at time 0. Recorded in darkness. (From Madachi-Yamamoto et al., 1984.)

al. (1991) have combined photic and nonphotic responses into a single protocol (Fig. 10-11). This allows recording within one 2-hour session of hyperosmolarity and acetazolamide responses, as well as the conventional EOG (light peak) and, if desired, the fast oscillation (Gupta and Marmor, 1994).

Mechanism. The effects of transepithelial hyperosmotic gradients have been studied in in vitro RPE preparations. In human RPE-choroid tissues separated from the neural retina, the transepithelial potential is reduced by a choroidal hyperosmotic gradient and increased by a retinal hyperosmotic gradient (Mukoh, 1985). Similar results were observed in animal studies, suggesting that a choroidal hyperosmotic load produces the EOG potential change (Mukoh, 1985; Shirao and Steinberg, 1987). This result might be expected since (1) blood flow through the choroidal circulation is many times greater than in the retinal circulation, (2) the diffusion pathway to the RPE is shorter from the choroidal circulation, and (3) the fenestrated choriocapillaris is much more permeable than the retinal capillaries (Shirao and Steinberg, 1987). In animal studies the TEP decrease was found to originate primarily from a hyperpolarization of the RPE basal membrane accompanied by a decrease in its apparent conductance (Mukoh et al., 1985; Shirao and Steinberg, 1987). The mechanism appears to involve a decrease in basal membrane Cl conductance (Gallemore and Steinberg, 1989a; 1989b) and could involve a volume-sensitive Cl channel (Botchkin and Matthews, 1993; Ueda and Steinberg, 1994; Gallemore

et al., 1996). Since the light peak voltage is generated by an increase in basolateral membrane Cl conductance (Gallemore and Steinberg, 1991b; 1992; 1993), suppression of this response by hyperosmolarity (Kawasaki et al., 1977) supports the involvement of the Cl conductance in the hyperosmolarity response.

We recently investigated the effects of hyperosmotic gradients in confluent monolayers of human RPE. This preparation exhibits electrical properties and ion transport mechanisms that are similar to those found in fresh mammalian RPE (Gallemore et al., 1995). Consistent

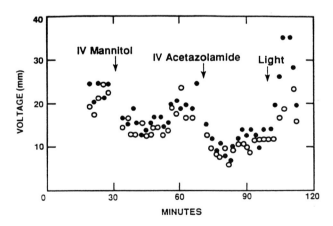

FIGURE 10-11. Combined recording of EOG, hyperosmolarity response, and acetazolamide response in a normal human subject. Intravenous infusion of hyperosmolar solution (25% mannitol) was followed by infusion of acetazolamide (8 mg/kg) and then exposure to light. The ordinate shows millimeters of pen-recorded deviation (proportional to the standing potential voltage). (From Marmor, 1991.)

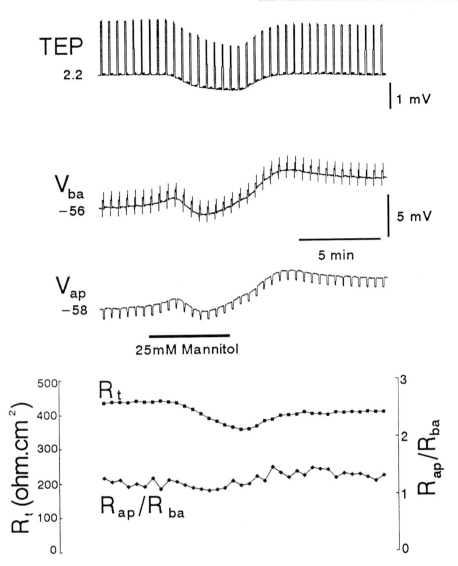

FIGURE 10-12. Effects of choroidal perfusion with hyperosmotic solution in preparation of cultured human RPE. Transepithelial current was passed to measure transepithelial resistance (R_t) and apical-to-basolateral membrane resistance ratio (R_{ap}/R_{ba}). The recording was made in a modified Ussing chamber (Hu et al., 1984). The transepithelial potential (TEP), apical membrane potential (V_{ap}) and basolateral membrane potential (V_{ba}) are recorded using conventional electrophysiological techniques. The osmolarity of the choroidal perfusate was increased from a control level of 272 to 295 mOsm by addition of 25 mM of mannitol.

with studies in fresh human and animal preparations, choroidal hyperosmotic loads decreased the TEP while retinal hyperosmotic loads increased it. As shown in Figure 10-12, while a monotonic decrease in TEP was observed during a choroidal hyperosmotic gradient, the membrane voltage changes were more complex and included membrane hyperpolarizations and depolarizations. Using selective ionic conductance blockers, we found that both a decrease in basal membrane Cl conductance and an increase in paracellular (tight junctional) resistance contributed to the voltage and resistance changes observed in choroidal hyperosmolarity (F. Maruiwa, R. Gallemore, J. Hu and D. Bok, unpublished observations). The membrane mechanisms that may contribute to the electrophysiologic effects of a choroidal hyperosmotic load are illustrated in Figure 10-13.

In vitro, the TEP decrease produced by a choroidal osmotic load appears to depend on both the basolateral membrane Cl conductance as well as the paracellular shunt pathway. Thus, the clinical hyperosmolarity response may assess primarily the integrity of the RPE tight junctions and the basolateral membrane. Selective

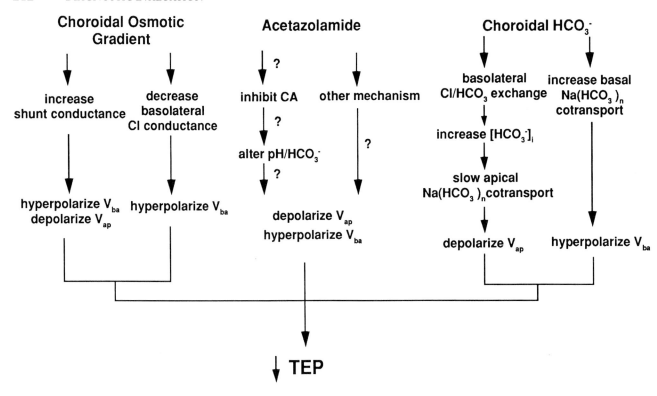

FIGURE 10-13. Diagram of the nonphotic response mechanisms. See text for details.

reductions in the hyperosmolarity response in comparison with other nonphotic RPE tests may be attributable, then, to differences in the origin of each response. It must be emphasized, however, that changes in any part of the RPE electrical circuit could alter the response amplitude of any of these tests. Thus, any factor altering apical or basolateral membrane resistance or paracellular (tight junctional) resistance will alter the amplitude of the hyperosmolarity response. This may explain why the hyperosmolarity response is affected clinically by a wide range of diseases, and is relatively nonspecific as a diagnostic test. Nevertheless, based on the apparent mechanism in vitro, a more pronounced diminution of the response might be expected when the tight junctional complexes or the basolateral membrane Cl-conductance are selectively affected.

Clinical experience. The hyperosmolarity response appears abnormal in a broad range of RPE disorders, including retinitis pigmentosa, Stargardt's disease, butterfly dystrophy, retinal detachment, senile disciform macular degeneration, the late stages of Harada's disease, select cases of high myopia, and pigmented paravenous atrophy (Kawasaki et al., 1984a; 1984b; Madachi-Yamamoto et al., 1984a; Yonemura et al.,

1979; 1982; 1983; 1984; Asai, 1993; Ushimura et al., 1990; Ushimura et al., 1992; Ushimura et al., 1993; Ushimura, 1993). It can also be abnormal in some disorders that are usually thought to be of retinal origin, such as diabetic retinopathy or central retinal artery occlusion (Shirao and Segawa, 1989; Segawa, 1994). This may reflect secondary RPE involvement or an unsuspected primary RPE-choroid abnormality. The hyperosmolarity response is abnormal even when the EOG is normal in fundus albipunctatas or butterfly dystrophy and after recovery from retinal detachment or central retinal artery occlusion. While these are interesting clinical observations, they are of limited clinical import because of the lack of specificity of the hyperosmolarity response (Marmor, 1991). It does not facilitate or modify the diagnosis of any of these diseases.

It is interesting that in central serous retinopathy (Fig. 10-14), the hyperosmolarity response is preserved (Gupta and Marmor, 1996). This may seem surprising since this condition involves a "defect" in the RPE barrier that allows fluid to pass into the subretinal space, and an impairment of transport across surrounding RPE that allows formation of a localized serous retinal detachment (Negi and Marmor, 1983; 1984; Marmor, 1988; 1997; Marmor and Yao, 1994; Bird, 1994). A lo-

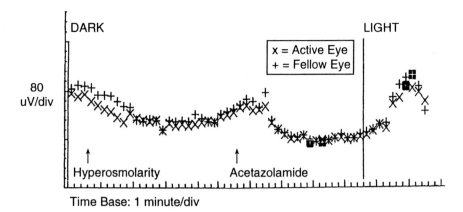

FIGURE 10-14. Recordings of photic and nonphotic EOG responses from a patient with active central serous chorioretinopathy. There was no difference between the eye with detachment (active) and the unaffected fellow eye. (From Gupta and Marmor, 1996.)

calized defect in RPE function would be insufficient to cause an abnormality in the hyperosmolarity response, which is a mass measure of RPE integrity. However, more recent studies with ICG angiography suggest that CSR may involve a broad abnormality in choroidal blood flow that could secondarily affect RPE transport physiology (Guyer et al., 1994; Marmor, 1997; see Chapter 21 and Chapter 22). The hyperosmolarity response is also normal in diffuse (hereditary) drusen (Gupta and Marmor, 1994).

The Acetazolamide Response

The acetazolamide (Diamox) response in humans is elicited by a slow intravenous infusion of acetazolamide (e.g., 8–10 mg/kg, given over 1 minute—Yonemura et al., 1978; Marmor, 1989). The response is similar to the hyperosmolarity response, consisting of a slow decrease in the standing potential, but the response is slightly more rapid and reaches a minimum in about 10 min (Fig. 10-15). The mechanisms by which acetazolamide

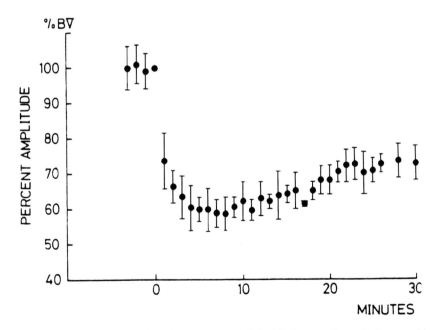

FIGURE 10-15. The clinical acetazolamide response recorded with electrooculography in normal human subjects. The intravenous injection of 500 mg acetazolamide was started at point 0, after the amplitude of the EOG had been stabilized in darkness. (From Madachi-Yamamoto et al., 1984.)

affects RPE voltage and transport are unclear. While the studies are limited, we review them in some detail here since acetazolamide is of particular clinical interest.

Mechanism. The one published study on the effects of acetazolamide on membrane potentials is in the in vitro frog RPE-choroid preparation (Kawasaki et al., 1986b). In frog, apical acetazolamide reduced the TEP by hyperpolarizing the basal membrane. A delayed depolarization of the apical membrane (as the TEP continues to fall) is seen in the published figure but may not have been a consistent finding. Basal acetazolamide hyperpolarized both membranes but produced little change in the TEP. On this basis, the authors concluded that systemic acetazolamide decreases the TEP by its effect on the apical membrane. In cultured human RPE, apical acetazolamide (1 mM) decreased the TEP and produced small changes in membrane voltage—typically an initial apical depolarization followed by membrane hyperpolarizations; basal acetazolamide produced small, inconsistent results (F Maruiwa, RP Galemore, J Hu, and D Bok, unpublished observations). In vivo, systemic acetazolamide probably reaches the RPE via the basal membrane. It may mediate its effects via diffusion to the apical membrane, since acetazolamide is a cell permeant inhibitor of carbonic anhydrase (Burckhardt and Burckhardt, 1988). It is significant, then, that membrane-bound carbonic anhydrase (CA IV) has been localized to the apical side of the RPE in fresh and cultured human preparations (Wolfensberger et al., 1994). Cytosolic carbonic anhydrase II has also been reported (Korte and Smith, 1993).

The mechanism by which acetazolamide alters RPE membrane potentials remains unclear. In the frog RPE-choroid preparation acetazolamide reduces net Cl absorption by stimulating the basal to apical transepithelial Cl flux (Miller and Steinberg, 1977a). How this effect on transport relates to the membrane voltage change awaits investigation. In addition, the effects may differ in mammalian RPE. In any event, the effect of acetazolamide on membrane transport presumably relates to inhibition of carbonic anhydrase. We can suggest that under normal conditions, RPE-associated carbonic anhydrase will function to combine H^+ generated by the photoreceptors with HCO_3 to produce CO_2 + H_2O, which can then diffuse into the blood stream. Consistent with this idea, systemic acetazolamide in the intact cat eye leads to acidification of the subretinal space, and the acidification is highest near the apical membrane of the RPE (Yamamoto and Steinberg, 1992). Photoreceptor metabolism will also generate CO_2, but this can diffuse directly to the circulation without action by carbonic anhydrase. The effect of acetazolamide on RPE transport, then, may be secondary to

its effect on pH regulation by the RPE. Several transport mechanisms have been identified in both amphibian and mammalian RPE that may contribute to pH regulation. As shown in Figure 10-2, these include apical membrane electrogenic $NaHCO_3$ cotransport, electroneutral Na/H exchange, and basal membrane electroneutral Cl/HCO_3 exchange. Effects on these transporters and secondary effects on other transport mechanisms may be involved. The net result should include apical membrane depolarizations and/or basolateral membrane hyperpolarizations producing a decrease in TEP (Fig. 10-13). The possible effects of acetazolamide on RPE transport physiology are considered further in Chapter 6.

While the significance is unclear, we should mention that the effect of acetazolamide on the standing potential appears to be species dependent. In frog, chick, monkey, and humans, acetazolamide reduces the standing potential (or TEP), while in cat and rabbit, an increase in standing potential is observed (Kawasaki et al., 1977; 1986; Miller and Steinberg, 1977b; Yonemura and Kawasaki, 1979; Heike and Marmor, 1991). Since the transepithelial potential is established by a delicate balance between the activity of transport mechanisms at the apical and basal membranes, the essential mechanism of the acetazolamide response may be similar in each case, with a different voltage response produced by differences in the balance of transport activities.

While the mechanism of the acetazolamide response remains unclear, the difference in its effect on the light peak differentiates it from the other nonphotic responses (Fig. 10-16). Acetazolamide does not suppress the light peak (Madachi et al., 1984b), while the hyperosmolarity response decreases it (Kawasaki et al., 1977) and choroidal bicarbonate increases it (Maruiwa et al., 1994). The acetazolamide response may assess different aspects of RPE function, which could facilitate its use in the differentiation and diagnosis of specific diseases involving the RPE. As with the other responses, it will also be affected nonspecifically by any conditions affecting the component resistances of the RPE.

Clinical experience. Initial comparisons of the hyperosmolarity and acetazolamide responses suggested that the hyperosmolarity response was most affected by diffuse or peripheral disease of the RPE, whereas the acetazolamide response was more indicative of macular involvement (Yonemura and Kawasaki, 1979). This would have been very valuable clinically, but later studies (Yonemura et al., 1982; 1983; 1984; Kawasaki et al., 1984; 1986a; Ushimura et al., 1990) have blurred this distinction.

In general, whereas the hyperosmolarity response is reduced rather nonspecifically in a wide range of retinal and RPE disorders, the acetazolamide response is rather

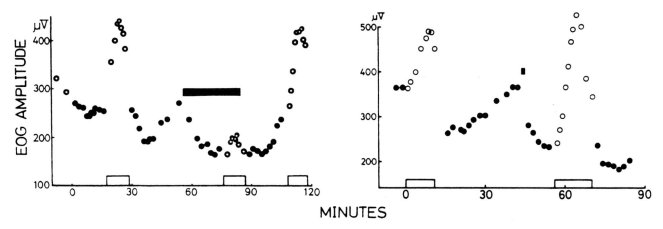

FIGURE 10-16. Interaction of nonphotic potentials with the human light response. The closed and open circles indicate the amplitude of the EOG in the dark and the light, respectively. *Left:* Reversible abolition of the light rise by hyperosmolarity. The black horizontal bar shows the intravenous injection of hypertonic solution. *Right:* Resistance of the light rise to acetazolamide. The small black bar (at 45 min) indicates the injection of acetazolamide. (From [left] Kawasaki et al., 1977 and [right] Madachi-Yamamoto et al., 1984.)

resistant to disease. It remains normal even in severe retinitis pigmentosa, choroideremia, retinal detachment, senile disciform macular degeneration, post-treatment stage of panretinal photocoagulation and central retinal artery occlusion. It may be reduced rather selectively in some cases of fundus flavimaculatus, retinal pigment epitheliopathy, Harada's disease, and central exudative chorioretinopathy (Yonemura et al., 1984; Kawasaki et al., 1984a; Asia 1993; Ushimura, 1993). In diabetic retinopathy, the acetazolamide response may be reduced slightly in advanced disease, but the change does not correlate well with the degree of retinopathy (Segawa, 1994). More recently, Sugawara and colleagues (1996) reported a selective reduction in the acetazolamide response in diabetics with "macular deposits," with normal amplitudes of the EOG L/D ratio and the hyperosmolarity response. Shirao et al. (1997) noted reduced acetazolamide responses in patients with idiopathic as opposed to age-related neovascular maculopathy. More studies are needed, however, to confirm and clarify the diagnostic specificity of these non-photic tests.

In vivo, acetazolamide appears to increase fluid absorption across the RPE. This has been demonstrated experimentally where serous detachments resorb more rapidly with acetazolamide (Marmor and Maack, 1982). Clinically, select cases of cystoid macular edema may respond dramatically to acetazolamide, consistent with this notion (Cox et al., 1988; Fishman et al., 1989; Marmor, 1990; Tripathi et al., 1991). An abnormal acetazolamide response, therefore, may reflect a defect in RPE fluid transport activity. Indeed, Asai (1993) reported a decreased acetazolamide response in Vogt-Koyanagi-Harada disease when associated with serous

retinal detachment. In contrast, however, a normal response was observed (Fig. 10-14) in central serous retinopathy (Gupta and Marmor, 1996), a disorder that may involve abnormality of RPE fluid transport (Marmor, 1997; see Chapter 21). This issue was discussed above in the section on clinical experience under hyperosmolarity response.

Bicarbonate Response

Intravenous infusion of sodium bicarbonate (7% soln, 0.83 ml/kg) also produces a fall in the human standing potential, readily recorded with the EOG (Fig. 10-17) (Segawa, 1987b).

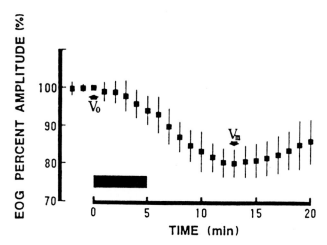

FIGURE 10-17. The clinical bicarbonate response recorded in normal human subjects to an intravenous infusion of 7% NaHCO₃ *(black horizontal bar).* (From Segawa, 1987.)

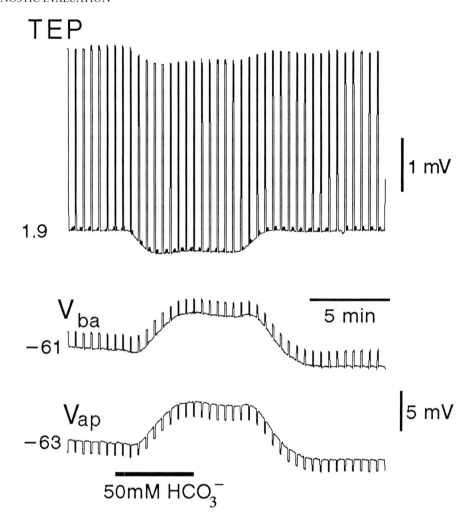

FIGURE 10-18. Effect of choroidal perfusion with high HCO_3 on the electrophysiology of cultured human RPE in vitro. A confluent monolayer of cultured human RPE was mounted in a modified Ussing chamber. The transepithelial potential (TEP), apical membrane potential (V_{ap}), and basal membrane potential (V_{ba}) were recorded using conventional electrophysiological techniques. Transepithelial current was passed to measure the transepithelial resistance (R_t) and apical/basal resistance ratio (R_{ap}/R_{ba}). The basolateral membrane was perfused with 50 mM HCO_3. $NaHCO_3$ was exchanged for NaCl.

Mechanism. A report on an in vitro preparation of cat RPE-choroid (Segawa, 1987a) revealed that basal HCO_3 produced a depolarization of both membranes along with a decrease in TEP, and this is consistent with the depolarization originating at the apical membrane. Basal HCO_3 has the opposite effect in chick RPE, depolarizing the basal membrane and increasing the TEP (Maruiwa et al., 1994). In bovine RPE (Joseph and Miller, 1991) and frog RPE (Miller and Steinberg, 1977b), basal HCO_3 had no significant effect on electrical parameters, while apical HCO_3 hyperpolarized the apical membrane and increased the TEP.

Recently, we studied the response to basal HCO_3 in confluent monolayers of cultured human RPE (F Maruiwa, RP Gallemore, J Hu, and D Bok, unpublished observations). As shown in Figure 10-18, we observed a decrease in transepithelial potential accompanied by depolarizations of both membranes. This indicates a depolarization of the apical membrane with passive shunting to the basal membrane. This is the same result as was observed in cat. We have evidence that this response results in part from inhibition of electrogenic Na/HCO_3 cotransport at the apical membrane. Blockade of apical $NaHCO_3$ cotransport with 4,4′-diisothiocyanostilbene-2,2′-disulfonate (DIDS; Hughes et al., 1989), blocked the membrane depolarizations. In addition, however, in the presence of apical DIDS, basal bicarbonate still produced a small decrease in TEP accompanied by membrane hyperpolarizations. This effect could be on basolateral electrogenic Na/HCO_3-cotransport for which there is now evidence in both cultured and fresh human RPE (Kenyon et al., 1994). Thus, high basal HCO_3 may decrease the TEP by stimulating basolateral $NaHCO_3$ cotransport and inhibiting apical $NaHCO_3$ cotransport. The apical effect may involve HCO_3 entry via basolateral Cl/HCO_3 exchange (Lin and Miller, 1994). The possible membrane contributions to the electrophysiological effects of choroidal HCO_3 are shown in Figure 10-13.

Thus, the HCO_3 response in humans may reflect the activity of electrogenic HCO_3 transport mechanisms. Since these mechanisms appear to be present in both membranes, the response may not test the function of a specific membrane. In addition, since HCO_3 transport functions in pH regulation (Lin and Miller, 1991; 1994; Edelman et al., 1994a; 1994b; Kenyon et al., 1994), any disease which affects pH homeostasis would be expected to alter the response. Any metabolic derangement, for example, affecting photoreceptor metabolism or causing retinal hypoxia could alter retinal pH and affect the RPE in this way (e.g., Yamamoto and Steinberg, 1992b). Finally, as in all of the nonphotic responses, any change in the relative resistance of the RPE could also alter the response amplitude.

Clinical experience. Clinical experience with the bicarbonate response reveals that it may be more sensitive than either the acetazolamide or hyperosmolarity responses to the presence of widespread RPE dysfunction (Segawa, 1987b). In patients with siderosis bulbi and select patients with retinitis pigmentosa and diabetic retinopathy, for example, the bicarbonate response may be severely depressed or absent while the other nonphotic responses show minimal or no reduction (Segawa, 1987b; 1994; Sugawara et al., 1996). The bicarbonate response may also be reduced in patients with neovascular maculopathy of various etiologies, high myopia with diffuse chorioretinal atrophy, Behcet's disease, and sarcoidosis. (Ushimura, 1993; Mori, 1992; Asai, 1993). By elucidating the underlying mechanism of the bicarbonate response, we may learn more about the pathophysiology of diseases where the response is selectively reduced. From our understanding to date, we can suggest that abnormalities in apical or basolateral membrane HCO_3 transport and pH regulation may be present in those conditions where the response is suppressed.

Hypoxia

Standing potential. The human standing potential has been known for decades to be very sensitive to mild lev-els of hypoxia (Fenn et al., 1949; Kolder, 1959). These mild levels are physiologic, comparable to those experienced at high altitudes on land (e.g., 60–80 mm Hg, see Steinberg, 1987 for review). The standing potential is increased by hypoxia and a series of studies by Linsenmeier, Steinberg, and colleagues have revealed many of the fundamental mechanisms underlying the effects of systemic hypoxia on the standing potential of the eye. The retinal pigment epithelium is the origin of the standing potential change in hypoxia. The RPE response is the result of an elevation in extracellular (subretinal) K produced by the slowing of the photoreceptor Na/K pump (Linsenmeier and Steinberg, 1986). The K increase produces a delayed depolarization of the basal membrane increasing the standing potential. (The initial apical depolarization is neutralized by a transretinal potential change, presumably a Müller cell response to the K increase—Linsenmeier and Steinberg, 1984b; 1986.) The basal response is analogous, but of opposite polarity, to the delayed basal membrane hyperpolarization of the fast oscillation, which originates from the light-evoked decrease in subretinal $[K]_o$ (Linsenmeier and Steinberg, 1984a; Griff and Steinberg, 1984; Chapter 9). By analogy, then, the $[K]_o$ increase in hypoxia may stimulate the apical Na,K,2Cl cotransporter, leading to an increase in intracellular Cl activity and depolarization of the basal membrane Cl channel. This hypothesis remains to be tested, and changes in intracellular K could also affect the basal membrane (Linsenmeier and Steinberg, 1986).

DC ERG. The RPE-dependent responses of the DC-ERG are also very sensitive to mild levels of hypoxia. As shown in Figure 10-19, hypoxia increases the c-wave amplitude, deepens the fast-oscillation trough, and suppresses the light peak. The c-wave increase originates from an apparent decrease in RPE basal membrane resistance (Linsenmeier and Steinberg, 1984b). This decrease in basal membrane resistance may be due to the presumed elevation of intracellular Cl activity during hypoxia, which could increase the relative Cl conductance of the basal membrane.

The increase (deepening) of the fast-oscillation trough by hypoxia reflects the change in the light-evoked K decrease that generates this response (Linsenmeier and Steinberg, 1984b; 1986). The slowed photoreceptor Na/K pump causes a slower recovery of the light-evoked $[K]_o$ decrease, resulting in a more sustained (larger) K decrease (Linsenmeier and Steinberg, 1984b). A larger K decrease results in a larger delayed basal hyperpolarization, presumably by slowing the Na,K,2Cl cotransporter to a greater extent in response to the larger, more sustained decrease in $[K]_o$ in hypoxia. This would pro-

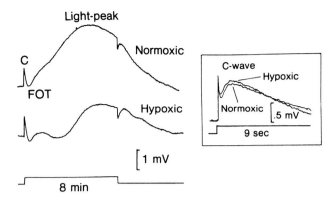

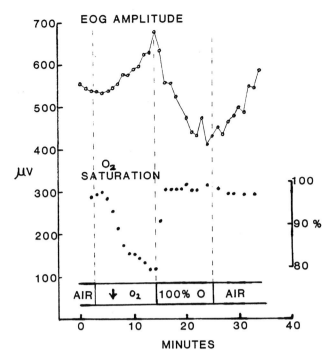

FIGURE 10-19. Effects of hypoxia on the amplitude and time course of the DC-ERG. The components that change during hypoxia are the c-wave *(inset)*, fast-oscillation trough (FOT), and light peak. These are vitreal recordings in response to 8 min of illumination at rod saturation. The hypoxic response was recorded 2 hr after the onset of hypoxia, when P_aO_2 was 30 mm Hg. Vitreal positive signals are shown with an upward polarity. (From Linsenmeier and Steinberg, 1986.)

FIGURE 10-20. Changes in the human standing potential with oxygen saturation. EOG recordings were made in the dark while breathing different concentrations of oxygen. The left-hand scale shows microvolts of EOG amplitude; the right-hand scale shows oxygen saturation. (From Marmor et al., 1985.)

duce a larger fall in intracellular Cl and hence, a larger hyperpolarization of the basolateral membrane.

Suppression of the light peak by hypoxia is perhaps the most complex and least well understood effect. As discussed earlier and in Chapter 9, the light peak does not depend directly on light-evoked $[K]_o$ changes (Steinberg and Niemeyer, 1981) and the paracrine signal between the photoreceptors and RPE remains unknown. The "light peak substance" may be released directly by the photoreceptors (Linsenmeier and Steinberg, 1982; Gallemore et al., 1988), thus the exquisite sensitivity of the light peak to hypoxia may reflect its dependence on photoreceptor metabolism. The sensitivity of the light peak to hypoxia has also been confirmed in EOG recordings in humans (Linsenmeier et al., 1987). A more complete understanding of the effects of hypoxia on the light peak will first require a greater understanding of the origin of this potential.

Clinical experience. The sensitivity of the standing potential to hypoxia has not been applied as a clinical test. Marmor and colleagues (1985) studied the effects of hypoxia and hyperoxia on the human standing potential. They used sequential exposure to hypoxia followed by hyperoxia to produce a substantial oscillation in the standing potential, an increase followed by a decrease (Fig. 10-20). In theory, this change could be applied as a clinical measure of RPE function, but the difficulty and risks of modulating oxygen would limit its application (Marmor et al., 1985). Linsenmeier et al. (1987) confirmed the effects of hypoxia on the EOG standing potential and light peak in human subjects using standardized EOG measurement protocols.

Ethanol

The human standing potential is also known to be sensitive to systemic administration of ethanol (Zrenner et al., 1986). A moderate oral dose of ethanol (Skoog et al., 1975) induces a large increase in the human standing potential within 10 minutes, in both the dark- and light-adapted state, and the potential will then oscillate slowly for one or two cycles. Experiments in bovine RPE-choroid preparations provide evidence that ethanol increases that TEP by increasing the basolateral membrane Cl conductance. Ethanol depolarizes the basolateral membrane and increases its apparent conductance (Bialek et al., 1996). Similar results have also been obtained in human RPE (Quinn and Miller, 1992).

CONCLUSIONS

Much progress has been made over the last two decades toward understanding the cellular origin of photic and nonphotic RPE responses. However, none of the RPE responses has been linked to functions that modify retinal health or vision. Until such linkage can be established, these tests will be of limited clinical value. They serve as nonspecific markers of diffuse RPE damage, but have little specificity for individual diseases or mechanisms of disease. Since most RPE diseases are visible ophthalmoscopically, electrophysiology is not needed unless the diagnosis is in question or additional information about pathogenesis will be revealed.

The photic responses—c-wave, fast oscillation, EOG light response—are most widely used at present, primarily the EOG light response. It is uniquely valuable for Best's disease because of its severe suppression in that disease. However, the complete functional normality (so far as we know at present) of some carriers of the Best gene, while the EOG is suppressed, highlights the limitation of the test as a provider of functional information about the health of RPE. All of the photic responses must be interpreted with caution, with respect to RPE specificity, since photoreceptor activity is needed to initiate the responses. Photoreceptor disease will affect the signals, and in fact any retinal or choroidal process that causes a release of humoral factors or an alteration in ionic environment may alter the responses by modifying the transport physiology of the RPE membranes.

The nonphotic responses have been used very little by clinicians, partly because of the time required and medical risks of intravenous injections, and partly for a lack of data on their specificity for diseases or disease processes. They have the theoretical advantage of being independent of photoreceptor activation, but they are not independent of retinal pathology such as ischemia, since diffusion of ionic effects or active metabolites from retinal and/or choroidal sites may alter RPE membrane function. As we learn more about the photic and nonphotic responses, their value will increase for determining mechanisms of disease, staging disease, and assessing response to treatment.

Additional tests are needed that would assess more specifically RPE health independent of the retina, for example, as markers of aging changes or toxic effects, to stage specific diseases of the RPE, and to evaluate RPE function relative to newer therapies such as RPE transplantation and nutrient supplementation. Other RPE functions to monitor include outer segment phagocytosis, transport of ions and metabolites, synthetic capability, adhesive properties, integrity of the interphotoreceptor matrix, and antioxidant activity. A challenge for the coming decades will be to find such tests.

REFERENCES

Abraham R, Hendy RJ. 1970. Irreversible lysosomal damage induced by chloroquine in the retinae of pigmented albino rats. Exp Mol Pathol 12:185–200.

Anderson WP, Sheppard DN, Berger HA, Welsh MJ. 1992. Chloride channels in the apical membrane of normal and cystic fibrosis airway and intestinal epithelia. Am J Physiol 263:L1–L14.

Arden GB. 1968. Recent work on the early receptor potential and related rapid responses. In: The Clinical Value of Electroretinography (ISCERG Symp Ghent 1966). Basel: Karger, 51–59.

Arden GB, Fojas MR. 1962. Electrophysiological abnormalities in pigmentary degenerations of the retina. Arch Ophthalmol 68:369–389.

Arden GB, Kelsey JH. 1962. Changes produced by light in the standing potential of the human eye. J. Physiol 161:189–204.

Arden GB, Barrada A, Kelsey JH. 1962a. New clinical test of retinal function based upon the standing potential of the eye. Br J Ophthalmol 46:449–467.

Arden GB, Friedman A, Kolb H. 1962b. Anticipation of chloroquine retinopathy. Lancet 1:1164–1165.

Arden GB, Ikeda H, Siegel IM. 1966. New components of the mammalian receptor potential and their relation to visual photochemistry. Vision Res 6:373–384.

Asai H. 1993. Electrophysiological analysis of uveitis. J Juzen Med Soc 102:605–626.

Bernstein HN. 1992. Ocular safety of hydroxychloroquine sulfate (Plaquenil). Southern Medical Journal 85:274–279.

Bernstein HN, Ginsberg J. 1964. The pathology of chloroquine retinopathy. Arch Ophthalmol 71:238–245.

Berson EL. 1993. Retinitis pigmentosa. The Friedenwald Lecture. Invest Ophthalmol Vis Sci 36:523–541.

Bialek S, Joseph D, Miller S. 1995. The delayed basolateral membrane hyperpolarization of the bovine retinal pigment epithelium: mechanism of generation. J Physiol 484:53–67.

Bialek S, Quong J, Yu K, Miller SS. 1996. Non-steroid anti-inflammatory drugs modulated Cl conductance and fluid transport in bovine pigment epithlium. Am J Physiol 27:C1175–1189.

Bird AC. 1994. Pathogenesis of serous detachment of the retina and pigment epithelium. In Ryan SJ ed, Retina, 2nd edition. St. Louis: Mosby, 63:1019–1026.

Bird AC. 1995. Retinal photoreceptor dystrophies LI. Edward Jackson Memorial lecture. Am J Ophthalmol 119:543–562.

Bishara SA, Matamoros N. 1989. Evaluation of several tests in screening for chloroquine maculopathy. Eye 3:777–782.

Blazynski C, Cohen AI, Fruh B, Niemeyer G. 1989. Adenosine: autoradiographic localization and electrophysiologic effects in the cat retina. Invest Ophthalmol Vis Sci 30:2533–2536.

Botchkin LM, Matthews G. 1993. Chloride current activated by swelling in retinal pigment epithelium cells. Am J Physiol 265:C1037–C1045.

Braun RD, Linsenmeier RA. 1995. Retinal oxygen tension and the electroretinogram during arterial occlusion in the cat. Invest Ophthalmol Vis Sci 36:523–541.

Brink H, Pinckers A, Verbeek A. 1989. The electro-oculogram as an aid in the diagnosis of uveal melanoma. Int Ophthalmol 13:305–309.

Brinkley JR Jr, Dubois EL, Ryan SJ. 1979. Long term course of chloroquine retinopathy after cessation of medication. Am J Ophthalmol 88:1–11.

Brown KT. 1965. An early potential evoked by light from the pigment epithelium-choroid complex of the toad. Nature 207:1249–1253.

Brown KT, Crawford JM. 1967. Intracellular recording of rapid light-evoked response from pigment epithelium cells of the frog eye. Vis Res 7:265–278.

Brown KT, Gage PW. 1966. An early phase of the light-evoked electrical response from the pigment epithelium-choroid complex of the eye of the toad. Nature 211:155–158.

Burckhardt R-Ch, Burckhardt G. 1988. Cellular mechanisms of proximal tubular acidification. In: Haüssinger D ed, pH Homeostasis: Mechanisms and Control. San Diego: Academic Press, 233–262.

Cox NH, Paterson WD. 1994. Ocular toxicity of antimalarials in dermatology: a recent survey of current practice. Br J Derm 131: 878–882.

Cox SN, Hay E, Bird AC. 1988. Treatment of chronic macular edema with acetazolamide. Arch Ophthalmol 106:1190–1195.

Cross HE. 1974. Electro-oculography in Best's macular dystrophy. Am J Ophthalmol 77:46–50.

Dawis SM, Niemeyer G. 1985. Dopamine influences the light peak in the perfused mammalian eye. Invest Ophthalmol Vis Sci 27: 330–335.

Dawis SM, Niemeyer G. 1987. Theophylline abolishes the light peak in perfused cat eyes. Invest Ophthalmol Vis Sci 28:700–706.

De Rouck A, Kayembe D. 1981. A clinical procedure for the simultaneous recording of fast and slow EOG oscillations. Int Ophthalmol 3:179–189.

Deutman AF. 1994. Macular dystrophies. In: Ryan SJ ed, Retina, 2nd edition. St Louis: Mosby, 1186–1240.

Du Bois-Reymond E. 1849. Untersuchungen uber thierische Elektricitat. Berlin: Teimer, 2:256–257.

Drenckhahn D, Lullmann-Rauch R. 1978. Drug-induced retinal lipidosis: differential susceptibilities of pigment epithelium and neuroretina towards several amphiphilic cationic drugs. Exp Mol Pathol 28:360–371.

Easterbrook M. 1984. The use of Amsler grids in early chloroquine retinopathy. Ophthalmology 91:1368–1372.

Easterbrook M. 1993. Screening for antimalarial toxicity. Can J Ophthalmol 28:51–52.

Ebrey TG, Cone RA. 1967. Melanin, a possible pigment for the photostable electrical responses of the eye. Nature 213:360–362.

Edelman JL, Miller SS. 1991. Epinephrine stimulates fluid absorption across bovine retinal pigment epithelium. Invest Ophthalmol Vis Sci 32:3033–3040.

Edelman JL, Lin H, Miller SS. 1994a. Acidification stimulates chloride and fluid absorption across frog retinal pigment epithelium. Am J Physiol 266:C946–C956.

Edelman JL, Lin H, Miller SS. 1994b. Potassium-induced chloride secretion across the frog retinal pigment epithelium. Am J Physiol 266:C957–C966.

Faber DS. 1969. Analysis of the slow transretinal potentials in response to light. Ph.D. dissertation. State University of New York, Buffalo.

Fenn WO, Galambos R, Otis AB, Rahn H. 1949. Corneo-retinal potential in anoxia and acapnia. J Appl Physiol 1:710–716.

Finbloom DS, Silver K, Newsome DA, Gunkel R. 1985. Comparison of hydroxychloroquine and chloroquine use and the development of retinal toxicity. J Rheumatol 12:692–694.

Fishman GA, Trimble S, Rabb MF, Fishman M. Pseudo-vitelliform macular degeneration. Arch Ophthalmol 95:73–76.

Fishman GA, Filbert COT, Fiscella RG, Kimura AE, Jampol LMM. Acetazolamide for treatment of chronic macular edema in retinitis pigmentosa. Arch Ophthalmol 1989; 107:1445–1452.

Frangieh GT, Green WR, Fine SL. 1982. A histopathologic study of Best's macular dystrophy. Arch Ophthalmol 100:1115–1121.

Fuller CM, Benos DJ. 1992. CFTR! Am J Physiol 263:C267–C286.

Fujii S, Gallemore RP, Hughes B, Steinberg RH. 1992. Direct evidence for a basolateral membrane Cl⁻ conductance in toad retinal pigment epithelium. Am J Physiol 262:C374–C383.

Gallemore RP. 1992. Ionic mechanism of the light-peak voltage of the DC electroretinogram. Ph.D. dissertation. University of California, San Francisco.

Gallemore RP, Steinberg RH. 1989a. Effects of DIDS on the chick retinal pigment epithelium. I. membrane potentials, apparent resistances and mechanisms. J Neurosci 9:1968–1976.

Gallemore RP, Steinberg RH. 1989b. Effects of DIDS on the chick retinal pigment epithelium. II. mechanism of the light peak and other responses originating at the basal membrane. J Neurosci 9:1977–1984.

Gallemore RP, Steinberg RH. 1990. Effects of dopamine on the chick retinal pigment epithelium: membrane potentials and light-evoked responses. Invest Ophthalmol Vis Sci 31:67–80.

Gallemore RP, Steinberg RH. 1991a. Cobalt increases photoreceptor-dependent responses of the chick retinal pigment epithelium. Invest Ophthalmol Vis Sci 32:3041–3052.

Gallemore RP, Steinberg RH. 1991b. The light peak of the DC ERG is associated with an increase in Cl⁻ conductance in chick RPE. Invest Ophthalmol Vis Sci (ARVO abstr). 32:837.

Gallemore RP, Steinberg RH. 1993. Light-evoked modulation of basal membrane Cl⁻ conductance in chick retinal pigment epithelium: the light peak and fast oscillation. J Neurophysiol 70:1669–1680.

Gallemore RP, Griff ER, Steinberg RH. 1988. Evidence in support of a photoreceptoral origin of the "light-peak substance." Invest Ophthalmol Vis Sci 29:566–571.

Gallemore RP, Hernandez E, Tayyanipour R, Fujii S, Steinberg RH. 1993. Basolateral membrane Cl⁻ and K⁺ conductances in the dark-adapted chick retinal pigment epithelium. J Neurophysiol 70:1656–1668.

Gallemore RP, Hue JG, Frambach DA, Bok D. 1995. Ion transport in cultured fetal human retinal pigment epithelium. Invest Ophthalmol Vis Sci (ARVO abstr). 36:216.

Gallemore RP, Maruiwa F, Takahira M, Hughes B, Hu JG, Bok D. 1996. Swelling-activated chloride conductance in cultured human retinal pigment epithelium. Invest Ophthalmol Vis Sci (ARVO abstr) 37:S230.

Gallemore RP, Hughes BA, Miller SS. 1997. Retinal pigment epithelial transport mechanisms and their contributions to the electroretinogram. Prog Ret Eye Res 16:509–566.

Gouras P, Carr RE. 1965. Light-induced DC responses of monkey retina before and after central retinal artery interruption. Invest Ophthalmol 4:316–317.

Griff E, Steinberg RH. 1982. Origin of the light peak: in vitro study of Gekko gekko. J Physiol (Lond) 331:637–652.

Griff E, Steinberg RH. 1984. Changes in apical $[K^+]_o$ produce delayed basal membrane responses of the retinal pigment epithelium in gecko. J Gen Physiol 83:193–211.

Gupta LY, Marmor MF. 1994. Sequential recording of photic and nonphotic electro-oculogram responses in patients with extensive extramacular drusen. Doc Ophthalmol 88:46–55.

Gupta LY, Marmor MF. 1996. Electrophysiology of the retinal pigment epithelium in the central serous chorioretinopathy. Doc Ophthalmol 91:101–107.

Hara A, Miura M. 1994. Decreased inner retinal activity in branch retinal vein occlusion. Doc Ophthalmol 88:39–47.

Hara A, Nagatomo M. 1995. Branch retinal vein occlusion decreases the potential of the inner retinal layer. Nippon Med School 62:50–54.

Hart WM Jr, et al. 1984. Static preimetry in chloroquine retinopathy: perifoveal patterns of visual field depression. Arch Ophthamol 102:377–380.

Hess F, Niemeyer G. EOG changes in dominantly inherited drusen (Malattia leventinese). Doc Ophthalmol 37:105–113.

Heckenlively JR. 1988. RP syndromes. In: Heckenlively JR, ed, Retinitis Pigmentosa. Philadelphia: Lippincott, 150–154.

Heike M, Marmor MF. 1991. Recovery of retinal pigment epithelial function after ischemia in the rabbit. Invest Ophthalmol Vis Sci 32:73–77.

Hock PA, Marmor MF. 1983. Variability of the human c-wave. Doc Ophthalmol Proc Series 37:151–157.

Hsieh RC, Fine BS, Lyons JS. 1977. Pattern dystrophies of the retinal pigment epithelium. Arch Ophthalmol 95:429–435.

Hughes BA, Segawa Y. 1993. cAMP-activated chloride currents in amphibian retinal pigment epithelial cells. J Physiol 466:746–766.

Hughes BA, Miller SS, Machen TE. 1984. Effects of cyclic AMP on fluid absorption and ion transport across frog retinal pigment epithelium: measurements in the open-circuit state. J Gen Physiol 83:875–899.

Hughes BA, Miller SS, Farber DB. 1987. Adenylate cyclase alters transport in frog retinal pigment epithelium. Am J Physiol 252:C385–C395.

Hughes BA, Adorante JS, Miller SS, Lin H. 1989. Apical electrogenic $NaHCO_3$ cotransport: a mechanism for HCO_3 absorption across the retinal pigment epithelium. J Gen Physiol 94:125–150.

Itabashi R, Katsumi O, Mehta MC, Wajima R, Tamiai M, Hirose T. 1993. Stargardt's disease/fundus flavimaculatus: psychophysical and electrophysiological results. Graefes Arch Clin Exp Ophthalmol 231:555–562.

Johnson MA, McPhee TJ. 1993. Electroretinographic findings in iris neovascularization due to acute central retinal vein occlusion. Arch Ophthalmol 111:806–814.

Joseph D, Miller S. 1991. Apical and basal membrane ion transport mechanisms in bovine retinal pigment epithelium. J Physiol 435:439–463.

Joseph D, Miller S. 1992. Alpha-1-adrenergic modulation of K and Cl transport in bovine retinal pigment epithelium. J Gen Physiol 99:263–290.

Kawasaki K, Yamamoto S, Yonemura D. 1977. Electrophysiological approach to clinical test for the retinal pigment epithelium. Acta Soc Ophthalmol Jpn 81:89–98.

Kawasaki K, Yonemura D, Madachi-Yamamoto S. 1984a. Hyperosmolarity response of ocular standing potential as a clinical test for retinal pigment epithelium activity: diabetic retinopathy. Doc Ophthalmol 58:375–384.

Kawasaki K, Madachi-Yamamoto S, Yonemura D. 1984b. Hyperosmolarity response of ocular standing potential as a clinical test for retinal pigment epithelium activity: rhegmatogenous retinal detachment. Doc Ophthalmol 57:175–180.

Kawasaki K, Yonemura D, Yanagida T, Segawa, Y, Wakabayashi K, Mukoh S, Ishida H, Fujii S, Takahara Y. 1986a. Suppression of hyperosmolarity response after cataract surgery. Doc Ophthalmol 63:367–373.

Kawasaki K, Mukoh S, Yonemura D, Fujii S, Segawa Y. 1986b. Acetazolamide-induced changes of membrane potentials of the retinal pigment epithelial cell. Doc Ophthalmol 63:375–381.

Kenyon E, Joseph D, Miller S. 1994. Evidence for electrogenic Cl-dependent Na-HCO_3 cotransport at the apical membrane of bovine RPE. Invest Ophthalmol Vis Sci (ARVO abstr) 35:1759.

Kolb H. 1965. Electro-oculogram findings in patients treated with antimalarial drugs. Br J Ophthalmol 59:573–590.

Kolder H. 1959. Spontane and experimentelle Angerungen des Bestandpotentials des menschlichen Auges. Pflugers Arch 268:258–272.

Kolder H, Brecker GA. 1966. Fast oscillations of the corneo-retinal potential in man. Arch Ophthalmol 75:232–237.

Kolder H, North AW. 1966. Oscillations of the corneo-retinal potential in animals. Ophthalmol 34:229–241.

Kris C. 1958. Corneo-fundal potential variations during light and dark adaptation. Nature 182:1027–1028.

Leguire LE, Pappa KS, McGregor ML, Bremer DL. 1992. Electro-oculogram in vitamin A deficiency associated with cystic fibrosis: short communication. Ophthalmic Paediatrics and Genetics 13:187–189.

Lessel MR, Thaler A, Scheiber V, Heilig P. 1993. Comparison of electro-oculogram recording methods. Ophthalmic Res 25:245–252.

Lim ATH, Goh KY, Lim SA, Khoo BK. 1996. Red saturation comparison charts a new semiquantitative color test for unilateral optic neuropathies. Invest Ophthalmol Vis Sci (ARVO abstr) 37:S1078.

Lin H, Miller S. 1991. pHi regulation in frog retinal pigment epithelium: two apical membrane mechanisms. Am J Physiol 261:C132–C142.

Lin H, Miller S. 1994. pH$_i$-dependent Cl-HCO_3 exchange at the basolateral membrane of frog retinal pigment epithelium. Am J Physiol 266:C935–C945.

Linsenmeier RA, Steinberg RH. 1982. Origin and sensitivity of the light peak in the intact cat eye. J Physiol (Lond) 331:653–673.

Linsenmeier RA, Steinberg RH. 1984a. Delayed basal hyperpolarization of the cat retinal pigment epithelium, and its relation to the fast-oscillation of the DC ERG. J Gen Physiol 83:213–232.

Linsenmeier RA, Steinberg RH. 1984b. Effects of hypoxia on potassium homeostasis and pigment epithelial cells in the cat retina. J Gen Physiol 84:945–970.

Linsenmeier RA, Steinberg RH. 1986. Mechanisms of hypoxic effects on the cat DC electroretinogram. Invest Ophthalmol Vis Sci 27:1385–1394.

Linsenmeier R, Smith VC, Pokorny J. 1987. The light rise of the electrooculogram during hypoxia. Clin Vis Sci 2:111–116.

MacKenzie AH. 1983. Dose refinements in long-term therapy of rheumatoid arthritis with antimalarials. Am J Med 75:40–45.

MacKenzie AH, Scherbel AL. 1968. A decade of chloroquine maintenance therapy: rate of administration governs incidence of retinotoxicity. Arthritis Rheum 11:496.

Madachi-Yamamoto S, Yonemura D, Kawasaki K. 1984a. Hyperosmolarity response of ocular standing potential as a clinical test for retinal pigment epithelial cell activity: normative data. Doc Ophthalmol 57:153–162.

Madachi-Yamamoto S, Yonemura D, Kawasaki K. 1984b. Diamox response of ocular standing potential as a clinical test for retinal pigment epithelium activity: normative data. Acta Soc Ophthalmol Jpn 88:1267–1272.

Marmor MF. 1979a. "Vitelliform" lesions in adults. Am Ophthalmol 11:1705–1712.

Marmor MF. 1979b. Dystrophies of the retinal pigment epithelium. In: Zinn K, Marmor MF, eds, The Retinal Pigment Epithelium. Cambridge, MA: Harvard University Press, 424–453.

Marmor MF. 1988. New hypothesis on the pathogenesis and treatment of serous retinal detachment. Graefes Arch Clin Exp Ophthalmal 226:548–552.

Marmor MF. 1989. Clinical electrophysiologic tests for evaluating the retinal pigment epithelium. In: Zingirian M, Piccolino FC, eds, Retinal Pigment Epithelium: Proceedings of the International Meeting of S. Margherita Ligure, Italy, 1988. Amsterdam: Kugler & Ghedini, 9–15.

Marmor MF. 1990. Hypothesis concerning carbonic anhydrase treatment of cystoid macular edema: example with epiretinal membrane. Arch Ophthalmol 108:1524–1525.

Marmor MF. 1991. Clinical electrophysiology of the retinal pigment epithelium. Doc Ophthalmol 76:301–313.

Marmor MF. 1997. On the cause of serous detachments and acute central serous chorioretinopathy. Brit J Ophthalmol 81:812–813.

Marmor MF, Byers B. 1977. Pattern dystrophy of the pigment epithelium. Am J Ophthalmol 84:32–44.

Marmor MF, Lurie M. 1979. Light-induced electrical responses of the retinal pigment epithelium. In: Zinn K, Marmor MF, eds, The Retinal Pigment Epithelium. Cambridge, MA: Harvard University Press, 226–244.

Marmor MF, Maack T. 1982. Enhancement of retinal adhesion and subretinal fluid resorption by acetazolamide. Invest Ophthalmol Vis Sci 23:121–124.

Marmor MF, Negi A. 1986. Pharmacologic modifications of subretinal fluid absorption by acetazolamide. Arch Ophthalmol 104:1674–1677.

Marmor MF, Yao XY. 1994. Conditions necessary for the formation of serous detachment: experimental evidence from the cat. Arch Ophthalmol 112:830–838.

Marmor MF, Zrenner E. 1993. Standard for clinical electro-oculography. Arch Ophthalmol 111:601–603.

Marmor MF, Donovan WJ, Gaba DM. 1985. Effects of hypoxia and hyperoxia on the human standing potential. Doc Ophthalmol 60:347–352.

Maruiwa F, Nao-i N, Nakazaki S, Sawada A. 1994. Effect of bicarbonate ion on chick retinal pigment epithelium: membrane potentials and light-evoked responses. Invest Ophthalmol Vis Sci (ARVO abstr). 35:2127.

Matsuura T, Miller WH, Tomita T. 1978. Cone-specific c-wave in the turtle retina. Vision Res 18:767–775.

Miles WR. 1940. Modification of the human-eye potential by dark and light adaptation. Science 91:456.

Miller SS, Steinberg RH. 1977a. Active transport of ions across retinal pigment epithelium. Exp Eye Res 25:235–248.

Miller SS and Steinberg RH. 1977b. Passive ionic properties of frog retinal pigment epithelium. J Membr Biol 36:337–372.

Miller SS, Rabin J, Strong T, Iannuzzi M, Adams A, Collins F, Reenstra W, McCray P Jr. 1992. Cystic fibrosis (CF) gene product is expressed in retina and retinal pigment epithelium. Invest Ophthalmol Vis Sci 33:1009 (Abstract).

Miller SS, Peterson WM, Meggyesy C, Lin H. 1996. P2-purinergic receptors modulate K and Cl transport across bovine RPE. Invest Ophthalmol Vis Sci (ARVO abstr) 37:S229.

Mori T, Marmor MF, Miyamoto K, Tazawa Y. 1991. Combined photic and nonphotic electrooculographic responses in clinical evaluation of the retinal pigment epithelium. Doc Ophthalmol 76:315–322.

Mukoh S. 1985. Electrical responses of the retinal pigment epithelium to hyperosmolarity. Acta Soc Ophthalmol Jpn 89:482–497.

Mukoh S, Kawasaki K, Yonemura D, Tanabe J. 1985. Hyperosmolarity-induced hyperpolarization of the membrane potential of the retinal pigment epithelium. Doc Ophthalmol 60:369–374.

Mori T. 1992. Evaluation of the electrophysiological examination for uveitis. Ganka 34:153–161.

Nao-i N, Neilson SE, Gallemore RP, Steinberg RH. 1989. Effects of melatonin on the chick retinal pigment epithelium: membrane potentials and light-evoked responses. Exp Eye Res. 49:1–17.

Nao-i N, Gallemore RP, Steinberg RH. 1990. Effects of cAMP and IBMX on the chick retinal pigment epithelium: membrane potentials and light-evoked responses. Invest Ophthalmol Vis Sci 31:54–66.

Negi A, Marmor M. 1983. The resorption of subretinal fluid after diffuse damage to the retinal pigment epithelium. Invest Ophthalmol Vis Sci 24:1475–1479.

Negi A, Marmor M. 1984. Experimental serous retinal detachment and focal pigment epithelial damage. Arch Ophthalmol 102:445–449.

Niemeyer G. 1989. Indications for electrophysiologic studies of the eye. Klinische Monatsblatter fur Augenheilkunde. 194:333–336.

Nilsson SE. 1985. Electrophysiology in pigment epithelial changes. Acta Ophthalmologica Supplementum 173:22–27.

Noell WK. 1952. Azide-sensitive potential difference across the eyebulb. Am J Physiol 170:217–238.

Noell WK. 1953. Studies on the electrophysiology and metabolism of the retina. Randolph Field, TX: USAF School of Aviation Med Project 21:1201–1204.

Oakley B II, Green DG. 1976. Correlation of light-induced changes in retinal extracellular potassium concentration with the c-wave of the electroretinogram. J Neurophysiol 39:1117–1133.

Olschwang S, Tiret A, Laurent-Puig P, Muleris M, Parc R, Thomas G. 1993. Restriction of ocular fundus lesions to a specific subgroup of APC mutations in adenomatous polyposis coli patients. Cell 75(5):959–968.

Papakostopoulos D, Bloom PA, Grey RH, Dean Hart JC. 1992. The electro-oculogram in central retinal vein occlusion. Br J Ophthalmol 76:515–519.

Pinckers A, van Aarem A, Brink H. 1994. The electrooculogram in heterozygote carriers of Usher syndrome, retinitis pigmentosa, neuronal ceroid lipofuscinosis, senior syndrome and choroideremia. Ophthalmic Genetics 15:25–30.

Ponte F, Anastasi M and Cillino S. 1986. Clinical patterns and electrophysiological findings in retinal pigment epithelium disease: does a correlation exist? Doc Ophthalmol. 62:73–79.

Priem HA, De Rouck A, De Laey JJ, Bird AC. 1988. Electrophysiologic studies in birdshot choroiretinopathy. Am J Ophthalmol 106:430–436.

Quinn RH, Miller SS. 1992. Ion transport mechanisms in native human retinal pigment epithelium. Invest Ophthalmol Vis Sci 33:3513–3527.

Raines M, Bhargava S, Rosen E. 1989. The blood-retinal barrier in chloroquine retinopathy. Invest Ophthalmol Vis Sci 30:1726–1731.

Rosenthal AR, Kolb H, Bergsma D, Huxsoll D, Hopkins JL. 1978. Chloroquine retinopathy in the rhesus monkey. Invest Ophthalmol Vis Sci 17:1158–1175.

Rubin M, Slonicki A. 1966. A mechanism for the toxicity of chloroquine. Arthritis Rheum 9:537.

Santos A, Morales L, Hernandez-Quintela E, Jimenez-Sierra JM, Villalobos JJ, Panduro A. 1994. Congenital hypertrophy of the retinal pigment epithelium associated with familial adenomatous polyposis. Retina. 14:6–9.

Segawa Y. 1987a. Electrical response of the retinal pigment epithelium to sodium bicarbonate. I: experimental studies in animals. J Juzen Med Soc 96:1008–1021.

Segawa Y. 1987b. Electrical response of the retinal pigment epithelium to sodium bicarbonate. II: Clinical use for electrophysiological evaluation of the retinal pigment epithelium activity. J Juzen Med Soc 96:1022–1041.

Segawa Y. 1994. Retinal pigment epitheliopathy in diabetes mellitus. J Juzen Med Soc 103:743–781.

Shirao Y, Segawa Y. 1989. Electrical response of the retinal pigment epithelium. In: Mishima S, Tsukahara I, Uemura Y, eds, Ganka Mook 41. Tokyo: Kinbara, 71–86.

Shirao Y, Steinberg RH. 1987. Mechanisms of effects of small hyperosmotic gradients on the chick RPE. Invest Ophthalmol Vis Sci 28:2015–2025.

Shirao Y, Ushimura S, Kawasaki K. 1997. Differentiation of neovascular maculopathies by nonphotic electroculogram responses. Jpn J Ophthalmol 41:174–179.

Skoog KO, Textorius O, Nilsson SEG. 1975. Effects of ethyl alcohol on the directly recorded standing potential of the human eye. Acta Ophthalmol 53:710–720.

Spalton DJ, Verdon Roe GM, Hughes GR. 1993. Hydroxychloroquine: dosage parameters and retinopathy. Lupus 2:355–358.

Spitznas M. 1986. Pathogenesis of central serous retinopathy: a new working hypothesis. Graefes Arch Clin Exp Ophthalmol. 224:321–324.

Steinberg RH, 1987. Monitoring communications between photoreceptors and pigment epithelial cells: effects of "mild" systemic hypoxia. Invest Ophthalmol Vis Sci 28:1888–1904.

Steinberg R, Niemeyer G. 1981. Light peak of cat DC electroretinogram: not generated by a change in $[K^+]_o$. Invest Ophthalmol Vis Sci 20:414–418.

Steinberg RH, Oakley B II, Niemeyer G. 1980. Light-evoked changes in $[K^+]_o$ in retina of intact cat eye. J Neurophysiol 44:897–921.

Steinberg RH, Linsenmeier RA, Griff ER. 1985. Retinal pigment epithelial cell contributions to the electrooculogram. In: Osborne N, Chader G, eds, Progress in Retinal Research, vol 4. New York: Pergamon Press, 33–66.

Sugawara T, Fukada A, Sasaki Y, Sasaki K, Takahashi Y, Tazawa Y. 1996. RPE fuction and macular deposits in diabetic retinopathy. Folia Ophthalmol Jpn 47:501–504.

Sunness JS, Massof RW. 1986. Focal electro-oculogram in age-related macular degeneration. Am J Optom and Physiol Optics 63:7–11.

Sunness JS, Massof RW, Johnson MA, Finkelstein D, Fine SL. 1985. Peripheral retinal function in age-related macular degeneration. Arch Ophthalmol 103:811–816.

Taumer R, Rhode N, Wollensak J. 1982. Course of disturbance of EOG in retinal vessel occlusion. Graefes Arch Clin Exp Ophthalmol 219:29–33.

Timmins N, Marmor MF. 1992. Studies on the stability of the clinical electro-oculogram. Doc Ophthalmol 81:163–171.

Tripathi RC, Fekrat S, Tripathi BJ, Ernest TJ. 1991. A direct correlation of the resolution of psudophakic cystoid macular edema with acetazolamide therapy. Ann Ophthalmol 23:127–129.

Tsuboi S, Pederson J. 1985. Experimental retinal detachment X. Effect of acetazolamide on vitreous fluorescein disappearance. Arch Ophthalmol 103:1557–1558.

Ueda Y, Steinberg R. 1994. Chloride currents in freshly isolated rat retinal pigment epithelial cells. Exp Eye Res 58:331–342.

Ushimura S. 1993. Electro-oculographical analysis of neovascular maculopathy. J Juzen Med Soc 102:92–123.

Ushimura S, Asai H, Wakabayashi K, Kawasaki K. 1990. Studies on retinal pigment epithelium activities in neovascular maculopathy. Folia Ophthalmol Jpn 41:1352–1557.

Ushimura S, Wakabayashi K, Kawasaki K. 1992. Electro-oculographical features of high myopia. Jpn J Clin Ophthalmol 46(6):449–453.

Ushimura S, Iwase T, Shirao Y, Tanabe J, Wakabayashi K. 1993. Electro-oculographic findings in retinal disease with macular hemorrhage. Folia Ophthalmol Jpn 44:610–615.

van Aarem A, Cremers CW, Pinkers AJ, Hombergen GC, Kimberling BJ. 1995. The Usher syndrome type 2A: climical findings in obligate carriers. Int J Ped Otorhinolaryngol 31:159–174.

Wajima R, Chater SB, Katsumi O, Mehta MC, Hirose T. 1993. Correlating visual acuity and electrooculogram recordings in Best's disease. Ophthalmologica. 207:174–181.

Wallis YL, McDonald F, Hulten M, Morton JE, McKeown CM, Neoptolemos JP, Keighley M, Morton DG. 1994. Genotype-phenotype correlation between position of constitutional APC gene mutation and CHRPE expression in familial adenomatous polyposis. Human Genetics 94:543–548.

Walter P, Brunner R, Heimann K. 1994. Atypical presentations of Best's vitelliform macular degeneration: clinical findings in seven cases. German J. Ophthalmol 3:440–444.

Weingeist TA, Kobrin JL, Watzke RC. 1982. Histopathology of Best's macular dystrophy. Arch Ophthalmol 100:1108–1114.

Weleber RG. 1989. Fast and slow oscillations of the electro-oculogram in Best's macular degeneration and retinitis pigmentosa. Arch Ophthalmol 107:530–537.

Witkovsky P, Dudek FE, Ripps H. 1975. Slow PIII component of the carp electroretinogram J Gen Physiol 65:119–134.

Yamamoto F, Steinberg RH. 1992a. Effects of intravenous acetazolamide on retinal pH in the cat. Exp Eye Res 54:711–718.

Yamamoto F, Steinberg RH. 1992b. Effects of systemic hypoxia on pH outside rod photoreceptors in the cat retina. Exp Eye Res 54:699–709.

Yonemura D, Kawasaki K. 1979. New approaches to ophthalmic electrodiagnosis by retinal oscillatory potential, drug-induced responses from retinal pigment epithelium and cone potential. Doc Ophthalmol 48:163–222.

Yonemura D, Kawasaki K, Uhukura H, Yanagida T, Yamamoto Y. 1977. Electroretinogram and electro-oculogram in occlusion of the central retinal artery. Acta Soc Ophthalmol Jpn 81:323–329.

Yonemura D, Kawasaki K, Tanabe J, Yamamoto S. 1978. Susceptibility of the standing potential of the eye to acetazolamide and its clinical application. Folia Ophthalmol Jpn 29:408–416.

Yonemura D, Kawasaki K, Wakabayashi K, Madachi-Yamamoto S, Kawaguchi I. 1982. New approach to electrophysiological analysis of flecked retina syndrome. Doc Ophthalmol 31:165–175.

Yonemura D, Kawasaki K, Wakabayashi K, Tanabe J. 1983. EOG application for Stargardt's disease and X-linked juvenile retinoschisis. Doc Ophthalmol 37:115–120.

Yonemura D, Kawasaki K, Madachi-Yamamoto S. 1984. Hyperosmolarity response of ocular standing potential as a clinical test for retinal pigment epithelium activity: chorioretinal dystrophy. Doc Ophthalmol 57:163–173.

Zrenner E, Riedel KG, Adamczyk R, Gilg T, Liebhardt E. 1986. Effects of ethyl alcohol on the electrooculogram and color vision. Doc Ophthalmol 63:305–312.

11. Autofluorescence imaging of the human fundus

ANDREA VON RÜCKMANN, FREDERICK W. FITZKE, AND ALAN C. BIRD

In vivo imaging of the retinal pigment epithelium (RPE) is difficult due to optical limitations of the eye combined with the small size of the cellular elements, and the low contrast and strong absorption by melanin pigments. Recent advances in ophthalmoscopic imaging based on new technologies such as confocal laser scanning and optical coherence tomography have resulted in improvements which have revealed previously invisible structures. The RPE contains lipofuscin, which has led to a novel means of imaging by taking advantage of its intrinsic autofluorescence. Autofluorescence imaging can provide highly detailed and quantitative information about the levels and distribution of lipofuscin of the RPE within the living eye.

Our understanding of lipofuscin levels in disease states has been based until recently on in vitro observations, which do not allow the recording of change with time or the correlation of autofluorescence with other funduscopic features. In vivo recording of pigment epithelial autofluorescence as an index of lipofuscin accumulation allows analysis of the sequence of pigment epithelial changes.

It is expected, based on histopathological observations, that the spatial distribution of lipofuscin in disease states may be complex. It is evident that accurate imaging of the distribution of autofluorescence in the pigment epithelium, quantitative measurements under direct viewing in specific areas, and studies of the dynamics of accumulation, degradation, and clearance would add a great deal of information regarding the relation between the pigment epithelial autofluorescence and retinal disease.

Recently, in vivo high-spatial-resolution images of the distribution of pigment epithelial autofluorescence as an index of lipofuscin has been achieved with a confocal scanning laser ophthalmoscope (von Rückmann et al., 1995; 1997a; 1997b).

The confocal laser scanning ophthalmoscope (cLSO) was a prototype SM 30-4024 donated by Zeiss (Zeiss, Oberkochen, Germany). Argon laser light (488 nm, 250 μW) was used for illumination, and to record autofluorescence a wide-band pass filter was inserted in front of the detector with a short wavelength cutoff at 521 nm extending beyond 650 nm for the longer wavelengths. The cLSO images were recorded either digitally or at standard video-scanning rates on SVHS videotape, using a frame grabber, and then processed by computer. An averaging procedure was used for all eyes as described previously, originally using manual alignment and subsequently with automatic computer alignment.

In vivo recordings of fundus autofluorescence show good evidence that the autofluorescence is derived from lipofuscin in the RPE (von Rückmann et al., 1995; 1997a; 1997b; Boulton et al., 1990; 1991; Dorey et al., 1989; 1993; Kitagawa et al., 1989; Delori et al., 1995). That the spectral characteristics of in vivo fundus autofluorescence are consistent with those of lipofuscin was demonstrated by Delori and colleagues (1995), with reference to the identification of individual lipofuscin fluorophores by Eldred (1988), and the demonstration that the excitation spectrum of the "orange-red" fluorophores extended in the visible range, making them accessible for in vivo excitation.

There is good evidence that the images are derived from RPE and Bruch's membrane, since the signal appears to be derived from anterior to the choriocapillaris and posterior to the neuroretina (von Rückmann et al., 1997a; Delori et al., 1995). In addition, the variation of intensity in disease accords with that found by microscopy (Farkas et al., 1971; Ishibashi et al., 1986; Burns et al., 1980; Sparks et al., 1988; O'Gorman et al., 1988; McFarland et al., 1955; Frangieh et al., 1982; Weingeist et al., 1982).

The normal fundi show a consistent pattern over the age of 6 years, with diffuse autofluorescence that is most intense between 5° and 15° from the fovea without focal variations other than the optic disc and retinal blood vessels, which are shown as dark structures in Figure 11-1 (von Rückmann et al., 1995; 1997a).

This pattern of distribution of fundus autofluorescence is consistent regardless of age. The autofluorescence intensity recorded at the fovea and temporal to the fovea at the site of maximal autofluorescence intensity increases significantly with age, which corresponds with

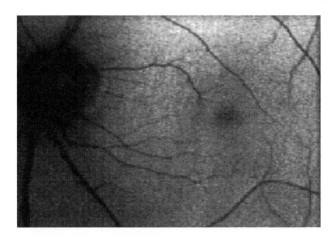

FIGURE 11-1. A 31-year-old man with normal fundus and a visual acuity of 20/20. Fundus autofluorescence imaging shows diffuse fundus autofluorescence with decreased intensity at the fovea; blood vessels and optic disc shown as dark structures.

the information derived from in vitro studies (von Rückmann et al., 1997a) (Fig. 11-2).

AGE-RELATED MACULAR DEGENERATION

It is widely believed that the changes leading to visual loss in age-related macular degeneration occur in response to accumulation of debris in Bruch's membrane, and there is good evidence that this material is derived from the RPE, which discharges cytoplasmic contents into the inner portion of Bruch's membrane in order to achieve cytoplasmic renewal (Pauleikhoff et al., 1990;

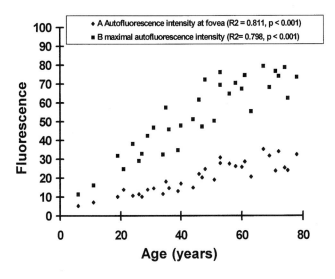

FIGURE 11-2. Fundus autofluorescence of normal subjects measured at the fovea (A) and at the site of maximum intensity, at 7–15 degrees of eccentricity (B). (Reprinted from von Rückmann et al. 1997a.)

Sheraidah et al., 1993; Holz et al., 1994). This material is believed to be cleared by the choroid, and incomplete clearance is related to thickening of Bruch's membrane. Thus a relation between accumulation of debris in RPE as shown by autofluorescence and in Bruch's membrane might be expected, and variation of both background and focal autofluorescence may bear some relationship to the outcome of disease.

The intensity of autofluorescence over hard and soft drusen is within or below the range of the background autofluorescence when compared with age-matched normal controls. That the autofluorescence over drusen can not be differentiated from that of the background was also demonstrated by spectral analysis (Arendt et al., 1995). Delori (1994) measured the fundus autofluorescence in vivo and showed that aging Bruch's membrane exhibits autofluorescence that may—at 620 nm, using an excitation wavelength of 510 nm—account for 10% of the total fundus autofluorescence. The background autofluorescence is no greater in those eyes with visible drusen than in fundi without drusen.

A striking finding was the consistent presence of localized high autofluorescence, which did not correspond with drusen but often appeared to be derived from areas of retinal pigment epithelial pallor (Fig. 11-3). Those areas of increased autofluorescence may correspond to a group of RPE cells containing higher quantities of lipofuscin than their neighbors. Over time, focal increased autofluorescence may demonstrate change or may remain stable (Fig. 11-3).

Pigment figures at the level of the RPE—whether detached or flat—which are hypofluorescent on fluorescein angiography may show intense autofluorescence (Fig. 11-4). It is likely that melanolipofuscin accounts for the high levels of autofluorescence. The significance of this focal pigment epithelial accumulation of fluorescent material to disease is uncertain, and may be elucidated by longitudinal studies.

RPE detachments older than 6 months may show a mild diffuse increased autoflourescence corresponding exactly with the detached area (Fig. 11-4), which is not readily explained. The mildly increased autofluorescence may persist for a period longer than 2 months after the detachment flattens, for example, after successful laser treatment.

In patients with choroidal neovascularization the autofluorescence is very irregular, with regions of greater and lesser fluorescence than the background. The distribution of fundus autofluorescence changes over time, and focal regions of increased autofluorescence may develop into regions of decreased autofluorescence (Fig. 11-5).

Elevated autofluorescence may often be seen extending beyond the edge of the lesion. Over disciform scars the autofluorescence intensity is less than background.

In subjects in whom there are areas of geographic atrophy, absence of autofluorescence corresponds well with the atrophy but is present in the adjacent regions where geographic atrophy is not evident. Often a band of increased autofluorescence around the edge of geo-

graphic atrophy may be seen (Figs. 11-3, 11-6). With time, new sites of geographic atrophy are associated with decreased autofluorescence, and these cases may be preceded by focal increases of autofluorescence (Fig. 11-3). Decreased autofluorescence occurs over areas which have undergone laser treatment for choroidal neovascularization; the treated areas, similar to sites of geo-

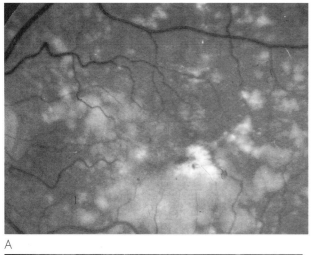

A

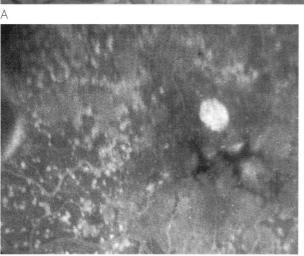

B

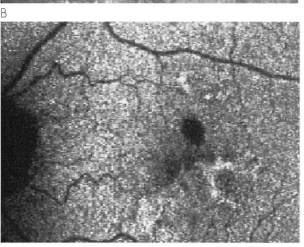

C

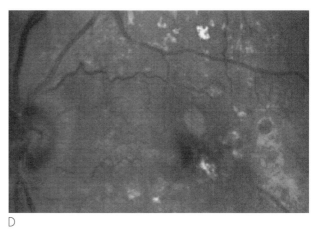

D

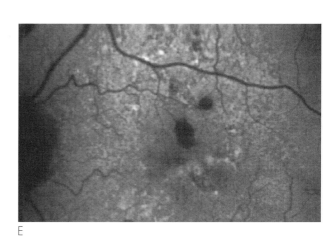

E

FIGURE 11-3. Reflectance image (A), fluorescein angiogram (B), and autofluorescence image (C) of a 68-year-old man with soft, scattered, subconfluent and confluent drusen; pigment clumping; retinal pigment epithelial hypopigmentation; and a small, central area of geographic atrophy. Visual acuity was 20/30. Focal changes show (1) the highest autofluorescence intensity corresponded with dark areas on fluorescein angiogram and was present in the areas with pigment clumping, adjacent to rather old-looking, resolving, and mineralized drusen areas; (2) in the areas of confluent drusen and retinal pigment epithelial pallor there was focal, mild increased autofluoresence that did not correspond to the drusen pattern; (3) there were no focal areas of increased autofluorescence in the scattered drusen areas; (4) the area of geographic atrophy showed decreased autofluorescence (C). (Reprinted from von Rückmann et al., 1997a.) Eighteen months later the patient developed new areas of geographic atrophy (D), and the distribution of fundus autofluorescence changed. The new areas of geographic atrophy corresponded with new areas of decreased autofluorescence which occurred at the site of focal increased autofluorescence (E).

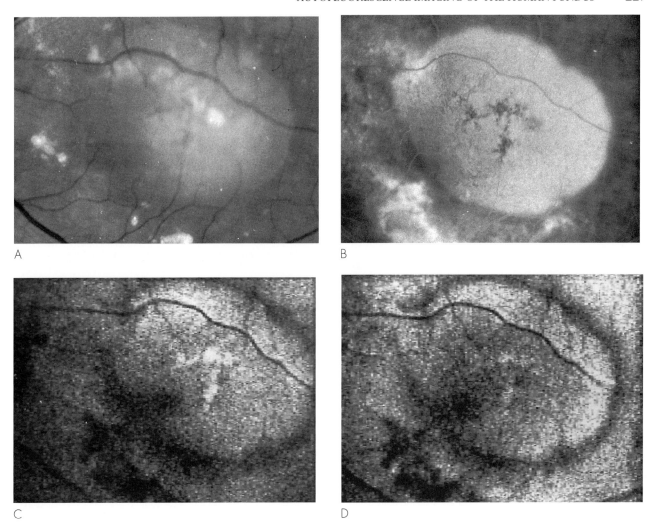

FIGURE 11-4. Reflectance image (A), fluorescein angiogram (B), and autofluorescence images (C, D) of a 71-year-old woman with a pigment epithelial detachment reducing the visual acuity in the left eye to 20/120 (A). Focusing on the surface of the PED on autofluorescence imaging (C), a highly autofluorescent area that corresponded with the pattern of blocked fluorescence in the angiogram (B) became evident.

Focusing closer to the area of attached retina (D), an area of low autofluorescence, containing focal highly autofluorescent features became evident inferiorly; the two spots of maximal fluorescence intensity corresponded with the dark spots on the angiogram and the low-autofluorescence area corresponded with atrophic retinal pigment epithelium. (Reprinted from von Rückmann et al., 1997a.)

graphic atrophy, may be preceded by focal increases of autofluorescence (Fig. 11-7). Crystalline drusen also show reduced autofluorescence (Fig. 11-3).

This observation might be expected if accumulation of fluorescent material in the RPE reflects the level of metabolic activity, which is largely determined by the quantity of photoreceptor outer segment renewal, and the residual bodies had a finite half-life. The first premise is widely believed to be true, and there is evidence to support the second. There appears to be constant degradation of residual bodies in the retinal pigment epithelium (Rungger-Branche et al., 1988; Feeney et al., 1978) so that progressive loss of lipofuscin in the RPE would be expected if metabolic demand were to be reduced by demise of photoreceptor cells. Alternatively,

it is possible that the RPE discharges material into Bruch's membrane prior to cell death or metabolic failure, which itself leads to photoreceptor loss.

The presence of areas of increased autofluorescence around disciform lesions and geographic atrophy may be due to the RPE becoming multilayered, a phenomenon well illustrated by histopathology (Sarks et al., 1988). Phagocytosis of debris derived from exudation from the new vessel complex may also contribute toward the accumulation of intracellular material.

The observation that the number of photoreceptor cells is reduced in the presence of increased lipofuscin content in the RPE led to the proposal that increased accumulation of autofluorescent material may occur prior to cell loss (Dorey et al., 1989). The observation that

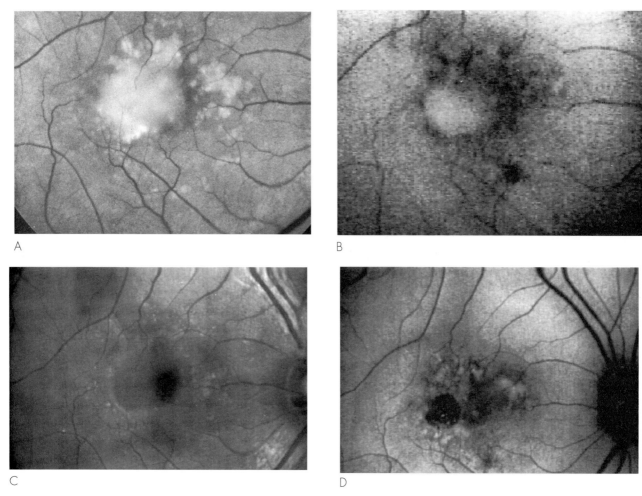

A   B

C   D

FIGURE 11-5. Reflectance image (A) and autofluorescence image (B, manual alignment) of a 67-year-old man with a retinal pigment epithelial detachment and occult neovascularization in the right eye reducing visual acuity to 20/100. Autofluorescence imaging shows diffuse mild increased autofluorescence over the detached area but not at the site of the drusen. (From von Rückmann et al., 1997.) Fourteen months later the distribution of fundus autofluorescence changed while the fundus appearance remained approximately the same (C). Areas of hypofluorescence occurred at the site of increased autofluorescence (D, automated alignment).

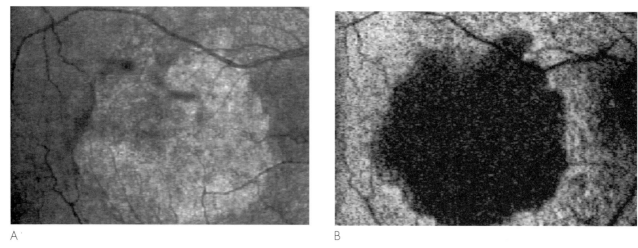

A   B

FIGURE 11-6. A 76-year-old woman with scattered drusen and geographic atrophy reducing visual acuity in the right eye to 20/120 (A). The low-autofluorescence areas on autofluorescence imaging (B) correspond with the area of geographic atrophy. The border of the geographic atrophy shows increased autofluorescence.

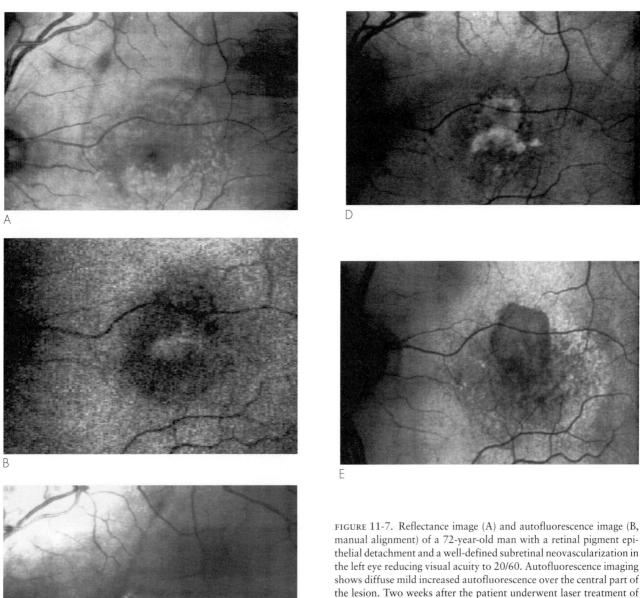

FIGURE 11-7. Reflectance image (A) and autofluorescence image (B, manual alignment) of a 72-year-old man with a retinal pigment epithelial detachment and a well-defined subretinal neovascularization in the left eye reducing visual acuity to 20/60. Autofluorescence imaging shows diffuse mild increased autofluorescence over the central part of the lesion. Two weeks after the patient underwent laser treatment of the subretinal neovascularization, the lesion flattened and the visual acuity was 20/40. On the reflectance image the laser scar could be seen (C), and on autofluorescence imaging focal increased autofluorescence corresponded well with the treated area (D, automated alignment). Focal increased autofluorescence could further be seen in the central part of the lesion that flattened. Autofluorescence image of the same fundus 12 months later showed decreased autofluorescence which corresponds with the treated area (E, automated alignment).

focal pigmentation indicates a high risk of visual loss in age-related macular disease would support this concept. Our findings imply that this does not occur evenly over the fundus but is focal. If high levels of autofluorescence presages geographic atrophy, its focal nature would be in keeping with clinical experience (Sarks et al., 1988). It has been conceived that the high volume of residual bodies may interfere with RPE function, although it could equally well be a consequence rather than a cause of dysfunction.

MACULAR DYSTROPHIES

It is well established that autofluorescent material accumulates in the retinal pigment epithelium in some mac-

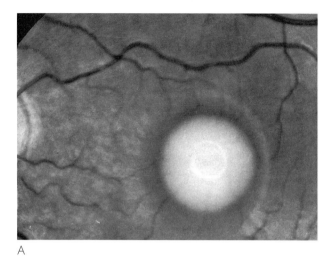
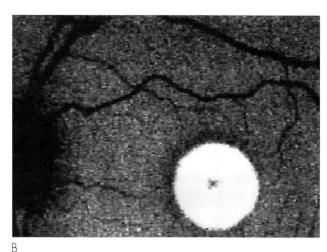

A   B

FIGURE 11-8. A 6-year-old boy with Best's disease with a well-defined white deposit at the level of the retinal pigment epithelium centrally (A). Left eye visual acuity was 20/20. Autofluorescence imaging showed
hyperfluorescence which corresponded with the deposit (B). The surrounding fundus was relatively more
fluorescent than in an age-matched normal. (Reprinted from van Rückmann et al., 1977b.)

ular dystrophies, and that the extracellular deposits may
also fluoresce (O'Gorman et al., 1988; McFarland et al.,
1955; Eagle et al., 1980; Frangieh et al., 1982; Weingeist
et al., 1982; Patrinely et al., 1985; Steinmetz et al., 1991;
Birnbach et al., 1994). Observations have been made as
a result of histological studies on a limited number of
eyes. It is not known if the finding is consistent from one
condition to another, and the time course of the acquisition of autofluorescent material has not been documented. Given that the many disorders are presumed to

have different basic metabolic defects, some variation
might be expected from one condition to another.

All dystrophies examined to date have in common accumulation of autofluorescent material in the RPE to a
greater degree than that seen with age (von Rückmann
et al., 1997b).

In all disorders with pale deposits at the level of
RPE/Bruch's membrane, such as Best disease, adult
vitelliform macular dystrophy, and fundus flavimaculatus, these deposits are consistently associated with high-

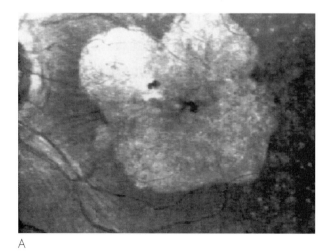
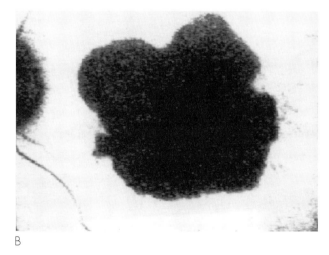

A   B

FIGURE 11-9. A 49-year-old man with dominantly inherited pattern dystrophy caused by a mutation in
the peripherin/rds gene; left eye vision was reduced to finger counting (A). Autofluorescence imaging
showed hypofluorescence of the site of outer retinal atrophy and increased autofluorescence of the surrounding area (B).

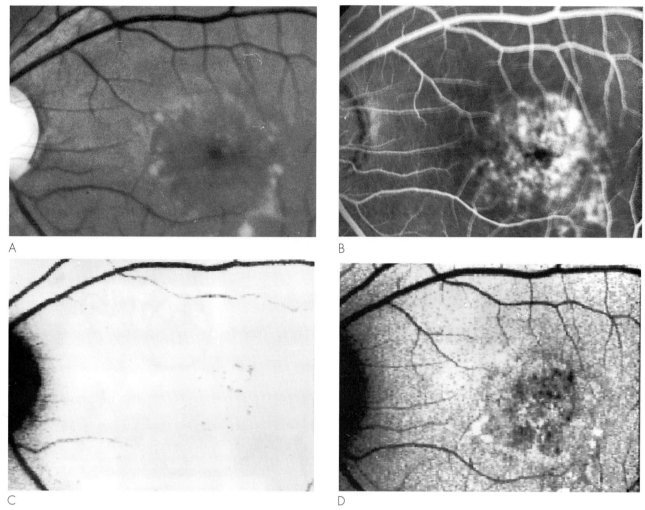

FIGURE 11-10. Fundus photograph of a 38-year-old man with macular dystrophy (A). Visual acuity was 20/30. There was no dark choroid on the fluorescein angiogram (B). There was high background autofluorescence (C), and when the gain was reduced by 0.8 log units, the white deposits appeared relatively more fluorescent than the background (D). (Reprinted von Rückmann et al., 1997b.)

er levels of autofluorescence than the background signal (Fig. 11-8) suggesting that the biochemical composition may be similar.

The entire fundus in patients with Best disease, fundus flavimaculatus, and pattern dystrophies (including pattern dystrophy due to a mutation in the *rds* gene—Fig. 11-9), and in the majority of patients with adult viteliform macular dystrophy, show abnormally intense autofluorescence, suggesting a generalized abnormality of the RPE even though on biomicroscopy the visible lesions are focal. Both these observations accord with findings in histopathological studies (von Rückmann et al., 1995; 1997b; Boulton et al., 1990; 1991; Dorey et al., 1989; 1993; Kitagawa et al., 1989).

It is surprising that high levels of background autofluorescence may be present whether or not there is a dark choroid on fluorescein angiography (Figs. 11-10,

11-11). The lack of choroidal fluorescence (dark choroid) in some macular dystrophies (Bonnin et al., 1971) has been ascribed to the presence of a short-wavelength-absorbing chromophore in the RPE (Fish et al., 1981); the most likely candidate was considered to be lipofuscin. The finding that a dark choroid is found in some families but not others had been seen as evidence of different mechanisms whereby lipofuscin accumulation occurred in some conditions but not in others (Uliss et al., 1987). Other results suggest that an excess of autofluorescent pigment exists whether or not there is a dark choroid. It is unlikely that different findings reflect different concentrations of the pigment, since the intensity of autofluorescence was similar in the two circumstances. This finding could be explained if the autofluorescent pigment in the two situations had different optical characteristics; it has been shown that species of

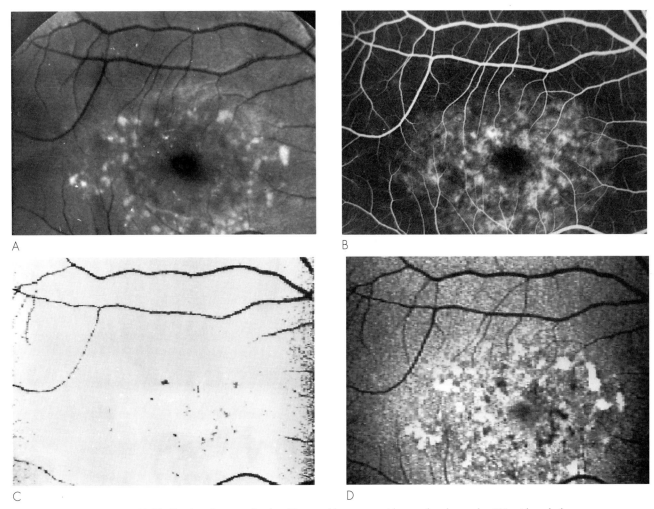

FIGURE 11-11. Fundus photograph of a 42-year-old woman with macular dystrophy (A) with a dark choroid on the fluorescein angiography (B). Visual acuity in the right eye was 20/30. Autofluorescence imaging showed high background autofluorescence (C). When reducing the gain by 0.8 log units, the white deposits appeared relatively more fluorescent than the background (D). (Reprinted from von Rückmann et al., 1997b.)

autofluorescent pigment have different absorption and emission characteristics in the retinal pigment epithelium (Eldred et al., 1988; Boulton et al., 1991; Gaillard et al., 1995). Alternatively, it is possible that a pigment other than autofluorescent pigment accounts for the blocking of choroidal fluorescence. The lack of correlation between autofluorescence and the presence of a dark choroid implies that there may be different fluorophores in different disorders.

We found increased levels of autofluorescence in subjects with a mutation known to cause macular dystrophy but in whom there were no manifest ophthalmoscopic or functional abnormalities. In two subjects from families with pattern dystrophy due to a mutation in the *rds* gene who were known to have the abnormal gene, abnormally high autofluorescence was evident at a time when there were no symptoms, the fundi were normal

by ophthalmoscopy, and there was no functional deficit as shown by electrophysiology and psychophysics. Three additional members who were at 50% risk of having the abnormal gene in families with autosomal disease have been shown to have abnormally high levels of autofluorescence, but no other signs of disease. Confirmation of their status depends on their developing phenotypic abnormalities or identification of the abnormal gene. The increased autofluorescence at a time when no other phenotypic expression is evident allows earlier identification of those with the abnormal gene.

RETINAL DYSTROPHIES

In inherited retinal dystrophies autofluorescence imaging can demonstrate retinal atrophy and areas of sur-

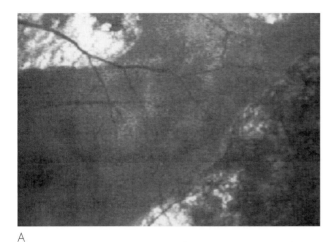
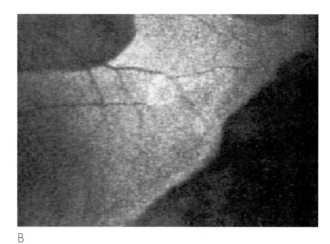

A   B

FIGURE 11-12. Reflectance image of a 46-year-old woman with autosomal-dominant retinitis pigmentosa with well-defined profound atrophy of the outer retina, retinal pigment epithelium, and inner choroid (A). Right eye visual acuity was 20/20. Autofluorescence imaging showed decreased autofluorescence at the site of atrophy and increased autofluorescence corresponding with the viable retina (B).

viving retina (Fig. 11-12). Variations in background autofluorescence in various cases of RP were noted. This appears to correlate with histopathologic studies demonstrating normal, reduced, or excessive lipofuscin content in the RPE. It would be expected that type I (diffuse) retinitis pigmentosa, in which the photoreceptors have a near normal complement of rhodopsin would have normal or excessive quantities of lipofuscin, whereas type II (regional) disease in which there is outer segment loss early would have reduced levels (Fish et al., 1981; Uliss et al., 1987; Gaillard et al., 1995; Massof et al., 1981; Arden et al., 1983; Lyness et al., 1985; Kemp et al., 1988).

A ring of increased autofluorescence occurs at 4–5 degrees eccentricity from the fovea in many forms of retinitis pigmentosa.

All forms of inherited drusen seen to date show increased levels of autofluorescence, in contrast to age-related drusen (Fig. 11-13).

It is evident that interpretable images of RPE autofluorescence can be obtained in retinal disease state. It will take time to realize the potential value of this new information to our understanding of the disease process, and its management. Incorporation of this technique in cross-sectional surveys and into longitudinal studies may add greatly to the value of these research efforts.

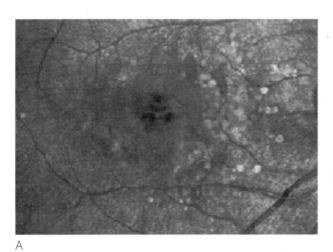
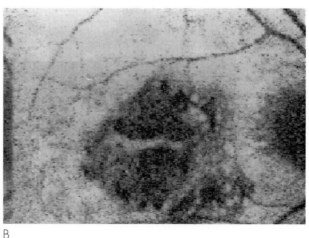

A   B

FIGURE 11-13. Reflectance image of a 52-year-old woman with malattia leventinese with soft drusen and a central pigmented linear figure (A). Right eye visual acuity was 20/40. Autofluorescence imaging showed increased background autofluorescence; the drusen and the central pigmented linear figure corresponded with focal areas of intense autofluorescence (B).

REFERENCES

Arden GB, Carter RM, Hogg CR, Powell DJ, Ernst WJK, Clover GM. 1983. Rod and cone activity in patients with dominantly inherited retinitis pigmentosa: comparison between psychophysical and electroretinographic measurements. Br J Ophthalmol 67:405–418.

Arendt OA, Weiter JJ, Goger DG, Delori FC. 1995. In vivo Fundus Fluoreszenz Messungen bei Patienten mit altersabhangiger Makuladegeneration. Ophthalmologe 92:647–653.

Birnbach CD, Järveläinen M, Possin DE, Milam AH. 1994. Histopathology and immunocytochemistry of the neurosensory retina in fundus flavimaculatus. Ophthalmology. 101:1211–1219.

Boulton M. 1991. Aging of the retinal pigment epithelium. In: Osborne NN, Chader GJ, eds. Progress in retinal research, vol 11. Oxford: Pergamon Press, 125–152.

Boulton M, Docchio F, Dayhaw-Barker P, Ramponi R, Cubbedu R. 1990. Age-related changes in the morphology, absorption and fluorescence of melanosomes and lipofuscin granules of the retinal pigment epithelium. Vis Res 30:1291–1303.

Burns RP, Feeney-Burns L. 1980. Clinico-morphological correlations of drusen and Bruch's membrane. Tr Amer Ophthalmol Soc 78: 206–225.

Delori FC, Dorey K, Staurenghi G, Arend O, Goger DG, Weiter JJ. 1995. In vivo fluorescence of the ocular fundus exhibits retinal pigment epithelial lipofuscin characteristics. Invest Ophthalmol Vis Sci 36:718–729.

Delori FC, Arend O, Staurenghi G, Goger D, Dorey CK, Weiter JJ. 1994. Lipofuscin and drusen fluorescence in aging and age related macular degeneration. Invest Ophthalmol Vis Sci 35:2145.

Dorey CK, Wu G, Ebenstein D, Garsd A, Weiter JJ. 1989. Cell loss in the ageing retina: relationship to lipofuscin accumulation and macular degeneration. Invest Ophthalmol Vis Sci 30:1691–1699.

Dorey CK, Staurenghi G, Delori FC. 1993. Lipofuscin in aged and AMD eyes. In: Holyfield JG, et al, eds, Retinal Degeneration. New York: Plenum Press, 3–14.

Eagle RC, Lucier AC, Bernadino VB, Yanoff M. 1980. Retinal pigment epithelial abnormalities in fundus flavimaculatus: a light and electron microscopic study. Ophthalmology 87:1189–1200.

Eldred GE, Katz ML. 1988. Fluorophores of the human retinal pigment epithelium: separation and spectral characterisation. Exp Eye Res 47:71–86.

Farkas T, Sylvester V, Archer D, Altona M. 1971. The histochemistry of drusen. Am J Ophthalmol 71:1206–1215.

Feeney L. 1978. Lipofuscin and melanin of human retinal pigment epithelium: fluorescence, enzyme cytochemical and ultrastructural studies. Invest Ophthalmol Vis Sci 17:583–600.

Fish G, Grey RHB, Sehmi KS, Bird AC. 1981. The dark choroid in posterior retinal dystrophies. Br J Ophthalmol 65:359–363.

Frangieh GT, Green R, Fine SL. 1982. A histopathological study of Best's macular dystrophy. Arch Ophthalmol 100:1115–1121.

Gaillard ER, Atherton SJ, Eldred G, Dillon J. 1995. Photophysical studies on human retinal lipofuscin. Photochem Photobiol 61: 448–453.

Holz FG, Sheriadah G, Pauleikhoff D, Bird AC. 1994. Analysis of lipid deposits extracted from macular and peripheral Bruch's membrane. Arch Ophthalmol 112:402–406.

Ishibashi T, Sorgente N, Patterson R, Ryan SJ. 1986. Pathogenesis of drusen in the primate. Invest Ophthalmol Vis Sci 27:184–193.

Kemp CM, Jacobson SG, Faulkner DJ. 1988. Two types of visual disfunction in autosomal dominant retinitis pigmentosa. Invest Ophthalmol Vis Sci 29:1235–1241.

Kitagawa K, Nishida S, Ogura Y. 1989. In vivo quantitation of autofluorescence in human RPE. Ophthalmologica 199:116–121.

Lyness AL, Ernst W, Quinlan MP, Clover GM, Arden GB, Carter R. 1985. A clinical, psychophysical and electroretinographic survey of patients with autosomal dominant retinitis pigmentosa. Br J Ophthalmol 69:326–339.

Massof RW, Finkelstein D. 1981. Two forms of autosomal dominant primary retinitis pigmentosa. Invest Ophthalmol Vis Sci 51: 289–346.

McFarland CB. 1955. Heredodegeneration of macula lutea: study of clinical and pathological aspects. Arch Ophthalmol 53:224–228.

O'Gorman S, Flaherty WA, Fishman GA, Berson EL. Histopathologic findings in Best's vitelliform macular dystrophy. Arch Ophthalmol 106:1261–1268.

Patrinely JR, Lewis RA, Font RL. 1985. Foveomacular vitelliform macular dystrophy, adult type. A clinicopathological study including electron microscopic observations. Ophthalmology 92:1712–1718.

Pauleikhoff D, Harper CA, Marshall J, Bird AC. 1990. Aging changes in Bruch's membrane: a histochemical and morphological study. Ophthalmology 97:171–178.

Rungger-Branche E, Englert U, Leuenberger PM. 1988. Exocytic clearing of degraded membrane material from pigment epithelial cells in frog retina. Invest Ophthalmol Vis Sci 28:2026–2037.

Sarks SH, Sarks J, Killingsworth C. 1988. Evolution of geographic atrophy of the retinal pigment epithelium. Eye 2:552–577.

Sheraidah G, Steinmetz R, Maguire J, Pauleikhoff D, Marshall J, Bird A. 1993. Correlation between lipids extracted from Bruch's membrane and age. Ophthalmology 100:47–51.

Steinmetz RL, McGuire J, Garner A, Bird AC. 1991. Histopathology of incipient fundus flavimaculatus. Ophthalmology 98:953–956.

Uliss AE, Moore AT, Bird AC. 1987. The dark choroid in posterior retinal dystrophies. Ophthalmology 95:1423–1427.

von Rückmann A, Fitzke FW, Bird AC. 1995. Distribution of fundus autofluorescence with a scanning laser ophthalmoscope. Br J Ophthalmol 119:543–562.

von Rückmann A, Fitzke FW, Bird AC. 1997. Fundus autofluorescence in age related macular disease imaged with a scanning laser ophthalmoscope. Invest Ophthalmol Vis Sci 38:478–486.

von Rückmann A, Fitzke FW, Bird AC. 1997b. In vivo fundus autofluorescence in macular dystrophies. Arch Ophthalmol 116: 609–615.

Weingeist TA, Kobrin JL, Watzke RC. 1982. Histopathology of Best's macular dystrophy. Arch Ophthalmol 100:1108–1114.

12. Optical coherence tomography imaging of the retinal pigment epithelium and its related disorders

JEFFREY G. COKER AND CARMEN A. PULIAFITO

Optical Coherence Tomography (OCT) is a recently introduced imaging technique which generates high-resolution cross-sectional images of the retina. Previous diagnostic instruments lacked sufficient resolution to provide useful cross-sectional images of retinal structure. The resolution of standard clinical ultrasound is limited by the wavelength of sound in ocular tissue to about 150 μm. High-frequency ultrasound biomicroscopy offers a resolution of about 20–40 μm; however, its penetration into the eye is limited to the first 4 mm of the anterior segment. Ocular aberrations and the maximum entrance pupil diameter of the eye limit the longitudinal resolution of confocal imaging techniques such as scanning laser ophthalmoscopy and scanning laser tomography to approximately 300 μm. OCT is analogous to ultrasonography except that optical, rather than acoustic, reflectivity is measured. Cross-sectional images of optical reflectivity in the retina are obtained, similar to ultrasound B-scan but with 10 μm longitudinal resolution. Unlike ultrasound, contact between the probe module and the eye is not required, so that slit-lamp biomicroscopy of the retina, simultaneous with image acquisition, is possible. The apparent reflectivity measured by OCT is a combination of the actual reflectivity and the scattering and absorption characteristics of the overlying media. Thus, the apparent reflectivity for retinal imaging may be affected by abnormalities in the cornea, aqueous, lens, vitreous, and anterior retinal layers (Hee et al., 1995a).

OCT has proven to be effective in analyzing a variety of macular diseases (Hee et al., 1995a; Hee et al., 1995b; Hee et al., 1995c; Hee et al., 1996; Puliafito et al., 1995). OCT may play a role in analyzing various diseases involving changes in the retinal pigment epithelium (RPE), such as age-related macular degeneration and central serous chorioretinopathy. Age-related macular degeneration (AMD) is the leading cause of blindness in the United States. The clinical presentation of AMD is varied, but may be classified as exudative or nonexudative. Choroidal neovascularization and its as-

sociated exudative maculopathy and nonexudative lesions, including drusen and geographic atrophy, can bring about changes in the RPE. Central serous chorioretinopathy is a common retinal disorder, which in its most prevalent form involves a detachment of the neurosensory retina secondary to one or more focal fluorescein angiographic leaks at the level of the RPE (Hee et al., 1996; Hee et al., 1995d). On OCT cross-sections, the RPE is seen as part of a highly reflective band that includes the choriocapillaris. This band defines the posterior boundary of the neurosensory retina.

SYSTEM AND TECHNIQUE OF OPTICAL COHERENCE TOMOGRAPHY

With optical coherence tomography, low-coherence light is coupled into a fiber-optic Michelson interferometer. A superluminescent diode light source (a laser diode containing an antireflection coated output facet) is used to provide a bright source of spatially uniform, low-coherence light. One of the two fiber-optic arms of the interferometer emits the probe beam and is used for both illumination of the retina and for collection of reflected light. Time-of-flight information is contained in the interference signal between this reflected probe beam and light returning from a reference optical delay path, and is detected by a photodiode followed by signal processing electronics and computer data acquisition. A constant refractive index of 1.36 is assumed to convert time-of-flight delay into a distance within the retina. The depth resolution of OCT imaging depends only on the source coherence length, which essentially describes the maximum optical path length mismatch between the sample and reference interferometer paths that will produce an interference signal at the detector. The source coherence length, which defines the ideal longitudinal point-spread-function of the OCT imaging system, was experimentally determined to be 14 μm full-width at half-maximum (FWHM) in air by measuring the width of the reflection from a mirror placed in the sample arm of the interferometer. This measurement agrees with theoretical calculations based on the spectral characteristics of the source and predicts a longitudinal resolution of 10 μm FWHM in the retina after accounting for the difference in refractive index between air and tissue. It is important to note that the temporal coherence property of the source, and consequently the longitudinal resolution, is independent of both the optical quality of the eye and the pupil aperture. The minimum achievable transverse resolution, determined by the probe beam diameter at the retina, was calculated to be 13 μm based on the Gullstrand schematic eye. Computer control and data acquisition enable arbitrary scanning patterns on the fundus and provide a real-time display of the tomograph in progress on a monitor. Less than 200 μW of 830 nm probe light is incident on the fundus, consistent with the ANSI-recommended exposure limit for permanent intrabeam viewing (Huang et al., 1991; Hee et al., 1995d; Swanson et al., 1992; Swanson et al., 1993).

A +78 diopter condensing lens mounted in front of the eye provides an indirect image of the retina that is used for both slit-lamp visualization of the fundus and OCT scanning. A single one-dimensional A-mode profile of optical reflectivity versus distance into the tissue is created by translating the reference arm mirror and measuring the magnitude of the interference signal at the detector. Two-dimensional, tomographic imaging of the retina is accomplished in a manner analogous to ultrasound B-scan. In ultrasound B-mode, a cross-sectional image of acoustic reflectivity is created by obtaining multiple, since A-mode scans while rapidly scanning the probe beam through tissue. Similarly, a B-scan OCT image is constructed from a sequence of uniaxial A-mode longitudinal profiles of optical reflectivity, obtained while transversely scanning the probe beam across the retina. The OCT tomographs are each composed of 100 A-mode scans (Huang et al., 1991; Hee et al., 1995d; Swanson et al., 1992; Swanson et al., 1993).

The technique is well tolerated by patients because it is noncontact and noninvasive. Scanning time is quick (2.5 sec) and the light delivered into the eye is near-infrared and thus not very bright. Each image is centered on the patient's fixation. For repeat visits, because each scan is saved as a pair of two-dimensional coordinates (1 for fixation, 1 for the scan), the examiner can acquire the same scan for follow-up by offsetting the probe and fixation to the same two points using keyboard controls. When the patient's visual acuity is less than approximately 20/300 in the eye being scanned, a standard externally mounted fixation light is used to fixate the gaze of the fellow eye. For such cases, the examiner uses

a video image of the fundus showing the probe location to place the scan in the desired location visually. The images are shown with a false color scheme, with dark colors corresponding to areas of decreased reflectivity and lighter colors corresponding to areas of increased reflectivity (Plates 12-I and II). The near-infrared probe light can penetrate mild to moderate cataracts but is limited by viterous hemorrhage, lens opacities, and cloudy vitreous (Puliafito et al., 1995). Image-processing techniques are used to compensate for longitudinal eye movement, but it is not possible to correct for transverse tracking or saccades. A commercial COT unit (Humphrey Instruments) utilizes faster scanning (1 sec) and allows the examiner to save a video image showing where the scan was taken in addition to the OCT image.

DIAGNOSTIC APPLICATION OF OCT IN THE RPE

While the RPE and choriocapillaris are difficult to distinguish on the OCT images, their combined reflection, which defines the posterior boundary of the neurosensory retina, provides useful information on chorioretinal pathologies such as age-related macular degeneration and central serous chorioretinopathy.

Hyperpigmentation of the RPE leads to increased backscatter, mild thickening of the posterior reflective boundary, and concomitant shadowing of the reflectivity from the choroid. With AMD, disciform scarring appears as a severely thickened posterior reflection from the high reflectivity and extension of fibrosis into the retina. Hypopigmentation of the RPE or pigment epithelial atrophy results in decreased reflectivity and an associated window defect, enabling increased penetration of the probe beam to the choroid, and higher reflectivity from the deeper layers (Fig. 12-1). Retinal thinning in the fovea is also often noted.

For eyes with AMD and choroidal neovascularization (CNV), laser photocoagulation treatment may be used to effectively reduce or delay severe vision loss (MPSG, 1982; 1990; 1991a; 1991b). However, many of the eyes with exudative AMD lack the fluorescein angiographic (FA) features required for treatment eligibility according to the Macular Photocoagulation Study Group (MPSG) guidelines (Bressler et al., 1987; Moisseiev et al., 1995; MPSG, 1991c). For this reason, OCT has been studied for purposes of better visualizing such occult neovascularization.

With exudative AMD, a classification of five categories was established from OCT: well-defined CNV, poorly defined CNV, serous (PED) fibrovascular PED, and hemorrhagic PED. A well-defined CNV was seen as a fusiform thickening and disruption of the RPE/chorio-

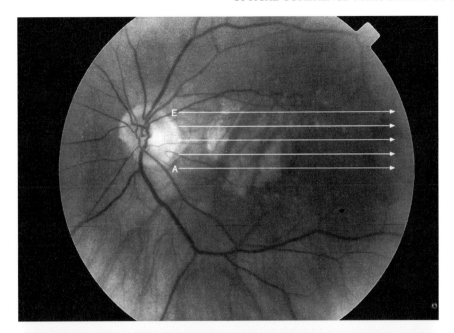

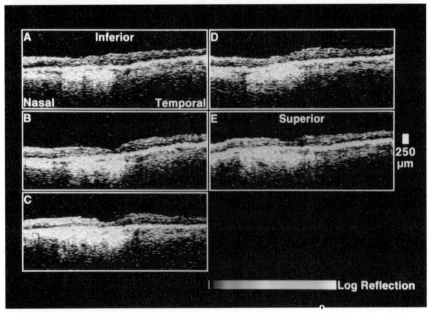

FIGURE 12-1. AMD/geographic Atrophy. An 85-year-old man with stable age-related macular degeneration had a visual acuity OS of counting fingers at four feet. *(top)* Fundus photograph of the left eye displays geographic atrophy involving the macula without associated subretinal fluid, hemorrhage, or exudate. *(bottom)* A sequence of horizontal OCT images displays increased penetration through an atrophic region, which is most prominent nasal to the fovea, leading to increased backscatter from the choroid due to increased penetration of both incident and reflected light through the atrophic pigment epithelium. Foveal scan B shows thinning of the neurosensory retina in the central macula.

capillaris complex with well-defined boundaries (Fig. 12-2 and Plate 12-I). The thickening extends upward in the OCT, creating a "bump" in the normal contour of the RPE which defines the boundaries of the CNV. Disciform scars and well-defined CNV can be difficult to distinguish just from viewing their size or uniformity of backscatter alone. However, disciform scars usually display retinal thinning, and the well-defined CNV most often is associated with intraretinal or subretinal fluid accumulation. Poorly defined CNV demonstrated enhanced choroidal reflectivity and disrupted reflections from the RPE and choriocapillaris with poorly defined

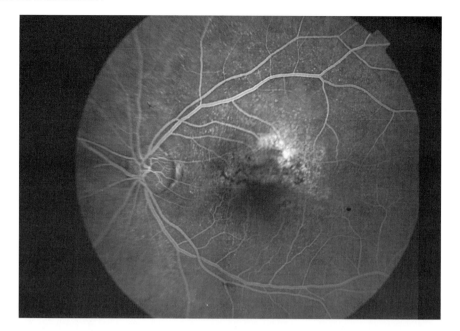

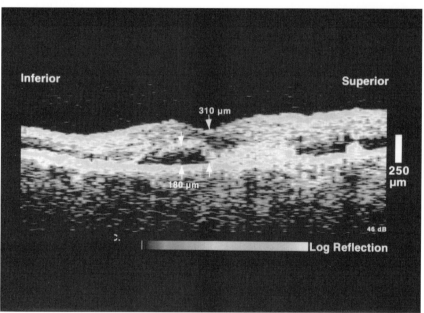

FIGURE 12-2. AMD/occult choroidal neovascularization well-defined on OCT. An 80-year-old woman complained of intermittent blurry vision in her left eye over several weeks. On examination, visual acuity OS was 20/25 and slit-lamp biomicroscopy revealed a shallow pigment epithelial detachment above fixation without hemorrhage or exudate *(not shown)*. *(top)* Fluorescein angiography shows early speckled hyperfluorescence superior and temporal to the fovea, and late leakage consistent with occult choroidal neovascularization. *(bottom)* Vertical OCT demonstrating thickening and disruption of the reflective band corresponding to the retinal pigment epithelium and choriocapillaris, with well-defined boundaries subfoveally and extending superiorly, consistent with a well-defined choroidal neovascular membrane. Inferior to the membrane, subretinal fluid is noted (180 μm). The false color appearance is shown in Plate 12-I.

boundaries and associated with subretinal or intraretinal fluid. The increased backscatter is confined below and blends into the normal contour of the RPE, which is unaffected. Subretinal or intraretinal fluid must be observed to distinguish this enhanced choroidal reflectivity from increased choroidal reflections due to pigmentary atrophy or RPE changes. In AMD, serous PED was seen on OCT as an elevation of the reflective band corresponding to the RPE and choriocapillaris above a region of decreased reflectivity, with shadowing of the choroid occurring (Fig. 12-3). Soft drusen, which cause a modulation in the RPE/choriocapillaris band, are con-

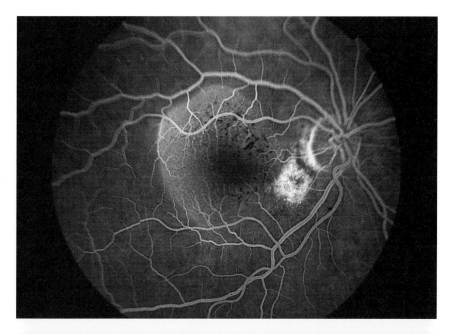

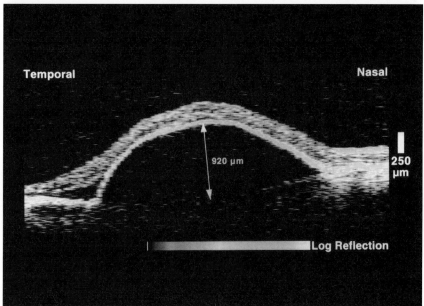

FIGURE 12-3. AMD/serous pigment epithelial detachment. A 70-year-old woman had a large serous detachment of the retinal pigment epithelium in her right eye associated with the clinical diagnosis of age-related macular degeneration. Visual acuity OD was 20/400. *(top)* Fluorescein angiography shows a placoid region of hyperfluorescence nasal to the fovea consistent with a neovascular membrane, and a large area of relative hyperfluorescence involving the macula corresponding to the pigment epithelial detachment. *(bottom)* Horizontal OCT image delineates a large elevation (920 μm) of the retina and retinal pigment epithelium above an optically clear space. The reflections from the choroid beneath the detachment were attenuated due to shadowing from the highly reflective detached pigment epithelium. A small pocket of subretinal fluid accumulation was noted temporal to the pigment epithelial detachment. The reflections from the nasal pigment epithelium and choriocapillaris appeared thicker than those at the temporal margin of the image, consistent with the leakage pattern of fluorescein dye observed clinically.

sistent with accumulation of material within or beneath Bruch's membrane (Fig. 12-4). These small elevations mimic small serous detachments of the RPE; however, unlike a PED, soft drusen display shallow margins and mild backscatter signal is noted which extends from the RPE into the choroid. A fibrovascular PED showed an elevation of the reflection corresponding to the RPE over a mild to moderately backscattering region between the detached pigment epithelium and choroid. A clear distinction is noted between the bright (red) re-

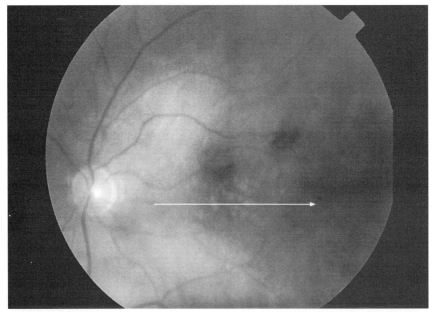

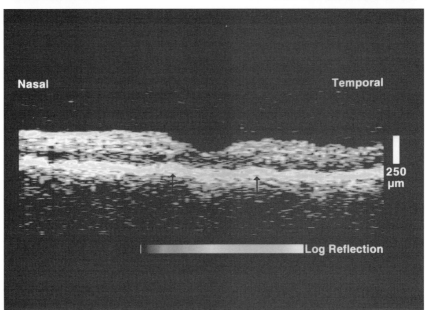

FIGURE 12-4. AMD/soft drusen. A 71-year-old man with age-related macular degeneration had a visual acuity of 20/40 in his left eye. *(top)* Fundus photograph displays soft drusen in the central macula OS. *(bottom)* Horizontal OCT shows small modulations *(black arrows)* in the contour of the RPE with moderate optical reflectivity below the lesions consistent with soft drusen.

flection from the RPE, and the moderate (green/yellow) sub-RPE reflections. No optical shadowing of the choroid is visible. Finally, hemorrhagic PEDs demonstrated an elevation of the reflection corresponding to the RPE over a highly backscattering region which attenuates rapidly toward the outer retina and completely shadows the choroidal reflection. Hemorrhagic neu-

rosensory detachments may be difficult to distinguish from hemorrhagic PEDs due to the similarity in reflectance between blood and detached pigment epithelium. Therefore, CNV can be categorized as well-defined, poorly defined, or as a fibrovascular PED (Hee et al., 1996).

These classifications did not necessarily correspond

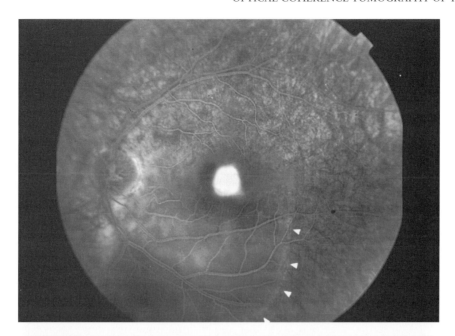

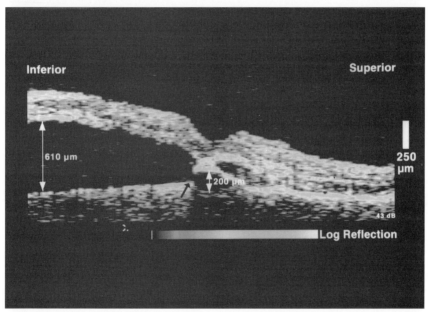

FIGURE 12-5. Central serous chorioretinopathy. The left eye of a 35-year-old man with a history of central serous chorioretinopathy in his right eye was examined. Indirect ophthalmoscopy revealed a small RPE detachment at the temporal edges of the macula *(not shown)*. *(top)* Fluorescein angiography shows pooling of dye within a neurosensory detachment surrounded by a large area of hyperfluorescence *(arrows)*. *(bottom)* A vertical OCT shows a subfoveal pigment epithelial detachment and a neurosensory retina detachment inferiorly (610 μm), consistent with central serous chorioretinopathy. An RPE break is noted *(black arrow)* allowing fluid leakage from the RPE detachment into the subretinal space. The false color appearance is shown in Plate 12-II.

to similar fluorescein angiographic findings. In general, angiographically classic CNV appeared as well-defined CNV on OCT, while angiographically occult neovascularization was characterized as either fibrovascular PED or poorly defined CNV. However, well-defined CNV sometimes presented as fibrovascular PED on OCT. In such cases, OCT may have been sensitive to the difference between predominantly subretinal versus predominantly sub-PRE neovascularization. Thus, well-defined CNV on OCT may represent new vessels which are penetrating through single or multiple breaks in Bruch's membrane. In contrast, the reflection from the RPE in a fibrovascular PED on OCT appears intact and suggests that neovascularization is confined to below the RPE. Consequently, OCT may provide useful structural information in evaluating patients for possible surgical removal of subfoveal CNV. Furthermore, the near-infrared wavelength and high detection sensitivity of OCT allowed enhanced penetration and imaging capability through blood compared to FA (Hee et al., 1996).

Both serous and hemorrhagic detachments of the RPE were successfully diagnosed with OCT. However, OCT was not able to detect CNV beneath serous PEDs because of optical shadowing and the absence of a RPE/choriocapillaris band. Since OCT is a cross-sectional imaging modality, a single OCT only provides information on CNV boundaries within a thin tissue slice. OCT also does not provide much additional information when there are angiographic features that obscure the boundaries of neovascular membranes. Moreover, OCT does not effectively image CNV beneath PEDs because of optical shadowing caused by the detached RPE. Similarly, blood often obscures the boundaries of CNV on angiography. While OCT can image CNV obscured on FA by thin hemorrhage, OCT probe light is attenuated by dense subretinal or intraretinal hemorrhage, which prevents adequate imaging of the choroid. Finally, it is important to note that reflections from the choroid on OCT were influenced by absorption and scattering properties of the RPE. The use of imaging wavelengths farther in the infrared should provide increased penetration of the probe beam through hemorrhage or a serous detachment of the RPE, allowing better imaging of CNV beneath these lesions (Hee et al., 1996).

As mentioned, neurosensory detachments occurring with central serous chorioretinopathy form secondary to one or more focal fluorescein angiographic leakages of fluid at the level of the RPE (Burton, 1972; Gass, 1967; Gass, 1987; Schatz, 1975; Yannuzzi et al., 1982). OCT provides a means for quantitatively monitoring the extent and height of retinal detachment and is more sensitive to small changes than biomicroscopy. Longitudinal examinations with OCT are able to track the resolution of the sensory retinal detachment, and reductions in subretinal fluid accumulation are often noticed before subsequent improvements is visual acuity (Hee et al., 1995d).

In contrast to serous PEDs, which show an elevation of the reflective band corresponding to the RPE, sharp margins, and shadowing of the reflections returning from the deeper choroid, neurosensory detachments appear as elevations of the sensory retina above an opti-

cally clear space, with well-defined boundaries at the fluid–RPE and fluid–retina interfaces, and shallow margins at the edges of the lesions. OCT appears to be highly sensitive to small elevations of the neurosensory retina because of the clear difference in reflectivity between retinal tissue and serous fluid. Figure 12-5 (see also Plate 12-II) clearly demonstrates a break in the RPE centrally which is allowing fluid to leak into the subretinal space inferiorly. Before the onset of symptoms occurring with central serous chorioretinopathy, patients usually develop areas of serous RPE detachment, which then leads to detachment of the overlying and surrounding retina (Hee et al., 1995d).

Although the disease typically affects adults between 20 and 50 years of age, central serous chorioretinopathy may be mistaken for AMD and subretinal neovascularization in older patients (Schatz et al., 1992). The occult form of choroidal neovascularization may show a similar angiographic appearance to central serous chorioretinopathy when a focal leakage point is present. OCT can distinguish between these two appearances by confirming the existence of a neurosensory detachment versus abnormalities in the RPE or choriocapillaris from neovascularization. OCT also has been able to detect detachments of the neurosensory retina that were undetected by slit-lamp biomicroscopy (Hee et al., 1995d).

In summary, OCT generates high-resolution cross-sectional tomograms of ocular tissue. OCT has found clinical application in the diagnosis and management of many macular diseases. This includes retinal disorders which involve disruption of the RPE, such as age-related macular degeneration and central serous retinopathy.

REFERENCES

Bressler NM, Bressler SB, Gragoudas ES. 1987. Clinical characteristics of choroidal neovascular membranes. Arch Ophthalmol 105: 209–213.

Burton TC. 1972. Central serous retinopathy. In: Blodi FC, ed, Current Concepts in Ophthalmology, vol. 3. St Louis: Mosby, 1–28.

Gass JDM. 1967. Pathogenesis of disciform detachment of the neuroepithelium. II: Idiopathic central serous choroidopathy. Am J Ophthalmol 63:587–615.

Gass JDM. 1987. Stereoscopic Atlas of Macular Diseases: Diagnosis and Treatment. 3rd ed. Vol 1. St Louis: Mosby, 46–65.

Hee MR, Izatt JA, Swanson EA, Huang D, Schuman JS, Lin CP, Puliafito CA, Fujimoto JG. 1995a. Optical coherence tomography of the human retina. Arch Ophthalmol 113:325–332.

Hee MR, Puliafito CA, Wong C, Duker JS, Reichel E, Schuman JS, Swanson EA, Fujimoto JG. 1995b. Optical coherence tomography of macular holes. Ophthalmology 102:748–756.

Hee MR, Puliafito CA, Wong C, Duker JS, Reichel E, Rutledge BK, Schuman JS, Swanson EA, Fujimoto JG. 1995c. Quantitative assessment of macular edema with optical coherence tomography (OCT). Arch Ophthalmol 113:1019–1029.

Hee MR, Puliafito CA, Wong C, Duker JS, Reichel E, Schuman JS, Swanson EA, Fujimoto JG. 1995d. Optical coherence tomography (OCT) of central serous chorioretinopathy. Am J Ophthalmol 120:65–74.

Hee MR, Baumal CR, Puliafito CA, Duker JS, Reichel E, Wilkins JR, Coker JG, Schuman JS, Swanson EA, Fujimoto JG. 1996. Optical coherence tomography of age-related macular degeneration and choroidal neovascularization. Ophthalmology 103:1260–1270.

Huang D, Swanson EA, Lin CP, Schuman JS, Stinson WG, Chang W, Hee MR, Flotte T, Gregory K, Puliafito CA, Fujimoto JG. 1991. Optical coherence tomography. Science 254:1178–1181.

Moisseiev NM, Alhalel A, Masuri R, Treister G. 1995. The impact of the macular photocoagulation study results on the treatment of exudative age-related macular degeneration. Arch Ophthalmol 113:185–189.

[MPSG] Macular Photocoagulation Study Group. 1982. Argon laser photocoagulation for senile macular degeneration: results of a randomized clinical trial. Arch Ophthalmol 100:912–918.

[MPSG] Macular Photocoagulation Study Group. 1990. Krypton laser photocoagulation for neovascular lesions of age-related macular degeneration: results of a randomized clinical trial. Arch Ophthalmol 108:816–824.

[MPSG] Macular Photocoagulation Study Group. 1991a. Argon laser photocoagulation for neovascular maculopathy: five-year results from randomized clinical trials. Arch Ophthalmol 109:1109–1114.

[MPSG] Macular Photocoagulation Study Group. 1991b. Subfoveal neovascular lesions in age-related macular degeneration: guidelines for evaluation and treatment in the Macular Photocoagulation Study. Arch Ophthalmol 1099:1242–1257.

[MPSG] Macular Photocoagulation Study Group. 1991c. Laser photocoagulation of subfoveal recurrent neovascular lesions in age-related macular degeneration: results of a randomized clinical trial. Arch Ophthalmol 109:1232–1241.

Puliafito CA, Hee MR, Lin CP, Reichel E, Schuman JS, Duker JS, Izatt JA, Swanson EA, Fujimoto JG. 1995. Imaging of macular diseases with optical coherence tomography (OCT). Ophthalmology 102:217–229.

Schatz H. 1975. Central serous chorioretinopathy and serous detachment of the retinal pigment epithelium. Int Ophthalmol Clin 15:159–168.

Schatz H, Madeira D, Johnson RN, McDonald HR. 1992. Central serous chorioretinopathy occurring in patients 60 years of age and older. Ophthalmology 99:63–67.

Swanson EA, Huang D, Hee MR, Fujimoto JG, Lin CP, Puliafito CA. 1992. High-speed optical coherence domain reflectometry. Opt Lett 17:151–153.

Swanson EA, Izatt JA, Hee MR, Huang D, Lin CP, Schuman JS, Puliafito CA, Fujimoto JG. 1993. In vivo retinal imaging by optical coherence tomography. Opt Lett 18:1864–1866.

Yannuzzi LA, Schatz H, Gitter KA. Central serous chorioretinopathy. In Yannuzzi LA, Gitter KA, Schatz H, eds: The Macula: A Comprehensive Text and Atlas. Baltimore: Williams & Wilkins, 1979. 145–165.

IV | INHERITED AND METABOLIC DISORDERS

13. Rodent models of retinal pigment epithelial disease

MICHAEL O. HALL

The critical relationship of the retinal pigment epithelium (RPE) to the neural retina is evident from a multitude of basic and clinical studies, which show that in the functioning vertebrate eye the RPE provides vital metabolic and functional support for the visual cells. The RPE has many complex functions, such as regulating the nutrition of the outer retina; absorption of stray light; uptake, conversion, storage, and transport of retinoids; synthesis of some components of the interphotoreceptor matrix; ion and fluid transport; phagocytosis of photoreceptor (PR) cell outer segments; and retinal adhesion. Under normal circumstances, the RPE does not renew itself, thus it must perform its many functions throughout the lifetime of the individual. If any of the above functions of the RPE are compromised, death of the underlying PR cells invariably follows.

A number of naturally occurring rodent models of retinal degeneration have been described and extensively studied. These models have provided critical information regarding the etiology of some retinal degenerations in humans. Thus, the defective gene in the *rd* mouse (rd-1) encodes an autosomal recessive mutation in the β-subunit of the rod-specific cGMP phosphodiesterase (for a review, see Farber et al., 1994). Studies by LaVail and Mullen (1976) have conclusively shown that the site of action of the *rd* gene is the neural retina, and that the RPE is uninvolved. Identification of the mutation in this mouse has resulted in the identification of the *rd* mutation in a subgroup of retinitis pigmentosa patients suffering from autosomal recessive RP (McLaughlin et al., 1995; Bayes et al., 1995; Danciger et al., 1995).

A second well-studied mouse model of retinal degeneration is the *rds* mouse (rd-2), in which the gene defect is also inherited as an autosomal recessive (for a review, see Molday, 1994). The normal gene encodes the protein peripherin, which is a structural component of the photoreceptor outer segment disk membranes, and thus the gene is also designated as *rds*/peripherin. Outer segments fail to develop in mice homozygous for the mutation, although inner segments persist for many months. As with the *rd* mutation, the *rds*/peripherin gene is not expressed in the RPE and no evidence exists to implicate the RPE in the retinal degeneration. Mutations in the *rds* gene have recently been shown to be responsible for retinal degeneration in humans suffering from autosomal-dominant RP (Farrar et al., 1991). Mutations in the *rds* gene have also been shown to be present in individuals suffering from autosomal-dominant retinitis punctata albescens (Kajiwara et al., 1993), vitelliform macular dystrophy (Wells et al., 1993), and butterfly macular dystrophy (Nicols, 1993). The absence of peripheral and night vision defects suggests that these mutations do not significantly affect rod photoreceptors. In the latter two diseases, although the gene is expressed in the photoreceptor cells, it has been suggested that excessive shedding and phagocytosis resulting from unstable cone outer segments, due to decreased amounts of *rds*/peripherin, may result in structural or metabolic changes in the RPE, leading to this form of macular degeneration.

Recently a number of other mouse models of inherited retinal degeneration have been identified (J. Heckenlively, personal communication). These are designated as rd-3, rd-4 and rd-5. Although these have all been mapped to their respective chromosomal locations, neither the site of expression of the mutant gene, nor the function which the mutation affects, have been identified.

Although studies of the above-mentioned models have provided clues which lead to the identification of mutations causing retinal degeneration in humans, none of these mutations are expressed in the RPE, or appear to directly affect the RPE. The only rodent model of retinal degeneration in which the primary genetic defect is unequivocally known to be expressed in the RPE is the RCS rat. A second rodent model in which the genetic defect may be expressed in the RPE, or may be primarily expressed elsewhere with a secondary effect on the RPE, is the vitiligo mouse. In both of these animal models, degeneration of the underlying PR cells is secondary to RPE cell dysfunction. These two animal models of RPE disease are thus discussed in some detail in this chapter.

THE RCS RAT

The Royal College of Surgeons (RCS) rat has provided researchers with an important model system for studying a number of physiological functions of the RPE and cellular interactions between the RPE and PR cells, and the pathological sequelae resulting from a defect in one of the normal interactions between these two cell layers. This animal exhibits a retinal dystrophy *(rdy)* which is inherited as an autosomal recessive gene (Bourne et al., 1938; Bourne and Gruneberg, 1939).

The retinal degeneration in the RCS rat was first studied in depth by Dowling and Sidman (1962). These investigators showed that the PR cells developed normally until 15 days of age, although subsequent ultrastructural studies showed that the photoreceptor tips are disorganized by 10 days of age (Bok and Hall, 1971). By 15 postnatal days a layer of disorganized "lamellar debris" began to accumulate at the apical surface of the RPE and the rhodopsin content of the eye started to increase. The electroretinogram (ERG) threshold also started to increase at day 15, and was completely extinguished by 60 days. At this age the PR cell layer had disappeared leaving only a layer of lamellar debris between the RPE and the inner nuclear layer, and the rhodopsin content of the retina had dropped to an undetectable level. Dowling and Sidman suggested that the lamellar debris might be elaborated by the RPE and that the increased rhodopsin, which they demonstrated was associated with the lamellar debris, must be synthesized by the photoreceptor cells.

The discovery that PR cells constantly renew their outer segments (Young, 1967; Young and Bok, 1969) led Herron and colleagues (1969) and Bok and Hall (1971) to study this process in the RCS rat, since it seemed likely that OS renewal was abnormal. Using autoradiography to follow the renewal of photoreceptor cell OS and the subsequent shedding of packets of discs from the tip of the OS, both groups of investigators clearly showed that RCS rats renew their PR cell outer segments in a fairly normal manner, but the shed tips of these cells are not phagocytized by the adjacent RPE. These shed tips accumulate at the apical surface of the RPE, leading to a buildup of OS-derived debris between the retina and the RPE (Fig. 13-1). These studies suggested that the process of phagocytosis was at fault in the RCS rat, but they did not define which cell type was expressing the mutant gene. Had the RPE lost its ability to phagocytize the shed tips of OS, or had the *rdy* gene modified the photoreceptor cell so that its outer segment membranes were not recognized and engulfed by the RPE cells? This question was elegantly and definitively answered by Mullen and LaVail (1976) using

tetraparental chimeric rats produced by fusing the eight-cell embryos derived from the mating of pigmented normal (+/+) rats with the eight-cell embryos derived from the mating of albino RCS *(rdy/rdy)* rats. The offspring produced by this fusion displayed mosaicism of the RPE, with patches of normal pigmented RPE interspersed with patches of albino RPE carrying the *rdy* gene. Analysis of ocular tissue sections from these chimeric rats revealed that degenerating retina always underlay mutant RPE, while retina underlying patches of normal RPE appeared normal (Fig. 13-2). Thus, the site of mutant gene expression in the RCS rat must be in the RPE. Taken together, these studies strongly suggested that the mutation affects the ability of these cells to ingest the shed tips of OS, causing a secondary loss of PR cells. These in vivo results were confirmed in vitro by Chaitin and Hall (1983), who showed that normal RPE cells grown in tissue culture were able to phagocytize OS from both normal or dystrophic rats, while RPE cells from dystrophic rats showed only limited phagocytosis of OS isolated from either animal. Additionally, these investigators showed that dystrophic RPE cells in tissue culture were able to bind OS as well as did normal RPE cells, but OS ingestion was greatly reduced. These studies confirmed and extended the earlier in vivo studies by showing that the mutation affects the ingestion phase of OS phagocytosis. Chaitin and Hall suggested that the phagocytosis of OS might be mediated by a specific receptor on the surface of the RPE.

Although the site of expression of the mutation has been elucidated, the defective gene has not been identified, nor has the molecular expression of the gene been described. A number of molecular sites are possible at which the mutation could be expressed.

The normal gene may express a receptor ("phagocytosis receptor") on the apical surface of the RPE, which is responsible for the phagocytosis of the shed tips of OS. There is an accumulating body of evidence that the phagocytosis of OS is a receptor-mediated process whereby a receptor on the RPE recognizes a ligand on the surface of the shed OS (for a review, see McLaughlin et al., 1994). After binding to the receptor, the shed OS is internalized by the RPE cells and subsequently digested by lysosomal enzymes. Numerous investigators have attempted to identify the phagocytosis receptor on the RPE, and a number of candidate molecules have been proposed. Boyle and colleagues (1991) have shown that the mannosylfucosyl (mannose) receptor is present on rat and human RPE cells. Incubation of cultured rat RPE cells with an antibody to the macrophage mannose receptor significantly inhibits the ingestion of OS, as does preincubation of OS with purified mannose receptor protein. A second molecule which has been pro-

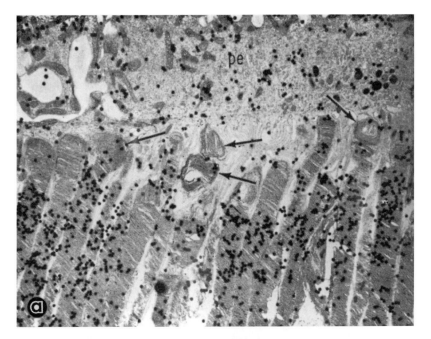

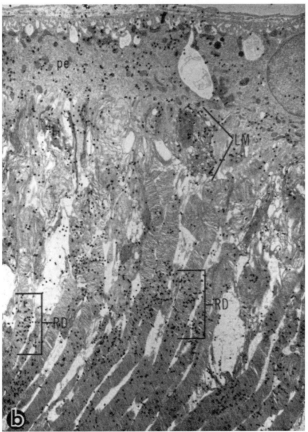

FIGURE 13-1. Electron micrograph autoradiograms of 16-day-old normal and RCS rat retinas. (a) In the normal rat retina, the OS are well aligned and are in close contact with the microvilli of the adjacent RPE. Packets of disks are in the process of being shed from the tips of OS and engulfed by the RPE *(arrows)*. (b) The OS of the RCS rat retina are the same length as those of the normal rat, but show disorganized disks in the OS tips and the accumulation of lamellar debris (LM) adjacent to the RPE. The microvilli do not appear to be in close contact with the OS. No evidence of organized shedding, or of OS phagocytosis is seen. The black dots represent radioactively labeled proteins and disks (RD). (Reproduced from Bok and Hall, 1971, by copyright permission of the Rockefeller University Press.)

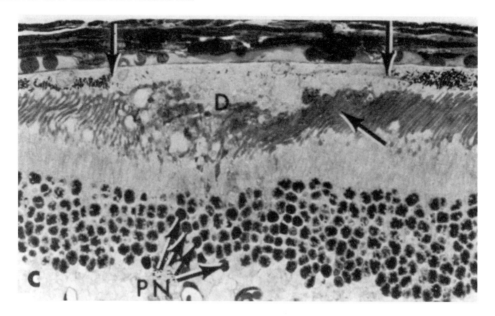

FIGURE 13-2. Light micrograph of a four-month-old chimeric rat retina produced by fusing the eight cell embryos derived from the mating of pigmented normal (+/+) rats with the eight cell embryos derived from the mating of albino RCS rats *(rdy/rdy)*. The RPE displays mosaicism, with patches of albino *rdy* RPE *(between vertical arrows)* interspersed between patches of pigmented normal RPE. Photoreceptors underlying and adjacent to the normal RPE cells appear normal *(hor-* *izontal arrow)*, while OS debris (D) and degenerating photoreceptors underlie the *rdy* pigment epithelium. The ONL beneath the *rdy* RPE is reduced in thickness and contains many pyknotic nuclei (PN). (Reproduced from Mullen and LaVail, 1976, by copyright permission of the American Association for the Advancement of Science, and with permission of the authors.)

posed is CD 36, an 88 kD multifunctional cell surface glycoprotein which serves as a scavenger receptor on macrophages (Ryeom et al., 1994; 1995). This molecule has been shown to be present on normal rat RPE cells, but absent on RCS rat RPE cells. When CD 36 was transfected into a nonphagocytic cell line, these cells gained the ability to bind OS; this binding was reduced when these cells were incubated with a monoclonal antibody to CD 36. However, neither of these cell surface receptors has conclusively been shown to be the specific phagocytosis receptor, which still remains unidentified at this time. This phagocytosis receptor may be defective in the RCS rat, allowing binding but not internalization of shed OS tips.

The normal gene may express a component of an intracellular signaling pathway which is linked to the phagocytosis receptor. It is quite possible that binding of shed OS tips to the receptor generates a transmembrane signal which activates the ingestion phase of OS phagocytosis. Such signaling pathways are usually composed of a number of discrete steps, any one of which might be the product of the defective gene in the RCS rat. Several intracellular signaling pathways which may be linked to the phagocytosis of OS have recently been investigated. The linkage of both the protein kinase C pathway (Hall et al., 1991) and the protein kinase A pathway (Hall et al., 1993; Kuriyama et al., 1994) to OS

ingestion have been studied. Activation of both of these pathways inhibits OS ingestion, thus eliminating them as potential sites of the mutation of the RCS rat, or of being primarily involved in the OS phagocytosis process. Recently Heth and colleagues (1995) suggested that OS ingestion in the RCS rat is upregulated by the generation of inositol trisphosphate (IP_3). These authors treated cultured rat RPE cells with carbachol to increase the intracellular concentration of IP_3 and reported that this overcame the phagocytosis defect in the mutant rat. However, recent studies by Hall and colleagues (1995) have cast doubt on this claim. Thus, the intracellular signaling pathway that is linked to OS phagocytosis remains a mystery.

RPE Cell Transplantation in the RCS Rat

In the mid-1980s a number of investigators showed that transplantation of RPE cells was feasible, and that the transplanted cells established themselves on the host Bruch's membrane, and appeared histologically normal. The success of these early experiments led these researchers to seek out an animal model in which the physiological competence of the transplanted RPE cells could be tested. The RCS rat was an obvious model for such studies, since the genetic defect had been clearly shown to reside in the RPE.

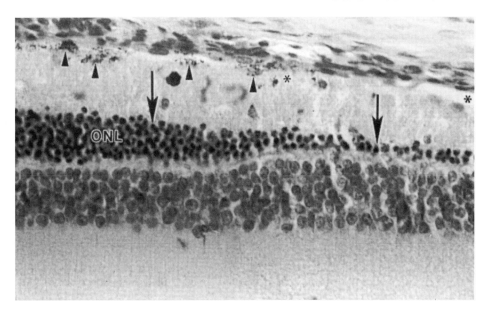

FIGURE 13-3. Light micrograph of a 60-day-old RCS rat retina grafted with normal RPE cells *(arrowheads)* at postnatal day 26. The area between the arrows shows a transition zone where the number of grafted normal RPE cells is reduced, with a concomitant thinning of the outer nuclear layer (ONL). No transplanted RPE cells are seen in the area of most severe degeneration *(between the asterisks)*. (Reproduced from Li and Turner, 1988b, with permission from the authors and by copyright permission from Academic Press Ltd.)

Li and Turner (1988a) reported the first successful transplantation of RPE cells into the eyes of RCS rats. RPE cells isolated from 6- to 8-day-old pigmented Long Evans control rats were injected into the subretinal space of 26-day-old albino RCS rats. At this age retinal degeneration in this animal is clearly evident, but is not so advanced as to cause extensive photoreceptor cell death. At 60 days of age, when most of the PR cells in the retinas of the RCS rat have degenerated, the eyes of the experimental animals and of control RCS rats were examined by light and electron microscopy. The transplanted normal RPE cells, which could be identified by their pigment granules, had established themselves on Bruch's membrane as a mosaic, either singly or in clusters, surrounded by the nonpigmented host RPE cells (Fig. 13-3). Astoundingly, it was found that photoreceptor cells underlying the transplanted normal RPE cells appeared normal, the thickness of the debris zone was markedly diminished beneath the transplanted cells, and the thickness of the outer nuclear layer (ONL) under the transplanted cells was comparable to that seen in control rats of the same age (10–11 cells). By contrast, photoreceptor cells underlying the nearby dystrophic host RPE cells had continued to degenerate, the thickness of the debris zone had increased, and the outer nuclear layer was reduced to 1–2 cells in thickness. Thus the transplanted cells had apparently "rescued" the PR cells which lay beneath them. This experiment

was subsequently independently confirmed (Lopez et al., 1989) and expanded (for a review, see Sheedlo et al., 1992). In subsequent experiments it was shown that the transplanted RPE cells established normal structural interactions with the underlying photoreceptor cells (Sheedlo et al., 1989) and assumed the phagocytic function, which is defective in the RCS pigment epithelial cells (LaVail et al., 1992). Importantly, the rescued PR cells displayed many normal metabolic functions, such as a normal rate and pattern of OS renewal, normal staining of the interphotoreceptor matrix (LaVail et al., 1992), normal opsin immunostaining and a normal distribution of Na^+, K^+-ATPase (Sheedlo et al., 1989; Li et al., 1990). The resumption of normal PR cell structure and function beneath transplanted RPE cells proves that the only site of expression of the mutation is the RPE cell. It also strongly implicates the RPE as an active participant in the shedding process (since normal OS shedding is resumed under normal RPE cells), as well as in the maintenance of normal OS structure.

It is significant that the rescue of photoreceptors caused by transplanted normal RPE cells is maintained for extended periods of time—up to one year when optimal parameters of the age of the host and of the transplanted cells are met (Li and Turner, 1991). This is most important when considering the transplantation of RPE cells into human eyes in order to reverse or halt some of the pathologies which are expressed in these cells, and which cause a secondary degeneration of the photoreceptors.

A further exciting application of RPE cell transplantation is in the prevention or treatment of neovascularization of the RPE. In the three-month-old RCS rat, when photoreceptors have completely degenerated, new blood vessels arising in the retina proliferate and invade the RPE cell layer (Matthes and Bok, 1985; Caldwell et al., 1989). If healthy RPE cells are transplanted into the subretinal space at this age, the proliferation of new vessels is significantly reduced. Additionally, when RPE cell transplantation is carried out at six months, the number of preexisting neovascular profiles is reduced by 40% two months later, suggesting that transplantation of healthy RPE cells causes the regression of previously existing new blood vessels (Seaton et al., 1994).

In summary, the genetic defect in the RCS rat has clearly been shown to reside in the RPE, and can be cured by replacing the mutant RPE cells with RPE cells carrying the normal gene. This is an example of successful "gene therapy," with the vector being the intact RPE cell.

bFGF Delays Photoreceptor Cell Degeneration in the RCS Rat

During many RPE cell transplantation studies, it was noticed that photoreceptors located beyond the boundaries of the transplanted cells are rescued. Additionally, control RCS rats eyes that were injected intraocularly with only phosphate buffered saline (PBS) (no RPE cells), showed a significant degree of PR cell rescue beneath the injection site (Li and Turner, 1988b). This suggested that a diffusible factor might be released by the normal transplanted RPE cells, as well as in response to the trauma caused to the host RPE cells during the injection, and that this factor might exert a trophic effect on the adjacent PR cells. Since basic fibroblast growth factor (bFGF) was known to act as a neurotrophic agent, Faktorovich and colleagues (1990) injected either bFGF, acidic fibroblast growth factor (aFGF), or PBS subretinally or intravitreally into 23-day-old RCS rats, and measured the thickness of the outer nuclear layer (ONL) by light microscopy two and three months later (Fig. 13-4). While PBS and aFGF caused localized rescue of PR cells near the injection site, bFGF caused a quantitatively greater, longer-lasting, and much more extensive PR cell rescue. Unfortunately, this effect was transient, as the thickness of the ONL three months after injection of bFGF was significantly reduced from that at two months. Thus, despite the partial preservation of photoreceptor cell viability, bFGF does not reverse the genetic defect in the RCS rat, as the zone of

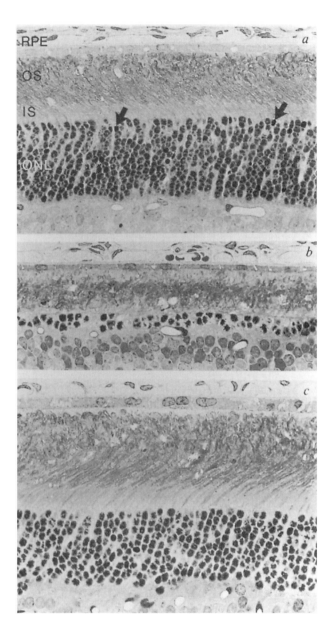

FIGURE 13-4. Light micrographs of RCS rat retinas at (a) postnatal day (P) 23, (b) P53, and (c) P53 after injection of bFGF subretinally at P23. At P23 (a), photoreceptor inner (IS) and outer (OS) segments are present. Some lamellar debris has accumulated adjacent to the apical surface of the RPE. The ONL is 10–13 rows thick. At P 53 (b), no IS or OS are present, and the area between the outer limiting membrane and the RPE consists entirely of lamellar debris. The ONL is reduced to one or two rows in thickness. At P53 (c), after injection of bFGF at P23, the retina appears generally unchanged from its appearance at the time of injection (compare [a] and [c]). Photoreceptor IS and OS are present, and the ONL is 10–11 rows in thickness. The thickness of the debris layer has increased. (Reproduced with permission from Faktorovich et al., 1990. Copyright 1990, Macmillan Magazines Limited, and with permission of the authors.)

lamellar debris was still present and no evidence of phagocytosis by the RPE cells was seen. That normal RPE cells do not secrete a factor which corrects the phagocytic defect in RCS cell was confirmed by Hall and Abrams (1991), who showed that when normal and dystrophic RPE cells are cocultured, no improvement is found in the ability of the dystrophic cells to ingest PR outer segments. Unfortunately, studies to find more efficacious and longer lasting trophic factors than bFGF have not been successful (LaVail, personal communication).

Since bFGF is synthesized by the RPE (Schweigerer et al., 1987), and PR outer segments have bFGF receptors (Mascarelli et al., 1987), it seemed possible that these tissues in the RCS rat might possess a relative deficit of this growth factor. However, recent immunohistochemical studies (Connolly et al., 1992; Rakoczy et al., 1993), showed no difference in either the distribution or concentration of bFGF, or its receptor, between the RPE or retinas of normal and RCS rats. It is therefore unlikely that bFGF plays a causative role in the retinal degeneration in the RCS rat. The trophic effect of bFGF may thus merely recapitulate an environment present during the early development of OS.

Since the injection of bFGF does not reverse the phagocytosis defect in the RCS rat, (Faktorovich et al., 1990), it is not surprising that the effect of bFGF on photoreceptor viability is transitory. RPE cell transplantation, by contrast, *cures* the retinal degeneration by providing healthy RPE cells, which appear to perform all of the functions of normal RPE cells. These transplanted RPE cells phagocytize the shed tips of OS which underlie them, and presumably allow the rescued PR cells to resume all of their normal functions. It is evident from these studies that normal phagocytosis of shed OS tips is mandatory for the maintenance of PR cell viability, or in a more general sense, the normal interaction of the RPE and PR cells is vital for the survival of the latter.

What are the implications of these discoveries in the RCS rat for the treatment of human ocular disease? A number of ocular diseases are thought to primarily affect the RPE, resulting secondarily in degeneration of the photoreceptors (e.g. age-related macular degeneration (AMD), Stargardt's disease, gyrate atrophy, chodoideremia, vitelliform macular degeneration, and possibly some forms of retinitis pigmentosa). Alterations in the retinal vasculature play a major role in ocular diseases such as the wet form of AMD and in proliferative diabetic retinopathy. All of these diseases are candidates for RPE cell transplantation. It has, however, been shown that RPE cells express class I and class II antigens of the MHC complex (Liversidge et al., 1988; Elner et al.,

1989), and thus their transplantation will require immunosuppression. Alternatively, improvements in methods for the biopsy of RPE cells from the anterior portion of the globe would allow histocompatible cells to be removed, grown in culture, and injected back into the host eye, thus eliminating the problems of immune rejection. However, if this approach is to be used, culture conditions which maintain the differentiated state of the RPE cells would have to be perfected, as it has been shown that passaged RPE cells, and RPE cells from older rats, rapidly lose their ability to rescue photoreceptors in the RCS rat (Sheedlo et al., 1993). RPE cells from fetal human eyes may well be the best source of RPE cells for transplantation (Gouras et al., 1994). Peyman and colleagues (1991), have reported the transplantation of either homologous or autologous RPE cells into the eyes of five patients with AMD.

The exciting observation that bFGF exerts a trophic effect on degenerating PR cells in the RCS rat may have important implications for the treatment of human diseases such as the family of inherited retinal degenerations classified as retinitis pigmentosa. Although the rescue effect in the RCS rat is temporary, alternative methods of delivery of this or other growth factors might allow for the preservation of vision past the time normally expected for patients suffering from this blinding disease.

In summary, the RCS rat has provided, and continues to provide, an important model for studying the interactions of the photoreceptor cells and the RPE, as well as the role played by the RPE in maintaining the functional homeostasis of the retina. Studies of the genetic defect in this animal have led to strategies for curing or slowing down the course of the retinal degeneration that accompanies the expression of the mutant gene. Such strategies may well be applicable to a number of diseases in humans which primarily affect the RPE, resulting in a secondary degeneration of the PR cells.

THE VITILIGO MOUSE

The vitiligo mouse was first described by Lerner and colleagues (1986). The vitiligo *(vit)* gene is inherited as an autosomal recessive and has been mapped to the microphthalmia (mi) locus on mouse chromosome 6 (Lamoreux et al., 1992). It is thus correctly designated as mi^{vit}/mi^{vit}. Since this mutant arose spontaneously from the inbred C57BL/6J strain, it is designated as C57BL/6-mi^{vit}/mi^{vit}. Phenotypically, the mi^{vit}/mi^{vit} (vitiligo) mouse is characterized by postnatal depigmentation of the pelage, skin, and eyes. Vitiligo mice also exhibit a slow progressive loss of photoreceptor cells

(Sidman and Neumann, 1988; Smirnakis et al., 1991; Smith, 1992), and it has been suggested that abnormalities of the pigment epithelium precede photoreceptor cell degeneration (Smirnakis et al., 1991). The choroid of the newborn vitiligo mouse is amelanotic, and acquires patchy pigmentation by three weeks. A central amelanotic patch surrounding the optic nerve is present in all animals, and persists through adulthood. The retinal pigment epithelium (RPE) appears continuous and contains areas of hyper- and hypopigmentation. Macrophages are present between the RPE and the photoreceptor (PR) cells by four weeks of age (Nir et al., 1995).

Extensive studies of the retinal degeneration affecting the vitiligo mouse have been carried out by Smith and her colleagues (Smith, 1992; Smith et al., 1994a; 1994b; 1994c; Smith and Hamasaki, 1994; Smith and Defoe, 1995; Nir et al., 1995; Smith et al., 1995).

The retinal degeneration in this mouse model proceeds slowly, with photoreceptor inner segments and nuclei persisting in the peripheral retina for eight months or longer, and is confined to the PR cells; the innermost portion of the neural retina is spared (Smith, 1992). Development of the PR cells proceeds normally over most of the retina for the first postnatal month, although abnormal PRs are seen in the posterior retina as early as 12 postnatal days (Nir et al., 1995). The outer plexiform layer (OPL) and the outer nuclear layer (ONL) are of normal thickness, the outer segments (OS) are of normal length, and the rhodopsin content of the retina is comparable to control animals of the same age (Smith, 1992). Thus the mi^{vit}/mi^{vit} mutation represents a degeneration of the PR cells and not a dysplasia. By two months of age, the number of rows of nuclei in the ONL has begun to decrease, as has the thickness of the OPL, indicative of PR cell death. While the rhodopsin content of the retina progressively decreases from two months of age, the length of the OS transiently increases between two and three months. This may indicate improper disk formation, faulty disk shedding, or impaired phagocytosis by the RPE. By four months of age, the PR outer segments have detached from the RPE in the posterior and equatorial retina, and numerous macrophages are seen in the subretinal space. In parallel with the OS degeneration, is a gradual loss of all components of the electroretinogram (ERG) (Smith and Hamasaki, 1994).

In a 1992 study Smith suggested that the increased length of OS observed at two to three months of age might be due to impaired OS shedding and/or phagocytosis by the RPE. In a subsequent study, Smith and colleagues (1994b) examined cyclic OS shedding and phagocytosis in the vitiligo mouse. They clearly showed that PR cells exhibited a light-activated shedding event,

but that at four weeks of age, the number of phagosomes was reduced to about 40% of that seen in control eyes, and to 20% or less at eight weeks or older. Phagosomes are observed in the RPE microvilli and in the cytoplasm of the RPE cells. Thus, the RPE is clearly capable of OS phagocytosis during the first two or three postnatal months, and the reduced number of phagosomes may be due to a reduced rate of OS shedding. However, in 20-week-old mice, the RPE microvilli present an abnormal appearance; instead of being elongated, they are composed of small vesiculated structures, which do not envelop the OS (Fig. 13-5). In areas where such abnormalities of the RPE are present, OS fragments are seen lying adjacent to the vesiculated microvilli, and they do not appear to be ingested. These vesiculated microvilli appear to form a barrier between the OS and the RPE in older animals. This suggests that, even if the RPE is not primarily involved in the disease process, as the disease progresses, RPE function is affected. No study has yet been made of the phagocytic ability of the melanotic versus amelanotic RPE cells seen in this mutant, although degeneration of the OS does not seem to correlate with RPE cell pigmentation.

Since reduced pigmentation of the RPE might lead to an increased susceptibility to light damage, Smith and colleagues (1994a) examined the effect of rearing vitiligo mice in the dark; this treatment did not affect the rate or extent of photoreceptor cell death.

In a recent study, Smith and Defoe (1995) examined OS renewal in the vitiligo mouse. It is of interest that they found a dramatic difference in both the rate and characteristics of renewal between the peripheral and posterior retina in six-week-old mutant mice. In the peripheral retina, a band of radioactivity was seen at the base of the OS one day after the injection of ³H-leucine. This radioactive band of OS disks was displaced sclerally at a slightly slower rate than in control mice; however, the band remained discrete and eventually reached the level of the RPE, where it presumably was lost due to disk shedding by 13 days. In the posterior retina of the mutant mouse, a discrete radioactive band was formed one day after injection. However, this band was not displaced further after three days, and by eight days no discernible band was present. Additionally, the OS in the posterior retina were elongated and detached from the RPE, and they appeared fragmented at their tips. Parallel studies of rhodopsin turnover showed that at 13 days after injection, the vitiligo mouse retina contained considerably more ³H-labeled rhodopsin that did control retinas. Thus, rhodopsin turns over more slowly in this mutant, possibly due to a reduced rate of disk shedding, particularly in the posterior pole of the eye. Both the reduced rate of shedding and the reduced rate of disk

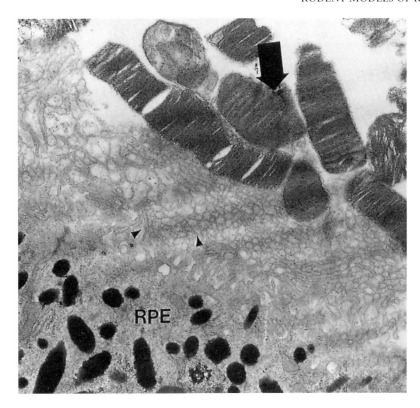

FIGURE 13-5. Electron micrograph of RPE and microvilli of 20-week-old mi^{vit}/mi^{vit} mouse. The microvilli *(arrowheads)* are short and vesiculated and appear to form a barrier between the RPE and the adjacent OS *(arrow)*. They do not surround the OS, as is seen in a normal mouse. (From Smith et al., 1994, with permission from the authors and by copyright permission of J. B. Lippincott Company.)

renewal may be a reflection of poor OS–RPE contact in the posterior retina.

The interesting posterior to peripheral gradient of photoreceptor degeneration has been further studied by Nir and colleagues (1995) Fig. 13-6). In the peripheral retinas of 14-month-old vitiligo mice PR cells with intact morphology are seen, whereas major RPE abnormalities and PR cell death are seen in the posterior retina of mice as young as 12 days old. In the posterior retina, pronounced abnormalities are also observed in RPE–PR interactions, particularly in the optic nerve head area, where RPE cells with very short microvilli are in direct contact with photoreceptor inner segments; no OS are present. RPE cells in this area are not present as a monolayer; rather several layers of cells of various shapes are observed, suggesting that RPE cell proliferation has occurred, possibly as a consequence of prior cell death. Further into the posterior and equatorial retina, short RPE microvilli appear separated from the PR layer, which displays shortened and disrupted OS. In the posterior area, the accumulation of an OS debris layer is observed, which appears to be a consequence of reduced phagocytosis of shed OS. In this area, RPE cells

manifest short microvilli, which do not envelop the accumulated OS debris (Fig. 13-6). However, the buildup of OS debris and the absence of phagocytosis is also seen in the equatorial area, where OS degeneration occurs later than in the posterior area. Macrophages are prominent in the posterior retina as early as four weeks, suggesting a removal of OS debris by a non-RPE route. By contrast, in the peripheral RPE normal-appearing microvilli enclose intact OS, phagocytosis of OS is seen, and macrophages are not observed. A distinct posterior-to-peripheral gradient of choroidal pigmentation, which closely approximates the gradient of OS degeneration, is also seen. Since choroidal melanocytes and RPE cells are derived from different embryonic sources (Nordlund, 1986), the mutation may affect these two cell layers quite differently. It is possible that the primary genetic defect may be in the choroidal melanocytes, secondarily affecting RPE function and OS survival. This suggestion is supported by the observation that the earliest and most severe evidence of PR degeneration, and abnormal RPE structure is seen around the optic nerve head, where choroidal pigmentation is absent (Nir et al., 1995).

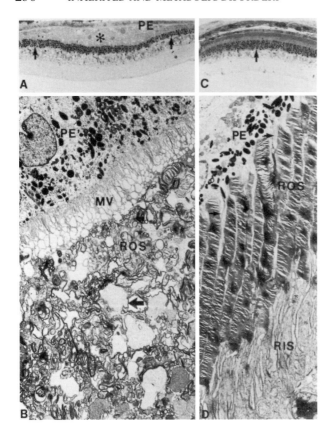

FIGURE 13-6. Seven-month-old vitiligo retina. (A) The section extends from the posterior *(right side)* to the equatorial region *(left side)*. Changes in the thickness of the photoreceptor nuclei layer are apparent *(arrows)*. The asterisk shows an area of lamellar debris buildup. (B) Ultrastructural details of the area shown by the asterisk in (A). This region is occupied by membranous debris derived from degenerating OS, and vesicles with fine granular material *(arrow)*, which might be derived from degenerated OS or from the interphotoreceptor matrix. PE cells appear intact, but the microvilli are short and swollen. (C) Section through the peripheral retina. An increase in the thickness of the ONL *(arrow)* is evident (compare to [A]). (D) Ultrastructure of photoreceptors in the area designated by the arrow in (C). Intact rod outer segments (ROS) and rod inner segments (RIS) are seen. Long RPE microvilli *(arrow)* appear to be in close apposition with the OS. (Reproduced from Nir et al., 1995, with permission from the authors and by copyright permission from Academic Press Ltd.)

Since vitamin A is so important to the functioning of the photoreceptor cells, Smith and colleagues (1994c) undertook a study of retinyl palmitate and retinol levels in the RPE, retina, liver, and plasma of control and mi^{vit}/mi^{vit} mice. Retinyl palmitate, which is the storage form of retinol in the body, was elevated in whole eyes of mutant mice at four weeks of age, and by ten weeks, was more than threefold higher than in controls. When retinoid levels of six-week-old rats are measured in separated RPE and neural retina, elevated levels of retinyl palmitate (threefold) and retinol (fourfold) are found in the RPE of vitiligo mice, while levels of both of these

retinoids are normal in the retina of this mutant. Levels of all-*trans* and 11-*cis* retinal are similar to controls in both retina and RPE. Since retinol is a potentially toxic compound, long-term exposure of RPE membranes to high concentrations of this vitamin could compromise RPE function. Liver retinyl palmitate levels, but not retinol levels, are twice as high in vitiligo as in control mice, while plasma levels of both these retinoids are unchanged. Since interphotoreceptor retinoid binding protein (IRBP) is important in the transport of retinoids between the retina and RPE, the levels of this glycoprotein were determined in mutant and normal mice (Smith et al., 1994c). While IRBP levels in vitiligo mice are normal up to 4 weeks of age, they are more than twice as high between 5 and 9 weeks, and then decrease to slightly higher levels than in normal animals by 14 weeks. Since the IRBP mRNA levels are not elevated above those found in control mice, it is likely that this elevation is due to a decreased rate of IRBP turnover. These results may point to a defect in retinoid metabolism that is common to RPE and liver, possibly in one or more factors that regulate the turnover and storage of vitamin A (Smith et al., 1994c).

In summary, the mi^{vit}/mi^{vit} mouse is a model of retinal degeneration in which the primary site of the lesion is not known. RPE cells show variable melanin content from birth and alterations in the posterior RPE precede the retinal degeneration. Based on these observations, it has been suggested that the mutation affects the RPE, and that degeneration of the PRs is secondary to a defect in the RPE. The observation that retinoid levels are increased in the RPE, but not in the retina, lends support to such a suggestion. However, no correlation is seen between the level of RPE cell pigmentation and the extent of OS degeneration. OS degeneration is most severe in the posterior retina, while the peripheral retina contains structurally normal OS and RPE cells. The posterior-to-peripheral gradient of OS survival does not correlate with lack of RPE pigmentation, but does strongly correlate with a gradient of increasing pigmentation of the choroid from the posterior to the periphery of the eye (Nir et al., 1995). Recent evidence supporting the suggestion that the RPE is affected by the mutation before the neural retina, comes from studies of the TRPM-2/clusterin gene (Smith et al., 1995), which is upregulated during membrane injury and repair. The TRPM-2/clusterin mRNA is elevated in the RPE of vitiligo mice as early as two postnatal weeks, an age which precedes OS loss, except in the optic nerve area. The gene is also upregulated in neural retina, but the increased expression of mRNA parallels photoreceptor cell loss, rather than preceding it.

The mi^{vit}/mi^{vit} mutation maps to mouse chromosome

6, at or near the microphthalmia locus (Lamoreux et al., 1992; Tang et al., 1992). Recently, mutations at this locus have been shown to be associated with a defect in a gene encoding a novel basic-helix-loop-helix-zipper protein, which is part of a family of DNA transcription factors (Hodgkinson et al., 1993; Hughes et al., 1993). The *mi* gene is expressed in the outer retina (including the RPE) in the normal mouse embryo at day $13\frac{1}{2}$ (Hodgkinson et al., 1993), thus a mutation in this gene could conceivably lead to abnormalities in either the RPE or the PR cells. The mi^{vit}/mi^{vit} mutation may affect a process common to a number of pigmented cells, including those of the skin, choroid, and RPE. If such is the case, then the RPE could be a primary site of expression of the mutation, or could react secondarily to a primary defect elsewhere in the body—such as the choroid. A defect in *mi* expression in the RPE could affect the function of these cells, and thus influence the viability of the underlying photoreceptors. These questions will undoubtedly be answered in the future. In the meantime, the slow progression of this retinal degeneration makes this an extremely attractive and important model for the study of retinal degeneration, and of RPE function.

ACKNOWLEDGMENTS

The author thanks Dr. Sylvia Smith and Dr. I Nir for making results available before publication, and Dr. Smith for reading parts of this manuscript and providing helpful suggestions for its improvement.

REFERENCES

Bayes M, et al. 1995. Homozygous tandem duplication within the gene encoding the beta-subunit of rod phosphodiesterase as a cause of autosomal recessive retinitis pigmentosa. Hum Mutat 5: 228–234.

Bok D, Hall MO. 1971. The role of the pigment epithelium in the etiology of retinal dystrophy in the rat. J Cell Biol 49:664–682.

Bourne MC, Gruneberg H. 1939. Degeneration of the retina and cataract, a new recessive gene in the rat (Rattus norvegicus). J Hered 30:130–136.

Bourne MC, Campbell DA, Tansley T. 1938. Hereditary degeneration of the retina. Br J Ophthalmol 22:613–623.

Boyle D, Tien L, Cooper NGF, Shepherd VL, McLaughlin BJ. 1991. A mannose receptor is involved in retinal phagocytosis. Invest Ophthalmol Vis Sci 32:1464–1470.

Caldwell RB, Roque RS, Soloman SW. 1989. Increased vascular density and vitreo-retinal membranes accompany vascularization of the pigment epithelium in the dystrophic retina. Curr Eye Res 8: 923–937.

Chaitin MH, Hall MO. 1983. Defective ingestion of rod outer segments by cultured dystrophic rat pigment epithelial cells. Invest Ophthalmol Vis Sci 24:812–820.

Connolly SE, Hjelmeland LM, LaVail MM. 1992. Immunohistochemical localization of basic fibroblast growth factor in mature and developing retinas of normal and RCS rat. Curr Eye Res 11:1005–1017.

Danciger M, Blaney J, Gao YQ, Zhao DY, Heckenlively JR, Jacobson SG, Farber DB. 1995. Mutations in the PDE6B gene in autosomal recessive retinitis pigmentosa. Genomics 30:1–7.

Dowling JE, Sigman RL. 1962. Inherited retinal dystrophy in the rat. J Cell Biol 14:73–107.

Elner VM, Nielsen JC, Elner SG, Franklin WA. 1989. Immunophenotypic modulation of cultured human retinal pigment epithelial cells by gamma-interferon and phytohemagglutinin-stimulated human T-lymphocytes. Invest Ophthalmol Vis Sci 30(suppl):118.

Faktorovich EG, Steinberg RH, Yasumura D, Matthes MT, Lavail MM. 1990. Photoreceptor degeneration in inherited retinal dystrophy delayed by basic fibroblast growth factor. Nature 347:83–86.

Farber DB, Flannery JG, Bowes-Rickman C. 1994. The *rd* mouse story: seventy years of research on an animal model of inherited retinal degeneration. In: Osborne N, Chader G, eds, Progress in Retinal and Eye Research, Oxford: Pergamon Press, 31–64.

Farrar GJ, Kenna P, Jardan SA, Kumar-Singh R, Humphries MM, Sharp EM, Sheils DM, Humphries P. 1991. A three base pair deletion in the *peripherin-rds* gene in one form of retinitis pigmentosa. Nature 354:478–480.

Gouras P, Flood MT, Kjeldbye H, Bilek MK, Eggers H. 1985. Transplantation of cultured human retinal epithelium to Bruch's membrane of the owl monkey's eye. Curr Eye Res 4:253–256.

Gouras P, Cao H, Sheng Y, Tanabe T, Efremova Y, Kjeldbye H. 1994. Patch culturing and transfer of human fetal retinal epithelium. Graefes Arch Clin Exp Ophthalmol 232:599–607.

Hall MO, Abrams TA. 1991. RPE cells from normal rats do not secrete a factor which enhances the phagocytosis of ROS by dystrophic rat RPE cells. Exp Eye Res 52:461–464.

Hall MO, Abrams TA, Mittag TW. 1991. ROS ingestion by RPE cells is turned off by increased protein kinase C activity and by increased calcium. Exp Eye Res 52:591–598.

Hall MO, Abrams TA, Mittag TW. 1993. The phagocytosis of rod outer segments is inhibited by drugs linked to cyclic adenosine monophosphate production. Invest Ophthalmol Vis Sci 34:2392–2401.

Hall MO, Burgess BL, Martinez MO. 1996. Carbachol does not correct the defect in phagocytosis of OS by RCS rat RPE cells. Invest Ophthalmol Vis Sci 37:1473–1477.

Herron WL, Riegel BW, Myers OE, Rubin ML. 1969. Retinal dystrophy in the rat: a pigment epithelial disease. Invest Ophthalmol 8:595–604.

Heth CA, Marescalchi PA, Ye L. 1995. IP$_3$ generation increases rod outer segment phagocytosis by cultured Royal College of Surgeons retinal pigment epithelium. Invest Ophthalmol Vis Sci 36:984–989.

Hodgkinson CA, Moore K, Nakayama A, Steingrimsson E, Copeland NG, Jenkins NA, Arnheiter H. 1993. Mutations at the mouse microphthalmia locus are associated with defects in a gene encoding a novel basic-helix-loop-helix-zipper protein. Cell 74:395–404.

Hughes MJ, Lingrel JB, Krakowsky JM, Anderson KP. 1993. A helix-loop-helix transcription factor-like gene is located at the *mi* locus. J Biol Chem 268:20687–20690.

Kajiwara K, Sandberg MA, Berson EL, Dryja TP. 1993. A null mutation in the human peripherin/*rds* gene in a family with autosomal dominant retinitis punctata albescens. Nature Genet 3:208–212.

Kuriyama S, Hall MO, Abrams TA, Mittag TW. 1994. Isoproterenol inhibits rod outer segment phagocytosis by both cAMP-dependent and independent pathways. Invest Ophthalmol Vis Sci 36:730–736.

Lamoreux ML, Boissy RE, Womack JE, Nordlund JJ. 1992. The vit gene maps to the mi (microphthalmia) locus of the laboratory mouse. J Heredity 83:435–439.

LaVail MM, Mullen RJ. 1976. Role of the pigment epithelium in inherited retinal degeneration analyzed with experimental rat chimeras. Exp Eye Res 23:227–245.

LaVail MM, Li L, Turner JE, Yasumura D. 1992. Retinal pigment epithelial cell transplantation in RCS rats: normal metabolism in rescued photoreceptors. Exp Eye Res 55:555–562.

Lerner AB, Shiohara T, Boissy RE, Jacobson KA, Lamoreux ML, Moellmann GE. 1986. A mouse model for vitiligo. J Invest Dermatol 87:299–304.

Li L, Turner JE. 1988a. Transplantation of retinal pigment epithelial cells to immature and adult rat hosts: short- and long-term survival characteristics. Exp Eye Res 47:771–785.

Li L, Turner JE. 1988b. Inherited retinal dystrophy in the RCS rat: prevention of photoreceptor degeneration by pigment epithelial transplantation. Exp Eye Res 47:911–917.

Li L, Turner JE. 1991. Optimal conditions for the long-term photoreceptor cell rescue in RCS rats: the necessity for healthy RPE transplants. Exp Eye Res 52:669–679.

Li L, Sheedlo HJ, Turner JE. 1990. Long-term rescue of photoreceptor cells in the retinas of RCS dystrophic rats by pigment epithelial cell transplants. Prog Brain Res 82:179–185.

Liversidge JM, Sewell HF, Forrester JV. 1988. Human retinal pigment epithelial cells differentially express MHC class II (HLA DP, DR and DQ) antigens in response to in vitro stimulation with lymphokine or purified IFN-gamma. J Exp Immunol 73:489–494.

Lopez R, Gouras P, Brittis M, Kjeldbye H. 1987. Transplantation of cultured rabbit retinal epithelium to rabbit retina using a closed eye method. Invest Ophthalmol Vis Sci 28:1131–1137.

Lopez R, Gouras P, Kjeldbye H, Sullivan B, Reppucci V, Brittis M, Wapner F, Goluboff E. 1989. Transplanted retinal pigment epithelium modifies the retinal degeneration in the RCS rat. Invest Ophthalmol Vis Sci 30:586–588.

Mascarelli F, Raulais D, Counis MF, Courtois Y. 1987. Characterization of acidic and basic fibroblast growth factors in brain, retina and vitreous of the chick embryo. Biochem Biophys Res Comm 146:478–448.

Matthes MT, Bok D. 1985. Blood vascular abnormalities in animals with inherited retinal degeneration. In: LaVail MM, Hollyfield JG. Anderson RE, ed, Retinal Degeneration: Experimental and Clinical Studies. New York: 209–219.

McLaughlin BJ, Cooper NGF, Shepherd VL. 1994. How good is the evidence to suggest that phagocytosis of ROS by RPE is receptor mediated? Prog Ret Eye Res 13:147–164.

McLaughlin ME, Erhart TL, Berson EL, Dryja TP. 1995. Mutation spectrum of the gene encoding the β-subunit of rod phosphodiesterase among patients with autosomal recessive retinitis pigmentosa. Proc Nat Acad Sci USA 92:3249–3253.

Molday RS. 1994. Peripherin/rds and rom-1: molecular properties and role in photoreceptor cell degeneration. In: Osborne N, Chader G, eds. Oxford: Pergamon Press, 271–299.

Mullen RJ, LaVail MM. 1976. Inherited retinal dystrophy: primary defect in pigment epithelium determined with experimental rat chimeras. Science 192:799–801.

Nicols BE, Sheffield VC, Vandenburgh K, Drack AV, Kimura AE, Stone EM. 1993. Butterfly-shaped pigment dystrophy of the fovea caused by a point mutation in codon 167 of the rds gene. Nature Genet 3:202–207.

Nir I, Ransom N, Smith SB. 1995. Ultrastructural features of retinal dystrophy in mutant vitiligo mice. Exp Eye Res 61:363–377.

Nordlund JJ. 1986. The lives of pigment cells. Dermatol Clin 4:404–418.

Peyman GA, Blinder KJ, Paris CL, Desai U, Alturki W, Nelson NC. 1986. A technique for retinal pigment epithelium transplantation for age-related macular degeneration secondary to extensive subfoveal scarring. Ophthal Surg 22:102–108.

Rakoczy PE, Humphrey MF, Cavaney DM, Chu Y, Constable IJ. 1993. Expression of basic fibroblast growth factor and its receptor in the retina of Royal College of Surgeons rats: a comparative study. Invest Ophthalmol Vis Sci 34:1845–1852.

Ryeom SW, Sparrow JR, Silverstein RL. 1994. CD 36 is expressed on retinal pigment epithelium (RPE) and mediates phagocytosis of photoreceptor outer segments (ROS). Invest Ophthalmol Vis Sci 35(suppl):2140.

Ryeom SW, Silverstein RL, Sparrow JR. 1995. The absence of CD 36, a molecule mediating phagocytosis of photoreceptor outer segments (OS) correlates with a lack of uptake of ROS by retinal pigment epithelial cells (RPE). Invest Ophthalmol Vis Sci 36(suppl): S815.

Schweigerer L, Malerstein B, Neufeld G, Gospodarowicz D. 1987. Basic fibroblast growth factor is synthesized in cultured retinal pigment epithelial cells. Biochem Biophys Res Comm 143:934–940.

Seaton AD, Sheedlo HJ, Turner JE. 1994. A primary role for RPE transplants in the inhibition and regression of neovascularization in the RCS rat. Invest Ophthalmol Vis Sci 35:162–169.

Sheedlo HJ, Li L, Turner JE. 1989. Functional and structural characteristics of photoreceptor cells rescued in RPE-cell grafted retinas of RCS dystrophic rats. Exp Eye Res 48:841–854.

Sheedlo HJ, Li L, Gaur VP, Young RW, Seaton AD, Stovall SV, Jaynes CD, Turner JE. 1992. Photoreceptor rescue in the dystrophic retina by transplantation of retinal pigment epithelium. Int Rev Cytol 138:1–49.

Sheedlo HJ, Li L, Turner JE. 1993. Effects of RPE age and culture conditions on support of photoreceptor cell survival in transplanted RCS dystrophic rats. Exp Eye Res 57:753–761.

Sidman RL, Neumann P. 1988. Vitiligo: a new retinal degeneration mutation. Mouse News Lett 81:60.

Smirnakis SM, Tang M, Sidman RL. 1991. Abnormalities of pigment epithelium precede photoreceptor cell degeneration in vitiligo mutant mice. Invest Ophthalmol Vis Sci 31(suppl):298.

Smith SB. 1992. C57BL/6J-vit/vit mouse model of retinal degeneration: light microscopic analysis and evaluation of rhodopsin levels. Exp Eye Res 55:903–910.

Smith SB, Defoe DM. 1995. Autoradiographic and biochemical assessment of rod outer segment renewal in the vitiligo (mi^{vit}/mi^{vit}) mouse model of retinal degeneration. Exp Eye Res 60:91–96.

Smith SB, Hamasaki DI. 1994. Electroretinographic study of the C57BL/6-mi^{vit}/mi^{vit} mouse mode of retinal degeneration. Invest Ophthalmol Vis Sci 35:3119–3123.

Smith SB, Cope BK, McCoy JR. 1994a. Effects of dark rearing on the retinal degeneration of the C57BL/6-mi^{vit}/mi^{vit} mouse. Exp Eye Res 58:77–84.

Smith SB, Cope BK, McCoy JR, McCool DJ, Defoe DM. 1994b. Reduction of phagosomes in the vitiligo (C57BL/6-mi^{vit}/mi^{vit}) mouse model of retinal degeneration. Invest Ophthalmol Vis Sci 35:3625–3632.

Smith SB, Duncan T, Kutty G, Kutty RK, Wiggert B. 1994c. Elevation of retinyl palmitate in eyes and livers and the concentration of interphotoreceptor retinoid-binding protein in eyes of vitiligo mutant mice. Biochem J 300:63–68.

Smith SB, Boca N, McCool DJ, Kutty G, Wong P, Kutty RK, Wiggert B. 1995. Photoreceptor cells in the vitiligo mouse die by apoptosis: TRPM-2/clusterin expression is elevated in the neural retina, and in the retinal pigment epithelium. Invest Ophthalmol Vis Sci 36:2193–2201.

Tang M, Neumann PE, Kosaras B, Taylor BA, Sidman RL. 1992. Vitiligo maps to mouse chromosome 6 within or close to the mi locus. Mouse Genome 90:441–443.

Wells J, Wroblewski J, Keen J, Ingelhearn C, Jull C, Eckstein A, Jay M, Arden G, Bhattaracharya S, Fitzke F, Bird A. 1993. Mutations in the human retinal degeneration slow (*rds*) gene can cause either retinitis pigmentosa or macular dystrophy. Nature Genetic 3:213–218.

Young RW. 1967. The renewal of photoreceptor cell outer segments. J Cell Biol 33:61–67.

Young RW, Bok D. 1969. Participation of the retinal pigment epithelium in the rod outer segment renewal process. J Cell Biol 42:392–403.

14. Diseases of the retinal pigment epithelium–photoreceptor complex in nonrodent animal models

GUSTAVO D. AGUIRRE, JHARNA RAY AND LAWRENCE E. STRAMM

The retinal pigment epithelium (RPE) is strategically situated between the photoreceptor cells and the choroid to mediate a number of activities which are essential for normal photoreceptor function and viability. Traditionally, these activities are considered to involve retinoid transport, esterification and isomerization, the phagocytosis and degradation of shed outer segments, and the regulation of ion and metabolite transport. Additionally, evidence for the critical role played by the RPE in sustaining the visual cells has been supported by studies carried out in the Royal College of Surgeons (RCS) strain of retinal-dystrophic rats. In these animals, postnatal retinal development is initially normal, but degeneration begins soon after photoreceptor cells have differentiated normally. Disease occurs because the mutant RPE is unable to internalize and degrade the outer segment membranes that are discarded on a daily basis from the distal tips of the photoreceptors (Herron et al., 1969). This material appears as whorls of membranes whose accumulation in the interphotoreceptor space presages the degeneration and death of the visual cells. Elegant studies by Mullen and LaVail (1976) have established that the target tissue for mutation is the RPE and not the photoreceptors, and the phagocytic defect can be examined in cell (Edwards and Szamier, 1977) or organ (Tamai and O'Brien, 1979) culture, and the photoreceptor disease prevented by the transplantation of genetically normal RPE cells (Li and Turner, 1988).

These and other studies carried out over the past twenty years have identified the critical photoreceptor-supportive roles played by the RPE. It has been established that primary dysfunction in the RPE can result in visual cell pathology and cell loss. Similarly, abnormalities in the photoreceptor cells can elicit a pathologic response in the RPE, either very early in the disease process or late, once the photoreceptor cells have degenerated and disappeared. In other cases, however, the RPE plays a passive role, demonstrating minimal response to the very severe disease that is occurring in its surround. An explanation for the varied repertoire of disease and responsiveness demonstrated by the RPE lies in its complexity and varied functional roles. The RPE can no longer be considered a simple epithelial monolayer with uniform function and behavior. Instead, it must be regarded as a highly complex cell whose cytologic and functional properties are determined or modified by positional and topographic factors. This chapter examines the role of the RPE in diseases of the pigment epithelial–photoreceptor complex in selected domestic animal species. In some cases, the diseases occur sporadically in animals, but the RPE response is so unique that it provides insights into RPE biology or pathology. In other cases, the diseases, which were once identified as naturally occurring primarily in the dog and cat, are now maintained in laboratory colonies. As a result, the models have the same gene defect and demonstrate a consistent disease phenotype that lends itself readily to experimental study and analysis.

NORMAL ANATOMY

The histology of the RPE of domestic animals is influenced by its relationship to the tapetum lucidum, a choroidal modification that is located between the large choroidal vessels and the choriocapillaris. In dog and cat, the tapetum consists of rows of multilayered, flat, often irregularly shaped cells (tapetum cellulosum; Fig. 14-1). Ultrastructurally, the cytoplasm of the tapetal cells contains groups of elongated membrane-bound rods that are electron-dense, are oriented parallel to each other, and are uniform in size and spacing. The rods are separated from each other by amorphous ground substance, and by very fine fibrils and filaments. Within each cell, there are several groups of rods, each group having its own characteristic and independent orientation (Bernstein and Pease 1959). However, the rods are all arranged in a plane parallel to the pigment epithelial basement membrane (Fig. 14-2).

Differences in tapetal structure, organization, and

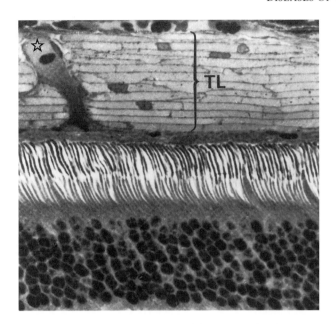

FIGURE 14-1. Anatomic relationship of the tapetum lucidum (TL), retinal pigment epithelium, and photoreceptor cells in the posterior pole of the dog eye. The outer retina is nourished by arterioles from the choroid *(open star, left)* which penetrate through the tapetum and spread horizontally between the tapetum and retinal pigment epithelium to form the choriocapillaris. Magnification ×650.

composition have been noted in the past by several investigators, and these differences appear to be species specific (see Pirie, 1966 for review). Recent studies have examined the tapetum lucidum in the dog and cat (Bussow, 1980; Burns et al., 1988; Wen et al., 1985) and found that, although superficially similar in the two species, there are many differences in structure, cell number, and chemical composition (Table 14-1). Unlike in the dog, the tapetal rodlets in the cat retain an electron-dense core after fixation, and have a single ring rather than concentric rings of zinc deposition, as visualized with a sulfide-silver histochemical method (Wen et al., 1982; 1985). The peripheral rather than internal distribution of zinc around the tapetal rodlets of the cat may account for the tenfold-lower concentration of this divalent cation in the tapetum in comparison to the dog. In the latter species, the zinc is complexed to cysteine, which occurs in higher concentration in the dog tapetum than in any other tissue (Wen et al., 1982).

In contrast to carnivores, herbivores have a fibrous tapetum (tapetum fibrosum), consisting of bundles of undulating collagenous fibers arranged somewhat concentrically and with an iridescent surface. Except for an occasional fibrocyte, the fibrous tapetum is basically

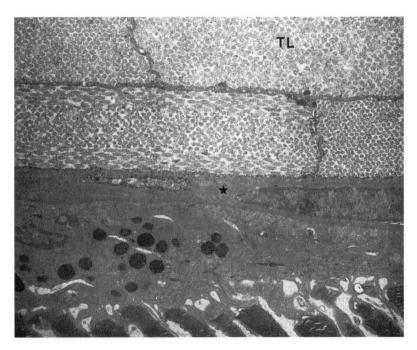

FIGURE 14-2. The tapetum lucidum (TL) consists of a multilayer of flattened cells. Each cell contains groups of membrane bound rods oriented parallel the basement membrane of the retinal pigment epithelium. Note the prominent choriocapillaris layer *(star)*. In the tapetal zone, the pigment epithelium is not pigmented; the cytoplasmic granules are lipofuscin. Magnification ×5,800.

TABLE 14-1. *Comparison of the morphological and histochemical parameters of the mature tapetum lucidum of the dog and cat*

Parameters	Dog	Cat
Number of tapetal cell layers (central)	9–11	16–20
Thickness of central tapetum	26–33 μm	61–67 μm
Thickness of retina from the area of center tapetum	151–184 μm	145–150 μm
Presence of a microtubule-like structure in each tapetal rod	present	absent
Presence of electron-dense cores in tapetal rods after prolonged glutaraldehyde fixation	absent	present
Distribution pattern of zinc in tapetal rod	two concentric rings	one outer ring
Zinc in tapetum (PPM)	26,000 ± 1,100	1,497 ± 152
Cysteine in tapetum (μM/g tissue) (n = 6–8)	241 ± 18	0

Modified from Wen et al., 1982; 1985

acellular (Bellairs et al., 1975). In the cow, this layer can be up to 50 μm thick, with the collagenous bundles oriented in a plane parallel to the RPE basement membrane (Nakaizumi 1964). Pig, rabbit, rat, guinea pig, and most higher primates lack a tapetum.

Blood supply to the RPE and outer retinal layer in the tapetal regions is derived from the large choroidal vessels external to the tapetum. Smaller vessels penetrate this layer and branch extensively under the tapetum, forming an incomplete choriocapillaris layer. In the dog and cat, the choriocapillaris forms a thin vascular zone interposed between the tapetal cells and the basal surface of the RPE. Occasionally, however, deep invaginations of the choriocapillaris into the basal RPE are seen. In the nontapetal regions, the choriocapillaris is adjacent to the larger choroidal vessels. In both tapetal and nontapetal regions, there are multiple fenestrations in the thin endothelial wall of the choriocapillaris adjacent to the RPE.

Unlike the human, the dog and cat lack a well-defined Bruch's membrane. The RPE and choriocapillaris basement membranes are apposed, with infrequent collagenous and elastic fibers present between the two. In the intercapillary space of the tapetal and nontapetal regions, more collagenous and elastic fibers are present, and a more classical Bruch's membrane is occasionally recognized. Of all the domestic species, the pig has the most prominent Bruch's membrane (Prince et al., 1960).

The topographic variation in tapetal distribution is reflected in the differing cytologic characteristics of the RPE. The most obvious of these is the presence of

melanin granules. Melanin is absent in areas overlying the tapetum, although sparse pigmentation begins to appear in junctional zones, either centrally or peripherally. In these areas, the tapetal thickness gradually decreases to one or two cells, and melanin granules are present. As the tapetal cells disappear, the degree of pigmentation increases. In general, RPE cells are smaller and have less-dense pigmentation in the posterior pole, and increase both in size and in extent of melanin pigmentation peripherally. The topographic distribution of pigmentation in relation to the tapetum is illustrated in Figure 14-3. However, the elegant studies of the human RPE, which examine the cell number and size, and the degree of pigmentation and lipofuscin accumulation in relation to age and topographic position have not been done in nonprimate species (see Dorey et al., 1989; Gao et al., 1992; Feeney-Burns and Ellersieck, 1985; Feeney-Burns et al., 1984). This limitation interferes with studies examining disease processes in the RPE–photoreceptor interface.

THE RPE IN DISEASES OF THE TAPETUM LUCIDUM

Hereditary Diseases

Hereditary abnormalities of the tapetum lucidum have been described in beagle dogs (Bellhorn et al., 1975; Burns et al., 1988) and Siamese cats (Wen et al., 1982; Collier et al., 1985a). In dogs, the disease is autosomal recessive, and affected animals lack the normal tapetal reflex visible on ophthalmoscopy; instead, the fundus has a uniform red appearance without the topographic separation of tapetal and nontapetal zones (Burns et al., 1988) (Plates 14-I, 14-2). Unlike the albino fundus, where the lack of RPE and choroidal pigmentation permit visualization of the choroidal vasculature overlying the white sclera (Plate 14-III), dogs with the hereditary tapetal defect have a light, uniform choroidal pigmentation which precludes visualization of the choroidal vessels. With the exception of the foveomacular region, which is not present in nonprimate species, the fundus appearance is quite similar to that of a lightly pigmented human.

In affected dogs, there are normal numbers of tapetal cells at birth, but, with time, there is a progressive degeneration of this layer; in adult animals, the remaining layer of dysmorphic tapetal cells is only 1–2 cells thick (Fig. 14-4; Burns et al., 1988). Ultrastructural disease is evident in cells as early as 46 days after birth by the loss of the normal complement of tapetal rodlets, and the accumulation of cytoplasmic membranous whorls (Fig. 14-5). At this age, the normal tapetal cells are in the

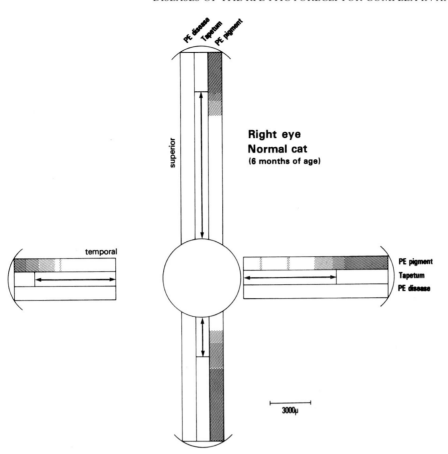

FIGURE 14-3. Schematic representation of the distribution of PE pigmentation and the presence of the tapetum lucidum in the eye of a normal cat. For comparison with the disease (MPS VI) see Figure 14-26. The eye is drawn to scale based on observations of sequential 150 μm fields extending from the disc to the ora serrata *(curved line)*. Note that the tapetum is present primarily in the superior, nasal, and temporal meridians. The pigment epithelium is not pigmented in areas where the tapetum is present. *Key:* arrows indicate the presence of tapetum; RPE pigmentation varies from absent (empty) to moderate (density present in the far periphery). (For details refer to Aguirre et al., 1983, from which this figure was reprinted.)

process of postnatal differentiation. By 13 weeks of age, the abnormal tapetal cells contain only membranous whorls and membrane-limited inclusions. These abnormalities are characteristic of the process of tapetal cell degeneration. Associated with the cytologic abnormalities, the tapetal rodlets fail to show an identifiable zinc signal by X-ray microanalysis, either in very young (21 days) or adult animals (17 months) (Burns et al., 1988). In spite of the severe disease that is occurring in the tapetal layer, the RPE remains normal, and retinal function and structure are preserved.

Similar tapetal degenerative changes have been identified in cats with Chediak-Higashi syndrome (CHS; Collier et al., 1985a), and, in both diseases, there is a striking absence of phagocytic cells during the active process of tapetal cell degeneration. As in the atapetal beagle, tapetal cells in CHS cats develop normally dur-

ing the early postnatal period. However, the intracellular rods begin to degenerate by four weeks of age, and are completely degenerated by two months of age, a time by which postnatal retinal differentiation is completed (Vogel, 1970). Thereafter, the disrupted tapetal cells begin to degenerate, and this choroidal layer is lost by one year of age.

The tapetal pathology identified in cats with CHS is presumably unrelated to abnormalities in the RPE, since these occur uniformly across the monolayer as well as in other tissues (Collier et al., 1984). The disease is characterized by greatly enlarged cytoplasmic granules, including melanosomes and lysosomes. In the RPE of young affected animals, very few melanosomes are present, and most of the melanin granules are giant sized. These giant granules are composed of several melanosomes and premelanosomes in different stages of

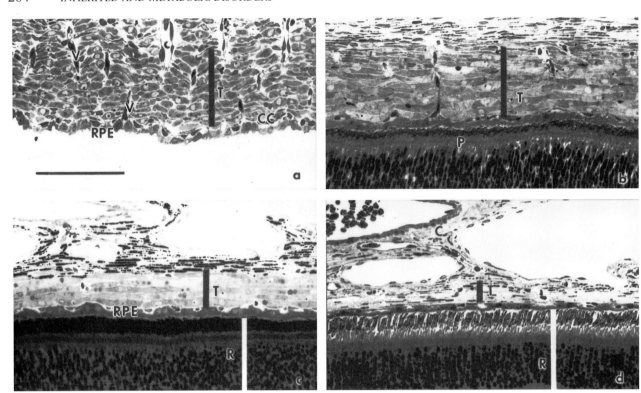

FIGURE 14-4. Tapetal region from beagles affected with a hereditary degeneration of the tapetum lucidum at different stages of the disease. (a) 7 days old. The tapetal cells (T) form a loose, irregular meshwork between the RPE and choroid (C). Vessels (V) penetrate the tapetum and form the choriocapillaris (CC). (b) 21 days. The tapetal layer (T) is more regular, and the photoreceptors (P) are differentiating. (c) 46 days. The retina (R) and RPE are normal. The tapetal layer (T) is thinner, but the remaining cells, although lightly staining, retain normal shape. (d) 17 months old. The tapetum (T) has almost disappeared, but the RPE and retina (R) are normal. Bar = 100 μm. (Reprinted from Burns et al., 1988.)

maturation, and contain lysosomal and melanosomal components (Collier et al, 1985b). The giant granules appear to form by inappropriate fusion of cytoplasmic structures, and the hypopigmentation of the RPE likely results from fusion of premelanosomes and lysosomes, with resultant destruction of the former. In the RPE of older animals (>7 years), numerous variably sized autofluorescent inclusions accumulate which, on ultrastructural examination, are identified as secondary lysosomes. Additionally, extracellular giant residual bodies form drusenoid accumulations beneath the basal lamina of the RPE. These abnormalities are associated with focal reactive and degenerative changes of the RPE, characterized as focal cells loss, detachment, and migration into the interphotoreceptor space (Collier et al., 1986).

Although the involvement of the lysosomal system in CHS is evident by the abnormal fusion of lysosomes, it is clear that lysosomal function is normal, at least in regards to the degradation of proteoglycans associated with the RPE extracellular matrices, or of glycoproteins internalized during phagocytosis of photoreceptor outer segments (see below). This has been confirmed by studies which demonstrate that there is little effect on endocytic and degradative functions, even though disease affects the late endosomes and lysosomes and may result in the abnormal secretion of some lysosomal enzymes into the media by cultured cells (Burkhardt et al., 1993; Zhao et al., 1994). Of interest have been the recent complementation studies using normal fibroblasts and fibroblasts from CHS-affected humans, mink, and mice. The normal human fibroblasts complemented the CHS fibroblasts regardless of the species, resulting in restoration of normal lysosomal size and distribution; this finding suggests the homology between the diseases occurring in the different species (Perou and Kaplan, 1993).

The tapetal defect described in the Siamese cats is not a specific hereditary defect within the breed, but appears to be part of the overall genetic makeup of the breed.

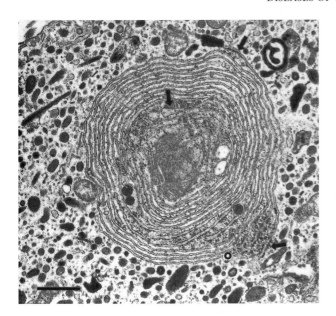

FIGURE 14-5. Degenerating tapetal cell from a 46-day-old beagle with hereditary tapetal degeneration. The tapetal rods have degenerated and the cell is filled with inclusions. The membrane whorl appears to have originated from the rough endoplasmic reticulum, and ribosomes are present inside or at the outer border *(arrows)* of the whorl. Bar = 1 μm. (Reprinted in part from Burns et al., 1988.)

Other breed-specific characteristics reported are differences in fur and ocular pigmentation, strabismus, and abnormalities in the retinogeniculate and cortical projections (see Wen et al., 1982 for review). Even though the ophthalmoscopic appearance of the tapetum is normal in Siamese cats, microscopic abnormalities have been identified in some animals, and consist of weakly staining tapetal cells on light microscopic examinations. On ultrastructural examination, the abnormal cells are filled with irregular and disoriented tapetal rods whose membranes are enlarged or disrupted. The cores of the tapetal rods appear empty, or are filled with an electron-dense material. These abnormalities are not present uniformly in all tapetal cells, but vary in different layers. Overall, however, disease of individual tapetal cells is most severe in the retinal aspect of the tapetum. Associated with the tapetal abnormality is a significant reduction in the amount of zinc in the tapetal rods (Wen et al., 1982). The causal association between the lower levels of zinc and the tapetal cell degeneration is not clear at this time. In spite of the damage to the tapetal cells, the RPE remains normal (Aguirre, unpublished).

Acquired Defects: Nutritional and Toxic Damage

Tapetal defects in cats have been reported secondary to a nutritional deficiency of taurine (Wen et al., 1979). In affected cats there is a marked reduction in thickness as-

sociated with a decrease in cell number. Additionally, there is a marked disorganization of the lattice arrangement of the tapetal rods. This abnormality is associated with a taurine-associated progressive degeneration of the cone and rod photoreceptors, with sparing of the RPE (Aguirre and Rubin, 1979: Fig. 19.23).

The most common causes of acquired tapetal defects have been reported in ophthalmic toxicology studies, particularly of dogs, where administration of various compounds results in dramatic changes in the tapetum which are visible on ophthalmoscopy, histopathology, and ultrastructural examination (Figs. 14-6, 14-7). The prototype compound to produce this effect is the antitubercular drug ethambutol. Administration of this compound to dogs causes a decoloration of the tapetum and a reversible disorientation of the tapetal rods with no RPE or retinal damage (Kaiser, 1963; Vogel and Kaiser, 1963). More-severe tapetal damage occurs in the dog following administration of the potent zinc chelator diphenylthiocarbazone (dithizone). There is retinal edema, pigmentary disruption, and end-stage retinal degeneration with intraretinal pigmentation at the higher doses. It appears, however, that the tapetum may play a protective role in ameliorating dithizone toxicity of the retina. In the tapetal area, dithizone causes tapetal necrosis while sparing the underlying RPE and retinal layers. In contrast, areas devoid of tapetum show severe RPE and retinal degeneration (Aguirre and Rubin, 1979). Similar neuroretinal damage has been reported in animals without a tapetum (Budinger, 1961, Butturini et al., 1953).

Tapetal lesions also have been reported with various classes of compounds, not all of which are known zinc chelators. For example, administration of zinc pyridinethione (Cloyd et al., 1978), selected beta-adrenergic blocking agents (Schiavo et al., 1984), macrolide antibiotics (Massa et al., 1984), aromatase inhibitors (Schiavo et al., 1988), and other compounds can cause varying degrees of tapetal damage in the dog or cat (Cloyd et al., 1978). Where damage is acute and severe, such as with zinc pyridinethione, the necrotic changes in the tapetum result in damage to the penetrating tapetal arterioles. This causes focal lesions, presumably infarcts in the RPE and retina, which are evident as focal areas of subretinal edema and hemorrhage. When the lesions are more severe, there is diffuse subretinal edema, retinal detachment, and blindness (Cloyd et al., 1978). In this case the RPE appears to be damaged secondarily by the severe changes occurring in the adjacent tapetal layer, and displays a breakdown of the outer blood–retina barrier. In other cases, for instance following the administration of an aromatase inhibitor (Schiavo et al., 1988), tapetal damage is selective and limited to this cell

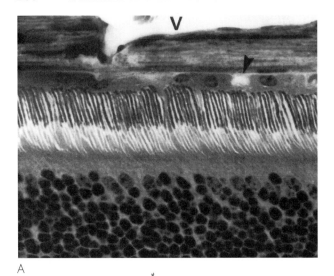

A

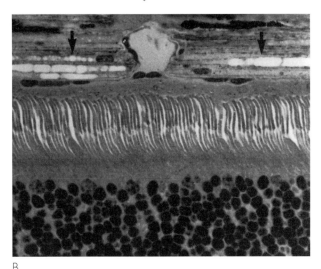

B

FIGURE 14-6. Chronic administration of a tapetotoxic compound results in tapetal degeneration in the dog. In some areas there is loss of tapetal cells (A) and the RPE abuts the vascular choroid (v). In other areas, the few remaining tapetal cells have vacuolated inclusions (arrows, B). Arrowhead indicates indentation of the normal RPE by the choriocapillaris. Magnification ×680.

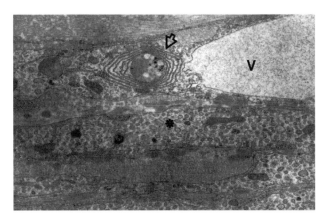

FIGURE 14-7. Ultrastructural appearance of tapetal degeneration induced by chronic administration of a tapetotoxic compound. There is loss of tapetal cells. Remaining cells have disorientation of the rodlets (*), and accumulation of vacuoles (V) and membrane whorls (open arrow). Magnification ×10,000. Compare with Figure 14-5.

layer; thus the RPE and retina remain normal. The differential expression of the compound-associated damage between the tapetal and nontapetal areas is intriguing, and raises concerns about the interpretation of tapetal lesions in animals used in toxicologic studies. For that reason, several studies of potentially tapetotoxic compounds also use atapetal dogs having the hereditary absence of this structure (Burns et al., 1988). It has been clearly demonstrated that, in contrast to the findings in normal dogs, these compounds cause no oc-

ular abnormalities in dogs lacking a tapetum (Cloyd et al., 1978; Massa et al., 1984; Schiavo et al., 1984).

THE RPE IN HEREDITARY PHOTORECEPTOR DISEASES

Hereditary diseases affecting the rods and cones, either primarily or secondary to an RPE defect, are recognized in a number of different species including man. Regardless of the underlying cause, the diseases appear to affect the photoreceptors early and progressively; in the advanced stages, the entire visual cell layer is destroyed, and there is damage also to the inner retinal layers and the RPE. In man, this class of diseases is referred to, collectively, as retinitis pigmentosa (RP). Multiple loci for RP have been recognized, but few genes have been identified (see Dryja and Li, 1995 for review). Recent studies of retinal degeneration in human patients and animal models have identified mutations in six different genes (rhodopsin, peripherin/rds, rom-1, a and β subunits of rod cyclic GMP-phosphodiesterase [PDEA and PDEB], and the cyclic GMP-gated channel) as causally associated with RP (Humphries et al., 1992; Kajiwara et al., 1991; 1994; Travis et al., 1989; Bowes et al., 1990; Suber et al., 1993; McLaughlin et al., 1993; Dryja et al., 1995; Huang et al., 1995). Some of these genes—rhodopsin, rom-1, PDEB—are expressed exclusively in the rod photoreceptor cells, yet the clinical and pathologic phenotype of RP and related diseases indicates that there is progressive rod and cone degeneration with a late and secondary involvement of the RPE. It appears that all defects that cause widespread disease and degeneration of rods, regardless of the selective expression of the gene product in rods, result in the concomitant loss of cones, and progressive retinal degenerative disease.

The manner in which cellular dysfunction, disease, and degeneration are expressed in the visual cell layer is dependent, to a large extent, on the gene affected and the nature of the mutation. However, different mutations of the same gene can result in a varied clinical phenotype, for example with opsin (Berson et al., 1991; Dryja et al., 1993) and peripherin/rds (Weleber et al., 1993) genes, and factors external to the visual cell may also play a modulatory role to influence the temporal, topographic, or cellular distribution of the disease. In this brief overview, we discuss different aspects of photoreceptor disease from the perspective of the RPE.

Progressive Retinal Atrophy (PRA) in the Dog

The PRA class of diseases represents a heterogeneous grouping of retinal disorders having similar disease phenotype. Like RP in man, the term PRA represents an aggregate of different genetic defects having a broadly similar clinical phenotype. All show the same general ophthalmoscopic abnormalities (Plate 14-IV) and visual deficits characterized initially by rod dysfunction followed by loss of day vision; in the late stages of the disease, the animals are blind, have end-stage retinal degenerative changes, and secondary cataracts. Excluding the absence of intraretinal pigmentation, which appears to be a property unique to the human retina with advanced photoreceptor disease, the clinical phenotype of PRA in dogs is similar to RP in man.

Within this general grouping, PRA is subdivided into developmental and degenerative diseases (Table 14-2). The developmental class represents a large grouping of genetically distinct disorders which are expressed cytologically in the postnatal period, at the time that visual cells are beginning to differentiate. These developmental disorders represent a dysplasia of the rod and/or cone photoreceptors, and each has its own unique disease course and phenotype, as assessed by functional and morphologic criteria (Aguirre, 1978; Acland and Aguirre, 1987; Acland et al., 1989; Parshall et al., 1991). Even though all dysplasias show rather severe structural alterations of the photoreceptor cells, the rate of progression to loss of cones, the hallmark criteria for loss of functional vision, is varied; e.g., this occurs early in the *erd, rcd1* and *rcd2* retinas, but not until the equivalent of middle age in *pd* and *rd*. In contrast, the degenerative class of diseases represents defects in which photoreceptor cells degenerate after having differentiated normally; this class includes diseases at the progres-

Data from Aguirre and Acland, 1988; Acland et al., 1989; 1994; 1995; Aguirre and Rubin 1974; Akhmedov et al., 1997; Ray et al., 1996, 1997; Wrigstad, 1994.

TABLE 14-2. *Gene loci for hereditary photoreceptor diseases in dogs*

Disease name	Gene locus	Genes excluded/*included*
Progressive Retinal Atrophy (PRA)		
I. Abnormal Photoreceptor Development		
Rod-cone dysplasia 1	rcd1	*PDEB (codon 807-stop)*
Rod-cone dysplasia 2	rcd2	PDEB, transducin α-1
Rod dysplasia	rd	
Early retinal degeneration	erd	RDS/peripherin, opsin, PDEB, transducin α-1
Photoreceptor dysplasia	pd	
II. Photoreceptor Degeneration		
Progressive rod-cone degeneration	prcd	RDS/peripherin, opsin, PDEB, transducin α-1
X-linked PRA	XLPRA	
Other Primary Photoreceptor Diseases		
Cone degeneration	cd	Transducin β3
Congenital stationary night blindness	csnb	

sive rod-cone degeneration *(prcd)* and XLPRA gene loci (Aguirre et al., 1982a; Aguirre and Acland, 1988; Acland et al., 1994). Here, disease occurs more slowly, and is modified by temporal and topographic factors (see below). Different alleles have been identified at the *prcd* locus (Aguirre and Acland, 1988), and these segregate independently to regulate the rate, but not the phenotype, of photoreceptor degeneration (Acland and Aguirre, unpublished). Examples are presented below.

Photoreceptor Dysplasias, Abnormal Retinal cGMP Metabolism and Retinal Degeneration

Rod-cone dysplasia 1. Rod-cone dysplasia1 *(rcd1)* in the Irish setter is a recessively inherited photoreceptor defect characterized by arrested differentiation of visual cells resulting from an abnormality in retinal cyclic GMP (cGMP) metabolism (Aguirre et al., 1978; 1982b). Beginning at ten days of age, deficient cGMP-phosphodiesterase (cGMP-PDE) activity causes the retinal levels of cGMP to rise sharply to concentrations up to tenfold higher than normal; these biochemical abnormalities are present before degenerative changes are observed in the photoreceptor cells (Fig. 14-8). The morphologic and biochemical phenotype of the disease is similar to that present in the *rd* mouse (Farber and Lolley, 1974). Homology between the dog and mouse diseases, as well as to some forms of RP in man, has been established by identification of mutations in the PDE-Beta (PDEB)

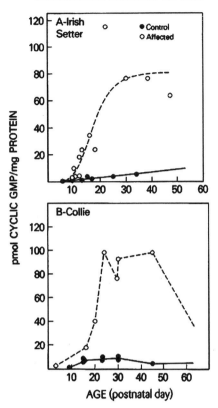

PATTERN OF CYCLIC GMP DEVELOPMENT IN CONTROL AND AFFECTED RETINAS

FIGURE 14-8. Developmental pattern of changes in cGMP concentration with age in retinas from dogs affected with *rcd1* (Irish setter, upper panel) and *rcd2* (collie, lower panel). Normal values (*solid circles*) from controls are included in each figure. In both *rcd1* and *rcd2*, levels of cGMP increase early in the postnatal period to values 8–10 times higher than normal. (Modified from Chader et al., 1985.)

subunit gene as being responsible for the diseases in the three different species (McLaughlin et al., 1993; Bowes et al., 1990; Farber et al., 1990; 1992; Suber et al., 1993). Not surprisingly, human RP patients with abnormalities in the PDEB gene show a varied mutation spectrum (McLaughlin et al., 1995). In contrast, the same two different abnormalities have been identified concurrently in all *rd* strains examined (Pittler and Baehr, 1991; Bowes et al., 1993), while all *rcd1*-affected dogs have the same mutation in codon 807 (TRP807X), which presumably results in the premature termination of the PDEB protein by 49 amino acid residues (Clement et al., 1993; Ray et al., 1994 and 1995).

A question arises about the specificity of the abnormal retinal cyclic nucleotide metabolism, and whether it is limited to the visual cells. In our original study, we found that retinal cGMP levels were elevated in retina, but not in the RPE/choroid complex or in nonocular tissues (Aguirre et al., 1978). Subsequently, using the reti-

nal layer microdissection method of Lowry, Barbehenn and colleagues (1988) found that the elevated retinal cGMP levels are confined to the photoreceptor cells. Since the outer segments of the affected visual cells are small, and degenerate early, the elevated cGMP levels are not located in this structure but, rather, are present in the outer nuclear and plexiform layers (Barbehenn et al., 1988). Such abnormally high levels of cGMP in the synaptic terminals are unexplained, but may indicate aberrant sites of synthesis or trafficking of newly synthesized cyclic nucleotides in the dysplastic rod photoreceptors. Additionally, more recent studies indicate that there are no abnormalities in cyclic nucleotide levels in cultured RPE cells of *rcd1*-affected dogs, further confirming the specificity of the defect to the visual cells (Table 14-3; Stramm, Fletcher, Aguirre, and Chader, unpublished).

In *rcd1*-affected dogs, there is normal retinal structure and opsin biosynthesis during the first two weeks of life. However, at the time when photoreceptors begin to differentiate in the normal retina (13–16 days), development of rods in the *rcd1* retina is arrested, and the diseased cells begin to degenerate; by 25 days after birth, photoreceptor cell death begins, and this process continues throughout the first year of life (Fig. 14-9) (Aguirre et al., 1982b; Schmidt and Aguirre, 1985). The degeneration initially affects the rods, and, as these cells degenerate, the proportion of cones in the visual cell layer increases. However, cone degeneration develops eventually, and results in collapse of the interphotoreceptor space, bringing into close apposition the apical surfaces of the RPE and Müller cells. In spite of the severe disease that is occurring in the apposing visual cell layer, the RPE remains normal and minimally reactive, and, as is characteristic of hereditary retinal diseases in nonprimate models, there is a lack of intraretinal pigment migration.

Photoreceptor–RPE interactions occur through the interphotoreceptor matrix (IPM). Until recently, this matrix was ill defined, and its structural and functional characteristics were not clear. The IPM is now known to be a complex and highly ordered structure consisting of soluble and insoluble constituents in which proteins,

TABLE 14-3. *Cyclic nucleotide levels (picomole/mg protein) in primary cultures of RPE cells from ten-week-old normal, carrier, and* rcd1-*affected dogs*

Nucleotide	Normal	Carrier	Affected
cAMP	3.1 ± 1.6	3.9 ± 2.9	2.2 ± 0.2
cGMP	1.8 ± 1.7	1.8 ± 1.1	1.2 ± 0

Unpublished data from Stramm, Fletcher, Aguirre, and Chader.

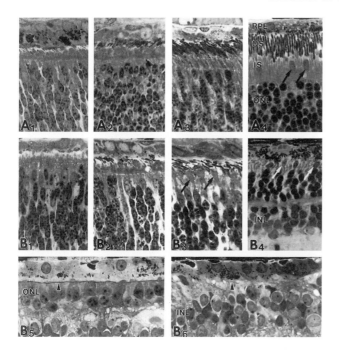

FIGURE 14-9. Retinas from normal (A_{1-4}) and *rcd1*-affected Irish setters (B_{1-6}) of different ages. Normal: A_{1-4} = 10 days, 13 days, 26 days, and adult. Affected: B_{1-4} = 9 days, 16 days, 33 days and 57 days; $B_{5,6}$ = 1 year. In the normal dog, the inner segments are distinct by 10 days, and outer segments have elongated to near adult proportions by 26 days. The adult retina has a high photoreceptor density, and the rods outnumber the cones (arrows in A_4). The *rcd1* retina shows normal development at 9 days of age. At 16 and 33 days of age, the rod inner segments have not elongated, and the outer segments are short and disorganized. Loss of rods results in increased prominence of cones (arrows in $B_{3,4}$), and thinning of the outer nuclear layer. By 1 year of age, photoreceptor loss is extensive. At all stages of the disease, the RPE is normal. Magnification ×400. (Reprinted from Farber et al., 1992.)

glycoproteins, enzymes (acid hydrolases, etc.), glycosaminoglycans (GAGs), proteoglycans, and other molecules are localized (see Hageman and Johnson, 1991 for review). Within the insoluble matrix, individual rods and cones are invested by photoreceptor type specific domains (Hageman and Johnson, 1991; Mieziewska et al., 1991). A matrix disorder that affects either its synthesis or maintenance could adversely affect these two cell layers; alternatively, disease in the photoreceptors or RPE layers could induce secondary changes in the matrix structure to modify the rate of visual cell degeneration.

The complexity of the IPM and the various cell types that border the matrix (rods, cones, RPE, and Müller cells) precludes establishing a cell-specific association between a given component and a cell. Similarly, the contribution of different cell classes to the development of the matrix is also not known. Because of the severe developmental arrest that occurs in *rcd1*-affected photoreceptors, we have examined the matrix to see if ab-

normalities in photoreceptor differentiation affect the development or maintenance of the insoluble IPM (Mieziewska et al., 1993a). The insoluble matrix domains of the IPM are characterized using lectin cytochemistry (wheat germ agglutinin [WGA] and peanut agglutinin [PNA] lectins) in cryosections of retinal tissues and in extracted insoluble matrix preparations, and examined by epifluorescence and scanning confocal laser microscopy.

In the normals, the insoluble matrix is extracted as a continuous sheet that comprises two photoreceptor-specific matrix domains distinguished both by the size of the domains, and by differential binding of WGA and PNA lectins (Mieziewska et al, 1991). Each domain encloses a photoreceptor inner and outer segment. The PNA lectin primarily labels galactose residues in the cone-associated matrix, with weak binding to the rod matrix; the WGA lectin labels equally the rod- and cone-associated matrices which contain N-acetyl glucosamine and sialic acid residues. The specific matrix domains identified with these lectins are present early in the postnatal developmental period, at the time that the two classes of photoreceptors are recognizable cytologically, and they mature in parallel with visual cell morphogenesis. Since the matrix conforms to the shape of the individual rods and cones it surrounds, the structural changes associated with normal photoreceptor development also occur in the matrix (Fig. 14-10$A_{1,2}$) (Mieziewska et al., 1993a).

As noted previously, the *rcd1* retina shows normal development of the photoreceptors during the first two weeks of life, and during this time period the IPM also develops normally. However, no change in matrix structure or carbohydrate specificity is found during the period of developmental arrest (13–24 days postnatal), or after the onset of photoreceptor degeneration (after 25 days of age; Schmidt and Aguirre, 1985). The only changes in the IPM that occur during this time are conformational, i.e. distortion, adherence of cellular debris, and loss of continuity, abnormalities that are presumably secondary to the severe pathology occurring in the visual cells within the individual domains. These occur in older affected retinas as the abnormally developed outer segments disappear and the inner segments shorten and broaden concomitant with cell loss in the photoreceptor layer (Fig. 14-10B_{1-4}, $C_{1,2}$). Survival of cones late in the disease is a feature of *rcd1*, and PNA labeled cone domains remain intact, even when surrounding severely degenerated cone cells (Mieziewska et al., 1993a).

The cellular origin of the matrix constituents has not been established (Mieziewska, 1993). Due to the close relationship between matrix and photoreceptor cells in

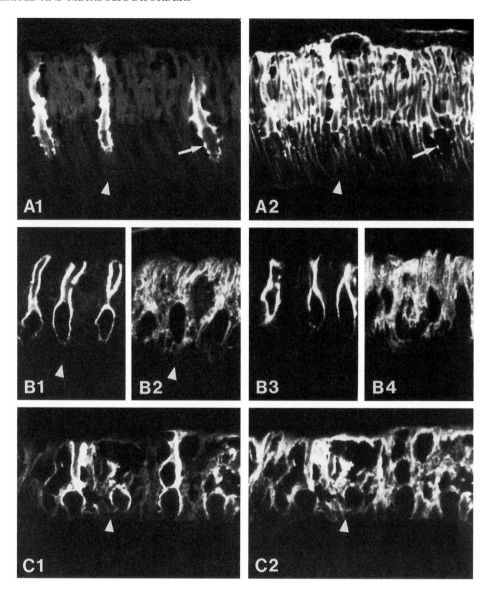

FIGURE 14-10. Optical sections normal and *rcd1*-affected retinas viewed with a confocal scanning laser microscope. Sections were collected in 0.5 μm increments, and each picture represents one section. Normal retina 60 days old shows the distribution of PNA (A$_1$) and WGA (A$_2$) label in both rod and cone matrices. A substructure of the cone matrix is labeled by both PNA and WGA *(arrow)*. The WGA matrix label is stronger in the OS layer than in the IS layer. In the 40-day-old *rcd1*-affected retina (B$_{1,3}$ = PNA, central [1] and peripheral [3] retina; B$_{2,4}$ = WGA, central [2] and peripheral [4] retina) the CIS appear to be displaced sclerally in relation to the small RIS. At 60 days (C1 = PNA, C2 = WGA) substantial cell loss has occurred and the cone inner segments are close to the OLM *(arrowhead)*, but label specificity is comparable to the normal retina (C$_1$). The WGA lectin labels a domain that is irregular and distorted secondary to the rod disease (C$_2$). Magnification ×1200. (Reprinted from Mieziewska et al., 1993a.)

normal and diseased retinas, it is reasonable to assume that the photoreceptor cell is synthesizing its own matrix domain. Studies have shown that photoreceptors are likely to synthesize chondroitin sulfate proteoglycans which are parts of the insoluble matrix (Landers et al., 1991). However, the close association between photoreceptor cells, matrix, and RPE does not preclude the involvement of RPE in synthesis of specific matrix components, either directly or via inductive factors. The studies with the *rcd1* mutant show that normal photoreceptor development is not a prerequisite for the insoluble IPM to develop normally. Similarly, normal maintenance of the matrix occurs even when the visual cells are undergoing very rapid and severe degeneration, and the matrix disappears only after there is photoreceptor loss. It is possible, therefore, that the RPE and/or

Müller cells are the principal cells involved in maintaining this elaborate and complex extracellular scaffold once it is synthesized. Alternatively, one could argue that the photoreceptor cells, although severely diseased, still are able to orchestrate the formation of the insoluble IPM, and this structure is maintained normally until the visual cells disappear. These are issues that cannot be resolved at present. What is known, however, is that the RPE plays a critical role in the remodeling and degradation of matrix constituents through the extracellular and intracellular pathways involved in the degradation of the GAG components of matrix proteoglycans. This will be discussed in subsequent sections (see below).

Rod-cone dysplasia 2. A second early-onset photoreceptor dysplasia has been identified which appears to share many phenotypic similarities with *rcd1*, and, as a result, has been given the disease designation of rod-cone dysplasia 2 (*rcd2*) to differentiate it from the disease present in the Irish setter dogs. Based on clinical, electrophysiological, morphological, and biochemical criteria, the two diseases are identical (Chader, 1991; Woodford et al., 1982). In both, there is an equally rapid increase in retinal cGMP levels early in the postnatal period; the magnitude of this elevation, as well as its time course, are the same (Fig. 14-8). In both *rcd1* and *rcd2* there also is deficient cGMP-PDE activity, although in the latter the activity is calmodulin independent (Chader et al., 1985; Chader, 1991). As in *rcd1*, the disease is expressed initially in the photoreceptor cells, and there is sparing of the RPE and inner retinal layers until the end-stages of the disease.

Although *rcd1* and *rcd2* are phenotypically and biochemically identical, there is considerable evidence that the disorders represent mutations of different genes. With the advent of a molecular diagnosis for *rcd1*, we have established that this mutation is *not* present in *rcd2*, and that the nucleotide sequence of exon 21 of the PDEB gene in *rcd2*-affected dogs is normal (Ray et al., 1994). This finding does not by itself rule out the PDEB gene involvement in *rcd2*, as a different mutation may be present elsewhere in the coding sequence, in an intron–exon junction or in the promoter or a regulatory region. The most compelling evidence for nonidentity of the two diseases comes from our group's previous work in which they performed crosses between dogs affected with *rcd1* and *rcd2* and found the progeny to be normal (Acland et al., 1989). Thus *rcd1* and *rcd2* represent nonallelic diseases that have similar effects on retinal cyclic GMP metabolism. It is likely, therefore, that the molecular defect in *rcd2* resides in one of the two remaining PDE subunits, or in the genes coding for proteins involved in PDE activation.

Other photoreceptor dysplasias. Table 14-2 summarizes the developmental and degenerative photoreceptor diseases of the dog. Two of these, *rcd1* and *rcd2* have been discussed above. Of the three remaining diseases, the mutant strain for one, rod dysplasia *(rd)*, has been lost, and the disease is no longer extant in the general population, nor is it maintained in experimental research colonies (Aguirre, 1978; Acland and Aguirre, 1987). In all of these diseases there is a minimal RPE response to the degenerative process occurring in the adjacent photoreceptor layer (Fig. 14-11). It is only in the late stages of the disease that the RPE undergoes atrophy and limited intraretinal migration into areas that are gliotic and disorganized (Fig. 14-12). These reactions are secondary and nonspecific. Of interest is the exclusion of abnormalities in retinal cyclic nucleotide metabolism as being causally associated with the diseases. This has been done biochemically in the case of *pd* and *erd* (Acland et al., 1989; Parshall et al., 1991). In the latter disease, mutations in the PDEB gene have been excluded, respectively, by breeding and molecular studies (Acland et al., 1989; Ray et al., 1994). This establishes that abnormalities in retinal cGMP metabolism in the retina are not the only causes of photoreceptor dysplasias, although they are likely to be involved in those diseases that have an early onset and a relatively rapid disease course.

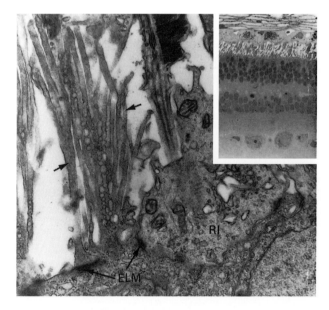

FIGURE 14-11. Müller fiber baskets *(arrows)* projecting through the external limiting membrane (ELM) become prominent after loss of photoreceptor cells in *rd*-affected retina. Inset shows the reduction in photoreceptor number and the shortening of rod inner segments (RI). The RPE is normal. Magnifications: ×17,000 for main figure, ×200 for inset. (Reprinted from Aguirre, 1978.)

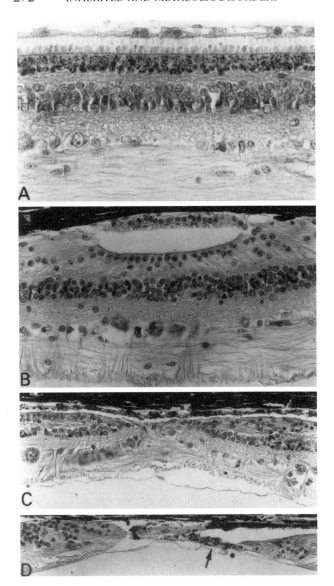

FIGURE 14-12. Different stages of disease in *rd* illustrate the RPE response to the photoreceptor degeneration. (A) In a high-cone-density area of the posterior pole, the loss of rods results in increased prominence of cones. The RPE is normal. (B) An isolated segment of RPE and outer nuclear layer remain. (C) Focal retinal gliosis with loss of retinal layer organization; the RPE is normal. (D) End stage atrophy. The RPE is absent to the left of atrophic focus, but is present to the right and has migrated intraretinally *(arrow)*. Magnifications: (A) ×370; (B) ×100; (C) ×200; (D) ×170. (Reprinted from Aguirre, 1978.)

Photoreceptor degenerations. Of the degenerative group of hereditary retinal diseases, mutations at the *prcd* gene locus account for all of the autosomal disorders recognized to date (Aguirre and Acland, 1988; 1991; unpublished). The *prcd* gene, as well as the different mutations responsible for the defined allelic variants, has yet to be identified. However, very recent studies in our lab have excluded the peripherin/rds, opsin, PDEB rod transducin α1 genes from the *prcd* gene locus (Acland et al., 1995; Wang et al., 1995; Ray et al., 1996; 1997). Thus, *prcd* may represent a mutation of one of the other genes or gene loci that have been identified to cause RP, or, alternatively, of a novel gene not previously associated with the disease.

Photoreceptor disease and degeneration-temporal and topographic factors. As a degenerative disease of the visual cells, structural and functional abnormalities in *prcd* become evident after the cells have developed normally. Pathology occurs first in the rod outer segments, and progresses, with time, to involve the inner segments, and the inner retinal layers. This highly characteristic sequence of disease has allowed us to stage the structural abnormalities into three major phases: a—disease (stages 1*–1); b—degeneration (stages 2–4); c—atrophy (stages 5–8) (Fig. 14-13; Aguirre and Acland, 1988; Long and Aguirre, 1991). Starting at approximately 12–14 weeks of age, all photoreceptor cells begin to develop the stage-specific pathology characteristic of the disease, but the rate of progression is dependent on topographic factors (Aguirre et al., 1982a). In all cases, pathology is more severe in the inferior quadrants, while the visual cells in the superior and temporal retinal quadrants are spared the ravages of the disease until later (Fig. 14-14). Throughout the three phases of the disease, the RPE remains normal and minimally reactive (Fig. 14-13). Only in very advanced disease will the RPE show the nonspecific atrophic and migratory responses illustrated in Figure 14-12D. An additional complexity is the selectivity of the disease, at least initially, for rods. Cone pathology develops late, after rods have begun to degenerate (stage 2 and later). With loss of rods, the cones become the predominant cell remaining in the photoreceptor layer (Fig. 14-15).

This topographic distribution of disease is not unique to *prcd*, but occurs also in other retinal degenerations, particularly in man. The inferior retina appears to be selectively affected in some forms of RP regardless of the molecular basis of the disease. Different rhodopsin mutations have been causally associated with RP, e.g. Pro23His and Gly106Arg (Heckenlively et al., 1991; Fishman et al., 1992), although not all patients with the same molecular defect show the same regionally selective damage to the inferior retina (compare Berson et al., 1991 and Heckenlively et al., 1991). The identification of the factors that modify the topographic expression of the photoreceptor pathology would provide important information on the interaction between the molecular defect, the visual cell, and the local retinal environment, and provide insights of the regulation of the disease phenotype. In order to identify such factors, we have ex-

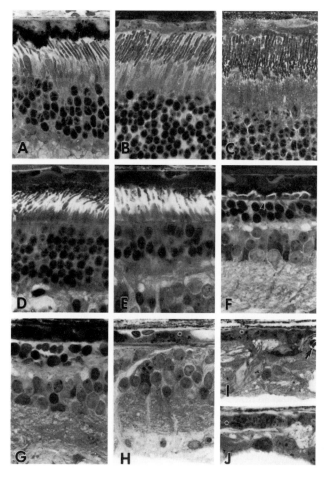

FIGURE 14-13. Disease stages in *prcd*: S-0 (A), S-1* (B), S-1 (C), S-2 (D), S-3 (E), S-4 (F), S-5 (G), S-6 (H), S-7 (I) and S-8 (J). Arrowhead (F) indicated RPE process contacting the external limiting membrane; * (H, I, J) indicate RPE; arrow (I) indicates retinal vessel. At all stages of the disease, the RPE remains structurally normal. Magnification ×430. (For details refer to Aguirre and Acland, 1988, from which this figure was reprinted with permission.)

amined several different parameters that could be involved in modulating the rate and severity of the photoreceptor degeneration. These include: RPE pigmentation (Aguirre and O'Brien, 1986), invasion of pha-gocytic cells into the interphotoreceptor space (Aguirre, 1986), visual cell renewal (Aguirre and O'Brien, 1986), the soluble and insoluble components of the IPM (Wiggert et al., 1991; Mieziewska et al., 1993b), and the expression of photoreceptor-specific proteins and transcripts (Huang et al., 1994). Thus far, no specific properties have been identified in the inferior retinal quadrant that selectively predisposes this area to earlier and more severe disease. Some of these issues are addressed below.

Photoreceptor degeneration, RPE pigmentation and interphotoreceptor space phagocytic cells. As noted in the

section on "Normal Anatomy," above, the dog RPE is not pigmented in the tapetal region (Fig. 14-1). Additionally, the density of pigmentation is also not uniform, with pigmentation density being greater in the periphery. Because of the presence of pigmented and nonpigmented RPE regions overlying the photoreceptor mosaic, it is essential to consider topographic effects when evaluating the influence of pigmentation on diseases of the photoreceptor–RPE complex.

We have developed a technique for sampling retinal tissues from topographically defined regions of the eye using tissues embedded either in plastic (following glutaraldehyde/osmium tetroxide fixation) or in diethylene glycol distearate (DGD) wax after paraformaldehyde fixation (Aguirre et al., 1983; 1986; Huang et al., 1993). This permits cutting 1 μm sections which extend from the optic disc to the ora serrata in all four quadrants; the tissue can then be examined by conventional light microscopy after staining (plastic sections), or following

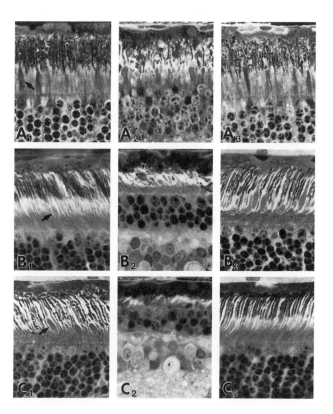

FIGURE 14-14. Variation of *prcd* disease severity by quadrant. All photographs taken 3000 μm from the edge of the optic disc in the superior (A_1, B_1, C_1), inferior (A_2, B_2, C_2) and temporal (A_3, B_3, C_3) quadrants of animals at 1.1 (A_{1-3}), 2.1 (B_{1-3}), and 2.5 (C_{1-3}) years. Disease progresses first in the inferior quadrant; visual cells degenerate, and macrophages *(arrowhead)* invade the interphotoreceptor space. Cones *(arrows)* are generally spared by the disease process and remain normal, particularly in the temporal quadrant. Magnification ×400. (Reprinted from Aguirre and Acland, 1988.)

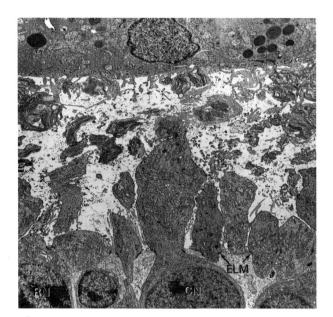

FIGURE 14-15. Stage 2 disease *(prcd)*. There is extensive rod outer and inner segment degeneration and loss which results in the increased prominence of the cones. The RPE is normal. RN = rod nucleus, CN = cone nucleus, ELM = external limiting membrane. Magnification ×4000. (Reprinted from Aguirre and O'Brien, 1986.)

lectin, immunocytochemical and/or *in situ* hybridization procedures carried out in the same tissue. In this manner, it is possible to correlate disease stage with any of the parameters that are potentially involved in modulating the severity of the visual cell degenerative process.

In young *prcd*-affected animals, the retinas show a central-to-peripheral gradation of disease severity (Fig. 14-16). Early disease (stages -1*, -1) is present throughout the posterior pole and equatorial regions, but stops abruptly in the periphery where the photoreceptors become normal. This change in disease severity could be associated with increasing RPE pigment density, since a gradual change in pigmentation also occurs in a central-to-peripheral gradient. This finding raises the possibility of a pigmentation associated protective effect. However, critical examination of the areas where pigmentation changes abruptly reveals that the change in disease severity (from stage-1 to stage-0) is not associated with a change in pigmentation. Thus, the improvement in disease severity appears to be dependent on topographic position of the visual cells in the photoreceptor mosaic rather than RPE pigmentation. With progression of the disease, the peripheral sparing effect is lost, and disease severity is of equal or greater magnitude to that present more centrally (Fig. 14-17).

In fact, it could be argued that the presence and density of RPE pigmentation *per se* enhances the disease process. After all, the transition from disease (stage-1)

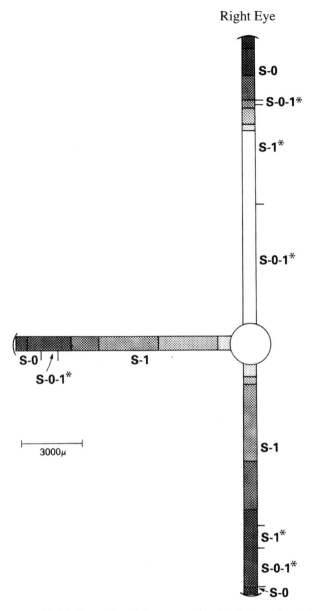

FIGURE 14-16. Illustration of the topographic distribution of retinal disease in the right eye of a 22-week-old *prcd*-affected dog (refer to Figure 14-13 for details of disease stages). The rectangles indicate the exact length of the section and retinal position *(refer to 3000 μm calibration marker)* in relation to the optic nerve *(central circle)* and ora serrata *(curved line)*. Rectangles above and below the optic disc represent, respectively, the superior and inferior retinal quadrants; the temporal quadrant is represented by a horizontal rectangle. The degrees of shading within the rectangles represent the extent of RPE pigment density. Note that the peripheral retina is normal, but the RPE pigmentation density does not ameliorate the severity of the disease. (Reprinted with modification from Aguirre and O'Brien, 1986.)

to degeneration (stages-2, -3, -4) occurs first in the inferior retinal quadrant, a region characterized by heavy pigmentation in the RPE monolayer (Fig. 14-17). It is this quadrant that shows the degeneration of the pho-

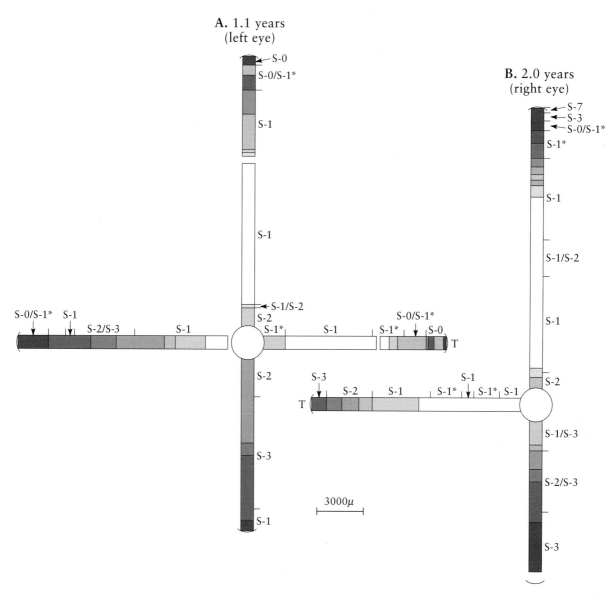

A. 1.1 years
(left eye)

B. 2.0 years
(right eye)

3000μ

FIGURE 14-17. Comparison of the topographic distribution and progression of retinal disease in both eyes of a *prcd*-affected dog at two different ages (1.1 and 2.0 years). Refer to Figure 14-13 for details of disease stages, and to Figure 14-16 for explanation of the schematic illustration. At the earlier time period (1.1 years), the peripheral reti- na is normal in the superior, temporal, and nasal quadrants. With time, the disease progresses to involve the periphery. Note that disease is more severe in the inferior quadrants, and that RPE pigmentation does not have a protective effect. (Reprinted with modification from Aguirre and Acland, 1988.)

toreceptors and loss of 75%–80% of the outer nuclear layer at the time that the visual cells in other quadrants of the eye show minimal disease. Thus, the selectivity of the disease process for the inferior retinal quadrant can not be explained on the basis of a protective effect of pigmentation. These results are different from those re- ported for the RCS rat, where light deprivation or pig- mentation have a protective effect, and reduce the rate of the retinal degeneration (LaVail and Battelle, 1975; LaVail, 1980).

A prominent feature of the degenerative phase of the disease is the presence of cells in the interphotoreceptor space (Fig. 14-14B$_2$). Initially, we suspected that these cells represented activated RPE cells that had detached and migrated into the interphotoreceptor space. How- ever, we found no area of the RPE monolayer that was devoid of RPE cells, or that showed breaks in the apical tight junctions that define the outer blood–retina barri- er. Cytological examination showed that these cells like- ly represented phagocytic rather than RPE cells, because

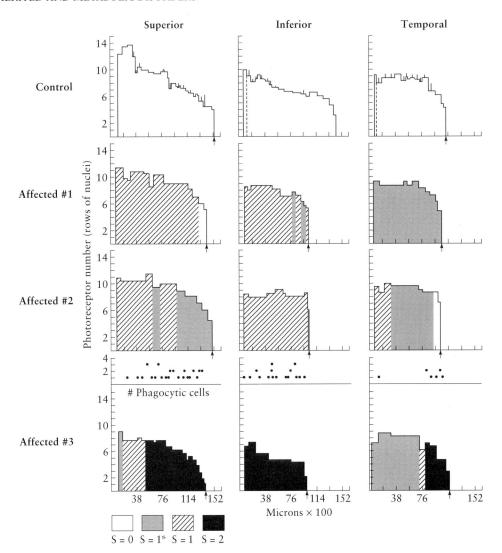

FIGURE 14-18. Histograms correlating photoreceptor numbers *(rows of nuclei)*, disease stage *(refer to shading key below)*, and number of phagocytic cells in the interphotoreceptor space for the superior, inferior and temporal retinal quadrants of control and *prcd*-affected dogs at 22 weeks (#1 and 2) and 36 weeks (#3) of age. In the younger affected dogs, disease is less severe in the periphery, the photoreceptor number remains within normal limits, and phagocytic cells are not present. The older affected dog (#3) shows more advanced disease (S-2), especially in the inferior quadrant. Phagocytic cells are present in the interphotoreceptor space, primarily in areas of S-2 disease. (Reprinted with modification from Aguirre and O'Brien, 1986, and Aguirre, 1986.)

they lacked pigmentation and had irregularly shaped, pale nuclei with dense peripheral chromatin condensation (Aguirre, 1986). Recent studies in the RCS rat indicate that the phagocytic cells that invade the interphotoreceptor space are of microglial origin (Roque et al., 1996).

We have examined the association between photoreceptor disease and the presence of phagocytic cells in the interphotoreceptor space. In young affected dogs, early disease (stages 1* and 1) is present uniformly throughout the eye, and phagocytic cells are absent. With progression to stage 2, however, phagocytic cells appear

(Fig. 14-18). It is at this stage of the disease that rod inner and outer segments begin to degenerate rapidly, and the number of outer nuclear layer nuclei decreases. The histogram illustrating disease severity with the number of phagocytic cells in the interphotoreceptor space indicates a direct correlation between the two processes. Almost all the phagocytic cells that are present are restricted to those areas having the more severe stage-2 disease. In the late degenerative (stage-4) and atrophic (stages-5 and -6) phases of the disease, the number of phagocytic cells decrease (Aguirre, unpublished). This would suggest that the debris accumulating in the inter-

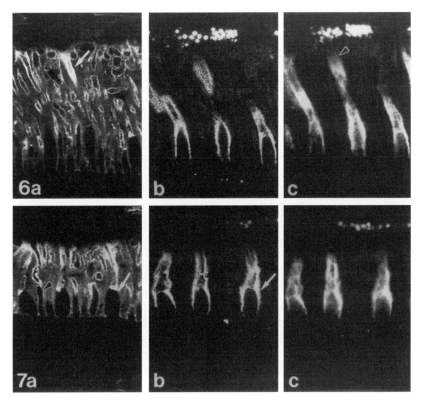

FIGURE 14-19. The central (6$_{a-c}$) and peripheral (7$_{a-c}$) retinal areas of a 3 year old *prcd*-affected dog with stage 3 disease. (6a) WGA strongly labels the IPM space adjacent to the outer segments; there is diffuse but weak labeling of the remaining IPM. The surviving photoreceptors are well organized, except for the whorls of OS debris located on the RPE apical surface. WGA labels the RPE cone sheaths strongly *(arrow)*. (6b) The PNA domain is thicker than normal, smooth and slightly "fluffy" in appearance. (6c) The composite shows the diminishing PNA label intensity at the RPE level *(arrowhead)*. RPE lipofus- cin granules were brightly labeled. The peripheral retina shows more advanced stage 3 disease. (7a) WGA label is strong immediately around the remaining cells *(rods = arrowhead, cones = white arrow)*. (7b) PNA label is prominent and thick around cone IS and OS *(arrow)*. Note that the cone matrix thickness differs when visualized with the WGA and PNA lectins *(compare Figures 14-7a and b, arrow)*. (7c) The composite shows the circumference and thickness of the PNA domain around the cones. Magnification ×1,000. (Reprinted from Mieziewska et al., 1993b.)

photoreceptor space secondary to photoreceptor degeneration may serve as the signal for the invasion of macrophages.

The interphotoreceptor matrix. Using the techniques of lectin cytochemistry, we have examined the molecular components of the insoluble IPM to determine if abnormalities are present in the *prcd*-affected retina, either before the development of the disease, or after the process of photoreceptor degeneration has been initiated (Mieziewska et al., 1993b; Mieziewska, 1993). Because of the topographic specificity for early degeneration in the inferior quadrant, we examined for differences between this quadrant and other retinal loci. We reasoned that degenerative changes in the visual cells could be initiated in response to a damaged matrix environment, irrespective of the nature of the primary defect that is responsible for the cell dysfunction. Because the slow degeneration present in the *prcd* mutant retina allows diseased photoreceptors to remain viable for a

relatively long period of time, the microenvironment of the IPM during degeneration may reflect more accurately that present in RP, the comparable disease in man.

With the exception of the late atrophic stages (stages 5–8) of the disease, the lectin specificity remains normal in all the ages and stages examined. However, a thickening of the rod and cone matrix domains is observed in some samples representing stages 2 and 3 (Fig. 14-19). Since the change in thickness was observed at a relatively advanced stage of degeneration, when substantial cell death had already occurred, the thickening may represent a secondary response of the surviving cells. This response would maintain the structural integrity of the IPM and prevent the disruption of molecular flow through the IPM resulting from discontinuity in the structure. The number of photoreceptors remaining in the IPM compartment has been severely reduced by the time stage 2 is reached. The extra space is presumably occupied by broadened photoreceptors and matrix domains, as seen in later stages. Additionally, we found that the cone domains terminated somewhat more vitreal to the RPE than normal, and, in the older affected animals with shorter PNA cone domains, WGA (wheat germ agglutin) strongly labeled the RPE cone sheath surrounding these cones. The significance of this finding is unclear, but it could be the result of outer segment debris accumulation below the apical surface of the RPE. Extreme displacement of IPM material due to debris accumulation has been shown in the RCS rats (LaVail et al., 1981; Porrello et al., 1986). Our findings in the *prcd* mutant indicates that the photoreceptor-specific IPM constituents which form the insoluble IPM are not primarily involved in this hereditary retinal degeneration.

Progressive Retinal Atrophy (PRA) in the Cat

Similar hereditary retinal disorders have been recognized in other animal species. Brief mention will be made only of the diseases occurring in the cat, where both early- and late-onset hereditary photoreceptor degenerations have been described. Three different early-onset disorders have been identified; two are dominantly inherited (mixed-breed cats [West-Hyde and Buyukmihci, 1982] and Abyssinians [Barnett and Curtis, 1985; Curtis et al., 1987]), and one is recessively inherited in the Persian breed (Rubin and Lipton, 1973; Gaarder and Aguirre, unpublished). Surprisingly, all three diseases have a very early onset and rapid degeneration, and end-stage retinal disease is evident on ophthalmoscopy by the time the animals are only a few months of age (Plates 14-V, 14-VI). This is different from what is found in dogs with the comparable developmental photoreceptor diseases (Table 14-2). A late-onset, slowly progressive disease, also recognized in the Abyssinian breed, is inherited as autosomal recessive (Narfström, 1983). Both of the diseases found in the Abyssinian breed are maintained in experimental colonies by different research groups, and confusion may arise in those not familiar with the profound differences that exist between the two disorders.

Heterozygous Abyssinian cats affected with the early onset rod-cone dysplasia (*Rdy*) show equal structural abnormalities in the rod and cone photoreceptors (Leon and Curtis, 1990). These remain rudimentary, and fail to form organized outer segments; in addition, there is delayed and incomplete photoreceptor synaptogenesis. Degeneration begins in the central retina and progresses to the periphery; by 30 weeks of age, two to five rows of nuclei remain in the outer nuclear layer. In the area centralis, the feline equivalent of the foveomacular region of primates, there is atrophy of the RPE and the choriocapillaris, and thinning of the overlying tapetal layer. These changes are presumably secondary, as they occur late in the disease process. Abnormalities in retinal cyclic nucleotide metabolism have been reported in abstract form for the *Rdy* model (Leon et al., 1988), but not published. In that brief abstract, the authors reported the presence of elevated retinal cGMP levels in affected animals in the earliest stages of the dystrophy, at a time when the cGMP-PDE activity was low.

The late-onset, recessive degenerative photoreceptor disorder is characterized initially by disorientation of the rod disc membranes (Narfström and Nilsson, 1989). This is followed at approximately six months of age by disintegration of the rod outer segments, appearing as vacuolization and clumping of disc material and accumulation of debris. Thereafter, rod cells are lost from the photoreceptor and outer nuclear layers. Cones develop and remain normal until two to three years of age, at which time degeneration begins (Narfström and Nilsson, 1986). In several respects, this disease has many similarities to *prcd* in the dog, among which are the clinical, cytological, and temporal characteristics of photoreceptor degeneration, as well as the presence of abnormalities in plasma lipids, particularly docosahexaenoic acid (22:6n-3; Anderson et al., 1991).

Retinal pigment epithelial defects have not been described in the Abyssinian cat with the late onset recessive disease. Based on normal rhodopsin regeneration as determined *in situ* by imaging fundus reflectometry, the normal participation by the RPE in this aspect of the rhodopsin cycle is implied (Jacobson et al., 1989). Similarly, normal RPE function has been established electrophysiologically by measurements of the DC-recorded c-wave and direct measurements of the standing potential (Narfström et al., 1985). Normal dark-adapted sensitivity (Narfström et al., 1988) and rhodopsin regeneration occur, even though a profound decrease in IRBP gene expression has been reported at both the message and protein levels (Narfström et al., 1989a; Wiggert et al., 1994). It is not clear how this finding relates to the retinal function, or its significance in terms of the identification of the molecular defect of the disease. To date, only the phosducin and peripherin/rds genes have been excluded from the disease (Gorin et al., 1993, 1995).

THE RPE IN INHERITED DEFECTS OF LYSOSOMAL FUNCTION

Our laboratories have been involved in studies of the RPE disease present in animals with lysosomal storage disorders. In both man and animals, these diseases are caused by the inherited deficiency of lysosomal enzymes, and represent generalized multisystemic abnormalities of which the ocular lesions are but one component. That selective deficiency of an enzyme results in substrate accumulation indicates that the degradative pathway involved, as well as the substrate accumulating, are critical for the normal function of the tissue studied. These aspects of the diseases lend themselves to be used to define specific catabolic pathways essential for normal RPE function. Disease in the RPE is dramatic, and underscores the importance of the lysosomal system in the function of this cell layer. This is not surprising, because compared with other tissues of the body the RPE shows a higher activity for most of the acid hydrolases and sulfatases (Hayasaka, 1974; Zimmerman et al., 1983; Stramm et al., 1983; Aguirre and Stramm, 1991). Of this group of diseases, our focus has been primarily on those disorders involved in the degradation of glycosaminoglycans (GAGs), known collectively as the *inherited mucopolysaccharidoses.*

Mucopolysaccharide (MPS) Storage Diseases

Severe RPE pathology with no photoreceptor disease. We have examined the RPE in animals with mutations of three different lysosomal enzyme gene loci: arylsulfatase B (ASB; cat), α-L-iduronidase (α-L-id; cat) and β-glucuronidase (GUSB; dog) (see Table 14-4 and Aguirre and Stramm, 1991 for review). The lysosomal enzymes encoded by these genes participate in the degradation of GAGs. Morphologic studies of the three mutations indicate that the accumulation of intracellular inclusions in secondary lysosomes serves as a distinct structural marker of the enzyme deficient RPE. By light microscopy, these inclusions appear vacuolated, or homogeneous and indistinct from the surrounding cytoplasm. Ultrastructurally, the inclusions can vary from electron lucent to granular, lamellar, or mixed (Fig. 14-20). The electron-lucent and granular vacuoles are believed to represent leached and stored GAGs, respectively, while

lamellar inclusions result from lipid accumulation secondary to inhibition of ganglioside degradative pathways by the stored GAGs (Rushton and Dawson, 1977).

Accumulation of secondary lysosomal inclusions in the enzyme-deficient RPE is the hallmark structural abnormality. Using the MPS–VI deficient mutant as the prototype disease, we have found that there is RPE hypertrophy subsequent to the accumulation of vacuolated inclusions. In the RPE, single cytoplasmic inclusions are present initially in the early postnatal period. Their number and size increase during the period of photoreceptor differentiation. Subsequently, the RPE cells enlarge, and the monolayer becomes uniformly hypertrophied. In older animals, some of the enlarged cells become massively hypertrophied, and have a uniformly rounded apical border. These hypertrophied cells, which can have an apical–basal height greater than 25 microns, occur either singly or in clusters, and result in loss of the uniformity that is characteristic of the RPE monolayer (Fig. 14-21). Similar disease is present in the MPS VII RPE (Stramm et al., 1990). In contrast, the MPS–I affected RPE accumulates homogeneous inclusions that are not distinct from the surrounding cytoplasm, and RPE hypertrophy is minimal or absent (Stramm et al., 1989). The inclusions represent stored GAGs that accumulate in the diseased RPE cells (Fig. 14-22).

In spite of the severe RPE pathology, there is complete preservation of neuroretinal structure and function. Examination of the ERG rod-and-cone system responses indicates maintenance of normal retinal function at a time when RPE storage is severe (Aguirre et al., 1986). Morphologic examination also shows that the internal lamellar organization of the rod outer segments is preserved, even though they appear disoriented when adjacent to massively hypertrophied RPE cells. In fact, outer segment lengths and renewal rate, an indication of the normal participation of the RPE in the outer segment renewal process, are normal when studied both early and late in the disease (Fig. 14-23). It is apparent, therefore,

TABLE 14-4. *Lysosomal storage diseases in animal models*

Number	Eponym	Animal	Enzyme	Stored GAGs
MPS I*	Hurler	Cat, dog	α-L-Iduronidase	DS, HS
MPS II	Hunter	Dog	Iduronate-2-sulfatase	HS, DS
MPS IIID	Sanfilippo	Goat	N-Acetylglucosamine 6-Sulfatase	HS
MPS VI*	Maroteaux-Lamy	Cat, dog, rat	Arylsulfatase B	DS
MPS VII*	Sly	Dog, mouse, cat	β-Glucuronidase	DS, HS, CS

DS = dermatan sulfate   HS = heparan sulfate   CS = chondroitin sulfate
*Extensive RPE storage of substrate has been reported; refer to text for details.

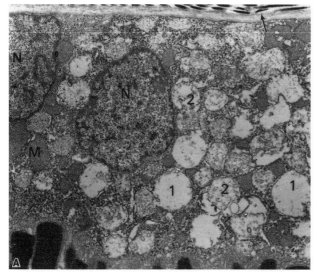

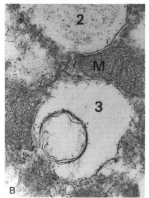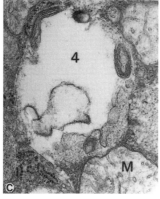

FIGURE 14-20. Nonpigmented RPE cell from the tapetal zone *(arrow)* of an MPS VI–affected cat (ASB deficiency) accumulates electron lucent (1), granular (2), lamellar (3), and mixed (4) inclusions in secondary lysosomes. The inclusions are membrane limited and distinct from mitochondria (M). N = nucleus. Magnifications: (A) ×5,700; (B) ×19,000; (C) ×17,500. (Reprinted from Aguirre et al., 1983.)

that the diseased RPE cells, in spite of their massive hypertrophy, are still able to maintain their photoreceptor-supportive functions. Similar preservation of photoreceptors occurs in both the MPS I (cat) and VII (dog) models, although, in the latter, there is disorientation of cone outer segment disc membranes (Aguirre et al., 1986; Aguirre and Stramm, 1991). Of all the MPS models reported, photoreceptor degeneration occurs only in the MPS VII mouse (Lazarus et al., 1993).

The interphotoreceptor matrix in MPS VII. β-glucuronidase, the enzyme deficient in MPS VII, is involved in the degradation of the three principal GAGs present in the RPE: chondroitin sulfate (CS), dermatan sulfate (DS), and heparan sulfate (HS). Of these, heparan and

chondroitin sulfates have important biological activities in, respectively, mediating cell-to-cell interaction and being an important molecular constituent of the main class of proteoglycans present in the IPM (Stramm et al., 1989; 1990). Of the cells bordering the interphotoreceptor space, it is only the RPE that is involved in the degradation of the CS component of IPM proteoglycans (Stramm et al., 1990). Because of the severe disease that occurs in the RPE from GUSB deficiency, it is plausible that an equally severe abnormality would occur in the IPM. For that reason, we have examined the matrix in normal and mutant animals using a series of antibodies and lectins directed at different molecular constituents of this structure. Surprisingly, we have found only a minor alteration in the matrix (Long et al., 1989; Long and Aguirre, unpublished). The distribution of chondroitin sulfate proteoglycan species (0-S, 4-S, and 6-S) is normal, although there is a condensation of the 6-S molecular species limited to the area of the cone matrix sheath. Within this sheath, some of the cone outer segments show a nonprogressive disorientation of the "coin-stack" organization of the discs. However, the major portion of the matrix and the rod photoreceptors are normal (Fig. 14-24). In contrast, the elegant studies of the MPS VII mouse retina by Lazarus and colleagues have shown that abnormalities of the IPM occur early, and that changes in its biochemical composition or physical structure may be causally associated with the subsequent photoreceptor degeneration (Lazarus et al., 1993).

The topography of RPE disease is not uniform. The lysosomal enzymes serve general "housekeeping" functions in the catabolism of complex macromolecules that are targeted to the lysosomal compartment during the remodeling and turnover of cell membranes and extracellular matrices. Because of their ubiquitous distribution in all tissues, including the RPE, and the presumably uniform function of this cell layer in the eye, one would expect that enzyme deficiency would result in uniform disease expression within the monolayer. However, this is far from the case.

In the MPS VI–deficient mutant, the number of RPE inclusions increases with time, but this increase cannot be considered strictly age dependent, as it is strongly modified by topographic factors which appear to regulate disease expression. A striking feature of the ASB-deficient RPE is the lack of uniformity in the expression of the disease phenotype. This is clearly demonstrated in Figure 14-25, which compares disease in nonpigmented (A) and pigmented (B) RPE cells from equivalent positions in the superior and inferior quadrants of the same adult eye; the nonpigmented RPE becomes massively

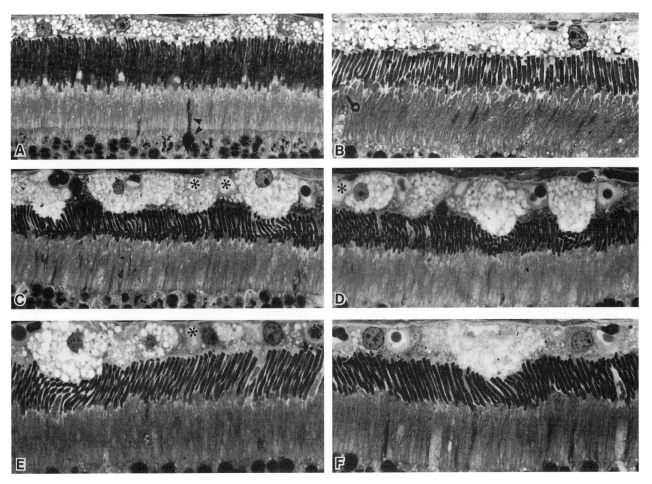

FIGURE 14-21. Nonpigmented RPE from the tapetal zone of MPS VI–affected cats of different ages. (A) 6 months; (B) 9.5 months; (C)–(F) 5 years. (A) vacuolated inclusions fill the cytoplasm without causing hypertrophy. (B) the height of the RPE cells increases concurrent with the accumulation of larger vacuoles. (C)–(F) Hypertrophy of the RPE cells, either singly or in clusters, results in focal disarray of the outer segment layer. Note that photoreceptor disorientation is not accompanied by disease. Arrowheads (A) indicate a necrotic cell that is not associated with the ASB deficiency; asterisks (C) denote normal choriocapillaris indentation of the basal RPE. Magnifications: (A), (B), (E), (F) ×830; (C), (D) ×650. (Reprinted from Aguirre et al., 1983.)

hypertrophied while the pigmented RPE remains normal. In general, two spatial gradients are present in the ASB-deficient RPE (Aguirre et al., 1983). These are (a) central-to-peripheral gradient within the same quadrant: The RPE disease always is more severe in the posterior pole than in the periphery although, with aging, disease in the periphery increases in severity; and (b) quadrant- (pigmentation-) specific distribution: The RPE abnormality is not distributed equally about the optic disc, but has the same disposition as that of nonpigmented RPE cells in the superior, temporal, and nasal meridians. That is, areas of the RPE monolayer that are nonpigmented and over the tapetum lucidum show marked RPE storage, while minimal-to-no storage is present in areas where the RPE is pigmented (Fig. 14-26; compare with Fig. 14-3). In older animals, the relationship between RPE pigmentation and absence of disease decreases in all quadrants, as progressively more pigmented cells accumulate secondary lysosomes and become hypertrophied. The disease phenotype, however, is always less severe in the pigmented RPE.

The lack of uniformity in the response of the RPE to an inherited lysosomal enzyme deficiency raises questions concerning topographic variability in the function and metabolism of the cell layer. It is possible that RPE ASB enzyme activity normally is not the same throughout the monolayer and, in the affected RPE cells, substrate accumulates in those regions having a

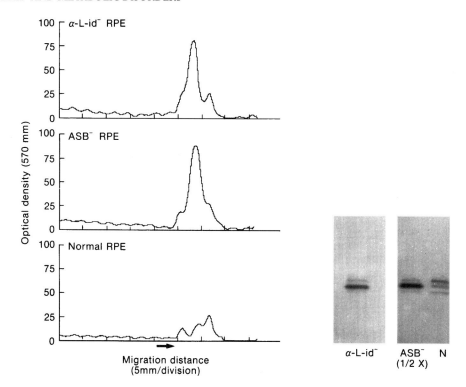

FIGURE 14-22. Scanning densitometry tracing of Alcian Blue–stained GAGs separated by cellulose acetate electrophoresis from freshly isolated RPE cells of a normal cat, and cats affected with MPS I (α-L-id⁻) and MPS VI (ASB⁻). The tracing of the normal RPE cell GAGs shows three distinct peaks, the faster migrating doublet of chondroitin sulfate/dermatan sulfate, and the slower isolated heparan sulfate peak. In both diseases there is an accumulation of GAGs, particularly dermatan sulfate. (Reprinted with modification from Aguirre and Stramm, 1991.)

more profound deficiency. This is not an unreasonable hypothesis, as the activities of several lysosomal enzymes have been shown to exhibit regional variations (Burke and Twining, 1988; Cabral et al., 1990). Other mechanisms that explain the milder disease phenotype of pigmented RPE may be the presence of alternate degradative pathways, a protective action by pigment, or regional differences in GAG metabolism (synthesis, secretion, and/or internalization). Recent in vitro studies, discussed below, indicate that regional differences in GAG metabolism determine the disease topography, and that these differences are not the result of the presence of the tapetum lucidum, but are dependent on the positional origin of the RPE cells.

A lack of spatial uniformity in RPE disease expression is also present in the MPS I feline model. However, because the disease phenotype is not as dramatic as in MPS VI (inclusions are homogeneous rather than vacuolated, and RPE cell hypertrophy is absent), it has been more difficult to ascertain the disease topography. As in the MPS VI model, we have found that accumulations of secondary lysosomes in the α-L-iduronidase-deficient RPE occur primarily in the superior quadrant where the RPE is not pigmented. In this area, the inclusions occupy approximately 18% of the cytoplasmic space. In contrast, RPE cells from the inferior quadrant accumulate a much smaller number of inclusions, and these occupy no more than 5%–6% of the cytoplasmic area. With the exception of melanin, which is not present in the superior (central and equatorial) quadrant, there are no differences in the presence and distribution of other cellular organelles (Stramm et al., 1989).

In vitro expression of RPE disease. Biochemical studies on the RPE are difficult to perform; only small quantities of tissue can be obtained from a single eyecup, and the material is often contaminated by other cell types. In vitro studies overcome these limitations by allowing the preparation and amplification of pure populations of RPE cells. The use of a controlled tissue culture environment allows for the precise determination of the role of metabolic/degradative pathways in normal RPE function. The in vitro systems also are amenable to studies of the regulation of selected pathways, both at the cel-

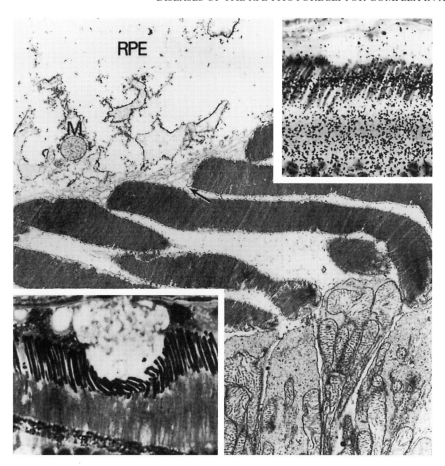

FIGURE 14-23. The RPE in feline MPS VI. Focal disorientation of outer segments opposite a massively hypertrophied RPE cell *(lower inset)*. The internal lamellar organization of the outer segments is normal *(main figure)*, but the RPE cytoplasm is full of vacuolated inclusions, and few organelles are recognizable (M = mitochondrion). Three days after the intravitreal injection of ^{3}H-leucine *(upper inset)*, a band of silver grains is present in the autoradiogram midway along the outer segment length in rods located opposite hypertrophied and diseased RPE cells. This indicates that renewal is normal in spite of severe RPE disease. Arrow in main figure indicates apical microvilli of the RPE. Magnification: ×10,000 for main figure; insets ×850. (Reprinted from Aguirre et al., 1986.)

lular and molecular level, and are useful for developing methodologies for correction of the metabolic defects at the gene level. Other chapters in this book discuss the use of tissue culture to study RPE function and metabolism. In this section, we address the use of in vitro methods in the study of inherited lysosomal deficiencies in the RPE; this topic has been reviewed previously (Aguirre and Stramm, 1991). Of the four lysosomal storage diseases studied in our laboratories (MPS I [dog and cat], VI [cat] and VII [dog]; α-mannosidase deficiency [cat]), all show in vitro retention of the morphologic, biochemical and molecular characteristics of the disease (Aguirre et al., 1995; Ray et al., 1996; Ray et al., 1997; Stramm et al., 1985, 1986, 1989, 1990). Studies presented in this section focus on the disease present in the MPS VI cat model.

MPS VI in vitro disease. Primary cultures of RPE cells initiated from the entire eyecup of cats with MPS VI show that there is a profound decrease of ASB activity, typically 5%–10% of normal (Stramm et al., 1985). This low level, termed *residual enzyme activity,* is insufficient to prevent the morphological manifestations of the disease, and the MPS VI–affected cells accumulate intracellular inclusions identical to those found in situ (Fig. 14-27). In RPE cultures from heterozygotes, the activity of ASB is reduced to approximately 50% of normal. Since these cells are phenotypically normal, both in vitro and in vivo, it appears that this level of enzyme activity is sufficient to prevent expression of the disease. One can conclude, therefore, that ASB activity must be reduced below some critical level in the MPS VI RPE before disease is expressed morphologically. One also may

CHONDROITIN SULFATE 6-S

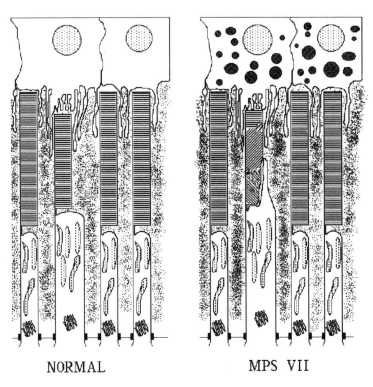

NORMAL   MPS VII

FIGURE 14-24. Schematic illustration of IPM layer immunocytochemical labeling with antibody directed against the 6–0 species of chondroitin sulfate proteoglycan in normal and MPS VII–affected dog retinal sections. In both there is diffuse and similar labeling throughout the IPM. In the MPS VII retina, however, there is a condensation also of immunoreactivity in the matrix around the cone inner and outer segments, and intense labeling of the inclusions present in the RPE. Note the disorientation of the cone outer segment discs, and the extension of a long calyceal process. (Long and Aguirre, unpublished.)

infer from these observations that it may not be necessary to restore 100% of the deficient enzyme activity to restore normal function to the diseased cells.

In a previous section, we showed that the topography of the RPE disease in MPS VI was not uniform, and that cells in the posterior pole exhibited massive intracellular storage while those in the far periphery showed little or no accumulation of undegraded substrate. Within the posterior pole, however, storage of undegraded substrate was more severe in the superior than in the inferior regions. To examine the factors that contribute to the region-specific distribution of RPE disease, we have studied the in vitro RPE isolated from regionally defined areas of the monolayer. In contrast to the isolation method that harvests cells from the entire eyecup (Stramm et al., 1983), regional cultures isolate cells from topographically preselected regions by using small glass cylinders or cloning rings to demarcate the sampled area (Stramm et al., 1985; see Aguirre and Stramm, 1991 for review). A limitation of the method is that only a small sample of cells can be harvested, but, when seeded at a high density, they are highly differentiated and remain pigmented if isolated from the nontapetal regions of the eye.

MPS VI-topographic preservation of disease in vitro. Regional cultures have been initiated from cells isolated from the superior and inferior regions of the eye. We have found that the accumulation of inclusions, representing stored substrate in secondary lysosomes, occurs primarily in cultures initiated from the posterior pole and superior equatorial regions, and not in those initiated from the inferior regions or periphery (Fig. 14-28). This region-specific in vitro disease phenotype is identical to what is observed in situ, and reflects differences in substrate accumulation that are topographically determined. However, disease is not the result of regional

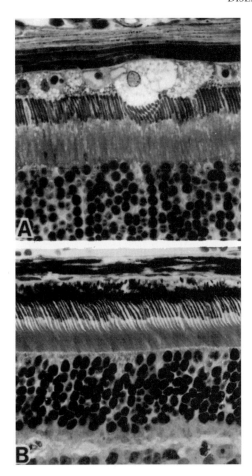

FIGURE 14-25. Sections from the tapetal (A—pigment epithelium not pigmented) and nontapetal (B—pigment epithelium pigmented) zones of a cat with MPS VI. As a result of arylsulfatase B deficiency, the non-pigmented RPE becomes massively hypertrophied (A) and accumulates cytoplasmic vacuolated inclusions. The pigmented RPE remains normal (B). Magnification ×420. (Reprinted from Aguirre et al., 1986.)

topographic origin of the cells. The accumulation of GAGs within the cell layer was much greater in cultures initiated from the superior region of the eye than in cultures from the inferior region (Fig. 14-29). This is in agreement with our in vivo and in vitro morphologic results (Aguirre et al., 1983; Stramm et al., 1986). In contrast to the cell layer, the media from affected cultures initiated from the inferior region of the eye contained much higher levels of DS/CS than cultures from the superior region, and this difference in the release of newly synthesized GAGs into the media between regions was sustained during the 72-hour chase period. Associated with the accumulation of GAGs, there was a significant increase of collagen production in nonpigmented cultures from the superior quadrant (Stramm et al., 1991).

Our studies show that the region-specific alterations in both cell layer storage of GAGs and the release of GAGs into the media are maintained in vitro in the presence of a lysosomal enzyme deficiency that uniformly affects both regions of the RPE. This finding indicates that additional pathways for GAG turnover exist in the RPE, and are more active in the less severely diseased regions. The alternate pathways do not appear to operate in a regionally selective manner in normal RPE, as evidenced by similar GAG synthesis and secretion profiles in cultures initiated from different areas of the eye. In the disease, however, the function of these pathways appears to be selectively increased in cells derived from specific regions of the eye. Such regionally selective processes indicate that the RPE, although a monolayer, must not be considered to be homogeneous in its function and metabolism. This is of critical importance for the studies of RPE diseases which are expressed in a topographically specified site, such as AMD.

α-Mannosidosis

Our studies of the RPE in the mucopolysaccharidoses have illustrated the importance of the lysosomal-degradative pathways for the turnover of GAGs located in the RPE cell coat, or in the extracellular matrices that surround this cell layer (see Aguirre and Stramm, 1991 for review). Our results emphasize also that RPE disease per se is not causally associated with visual cell disease and neuroretinal degeneration. It could be argued that lysosomal degradation of RPE GAGs, although important for the turnover and remodeling of cell surface and matrix proteoglycans, is not sufficient by itself to cause visual cell disease when a degradative pathway is impaired by an inherited disease. However, similar preservation of photoreceptor integrity is main-

differences in expression of the deficient (ASB) enzyme. For example, cell cultures initiated from the inferior and peripheral regions of the eye, which show no substrate storage, have equally deficient ASB activity as cultures from the superior regions and posterior pole, areas which exhibit massive substrate accumulation. This is similar to what occurs in normals, where ASB activity is uniform, but high, throughout the monolayer (Stramm et al., 1986).

Regional differences in RPE metabolism of GAGs determine disease topography. To determine the factors that regulate the topography of disease expression in MPS VI, we have examined the regional metabolism of GAGs in the RPE using an in vitro approach. The extent of radiolabeled GAG accumulation was dependent on the

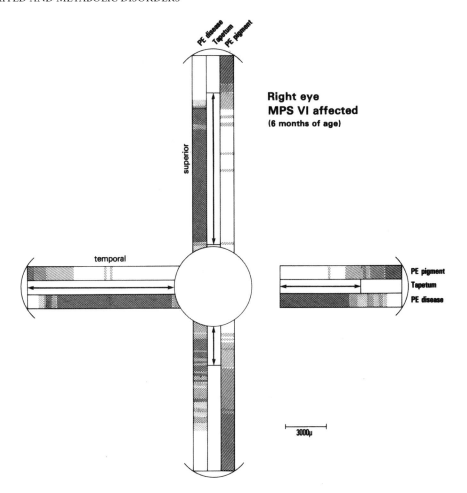

FIGURE 14-26. Schematic representation of the distribution of PE disease, pigmentation and the presence of the tapetum lucidum in the eye of a young MPS VI–affected cat. For comparison with the normal see Figure 14-3. The eye is drawn to scale based on observations of sequential 150 μm fields extending from the disc to the ora serrata *(curved line)*. Note that the tapetum is present primarily in the superior, nasal, and temporal meridians. The pigment epithelium is not pigmented in areas where the tapetum is present. Disease in the pigment epithelium, characterized by the accumulation of vacuolated inclusions and cellular hypertrophy, is more severe in areas where the cell layer is not pigmented. This is most dramatic in the superior meridian. *Key:* arrows indicate the presence of tapetum; RPE pigmentation varies from absent (empty) to moderate (density present in the far periphery); RPE disease varies from normal (empty) to moderate (darker shading indicates that >50% of the cell volume is occupied by vacuolated inclusions and hypertrophy is present). (For details refer to Aguirre et al., 1983, from which this figure was reprinted.)

tained in another lysosomal-storage disorder which is critically involved in rhodopsin degradation.

Acidic α-mannosidase is one of several lysosomal exoglycosidases which sequentially remove sugars from the nonreducing ends of glycoproteins (see Aguirre et al., 1986 for review of animal models of mannosidosis and fucosidosis). Since rhodopsin is the predominant mannose-containing glycoprotein presented to the RPE for degradation, enzyme deficiency results in the progressive accumulation of complex N-linked mannose pentasaccharides (DeGasperi et al., 1991; Alroy et al., 1991). The RPE disease in this mutant is far more severe

and far more rapidly progressive than in the comparable mutants with defects in GAG degradation. The cytoplasm is full of secondary lysosomal inclusions, and, other than compacted and often distorted nuclei, it is difficult to identify cellular organelles (Fig. 14-30). In all other respects, however, the RPE appears to function normally. The participation of the RPE in the outer segment renewal process is evident by the accumulation of phagosomes in the apical cytoplasm, even though the degradation of rhodopsin containing outer segment material is incomplete (Aguirre, Haskins, and Ray, unpublished; Aguirre et al., 1995). The outer segments are

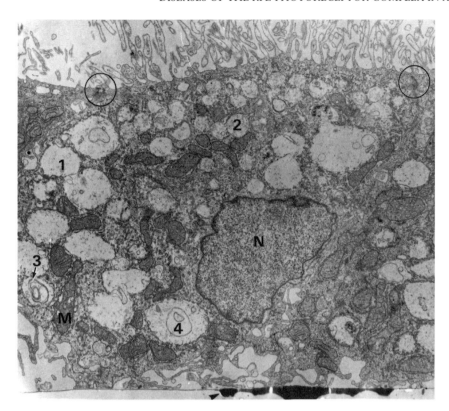

FIGURE 14-27. MPS VI–affected cat RPE after 14 days in tissue culture retains a differentiated phenotype as well as the essential features of the disease (compare with Figure 14-20). There is accumulation of storage in secondary lysosomes; the inclusions appear electron lucent (1), granular (2), lamellar (3), or mixed (4). N = nucleus, M = mitochondria, circle = apicolateral junctions, arrowhead = culture plate. Magnification ×9,400. (Reprinted from Stramm et al., 1985.)

structurally normal, but their average length is reduced by approximately 40%–50%. Similar changes in the RPE have been described in cattle with hereditary α-mannosidase deficiency (Jolly et al., 1987).

The α-mannosidase-deficient mutant has a short lifespan, and most animals die in their first year. It is likely that such a severe deficiency, if sustained for years in an animal or for decades in a human, would eventually result in photoreceptor degeneration secondary to RPE disease. What is more difficult to evaluate, however, is the effect of a less severe but long-term change in the activity of α-mannosidase or another RPE lysosomal enzyme as the result of aging (Wyszynski et al., 1989; Boulton et al., 1994). While there may be an effect on the RPE and neuroretina, our studies in the mutant animals would suggest that the effect is likely to be complex, and modified by other factors, both genetic and environmental, which play a role in the aging eye. Such issues are particularly relevant to a complex disorder such as AMD in man, and continuing studies of the RPE system in these animal models are crucial to clearly defining the importance of the lysosomal degradative pathways in the metabolic pathways of this cell layer.

Experimental Therapy of the RPE in Lysosomal Storage Disorders

Following the in vitro demonstration that soluble "corrective factors" are released into the media and reverse substrate storage in diseased cells (Fratantoni et al., 1968), various strategies have been used to treat the lysosomal storage disorders. Therapy has been directed toward restoring the deficient enzyme function by enhancing residual activity (Vine et al., 1982), by providing normal enzyme directly, or, indirectly, by transplanting bone marrow or other cells (Krivit et al., 1984; Summers et al., 1989; Wenger et al., 1986; Haskins et al., 1991; Akle et al., 1985). More recently, gene therapy using in vivo or ex vivo correction has been accomplished experimentally and in clinical trials. Because the disease may be variable within and between the different clinical entities, and most patients show the disease pheno-

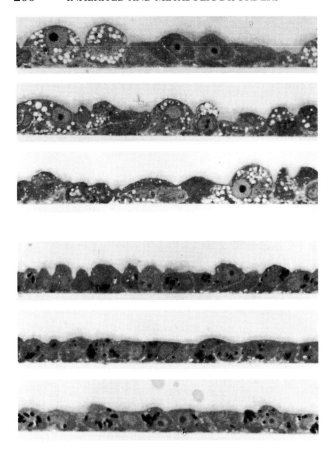

FIGURE 14-28. MPS VI–affected cat RPE cells after 14 days in primary culture. The cells were isolated from defined regions of the eye. The top three sections are of cultures initiated from the superior equatorial region; the three lower sections are from the inferior equatorial region. Although the cultures have equal and deficient levels of ASB activity, only the cells isolated from the superior region are diseased. Magnification ×800. (Reprinted from Aguirre and Stramm, 1991.)

type at the time therapy is initiated, it has been difficult to establish criteria by which the success of therapy can be evaluated. Determination of enzyme activity in the serum or leukocytes provides an objective measurement, but one that may not be appropriate, as the assays generally are made using artificial rather than natural substrates. Consequently, the presence of normal activity in the blood does not necessarily mean that normal degradative function is occurring in the lysosomal compartment of the other affected tissues. In collaboration with associates (M. Haskins and J. Wolfe) at the University of Pennsylvania, our laboratories have examined the effect of bone marrow transplantation (BMT) on the RPE disease phenotype, and have begun experimental gene therapy studies. These areas are discussed below.

Correction of RPE disease phenotype following bone marrow transplantation. Our laboratories have examined the RPE in animal models of MPS VI (cat), VII (dog), and α-mannosidosis (cat) following successful BMT (see Haskins et al., 1991 for review). Within each disease, the results were consistent, but demonstrated that the response to BMT was disease specific. This response appears to be dependent on the amount of enzyme that is

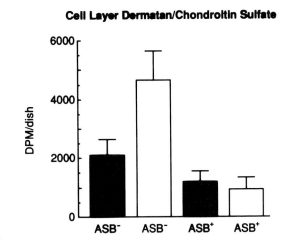

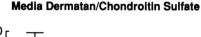

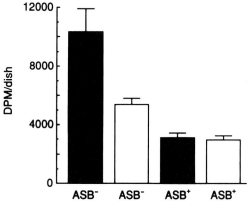

FIGURE 14-29. Cell layer (A) and media (B) GAGs (dermatan sulfate/chondroitin sulfate; DS/CS) at the end of a 72-hour period of labeling with $^{35}SO_4$. Accumulation of radio-labeled DS/CS in the RPE is significantly elevated in MPS VI–affected (ASB⁻) cultures initiated from the superior region of the eye (P < 0.02). No regional differences are present in the normal (ASB⁺) RPE. Release to the media of radio-labeled DS/CS at the end of a 72-hour labeling period is significantly elevated in MPS VI–affected (ASB⁻) cultures initiated from the inferior region of the eye (P < 0.0005). Although not as dramatic, release of ^{35}S-DS/CS also was significantly elevated in affected cultures initiated from the superior region of the eye (P < 0.01). No regional differences were present in the normal (ASB⁺) cultures. Mean ±SEM. Cultures from superior (nonpigmented) region = open bars; cultures from inferior (pigmented) regions = dark bars. (Reprinted from Stramm et al., 1991.)

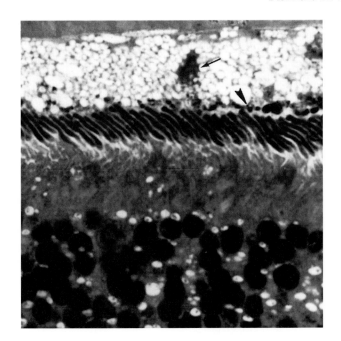

FIGURE 14-30. RPE disease is severe in a young cat affected with α-mannosidase deficiency. The RPE cells are hypertrophied, and the cytoplasm is full of vacuolated inclusions representing incompletely digested substrate that has been leached during tissue processing. The RPE nucleus is indented *(arrow)* by the inclusions that surrounded it; phagosomes *(arrowhead)* are prominently located in the RPE apical region. Although the rod outer segments are shortened, the photoreceptors are intact, but they accumulate inclusions in the inner segment and perinuclear region. Magnification ×1,250. (Aguirre, Haskins and Ray, unpublished.)

normally present extracellularly, and released by the transplanted cells.

Even though MPS VI–affected animals have shown improvement in some tissues after BMT (Gasper et al., 1984), we have not observed any modification of the RPE disease phenotype (Aguirre, Haskins, and Thrall, unpublished). In these animals, the RPE cells continue to hypertrophy as they progressively accumulate cytoplasmic vacuolated inclusions. A similar lack of correction has been found in the cornea, either following BMT (Aguirre, unpublished) or after reciprocal corneal transplantation where MPS VI–affected corneal buttons were transplanted to corneas of genetically normal animals (Aguirre et al., 1992). In order to correct the disease in the RPE and other tissues following BMT, the normal enzyme has to be released from the hematopoietically derived donor cells and has to enter the target cells by a receptor-mediated internalization process with subsequent targeting to the lysosomal compartment. There, the active enzyme is able to degrade stored substrate and prevent the subsequent GAG accumulation in the secondary lysosomes. Lack of correction of the RPE disease

could result from one or a combination of different mechanisms: low levels of enzyme in the extracellular compartments, failure of diffusion of enzyme from the vascular compartment to the RPE, or failure of the affected RPE cells to internalize the secreted extracellular enzyme. Based on in vitro studies of the RPE, it appears that lack of correction results from the extremely low availability of ASB in the extracellular compartment. Unlike other lysosomal enzymes, ASB activity is primarily intracellular, with very little release to the extracellular compartment (Ray, unpublished).

In contrast, MPS VII–affected dogs show moderate correction of the RPE disease phenotype after long-term BMT. Many areas of the RPE monolayer show absence of storage, while others show small clusters of cells with cytoplasmic vacuolated inclusions (Fig. 14-31, B). Overall, there is no cellular hypertrophy, and BMT results in marked improvement of the RPE disease (Aguirre, Ray, and Haskins, unpublished). Associated with the BMT, there is a dramatic clearing of the cornea, and generalized improvement of the multiorgan disease that is normally present in canine MPS VII (Haskins et al., 1992). Similar studies have been carried out in the mouse model of MPS VII. Dramatic improvement of the disease phenotype was observed in all tissues except the RPE and retina, presumably because the high doses of irradiation given in the perinatal period prior to BMT resulted in complete retinal degeneration (Sands et al., 1993).

We have found that the most remarkable correction of RPE storage occurs following BMT in the feline model of α-mannosidosis. Eighteen months after transplantation, the RPE disease is completely reversed—the cytoplasmic inclusions disappear, cell size returns to normal, and cellular contours are restored (Fig. 14-31, A). As a result of the correction of the RPE disease, the photoreceptor outer segments resume normal orientation and elongate (Aguirre and Haskins, unpublished). As in the MPS VII–treated animals, there is correction of the storage in other organs, particularly the CNS, and the severe, progressive neurologic disease is prevented (Haskins, unpublished; Walkley et al., 1994). The success of correction of the RPE disease phenotype in both models probably results in part from the high levels of extracellular enzyme present following BMT. We have found that the RPE in culture has a very high level of cellular GUSB and α-mannosidase activity, and that it releases into the media catalytically active protein (Ray et al., 1997; Ray, unpublished). It is this extracellular enzyme that presumably is involved in the correction of disease in distant target tissues. These studies demonstrate that RPE disease can be treated by the systemic route as long as the corrective factor being supplied to the diseased cells is available in the extracellular environment.

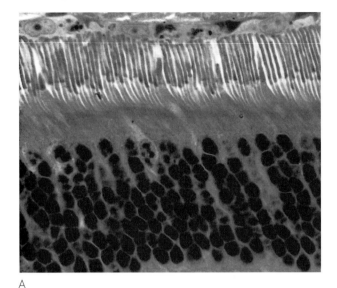

A

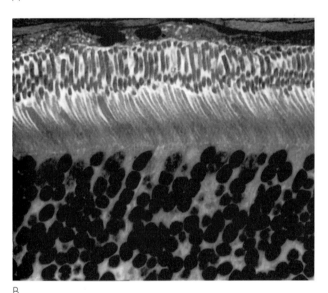

B

FIGURE 14-31. Improvement of RPE disease following long term bone marrow transplantation in a cat with α-mannosidosis *(A)*, and a dog with MPS VII *(B)*; the transplantation intervals are 2 years and 18 months, respectively. In α-mannosidosis *(A)*, the RPE is normal and the photoreceptors have elongated and are now of normal length (compare with Figure 14-30). In contrast, the treated MPS VII dog still shows some accumulation of vacuolated inclusions in the RPE, but no hypertrophy. At this stage the RPE would show marked hypertrophy and the cytoplasm would be full of vacuolated inclusions. Magnification ×800. (Aguirre and Haskins, unpublished.)

Gene therapy of RPE disease in lysosomal storage disorders. The prospects of genetically altering cells and/or organisms that have inherited defects have been improved by the recent advances in molecular biology. In order to genetically engineer the cells, the foreign DNA sequence or gene must not only be introduced into the

cell, but also needs to be expressed. Microinjection, electroporation, and calcium phosphate (or dextran sulfate) coprecipitation of DNA have been the traditional methods by which foreign DNA has been transferred into cells. However, each of these methods has inherent limitations. In some cases, a large number of cells need to be injected; in others, the efficiency of transfection and/or expression is low.

The use of retroviral vectors to mediate gene transfer has overcome many of the limitations inherent in other methods of DNA transfer. By altering the structure of internal retroviral sequences, these vectors lack the polymerase and glycoprotein genes essential for replication, and contain instead the foreign DNA that is to be transferred. The deleted sequences, or *trans* acting functions, are provided by a packaging cell line which determines the host range and viral titers produced (Miller and Buttimore, 1986). These retroviral vectors are infective but replication incompetent, and they usually result in the high-efficiency transfer of the foreign DNA. Their disadvantage, however, is that the transferred DNA integrates randomly into the host cell chromosomes.

For most of our studies we have used retroviral vectors which have internal promoters and the cDNA sequences to be transferred (Armentano et al., 1987; Wolfe et al., 1990) (Fig. 14-32) These vectors are designed to use two different promoters (the strong promoter from the retroviral 5' long-terminal repeat [LTR] and an independent internal promoter) to regulate the expression of two different genes: the *neo* gene and the transferred cDNA. The *neo* gene confers resistance to the neomycin analog G-418, and provides a means for selecting in vitro those cells infected and transduced by the retroviral vector; that is, only transduced cells will survive when G-418 is added to the culture media. We also have used other vectors without internal promoters or selectable marker genes, and have found them to be

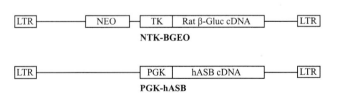

FIGURE 14-32. Retroviral vectors used to mediate cDNA transfer to the RPE. The NTK-BGO vector contains the rat β-glucuronidase cDNA driven by the herpes simplex thymidine kinase (TK) promoter, and the *neo* gene is used for selection of the transduced cells. A similar vector contains the SV-40 promoter to regulate the rat GUSB cDNA expression (see Wolfe et al., 1990, for details). The PGK-hASB vector has the human arylsulfatase B cDNA under the control of the mouse phosphoglucokinase-1 (PGK) promoter, but no selectable marker. (LTR) = long terminal repeat. (Ray et al., 1995.)

equally effective in transferring and expressing a foreign DNA in cultured RPE cells (Fig. 14-32).

In vitro correction of RPE disease in MPS VII (dog) and MPS VI (cat). The rat GUSB cDNA has been transferred in vitro to the RPE of MPS VII–affected dogs using one of two different N2–derived retroviral vectors that contain the entire coding sequence of the rat GUSB cDNA (Nishimura et al., 1986; Wolfe et al., 1990). The difference between the vectors is in the internal promoter used to drive the heterologous cDNA; these are the simian virus 40 (SV-40) and the herpes simplex thymidine kinase (TK) promoters, which are cloned upstream from the rat GUSB cDNA (Fig. 14-32). Both the SV-40 and TK promoters are constitutive promoters with no RPE specificity, yet the level of expression of the gene they regulate is sufficient to correct the inherited RPE defect (see below). It appears, therefore, that nonspecific promoters can be used in the RPE to regulate the expression of a gene that subserves a critical degradative function. Use of these vectors in high concentration (2×10^6 CFU/ml) results in high efficiency of RPE cell transduction without any impairment of cellular growth, metabolism, or viability (Stramm et al., 1990; Wolfe et al., 1990; Ray et al., 1992).

Following retroviral mediated GUSB cDNA transfer, the MPS VII–affected RPE cells show complete restoration of GUSB activity. This represents approximately a three- to five-hundred-fold increase in activity from the levels measured in untreated affected cells. The effect is specific, as the activity of other lysosomal enzymes remains normal and unchanged (Table 14-5; Ray, unpublished). These results have been confirmed in separate experiments using RPE cells from different affected dogs and the same vector constructs. We have found that the GUSB activity present in the vector-treated RPE cells is catalytically active on the natural substrate, and corrects the block in GAG degradation. Following 72 hours of continuous labeling with $^{35}SO_4$, the synthesized GAGs retained by the cell layer of the vector-treated cells are the same as in normal. In contrast, the untreated, affected cells accumulate heparan and chondroitin sulfates (Figs. 14-33, 14-34). The restoration of normal GAG-degradative function in the vector-treated cells occurs specifically in the cell layer compartment, as there are no changes in the media GAGs to indicate increased secretion or enhanced extracellular degradation. The localization of GUSB activity in the lysosomal compartment of the MPS VII vector-treated cells has been demonstrated histochemically (Wolfe et al., 1990).

Similar studies have been carried out in MPS VI cat RPE cells having a deficiency of ASB (Ray et al., 1995). Transduction of RPE cells was done using a retroviral vector containing the human ASB cDNA driven by the

TABLE 14-5. *Lysosomal enzyme activities in cultured MPS VII–affected and vector-treated RPE cells*

Group	β-glucuronidase	α-L-iduronidase (α-mannosidase)
Experiment # 1		
MPS VII	5%*	(88%)
Experiment # 2		
MPS VII	0.3%*	107%
MPS VII/TK1	117%	103%
Experiment # 3		
MPS VII	0.2%*	88%
MPS VII/TK1	71%	84%
MPS VII/SV8	102%	118%

Table reproduced from Aguirre and Stramm, 1991 and contains data from Wolfe et al., 1990 and Stramm et al., 1990.

Enzyme activities determined as nmol of substrate cleaved/hour/mg protein and expressed as % of normal control values. Each determination is based on four to ten different samples of three separate experiments: Experiment 1—primary cultures; Experiments 2 and 3—second passage cultures.

*Within experiment comparison between affected and normal or treated cells, $p < 0.001$, t-test. TK1 and SV8-cells infected with vectors NTK-BG-A1 and NSV-BG-A8 having the rat GUSB cDNA under the control, respectively, of the thymidine kinase and SV-40 promoters (Wolfe et al., 1990).

mouse phosphoglucokinase-1 promoter (Fig. 14-32). In the affected cells, the ASB activity was only 5%–10% of normal, but, following transduction, there was a hundredfold increase in enzymatic activity. Restoration of ASB activity resulted in a remarkable decrease in the storage of dermatan sulfate, the GAG that accumulates in the MPS VI RPE and other tissues.

In vivo correction of RPE disease in the MPS VII mouse. The MPS VII mouse model has been used extensively to explore different treatment modalities aimed at correcting the lysosomal enzyme deficiency, and arresting or reversing the pathologic sequela. Transgenic MPS VII mice that overexpress the human GUSB cDNA in a heterozygous manner show complete reversal of the storage disease (Kyle et al., 1990). Retroviral vectors also have been used to transduce enzyme deficient hematopoietic stem cells or fibroblasts with the normal GUSB cDNA, followed by transplantation of these cells into MPS VII mice. Treatment results in variable degrees of tissue-specific correction of the disease phenotype, but there have been no reports of the correction of the ocular lesions (Wolfe et al., 1992; Maréchal et al., 1993; Moullier et al., 1993). In regards to the eye, the most dramatic correction of the RPE disease in vivo has been effected by the adenoviral-mediated transfer of the human GUSB cDNA to ocular tissues following the intravitreal injection of the viral vector. In short-term ex-

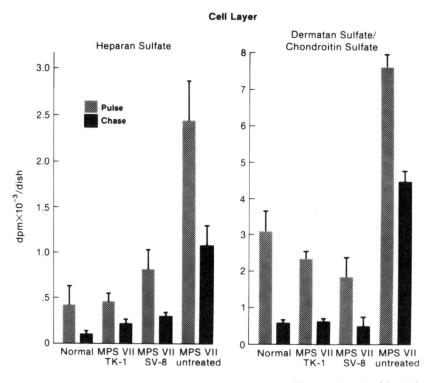

FIGURE 14-33. Cell layer GAGs in normal, MPS VII–affected, and vector-treated affected cells (MPS VII/TK-1, MPS VII/SV-8) following a 72-hour labeling period (pulse) with $^{35}SO_4$, or after a 24-hour chase. The two vector constructs were similar except for the internal promoter driving the rat GUSB cDNA: TK-1 = herpes simplex thymidine kinase promoter, SV-8 = simian virus 40 promoter (see Wolfe et al., 1990, for details). In the MPS VII–untreated cells, newly synthesized radio-labeled GAGs (heparan sulfate and chondroitin sulfate) accumulate in the cell layer at the end of the 72-hour pulse and remain elevated after a 24-hour chase period. In contrast, the vector-treated cells have normal levels of GAGs in the cell layer at the two time periods examined. Enzyme digestion and deamination indicates that the increased radioactivity in the dermatan sulfate/chondroitin sulfate peak of the MPS VII cells is only in chondroitin sulfate. (Reprinted from Aguirre and Stramm, 1991.)

periments that lasted up to three weeks, reversal of the RPE storage began after one week, and, by three weeks, the MPS VII RPE was indistinguishable from normal (Li and Davidson, 1995). It is not clear from these studies if the adenoviral-vector-mediated cDNA transfer directly corrected the affected RPE cells, or whether cells located outside the RPE–photoreceptor interface were corrected, and secreted GUSB enzyme that diffused into the subretinal space and cross-corrected the diseased RPE. Another issue not established from these studies is the duration of correction. Since adenoviral vectors do not stably integrate into the host cell's genetic material, it is likely that long-term stability of expression will not occur, thus necessitating repeated treatments.

These studies indicate the feasibility of using vector mediated cDNA transfer to correct inherited defects of the RPE. In vitro, there is high efficiency of transduction of RPE cells, and the retroviral-vector-corrected cells show stable and long-term expression of the transferred cDNA (J. Ray, unpublished). In vivo, the recent studies using adenoviral vectors are extremely encouraging, and illustrate the possibilities of gene therapy for the treatment of diseases of the RPE and other posterior segment structures. Some of the issues of gene therapy in the RPE have been discussed previously (Aguirre and Stramm, 1991).

RPE LIPOIDAL EPITHELIOPATHY

Aging Monkey

We and others have noted the presence of clusters of yellow flecks and dots present in the foveomacular region of aged rhesus monkeys that are maintained in long-term toxicologic studies (Fine and Kwapien, 1978; Bellhorn et al., 1981). These abnormalities have been described clinically as "pigmentary abnormalities of the macula" or "lipoidal degeneration" and represent a common aging response of the rhesus monkey RPE. Similar lesions have been described in cynomolgus monkeys (Feeney-Burns et al., 1981). In the rhesus monkey,

RPE Cell Layer ^{35}S-Labeled GAGs

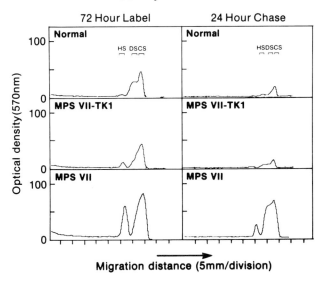

FIGURE 14-34. Scanning densitometer tracings of $^{35}SO_4$-labeled RPE cell layer GAGs after continuous labeling for 72 hours or after a 24-hour chase period. Each densitometer tracing represents the cell layer GAGs of one culture of normal, MPS VII–affected, or TK 1–vector-treated affected cells (MPS VII–TK1) for each labeling period. The markers indicate where the different GAGs run on the scan. The MPS VII–affected RPE shows two prominent peaks of radioactivity consisting of HS and a DS/CS doublet. After the 24-hour chase period, the levels of radioactivity decrease, but never approximate those of the normal or treated cells. (Reprinted with modification from Stramm et al., 1990.)

the lesions are found in both males and females, and appear to increase in severity with aging. The mildest form is characterized by a slight unevenness in macular pigmentation. Later, the macula has a finely stippled or a salt-and-pepper appearance. In the most severe form, the foveomacular region has variable numbers of yellowish flecks (hypopigmented spots) which result in loss of the foveal reflex (Bellhorn et al., 1981). Fluorescein angiographic studies have reported conflicting findings. One study indicates that the hypopigmented spots result in window defects visible on angiography; the window effect being caused by vacuolization of individual RPE cells (Fine and Kwapien, 1978). A second study has not been able to confirm these findings, and no association between the location and extent of the hypopigmented spots and angiographically visible fluorescent foci has been established (Bellhorn et al., 1981). These foveomacular pigmentary abnormalities cause no impairment of function as assessed by retinal testing with electroretinography and visual evoked responses (Bellhorn et al., 1981). Morphologically, the affected RPE cells and adjacent photoreceptors remain intact (Fine and Kwapien, 1978; Fine, 1981; Aguirre and Bellhorn, unpublished).

In glutaraldehyde/osmium-fixed retinas embedded in plastic, light microscopic abnormalities are readily apparent in some RPE cells located in the foveomacular region. The affected cells contain light brown to dark brown inclusions which, when numerous, completely fill the cell. These abnormalities are extremely difficult to detect in eyes that are conventionally fixed, embedded in paraffin, and sectioned at 5–6 μm. By electron microscopy, the affected RPE cells accumulate intracytoplasmic inclusions (Fine and Kwapien, 1978; Fine, 1981; Aguirre and Bellhorn, unpublished). The vacuoles have a distinct limiting membrane, and, in most cases, have low electron density and a homogeneous appearance; in some cells, the inclusions are electron lucent and empty (Fig. 14-35). When few in number, they usually are located basally. As their number increase, the inclu-

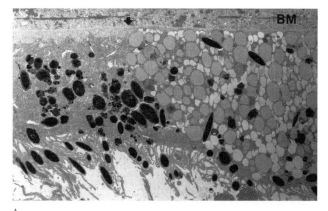

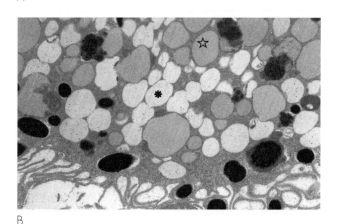

FIGURE 14-35. Macular RPE of an aged rhesus monkey. Upper panel (A) shows an RPE cell *(right of vertical arrow)* whose cytoplasm is full of lipoidal inclusions of varying electron density. The cell on the left is unaffected, and contains melanin granules and lipofuscin and melano-lipofuscin inclusions. The lower panel (B) shows that the lipoidal inclusions are homogeneous *(open star)* or vacuolated (*). BM = Bruch's membrane. Magnifications: upper panel ×3,500; lower panel ×8,600. (Aguirre and Bellhorn, unpublished.)

sions are located in the basal and central zones, often in close proximity to lysosomal and/or lipofuscin granules. The lipid origin of these inclusions has been confirmed by using osmium tetroxide fixation for electron microscopy, or glutaraldehyde fixation prior to cryosectioning and oil red O staining (Fine, 1981). It is likely that these lipid inclusions have a similar origin to those identified in the RPE of human eyes (El Baba, et al., 1986).

Congenital Stationary Night Blindness (CSNB) in the Dog

Lipoidal epitheliopathy also has been described in the RPE of Swedish briard dogs having congenital night blindness (Narfström et al., 1994). The disease, initially described as a stationary disorder analogous to human CSNB, is now considered to have a progressive component (Narfström et al., 1989b; Wrigstad, 1994). In general, affected dogs have an ERG of normal waveform, but showing a marked diminution of the response amplitudes, similar to a "Riggs-type" ERG in man. The ERG recorded under DC conditions shows complete absence of the a-, b-, and c-waves, with the latter waveform being replaced by a very slow negative potential which develops when the stimulus intensity is greater than 3 log units above the normal b-wave threshold. The authors interpret the abnormalities in the a- and b-waves as representing a delay in rod phototransduction, while the lack of a c-wave was ascribed to the morphologic abnormalities identified in the RPE (Nilsson et al., 1992).

Microscopic examination of the RPE showed the presence of large inclusions in the central and midperipheral tapetal regions in dogs as early as 3.5 months of age. By light microscopy, the inclusions are single to multiple; depending on the fixative used, they are vacuolated or appear homogeneous and stain intensely with crystal violet or other lipid stains (R. Riis, personal communication, 1995). Ultrastructurally, the inclusions are electron lucent vacuoles with a more homogeneous cortex which often contains membranous debris (Wrigstad et al., 1992; 1994). Unlike the lipoidal inclusions found in the aging monkey RPE, a single limiting membrane was absent or not distinct in some of the vacuoles. With aging, the inclusions increase in number and are found in the peripheral RPE cells. The striking feature of some of the lipid inclusions is their immense size (Fig. 14-36).

At this time, the association between the lipoidal changes in the RPE and the primary photoreceptor defect is unknown. That this interesting RPE abnormality

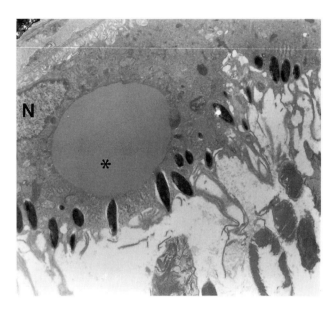

FIGURE 14-36. Nontapetal RPE of adult briard dog with congenital stationary night blindness. Note the extremely large and homogeneous lipid inclusion (*) present in the RPE which dwarfs the cell nucleus (N). The retina is artifactually detached. Magnification ×5,200. (Photograph courtesy of Dr. Ron Riis.)

is not an incidental finding is demonstrated by the presence of similar RPE lesions in unrelated briard dogs with CSNB, both in France and the United States. However, the causal association between the RPE and photoreceptor pathology is not clear. The ERG results indicate a widespread transduction disorder of all photoreceptors. In contrast, the RPE lipid storage, although prominent, is not present uniformly in all cells, and the severity of the RPE pathology and photoreceptor dysfunction are not correlated.

RPE AUTOFLUORESCENT INCLUSION EPITHELIOPATHY

Retinal Pigment Epithelial Dystrophy (RPED)

Central progressive retinal atrophy (CPRA) is a specific pigment epithelial dystrophy recognized in several breeds of dogs (Parry, 1954; Aguirre and Laties, 1976), which is now termed *retinal pigment epithelial dystrophy* (RPED) (Bedford, 1984). Ophthalmoscopically, the disease is characterized by the accumulation of irregular foci of light brown pigment over the tapetal zone; with time, these foci increase in size and become distributed throughout the tapetal fundus (Plate 14-VII). In the end stages of the disease, the pigmentation decreases or forms clusters around the margins of foci of retinal atrophy.

Using conventional histologic methods, the earliest

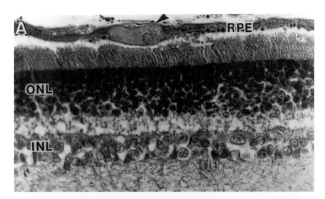

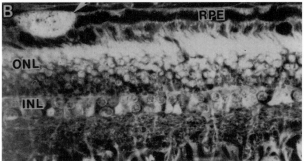

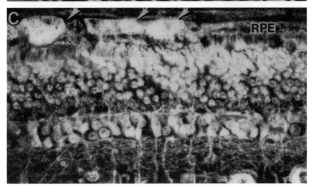

FIGURE 14-37. Retinal pigment epithelial dystrophy (RPED) in the dog. (A) In the early stages of the disease, there is focal hypertrophy of the RPE *(arrowhead)* with accumulation of granular light brown material in the cytoplasm. (B) This material is intensely autofluorescent *(white arrow)*. Note that the rest of the RPE layer is normal. (C) With time, more cells in the monolayer become diseased *(white arrowheads)*. Opposite the hypertrophied cells, the photoreceptor inner and outer segments are disoriented and compressed. The outer and inner nuclear layers (ONL and INL) show normal levels of autofluorescence for fixed tissues. Magnifications: (A) and (B) ×280; (C) ×225.

recognizable lesion is in the RPE. Individual cells become hypertrophied and accumulate a light brown granular material in the cytoplasm. Opposite the hypertrophied cells, the photoreceptor outer segments are shortened. Gradually, the focal lesion spreads in the RPE monolayer, and more cells become hypertrophied (Fig. 14-37). In the end stages of the disease, the hypertrophied RPE cells form multicellular cell nests; at this

time, there is focal degeneration of the photoreceptors followed by complete retinal degeneration with intraretinal migration of non-melanin-containing cells. Fluorescent microscopy of unstained retinal sections indicates that the diseased RPE cells, either located on Bruch's membrane or migrating intraretinally, contain a bright autofluorescent lipopigment similar to ceroid or lipofuscin (Fig. 14-37B, C). Recent studies reported in abstract form suggest that the pigments that accumulate in the disease vary by breed, and differ from those that accumulate in the aging human RPE in that they are the result of peroxidation of rod outer segment lipids (Watson and Bedford, 1992; P. Watson, personal communication, 1993).

Most current studies of RPED have been carried out in the briard dog breed in the United Kingdom (Bedford, 1984; Lightfoot, 1988) (Note that RPED differs from the CSNB, which also is reported in briards.). These have demonstrated that rod outer segment renewal is normal, as is acid phosphatase activity in the RPE. In contrast, affected dogs are hypercholesterolemic and systemically deficient in vitamin E and taurine (P. Bedford, personal communication, 1996; Watson et al., 1993).

The clinical and histologic features of RPED are similar to vitamin E deficiency retinopathy in dogs, either naturally acquired (Hayes et al., 1970) or produced experimentally (Riis et al., 1981). In all three diseases, the RPE cells become hypertrophied and accumulate lipofuscin inclusions. In the experimental deficiency, however, lipofuscin accumulation and RPE hypertrophy occur after there is the beginning of photoreceptor outer segment degeneration visible by electron microscopy, and the disease course is much more rapid (Riis et al., 1981). This suggests that the target cell for the disease may be the photoreceptor, even though the most dramatic manifestation of the disease is in the RPE.

The similarities between RPED and vitamin E deficiency may explain its unique geographic distribution. The disease was once prevalent in the United States, but now is extremely rare, and only sporadic cases are identified. In Western Europe, particularly the United Kingdom, by contrast, the disease has had a very high prevalence until recently, and many breeds of dogs have been affected. Because of the possibility that RPED is associated with antioxidant deficiency, the disease frequency in young dogs has been markedly reduced with the widespread use of vitamin E supplementation (P. Bedford, personal communication, 1996). It is not clear at this time, however, whether the disease represents a strictly nutritional deficiency, or is an inherited defect that becomes manifested clinically by inadequate diets.

Equine Motor Neuron Disease (EMND)

A spontaneous neuronopathy has been recently identified in adult horses which bears a striking resemblance to the sporadic form of amyotrophic lateral sclerosis of man (Cummings et al., 1990). The disease is a progressive degeneration of motor neurons of the spinal cord and brainstem which results in muscle atrophy, weakness, and wasting; it is generally fatal. Studies have suggested an association between vitamin E deficiency and EMND, since affected animals have been found to have marked decreases in plasma vitamin E levels (Divers et al., 1994), and they have demonstrated ceroid lipopigment accumulation in the endothelial cells of small vessels in the spinal cord (Cummings et al., 1995).

Characteristic lesions of the RPE have been found in most animals with clinical abnormalities indicative of EMND; in all cases, the ocular abnormalities have always been found in association with the neurologic disease. Fundus examination reveals a horizontal linear or mosaic pattern of pigmentation, located either close to the optic disc or throughout the fundus. These lesions are bilateral, but may vary in severity between the two eyes (Riis et al., 1995). The fundus abnormalities are the result of accumulation of an autofluorescent lipopigment within hypertrophied RPE cells. Initially, the hypertrophied cells occur in foci with no apparent photoreceptor disease. Later, there is degeneration of the photoreceptor cells and inner retinal layers, and macrophages accumulate in the interphotoreceptor space and migrate intraretinally. Autofluorescent lipopigments are found in the hypertrophied RPE and in macrophages. By electron microscopy, the RPE lipopigments are typical of lipofuscin and ceroid (Fig. 14-38) (Cummings et al., in press; R. Riis, personal communication, 1995)

Neuronal Ceroid Lipofuscinosis (NCL)

The neuronal ceroid lipofuscinoses in man are a group of diseases divided into distinct syndromes based on clinical and pathologic criteria; in general, four syndromes have been recognized (infantile, late infantile, juvenile, and adult), and each has a complex of eponyms. Although the diseases have a broad spectrum of neurologic abnormalities, the common denominator is the accumulation of autofluorescent lipopigments in neurons and other cells (Jolly and Palmer, 1995). Except for the infantile form of the disease, which is caused by mutations in the palmitoyl protein thioesterase gene, the molecular basis of NCL is unknown (Vesa et al., 1995). The same diversity of clinical disease and ocular abnormalities also occurs in animals with NCL (Aguirre et al.,

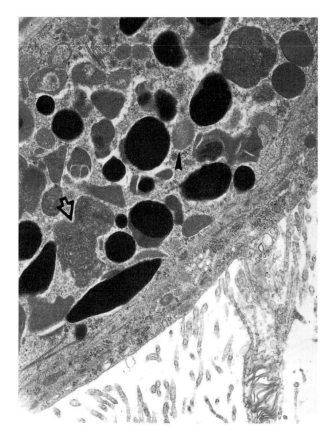

FIGURE 14-38. RPE cell from horse affected with equine motor neuron disease (EMND). Melanin granules and numerous lipofuscin *(arrowhead)* and ceroid *(open arrow)* inclusions are present in the cytoplasm. Magnification ×8500. (Photograph courtesy of Drs. R. Riis and J. Cummings.)

1986; Jolly and Palmer, 1995; Jolly et al., 1994). A common clinical manifestation in both man and animals is the presence of blindness, which occurs at approximately the same time as the clinical syndrome with which it is associated. With some exceptions (see below), the blindness is cortical in origin, since photoreceptor structure and function generally are preserved.

In sheep, an early adult onset, acute form of NCL has been described. Animals develop normally for several months after birth, and then show progressive neurologic abnormalities, visual deficits, and blindness; death occurs by approximately two years of age. Blindness in sheep is the result of a progressive degeneration of the photoreceptor cells, particularly the rods. In affected animals, there is a marked loss of rod-mediated ERG responses until they disappear soon after one year of age; cone responses, on the other hand, remain normal until that time and decay thereafter. These functional abnormalities are reflected in the pathology of the retina, which demonstrates a progressive rod-cone degenerative process. The RPE remains relatively normal throughout the disease, but accumulates numerous electron-dense membranous cytoplasmic structures which are autofluorescent. However, these inclusions are smaller and less numerous than elsewhere in the retina (Graydon and Jolly, 1984). Additionally, RPE function, as determined by the response to azide, remains normal even in blind, terminal animals (R. Jolly, personal communication, 1984). Extensive photoreceptor degeneration with preservation of the RPE also has been found in Devon cattle with NCL (Jolly et al., 1992).

In contrast, most canine forms of NCL are distinguished by blindness of nonretinal origin (see Jolly et al., 1994 for review). Of these, the best characterized disease is that found in the English setter which has an early adult onset with an acute course (see Koppang, 1992 for review). In this breed, retinal function is initially normal at a time when neurologic abnormalities are present. Thereafter, ERG responses become reduced (Berson and Watson, 1980; Aguirre et al., 1986), and, in the very late stages of the disease, the DC recorded ERG shows a severe depression of the responses. At this time, there is a decrease in amplitude and eventual disappearance of the ERG c-wave, and a reduction in the standing potential (Nilsson et al., 1983). These findings suggest an impairment of RPE function.

Retinal abnormalities associated with NCL have been reported in the Tibetan terrier (Riis et al., 1992), miniature schnauzer (Smith et al., 1996) and Polish Owczarek Nizinny (Wrigstad et al., 1995) dog breeds. In Tibetan terriers night blindness is the primary clinical abnormality recognized in young animals. In contrast, NCL in the Nizinny breed appears clinically similar to RPED, and the fundus shows the accumulation of irregular foci of light brown pigment over the tapetal zone which, histologically, reflects the storage of autofluorescent lipopigments in hypertrophied RPE cells . In these three breeds, the clinical manifestations of NCL are initially retinal (photoreceptor or RPE), with neurological abnormalities occurring later in life.

As in humans and other animal models of NCL, autofluorescent lipopigment inclusions accumulate in the RPE cells and other retinal and CNS neurons of affected English setter dogs. However, the association between neuronal lipopigment storage and cell death is not known. Since there is no degeneration of the retina or RPE cells in many different animals with this disease, even though significant storage is present (Neville et al., 1980), the causal association between lipopigment storage, cell dysfunction, and cell death is not clear at this time. This will require identification of the molecular defects present in these different diseases, and characterization of the biochemical abnormalities resulting from the gene defect(s).

MACULAR ABNORMALITIES AND DRUSEN IN MONKEYS

Macular degeneration is uncommon in the subhuman primate. With few exceptions, abnormalities of the macula occur sporadically, and are reported as single case studies. Attempts to determine if macular degeneration occurs naturally in primates have resulted in surveys of monkey colonies (Stafford, 1974; El-Mofty et al., 1978; Nicolas et al., 1996), the most extensive of these undertaken at the Cayo Santiago colony, a part of the Caribbean Primate Center (El-Mofty et al., 1978; 1980; Engel et al., 1988; Dawson et al., 1989). In their initial survey, El-Mofty and colleagues (1978) reported two types of macular anomalies which were age related and affected approximately half of the 105 animals examined: (a) a macular pigmentary disorder showing various degrees of irregularity in the distribution and intensity of pigmentation, and (b) multiple discrete small white spots that mainly clustered in the paramacular area. The pigmentary abnormalities probably are the lipoidal epitheliopathy described in a preceding section, while the paramacular white spots were interpreted by the authors as drusen. A repeat study of a larger group of animals confirmed the previous observations and found that over 80% of old animals had macular lesions (El-Mofty et al., 1980). However, some young animals one to three years of age also showed similar lesions of equal severity, suggesting a heritable component to the disorder. A separate and independent survey of this colony has been undertaken, and confirmed the presence of macular drusen which, histologically, are nearly identical to similar lesions found in the human eye. Although this limited sample did not show any animals with the exudative form of AMD or disciform scars (Engels et al., 1988), a larger sampling reported older animals with end-stage disciform changes (Dawson et al., 1989).

In a study by Feeney-Burns and colleagues (1981), the authors examined the retinas of cynomolgus monkeys with macular abnormalities visible by ophthalmoscopy or fluorescein angiography. Lipoidal epitheliopathy, misshapen foveal depressions, RPE depigmentation, and exudative foci underneath the RPE were found. Surprisingly, morphologic examination of the macular region of animals considered clinically normal showed retinal pathology limited to the macular region. These consisted of degeneration of parafoveal cones, ballooning and disarray of foveolar cone outer segment disc membranes, and accumulation of lamellar, osmiophilic material in the inner and outer segments. The authors emphasized the importance of thoroughly characterizing the normalcy of primate populations before their use in experimental studies.

Drusen have been reported in monkeys, either limited to the macular region, or uniformly distributed throughout the fundus (Barnett et al., 1972; Stafford, 1974; El-Mofty et al., 1980; Ishibashi et al., 1986). The histologic appearance of the lesions is quite characteristic, and similar to comparable abnormalities in man. As noted previously, the incidence of macular and paramacular druse increases with aging. Generalized drusen of the fundus have been found in baboons and rhesus monkeys, usually at a young age, suggesting that these lesions may be present congenitally or develop in the perinatal period. They occur as large, single or multiple nodules which are overlaid by an extremely thin and attenuated RPE. Other than disorientation of the apposed photoreceptor cells, there is surprisingly minimal pathology of the retina (Barnett et al., 1972; Aguirre, unpublished).

A bilateral macular degeneration associated with widespread outer retinal disease has been reported in a colony of captive reared Guinea baboons (Vainisi et al., 1974). In the propositus, the maculae were atrophic, with a reticular yellow metallic appearance, and prominent window defects were evident on angiography (Plate 14-VIII). The RPE and retina were absent in the macular region; more peripherally, there was photoreceptor degeneration with RPE preservation. Additional studies on animals from this colony have shown that the disease is likely to be hereditary, but the mode of inheritance has not been established. In young animals, the initial clinical abnormalities are restricted to the macula (subtle depigmentation in the fovea surrounded by a hyperpigmented ring); histologically, the RPE is normal, but disease is present in the photoreceptors and is more widespread. There is initially degeneration of parafoveal rods and cones which subsequently spreads to involve those photoreceptors in the equator and periphery. In animals with advanced macular degeneration, there is extensive degeneration and loss of the photoreceptor and outer nuclear layers in the equator and periphery (Tso et al., 1983; Santos-Anderson et al., 1983). Unfortunately, a colony of this potentially important animal model for human retinal disease is no longer extant.

ORNITHINE-δ-AMINO TRANSFERASE DEFICIENCY IN CATS

Deficiency of the mitochondrial matrix enzyme ornithine-δ-amino transferase (OAT) causes a retinal degeneration in man and cats. In man, the disease is termed *gyrate atrophy of the choroid and retina* because of the characteristic fundus lesions. In contrast, cats with OAT deficiency have a generalized retinal degen-

eration (Plate 14-IX) that is clinically indistinguishable from that present in animals affected with PRA, the group of primary photoreceptor degenerative diseases.

In cats the disease has been found sporadically, and is characterized by hundredfold elevation in plasma ornithine levels with overflow ornithinuria (Valle et al., 1981; 1983; Rosenzweig et al., 1990). This results from deficiency of OAT in tissues, and enzyme deficiency is confirmed in cultured fibroblasts. A suggestion of autosomal recessive inheritance is based on the finding that presumably heterozygous animals have reduced OAT activity levels that are intermediate between affected and normal cats (Giger, personal communication, 1995). In one animal, OAT was pyridoxine responsive, but long-term oral supplementation with this vitamin did not affect the progression of retinal degeneration (Aguirre, unpublished). Histologic examination of the retina shows complete atrophy of the RPE and photoreceptor cells, and end-stage retinal degeneration (Fig.

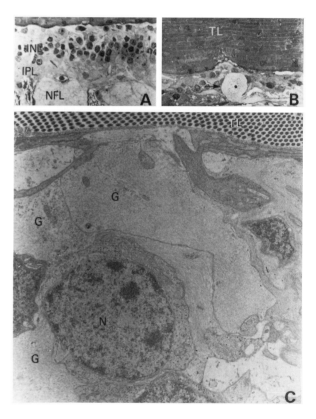

FIGURE 14-39. Light (A and B) and electron (C) micrographs of the tapetal retina from an adult cat with ornithine-δ-amino transferase deficiency. (A) Retina in the posterior pole shows loss of RPE and photoreceptor layers, with preservation of inner retina (INL, IPL, NFL). (B) Tapetal region (TL) showing a very thin and gliotic retina with a prominent ganglion cell. (C) Unidentified neuron (N) surrounded by prominent glial fibers (G) is located adjacent to the tapetum lucidum (TL). Magnifications: (A) and (B) ×400, (C) ×9,600. (Reprinted from Valle et al., 1981.)

14-39) (Valle et al., 1981). Such extensive atrophy of the outer retina is unusual for retinal-degenerative disorders in cats or other animals.

THE RPE AND ECTOPIC PHOTORECEPTOR NUCLEI

Subretinal displacement of photoreceptor nuclei has been found in many different animal species. In the rat, the displacement reflects a general mechanism of cell loss that is influenced, to some extent, by aging and environmental exposure to high ambient light intensities (Lai et al., 1978; Lai 1980). A similar process occurs in humans and has been associated with age-related degenerative disorders of the eye, diabetes, or systemic infections (Lai et al., 1982). In most cases, the distinct cytologic characteristics of the photoreceptor nuclei help to distinguish them from the phagocytic cells that invade the subretinal space during the degenerative phase of primary photoreceptor diseases (see "Photoreceptor degeneration, RPE pigmentation, and interphotoreceptor space phagocytic cells," above).

The presence of ectopically located photoreceptor nuclei in the subretinal space is supposed to represent two different cell death mechanisms: in situ death followed by displacement, and the outward movement of photoreceptors with their subsequent death in the subretinal space (Lai et al., 1982). Recent studies in dogs with inherited cone degeneration question the loss of viability of the ectopically located photoreceptor cell nuclei, particularly cones (Gropp et al., 1996).

We have previously identified a canine model for rod monochromatism in man (Aguirre and Rubin, 1974; 1975). The disease was initially termed *hemeralopia*, but, in order to prevent etymological controversy, the name and gene locus identification were changed to *cone degeneration* (Long and Aguirre, 1991). Cone degeneration *(cd)* is a rare, autosomal recessive disorder found originally in the Alaskan malamute breed, and characterized by specific functional and structural abnormalities limited to the cone photoreceptors. The disease is unique in being the only model for selective cone degeneration in man. In the *cd* retina, cones become dysfunctional early in life, show disorganization and loss of outer segments, and accumulate 100 Å neurofilament bundles in the inner segment and perinuclear cytoplasm; degeneration of cones occurs subsequently.

An unusual feature of *cd* is the manner in which cone

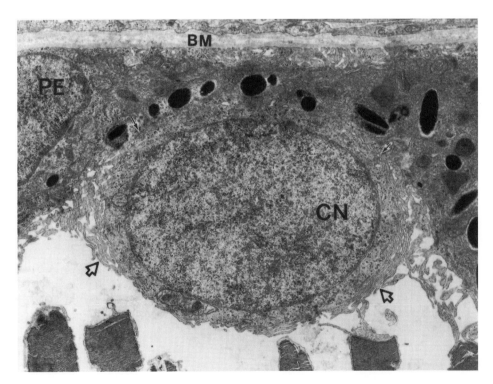

FIGURE 14-40. Ectopically located cone nucleus (CN) adjacent to the retinal pigment epithelium (PE) in an adult dog with hereditary cone degeneration *(cd)*. The ectopic nucleus is surrounded by a rim of cytoplasm, and indents the apical border of the PE, bringing the apically located melanin granules closer to the basal PE surface and Bruch's membrane (BM). The ectopic nucleus is surrounded by the apical microvilli of the PE *(open arrows)*. Note the distinct separation between the cytoplasmic membranes of the PE and the ectopic cone nucleus *(black/white arrows)*. Magnification ×10,500. (Reprinted from Gropp et al., 1996.)

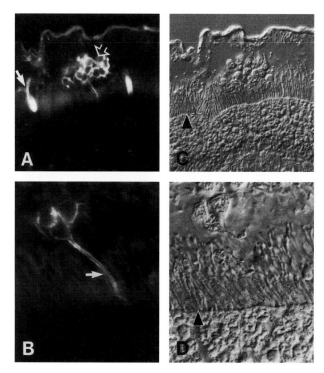

FIGURE 14-41. Paired PNA fluorescence and Nomarski (A, C and B, D) photomicrographs of the *cd* retina from an adult affected dog. Groups of PNA-positive cone somata are clustered ectopically in the subretinal space (A) *(open arrow)*. Some cells extend PNA positive processes (B) *(arrow)* proximally to the external limiting membrane (marked by arrowheads in C and D). Distinct cone matrix sheaths are still present (A) *(arrow)*. Artefactual detachment of the retinal pigment epithelial layer accentuates the ectopically located cone nuclei. Magnifications: (A) and (C) ×250; (B) and (D) ×750. (Reprinted from Long and Aguirre, 1991.)

loss evolves. Unlike other models of photoreceptor degeneration, where nuclear pyknosis and apoptotic cell death follow disease and degeneration of the outer and inner segments (Chang et al., 1993; Portera-Cailliau et al., 1994), this process does not occur, at least initially, in the *cd* retina. Diseased cones undergo slow extrusion of the nucleus into the inner segment, displacement into the interphotoreceptor space, and final placement adjacent to the RPE (Fig. 14-40). In this position, the ectopically located nuclei indent the RPE surface, but cause no further response (Gropp et al., 1996). Cone extrusion also occurs in complete typical rod monochromatism in man, the disease for which *cd* serves as an animal model (Larsen, 1921; Harrison et al., 1960; Falls et al., 1965). In the retinas of humans affected with this disorder, there is loss of cones as well as the presence of ectopic cone nuclei which are located in the inner segment, in the interphotoreceptor space, and adjacent to the RPE (Falls et al., 1965).

Examination of *cd*-affected retinas embedded in plastic and sectioned at 1 μm suggests that the ectopic cone

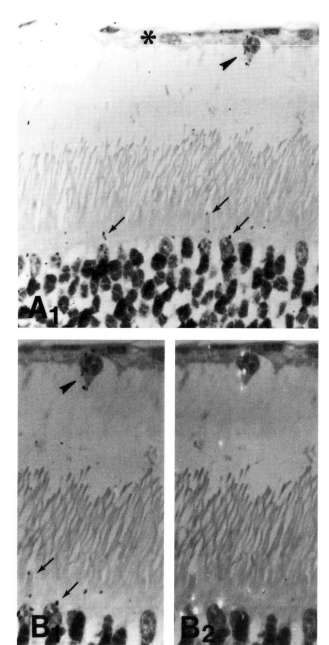

FIGURE 14-42. Brightfield (A$_1$, B$_1$) and combined brightfield/epipolarization (B$_2$) photomicrographs of the *cd* retina from a young affected dog hybridized with ^{3}H-labeled antisense human red/green cone opsin cRNA probe. The ectopically located cone nuclei *(arrowheads)* are located adjacent to the retinal pigment epithelium (A$_1$, *; see B$_1$ for higher magnification), and have an accumulation of silver grains in the perinuclear cytoplasm. The remaining cones in the photoreceptor layer *(arrows,* A$_1$, B$_1$) have silver grains that cluster in the perinuclear cytoplasm or the proximal inner segment. The intensity of the hybridization signal in all cones is normal. Magnifications: (A$_1$) ×800; (B$_1$) and (B$_2$) ×1000. (Reprinted from Gropp et al., 1996.)

nuclei are separated from the photoreceptor layer. However, in thicker sections (10 μm) reacted with peanut agglutinin (PNA) lectin to identify the extracellular cone matrix domains, some of the subretinal nuclei appear to be connected to the external limiting membrane, and, in some cases, form cellular aggregates in the subretinal space (Fig. 14-41—Long and Aguirre, 1991). Additionally, in situ hybridization using a red/green cone pigment cRNA probe indicates normal cone opsin gene expression (Fig. 14-42). Based on the presence of cone pigment mRNA transcripts, and immunoreactivity (using cone-specific antibodies) of intensity equal to that found in normally placed cone cells, we consider these ectopic cone nuclei viable (Gropp et al., 1996). With aging, there is progressive loss of cone nuclei from their normal position in the photoreceptor layer, and the oldest retina examined had the greatest number of ectopic cone nuclei located at the level of the RPE. Whether the ectopically located cone nuclei eventually degenerate or remain viable is not known at this time. However, their position adjacent to the RPE monolayer fails to elicit any histologically evident cellular response.

ACKNOWLEDGMENTS

The studies presented in this chapter have been supported in part by NIH grants EY-01244, -06855, -07705 and -11,142, DK-25759 and NS-33526, The Foundation Fighting Blindness, The Morris Animal Foundation, The Seeing Eye, Inc., the American Federation for Aging Research and the Starr Foundation.

REFERENCES

Acland GM, Aguirre GD. 1987. Retinal degenerations in the dog: IV. Early retinal degeneration (erd) in Norwegian elkhounds. Exp Eye Res 44:491–521.

Acland GM, Ray K, Aguirre GD. 1995. Exclusion of the cyclic GMP-PDE beta subunit gene as a candidate in the prcd-dog. Invest Ophthalmol Vis Sci 36:S891.

Acland G, Fletcher RT, Gentleman S, Chader G, Aguirre G. 1989. Non-allelism of three genes (rcd 1, rcd 2 and erd) for early-onset hereditary retinal degeneration. Exp Eye Res 49:983–998.

Acland G, Blanton SH, Hershfield B, Aguirre G. 1994. XLPRA: A canine retinal degeneration inherited as an x-linked trait. Am J Med Gen 52:27–33.

Aguirre GD. 1978. Retinal degenerations in the dog. I. Rod dysplasia. Exp Eye Res 26:233–253.

Aguirre G. 1986. Phagocytic cells in the interphotoreceptor space: correlation with disease stage in canine progressive rod-cone degeneration. In: Agardh E, Ehinger B, eds, Retinal Signal Systems, Degenerations and Transplants. New York: Elsevier, 193–200.

Aguirre GD, Acland GM. 1988. Variation in retinal degeneration phenotype inherited at the prcd locus. Exp Eye Res 46:663–687.

Aguirre G, Acland G. 1991. Inherited retinal degeneration in the Labrador retriever dog. a new animal model of RP? Invest Ophthalmol Vis Sci 32(Suppl):889.

Aguirre GD, Laties A. 1976. Pigment epithelial dystrophy in the dog. Exp Eye Res 23:247–256.

Aguirre G, O'Brien P. 1986. Morphological and biochemical studies of canine progressive rod-cone degeneration: ³H-fucose autoradiography. Invest Ophthal Vis Sci 27:635–655.

Aguirre GD, Rubin LF. 1974. Pathology of hemeralopia in the Alaskan malamute dog. Invest Ophthalmol 13:231–235.

Aguirre GD, Rubin LF. 1975. The electroretinogram in dogs with inherited cone degeneration. Invest Ophthalmol 14:840–847.

Aguirre GD, Rubin LF. 1979. Diseases of the retinal pigment epithelium in animals. In: Zinn K, Marmor M, eds, The Retinal Pigment Epithelium. Cambridge (MA): Harvard University Press; 334–356.

Aguirre G, Stramm L. 1991. The RPE: a model system for disease expression and disease correction. Prog Retinal Res 11:153–191.

Aguirre GD, Lolley R, Farber D, Fletcher T, Chader G. 1978. Rod-cone dysplasia in Irish setter dogs: a defect in cyclic GMP metabolism in visual cells. Science 201:1133–1134.

Aguirre G, Alligood J, O'Brien P, Buyukmihci N. 1982a. Pathogenesis of progressive rod-cone degeneration in miniature poodles. Invest Ophthal Vis Sci 23:610–630.

Aguirre G, Farber D, Lolley R, O'Brien P, Alligood J, Fletcher RT, Chader G. 1982b. Retinal degenerations in the dog: III. Abnormal cyclic nucleotide metabolism in rod-cone dysplasia. Exp Eye Res 35:625–642.

Aguirre G, Stramm L, Haskins, M. 1983. Feline mucopolysaccharidosis: VI. General ocular and pigment epithelial pathology. Invest Ophthal Vis Sci 24:991–1007.

Aguirre G, Stramm L, Haskins M, Jezyk P. 1986. Animal models of metabolic eye disease. In: Renie W, Goldberg M, eds, Goldberg's Genetic and Metabolic Eye Disease. Boston: Little, Brown 139–167.

Aguirre G, Raber I, Yanoff M, Haskins M. 1992. Reciprocal corneal transplantation fails to correct mucopolysaccharidosis VI corneal storage. Invest Ophthalm Vis Sci 33:2702–2713.

Aguirre G, Ray J, Pearce-Kelling S, Stramm L, Haskins M. 1995. Lysosomal α-mannosidase is essential for retinal pigment (RPE) degra-dative function. Invest Ophthal Vis Sci 36:S816.

Akle C, McColl I, Dean M, Adinolfi M, Brown S, Fensom A, Marsh J, Welsh K. 1985. Transplantation of amniotic epithelial membranes in patients with mucopolysaccharidoses. Expl Clin Immunogenet 2:43.

Akhmedov NB, Piriev NI, Ray K, Acland, GM, Aguirre GD, Farber DB. 1997. Structure and analysis of transducin β3-subunit, a candidate for inherited cone degeneration (cd) in the dog. Gene 194:47–56.

Alroy J, Bachrach A Jr, Thalhammer JC, Panjwani N, Richard R, DeGasperi R, Warren CD. 1991. Clinical, neurophysiological biochemical and morphological features of eyes in Persian cats with mannosidosis. Virchows Archiv B Cell Pathol 60:173–180.

Anderson R, Maude M, Alvarez R, Nilsson SE, Narfstrom K, Acland G, Aguirre G. 1991. Plasma lipid abnormalities in prcd-affected miniature poodles and Abyssinian cats. In: Hollyfield JG, Anderson RE, Lavail MM, eds, Degenerative Retinal Disorders: Clinical and Laboratory Investigations. Boca Raton, Fla.:CRC Press, 131–142.

Armentano D, Yu S-F, Kantoff PW, von Ruden T, Anderson WF, Gilboa E. 1987. Effect of internal viral sequences on the utility of retroviral vectors. J Virol 61:1647–1650.

Barbehenn E, Gagnon C, Noelker D, Aguirre G, Chader G. 1988. Inherited rod-cone dysplasia: abnormal distribution of cyclic GMP in visual cells of affected Irish setters. Exp Eye Res 46:149–159.

Barnett KC, Curtis R. 1985. Autosomal dominant progressive retinal atrophy in Abyssinian cats. J Hered 76:168–170.

Barnett KC, Heywood R, Hague P. 1972. Colloid degeneration of the retina in a baboon. J Comp Pathol 82:117–118.

Bedford PGC. 1984. Retinal pigment epithelial dystrophy (CPRA): a study of the disease in the briard. J Small Anim Pract 25:129–138.

Bellairs R, Harkness LR, Harkness RD. 1975. The structure of the tapetum in the eye of the sheep. Cell Tiss Res 157:73.

Bellhorn RW, Bellhorn MB, Swarm RL, Impellizzeri CW. 1975. Hereditary tapetal abnormality in the beagle. Ophthal Res 7:250–260.

Bellhorn RW, King CD, Aguirre GD, Ripps H, Siegel IM, Tsai HC. 1981. Pigmentary abnormalities of the macula in rhesus monkeys: clinical observations. Invest Ophthalmol Vis Sci 21(6):771–781.

Bernstein MH, Pease DC. 1959. Electron microscopy of the tapetum lucidum of the cat. J Biophys Biochem Cytol 5:35–53.

Berson EL, Rosner B, Sandberg MA, Dryja TP. 1991. Ocular findings in patients with autosomal dominant retinitis pigmentosa and a rhodopsin gene defect (PRO-23-HIS). Arch Ophthalmol 109:92–101.

Berson EL, Watson G. 1980. Electroretinograms in English setters with neuronal ceroid lipofuscinosis. Invest Ophthalmol Vis Sci 19:87–89.

Boulton M, Moriarty P, Jarvis-Evans J, Marcyniuk B. 1994. Regional variation and age-related changes of lysosomal enzymes in the human retinal pigment epithelium. Br J Ophthalmol 78:125–129.

Bowes C, Li T, Danciger M, Baxter LC, Applebury ML, Farber DB. 1990. Retinal degeneration in the rd mouse is caused by a defect in the β subunit of rod cGMP-phosphodiesterase. Nature 347:677–680.

Bowes C, Li T, Frankel WN, Danciger M, Coffin JM, Applebury ML, Farber DB. 1993. Localization of a retroviral element within the rd gene coding for the beta subunit of cGMP phosphodiesterase. Proc Nat Acad Sci USA 90:2955–2959.

Budinger JM. 1961. Diphenylthiocarbazone blindness in dogs. Arch Pathol 71:304.

Burke J, Twining S. 1988. Regional comparisons of cathepsin D activity in bovine retinal pigment epithelium. Invest Ophthalmol Vis Sci 29:1789–1793.

Burkhardt JK, Wiebel FA, Hester S, Argon Y. 1993. The giant organelles in beige and Chediak-Higashi fibroblasts are derived from late endosomes and mature lysosomes. J Exp Med 178:1845–1856.

Burns MS, Bellhorn RW, Impellizzeri CW, Aguirre GD, Laties AM. 1988. Development of hereditary tapetal degeneration in the beagle dog. Curr Eye Res 7:103–114.

Bussow H. 1980. The tapetal cell: a unique melanocyte in the tapetum lucidum cellulosum of the cat (Felis domestica L): an electron microscopic, cytochemical and chemical study. Anat Embryol 158:289–302.

Butturini U, Grignolo A, Baronchelli A. 1953. "Diabete" da ditizone aspetti metabolici oculari ed istologici. G Clin Med 34:1253–1347.

Cabral L, Unger W, Boulton M, Lightfoot R, McKechnie N, Grierson I, Marshall J. 1990. Regional distribution of lysosomal enzymes in the canine retinal pigment epithelium. Invest Ophthalmol Vis Sci 31:670–676.

Chader GJ. 1991. Animal mutants of hereditary retinal degeneration: General considerations and studies on defects in cyclic nucleotide metabolism. Prog Vet Comp Ophthalmol 1:109–126.

Chader GJ, Fletcher RT, Sanyal S, Aguirre G. 1985. A review of the role of cyclic GMP in neurological mutants with photoreceptor dysplasia. Curr Eye Res 4:811–819.

Chang GQ, Hao Y, Wong F. 1993. Apoptosis: final common pathway of photoreceptor death in rd, rds, and rhodopsin mutant mice. Neuron 11:595–605.

Clements PJM, Gregory CY, Petersoe-Jones SM, Sargan DR, Bhattacharya SS. 1993. Confirmation of the rod cGMP phosphodiesterase β subunit (PDEβ) nonsense mutation in affected rcd-1 Irish

setters in the UK and development of a diagnostic test. Curr Eye Res 12:861–866.

Cloyd GG, Wyman M, Shadduck JA, Winrow MJ, Johnson GR. 1978. Ocular toxicity studies with zinc pyridinethione. Toxicol Appl Pharmacol 45:771–782.

Collier LL, Prieur DJ, King EJ. 1984. Ocular melanin pigmentation anomalies in cats, cattle, mink, and mice with Chediak-Higashi syndrome: histologic observations. Curr Eye Res 3:1241–1251.

Collier LL, King EJ, Prieur DJ. 1985a. Tapetal degeneration in cats with Chediak-Higashi syndrome. Curr Eye Res 4:767–773.

Collier LL, King EJ, Prieur DJ. 1985b. Aberrant melanosome development in the retinal pigmented epithelium of cats with Chediak-Higashi syndrome. Exp Eye Res 41:305–311.

Collier LL, King EJ, Prieur DJ. 1986. Age-related changes of the retinal pigment epithelium of cats with Chediak-Higashi syndrome. Invest Ophthalmol Vis Sci 27:702–707.

Cummings JF, DeLahunta A, George C, Fuhrer L, Valentine BA, Cooper BJ, Summers BA, Huxtable CR, Mohammed HO. 1990. Equine motor neuron disease. Cornell Vet 80:357–379.

Cummings JF, DeLahunta A, Mohammed HO, Divers TJ, Summers BA, Valentine BA, Jackson CA. 1995. Endothelial lipopigment as an indicator of α-tocopherol deficiency in two equine neurodegenerative diseases. Acta Neuropathol 90:262–272.

Cummings JF, DeLahunta A, Mohammed HO, Divers TJ. In press. The histopathology of equine motor neuron disease (ENMD). Equine Vet J.

Curtis R, Barnett KC, Leon A. 1987. An early-onset retinal dystrophy with dominant inheritance in the Abyssinian cat. Invest Ophthalmol Vis Sci 28:131–139.

Dawson WW, Engel HM, Hope GM, Kessler MJ, Ulshaffer RJ. 1989. Adult-onset macular degeneration in the Cayo Santiago macaques. PR Health Sci J 8:111–115.

DeGasperi R, Daher SA, Daniel PF, Winchester BG, Jeanloz RW, Warren CD. 1991. The substrate specificity of bovine and feline lysosomal alpha-D-mannosidases in relation to alpha-mannosidosis. J Biol Chem 266:16556–16563.

Divers TJ, Mohammed HO, Cummings JF, Valentine BA, deLahunta A, Jackson CA, Summers BA. 1994. Equine motor neuron disease: findings in twenty-eight horses and proposal of a pathophysiological mechanism for the disease. Equine Vet J 26:409–415.

Dorey C, Wu G, Ebenstein D, Garsd A, Weiter J. 1989. Cell loss in the aging retina: relationship to lipofuscin accumulation and macular degeneration. Invest Ophthalmol Vis Sci 30:1691–1699.

Dryja TP, Li T. 1995. Molecular genetics of retinitis pigmentosa. Hum Mol Genet 4:1739–1743.

Dryja TP, Berson EL, Rao VR, Oprian DD. 1993. Heterozygous missense mutation in the rhodopsin gene as a cause of congenital stationary night blindness. Nat Genet 4:280–283.

Dryja TP, Finn JT, Peng YW, McGee TL, Berson EL, Yau KW. 1995. Mutations in the gene encoding the α subunit of the rod cGMP-gated channel in autosomal recessive retinitis pigmentosa. Proc Natl Acad Sci USA 92:10177–10181.

Edwards RB, Szamier RB. 1977. Defective phagocytes of isolated rod outer segments by RCS rat retinal pigment epithelium in culture. Science 197:1001–1003.

El Baba FE, Green WR, Fleischmann J, Finkelstein D. 1986. Clinicopathologic correlation of lipidization and detachment of the retinal pigment epithelium. Am J Ophthalmol 101:576–583.

El-Mofty A, Gouras P, Eisner G, Balazs EA. 1978. Macular degeneration in rhesus monkey (Macaca mulatta). Exp Eye Res 27:499.

El-Mofty AAM, Eisner G, Balazs EA, Denlinger JL, Gouras P. 1980. Retinal degeneration in rhesus monkeys, Macaca mulatta: survey of three seminatural free-breeding colonies. Exp Eye Res 31:146–166.

Engel HM, Dawson WW, Ulshafer RJ, Hines MW, Kessler MJ. 1988. Degenerative changes in maculas of rhesus monkeys. Ophthalmologica 196:143–150.

Falls HF, Wolter JR, Alpern M. 1965. Typical total monochromacy: a histological and psychophysical study. Arch Ophthal 74:610–616.

Farber DB, Lolley RN. 1974. Cyclic guanosine monophosphate: Elevation in degenerating photoreceptor cells of the C3H mouse retina. Science 186:449–451.

Farber DB, Danciger JS, Aguirre G. 1990. Early mRNA defect in Irish setter dog retina. Invest Ophthalmol Vis Sci (Supp). 31:310.

Farber D, Danciger JS, Aguirre G. 1992. The β-subunit of cyclic GMP phosphodiesterase is deficient in canine rod-cone dysplasia 1. Neuron 9:349–356.

Feeney-Burns L, Ellersieck MR. 1985. Age-related changes in the ultrastructure of Bruch's membrane. Am J Ophthalmol 100:686–697.

Feeney-Burns L, et al. 1981. Maculopathy in cynomolgus monkeys: a correlated fluorescein angiographic and ultrastructural study. Arch Ophthalmol 99:664–672.

Feeney-Burns L, Hilderbrand ES, Eldridge S. 1984. Aging human RPE: morphometric analysis of macular, equatorial and peripheral cells. Invest Ophthalmol Vis Sci 25(1):195–200.

Fine BS. 1981. Lipoidal degeneration of the retinal pigment epithelium. Am J Ophthalmol 91:469–473.

Fine BS, Kwapien RP. 1978. Pigment epithelial windows and drusen: an animal model. Invest Ophthalmol Vis Sci 17:1059.

Fishman GA, Stone EM, Gilbert LD, Sheffield VC. 1992. Ocular findings associated with a rhodopsin gene codon 106 mutation: glycine-to-arginine change in autosomal dominant retinitis pigmentosa. Arch Opthhalm 110:646–653.

Fratantoni J, Hall C, Neufeld E. 1968. Hurler and Hunter syndromes: mutual correction of the defect in cultured fibroblasts. Science 612:500.

Gao H, Hollyfield JG. 1992. Aging of the human retina. Invest Ophthalmol Vis Sci 33(1):1–17.

Gasper PW, Thrall MA, Wenger DA, Macy DW, Ham L, Dornsife RE, McBiles K, Quackenbush SL, Kesel ML, Gillette EL, Hoover EL. 1984. Correction of feline arylsulfatase B deficiency (mucopolysaccharidosis VI) by bone marrow transplantation. Nature 312:467–469.

Gorin MB, To AC, Narfström K. 1995. Sequence analysis and exclusion of phosducin as the gene for the recessive retinal degeneration of the Abyssinian cat. Bioch Biophys Acta 1260:323–327.

Gorin MB, Snyder S, Narfstrom K, Curtis R. 1993. The cat RDS transcript: candidate gene analysis and phylogenetic sequence analysis. Mamm Genome 4:544–548.

Graydon RJ, Jolly RD. 1984. Ceroid-lipofuscinosis (Batten's disease): sequential electrophysiologic and pathologic changes in the retina of the ovine model. Invest Ophthalmol Vis Sci 25:294–301.

Gropp KE, Szél A, Huang JC, Acland GM, Farber DB, Aguirre GD. Selective absence of cone outer segment β3-transducin immunoreactivity in hereditary cone degeneration (cd). Exp Eye Res 63:285–296.

Hageman GS, Johnson LV. 1991. Structure, composition and function of the retinal interphotoreceptor matrix. In: Osborne N, Chader GJ, eds, Progress in Retinal Research, vol. 10 Oxford: Pergamon Press.

Harrison R, Hoefnagel D, Hayward JN. 1960. Congenital total color blindness: a clinicopathological report. Arch Ophthalmol 64:685–692.

Haskins M, Baker H, Birkenmeier E, Hoogerbrugge P, Poorthuis B, Sakiyama T, Shull R, Taylor R, Thrall M, Walkley S. 1991. Transplantation in animal model systems. In: Desnick R, ed, Therapy of Genetic Disease. New York: Churchill Livingston.

Haskins M, Chieffo C, Wang P, Just C, Evans S, Aguirre G. 1992. Bone marrow transplantation in canine mucopolysaccharidosis VII (beta-glucuronidase deficiency). Am J Hum Genet 49:435.

Hayasaka S. 1974. Distribution of lysosomal enzymes in the bovine eye. Jpn J Ophthalmol 18:233–239.

Hayes KC, Rousseau JE, Hegsted DM. 1970. Plasma tocopherol concentrations and vitamin E deficiency in dogs. J Am Vet Med Assoc 157(1):64–71.

Heckenlively JR, Rodriguez JA, Daiger SP. 1991. Autosomal dominant sectoral retinitis pigmentosa: two families with transversion mutation in codon 23 of rhodopsin. Arch Ophthalmol 109:84–91.

Herron WL, Riegel BW, Myers OE, Rubin ML. 1969. Retinal dystrophy in the rat—a pigment epithelial disease. Invest Ophthal 8:595–604.

Huang J, Mieziewska K, Philp N, van Veen T, Aguirre G. 1993. Diethylene glycol distearate (DGD): a versatile embedding medium for retinal cytochemistry. J Neurosci Meth 47:227–234.

Huang J, Chesselet M-F, Aguirre G. 1994. Decreased opsin mRNA and immunoreactivity in progressive rod-cone degeneration (prcd): Cytochemical studies of early disease and degeneration. Exp Eye Res 58:17–30.

Huang SH, Pittler SJ, Huang X, Oliveira L, Berson EL, Dryja TP. 1995. Autosomal recessive retinitis pigmentosa caused by mutations in the α subunit of rod cGMP phosphodiesterase. Nature Genetics 11:468–471.

Humphries P, Kenna P, Farrar GJ. 1992. On the molecular genetics of retinitis pigmentosa. Science 256:804–808.

Ishibashi T, Sorgente N, Patterson R, Ryan SJ. 1986. Pathogenesis of drusen in the primate. Invest Ophthalmol Vis Sci 27:184–193.

Jacobson SG, Kemp CM, Narfstrom K, Nilsson SE. 1989. Rhodopsin levels and rod-mediated function in Abyssinian cats with hereditary retinal degeneration. Exp Eye Res 49:843–852.

Jolly RD, Palmer DN. 1995. The neuronal ceroid-lipofuscinoses (Batten disease): comparative aspects. Neuropathol Appl Neurobiol 21:50–60.

Jolly RD, Shimada A, Dalefield RR, Slack PM. 1987. Mannosidosis: ocular lesions in the bovine model. Curr Eye Res 6:1073–1079.

Jolly RD, Gibson AJ, Healy PJ, Slack PM, Birtles MJ. 1992. Bovine ceroid-lipofuscinosis: pathology of blindness. New Zealand Vet J 40:107–111.

Jolly RD, Palmer DN, Studdert VP, Sutton RH, Kelly WR, Koppang N, Dahme G, Hartley WJ, Patterson JS, Riis RC. 1994. Canine ceroid-lipofuscinoses: a review and classification. J Sm Anim Pract 35:299–306.

Kaiser JA. 1963. Tapetal depigmentation in dogs produced by ethylenediamines. Fed Proc 22:369.

Kajiwara K, Berson EL, Dryja TP. 1994. Digenic retinitis pigmentosa due to mutations at the unlinked peripherin/RDS and ROM1 loci Science 264:1604–1608.

Kajiwara K, Hahn LB, Mukai S, Travis GH, Berson EL, Dryja TP. 1991. Mutations in the human retinal degeneration slow gene in autosomal dominant retinitis pigmentosa. Nature 354:480–484.

Koppang N. 1992. English setter model of neuronal ceroid-lipofuscinosis in man. Am J Med Genet 42:599–604.

Krivit W, et al. 1984. Bone-marrow transplantation in the Maroteaux-Lamy syndrome (mucopolysaccharidosis type VI). New Eng J Med 311:1606–1611.

Kyle JW, Birkenmeier EH, Gwynn B, Vogler C, Hoppe PC, Hoffman JW, Sly WS. 1990. Correction of murine mucopolysaccharidosis VII by a human B-glucuronidase transgene. Proc Nat Acad Sci USA. 87:3914–3918.

Lai Y-L. 1980. Outward movement of photoreceptor cells in normal rat retina. Invest Ophthalmol Vis Sci 19:849–856.

Lai Y-L, Jacoby RO, Jonas AM. 1978. Age-related and light-associated retinal changes in Fischer rats. Invest Ophthalmol Vis Sci 17:634–638.

Lai Y-L, Masuda K, Mangum RL, Macrae DW, Fletcher G, Yung-Pin L. 1982. Subretinal displacement of photoreceptor nuclei in human retina. Exp Eye Res 34:219–228.

Landers RA, Tawara A, Varner HH, Hollyfield JG. 1991. Proteoglycans in the mouse interphotoreceptor matrix. IV. Retinal synthesis of chondroitin sulfate proteoglycan. Exp Eye Res 52:65–74.

Larsen H. 1921. Demonstration mikroskopischer Präparate von einem monochromatischen Auge. Z Augenheilkunde 46:228–229.

LaVail MM. 1980. Degenerate retinal disorders: interaction of environmental light and pigmentation with inherited retinal degenerations. Vision Res 20:1172–1177.

LaVail MM, Battelle B. 1975. Influence of eye pigmentation and light deprivation on inherited retinal dystrophy in the rat. Exp Eye Res 21:167–192.

LaVail MM, Pinto LH, Yasumura D. 1981. The interphotoreceptor matrix in rats with inherited retinal dystrophy. Invest Ophthalmol Vis Sci 21:658–668.

Lazarus HS, Sly WS, Kyle JW, Hageman GS. 1993. Photoreceptor degeneration and altered distribution of interphotoreceptor matrix proteoglycans in the mucopolysaccharidosis VII mouse. Exp Eye Res 56:531–541.

Leon A, Curtis R. 1990. Autosomal dominant rod-cone dystrophy in the *rdy* cat. 1. Light and electron microscopic findings. Exp Eye Res 51:361–381.

Leon A, Hussain AA, Curtis R. 1988. Rod-cone dysplasia in the *rdy* cat: electrophysiology and biochemistry. Invest Ophthalm Vis Sci 29(suppl):143.

Li T, Davidson B. 1995. Phenotype correction in retinal pigment epithelium in murine mucopolysaccharidosis VII by adenovirus-mediated gene transfer. Proc Nat Acad Sci USA 92:7700–7704.

Li L, Turner JE. 1988. Inherited retinal dystrophy in the RCS rat: prevention of photoreceptor degeneration by pigment epithelial cell transplantion. Exp Eye Res 47:911–917.

Lightfoot, RM. 1988. Retinal pigment epithelial dystrophy in the dog. PhD dissertation. University of London.

Long KO, Haskins ME, Aguirre GD. 1989. Photoreceptor-RPE interface in β-glucuronidase deficiency: an anatomical and immunocytochemical study. Invest Ophthalmol Vis Sci 30(suppl):3.

Long K, Aguirre G. 1991. The cone matrix sheath in the normal and diseased retina. Exp Eye Res 52:699–713.

Maréchal V, Naffakh N, Danos O, Heard JM. 1993. Disappearance of lysosomal storage in spleen and liver of mucopolysaccharidosis VII mice after transplantation of genetically modified bone marrow cells. Blood 82:1358–1365.

Massa T, Davis GJ, Schiavo D, Sinha DP, Szot RJ, Black HE, Schwartz E. 1984. Tapetal changes in beagle dogs. II. Ocular changes after intravenous administration of a macrolid antibiotic rosaramicin. Toxicol Appl Pharmacol 72:195–200.

McLaughlin ME, Sandberg MA, Berson EL, Dryja TP. 1993. Recessive mutations in the gene encoding the β-subunit of rod phosphodiesterase in patients with retinitis pigmentosa. Nat Genet 4:130–134.

McLaughlin ME, Ehrhart TL, Berson EL, Dryja TP. 1995. Mutation spectrum of the gene encoding the β subunit of rod phosphodiesterase among patients with autosomal recessive retinitis pigmentosa. Proc Nat Acad Sci USA 92:3249–3253.

Mieziewska K. 1993. The interphotoreceptor matrix: a study of structure and composition in normal and degenerating retinas. PhD dissertation. University of Göteborg, Faculty of Natural Sciences.

Mieziewska K, vanVeen T, Murray J, Aguirre G. 1991. Rod and cone specific domains in the interphotoreceptor matrix. J Comp Neurol 308:371–380.

Miewziewska K, van Veen T, Aguirre G. 1993a. Development and fate of interphotoreceptor matrix components during dysplastic photoreceptor differentiation: a lectin cytochemical study of rod-cone dysplasia 1. Exp Eye Res 56:429–441.

Mieziewska K, van Veen T, Aguirre G. 1993b. Structural changes of the interphotoreceptor matrix in an inherited retinal degeneration: A lectin cytochemical study of progressive rod-cone degeneration (*prcd*). Inv Ophthalm Vis Sci 34:3056–3066.

Miller AD, Buttimore C. 1986. Redesign of retrovirus packaging cell lines to avoid recombination leading to helper virus production. Mol Cell Biol 6:2895–2902.

Moullier P, Bohl D, Heard J-M, Danos O. 1993. Correction of lysosomal storage in the liver and spleen of MPS VII mice by implantation of genetically modified skin fibroblasts. Nat Genet 4:154–159.

Mullen RJ, LaVail MM. 1976. Inherited retinal dystrophy: primary defect in pigment epithelium determined with experimental rat chimeras. Science 192:799–801.

Nakaizumi Y. 1964. The ultrastructure of Bruch's membrane. II. Eyes with a tapetum. Arch Ophthalmol 77:388–394.

Narfström K. 1983. Hereditary progressive retinal atrophy in the Abyssinian cat. J Hered 74:273–276.

Narfström K, Nilsson SE. 1986. Progressive retinal atrophy in the Abyssinian cat. Invest Ophthalmol Vis Sci 27:1569–1576.

Narfström K, Nilsson SE. 1989. Morphological findings during retinal development and maturation in hereditary rod-cone degeneration in Abyssinian cats. Exp Eye Res 49:611–628.

Narfström KL, Nilsson SE, Andersson BE. 1985. Progressive retinal atrophy in the Abyssinian cat: studies of the DC-recorded electroretinogram and the standing potential of the eye. Br J Ophthalmol 69:618–623.

Narfström K, Wilen M, Andersson BE. 1988. Hereditary retinal degeneration in the Abyssinian cat: developmental studies using clinical electroretinography. Doc Ophthalmol 69(2):111–118.

Narfström K, Nilsson SE, Wiggert B, Lee L, Chader GJ, van Veen T. 1989. Reduced level of interphotoreceptor retinoid binding protein (IRBP) a possible cause for retinal degeneration in the Abyssinian cat. Cell Tissue Res 257:631–639.

Narfström K, Wrigstad A, Nilsson SEG. 1989. The Briard dog: a new animal model of congenital stationary night blindness. Br J Ophthalmol 73:750–756.

Narfström K, Wrigstad A, Ekesten B, Nilsson SEG. 1994. Hereditary retinal dystrophy in the Briard dog: clinical and hereditary characteristics. Vet Comp Ophthalmol 4(2):85–92.

Neville H, Armstrong D, Wilson B, Koppang N, Wehling C. 1980. Studies on the retina and the pigment epithelium in hereditary canine ceroid lipofuscinosis III. Morphologic abnormalities in retinal neurons and retinal pigmented epithelial cells. Invest Ophthalmol Vis Sci 19:75–86.

Nicolas MG, Fujiki K, Murayama K, Suzuki MT, Mineki R, Hayakawa M, Yoshikawa Y, Cho F, Kanai A. 1996. Studies on the mechanism of early onset macular degeneration in cynomolgus (Macaca fascicularis) monkeys. I. Abnormal concentrations of two proteins in the retina. Exp Eye Res 62:211–219.

Nilsson SEG, Armstrong D, Koppang N, Persson P, Milde K. 1983. Studies on the retina and the pigment epithelium in hereditary canine ceroid lipofuscinosis. IV: Changes in the electroretinogram and the standing potential of the eye. Invest Ophthalmol Vis Sci 24:77–84.

Nilsson SEG, Wrigstad A, Narfström K. 1992. Changes in the DC electroretinogram in briard dogs with hereditary congenital night blindness and partial day blindness. Exp Eye Res 54:291–296.

Nishimura Y, Rosenfeld MG, Kreibich G, Gubler U, Sabatini DD, Adesnik M, Andy R. 1986. Nucleotide sequence of rat preputial gland β-glucuronidase cDNA and in vitro insertion of its encoded polypeptide into microsomal membranes. Proc Nat Acad Sci USA 83:7292–7296.

Parry HB. 1954. Degenerations of the dog retina VI. Central progressive atrophy with pigment epithelial dystrophy. Br J Ophthal 38:653–668.

Parshall C, Wyman M, Nitroy S, Acland G, Aguirre G. 1991. Photoreceptor dysplasia: an inherited progressive retinal atrophy of miniature schnauzer dogs. Prog Vet Comp Ophtholmol 1:187.

Perou CM, Kaplan J. 1993. Complementation analysis of Chediak-Higashi syndrome: the same gene may be responsible for the defect in all patients and species. Somat Cell Mol Genet 19:459–468.

Pirie A. 1966. Chemistry and structure of the tapetum lucidum. In: Graham-Jones O, ed, Aspects of Comparative Ophthalmology. London: Pergamon Press, 57–68.

Pittler SJ, Baehr W. 1991. Identification of a nonsense mutation in the rod photoreceptor cGMP phosphodiesterase β-subunit gene of the rd mouse. Proc Nat Acad Sci USA 88:8322–8326.

Porrello K, Yasumura D, LaVail MM. 1986. The interphotoreceptor matrix in RCS rats: histochemical analysis and correlation with the rate of retinal degeneration. Exp Eye Res 43:413–429.

Portera-Cailliau C, Sung C-H, Nathans J, Adler R. 1994. Apoptotic photoreceptor cell death in mouse models of retinitis pigmentosa. Proc Nat Acad Sci USA 91:974–978.

Prince JH, Diesem CD, Eglitis I, Ruskell GL. 1960. Anatomy and Histology of the Eye and Orbit in Domestic Animals. Springfield, Charles C. Thomas, page 219.

Ray J, Wolfe J, Haskins M, Aguirre G. 1992. Specificity of β-glucuronidase cDNA to correct inherited defects of the lysosomal system in the RPE. Invest Ophthalmol Vis Sci 33(suppl):909.

Ray J, Wu Y, Haskins M, Salvetti A, Heard JM, Aguirre G. 1995. Enhanced degradation of accumulating GAGs in MPS VI-affected retinal pigment epithelium by arylsulfatase B cDNA transfer. Inv Ophthalmol Vis Sci 36(suppl):S918.

Ray J, DeSanto CM, Sun W, Haskins M, Aguirre G. 1996. Studies on the molecular basis of β-glucuronidase deficiency in mucopolysaccharidosis VII (MPS VII) in the retinal pigment epithelium. Invest Ophthalmol Vis Sci (suppl) 37:5379.

Ray J, Wu Y, Aguirre GD. 1997. Characterization of β-glucuronidase in the retinal pigment epithelium. Curr. Eye Res. 16:131–143.

Ray K, Baldwin V, Acland G, Blanton S, Aguirre G. 1994. Co-segregation of codon 807 mutation of the rod cGMP phosphodiesterase β gene (PDEB) in rcd1. Invest Ophthalmol Vis Sci 35:4291–4299.

Ray K, Baldwin V, Acland G, Aguirre G. 1995. Molecular diagnostic tests for ascertainment of genotype at the rod cone dysplasia 1 (rcd1) locus in Irish setters. Curr Eye Res 14:243–247.

Ray K, Acland GM, Aguirre GD. 1996. Nonallelism of erd and prcd and exclusion of the canine RDS/peripherin gene as a candidate for both retinal degeneration loci. Inv Ophthalm Vis Sci 37:783–794.

Ray K, Baldwin VJ, Zeiss C, Acland GM, Aguirre GD. In press. Canine rod transducin α-1: cloning of the cDNA and evaluation of the gene as a candidate for progressive retinal atrophy. Curr Eye Res 16:71–77.

Riis RC, Sheffy BE, Loew E, Kern TJ, Smith JS. 1981. Vitamin E deficiency retinopathy in dogs. Am J Vet Res 42:74–86.

Riis RC, Cummings JF, Loew ER, de Lahunta A. 1992. Tibetan terrier model of canine ceroid lipofuscinosis. Am J Med Gen 42:615–621.

Riis RC, Rebhun WC, Jackson CA, Loew E, Katz ML, Cummings JF, Mohammed HO, Divers TJ, deLahunta A, Valentine BA. 1995, Fundic lesions in horses affected with equine motor neuron disease. Proc Am Coll Vet Ophthalm 43.

Roque RS, Imperial CJ, Caldwell R. 1996. Microglial cells invade the outer retina as photoreceptors degenerate in Royal College of Surgeons rats. Invest Ophthalmol Vis Sci 37:196–203.

Rosenzweig M, Giger U, Metzler J, Valle DL, Aguirre G. 1990. Ornithine aminotransferase deficiency in a domestic short hair cat. J Vet Int Med 4:116.

Rubin LF, Lipton DE. 1973. Retinal degeneration in kittens. J Am Vet Med Assoc 162:467–469.

Rushton A, Dawson G. 1977. The effect of glycosaminoglycans on the in vitro activity of human skin fibroblast glycosphingolipid B-galactosidases and neuraminidases. Clin Chim Acta 80:133–139.

Sands MS, Barker JE, Vogler C, Levy B, Gwynn B, Galvin N, Sly WS, Birkenmeier E. 1993. Treatment of murine mucopolysaccharidosis type VII by syngeneic bone marrow transplantation in neonates. Lab Invest 68:676–686.

Santos-Anderson RM, Tso MOM, Vainisi SJ. 1983. Heredofamiliar retinal dystrophy in Guinea baboons. II. Electron microscopic observations. Arch Ophthalmol 101:1762–1770.

Schiavo DM, Sinha DP, Black HE, Arthaud L, Massa T, Murphy BF, Szot RJ, Schwartz E. 1984. Tapetal changes in beagles dogs. I. Ocular changes after oral administration of a beta-adrenergic blocking agent, SCH 19927. Toxicol Appl Pharmacol 72:187–194.

Schiavo DM, Green JD, Traina VM, Spaet R, Zaidi I. 1988. Tapetal changes in beagle dogs following oral administration of CGS 14796C, a potential aromatase inhibitor. Fundam Appl Toxicol 10:329–334.

Schmidt SY, Aguirre GD. 1985. Reductions in taurine secondary to photoreceptor loss in Irish setters with rod-cone dysplasia. Invest Ophthalmol Vis Sci 26:679.

Smith RIE, Sutton RH, Jolly RD, Smith KR. 1996. A retinal degeneration associated with ceroid-lipofuscinosis in adult miniature schnauzers. Vet Comp Ophthalmol 6:187–191.

Stafford TJ. 1974. Maculopathy in an elderly sub-human primate. Mod Probl Ophthal 12:214–219.

Stramm LE, Haskins ME, McGovern M, Aguirre G. 1983. Tissue culture of cat retinal pigment epithelium. Exp Eye Res 36:91–101.

Stramm L, Haskins M, Desnick RJ, Aguirre G. 1985. Disease expression in cultured pigment epithelium: feline mucopolysaccharidosis VI. Invest Ophthalmol Vis Sci 26:182.

Stramm LE, Desnick RJ, Haskins ME, Aguirre GD. 1986. Arylsulfatase B activity in cultured retinal pigment epithelium: regional studies in feline mucopolysaccharidosis VI. Invest Ophthalmol Vis Sci 27:1050.

Stramm LE, Haskins ME, Aguirre GD. 1989. Retinal pigment epithelial glycosaminoglycan metabolism: intracellular versus extracellular pathways. Invest Ophthalmol Vis Sci 30:2118.

Stramm L, Wolfe J, Schuchman E, Haskins M, Patterson DF, Aguirre G. 1990. β-glucuronidase mediated pathway essential for retinal pigment epithelial degradation of glycosaminoglycans. Disease expression and in vitro disease correction using retroviral mediated cDNA transfer. Exp Eye Res 50:521–532.

Suber ML, Pittler SJ, Qin N, Wright GC, Holcombe V, Lee RH, Craft CM, Lolley RN, Baehr W, Hurwitz RL. 1993. Irish setter dogs affected with rod/cone dysplasia contain a nonsense mutation in the rod cGMP phosphodiesterase β-subunit gene. Proc Natl Acad Sci USA 90:3968–3972.

Summers G, Purple R, Krivit W, Pineda R, Copland G, Ramsay N, Kersey J, Whitley C. 1989. Ocular changes in the mucopolysaccharidoses after bone marrow transplantation. Ophthalmol 96:977.

Tamai M, O'Brien PJ. 1979. Retinal dystrophy in the RCS rat: in vivo and in vitro studies of phagocytic action of the pigment epithelium on the shed rod outer segments. Exp Eye Res 28:399–411.

Travis GH, Brennan MB, Danielson PE, Kozak CA, Sutcliffe JG. 1989. Identification of a photoreceptor-specific mRNA encoded by the gene responsible for retinal degeneration slow (rds). Nature 338:70–73.

Tso MOM, Santos-Anderson RM, Vanisi SJ. 1983. Heredofamilial retinal dystrophy in Guinea baboons. I. A histopathologic Study. Arch Ophthalmol 101(10):1597–1603.

Vainisi S, Beck B, Apple D. 1974. Retinal degeneration in a baboon. Am J Ophthalmol 78(2):279–284.

Valle D, Boison A, Jezyk P, Aguirre G. 1981. Gyrate atrophy of the choroid and retina in a cat. Invest Ophthalmol Vis Sci 20:251.

Valle D, Jezyk P, Aguirre G. 1983. Gyrate atrophy of the choroid and retina. Comp Pathol Bull 15:2.

Vesa J, Hellsten E, Verkruyse LA, Camp LA, Rapola J, Santavuori P, Hofmann SL, Peltonen L. 1995. Mutations in the palmitoyl protein thioesterase gene causing infantile neuronal ceroid lipofuscinosis. Nature 376:584–587.

Vine D, McGovern M, Schuchman E, Haskins M, Desnick R. 1982. Enhancement of residual arylsulfatase B activity in feline mucopolysaccharidosis VI by thiol-induced subunit association. J Clin Invest 69:294.

Vogel M. 1978. Postnatal development of the cat's retina. Adv Anat Embryol Cell Biol 54(4):7–66.

Vogel AW, Kaiser JA. 1963. Ethambutol induces transient change and reconstruction (in vivo) of the tapetum lucidum color in the dog. Exp Mol Pathol 2(suppl):136–149.

Walkley SU, Thrall MA, Dobrenis K, Huang M, March PA, Siegel DA, Wurzelmann S. 1994. Bone marrow transplantation corrects the enzyme defect in neurons of the central nervous system in a lysosomal storage disease. Proc Nat Acad Sci USA 91:2970–2974.

Wang W, Acland GM, Aguirre GD, Ray K. 1995. Exclusion of rhodopsin, and probable exclusion of rds/peripherin, as candidates for canine progressive rod cone degeneration (prcd). Invest Ophthalmol Vis Sci 36(suppl):S772.

Watson P, Bedford PGC. 1992. The pigments of retinal pigment epithelial dystrophy in dogs. Vet Pathol 29:5.

Watson P, Simson, KW, Bedford, PGC. 1993. Hypercholesterolaemia in briards in the United Kingdom. Res Vet Sci 54:80–85.

Weleber RG, Carr RE, Murphey WH, Sheffield VC, Stone EM. 1993. Phenotypic variation including retinitis pigmentosa, pattern dystrophy, and fundus flavimaculatus in a single family with a deletion of codon 153 or 154 of the peripherin/RDS gene. Arch Ophthalmol 111:1531–1542.

Wen GY, Sturman JA, Wisniewski HM, Lidsky AA, Cornwell AC, Hayes KC. 1979. Tapetum disorganization in taurine-depleted cats. Invest Ophthalmol Vis Sci 18:1201–1206.

Wen GY, Wisniewski HM, Sturman JA. 1982. Hereditary abnormality in tapetum lucidum of the Siamese cats: A histochemical and quantitative study. Histochemistry 75:1–9.

Wen GY, Sturman JA, Shek JW. 1985. A comparative study of the tapetum, retina and skull of the ferret, dog, and cat. Lab Anim Sci 35:200–210.

Wenger D, Gasper P, Thrall M, Dial S, LeCoteur R, Hoover E. 1986. Bone marrow transplantation in the feline, model of arylsulfatase B deficiency. In: Krivit W, Paul N, eds. Bone Marrow Transplantation for Treatment of Lysosomal Storage Diseases. New York: Liss, 177.

West-Hyde Leigh DVM, Buyukmihci N. 1982. Photoreceptor degeneration in a family of cats. J Am Vet Med Assoc 181:243–248.

Wiggert B, Kutty G, Long K, Inouye L, Gery I, Chader G, Aguirre G. 1991. Interphotoreceptor retinoid-binding protein (IRBP) in progressive rod-cone degeneration (prcd). Exp Eye Res 53:389–398.

Wiggert B, van Veen T, Kutty G, Lee L, Nickerson J, Si J-S, Nilsson SEG, Chader GJ, Narfström K. 1994. An early decrease in interphotoreceptor retinoid-binding protein gene expression by Abyssinian cats homozygous for hereditary rod-cone degeneration. Cell Tissue Res 278:291–298.

Wolfe J, Schuchman E, Stramm L, Concaugh E, Haskins M, Aguirre G, Patterson D, Desnick R, Gilboa E. 1990. Restoration of normal lysosomal function in mucopolysaccharidosis type VII cells by retroviral vector-mediated gene transfer. Proc Nat Acad Sci USA 87: 2877–2881.

Wolfe JH, Sands MS, Barker JE, Gwynn B, Rowe LB, Vogler CA, Birkenmeier EH. 1992. Reversal of pathology in murine mucopolysaccharidosis type VII by somatic cell gene transfer. Nature 360: 749–753.

Woodford BJ, Liu Y, Fletcher RT, Chader GJ, Farber DB, Santos-Anderson R, Tso MOM. 1982. Cyclic nucleotide metabolism in inherited retinopathy in collies: A biochemical and histochemical study. Exp Eye Res 34:703–714.

Wrigstad A. 1994. Hereditary dystrophy of the retina and the retinal pigment epithelium in a strain of briard dogs: a clinical, morphologic and electroretinographic study. Linköping University Medical Dissertation #423.

Wrigstad A, Nilsson SEG, Narfström K. 1992. Ultrastructural changes of the retina and the retinal pigment epithelium in briard dogs with hereditary congenital night blindness and partial day blindness. Exp Eye Res 55:805–818.

Wrigstad A, Narfström K, Nilsson SEG. 1994. Slowly progressive changes of the retina and retinal pigments epithelium in briard dogs with hereditary retinal dystrophy: a morphologic study. Doc Ophthalmol 87:337–354.

Wrigstad A, Nilsson SEG, Dubielzig R, Narfström K. 1995. Neuronal ceroid lipofuscinosis in the Polish Owczarek Nizinny (PON) dog. Doc Ophthalmol 91:33–47.

Wyszynski RE, Bruner WE, Cano DB, Morgan KM, Davis CB, Sternberg P. 1989. A donor-age-dependent change in the activity of alpha-mannosidase in human cultured RPE cells. Invest Ophthalmol Vis Sci 30:2341–2347.

Zhao H, Boissy YL, Abdel-Malek Z, King RA, Nordlund JJ, Boissy RE. 1994. On the analysis of the pathophysiology of Chediak-Higashi syndrome: defects expressed by cultured melanocytes. Lab Invest 71:25–34.

Zimmerman W, Godchaux W, Belkin M. 1983. The relative proportions of lysosomal enzyme activities of bovine retinal pigment epithelium. Exp Eye Res 36:151–158.

15. Congenital abnormalities of the retinal pigment epithelium

ARTURO SANTOS AND ELIAS I. TRABOULSI

During the fifth week of embryogenesis and after the optic vesicle has formed and invaginated to become the optic cup, the outer wall of the optic cup is composed of a mitotically active, pseudostratified, columnar epithelium. With the expansion of the cup, the outer cells arrange themselves in a monolayer and take on a cuboidal appearance. The apical surface of these future retinal pigment epithelium (RPE) cells are reflected into short projections against the future photoreceptor outer segments. The RPE cells are the site of earliest melanin production in the body. Melanization of the RPE begins in the posterior pole of the developing eye, proceeds anteriorly, and is completed by the end of gestation. The RPE cells produce a basement membrane which becomes the inner portion of Bruch's membrane (Mund et al., 1972).

The RPE is one of the most reactive human tissues. It can undergo hyperplasia, hypertrophy, migration, metaplasia, and atrophy. Examples of all these morphologic changes are encountered in congenital abnormalities that affect this layer of tissue (Gass, 1989). Congenital abnormalities of the RPE may be divided into focal, diffuse, and mixed categories. In focal lesions, such as congenital hypertrophy of the retinal pigment epithelium (CHRPE), only a circumscribed group of cells are morphologically different from the rest of the RPE. On the other hand, in some metabolic diseases such as albinism, all RPE cells are abnormal. In still other conditions, such as familial adenomatous polyposis, there are focal lesions in addition to a diffuse RPE involvement. A clinicopathologic classification of these abnormalities is given in Table 15-1.

FOCAL ABNORMALITIES

Congenital Hypertrophy of the Retinal Pigment Epithelium

Patches of congenital hypertrophy of the retinal pigment epithelium (CHRPE) are present at birth (Champion and Daicker, 1989) and have no malignant potential.

CHRPE was first described by Reese and Jones in nine patients as "benign melanoma" of the RPE (Reese and Jones, 1956). The hypertrophic nature of the pigment epithelial cells in these lesions was demonstrated by Kurz and Zimmerman (1962) and by Buettner (1975). The term *congenital hypertrophy of the retinal pigment epithelium* was introduced by Buettner and has become widely accepted (Buettner, 1975). Gass (1989) classified focal congenital anomalies of the retinal pigment epithelium and proposed to call CHRPE "solitary melanotic nevi of the retinal pigment epithelium". Although some of the fundus lesions in intestinal polyposis are histologically similar to CHRPE, we reserve the term CHRPE for the solitary non-polyposis-related lesion. We chose the term POFL-FAP, or simply POFL (pigmented ocular fundus lesion of familial adenomatous polyposis) to describe any of the pleomorphic morphologic or histopathologic types of pigmented ocular lesion in patients with polyposis (see below).

Clinical features

Symptoms. Patients are generally asymptomatic and CHRPE lesions are incidental findings on routine ophthalmoscopy. In a case-control study of pigmented fundus lesions in polyposis, Traboulsi and colleagues (1987) found that an isolated patch of CHRPE of any size was present in about one-third of normal individuals. Only 2% or less of individuals have bilateral patches of CHRPE (Purcell and Shields, 1975; Lewis et al., 1984).

Ophthalmoscopy. CHRPE typically appears as an isolated, dark gray to black, flat or minimally elevated, round lesion located at the level of the RPE. The lesion has well-demarcated smooth or scalloped margins (Gass, 1974; Purcell and Shields, 1975; Buettner, 1975). The dark lesion is almost always surrounded by a white halo that is inside a darker rim, producing a double outline (Fig. 15-1). In some cases, punched-out areas of depigmentation develop in the center of the lesion and coalesce in a cauliflower-like fashion. CHRPE varies from 100 μm to 5 mm in diameter. Rare large lesions may in-

TABLE 15-1. *Classification of congenital abnormalities of the retinal pigment epithelium*

Focal abnormalities
   Congenital hypertrophy of the retinal pigment epithelium
   Congenital grouped pigmentation of the retinal pigment epithelium
   Solitary albinotic spot of the retinal pigment epithelium
   Congenital grouped albinotic spots of the retinal pigment epithelium

Diffuse abnormalities
   Albinism
   Albinoidism

Diffuse and focal abnormalities
   Familial adenomatous polyposis

volve almost one-quarter of the fundus (Gass, 1989). CHRPE is typically located in the retinal periphery but may surround part of the optic nerve head. There is no apparent predilection for any particular fundus quadrant (Buettner, 1975). Uncommon clinical findings include pigmented areas adjacent to the anterior border of the lesion, and the presence or the appearance of linear streaks near or across the CHRPE (Chamot et al., 1993). The retina and retinal vessels overlying the CHRPE appear normal. There may be occasional focal intraretinal pigmentation near the margin of the lesion (Buettner, 1975). Enlargement of the depigmented areas inside these lesions has been well described (Buettner,

1975; Gass, 1989; Chamot et al., 1993) (Fig. 15-2). Concentric enlargement of the whole lesion has also been observed (Norris and Cleasby, 1976; Gass, 1989; Boldrey and Schwartz, 1982; Chamot et al., 1993). Chamot and colleagues (1993) reported the clinical characteristics of CHRPE in 35 patients followed from 1 to 14 years with serial fundus photographs. Progressive enlargement of the depigmented area inside the lesions was observed in 83% of patients, and concentric enlargement was documented in 74%. This progression is very slow and may be detected only after careful examination of serial fundus photographs. Norris and Cleasby (1976) reported a patient in whom a CHRPE lesion doubled in surface area over a period of 13 years. Slight widening of the margins of CHRPE lesions was documented in two patients who were followed up for more than 7 years (Boldrey and Schwartz, 1982).

Ancillary diagnostic tests. Patients with CHRPE may have visual-field defects that correspond to the location and size of the fundus abnormality. In younger patients the scotoma tends to be relative, while in older patients it is absolute (Buettner, 1975). These scotomas are generally asymptomatic. Electroretinographic and electrooculographic responses are normal (Buettner, 1975). On angiography CHRPE lesions totally block the normal background choroidal fluorescence. The normal choriocapillaris flush can be observed through the central depigmented areas. Choroidal fluorescence has also been observed through the hypopigmented halo that

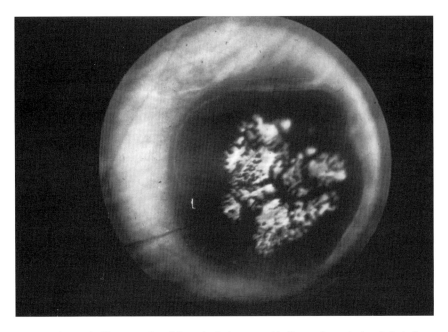

FIGURE 15-1. Congenital hypertrophy of the retinal pigment epithelium: a large, isolated, dark flat round lesion with well demarcated smooth margins, and surrounded by a white halo. There are multiple areas of depigmentation in the center of the lesion.

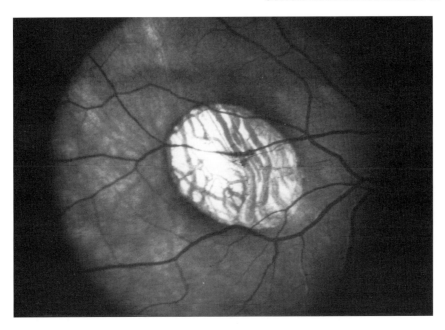

FIGURE 15-2. Completely depigmented patch of CHRPE.

surrounds some of the lesions. The retina and the retinal vasculature that overlie patches of CHRPE, as well as the RPE and choroid in these areas, usually exhibit a normal fluorescein angiographic pattern (Buettner, 1975). However, Cleary and colleagues (1976) described vascular nonperfusion with obliteration of the retinal capillary bed, retinal capillary leakage, and presumed neovascularization in five cases.

Associated findings. Solitary patches of congenital hypertrophy of the RPE are not associated with systemic diseases such as familial adenomatous polyposis (Purcell and Shields, 1975; Blair and Trempe, 1980; Buettner, 1986). However, patches of CHRPE have been observed in a newborn with multiple abnormalities of the spinal cord, thorax, and skull; these findings were thought to be consistent with a diagnosis of spondylothoracic dysplasia (Champion and Daicker, 1989). Champion and Daicker reported a six-year-old girl with microcephaly, epilepsy, spastic tetraparesis, persistent left upper vein, dysplastic fingernails and toenails and congenital glaucoma; a diagnosis of Donohue syndrome was considered (Champion and Daicker, 1989). Kurz and Zimmerman reported a 19-year-old woman with syringomyelia, a history of poliomyelitis, spinal fusion for scoliosis, several scattered cutaneous nevi, and "café-au-lait" spots (Kurz and Zimmerman, 1962). A possible association of CHRPE with neurofibromatosis has also been suggested (Shields, 1983). Patients with isolated CHRPE are not at a greater risk of developing intestinal cancer (Shields et al., 1992).

Histopathology. CHRPE lesions consist of a single layer of hypertrophied (tall), maximally pigmented RPE cells (Buettner, 1975; Lloyd et al., 1990; Gass, 1989; Wirz et al., 1982; Champion and Daicker, 1989) (Fig. 15-3). Segmental hyperplasia and focal atrophy of the RPE cells have also been observed in these lesions (Wirz et al., 1982). In a morphometric analysis of a CHRPE lesion performed by Lloyd and colleagues (1990) the density of the RPE cells that constituted the lesion was found to be 1.7 times greater than the density of adjacent normal peripheral RPE cells. The hypertrophic RPE cells contain an increased number of large, round pigment granules instead of the football-shaped melanin granules of normal RPE (Kurz and Zimmerman, 1962; Buettner, 1975) (Fig. 15-4). Initially, these granules were thought to be lipofuscin (Buettner, 1975), however, several authors (Wirz et al., 1982; Champion and Daicker, 1989; Lloyd et al., 1990) have excluded the presence of lipofuscin in CHRPE lesions using fluorescence microscopy, and identified these granules as enlarged melanin granules. Retinal photoreceptors that overlie CHRPE are variably degenerated (Buettner, 1975; Kurz and Zimmerman, 1962; Wirz et al., 1982; Lloyd et al., 1990). Bruch's membrane is thickened as a result of thickening of the basement membrane of the hypertrophied RPE cells. The choriocapillaris and choroid underneath the lesion are normal (Buettner, 1975). The inner retinal layers and retinal vasculature are unremarkable. The hypopigmented halo that surrounds some of the lesions consists of less pigmented

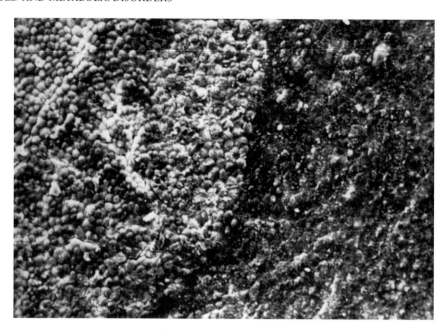

FIGURE 15-3. Abrupt transition is shown between the CHRPE *(left)* and adjacent normal RPE at the lesion's smoothly curved temporal margin. Compared with the cobblestoned surface of the lesion, the adjacent RPE is relatively flat (scanning electron microscopy; original magnification × 160). (Reprinted by permission from Lloyd, et al. 1990.)

hypertrophied RPE cells. In the central depigmented areas, both hypertrophied RPE cells and retinal photoreceptors are absent and are replaced by glial cells (Buettner, 1975).

Pathogenesis. The congenital nature of CHRPE was confirmed by Champion and Daicker (1989). These authors reported a term neonate with multiple congenital anomalies, including CHRPE, who died shortly after

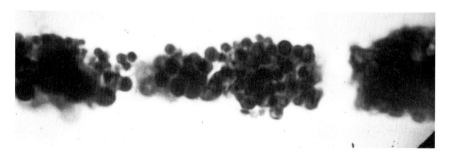

FIGURE 15-4. Pigment granules within CHRPE lesions are more spheroidal and more variable in size than in normal pigment epithelium (magnification × 900. AFIP neg 61-3087). (Reprinted by permission from Kurz and Zimmerman, 1962.)

birth. Based on the absence of lipofuscin pigment in CHRPE, it has been hypothesized that the abnormal RPE cells comprising the lesion lack the capacity to phagocytose and digest photoreceptor outer segments leading to degeneration of rods and cones and to visual-field defects (Lloyd et al., 1990). The pathogenic mechanisms for the enlargement of some lesions and for the development of pigmented areas and linear streaks adjacent to or overlying lesions remain unknown. Some histopathologic features, such as hypertrophy, segmental hyperplasia, and focal atrophy of the RPE cells found in CHRPE, may help explain the slow growth of some of these lesions (Champion and Daicker, 1989). In view of the benign clinical course of CHRPE, such changes in pigmentation and increases in size of the lesion should not be considered signs of malignant degeneration (Chamot et al., 1993).

Differential diagnosis. The ophthalmoscopic characteristics of CHRPE, and the occasional use of fluorescein angiography and ultrasonography, aid in differentiating this lesion from other pigmented retinal, RPE, and choroidal lesions (Purcell and Shields, 1975; Shields et al., 1992). The differential diagnosis includes choroidal melanoma, choroidal nevus, melanocytoma, hyperplasia of the RPE, pigmented ocular fundus lesions (POFLs) associated with familial adenomatous polyposis (FAP), congenital grouped pigmentation of the retinal pigment epithelium, sunburst lesions of sickle cell disease, hemorrhage beneath the RPE, old chorioretinitis, paving-stone degeneration, and enclosed bays of the ora serrata. In contradistinction to choroidal melanoma, CHRPE lesions are flat and have well-demarcated margins and characteristic depigmented changes (Shields et al., 1992; Buettner, 1975; Purcell and Shields, 1975; Lloyd et al., 1990). Choroidal melanomas have tapering boundaries, may hyperfluoresce on angiography, and may show low internal reflectivity on ultrasonography (Shields, 1983). The POFLs associated with intestinal polyposis are pleomorphic and have different ophthalmoscopic characteristics from solitary CHRPE; they are multiple and bilateral.

Congenital Grouped Pigmentation of the Retinal Pigment Epithelium

Congenital grouped pigmentation of the RPE, characterized by multiple well-circumscribed, flat lesions that are arranged in clusters, with an animal paw print appearance, was initially recognized by Mauthner (1868). The term grouped pigmentation of the fundus was first used by Hoeg (1911) to describe lesions that resembled animal tracks. Egerer (1976) reviewed all cases report-

ed before 1976, finding that 84% of lesions were unilateral; 59% involved a single quadrant of the fundus; and none were inherited. Two familial instances have been described. De Jong and Delleman (1988) described a father and son with grouped pigmentation of the RPE, suggesting autosomal dominant inheritance with variable expressivity. Renardel de Lavalette and colleagues (1991) reported on a mother and daughter, also suggesting dominant inheritance. Of patients examined in a general ophthalmic practice, 0.12% have grouped pigmentation of the RPE (de Jong and Delleman, 1988). The entity has also been called melanosis retinae, bear or animal tracks, nevoid pigmentation of the fundus, familial grouped pigmentation of the retinal pigment epithelium (de Jong and Delleman, 1988), grouped pigmentation of the retina (Mann, 1932), and congenital grouped pigmentation of the retina (Blake, 1926).

Clinical Features

Symptoms. Congenital grouped pigmentation of the RPE is asymptomatic and is detected during routine examinations of the eye (Yoshida et al., 1995).

Ophthalmoscopy. Grouped pigmentation of the RPE consists of multiple, small, well-circumscribed, uniformly pigmented flat lesions (Blake, 1926; Mann, 1932; Kurz and Zimmerman, 1962; Shields, 1975) that vary in size from 0.1 to 0.5 disc diameter and that are arranged in clusters in one or more sectors of the fundus. The smaller spots are usually located at the apex of each cluster and closer the posterior pole; this leads to the appearance of so-called animal paw prints or bear tracks (Hoeg, 1911; Mauthner, 1868; Parsons, 1905; Shields and Tso, 1975) (Fig. 15-5).

Ancillary diagnostic tests. Visual field, color vision, and dark-adaptation tests are normal (de Jong and Delleman, 1988; Yoshida et al., 1995). Similarly, electroretinography, electrooculography, and visually evoked cortical potentials have been found to be normal in patients with grouped pigmentation of the RPE (de Jong and Delleman, 1988; Yoshida et al., 1995). Fluorescein angiography shows blocked choroidal fluorescence by the RPE lesions in the early arteriovenous phase. The boundaries of larger lesions may hyperfluoresce. No leakage of dye is observed during any phase of the angiogram. The choroid, RPE, and retinal vasculature are not involved and show normal fluorescein angiographic pattern (Yoshida et al., 1995).

Associated findings. Congenital grouped pigmentation of the RPE occasionally occurs in association with other anomalies of the eye, such as convergent strabismus (Hoeg, 1911), macular coloboma (McGregor, 1945), Rieger's anomaly (de Jong et al., 1979), and

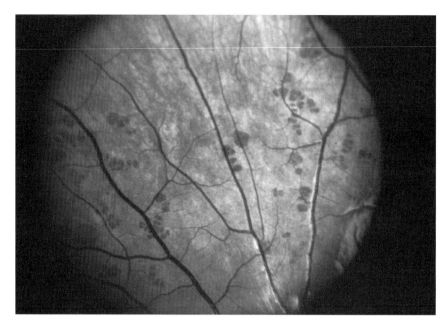

FIGURE 15-5. Grouped pigmentation of the RPE. Multiple small, uniformly pigmented, flat lesions arranged in clusters, producing so-called animal paw prints or bear tracks.

retinoblastoma (Regillo et al., 1993). No association has been reported with extraocular abnormalities. Patients with grouped pigmentation of the RPE are not at a greater risk of developing intestinal cancer (Shields et al., 1992).

Histopathology. The histopathologic features of grouped pigmentation of the RPE were mentioned in the French literature in 1904 (Parsons, 1905) and in the Italian literature in 1938 (Ciotola, 1938). In a light microscopic study by Shields and Tso (1975) the pigmented lesions were formed of focal areas of increased concentration of pigment granules in otherwise normal RPE cells. Pigment granules were large and football-shaped. The overlying photoreceptors were normal. Regillo and colleagues (1993) described the histopathologic and ultrastructural features of grouped pigmentation of the RPE in one eye of a two-year-old child with retinoblastoma. There was an abrupt transition between hyperpigmented and surrounding normal RPE. The height of RPE cells in the pigmented lesions did not differ significantly from that of uninvolved cells. The pigment granules, however, were 1.6 times larger in greatest dimension in the involved cells compared to normal cells. Melanosomes were larger in the hyperpigmented cells, but retained their normal football-shaped configuration. The basement membrane of the RPE under the lesion and in uninvolved areas was not thickened.

Pathogenesis. This benign condition of unknown etiology is congenital and nonprogressive (Shields and Tso,

1975). The presumed normal function of the RPE cells may explain the normal electrophysiological responses and visual fields usually reported in patients with this condition.

Differential diagnosis. The differential diagnosis of grouped pigmentation of the RPE includes sector retinitis pigmentosa, inflammatory conditions such as rubella retinopathy, pigment proliferation secondary to trauma or hemorrhage (Shields and Tso, 1975), congenital hypertrophy of the RPE, and pigmented ocular fundus lesions associated with familial adenomatous polyposis.

Solitary Albinotic Spot of the Retinal Pigment Epithelium

This condition was described as peripheral retinal albinotic spots (Schlernitzauer and Green, 1971). The lesions were noted during the routine processing of two autopsy eyes. Later, Gass noted an identical lesion during a gross examination of a fresh autopsy eye of an adult patient and labeled this *congenital amelanotic freckle of the RPE* (Gass, 1987). These lesions were documented in six of 842 individuals examined during a mass screening of members of a small Maryland community (Schlernitzauer and Green, 1971).

Clinical features. Solitary albinotic spots of the RPE are discovered during routine ophthalmic examinations and are asymptomatic. These lesions are focal, round, sharply circumscribed white spots, .25 to 1 disc diame-

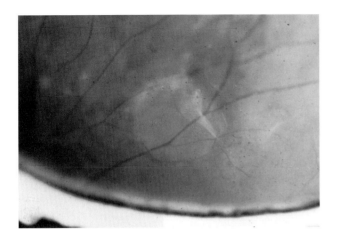

FIGURE 15-6. Gross photograph of the hypopigmented area noted in one autopsy eye of a 59-year-old man. (Reprinted by permission from Schlernitzauer and Green, 1971.)

ter in size, usually located in the midperiphery of the fundus (Fig. 15-6). Underlying large choroidal vessels are usually visible within the lesions (Gass, 1989).

Histopathology. On microscopic examination, there is an abrupt transition between the lesion and the normal surrounding RPE. The retinal pigment epithelial cells that form the lesion are slightly flatter than those in adjacent areas. These cells have virtually no pigment granules. The pigment granules observed at the borders of the lesion are football-shaped. The underlying Bruch's membrane, choriocapillaris, and choroid are normal. The overlying photoreceptors and internal retinal layers are also normal (Schlernitzauer and Green, 1971) (Fig. 15-7).

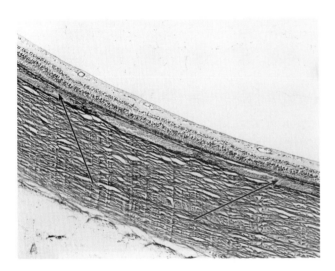

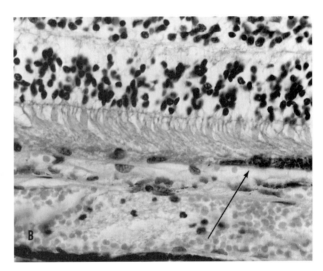

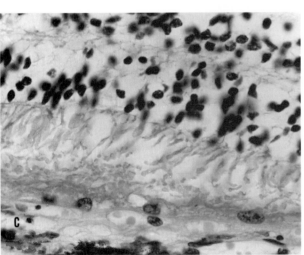

FIGURE 15-7. Photographs of the retinal pigment abnormality. (A) Overall view showing the extent of the lesion *(arrows indicate the borders)* (PAS, magnification × 45). (B) Higher-power view of the border of the lesion, showing the abrupt transition from normal-appearing retinal pigment epithelial cells to the abnormal cells *(arrow)* (hematoxylin and eosin, magnification × 575). (C) View of the center of a lesion showing the somewhat flattened retinal pigment epithelial cells which lack pigment and which rest on a normal-appearing Bruch's membrane and choriocapillaris (hematoxylin and eosin, magnification × 800). (Reprinted by permission from Schlernitzauer and Green, 1971.)

Pathogenesis. This lesion is thought to be congenital. The absence of all pigment in the RPE cells suggest that these lesions contain no melanin or white pigment from birth (Gass, 1989).

Differential diagnosis. The differential diagnosis of this condition includes a completely depigmented CHRPE, and nonpigmented choroidal nevi (Gass, 1989).

Congenital Grouped Albinotic Spots of the Retinal Pigment Epithelium

This is a very rare abnormality of the RPE. To date, only nine cases have been reported (Gass, 1989; Fuhrmann et al., 1992). Because of its ophthalmoscopic appearance, it is also known as *polar bear tracks* (Gass, 1989).

Clinical features

Symptoms. This condition may be observed in one or both eyes of typically asymptomatic healthy children or adults.

Ophthalmoscopy. Gass (Gass, 1989) described the grouped albinotic spots of the RPE as sharply circumscribed, placoid, chalky white lesions of the same size, shape, and distribution as congenital grouped pigmentation of the RPE. The spots appear to be slightly elevated and to lie at the level of the RPE. They may be uniformly thick or have a dimpled appearance. There is a focal narrowing of the major retinal vessels as they course over some of the larger lesions. Choroidal vessels may be visible beneath some lesions. Melanotic or partially melanotic spots may accompany albinotic ones. The lesions may be widely scattered in both eyes, or centered in one quadrant or less of the fundus. In some patients, small albinotic spots are present in the macular areas (Gass, 1989; Fuhrmann et al., 1992).

Ancillary diagnostic tests. The electroretinographic and electrooculographic recordings are normal in patients with this condition (Gass, 1989; Fuhrmann et al., 1992). Dark adaptation is also normal (Gass, 1989). Fluorescein angiography shows early hyperfluorescence corresponding to most of the albinotic spots. There is no leakage of dye or staining of the lesions (Gass, 1989).

Associated findings. Gass reported the case of an 11-year-old girl with bilateral widespread albinotic spots, who, at the age of 14 years, had severe visual loss from subretinal neovascularization in one eye (Gass, 1989).

Histopathology. To date, there is no histopathologic information about these lesions.

Pathogenesis. The biomicroscopic and angiographic findings locate these lesions at the level of the RPE

(Gass, 1989). Based on this clinical appearance, Gass postulated that polar bear tracks could consist of hypertrophied RPE cells packed with white pigment (Gass, 1989). Since choroidal neovascularization is uncommon in children, it is possible that this complication, reported in a 14-year-old patient with this condition, occurred at the site of one of the lesions (Gass, 1989).

Differential diagnosis. The ophthalmoscopic appearance and the fluorescein angiographic findings in grouped albinotic spots of the RPE are similar to those of nonfamilial stationary night blindness of Kandori. In this disorder, the retinal flecks are described as "dirty yellow" in color, and they do not affect the peripapillary or macular areas. In addition, mild changes are found in the dark-adaptation tests (Kandori et al., 1960). All eight patients reported by Gass denied nyctalopia, and in two of them the dark-adaptation test was normal (Gass, 1989).

DIFFUSE ABNORMALITIES

Familial Adenomatous Polyposis

Familial adenomatous polyposis (FAP) is an autosomal dominant condition characterized by the development of hundreds of adenomatous colonic polyps and the inevitable progression to colon cancer if a colectomy is not performed (Gebert et al., 1986) (Fig. 15-8). When FAP is associated with extracolonic manifestations, such as benign soft-tissue and bony tumors, jaw lesions, and desmoid tumors, the condition is termed *Gardner's syndrome* (Gardner, 1951). Patients with FAP are also at higher risk for developing extracolonic cancers of the thyroid, adrenal glands, and liver (Krush et al., 1988). The association of pigmented ocular fundus lesions (POFLs) with Gardner's syndrome and the clinical significance of these lesions in identifying patients at risk of developing polyps was first described by Blair and Trempe (1980). These lesions were first labeled as *congenital hypertrophy of the retinal pigment epithelium* (CHRPE) because of their similarity to the isolated CHRPE. Histopathologic and clinical studies have, however, allowed the differentiation of CHRPE from the polymorphic POFLs of FAP. The use of multiple POFLs as specific and reliable markers of FAP with extracolonic manifestations has been demonstrated in a number of studies (Lewis et al., 1984; Traboulsi et al., 1987; 1990a). Traboulsi and colleagues (1987; 1988) have shown that the presence of four or more POFLs predicts a carrier status of the FAP gene in family members at risk of the disease.

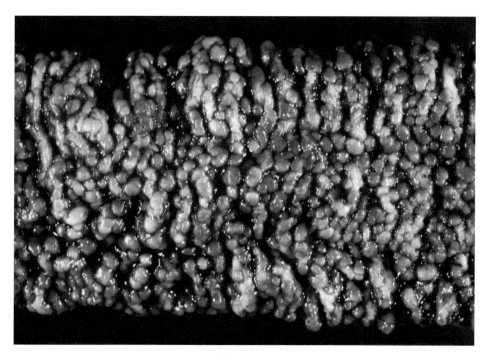

FIGURE 15-8. Colectomy specimen from a patient with FAP. Hundreds of adenomatous colonic polyps are present on mucosal aspect of colon.

Clinical features

Symptoms. Although multiple POFLs are usually present in patients with FAP, they do not cause symptoms unless the macula is involved, in which case visual acuity may be reduced (Traboulsi et al., 1987).

Ophthalmoscopy. These lesions are multiple and bilateral. The vast majority are less than 0.5 DD in size. Various morphologic forms can be observed in combination in the same subject. The most common type of lesion is small, flat, round, and hyperpigmented. This type of POFL occurs predominately in the equator and fundus midperiphery. Larger lesions, usually ovoid to round in shape, are present close to the posterior pole and vary in color from light gray-brown to black. Other POFLs are tear-shaped, coffee-bean-shaped, pencil-shaped, or irregular. The larger lesions exhibit variable degrees of hypopigmentation and lacunae formation. Some have a hypopigmented halo or a hypopigmented tail (Fig. 15-9). Most of the lesions appear flat with binocular biomicroscopy; others, however, are minimally elevated (Santos et al., 1994). Schmidt and colleagues (1994) described hyperpigmentation of the RPE underlying retinal vessels and longitudinally oriented RPE changes that followed the course of retinal vessels. The number of POFLs is variable among families but appears to be consistent within a kindred (Romania et al., 1989; Traboulsi, personal observation). Some of the lesions are difficult to identify by indirect ophthalmoscopy. Three-mirror contact lens examination has been recommended.

Ancillary diagnostic tests. Visual field scotomas corresponding to large lesions have been reported (Santos et al., 1994). Electroretinographic and electrooculographic studies in patients with Gardner's syndrome reveal no abnormalities (Stein and Brady, 1988; Santos et al., 1994). On fluorescein angiography, the hyperpigmented RPE totally blocks background choroidal fluorescence. A normal choriocapillaris flush is observed through the hypopigmented or depigmented lacuna present in some lesions (Santos et al., 1994). Retinal vascular abnormalities such as capillary nonperfusion, microaneurysm formation, and chorioretinal anastomoses are occasionally present in association with POFLs (Cohen et al., 1993).

From a systemic perspective, examination of the colon for polyps should be performed annually, commencing at ten years of age, in patients at risk for the disease (Jagelman, 1986). Determination of disease status in children is done by ocular examination, panoramic X-rays of the mandible (used to detect opaque jaw lesions—Offerhause et al., 1987), testing of the APC

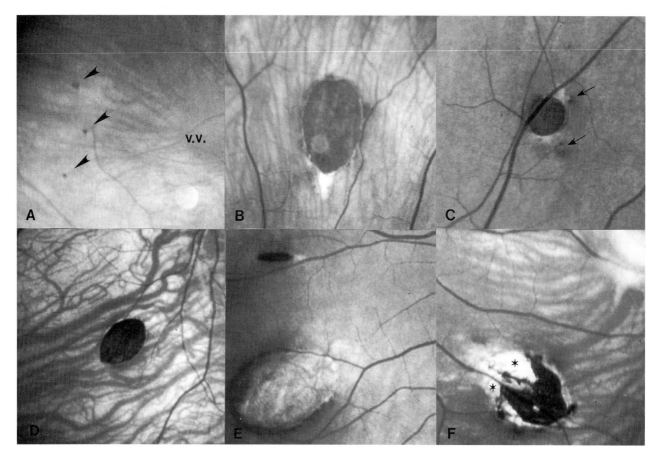

FIGURE 15-9. Various types of POFLs in FAP: (A) Midperiphery of retina with three small pigmented lesions *(arrowheads)* v.v. = vortex vein. (B) An oval, dark lesion with a hypopigmented tail. (C) A round lesion with mild pigmentary disturbance at edges. Two satellite lesions are present *(arrows)*. (D) An oval lesion in a blond fundus. (E) A large, lightly pigmented lesion and one smaller pen-shaped lesion. (F) A lesion with two areas of hypopigmentation (*) and a hypopigmented halo.

(adenomatous polyposis coli) gene for mutations, or a combination of the above.

Syndromes with POFLs. Gardner's syndrome is FAP with extracolonic manifestations such as POFLs, benign soft-tissue and bony tumors, jaw lesions, and desmoid tumors. Orbital osteomas have been reported in a few patients with Gardner's syndrome (Jones and Cornell, 1966; Whitson et al., 1986), and epidermal cysts of the eyelid skin may occur in these patients (Gardner, 1953).

Turcot syndrome is a variant of FAP in which patients develop brain tumors. Patients with Turcot syndrome may also have multiple POFLs (Munden et al., 1991; Traboulsi, personal observation).

Sheriff and Hegab (1988) reported three siblings with microcephaly and retinal/RPE abnormalities that included some lesions described as similar to those of FAP. Two had focal areas of chorioretinal atrophy and one had whitish round lesions in front of retinal vessels. None of these three patients had stigmata of intestinal polyposis.

Histopathology. The focal hyperpigmented lesions of FAP are present on a background of diffuse involvement of the RPE (Traboulsi et al., 1990; Kasner et al., 1992). RPE cells outside focal lesions are slightly enlarged and contain large, round melanin granules. These large round granules are different from the football-shaped melanin granules of normal RPE. Melanin and lipofuscin granules are also present in the hypertrophied RPE cells of patients with Gardner's syndrome (Traboulsi et al., 1990b). There is a thickening of Bruch's membrane under the focal lesions (Figs. 15-10–12). Traboulsi and colleagues (1990b) classified POFLs-FAP into four histopathological categories: (1) lesions formed of a single layer of hypertrophic RPE cells, (2) lesions consisting of a small mound of two to three cell layers of RPE located between the inner collagenous layer of Bruch's membrane and thickened RPE basement membrane, (3) thicker lesions composed of seven to eight cell layers of hyperplastic RPE cells, and (4) hyperplastic, darkly pigmented lesions that occupy the full thickness of the reti-

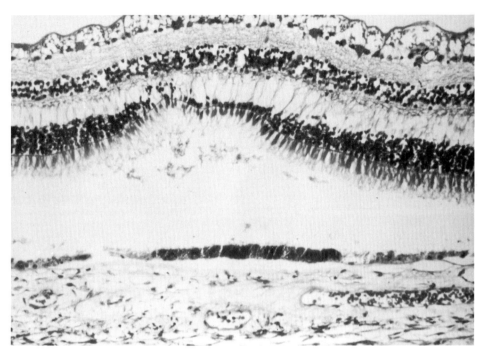

FIGURE 15-10. A 0.3 mm posterior pole lesion consists of tall darkly pigmented retinal pigment epithelial cells. There is partial loss of outer and inner photoreceptors and of the outer nuclear layer (hematoxylin and eosin, magnification × 175). (Reproduced by permission from Traboulsi et al., 1990.)

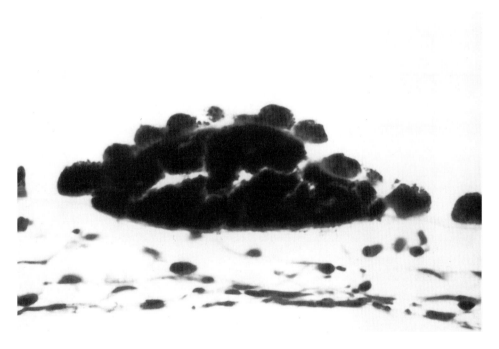

FIGURE 15-11. This lesion measured 0.15 mm in diameter and was located 6.5 mm posterior to the temporal ora serrata. This mound-shaped lesion consists of an aggregate of large, densely pigmented cells containing spherical pigment granules located between Bruch's membrane and the basement membrane of the overlying hypertrophic retinal pigment epithelium (periodic acid Schiff, magnification × 725). (Reproduced by permission from Traboulsi et al., 1990.)

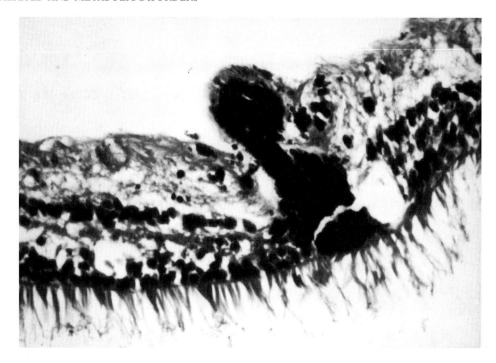

FIGURE 15-12. A 0.5 mm area of full-thickness intraretinal involvement by pigmented cells located 4 mm posterior to the inferonasal ora serrata (hematoxylin and eosin, magnification × 480). (Reproduced by permission from Traboulsi et al., 1990.)

na (Fig. 15-13. These authors also proposed that POFLs are best classified as adenomas of the RPE.

Molecular Genetics of FAP. Herrera and colleagues (1986) reported a patient with Gardner's syndrome and a deletion involving the long arm of chromosome 5. Following this report, the gene for FAP, designated as APC, was mapped to chromosome 5q21-q22 (Bodmer et al., 1987; Leppert et al., 1987; Meera Khan et al., 1988; Dunlop et al., 1991) and was later cloned (Groden et al., 1991; Kinzler, 1991), allowing mutation analysis of patients with this condition. Several reports describe the correlation between the type of mutation and the clinical phenotype of FAP (Spirio, 1993; Paul et al., 1993; Koorey et al., 1994; Giardiello et al., 1994; Caspari et al., 1994). Mutations in exons 1–8 of the APC gene are associated with POFL-negative phenotype, while those in exons 10–15 are generally associated with a POFL-positive phenotype (Olschwang et al., 1993; Wallis et al., 1994; Traboulsi et al., 1996).

Pathogenesis of ocular abnormalities in FAP. POFLs are congenital and have been observed in a premature neonate (Aiello, 1993). These lesions presumably do not increase in number of in size with age. Based on the histopathologic findings of diffuse and focal RPE abnormalities, Traboulsi and colleagues (1990b) and Kas-

ner and colleagues (1992) have suggested a generalized effect of the FAP gene on the RPE. The visual-field scotomas corresponding to the location of some of the focal lesions are explained by the overlying photoreceptor atrophy. The electroretinogram and the electrooculogram measure mass responses of the photoreceptors and RPE; the normal values recorded in patients with Gardner's syndrome indicate the absence of a detectable functional diffuse abnormality. Further studies on the role of the protein product of the APC gene in the RPE are needed to determine the pathology of the diffuse and focal abnormalities.

POFLs as clinical marker for FAP. The presence of four or more POFLs is a reliable presymptomatic, highly specific (>90%), and relatively sensitive (70%–80%) clinical marker for FAP. This biomarker is especially helpful in families where several affected individuals have numerous POFLs, because of the intrafamilial consistency of expression of the ocular trait. The absence of the ocular trait, however, does not rule out the disease in any family.

Differential diagnosis. The differential diagnosis of POFLs-FAP includes solitary CHRPE, choroidal nevus or melanoma, melanocytoma, hyperplasia of the RPE, congenital grouped pigmentation of the RPE, sunburst

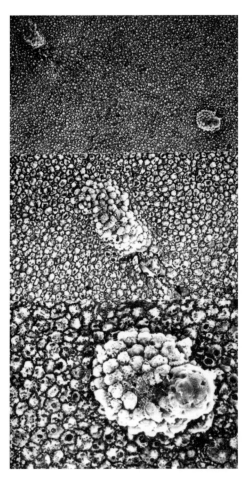

FIGURE 15-13. Top, scanning electron microscopic appearance of two discrete lesions composed of a cluster of enlarged retinal pigment epithelium surrounded by normal appearing 10.0 μm hexagonal retinal pigment epithelial cells. One lesion has a posterior trail of enlarged retinal pigment epithelial cells (magnification × 100). Middle, the first lesion is 140.0 μm in diameter, elevated, and consists of large, 15.0–17.0 μm cells that appear multilayered. A linear trail of large, 20.0–50 μm retinal pigment epithelial cells extends posteriorly for about 100 μm (magnification × 250). The second lesion is 100.0 μm in diameter and similar to the first except for a posterior trail of only one cell (magnification × 500). (Reproduced by permission from Traboulsi et al. 1990.)

lesions of sickle cell disease, hemorrhage beneath the RPE, old chorioretinitis, paving-stone degeneration, and enclosed oral bays.

Patients with Peutz-Jeghers syndrome and hereditary nonpolyposis colorectal cancer also have colonic polyps but no POFLs (Traboulsi et al., 1988).

Albinism

Albinism refers to a group of genetically determined disorders of melanin biogenesis characterized by congenital reduction or total absence of pigment in hair, skin, and eyes. The prevalence of all types of albinism has been estimated at 1:10,000 in Northern Ireland (Froggatt, 1960). Witkop (1979) found that 9% of partially sighted individuals attending special institutions in five states in the United States had some form of oculocutaneous albinism. Albinism has been classically divided into ocular and oculocutaneous categories. However, all albinos have some degree of cutaneous hypopigmentation. The current knowledge of the enzymes and genes involved in the production of melanin from tyrosine allows a better understanding of disorders of pigmentation. The cloning and mutation analysis of the tyrosinase gene (Kwon et al., 1987; Oetting and King, 1993; King et al., 1994), the P gene (Rinchik et al., 1993; Lee et al., 1994), and the tyrosinase-related protein gene (Jackson, 1989; Wagstaff, 1993; Boissy et al., 1993), and the recent mapping of the Hermansky-Pudlak gene (Wildenburg, 1995) and the Chediak-Higashi syndrome (Barrat, 1996; Fukai, 1996; Nagle, 1996) have provided the means to classify albinism on the basis of molecular genetic defects, complementing and modifying the classical clinical classification scheme (Spritz, 1994). Several forms of oculocutaneous albinism, previously thought to be clinically distinct, have been shown to be due to allelic mutations in the tyrosinase gene (Table 15-2).

Clinical Features. The severity of pigmentary dilution depends on the genetic subtype, the constitutive pigmentation, and age. There are several consistent features present in all forms of albinism. These include nystagmus, decreased visual acuity, hypopigmentation of the uvea and RPE, foveal hypoplasia, and abnormal decussation of optic nerve fibers at the chiasm.

Symptoms. Patients are generally photophobic. Visual acuity is impaired and ranges from 20/80 to 20/400 in most patients. Nystagmus tends to vary, depending on the type of albinism. It is detectable within the first few months of life, but often lessens somewhat as the child becomes older.

Slit-lamp biomicroscopy. A pink reflex is observed through the undilated iris. Diffuse transillumination of the iris and the globe can be elicited by retroillumination, revealing the outline of the lens (Abrams, 1964; Donaldson, 1974) (Fig. 15-14, and Plate 15-I).

Ophthalmoscopy. The hypopigmentation of the fundus is a striking feature in albinism (Fig. 15-15 and Plate 15-I). The degree of hypopigmentation varies considerably. Some patients lack all pigment in the RPE and choroid, while others have a fundus pigmentation that resembles that of a normal blond fundus. There is prominence of the choroidal vasculature because of the absence or paucity of pigment in the overlying RPE and surrounding choroidal stroma. Generally, there is an ab-

TABLE 15-2. *Classification of human albinism*

Clinical type	Defective gene	Gene map
Tyrosinase-negative oculocutaneous albinism	Tyrosinase (TYR)	11q14–q21
Yellow mutant type of oculocutaneous albinism	Tyrosinase (TYR)	11q14–q21
Temperature-sensitive oculocutaneous albinism	Tyrosinase (TYR)	11q14–q21
Rufous albinism, (xanthism)		
Brown albinism, (albinism with only moderate reduction in pigment)	Tyrosinase-related protein (TYRP)	9p
Tyrosinase-positive oculocutaneous albinism	Some cases due to mutations in tyrosinase, others to mutations in P gene.	15q11.2–q12 11q14–q21
Nettleship-Falls ocular albinism, X-linked ocular albinism		Xp22.3
Forsius-Eriksson disease, (Aland island eye disease)		Xp11.4–p11.2
Autosomal recessive ocular albinism	Some cases due to mutations in tyrosinase, others to mutations in P gene.	11q14–q21 15q11.2–q12
X-linked albinism with late-onset deafness		Xp22.3
Hermansky-Pudlak syndrome		10q23.1–q23.3
Chediak-Higashi syndrome	Lysosomal trafficking regulator (LYST)	1q42.1–q42.2

sence of the normal hyperpigmentation of the RPE in the macular area. In some cases, mild pigmentation may be present in the macular area, obscuring the view of the submacular choroidal vasculature. Macular hypoplasia associated with absence of the foveal pit is always present. The retinal vessels fail to wreathe the fovea.

Ancillary diagnostic tests. Color vision is generally normal. Electroretinographic (Krill and Lee, 1963) and electrooculographic (Reeser et al., 1970) responses have been recorded as supernormal in patients with albinism. The defect of the optic pathways present in patients with albinism can be detected with a high degree of accuracy by visually evoked potentials (Apkarian et al., 1983). The asymmetry which reflects the albino feature is contralateral and corresponds to the latency of the early

component (Apkarian et al., 1984). The tyrosinase test determines the activity of the enzyme tyrosinase in the hair bulb, and has been used to divide oculocutaneous albinism into two major groups: tyrosinase negative and positive.

Associated findings. Patients with albinism have a high incidence of strabismus (Fonda, 1962; Simon et al., 1984) and astigmatic errors of refraction (Silver, 1977). Cases of albinism associated with anterior segment dysgenesis and glaucoma have been reported (van Dorp et al., 1984; Larkin and O'Donoghue, 1988; Catalano et al., 1988), but the association between albinism and these conditions may be fortuitous. In some patients, albinism is only one of the clinical features that constitute a syndrome. In the Hermansky-Pudlak syndrome, albinism is associated with storage of ceroidlike material,

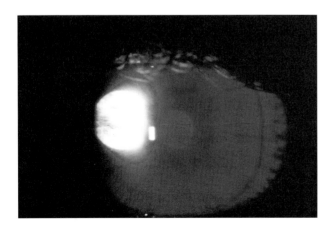

FIGURE 15-14. Diffuse transillumination of the iris elicited by retroillumination.

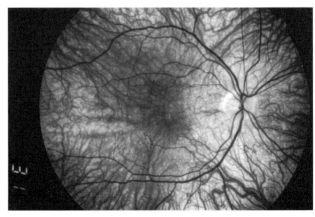

FIGURE 15-15. Hypopigmentation of the fundus in albinism.

platelet dysfunction with bleeding diathesis, and restrictive lung disease. Chediak-Higashi syndrome is characterized by variable oculocutaneous pigmentary dilution, susceptibility to pyogenic infections, and a predisposition to develop a lymphoma-like condition in adolescence (Blume and Wolff, 1972). Cross syndrome, described in an Amish family, is characterized by mental retardation, athetosis, spastic diplegia, cutaneous hypopigmentation, gingival fibromatosis, nystagmus, microphthalmos, and cloudy vascularized corneas (Cross et al., 1967).

Histopathology. Several electron microscopic studies have shown that the ocular structures contain various small amounts of melanin in most patients with albinism. Wong and colleagues (1983) demonstrated the presence of normal-sized type II, III, and IV melanosomes in retinal pigment epithelial cells of a 21-week old fetus with X-linked ocular albinism. O'Donnell and colleagues (1983) observed macromelanosomes in the RPE in one 22-year-old patient with the Nettleship-Fall type of X-linked ocular albinism. Fulton and colleagues (1978) reported the presence of premalanosomes and melanosomes in RPE cells. Naumann and colleagues (1976) described type III melanosomes in the eye of a patient with tyrosinase-positive oculocutaneous albinism. Mietz and colleagues (1992) reported the histopathologic and ultrastructural findings in an eye from a 99-year-old tyrosinase-negative albino woman. These authors demonstrated the absence of melanin throughout ocular tissues. Examination of the RPE revealed intracytoplasmic granules containing lipofuscin. No melanosomes or premelanosomes were present. The histopathologic confirmation of foveal hypoplasia in albinism was also reported (Mietz et al., 1992). Serial sec-

tions through the posterior pole failed to disclose the presence of a foveal pit (Fig. 15-16). In the normal anatomical location of the foveola, the retina was of normal thickness, with five to seven ganglion cell layers (Mietz et al., 1992). Foveal hypoplasia has been also described and proven in several histopathologic studies by other authors (Naumann et al., 1976; Fulton et al., 1978).

Pathogenesis. Albinism results from the defective production of melanin from tyrosine through a complex pathway of metabolic reactions. Melanogenesis is a transient activity of RPE cells. Retinal pigment cell melanogenesis begins by the third or fourth week of gestation (Wolff, 1976) and is thought to be completed shortly after birth. Retinal pigment epithelial cells are very reactive to a number of stimuli but do not seem to be able to resume melanogenesis. Evidence of misdirected optic nerve fibers in albinism has been demonstrated by the presence of significant hemispheric asymmetry to monocular stimulation (Creel et al., 1978; Boylan and Harding, 1983). A possible explanation for the anomalous crossing of optic nerve fibers in albinos is that melanin pigment is important for axonal guidance during the development of the optic nerve in mice and rats (Silver and Sapiro, 1981). Wack and colleagues postulated that the supernormal electroretinographic responses recorded in patients with albinism result from the increased amount of stimulating light entering the eye through a hypopigmented anterior ocular segment (Wack et al., 1989). This electrophysiologic finding should not be considered as diagnostic of albinism. The pathogenesis of foveal hypoplasia in albinism is unknown, but may be related to the decreased amount of melanin in the RPE.

Differential diagnosis. The congenital nystagmus almost invariably present in albinism should be differentiated from congenital motor nystagmus and nystagmus secondary to retinal dystrophy. Patients with congenital motor nystamus typically have a visual acuity of about 20/40 to 20/60 (Cogan, 1967). Some patients with this condition assume a compensatory head position. Albinos only occasionally assume such head position. In patients with retinal dystrophies such as Leber's congenital amaurosis and achromatopsia, the family history, clinical appearance, and psychophysical and electrophysiological tests are useful to establish the diagnosis.

The diagnosis of the patient with tyrosinase-negative oculocutaneous albinism is made on clinical grounds (Witkop et al., 1989). Patients with tyrosinase-positive oculocutaneous albinism are more difficult to diagnose if they are seen in childhood. A history of light cuta-

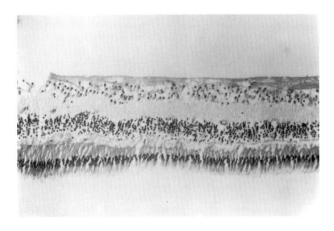

FIGURE 15-16. Section through the center of the anatomical location of the fovea with no foveal pit (hematoxylin-eosin; original magnification × 220). (Reproduced by permission from Mietz et al., 1992.)

neous pigmentation at birth and increasing pigmentation thereafter usually suggests this diagnosis, if the characteristic biomicroscopic and ophthalmoscopic features are present. X-linked ocular albinism is probably the most common cause of nystagmus in boys and should be suspected in all patients with nystagmus. Examination of the fundus and iris of the carrier mothers is helpful in those patients. Puerto Rican albinos should be screened for a bleeding diathesis, and for the Hermansky-Pudlak syndrome. Albinos with recurrent infections should be suspected of having Chediak-Higashi syndrome.

Albinoidism

In albinoidism there is generalized hypopigmentation of the skin, or the skin and eyes, but this may be mild. As in ocular albinism, cutaneous pigmentation falls within the normal range, but when compared with unaffected siblings, these patients have light complexion. The hypomelanosis usually involves the central frontal lock of hair and the ventral part of the trunk and extremities. This disease is differentiated from oculocutaneous and ocular albinism by the lack of nystagmus, photophobia, and significant visual impairment. There are several forms of, and syndromes that feature, albinoidism; some of these are discussed in the remainder of this section.

Autosomal dominant albinoidism. In this condition the skin is very fair, but it may tan. There is no nystagmus and visual acuity is normal. There is translucency of the irides and fundus hypopigmentation. The foveal reflex is present (Donaldson, 1974).

Ocular depigmentation and Apert syndrome. Pigmentary dilution of the skin and hair associated with fundus hypopigmentation and translucent irides have been observed in some patients with Apert syndrome (Margolis, 1978).

Waardenburg syndrome. This autosomal dominant disorder, described in 1951 by Waardenburg is characterized by heterochromia irides, deafness, albinoidism with a white forelock in some patients, and dystopia canthorum in most patients. The irides may be bright blue in both eyes. There are at least two types of Waardenburg syndrome. In type I there is dystopia canthorum with a normal interpupillary distance. Patients with type II do not have dystopia canthorum (Arias, 1971). Waardenburg syndrome type I was mapped to 2q35 (Foy et al., 1990). Mutations in the paired-box containing developmental gene PAX-3 that maps to the

same chromosomal region were later identified in families with Waardenburg syndrome types I and III (Tassabehji et al., 1993a; 1993b; Baldwin et al., 1993; Hoth et al., 1993). Waardenburg syndrome type II was mapped to 3q near the presumed locus for the human homolog of the murine microphthalmia gene (Hughes et al., 1994).

Waardenburg-like syndrome of Bard. Patients with this condition variably manifest a congenital sensorineural deafness, broad nasal root, white forelock, light complexion, premature graying of the scalp hair, segmental iris heterochromia, and fundus heterochromia (Bard, 1978). Visual acuity is 20/30 to 20/40 in the preferred eye. Hyperopia with esotropia and amblyopia and iris transillumination are often present. On ophthalmoscopy, there is severe fundus hypopigmentation and a hypopigmented fovea with a hypoplastic appearance.

Griscelli syndrome. This condition was described by Griscelli and colleagues (1978) as an autosomal recessive syndrome characterized by depigmentation of the hair, frequent pyogenic infections, acute episodes of fever, neutropenia, and thrombocytopenia.

ACKNOWLEDGMENTS

Dr Santos was supported in part by the Gillingham Pan-American Fellowship and the Retina Research Foundation and the Cleveland Clinic Eye Institute, Cleveland, Ohio.

REFERENCES

Abrams JD. 1964. Transillumination of the iris during routine slit lamp examination. Br J Ophthalmol 48:42–44.
Aiello LP, Traboulsi EI. 1993. Pigmented fundus lesions in a preterm infant with familial adenomatous polyposis. Arch Ophthalmol 111:302–303.
Apkarian P, Reits D, Spekreijse H. 1984. Component specificity in albino VEP asymmetry: maturation of the visual pathway anomaly. Exp Brain Res 53:285–294.
Apkarian P, Reits D, Spekreijse H, van Dorp D. 1983. A decisive electrophysiological test for human albinism. Electroencephalogr Clin Neurophysiol 55:513–531.
Arias S. 1971. Genetic heterogeneity in the Waardenburg syndrome. Birth Defects 7(4):87–101.
Baldwin CT, Hoth CF, Amos JA, et al. 1993. An exonic mutation in the HuP2 paired domain gene causes Waardenburg's syndrome. Nature 355:637–638.
Bard LA. 1978. Heterogeneity in Waardenburg's syndrome: report of a family with ocular albinism. Arch Ophthalmol 96:1193–1198.
Barrat FJ, et al. 1996. Genetic and physical mapping of the Chediak-Higashi syndrome on chromosome 1q42-43. Am J Hum Genet 59:625–632.
Blair NP, Trempe CL. 1980. Hypertrophy of the retinal pigment epithelium associated with Gardner's syndrome. Am J Ophthalmol 90:661–667.

Blake EM. 1926. Congenital grouped pigmentation of the retina. Trans Am Ophthalmol Soc 24:223–233.

Blume RS, Wolff SW. 1972. The Chediak Higashi syndrome: studies in 4 patients and a review of the literature. Medicine 51:247–280.

Bodmer WF, Bailey CS, Bodmer J, et al. 1987. Localization of the gene for familial adenomatous polyposis on chromosome 5. Nature 328:614–616.

Boissy RE, Zhao H, Austin LM, et al. 1993. Melanocytes from individual with brown oculocutaneous albinism lack expression of TRP-1, the product of the human homologue of murine brown locus. Am J Hum Genet 53(suppl):abstract 160.

Boldrey EE, Schwartz A. 1982. Enlargement of congenital hypertrophy of the retinal pigment epithelium. Am J Ophthalmol 94:64–66.

Boyland C, Harding GFA. 1983. Investigation of visual pathway abnormalities in human albinos. Ophthalmol Physiol Opt 3:273–285.

Buettner H. 1975. Congenital hypertrophy of the retinal pigment epithelium. Am J Ophthalmol 79:177–189.

Caspari R, et al. 1994. Familial adenomatous polyposis: mutation at codon 1309 and early onset of colon cancer. Lancet 343:629–632.

Catalano RA, Nelson LB, Schaffer DB. 1988. Oculocutaneous albinism associated with congenital glaucoma. Ophthalmic Paediatr Genet 9:5–6.

Cleary PE, Gregor Z, Bird AC. 1976. Retinal vascular changes in congenital hypertrophy of the retinal pigment epithelium. Br J Ophthalmol 60:499–503.

Chamot L, Zografos L, Klainguti G. 1993. Fundus changes associated with congenital hypertrophy of the retinal pigment epithelium. Am J Ophthalmol 115:154–161.

Champion R, Daicker BC. 1989. Congenital hypertrophy of the retinal pigment epithelium: light microscopic and ultrastructural findings in young children. Retina 9:44–48.

Ciotola G. 1938. Melanosi della retina. Ann Ottalmol Clin Ocul 66:543–552.

Cogan DG. 1967. Congenital nystagmus. Can J Ophthalmol 2:4–10.

Cohen SY, Quentel G, Guiberteau B, Coscas GJ. 1993. Retinal vascular changes in congenital hypertrophy of the retinal pigment epithelium. Ophthalmology 100:471–474.

Creel D, O'Donnell FE Jr, Witkop CJ Jr. 1978. Visual system anomalies in human ocular albinos. Science 201:931–933.

Cross HE, McKusick VA, Breen W. 1967. A new oculocerebral syndrome with hypopigmentation. J Pediatr 70:398–406.

de Jong PTVM, Delleman JW. 1988. Familial grouped pigmentation of the retinal pigment epithelium. Br J Ophthalmol 72:439–441.

de Jong PTVM, Delleman JW, Witmer JP, Zeilstra C. 1979. Riegers' anomaly with retinal pigmentations. Ophthalmologica 178:107–108.

Donaldson DD. 1974. Transillumination of the iris. Trans Am Ophthalmol Soc 72:89–104.

Dunlop MG, et al. 1991. Linked DNA markers for presymptomatic diagnosis of familial adenomatous polyposis. Lancet 337:313–316.

Egerer I. 1976. Die gruppierte (oder navoide) Pigmentation des Augenhintergrundes. Klin Monatsbl Augenheilkd 168:672–677.

Fonda G. 1962. Characteristics and low-vision corrections in albinism. Arch Ophthalmol 68:754–761.

Foy C, et al. 1990. Assignment of WS1 locus to human 2q37 and possible homology between Waardenburg syndrome and the Splotch mouse. Am J Hum Genet 46:1017–1023.

Froggat P. 1960. Albinism in Northern Ireland. Ann Hum Genet 24:213–238.

Fuhrmann C, Bopp S, Laqua H. 1992. Congenital grouped albinotic spots: a rare anomaly of the retinal pigment epithelium. Ger J Ophthalmol 1:103–104.

Fukai K, et al. 1996. Homozygosity mapping of the gene for Chediak-Higashi syndrome to chromosome 1q42-q44 in a segment of conserved synteny that includes the mouse beige locus (bg). Am J Hum Genet 59:620–624.

Fulton AB, Albert DM, Craft JL. 1978. Human albinism: light and electron microscopy study. Arch Ophthalmol 96:305–310.

Gass JDM. 1987. Stereoscopic Atlas of Macular Diseases: Diagnosis and Treatment. 3rd ed. St Louis: Mosby, 606–624.

Gass JDM. 1989. Focal congenital anomalies of the retinal pigment epithelium. Eye 3:1–18.

Gardner EJ. 1951. A genetic and clinical study of intestinal polyposis, a predisposing factor for carcinoma of the colon and rectum. Am J Hum Genet 3:167–176.

Gardner EJ, Richards RC. 1953. Multiple cutaneous and subcutaneous lesions occurring simultaneously with hereditary polyposis and osteomatosis. Am J Hum Genet 5:139.

Gebert HF, Jagelman DG, McGannon E. 1986. Familial polyposis coli. Am Fam Physician 33:127–137.

Giardiello FM, et al. 1994. Phenotypic variability of familial adenomatous polyposis in 11 unrelated families with identical APC gene mutation. Gastroenterology 106:1542–1547.

Griscelli C, et al. 1978. A syndrome associating partial albinism and immunodeficiency. Am J Med 65:691–702.

Groden J, et al. 1993. Mutational analysis of patients with adenomatous polyposis: identical inactivating mutations in unrelated individuals. Am J Hum Genet 52:263–272.

Herrera L, et al. 1986. Gardner syndrome in a man with interstitial deletion of 5q. Am J Med Genet 25:473–476.

Hoeg N. 1911. Die Gruppierte Pigmentation des Augengrundes. Klin Monastsbl Augenheilkd 49:49–77.

Hoth CF, et al. 1993. Mutations in a paired domain of the human PAX3 gene cause Klein-Waardenburg syndrome (WS-III) as well as Waardenburg syndrome type I (WS-1). Am J Hum Genet 52:455–462.

Hughes AE, et al. 1994. A gene for Waardenburg syndrome type 2 maps close to the human homologue of the microphthalmia gene at chromosome 3p12-p14.1. Nat Genet 7:509–512.

Jackson IJ. 1988. A cDNA encoding tyrosinase-related protein maps to the brown locus in mouse. Proc Nat Acad Sci USA 85:4392–4396.

Jagelman DG. 1986. Familial polyposis coli and hereditary cancer of the colon. Curr Ther Gastroenterol Liver Dis 2:228–233.

Jones EL, Cornell WP. Gardner's syndrome: review of the literature and report on a family. Arch Surg 92:287–300.

Kandori F, Setogawa T, Tamai A. 1966. Electroretinographical studies on "fleck retina with congenital nonprogressive nightblindness." Yonago Acta Med 10:98–108.

Kasner L, Traboulsi EI, De la Cruz Z, Green WR. 1992. A histopathologic study of the pigmented fundus lesions in familial adenomatous polyposis. Retina 12:35–42.

King RA, Summers CG, Creel D, Weleber R, Fryer JP, Oetting WS. 1994. Mutations of the tyrosinase gene produce autosomal recessive ocular albinism. Am J Hum Genet 55(suppl):A226.

Kinzler KW, et al. 1991. Identification of FAP locus genes from chromosomes 5q21. Science 253:661–665.

Koorey DJ, McCaughan GW, Trent RS, Gallagher ND. 1994. Exon eight APC mutation account for a disproportionate number of familial adenomatous polyposis families. Hum Mutat 3:12–18.

Krill AE, Lee GB. 1963. The electroretinogram in albinos and carriers of the ocular albino trait. Arch Ophthalmol 69:32–38.

Krush AJ, et al. 1988. Hepatoblastoma, pigmented ocular fundus lesions, and jaw lesions in Gardner syndrome. Am J Med Genet 29:323–332.

Kurz GH, Zimmerman LE. 1962. Vagaries of the retinal pigment epithelium. Int Ophthalmol Clin 2:441–464.

Kwon BS, Haq AK, Pomerantz SH, Halaban R. 1987. Isolation and sequence of a cDNA clone for human tyrosinase that maps at the mouse c-albino locus. Proc Nat Acad Sci 84:7473–7477.

Larkin DFP, O'Donoghue HN. 1988. Developmental glaucoma in oculocutaneous albinism. Ophthalmic Paediat Genet 9:1–4.

Lee S-T, et al. 1994. Mutations of the P gene in oculocutaneous albinism, ocular albinism and Prader-Willi syndrome plus albinism. N Eng J Med 330:529–534.

Leppert M, et al. 1987. The gene for familial polyposis coli maps to the long arm of chromosome 5. Science 238:1411–1413.

Lewis RA, et al. 1984. The Gardner syndrome: Significance of ocular features. Ophthalmology 91:916–925.

Lloyd WC III, et al. 1990. Congenital hypertrophy of the retinal pigment epithelium: electron microscopic and morphometric observations. Ophthalmology 97:1052–1060.

McGregor IS. 1945. Macular coloboma with bilateral grouped pigmentation of the retina. Br J Ophthalmol 39:132–136.

Mann WA Jr. 1932. Grouped pigmentation of the retina. Arch Ophthalmol 8:66–71.

Margolis S, Siegel IM, Choy A, Breinin GM. 1978. Depigmentation of hair, skin, and eyes associated with the Appert syndrome. Birth Defects 14:341–360.

Mauthner L. 1868. Lehrbuch der Ophthalmoscopie. Vienna: Tendler, 388.

Meera Khan P, et al. 1988. Close linkage of a highly polymorphic marker (D5S37) to familial adenomatous polyposis (FAP) and confirmation of FAP localization on chromosome 5q21-q22. Hum Genet 79:183–185.

Mietz H, Green WR, Wolff SM, Abundo GP. 1992. Foveal hypoplasia in complete oculocutaneous albinism: a histopathologic study. Retina 12:254–260.

Mund M, Rodriguez M, Fine B. 1972. Light and electron microscopic observations on the pigmented layers of the developing human eye. Am J Ophthalmol 73:167–182.

Munden PM, Sobol WM, Weingeist TA. 1991. Ocular findings in Turcot syndrome (glioma-polyposis). Ophthalmology 98:111–114.

Nagle DL, et al. 1996. Identification and mutation analysis of the complete gene for Chediak-Higashi syndrome. Nature Genet 14:307–311.

Naumann GOH, Lerche W, Schroeder W. 1976. Foveola-aplasie bei tyrosinase-positivem oculocutanem Albinismus. Graefes Arch Clin Exp Ophthalmol 200:39–50.

Norris JL, Cleasby GW. 1976. An unusual case of congenital hypertrophy of the retinal pigment epithelium. Arch Ophthalmol 94:1910–1911.

O'Donnell FE Jr, et al. 1976. X-linked ocular albinism: an oculocutaneous macromelanosomal disorder. Arch Ophthalmol 94:1883–1892.

Oetting WS, King RA. 1993. Molecular basis of type I (tyrosinase-related) oculocutaneous albinism: mutations and polymorphisms of the human tyrosinase gene. Hum Mutat 2:1–6.

Offerhaus GJ, et al. 1987. Occult radiopaque jaw lesions in familial adenomatous polyposis coli and hereditary nonpolyposis colorectal cancer. Gastroenterology 93:490–497.

Olshwang S, et al. 1993. Restriction of ocular fundus lesions to a specific subgroup of APC mutations in adenomatous polyposis coli patients. Cell 75:959–968.

Parsons JH. Some anomalies of pigmentation, in Dixieme congrès international d'ophtalmologie. Lausanne: Bridel, 152.

Paul P, et al. 1993. Identical APC exon 15 mutations result in a variable phenotype in familial adenomatous polyposis. Hum Mol Genet 2:925–931.

Purcell JJ Jr, Shields JA. 1975. Hypertrophy with pigmentation of the retinal pigment epithelium. Arch Ophthalmol 93:1122–1126.

Reese AB, Jones IS. 1956. Benign melanomas of the retinal pigment epithelium. Am J Ophthalmol 42:207–212.

Reeser F, Weinstein GW, Feiock KB. 1970. Electrooculography as a test of retinal function. Am J Ophthalmol 70:505–514.

Regillo CD, et al. 1993. Histopathologic findings in congenital grouped pigmentation of the retina. Ophthalmology 100:400–405.

Renardel de Lavalette VW, Cruysberg JRM, Deutman AF. 1991. Familial congenital grouped pigmentation of the retina. Am J Ophthalmol 112:406–409.

Rinchik EM, et al. 1993. A gene for the mouse pink-eyed dilution locus and for human type II oculocutaneous albinism. Nature 361:72–76.

Romania A, et al. 1989. Congenital hypertrophy of the retinal pigment epithelium in familial adenomatous polyposis. Ophthalmology 96:879–884.

Santos A, et al. 1994. Congenital hypertrophy of the retinal pigment epithelium associated with familial adenomatous polyposis. Retina 14:6–9.

Schlernitzauer DA, Green WR. 1971. Peripheral retinal albinotic spots. Am J Ophthalmol 72:729–732.

Schmidt D, Jung CE, Wolff G. 1994. Changes in the retinal pigment epithelium close to retinal vessels in familial adenomatous polyposis. Graefes Arch Clin Exp Ophthalmol 232:96–102.

Sheriff SMM, Hegab S. 1988. A syndrome of multiple fundal anomalies in siblings with microcephaly without mental retardation. Ophthalmic Surg 19:353–355.

Shields JA. 1983. Tumors and related lesions of the pigment epithelium. Diagnosis and Management of Intraocular Tumors. St Louis: Mosby, 389–400.

Shields JA, Tso MOM. 1975. Congenital grouped pigmentation of the retina. Arch Ophthalmol 93:1153–1155.

Shields JA, et al. 1992. Lack of association among typical congenital hypertrophy of the retinal pigment epithelium, adenomatous polyposis, and Gardner's syndrome. Ophthalmology 99:1709–1713.

Silver J. 1977. Low vision aids in the management of visual handicap. Br J Physiol Optics 31:47–87.

Silver J, Sapiro J. 1981. Axonal guidance during development of the optic nerve: the role of the pigment epithelia and other extrinsic factors. J Comp Neurol 202:521–538.

Simon JW, Kandel GL, Krohel GB, Nelson PT. 1984. Albinotic characteristics in congenital nystagmus. Am J Ophthalmol 97:320–327.

Spirio L, et al. 1993. Alleles of the APC gene: an attenuated form of familial polyposis. Cell 75:951–957.

Spritz RA. 1994. Molecular genetics of oculocutaneous albinism. Hum Mol Genet 3:1469–1475.

Stein EA, Brady KD. 1988. Ophthalmologic and electrooculographic findings in Gardner's syndrome. Am J Ophthalmol 106:326–331.

Tassabehji M, et al. 1993a. Waardenburg syndrome patients have mutations in the human homologue of the PAX3 paired box gene. Nature 355:635.

Tassabehji M, et al. 1993b. Mutations in the PAX3 gene causing Waardenburg syndrome Type 1 and Type 2. Nat Genetl 3:26.

Traboulsi EI, et al. 1987. Prevalence and importance of pigmented ocular fundus lesions in Gardner's syndrome. N Eng J Med 316:661–667.

Traboulsi EI, et al. 1988. Pigmented ocular fundus lesions in the inherited gastrointestinal polyposis syndromes and in hereditary nonpolyposis colon cancer. Ophthalmology 95:964–969.

Traboulsi EI, et al. 1990a. Congenital hypertrophy of the retinal pigment epithelium predicts colorectal polyposis in Gardner's syndrome. Arch Ophthalmol 108:525–526.

Traboulsi EI, et al. 1990b. A clinicopathologic study of the eyes in familial adenomatous polyposis with extracolonic manifestations (Gardner's syndrome). Am J Ophthalmol 110:550–561.

Traboulsi EI, et al. 1996. Pigmented ocular fundus lesions and APC mutations in familial adenomatous polyposis. Ophthalm Genet 17:167–174.

van Dorp DB, Delleman JW, Loewer-Sieger DH. 1984. Oculocutaneous albinism and anterior chamber cleavage malformations: not a coincidence. Clin Genet 26:440–444.

Waardenburg PJ. 1951. New syndrome combining developmental anomalies of the eyelids, eyebrows, and nose root with pigmentary defects of iris and head hair and with congenital deafness. Am J Hum Genet 3:195.

Wack MA, Peachy NS, Fishman GA. 1989. Electroretinographic findings in human oculocutaneous albinism. Ophthalmology 96:1778–1785.

Wagstaff J. 1993. A translocation-associated deletion defines a critical region for the 9p- syndrome. Am J Hum Genet 53(suppl):Abstract 619.

Wallis YL, et al. 1994. Genotype-phenotype correlation between position of constitutional APC gene mutation and CHRPE expression in familial adenomatous polyposis. Hum Genet 94:543–548.

Whitson WE, Orcutt JC, Walkinshaw MD. 1986. Orbital osteoma in Gardner's syndrome. Am J Ophthalmol 101:236–241.

Wildenburg SC, Oetting WS, Almodovar C, Krumwiede M, White JG, King RA. 1995. A gene causing Hermansky-Pudlak syndrome in a Puerto Rican population maps to chromosome 10q2. Am J Hum Genet 57:755–765.

Wirz K, Lee WR, Coaker T. 1982. Progressive changes in congenital hypertrophy of the retinal pigment epithelium: an electron microscopic study. Graefes Arch Clin Exp Ophthalmol 219:214–221.

Witkop CJ Jr. 1979. Depigmentations of the general and oral tissues and their genetic foundations. Ala J Med Sci 16:330.

Witkop CJ Jr. 1989. Albinism. Clin Dermatol 7:80–91.

Witkop CJ Jr, et al. 1973. Ophthalmologic, biochemical, platelet, and ultrastructural defects in the various types of oculocutaneous albinism. J Invest Dermatol 60:443–456.

Wolff E. 1976. Anatomy of the Eye and Orbit. 7th ed. Philadelphia: Saunders, 434.

Wong L, O'Donnell FE Jr, Green WR. 1983. Giant pigment granules in the retinal pigment epithelium of a fetus with X-linked ocular albinism. Ophthalmic Paediatr Genet 2:47–65.

Yoshida T, Adachi-Usami E, Kimura T. 1995. Three cases of grouped pigmentation of the retina. Ophthalmologica 209:101–105.

16. Dystrophies of the retinal pigment epithelium

MICHAEL F. MARMOR AND KENT W. SMALL

The classification of dystrophies and metabolic disorders of the fundus is difficult for several reasons. The pathologic examination typically reveals abnormalities in the retina, retinal pigment epithelium (RPE), and choroid. Therefore the tissue which is the primary seat of the disease is difficult to discern. Additionally, the phenotypic expression in the eye does not necessarily reveal or correlate in obvious ways with the primary site of pathology or the genetic defect. This current void in our knowledge makes any organization of this material somewhat arbitrary.

Because the focus of this book is the RPE, we have divided the dystrophic and metabolic diseases into two groups: (1) disorders which appear to involve the RPE (and choroid) primarily either as the site of disease or at least the major site of manifestation of the disease, (2) disorders of the retina primarily in which RPE involvement either complicates the disease or contributes to the clinical appearance and recognition. This chapter will consider the first of these categories; Chapter 17 will consider the second.

We recognize that this classification is imperfect because of overlap between retinal and RPE pathophysiology, and overlap between the expression in retina or RPE of genetic abnormalities. For example, one may think of retinitis pigmentosa (considered in Chapter 17) as a photoreceptor disorder, particularly those forms in which there is a genetic defect in the rhodopsin molecule. However, the mechanism by which this rhodopsin defect leads to photoreceptor death and RPE damage is unknown, and may involve interaction of the abnormal outer segment membranes with the RPE that must phagocytize, metabolize, and recycle outer segment material. Furthermore, at least two forms of RP are caused by genes that are expressed only in RPE, coding for retinoid transport and metabolism (Gu et al., 1997; Marlhens et al., 1997; Maw et al., 1997). Conversely, we think of vitelliform dystrophy, which histologically shows an accumulation of lipofuscin-like material in the RPE and abnormality of the electrooculogram, to be an RPE dystrophy, but the abnormal material could represent metabolic products from abnormal outer segment membranes. As an example, dystrophies involving an abnormality in peripherin, an outer segment protein, may manifest clinically as either variants of retinitis pigmentosa, variants of Stargardt's disease or as a pattern dystrophy.

It would be nice to organize material, in this dawning era of genetic and molecular biological knowledge about the retina, in terms of the genes or proteins involved, and undoubtedly such classifications will guide us in the future (Wright and Jay, 1994). However, it is difficult to survey the field of retina and RPE disease from this vantage point now because as yet, only a limited number of disorders have been genetically classified, our understanding of why phenotypic expression may vary is still fragmentary, and the known clinical entities are still recognized primarily in terms of clinical characteristics that are empirically relevant to their course and prognosis.

GENETIC FUNDAMENTALS

Considering the recent developments in our understanding of the molecular genetics of retinal and macular dystrophies, it is important to review briefly the different gene-mapping strategies and terminologies, in order to fully appreciate subsequent discussions. In essence, there are three major gene-mapping techniques: (1) linkage analysis, (2) candidate gene analysis, and (3) FISH (fluorescent in situ hybridization). All three methods are useful, and they are not necessarily mutually exclusive but build one upon the other, delineating the basic molecular genetics of different diseases.

In linkage analysis, families are the basic substrate. Individuals within the families are identified as to who is affected and not affected. Then polymorphic genetic markers in the family are analyzed to discern if one allele of a particular marker segregates with or is associated with the disease. This is an exceptionally powerful tool, which can be performed quite efficiently now, using new microsatellite markers (also called CA repeats, short tandem repeats [STRs], and tetra nucleotide re-

326

peats). While this is an extremely powerful technique, the weakness is that, typically, large families are necessary or many small families are necessary in order to be successful with this gene-mapping strategy. Another weakness of this strategy is that it does not discern directly what protein is mutated in the disease and is therefore causing the disease. Linkage analysis defines or narrows the genomic region in which the disease-causing gene is present. It is important to note that, typically, linkage analysis can only narrow the region down to 1–2 cM. This is an extremely large area. Linkage analysis is a statistical probability test that evaluates the likelihood of a gene being located within a certain genomic region. As with all statistical analyses, there are levels of confidence intervals around these likelihoods. In relatively small families, these confidence intervals are quite large (many centiMorgans).

In linkage analysis, the researcher has found a family with a particular disease phenotype. Without any knowledge of the mutated protein involved, the goal is to find the mutation in a gene. In candidate gene analysis, the researcher has a known gene and speculates what the disease phenotype would be like if it were mutated. Therefore, in gene analysis, families are not as necessary as isolated affected individuals. However, it is always useful to show that the mutation in the candidate gene segregates in the family with those who are affected and not with the unaffected. Candidate gene analysis is not necessarily mutually exclusive of linkage analysis. Frequently, a gene is mapped by linkage to a particular region. Within this genomic region, a reasonable candidate gene may be found, which then can be specifically analyzed for a mutation.

The third type of mapping technique is "physical mapping" or positional cloning. This technique may involve FISH, in which the candidate gene is labeled with a fluorescent tag and then binds to the specific region of the chromosome. Then the chromosome is examined under the microscope. With this technique, the actual gene and its location on the chromosome are visualized. However, FISH generally gives relatively crude localization. Newer techniques have been developed within the last several years, in which two or three loci can be very closely delineated. These techniques have been recently used to order a series of markers on a chromosome. Another aspect of physical mapping is positional cloning. With this technique, which is extremely labor intensive, chromosomal "walking and hopping" can be used in order to identify the disease-causing gene. It is interesting to note that only one ophthalmic disease, choroideremia, has been mapped by positional cloning strategies. Essentially, all other ophthalmic diseases have been mapped, either by linkage or by candidate gene analysis

after linkage had directed the search to a particular region.

MACULAR AND RPE DYSTROPHIES

We have grouped together disorders that are characterized by ophthalmoscopic changes in the macula and in the RPE because many "macular dystrophies" show an accumulation of yellowish material within or beneath the RPE, associated with the loss of macular and RPE cells. Conversely, most of the disorders that appear predominantly to involve the RPE also have a predilection for the macula. We will consider the major categories of disease that are presently recognized clinically, but the distinctions are not absolute and in some respects may not be accurate. Different genetic disorders may have overlapping expression phenotypically and several genes for "pattern dystrophy" have already been identified. Conversely, the same genetic abnormality or family may show different phenotypes. Peripherin abnormalities may manifest as a Stargardt's-like disease or a pattern dystrophy, and some families with pattern dystrophy have been identified in which some affected individuals show vitelliform rather than pattern lesions. Even the distinction from photoreceptor dystrophies such as RP is not absolute, since some individuals with Stargardt's disease or fundus flavimaculatus have a markedly reduced electroretinogram (ERG) and diffuse rod-cone dysfunction.

Many of these disorders have yellowish flecks or spots in the fundus, a finding which seems to characterize RPE involvement and degeneration. The old term *fleck retina syndrome*, which was used to group these disorders, has largely been abandoned, because we know from physiologic test results and genetic findings that disorders such as fundus flavimaculatus, drusen, and fundus albipunctatus may have little to do with one another pathophysiologically or symptomatically.

Fundus Albipunctatus

Clinical review. Fundus albipunctatus is a congenital disorder of visual pigment regeneration, a process which is thought to take place largely in the RPE. It is often grouped clinically with the stationary night-blinding disorders (Carr, 1969). Affected individuals are symptomatically night blind. However, they can regain normal sensitivity given a long enough period of time in the dark. With conventional ERG recordings and dark adaptometry they will have absent rod function and very poor dark adaptation; but after three to four hours of dark adaptation, the ERG and dark-adaptation results may be normal (Fig. 16-1). There is some variability in the clinical expression (Margolis et al., 1987). Fundus albipunctatus is characterized clinically by striking yellowish-white dots that are prevalent in the posterior pole (except the fovea) and radiate out toward the periphery (Fig. 16-2) (Marmor, 1977). Beyond the arcades the dots become more diffuse and fleck-like, and the disease must be distinguished from fundus flavimaculatus and from retinitis punctata albescens (a name which is used for variants of progressive retinitis pigmentosa showing white fundus spots). Visual acuity and color vision are typically very good, although mild abnormalities may be present. The symptoms and fundus findings are essentially stable (Marmor, 1990).

The physiologic basis of this disorder has been demonstrated by fundus reflectometry (Carr et al., 1974). Dark adaptometry shows both cone and rod sensitivity to be exceedingly slow in fundus albipunctatus. Fundus reflectometry shows that the regeneration of rhodopsin follows the same time course as psychophysical recovery. Thus, the process of visual pigment re-

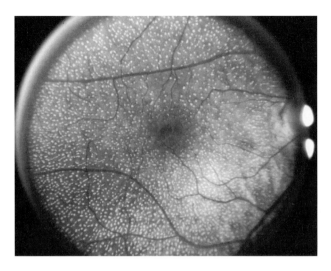

FIGURE 16-2. Fundus albipunctatus. Note that the punctate RPE lesions have a radial pattern beyond the arcades, and spare the fovea centrally. Vessels and disc are normal.

generation is abnormal in this disease; although the gene involved and the metabolic basis for this abnormality remains obscure, the RPE may well be the primary site of the metabolic abnormality.

Genetic and molecular considerations. A possible molecular relationship has been found in a single family with findings that resemble retinitis punctata albescens (RPA) and fundus albipunctatus (FA). Kajiwara and colleagues (1993) described a 59-year-old man with clinical signs of RPA in whom a peripherin mutation was found causing a truncated protein. This man's daughter also had the mutation and was asymptomatic but on fundus examination was found to have the appearance of FA and an abnormal ERG. However, it should be noted that FA and RPA are thought to be autosomal recessive, not autosomal dominant as in the family reported by Kajiwara and colleagues. Therefore the significance of this report to FA remains obscure.

Stargardt's Disease/Fundus Flavimaculatus

Clinical review. From the vantage point of a clinician, Stargardt's disease or fundus flavimaculatus is an inherited disorder characterized by discrete round or pisciform flecks at the level of the RPE (Noble and Carr, 1979; Weleber, 1994). When the flecks are scattered throughout the fundus, the term *fundus flavimaculatus* is usually applied (Fig. 16-3); when they are confined largely to the posterior pole, the condition is usually called Stargardt's disease (Fig. 16-4 and Plate 16-I). The major symptom is central visual loss, which may begin in the early teens or sometimes as late as the thirties or

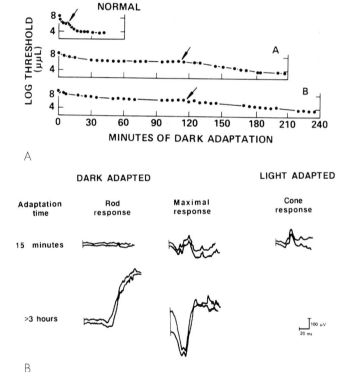

FIGURE 16-1. Functional abnormalities in fundus albipunctatus. (A) Dark-adaptation curves from a normal subject and two patients. Both cone and rod adaptation is markedly delayed in the patients. (B) Electroretinogram (ERG) from one patient, corresponding to lower curve in (A). After 15 minutes of dark adaptation (enough to produce a normal-appearing scotopic ERG), there was no rod response and the maximal response showed only cone activity. However, after more than 3 hours of dark adaptation, the scotopic ERG became normal. (From Marmor, 1977.)

forties. Visual acuity decreases as the macula becomes more atrophic, but most patients retain moderate (e.g., 20/70–20/100) acuity in at least one eye (Fishman et al., 1987). Visual loss below 20/200, or significant peripheral loss, is unusual. The vast majority of cases are autosomal recessive, but some dominant pedigrees have been reported.

There is quite a range of findings among families with Stargardt's disease. Some patients present in the first decade of life with decreased visual acuity but rather minimal ophthalmoscopic abnormalities. The characteristic yellow flecks may appear later in the macula, and patches of central atrophy sometimes develop in the later stages of the disease. Some temporal optic nerve pallor may be present (Newman et al., 1987). At the other extreme, patients may not become symptomatic until mid-adult life. Some patients have only peripheral flecks with little macular involvement, but it is more typical to see flecks in the perimacular area.

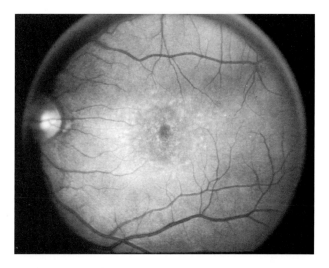

FIGURE 16-4. Stargardt's disease. The yellow flecks are limited to the central macula, and the periphery is normal. (See also Plate 16-I.)

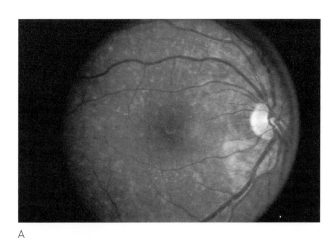

A

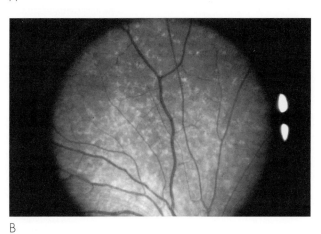

B

FIGURE 16-3. Fundus flavimaculatus. The macula (A) shows central atrophic changes; numerous small yellow flecks extend into the periphery (B).

In most patients with primarily central involvement, the ERG is normal; with increasing amounts of peripheral flecks and atrophy, the ERG may be moderately reduced. This is especially true of patients with diffuse flecks and visual loss beginning in childhood (Itabashi et al., 1993). The EOG is mildly reduced when extensive RPE changes are present. Dark adaptation may be delayed in Stargardt's patients, possibly as a result of altered RPE metabolism (Fishman et al., 1991).

Flecks in the early stages do not show well in fluorescein angiography, presumably because they represent an accumulation of material that is not very dense. As RPE atrophy develops and chronic flecks are in the macula, transmission defects become prominent. There is also a very characteristic phenomenon, called the *dark choroid*, which is seen in roughly half the cases with Stargardt's disease (Fig. 16-5) (Fish et al., 1981). The choroid appears dark and hypofluorescent throughout the angiogram, highlighting the retinal circulation. Until recently, this phenomenon was thought to reflect a blockage of choroidal fluorescence by lipofuscin-laden RPE cells. However, recent measurements of lipofuscin by autofluorescence (see Chapter 11) have shown that while Stargardt's eyes show increased autofluorescence, there was little or no correlation between Stargardt's eyes having or lacking a dark choroid (Delori et al., 1995; von Rückmann et al., 1997). Therefore some other pigment may be responsible for the blocked fluorescence.

Genetic and metabolic considerations. Pathologic studies on a few patients with this disease have shown an accumulation of a lipofuscin-like pigment throughout the

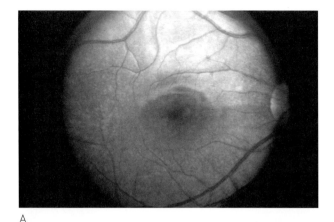

A

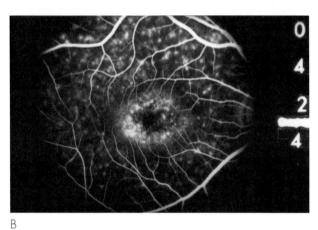

B

FIGURE 16-5. Patient with Stargardt's disease/fundus flavimaculatus. (A) Fundus photograph. (B) Fluorescein angiogram, showing a choroid that appears dark as if its normal fluorescence were obscured.

RPE, although its origin and functional significance is unknown (Eagles et al., 1980; McDonnell et al., 1986; Steinmetz et al., 1991). One group has suggested that the primary defect may be the retinal enzyme all-*trans*-retinal dehydrogenase (Birnbach et al., 1994).

Stargardt's disease is typically inherited in an autosomal-recessive fashion, although there are some families with an autosomal-dominant form. The autosomal-recessive Stargardt's disease was mapped to the short arm of chromosome 1 in 1993 by the French group led by Kaplan and colleagues. This same group subsequently demonstrated that the later-onset disease known as *fundus flavimaculatus* mapped precisely to the same region (Gerber et al., 1995). These two studies provide further evidence that fundus flavimaculatus and Stargardt's disease are most likely the same disease and are only allelic disorders of each other (i.e. same gene with different mutations). Recently the Stargardt's gene was identified by Allikmets et al., (1997a). It is called ABCR (ATP-binding casette, retina specific) and

is expressed in rod photoreceptors but not RPE. This suggests that our clinical impression of the primary site of a disease is not accurate. Additionally 16% of age related macular degeneration patients have been found to carry a base-pair change on one copy of this gene. (Allikmets et al., 1997b). However, some base-pair changes occur in a normal population so that the pathologic significance for age-related macular degeneration remains to be determined (Dryja et al., 1998). The ABCR gene appears to code for photoreceptor rim protein, which is localized to the ring of outer segment discs in rods and possibly cones (Azarian and Travis, 1997). Although the function of rim protein is unknown, it appears that the primary defect in Stargardt's disease is in the photoreceptors, rather than the RPE, and the accumulation of abnormal material in the RPE is secondary.

The autosomal-dominant form of Stargardt's macular dystrophy was mapped in 1994 by Zhang and colleagues to chromosome 13q34. A gene that encodes lysosome-associated membrane protein was mapped by FISH and somatic cell hybrid panel to chromosome 13q. Zhang and colleagues have subsequently (personal communication) shown that autosomal-dominant Stargardt's is not due to a mutation in this gene. Therefore, the search continues for the genetic defect of Stargardt's disease.

Best's Disease or Vitelliform Dystrophy

Clinical review. Vitelliform dystrophy gets its name from the appearance in some affected patients of a large yellow yolk-like (vitelliform) macular lesion (Fig. 16-6A and Plate 16-II). This is found most often in childhood, because it tends to break down over the years with resultant scarring and atrophy. The late lesions (Fig. 16-7) often have some gliosis of some longstanding deposits of yellowish material which may give clues to Best's disease as the underlying disorder; however, the identification of these scars in an adult is very difficult on clinical grounds alone. The definitive diagnosis is made on the grounds of an electrophysiological test (the electrooculogram or EOG) and documentation of a dominant family history.

Expression of this disease is variable, and some individuals who carry the gene (by necessity of the pedigree, and the finding of an abnormal EOG) have perfectly normal visual function and fundus appearance (Fig. 16-6B) (Maloney et al., 1977; Bard and Cross, 1975). The age of onset, the size, and the appearance of the macular lesions are also moderately variable and extramacular lesions are occasionally seen (Noble et al., 1978; Mohler and Fine, 1981; Fishman et al., 1993). Visual acuity is usually good as long as the yolk remains intact,

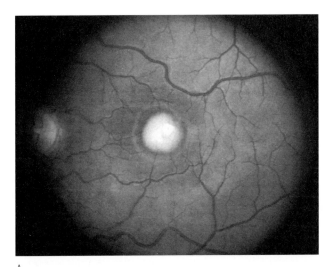

A

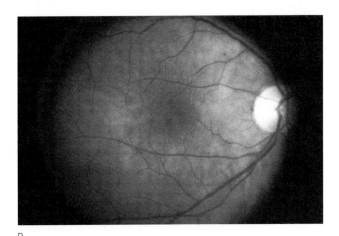

B

FIGURE 16-6. Best's vitelliform dystrophy. (A) Teenage boy with typical yolk. (See also Plate 16-II.) (B) His father who carries the gene (see Fig. 16-8) but has no visual or fundus abnormalities.

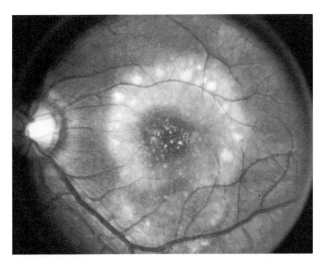

FIGURE 16-7. Best's vitelliform dystrophy. Macular appearance after a yolk has broken up, leaving a zone of atrophy surrounded by irregular yellow deposits.

RPE (Skoog and Nilsson, 1981; Rover and Bach, 1987). Curiously, the fast oscillation (which is a late RPE manifestation of the potassium concentration changes that generate the c-wave) has been reported to be normal (Weleber, 1989). The nonphotic hyperosmolarity response may be abnormal (Wakabayashi et al., 1983). The mechanism by which the light response and c-wave are abnormal in this disorder is unknown, and this diffuse electrophysiologic abnormality does not correlate with any known deficit of retinal or visual function. Nevertheless, because of its specificity for this disorder and its ready clinical availability, the EOG is useful for the evaluation of any poorly defined central macular

but once disruption and scarring occurs, visual acuity falls, typically to the range of 20/200 (Mohler and Fine, 1981; Fishman et al., 1993). There is no peripheral involvement on clinical examination. Most affected individuals retain reasonable vision for reading and driving in at least one eye, well into adult life. Rarely, choroidal neovascularization develops in an old vitelliform scar (Noble et al., 1978).

The critical diagnostic test is the EOG, which shows a severe and characteristic loss of the light response of the standing potential (Fig. 16-8) (see Chapter 10). The light/dark (Arden) ratio in Best's disease is typically < 1.5 and often near 1.1. This EOG abnormality is a constant finding, even with individuals who carry the gene and have normal fundi. The c-wave of the ERG is also severely reduced, consistent with its origin in the

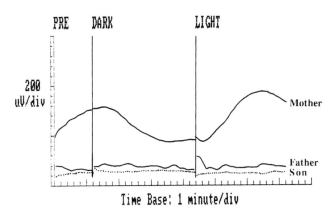

FIGURE 16-8. Electrooculograms (EOGs) from a family with Best's vitelliform dystrophy (see fundus photographs in Fig. 16-6). The light response was severely depressed in the genetically affected patients (father and son), although the father did not have a macular lesion. The mother's EOG was normal.

scar, to determine whether or not Best's disease is at fault.

We have a limited understanding of the pathophysiology of Best's disease. Eyes with Best's disease show increased background autofluorescence throughout the fundus (von Rückmann et al., 1997). The few histopathologic specimens that have been obtained show an accumulation of a lipofuscin-like material throughout the RPE cells everywhere in the fundus (Weingeist et al., 1982; Frangieh et al., 1982; O'Gorman et al., 1988). However, we have no direct knowledge about the configuration of the central vitelliform lesion that gives the disease its name. It is also interesting that a "dark-choroid effect" has not been observed, despite the abnormal material present in the RPE. The significance of the accumulated substance is also unclear, since patients with Best's disease have no functional abnormalities outside of the central macula, and even the macular dysfunction (poor visual acuity) is a result of atrophy and scarring rather than the material accumulated in and around the RPE.

Genetic and Metabolic Considerations. Best's macular dystrophy was mapped simultaneously by a Swedish group led by Forsman and colleagues and Stone and colleagues to chromosome 11q13 in 1992. A gene encoding the protein known as ROM1 (an integral membrane protein in the rod photoreceptor outer segment) has the same genomic localization as the Best's locus and was therefore a reasonable choice for a candidate gene. Subsequently, multiple groups have demonstrated that no ROM1 mutations exit in Best's macular dystrophy patients.

Because of the clinical appearance of Best's disease, along with the histopathologic findings of lipofuscin in the RPE and abnormal EOG, it has been assumed that Best's disease is primarily an RPE disease. However, it may turn out that it is a retinal membrane abnormality which causes the RPE to accumulate an aberrant breakdown product. Once the gene is cloned, we will be able to answer this question.

Vitelliform Lesions in Adults

Clinical review. A somewhat ill-defined group of disorders have been termed *adult vitelliform degeneration,* because affected patients show symmetric yellowish foveal deposits (Fig. 16-9, 16-10) that bear a resemblance to the lesions in Best's disease (Marmor, 1979; Epstein and Rabb, 1980; Sabates et al., 1982). However, the term has been used for patients with large yolk-like lesions from coalesced fine drusen, as well as for patients who show merely a fleck of yellow material in the

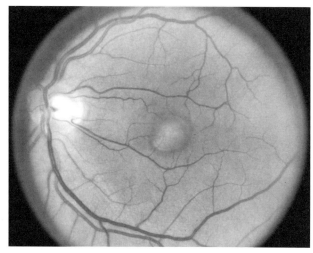

A

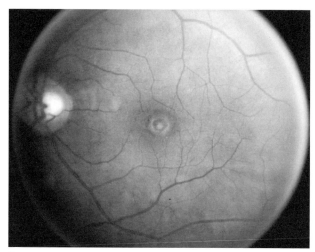

B

FIGURE 16-9. Adult vitelliform degeneration. (A) Patient with a cystic foveal lesion and normal EOG. (B) Patient with a flat lesion and a central pigment spot. This pattern has been called *fovemacular dystrophy* (Gass, 1974). The EOG was normal.

central foveola. The one cardinal feature of these disorders is that they are not Best's disease, and invariably show a normal or only minimally reduced EOG. They also have a presumed adult presentation, typically, and fundus changes which would at best be called atypical for Best's disease. The family history is variable.

An example of an adult vitelliform degeneration is the "foveo-macular dystrophy" (Fig. 16-9B) described by Gass (1974). The disorder is characterized by small bilateral, round, or oval yellow subfoveal lesions roughly one-third disc diameter in size, generally with a central pigmented spot. These findings are usually noticed in the fourth to sixth decade, and visual symptoms are ei-

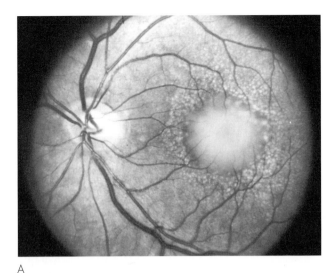

A

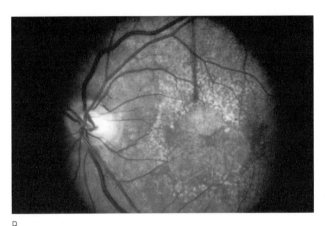

B

FIGURE 16-10. Adult vitelliform degeneration. (A) Diffuse tiny (cuticular) drusen causing a yolk-like central cyst (see also Plate 16-III). (B) A few years later, visual acuity worsened when the cyst absorbed leaving central geographic atrophy. The EOG was normal.

ther absent or limited to mild blurring or metamorphopsia. Some authors have classed this disorder among the pattern dystrophies. Histopathologic examination has shown damage centered at the level of the RPE (Gass, 1974; Patrinely et al., 1985; Jaffe and Schatz, 1988).

The most prominent "yolks" other than Best's disease occur in adults who have widespread, fine, cuticular drusen (Fig. 16-10 and Plate 16-III) (see below). These extensive drusen seem capable of coalescing into a vitelliform lesion, and the distinction from Best's disease is usually on the basis of a normal or only minimally abnormal EOG and observation of the drusen (Marmor, 1979; Gass et al., 1985).

Even though these adult vitelliform degenerations are pathophysiologically distinct from Best's disease, their prognosis is in some respects similar. Prominent yolk-like accumulations of material tend to be absorbed and break down over time, leaving atrophy (Fig. 16-10) and sometimes gliotic scar. As this occurs, visual acuity will fall, regardless of the primary cause of the disease.

Genetic and metabolic considerations. A few cases of Gass's "adult foveal macular dystrophy" have been found to be an autosomal-dominant trait with mutations in the peripherin/*rds* gene. This would suggest that Gass's adult foveal macular dystrophy is indeed a variant of pattern dystrophy, which was previously suspected (Feist et al., 1994; Wells et al., 1993).

Diffuse Drusen

Clinical review. This section concerns patients who have drusen present at an early age and extending beyond the macula—in other words, distinct from the typical pattern of age-related hard or soft drusen (Marmor, 1991a). These "diffuse" drusen are often termed *hereditary drusen*, although documentation of the family history is often difficult to obtain because many affected individuals are not identified until middle age. The characteristics of diffuse drusen are quite variable, and the term probably incorporates a variety of genetic conditions. Diffuse drusen typically extend beyond the arcades, and characteristically involve the retina nasal to the disc (Fig. 16-11). They may be rather large and sparse in number, or show as myriad tiny dots (cuticular or basal laminar drusen) which occasionally coalesce into a vitelliform detachment (Marmor, 1979; Gass et al., 1985). These different appearances have occasioned a variety of names in the older literature, such as *Doyne's honeycomb dystrophy, malattia Leventinese, guttate choroiditis,* and others (Deutman and Hansen, 1970).

Central vision is usually good in patients with diffuse drusen, as long as the lesions remain discrete and extrafoveal. It is unclear whether these patients may be at greater-than-normal risk for macular degenerative changes as they age. Fluorescein angiography often shows the drusen and RPE changes to be much more extensive than is evident on ophthalmoscopy. Functional testing, including the ERG and the EOG, are typically normal, although both may be affected to a mild degree in extensive cases (Hess and Niemeyer, 1983, Niemeyer, 1978; Fishman et al., 1976; Marmor, 1991a). The c-wave may also be subnormal (Rover and Bach, 1987).

The metabolic dysfunction that leads to these RPE lesions is unknown, and may be similar to the processes that underlie age-related drusen. It may be relevant that drusen-like deposits are seen in some hereditary renal

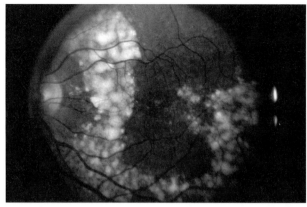

A

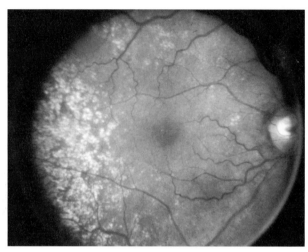

B

FIGURE 16-11. Two patients with different patterns (and sizes) of diffuse and presumably hereditary drusen.

disorders that involve basement membrane abnormalities, such as Alport's syndrome and glomerulonephritis type II (Govan, 1983; Kim et al., 1992).

Genetic and molecular considerations. Recently, autosomal dominant drusen has been mapped by linkage to chromosome 2p. Gregory and colleagues (1996) independently and simultaneously ascertained the original family with Doyne's honeycomb maculopathy while Heon and colleagues (1996) ascertained the originally described Swiss family with malattia Leventinese; both mapped to the same chromosome, 2p. This strongly suggests that these diseases are the same. It is suspected that the defect is probably an intercellular matrix protein or collagen or other structural protein mutation.

In Alport's syndrome, genes for collagen-type 4 alpha 3, collagen-type 4 alpha 6, and collagen-type 4 alpha 4

have been found to be mutated (Govan, 1993). There may be many structural or basement-membrane-type proteins that could account for the diffuse drusen diseases.

Pattern Dystrophies

Clinical review. The pattern dystrophies are a group of disorders characterized by patterns of granular or reticular black pigmentation at the level of the RPE (Fig. 16-12) (Marmor and Byers, 1977; Hsieh et al., 1977). Drusen or yellow flecks seen in other RPE dystrophies are not found, and visual acuity is usually good, at least through the first five or six decades of life. Some of these disorders have acquired descriptive names such as *Sjogren's reticular dystrophy* or *butterfly dystrophy*. However, many families have been described who do not clearly fit into these categories, and, within families, individuals can differ considerably in their pattern of pigmentation. This is a heterogeneous group of diseases, and a number of hereditary patterns have been documented. The grouping of these entities under the term *pattern dystrophy* is useful primarily as a way of segregating these disorders from other maculopathies that have a poorer prognosis or distinctive fundus findings.

Most patients with pattern dystrophy are asymptomatic or have minimal changes in visual acuity. A diagnosis is often made because unusual fundus lesions are discovered on ophthalmoscopy or angiography. Functional and electrophysiologic testing through middle age is typically normal except for a borderline EOG (Fig. 16-13) that may be considered consistent with a diffuse RPE disorder (Marmor, 1991b). Affected patients may develop geographic macular atrophy in old age that mimics age-related macular degeneration (Fig. 16-14) (Marmor and McNamara, 1996). The ERG may also become mildly subnormal in elderly individuals, suggesting diffuse damage to photoreceptors late in the disease (Fig. 16-15).

Genetic and molecular considerations. Peripherin, a protein encoded by a gene on the short arm of chromosome 6, has a mouse homolog called *rds* (retinal degeneration slow). It has been shown to have mutations associated with pattern dystrophy, adult foveal macular dystrophy of Gass, butterfly dystrophy of the retinal pigment epithelium, and adult vitelliform macular dystrophy. These disorders are generally seen in families with an autosomal-dominant pattern of inheritance. What is more interesting is that each mutation is not necessarily responsible for a particular phenotype. Indeed, Weleber and colleagues (1993) demonstrated in a single family a three-based pair deletion in periph-

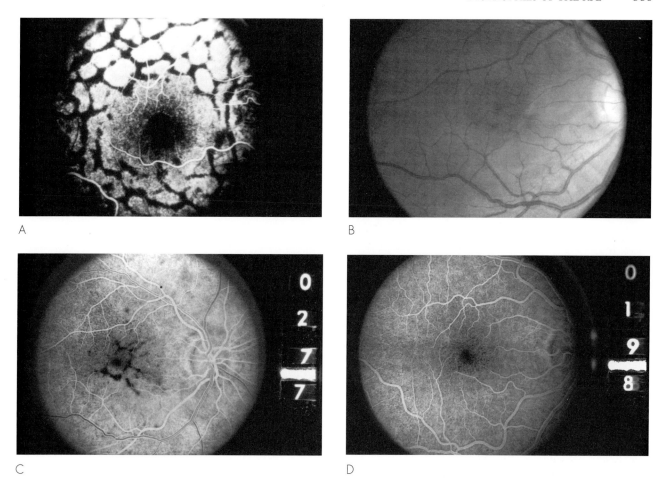

FIGURE 16-12. Pattern dystrophy. (A) Reticular dystrophy. The striking gridwork pattern of RPE pigment is highlighted in angiography. (B and C) Fundus photograph and fluorescein angiogram from a young man with a dominantly inherited pattern dystrophy. The pigment pattern is seen only faintly with the ophthalmoscope, but is striking on angiography. (D) Sister of this patient, showing coarse granular pigmentation rather than a reticular pattern. (Parts [B]–[D] from Marmor and McNamara, 1996.)

erin/*rds* gene, which caused the three different phenotypes of retinitis pigmentosa, pattern dystrophy, and fundus flavimaculatus. It is interesting to note that, within this family, there were varying degrees of ERG abnormalities. With all these different manifestations present in a single family, this clearly indicates that the genotype-to-phenotype correlation is not specific.

The history of our understanding of the peripherin/*rds* gene is a review of classic applications of molecular genetic techniques and a confluence of efforts from many directions, culminating in a brief period of continuity of understanding. Travis and colleagues (1989) identified a photoreceptor-specific gene which was responsible for a mouse model of retinal degeneration known as *rds* (retinal degeneration slow), with its human homolog on chromosome 6p. Subsequently, Jordan and colleagues found linkage of an autosomal dominant retinitis pigmentosa family to chromosome 6p. Simultaneously with Kajiwara and colleagues (1991), they found mutations in the peripherin/*rds* gene to be associated with retinitis pigmentosa. Because the peripherin/*rds* protein is thought to be expressed in cones as well, the search began to identify mutations in macular diseases. Wells and colleagues (1993), followed by Nichols and colleagues (1993), found mutations in the peripherin/*rds* to be associated with a variety of these pattern-type dystrophies.

The mechanisms by which peripherin abnormalities lead to pattern dystrophy (among other phenotypes) is unknown, but is of considerable interest insofar as the protein is considered a component of the photoreceptor outer segment while the typical manifestation of pattern

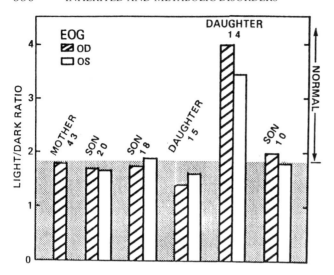

FIGURE 16-13. Electrooculograms (EOGs) from a family with dominantly inherited pattern dystrophy (see Figs. 16-12, 16-14 and 16-15). The mother and four of five children were affected, and had borderline Arden ratios. One unaffected daughter had a normal EOG. (After Marmor and Byers, 1979.)

dystrophy is RPE pigmentary changes with little or no abnormality in visual function. It is possible that some of the peripherin abnormalities have little direct effect on photoreceptor function, but interfere in some way with RPE metabolism after phagocytosis of the outdated outer segment material. Many eyes with pattern dystrophy show increased background autofluorescence that suggests RPE accumulation of a lipofuscin-like material (von Rückmann et al., 1997).

Other Maculopathies

There are many rare macular dystrophies, described in only one or a few families, such as *fenestrated sheen dystrophy, bull's-eye maculopathy, cystoid edema,* or *crystalline deposits.* Some of these may provide unique models of RPE involvement in disease, but most are characterized only clinically and have been neither mapped nor cloned.

Cystoid macular edema, which was first reported by Deutman and colleagues (1976) as an autosomal-dominant trait, has recently been studied. Kremer and colleagues (1994) mapped autosomal-dominant cystoid macular edema to chromosome 7p, using linkage analysis. The genomic region to which this is mapped is rather broad, encompassing 20 cM. However, autosomal-dominant retinitis pigmentosa, known as RP9, also maps this similar region (Inglehearn et al., 1994). Although cystoid macular edema is not thought to be primarily a disease of the RPE, until the gene is cloned and

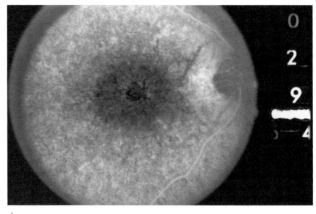

A

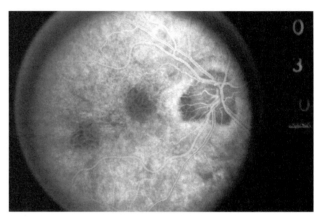

B

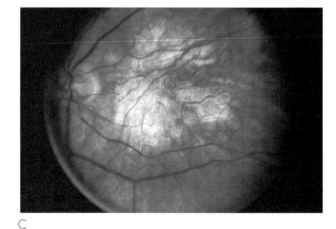

C

FIGURE 16-14. Progression of pattern dystrophy with age. (A) Mother (age 42) of the subjects illustrated in Figure 16-12B–D. Her fluorescein angiogram shows an irregular pigment pattern but no geographic atrophy. (B) The same eye at age 62. The pigment patterns have dispersed, and there are discrete parafoveal zones of RPE and choriocapillary atrophy. (C) Fundus photograph of her aunt at age 80. She had extensive atrophic macular degeneration and visual acuity reduced to 20/200. (From Marmor and Byers, 1979; Marmor and McNamara, 1996.)

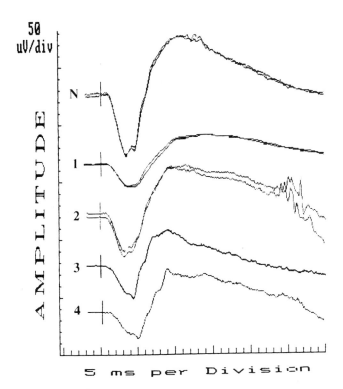

FIGURE 16-15. Dark-adapted electroretinograms from a family with dominantly inherited pattern dystrophy (see Figs. 16-12 to 16-14). A normal electroretinogram (N) from a 61-year-old subject is shown for comparison. Tracings (1)–(4) are from affected family members aged 62, 35, 73, and 61, respectively. The responses are all borderline or slightly below the range of normal values. (From Marmor and Mc-Namara, 1996.)

its expression in RPE is specifically evaluated, this could still be a possibility.

BRUCH'S MEMBRANE ABNORMALITIES

Angioid Streaks

Clinical review. Angioid streaks are characterized by diffuse abnormality of Bruch's membrane and the overlying RPE (Clarkson and Altman, 1982). In youth or early adulthood, the fundus takes on a peculiar mottled *"peau d'orange"* appearance that is quite characteristic, but sometimes hard to recognize if not specifically considered (Fig. 16-16A and Plate 16-IV). As individuals age, "cracks" in Bruch's membrane develop (Fig. 16-16B and C and Plate 16-V) that most often radiate from the disc in a manner that may mimic blood vessels (hence the name "angioid streaks"). These defects in Bruch's membrane tend to radiate toward the macula, where they are a frequent site of neovascular growth from the choroid. The disease does not affect vision primarily, but the neovascularization, hemorrhage, and scarring that occurs with macular involvement is fre-

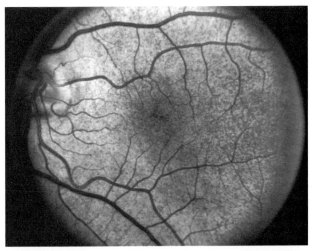

A

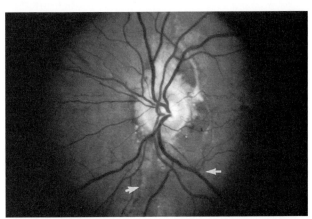

B

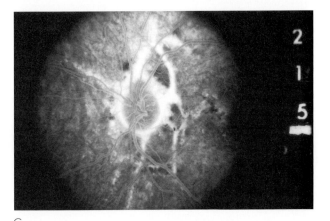

C

FIGURE 16-16. Angioid streaks. (A) Diffuse pigment stippling (peau d'orange) that characterizes affected fundi even before streaks appear. (See also Plate 16-IV). (B) Peripapillary region in a different patient. Note that some of the streaks are subtle *(arrows)* and have a "vascular" appearance in the fundus photograph. (See also Plate 16-V). (C) Fluorescein angiogram from the same patient. The extent of the Bruch's membrane defects is more apparent.

quently devastating to central vision. Laser photocoagulation can effectively destroy a leaking neovascular net, but recurrence near the treatment site or at a new area of Bruch's membrane abnormality is more the rule than the exception, and the long-term prognosis once neovascular breakdown begins in or around the macula is poor (Lim et al., 1993). However, visual loss is limited to the macula.

A large percentage of individuals with angioid streaks have the associated systemic abnormality of pseudoxanthoma elasticum (estimates range from 50% to 80%). Conversely, a high percentage of individuals with pseudoxanthoma have angioid streaks if they are sought. A skin biopsy is recommended for anyone with angioid streaks, since the skin findings may be subtle and not always evident upon clinical examination. Association with other disorders such as B-thalassemia and sickle cell disease (Aessopos et al., 1989; Hamilton et al., 1981) have been reported.

The association of angioid streaks with pseudoxanthoma elasticum suggests that the Bruch's membrane abnormality relates to an elastic tissue dysfunction. Despite the diffuse (*peau d'orange*) and focal (angioid streaks) RPE changes, the EOG is generally normal (Weinstein and Reeser, 1975), as is dark adaptation (Holtz et al., 1994).

Genetic and molecular considerations. The inheritance pattern of pseuodoexanthoma elasticum has in itself been controversial. Several researchers have proposed an x-linked recessive or even x-linked dominant form; others, autosomal recessive. Electron microscopy demonstrates changes in the elastic fibers involving elastin, whereas the microfibrillar component is unchanged. Raybould and colleagues (1994) evaluated patients with pseudoxanthoma elasticum for mutations or for linkage with an entronic polymorphism in the elastin gene. The elastin gene was excluded as the site of mutation in pseudoexanthoma elasticum. Additionally, the elastin gene has been evaluated for gross rearrangements, and none have been found. Recently an autosomal recessive form was mapped to chromosome 16p13 by van Soest and colleagues (1997).

Sorsby's Macular Dystrophy

Clinical review. This is a dominantly inherited disorder characterized by the development of bilateral choroidal neovascularization in the macula at an early age (typically around 40 years) (Carr et al., 1978; Hamilton et al., 1989; Polkinghorne et al., 1989). Numerous fine drusen or a confluent plaque of faintly yellowish material may be noted beneath the central RPE early in the

disease (see Chapter 35). Late in the disease one sees heavily pigmented macular scars and areas of geographic atrophy corresponding to the region of exudative maculopathy. The ERG and EOG are usually normal until very late in the disease. Histopathology of this disease shows a lipid-containing deposit between the basement membrane of the RPE and the inner collagenous layers of Bruch's membrane (Capon et al., 1989). It has been postulated that this lipid material impedes nutrient transport to the RPE, and thus may contribute to the pathogenesis of the drusen, RPE breakdown, and neovascularization and may account for functional changes such as abnormal dark adaptation (Steinmetz et al., 1992). It is not clear how to relate these pathologic findings to the recent isolation of a gene for Sorsby's dystrophy which codes for a tissue inhibitor of metalloproteinase.

Genetic and molecular considerations. The human tissue inhibitor of metalloproteinase-3 (TIMP-3) was cloned, characterized, and localized to human chromosome 22. This protein is involved in the regulation and composition of the extracellular matrix, assembly of supramolecular aggregates, and degradation of the extracellular matrix. This remodeling is felt to be important in organ hypertrophy and involution, bone adaptation, and wound healing. TIMP-3 is expressed by RPE, and is localized immunohistochemically to Bruch's membrane with minimal staining elsewhere in the retina (Vranka et al., 1996). Almost simultaneous to the localization to chromosome 22, Weber and colleagues (1994a) mapped Sorsby's fundus dystrophy using linkage analysis to the same region. TIMP-3 was an appealing candidate gene, and shortly thereafter they (Weber et al., 1994b) reported several mutations in TIMP-3 causing Sorsby's fundus dystrophy. Because of the many similarities of Sorsby's fundus dystrophy to age-related macular degeneration, Weber and colleagues (personal communication) then screened approximately two hundred random patients with age-related macular degeneration for mutations in TIMP-3. Disappointingly, none were found.

CHOROIDAL DYSTROPHIES: DIFFUSE DEGENERATIONS

Choroideremia

Clinical review. Choroideremia is an X-linked condition characterized by progressive degeneration of the choroid, choriocapillaris, and overlying RPE (Cameron et al., 1987; Flannery et al., 1990). In childhood, the findings may appear like mild RP, but by the adult years one

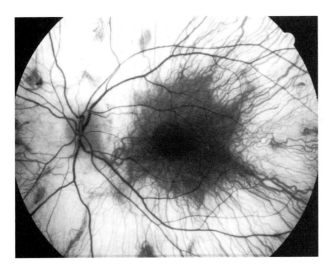

FIGURE 16-17. Fundus appearance in advanced choroideremia.

typically sees striking atrophy of the RPE and choroid quite distinct from the changes of RP (Fig. 16-17). Most males who are affected are aware of night blindness in the first or second decade of life, but more serious visual loss (acuity and peripheral vision) becomes prominent by early to mid-adulthood. By middle age, most affected patients have significant central and peripheral visual loss, much like patients with advanced RP.

The ERG begins to show abnormalities early in the course of disease, although not as severely as in typical RP (Sieving et al., 1986). However, by mid-adulthood, the ERG is typically unrecordable. Female carriers may have a mosaic fundus appearance, with focal areas of abnormality, but they are usually asymptomatic and electrophysiologically normal.

Genetic and molecular considerations. Choroideremia is the first retinal disease which was mapped and cloned by straight positional cloning strategies. All other retinal and macular diseases were mapped and cloned using either candidate gene analysis or a linkage analysis directing a candidate gene strategy. Early in the mapping of choroideremia, several patients were found with translocations at Xq21.2. Eventually, a series of such patients were found with a common chromosomal region deleted or abnormal, consisting of only 45 kb of DNA. Van Bokhoven and colleagues (1994) identified new DNA markers around the region to define the minimal region of overlap. From this region, genes were found expressed in the retina and RPE which were evolutionarily conserved. This gene was found to be geranylgeranyl transferase (Seabra et al., 1993). Today, there are nine different mutations in the geranylgeranyl transferase gene, which result in a termination codon, resulting in a truncated protein.

Gyrate Atrophy

Clinical review. Gyrate atrophy is a rare autosomal-recessive disorder caused by defects in the enzyme ornithine aminotransferase (OAT) (Takki, 1974). The disease gets its name because of the progression of large gyrate patches of atrophy that begin in the peripheral retina and gradually expand and coalesce as it progresses (Fig. 16-18) (Takki and Milton, 1981). Late in the disease, the fundus appearance may be indistinguishable from that in choroideremia. Although the large, scalloped paving-stone areas of atrophy are characteristic in young patients, the pathognomonic finding is the presence of elevated serum ornithine. Dietary restriction of ornithine may slow the progression but is difficult to maintain (Kaiser-Kupfer et al., 1991).

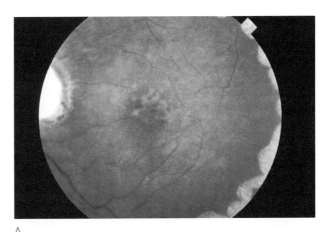

A

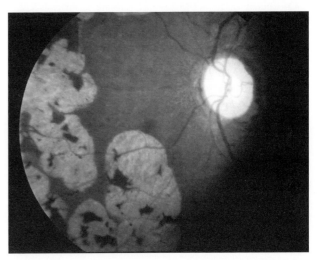

B

FIGURE 16-18. Gyrate atrophy. (A) The central macula is largely spared and shows only some central pigmentary disturbance. (B) The periphery shows characteristic scalloped zones of degeneration and atrophy.

Genetic and molecular counseling. Ornithine aminotransferase is the major enzyme involved in the catalysis for ornithine. Hyperornithinemia was first found to be due to deficiency in ornithine ketoacid aminotransferase in 1973 by Simell and Takki. The main source of ornithine is dietary arginine, and arginine-low diets have been shown to be of some therapeutic value by Kaiser-Kupfer and colleagues (1991). The gene encoding OAT was mapped to human chromosome 10q23, by O'Donnell and colleagues (1988). Family linkage analysis of gyrate atrophy families additionally linked to chromosome 10q, thus substantiating OAT as the mutated gene. Subsequently, 39 mutations associated with gyrate atrophy have been found in OAT. Recently, a knockout mouse in which OAT was deficient was engineered by Wang and colleagues (1995). Interestingly, the neonatal mouse had hypoornithinemia (in contrast to hyperornithinemia, which was expected) and was lethal. They subsequently showed that neonatal arginine supplementation allowed the mice to survive, then later in life the mice developed hyperornithinemia, similar to human gyrate atrophy patients. Subsequently, these researchers showed that human gyrate atrophy infants also have transient hypoornithinemia. This suggests that OAT expression varies with maturity. The OAT-1-deficient mouse also developed retinal degeneration involving the photoreceptors and pigment epithelium. Therefore, the OAT-deficient mouse is an excellent animal model of gyrate atrophy and will be a useful resource for future gene therapy studies.

CHOROIDAL DYSTROPHIES: REGIONAL AND CENTRAL CHOROIDAL DYSTROPHIES

A number of disorders have been described that exhibit a macular or regional choroidal degeneration. The central atrophies include disorders described as *central areolar choroidal dystrophy, central pigment epithelial and choroidal degeneration, North Carolina macular dystrophy, progressive bifocal chorioretinal atrophy* (PBCRA), and *atrophia areata.*

North Carolina Macular Dystrophy (MCDR1)

Clinical review. North Carolina macular dystrophy was first described by Lefler, Wadsworth, and Sidbury (1971) as an autosomal-dominant macular degeneration associated with amino aciduria. Shortly thereafter, the amino aciduria was found not to be associated with the maculopathy. However, subsequent studies on the single large family in North Carolina, Frank and colleagues (1974) published a larger portion of this pedi-

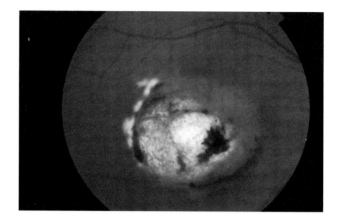

FIGURE 16-19. North Carolina macular dystrophy. (See also Plate 16-VI). The macular lesions can vary from mild to severe. This patient would be classed as grade III with a macular coloboma. (From Small, 1996.)

gree, calling it *dominant progressive foveal dystrophy.* More recently, Gass (1987) named it, North Carolina macular dystrophy. The original family was studied more recently by Small (Small, 1989; Small et al., 1992a) and was found to be a congenital maculopathy with highly variable phenotypic expression. Some individuals exhibit only a few drusen in the central macular region with normal vision, while others have a disciform scar and others have a central macular coloboma (Fig. 16-19 and Plate 16-VI). In general, the visual acuity is much better than one would predict from the ophthalmoscopic appearance. Generally, the disease is not progressive, except for individuals who develop a choroidal neovascular membrane. Small (1989) has found seven separate families in the United States, Europe, and Central America.

Genetic and molecular consideration. North Carolina macular dystrophy is now known as MCDR1 (MC = macular; D = dystrophy; R = subtype retina, to distinguish it from corneal macular dystrophy; and 1 for the first macular degeneration genetically mapped). Because of the large single family, Small and colleagues (1992b) used linkage analysis to map the diseased gene to chromosome 6q. Small had excluded approximately 95% of the entire human genome before finally obtaining linkage. Additionally, using genetic molecular techniques, as well as extensive genealogic studies, Small and colleagues (1992a) demonstrated that central areolar pigment epithelial dystrophy reported from Iowa and central pigment and choroidal degeneration reported in Chicago were actually branches of the same North Carolina dystrophy family. Additionally, of the seven families with North Carolina macular dystrophy ascertained by Small, all of the American families but one have the haplotype associated with the original MCDR1 family in North Carolina. This suggests a common founder effect, although the genealogic tie cannot be made despite ten generations of genealogic records.

Progressive Bifocal Chorioretinal Atrophy (PBCRA)

Progressive bifocal chorioretinal atrophy (PBCRA), has been restudied in a single five-generation British pedigree (Kelsell et al., 1995). This trait is inherited in an autosomal-dominant fashion, is considered to be completely penetrant, and is characterized by an onset in the first or second decade of life by macular atrophy, and then later on by nasal retinal atrophy (Douglas et al., 1968). The ERG and EOG, like in North Carolina macular dystrophy, are normal.

Most interestingly, this disease has been mapped to the precise genetic location overlapping North Carolina macular dystrophy (Kelsell et al., 1995). This suggests that PBCRA and North Carolina macular dystrophy may be allelic disorders or part of a gene family. The role these diseases have in interacting with RPE is unknown.

Atrophia Areata

Atrophia areata, also known as *peripapillary chorioretinal degeneration of Iceland,* and also called the *helicoidal peripapillary chorioretinal degeneration,* was first reported by Sveinsson (1939, 1979) in a single Icelandic pedigree. This was on subsequent examinations shown to be a slowly progressive disorder that begins in the RPE and usually combines with myopia and astigmatism.

In the past, there was a question whether this was an autosomal dominant or X-linked, dominantly inherited trait. Recently, Fossdal and colleagues (1995), using linkage analysis in this single large Icelandic family, mapped the gene to chromosome 11p15.

ACKNOWLEDGMENTS

Supported in part by The Foundation Fighting Blindness (KWS), National Eye Institute NIH/NEI RO1-EY12039 (KWS) and The Mc-Cone Endowment (KWS).

REFERENCES

Aessopos A, Stamatelos G, Savvides P, Kavouklis E, Gabriel L, Rombos I, Karagiorga M, Kaklamanis P. 1989. Angioid streaks in homozygous]3 thalassemia. Am J Ophthalmol 108:356–359.

Allikmets R, Singh N, Sun H, Shroyer NF, Hutchinson A, Chidambaram A, Gerrard B, Baird L, Stauffer D, Peiffer A, Rattner A, Smallwood P, Li Y, Anderson KL, Lewis RA, Nathans J, Leppert M,

Dean M, Lupski JR. 1997a. A photoreceptor cell-specific ATP-binding transporter gene (ABCR) is mutated in recessive Stargardt macular dystrophy. Nat Genet 15:236–246.

Allikmets R, Shroyer N, Singh N, Seddon J, Lewis RA, Bernstein P, Peiffer A, Zabriskie N, Li Y, Hutchinson A, Dean M, Lupski JR, Leppert M. 1997b. Mutations of the Stargardt gene (ABCR) in age related macular degeneration. Science 277:1805–1807.

Azarian SM, Travis GH. 1997. The photoreceptor rim protein is an ABC transporter encoded by the gene for recessive Stargardt's disease (ABCR). FEBS Letters 409:247–252.

Bard LA, Cross HE. 1975. Genetic counseling of families with Best macular dystrophy. Trans Amer Ophthalmol Otol 70:OP-865–OP-873.

Birnbach CD, Jarvelainen M, Possin DE, Milam AH. 1994. Histopathology and immunocytochemistry of the neurosensory retina in fundus flavimaculatus. Ophthalmology 101:1211–1219.

Cameron JD, Fine BS, Shapiro I. 1987. Histopathologic observations in choroideremia with emphasis on vascular changes of the uveal tract. Ophthalmology 94:187–196.

Capon MRC, Marshall J, Krafft JI, Alexander RA, Hiscott PS, Bird AC. 1989. Sorsby's fundus dystrophy. Ophthalmology 96:1769–1777.

Carr RE. 1969. The night-blinding disorders. Int Ophthalmol Clinics 9:971–1003.

Carr RE, Ripps H, Siegel IM. 1974. Visual pigment kinetics and adaptation in fundus albipunctatus. In Documenta Ophthalmol. Proceedings Series, Vol. IV. The Hague: Dr W Junk BV, 193–204.

Carr RE, Ripps H, Siegel IM, Weale RA. 1966. Rhodopsin and the electrical activity of the retina in congenital night blindness. Invest Ophthalmol 5:497–705.

Carr RE, Noble KG, Nasaduke I. 1978. Hereditary hemorrhagic macular dystrophy. Am J Ophthalmol 85:315–328.

Clarkson JG, Altman RD. 1982. Angioid streaks. Surv Ophthalmol 26:235–246.

Delori FC, Stavrenghi G, Arend O, Dorey CK, Goger DG, Weiter JJ. 1995. In vivo measurement of lipofuscin in Stargardt's disease - *fundus flavimaculatus.* Invest Ophthalmol Vis Sci 36:2327–2331.

Deutman AF, Hansen LMAA. 1970. Dominantly inherited drusen of Bruch's membrane. Br J Ophthalmol 34:373–382.

Deutman AF, Pinckers AJL, Aan de Kerk AL. 1976. Dominantly inherited cystoid macular edema. Am J Ophthalmol 82:540–548.

Douglas AA, Waheed I, Wyse CT. 1968. Progressive bifocal chorioretinal atrophy: a rare familial disease of the eyes. Brit J Ophthalmol 52:742–751.

Dryja TP, Briggs CE, Berson EL, Rosenfeld PJ, Abitol M. 1998. ABCR gene and age-related macular degeneration (letter). Science 279:1107.

Eagle RC, Lucier AC, Bernardino VG Jr, Yanoff M. 1980. Retinal pigment epithelial abnormalities in fundus flavimaculatus. Ophthalmology 87:1189–1200.

Epstein GA, Rabb MF. 1980. Adult vitelliform macular degeneration: diagnosis and natural history. Br J Ophthalmol 64:733–740.

Feist RM, White MF Jr, Skalka H, Stone EM. 1994. Choroidal neovascularization in a patient with adult foveomacular dystrophy and a mutation in the retinal degeneration slow gene. Am J Ophthalmol 118:259–260.

Fish G, Grey R, Sehmi KS, Bird AC. 1981. The dark choroid in posterior retinal dystrophies. Br J Ophthalmol 65:359–363.

Fishman GA, Carrasco C, Fishman M. 1976. The electro-oculogram in diffuse familial drusen. Arch Ophthalmol 94:231–233.

Fishman GA, Farber M, Patel BS, Derlacki DJ. 1987. Visual acuity loss in patients with Stargardt's macular dystrophy. Ophthalmology 94:809–814.

Fishman GA, Farbman JS, Alexander KR. 1991. Delayed rod dark adaptation in patients with Stargardt's disease. Ophthalmology 98: 957–962.

Fishman GA, Baca W, Alexander KR, Derlacki DJ, Glenn AM, Viana M. 1993. Visual acuity in patients with Best vitelliform macular dystrophy. Ophthalmology 100:1665–1670.

Flannery JG, Bird AC, Farber DB, Weleber RG, Bok DA. 1990. A histopathologic study of a choroideremia carrier. Invest Ophthalmol Vis Sci 31:229–236.

Forsman K, Graff C, Nordstrom S, Johansson K, Westermark E, Lundgren E, Gustavson K-H, Wadelius C, Holmgren G. 1992. The gene for Best's macular dystrophy is located at 11q13 in a Swedish family. Clin Genet 42:156–159.

Fossdal R, Magnusson L, Weber JL, Jensson O. 1995. Mapping the locus of atrophia areata, a helicoid peripapillary chorioretinal degeneration with autosomal dominant inheritance, to chromosome 11p15. Hum Molec Genet 4:479–483.

Frangieh GT, Green WR, Fine SL. 1982. A histopathologic study of Best's macular dystrophy. Arch Ophthalmol 100:1115–1121.

Frank HR, Landers MB III, Williams RJ, Sidbury JB Jr. 1974. A new dominant progressive foveal dystrophy. Am J Ophthalmol 78:903–916.

Gass JDM. 1974. A clinicopathologic study of a peculiar foveomacular dystrophy. Trans Am Ophthalmol Soc 72:139–156.

Gass JDM, Fallow S, Davis B. 1985. Adult vitelliform macular detachment occurring in patients with basal laminar drusen. Am J Ophthalmol 99:445–459.

Gass JDM. 1987. Stereoscopic Atlas of Macular Diseases: Diagnosis and Treatment. 3rd ed. St Louis: CV Mosby, 98–99.

Gerber S, Rozet J-M, Bonneau D, Souied E, Camuzat A, Dufier J-L, Amalric P, Weissenbach J, Munnich A, Kaplan J. 1995. A gene for late-onset fundus flavimaculatus with macular dystrophy maps to chromosome 1p13. Am J Hum Genet 56:396–399.

Govan JAA. 1983. Ocular manifestations of Alport's syndrome: a hereditary disorder of basement membranes? Br J Ophthalmol 67:493–503.

Gregory CY, Evans K, Wijesuriya SD, Kermani S, Jay MR, Plant C, Cox N, Bird AC, Bhattacharya SS. 1996. The gene responsible for autosomal dominant Doyne's honeycomb retinal dystrophy (DHRD) maps to chromosome 2p16. Hum Molec Genet 5:1055–1059.

Gu S, Thompson DA, Srikumari CRS, Lorenz B, Finckh U, Nicoletti A, Murthy KR, Rathmann M, Kumaramanickavel G, Denton MJ, Gal A. 1997. Mutations in RPE65 cause autosomal recessive childhood-onset severe retinal dystrophy. Nature Genet 17:194–197.

Hamilton AM, Pope FM, Condon PI, Slavin G, Sowter C, Ford S, Hayes JR, Serjeant GR. 1981. Angioid streaks in Jamaican patients with homozygous sickle cell disease. Br J Ophthalmol 65:341–347.

Hamilton WK, Ewing CC, Ives EJ, Carruthers JD. 1989. Sorsby's fundus dystrophy. Ophthalmology 96:1755–1762.

Hess F, Niemeyer G. 1983. EOG changes in dominantly inherited drusen (Malattia Leventinese). In: Kolder HEJW, ed, Slow Potentials, and Microprocessor Applications: Proceedings of the 20th I S C.E.V. Symposium. Boston: Junk, 105–113.

Heon E, et al. 1996. Linkage of autosomal dominant radial drusen (malattia leventinese) to chromosome 2p16-21. Arch Ophthalmol 114:193–198.

Holtz FG, Judd C, Fitzke FW, Bird AC, Pope FM. 1994. Dark adaptation and scotopic perimetry over peau d'orange in pseudoxanthoma elasticum. Br J Ophthalmol 78:79–80.

Hsieh RC, Fine BS, Lyons JS. 1977. Patterned dystrophies of the retinal pigment epithelium. Arch Ophthalmol 95:429–435.

Inglehearn C, Keen TJ, Al-Maghtheh M, Bhattacharya S. 1994. Loci for autosomal dominant retinitis pigmentosa and dominant cystoid macular dystrophy on chromosome 7p are not allelic. (Letter) Am J Hum Genet 55:581–582.

Itabashi R, Katsumi O, Mehta MC, Wajima R, Tamai M, Hirose T. 1993. Stargardt's disease/fundus flavimaculatus: psychophysical and electrophysiological results. Graefe's Arch Clin Exp Ophthalmol 231:555–562.

Jaffe GJ, Schatz H. 1988. Histopathologic features of adult-onset foveomacular pigment epithelial dystrophy. Arch Ophthalmol 106:958–960.

Jordan SA, Farrar GJ, Kumar-Singh R, Kenna P, Humphries MM, Allamand V, Sharp EM, Humphries P. 1992. Autosomal dominant retinitis pigmentosa (adRP;RP6): cosegregation of RP6 and the peripherin-RDS locus in a late-onset family of Irish origin. Am J Hum Genet 50:634–639.

Kaiser-Kupfer MI, Caruso RC, Valle D. 1991. Gyrate atrophy of the choroid and retina. Arch Ophthalmol 109:1539–1548.

Kajiwara K, Hahn LB, Mukai S, Travis GH, Berson EL, Dryja TP. 1991. Mutations in the human retinal degeneration slow gene in autosomal dominant retinitis pigmentosa. Nature 354:480–483.

Kajiwara K, Sandberg MA, Berson EL, Dryja TP. 1993. A null mutation in the human peripherin/RDS gene in a family with autosomal dominant retinitis punctata albescens. Nature Genet 3:208–212.

Kaplan J, et al. 1993. A gene for Stargardt's disease (fundus flavimaculatus) maps to the short arm of chromosome 1. Nature Genet 5:308–311.

Kelsell RE, Godley BF, Evans K, Tiffin PAC, Gregory CY, Plant C, Moore AT, Bird AC, Hunt DM. 1995. Localization of the gene for progressive bifocal chorioretinal atrophy (PBCRA) to chromosome 6q. Hum Molec Genet 4:1653–1656.

Kim DD, Mieler WF, Wolf WF. 1992. Posterior segment changes in membranoproliferative glomerulonephritis. Am J Ophthalmol 114:593–599.

Kremer H, Pinckers A, van den Heim B, Deutman AF, Ropers H-H, Mariman ECM. 1994. Localization of the gene for dominant cystoid macular dystrophy on chromosome 7p. Hum Molec Genet 3:299–302.

Lefler WH, Wadsworth JAC, Sidbury JB Jr. 1971. Hereditary macular dystrophy and amino-aciduria. Am J Ophthal 71(suppl):224–230.

Lim JI, Bressler NM, Marsh MJ, Bressler SB. 1993. Laser treatment of choroidal neovascularization in patients with angioid streaks. Am J Ophthalmol 116:414–423.

Maloney WF, Robertson DM, Duboff SM. 1977. Hereditary vitelliform macular degeneration. Arch Ophthalmol 95:979–983.

Margolis S, Siegel IM, Ripps H. 1987. Variable expressivity in fundus albipunctatus. Ophthalmology 94:1416–1422.

Marlhens F, Bareil C, Griffoin J-M, Zrenner E, Amalric P, Eliaou C, Liu S-Y, Harris E, Redmond TM, Arnaud B, Claustres M, Hamel CP. 1997. Mutations in RPE65 cause Leber's congenital amaurosis. Nature Genet 17:139–141.

Marmor MF. 1977. Fundus albipunctatus: a clinical study of the fundus lesions: the physiologic deficit and the vitamin A metabolism. Doc Ophthalmol 43:277–302.

Marmor MF. 1979. "Vitelliform" lesions in adults. Ann Ophthalmol 11:1705–1712.

Marmor MF. 1990. Long-term follow-up of the physiologic abnormalities and fundus changes in fundus albipunctatus. Ophthalmology 97:380–384.

Marmor MF. 1991a. Dominant drusen. In: Heckenlively JR, Arden GB, eds, Principles and Practice of Clinical Electrophysiology of Vision. St Louis: Mosby Year Book, 664–668.

Marmor MF. 1991b. Pattern dystrophies. In: Heckenlively JR, Arden

GB, eds, Principles and Practice of Clinical Electrophysiology of Vision. St Louis: Mosby Year Book, 700–704.

Marmor MF, Byers B. 1977. Pattern dystrophy of the pigment epithelium. Am J Ophthalmol 84:32–44.

Marmor MF, McNamara JA. 1996. Pattern dystrophy of the retinal pigment epithelium and geographic atrophy of the macula. Am J Ophthalmol 122:382–392.

Maw MA, Kennedy B, Knight A, Bridges R, Roth KE, Mani EJ, Mukkadan JK, Nancarrow D, Crabb JW, Denton MJ. 1997. Mutation of the gene encoding cellular retinaldehyde-binding protein in autosomal recessive retinitis pigmentosa. Nature Genet 17:198–200.

McDonnell PJ, Kivlin JD, Maumenee IH, Green WR. 1986. Fundus flavimaculatus without maculopathy. Ophthalmology 93:116–119.

Mohler CW, Fine SL. 1981. Long-term evaluation of patients with Best's vitelliform dystrophy. Ophthalmology 88:688–692.

Newman NM, Stevens RA, Heckenlively JR. 1987. Nerve fiber layer loss in diseases of the outer retinal layer. Br J Ophthalmol 71:21–26.

Nichols BE, Sheffield VC, Vandenburgh K, Drack AV, Kimura AE, Stone EM. 1993. Butterfly-shaped pigment dystrophy of the fovea caused by a point mutation in codon 167 of the RDS gene. Nature Genet 3:202–207.

Niemeyer G. 1978. Rod- and cone-function in malattia leventinese and in retinitis pigmentosa. Doc Ophthalmol Proc Series 17:337–344.

Noble KG, Carr RE. 1979. Stargardt's disease and fundus flavimaculatus. Arch Ophthalmol 97:1281–1285.

Noble KG, Scher BM, Carr RE. 1978. Polymorphous presentations in vitelliform macular dystrophy: subretinal neovascularisation and central choroidal atrophy. Br J Ophthalmol 62:561–570.

O'Donnell JJ, Vannas-Sulonen K, Shows TB, Cox DR. 1988. Gyrate atrophy of the choroid and retina: assignment of the ornithine aminotransferase structural gene to human chromosome 10 and mouse chromosome 7. Am J Hum Genet 43:922–928.

O'Gorman S, Flaherty WA, Fishman GA, Berson EL. 1988. Histopathologic findings in Best's vitelliform macular dystrophy. Arch Ophthalmol 106:1261–1268.

Patrinely JR, Lewis RA, Font RL. 1985. Foveomacular vitelliform dystrophy: adult type. Ophthalmology 92:1712–1718.

Polkinghome PJ, Capon MRC, Berninger R, Lyness AL, Sehmi K, Bird AC. 1989. Sorsby's fundus dystrophy: a clinical study. Ophthalmology 96:1763–1768.

Raybould MC, Birley AJ, Moss C, Hulten M, McKeown CME. 1994. Exclusion of an elastin gene (ELN) mutation as the cause of pseudoxanthoma elasticum (PXE) in one family. Clin Genet 45:48–51.

Rover J, Bach M. 1987. C-wave versus electrooculogram in diseases of the retinal pigment epithelium. Doc Ophthalmol 65:385–391.

Sabates R, Pruett RC, Hirose T. 1982. Pseudovitelliform macular degeneration. Retina 2:197–205.

Seabra MC, Brown MS, Goldstein JL. 1993. Retinal degeneration in choroideremia: deficiency of Rab geranylgeranyl transferase. Science 259:377–381.

Sieving PA, Niffenegger JH, Berson EL. 1986. Electroretinographic findings in selected pedigrees with choroideremia. Am J Ophthalmol 101:361–367.

Simell O, Takki K. 1973. Raised plasma ornithine and gyrate atrophy of the choroid and retina. Lancet 1:1031–1033.

Skoog K-O, Nilsson SEG. 1981. The c-wave of the electroretinogram in vitelliruptive macular degeneration (alvdalssjukan). Acta Ophthalmologica 59:756–758.

Small KW. 1989. North Carolina macular dystrophy, revisited. Ophthalmology 96:1747–1754.

Small KW, Hermsen V, Gurney N, Fetkenhour CL, Folk JC. 1992a.

North Carolina macular dystrophy and central areolar pigment epithelial dystrophy: one family, one disease. Arch Ophthalmol 110:515–518.

Small KW, Weber JL, Roses A, Lennon F, Vance JM, Pericak-Vance MA. 1992b. North Carolina macular dystrophy is assigned to chromosome 6. Genomics 13:681–685.

Steinmetz RL, Garner A, Maguire JI, Bird AC. 1991. Histopathology of incipient fundus flavimaculatus. Ophthalmology 98:953–956.

Steinmetz RL, Polkinghome PC, Fitzke FW, Kemp CM, Bird AC. 1992. Abnormal dark adaptation and rhodopsin kinetics in Sorsby's fundus dystrophy. Invest Ophthalmol Vis Sci 33:1633–1636.

Stone EM, Nichols BE, Streb LM, Kimura AE, Sheffield VC. 1992. Genetic linkage of vitelliform macular degeneration (Best's disease) to chromosome 11q13. Nature Genet 1:246–250.

Sveinsson K. 1939. Chorioiditis areata. Acta Ophthal 17:73–80.

Sveinsson K. 1979. Helicoidal peripapillary chorioretinal degeneration. Acta Ophthal 57:69–75.

Takki KK. 1974. Gyrate atrophy of the choroid and retina associated with hyperornithinaemia. Br J Ophthalmol 58:3–23.

Takki KK, Milton RC. 1981. The natural history of gyrate atrophy of the choroid and retina. Ophthalmology 88:292–301.

Travis GH, Brennan MB, Danielson PE, Kozak CA, Sutcliffe JG. 1989. Identification of a photoreceptor-specific mRNA encoded by the gene responsible for retinal degeneration slow (rds). Nature 338:70–73.

van Bokhoven H, van den Hurk JAJM, Bogerd L, Philippe C, Gilgenkrantz S, de Jong P, Ropers H-H, Cremers FPM. 1994. Cloning and characterization of the human choroideremia gene. Hum Molec Genet 3:1041–1046.

von Rückmann A, Fitzke FW, Bird AC. 1997. In vivo fundus autofluorescence in macular dystrophies. Arch Ophthalmol 115:609–615.

van Soest S, Swart J, Tijmes N, Sandkuijl LA, Rommers J, Bergen AAB. 1997. A locus for autosomal recessive pseudoxanthoma elasticum, with penetrance of vascular symptoms in carriers, maps to chromosome 16p13.1. Genome Res 7:830–834.

Vranka JA, Johnson E, Zho X, Shepardson A, Alexander JP, Bradley JMB, Wirtz MK, Weleber RG, Klein ML, Acott TS. 1997. Discrete expression and distribution pattern of TIMP-3 in the human retina and choroid. Curr Eye Res 16:102–110.

Wakabayashi K, Yonemura D, Kawasaki K. 1983. Electrophysiological analysis of Best's macular dystrophy and retinal pigment epithelial pattern dystrophy. Ophthalmic Paediatrics and Genetics 3:13–17.

Wang T, Lawler AM, Steel G, Sipila I, Milam AH, Valle D. 1995. Mice lacking ornithine-delta-amino-transferase have paradoxical neonatal hypoornithinaemia and retinal degeneration. Nature Genet 11:185–190.

Weber BHF, Vogt G, Wolz W, Ives EJ, Ewing CC. 1994a. Sorsby's fundus dystrophy is genetically linked to chromosome 22q13-qter. Nature Genet 7:158–161.

Weber BHF, Vogt G, Pruett RC, Stohr H, Felbor U. 1994b. Mutations in the tissue inhibitor metalloproteinases-3 (TIMP3) in patients with Sorsby's fundus dystrophy. Nature Genet 8:352–356.

Weingeist TA, Kobrin JL, Watzke RC. 1982. Histopathology of Best's macular dystrophy. Arch Ophthalmol 100:1108–1114.

Weinstein GW, Reeser F. 1975. The electro-oculogram, angioid streaks, and the R-membrane. Eye, Ear, Nose and Throat Monthly 54:182–187.

Weleber RG. 1989. Fast and slow oscillations of the electro-oculogram in Best's macular dystrophy and retinitis pigmentosa. Arch Opthalmol 107:530–537.

Weleber RG. 1994. Stargardt's macular dystrophy. Arch Ophthalmol 112:752–754.

Weleber RG, Carr RE, Murphey WH, Sheffield VC, Stone EM. 1993. Phenotypic variation including retinitis pigmentosa, patter dystrophy, and fundus flavimaculatus in a single family with a deletion of codon 153 or 154 of the peripherin/RDS gene. Arch Ophthalmol 111:1531–1542.

Wells J, Wroblewski J, Keen J, Inglehearn C, Jubb C, Eckstein A, Jay M, Arden G, Bhattacharya S, Fitzke F, Bird A. 1993. Mutations in the human retinal degeneration slow (RDS) gene can cause either retinitis pigmentosa or macular dystrophy. Nature Genet 3:213–218.

Wiznia RA, Perina B, Noble KG. 1981. Vitelliform macular dystrophy of late onset. Br J Ophthalmol 65:866–868.

Wright AF, Jay B, eds. 1994. Molecular Genetics of Inherited Eye Disorders. Vol 2 of Modern Genetics. Chur (Switzerland): Harwood.

Zhang K, Bither PP, Park R, Donoso LA, Seidman JG, Seidman CE. 1994. A dominant Stargardt's macular dystrophy locus maps to chromosome 13q34. Arch Ophthalmol 112:759–764.

17. Retinal heredodegenerations with retinal pigment epithelial involvement

KENT W. SMALL AND MICHAEL F. MARMOR

The retinal pigment epithelium (RPE) is involved in many disorders that represent primary dysfunction of the photoreceptors or other retinal cells. In some of these conditions the RPE may simply respond with scarring as the overlying retina degenerates. In others, the RPE may participate in the disease process through mechanisms such as pigment regeneration and photoreceptor renewal. As noted in Chapter 16, it is difficult to separate diseases that involve retina or RPE because abnormality of one tends to involve the other. Genes (i.e. peripherin) have already been found that can produce phenotypes of both retinal disease (retinitis pigmentosa) and RPE disease (pattern dystrophy). And while most retinitis pigmentosa (RP) appears to be photoreceptor disease with secondary RPE involvement, at least two forms of RP are caused by genes that are only expressed in RPE.

We have limited information, unfortunately, about the pathophysiology of most inherited retinal disorders at the level of RPE involvement. Therefore, much that follows will be clinical and genetic descriptions rather than mechanistic analyses. Nevertheless, we hope that this review will serve to show the breadth of inherited retinal disorders that clinically manifest with RPE abnormalities, and will encourage readers to think about why this occurs even where the current literature may not have answers. An introduction to the type of genetic analysis discussed herein is provided in Chapter 16.

PHOTORECEPTOR DYSTROPHIES

Rod-Cone Dystrophies (Retinitis Pigmentosa)

Clinical review. The term *retinitis pigmentosa* (RP) defines a large group of inherited retinal disorders which are characterized clinically by poor night vision, constricted visual fields, bone-spicule-like pigmentation of the fundus, and ERG evidence of photoreceptor dysfunction (Weleber, 1994; Kimura et al., 1995; Berson, 1994). The earliest symptom is usually night blindness, which is sometimes not recognized in childhood or youth. As the disease progresses, midperipheral sco-

tomas develop, which typically coalesce into a ring that spares a central island of vision and some far peripheral vision (most often temporal). Visual acuity usually remains good during youth and early adult life, but acuity loss may occur somewhat unpredictably, and older individuals with RP frequently have poor reading vision.

The typical clinical findings in RP include arteriolar narrowing, variable waxy pallor of the disc, and bone spicule pigment changes in the midperiphery which may be quite dense or extremely sparse (Fig. 17-1). The peripheral retina in RP appears atrophic even when spicules are absent. The macula is invariably abnormal, although the changes may be subtle—loss of a foveal reflex or irregularity of the vitreoretinal interface. Cystoid changes are sometimes present in the macula, although angiographic leakage is present in only a small percentage of RP patients. Vitreous cells are commonly observed, and posterior subcapsular cataracts develop in many patients, although they are infrequently the primary cause of visual loss.

Although these clinical findings are typical, they are not pathognomonic and may be mimicked by degeneration from other causes, including ischemia, chronic inflammation, or metabolic disease. Also, the clinical findings in RP vary enormously among patients, in large measure because this group of diseases comprises a large diversity of genetic entities which differ in the mechanism, rate, and severity of their effects on the retina. It is important in evaluating RP to consider this variability, and look carefully for milder variants of the disease.

The most critical diagnostic test for RP is the electroretinogram (ERG), which provides an objective measure of rod and cone function across the retina. The full-field ERG in RP typically shows a marked reduction of both rod and cone signals, although rod loss generally predominates. Both a- and b-waves are reduced, since the primary site of disease is at the photoreceptors or RPE. The ERG is usually abnormal in infancy or early childhood, except for some of the very mild and regional forms of RP.

Abnormalities in dark adaptation and color vision are

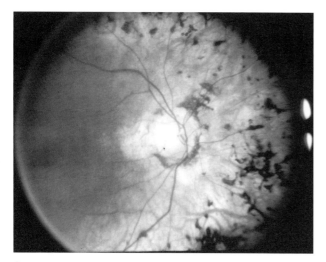

A

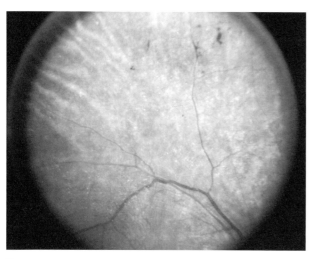

B

FIGURE 17-1. Retinitis pigmentosa. The syndrome is actually defined by progressive retinal dysfunction rather than pigment deposition (which can be quite variable). (**A**) Patient with typical bone corpuscular pigmentation, and (**B**) patient with minimal pigment deposition, although the typical vascular narrowing and RPE atrophy are evident.

also present. Mild blue-yellow axis color defects are common, although most RP patients do not clinically complain of major difficulty with color perception. The visual field is the most useful measure for ongoing follow-up of RP patients, since a progressive loss of side vision is often the major symptom (along with visual acuity changes). Goldmann (kinetic) perimetry is recommended to reach the far periphery. Contrast sensitivity is often reduced out of proportion to visual acuity (Marmor, 1986) and patients are usually hypersensitive to bright light (Gawande et al., 1986).

There is no accepted classification of RP variants, and

indeed the existing clinical distinctions will probably be superseded soon by schemata based on genetic subtypes. Clinicians have divided progressive adult RP into two broad types (Marmor, 1979; Massof and Finklestein, 1981), to distinguish (1) cases that have severe diffuse involvement of both rods and cones and a rather poor prognosis, from (2) cases in which the disease is somewhat regionalized, slower to progress, and less likely to affect macular function (Fig. 17-2). Infantile-onset RP blends into the group of disorders called Leber's congenital amaurosis; late adult-onset RP may be genetic but should raise concern about acquired entities such as cancer-associated retinopathy.

Specific drugs to modify the retinal degeneration of RP have not yet been found. Patients need to be educated about the disease, and be made aware of their field defects in order to make wise decisions about driving or vocational rehabilitation. In a small percentage of RP patients, cystoid edema may respond to oral carbonic anhydrase inhibitors such as acetazolamide, with some subjective improvement in visual function (Fishman et al., 1989; 1994). These may be patients in whom the macular RPE is relatively uninvolved by disease, since carbonic anhydrase inhibitors must act upon functional RPE to enhance water transport (Marmor, 1990).

In recent years therapeutic interest has centered on broader strategies for modifying the disease. The first, of course, is understanding the specific genetic defect, which might then become amenable to genetic or pharmacologic therapy. The second strategy is to look for "final common pathways" that may contribute to cellular dysfunction (such as light damage) or cellular

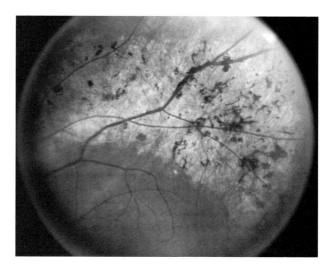

FIGURE 17-2. Delimited retinitis pigmentosa. There is a relatively sharp junction between the region of degeneration and the area of fundus that appears unaffected. The ERG can be moderately preserved in such patients, with normal b-wave implicit time.

death (such as the process of apoptosis), and that might be interrupted. For example, stressful light exposure, with its generation of free radicals and strain upon the regenerative capacity of the eye, might put dystrophic retinas at a disadvantage. However, there is little direct or epidemiologic evidence that the disease is modified by light.

The use of antioxidants might be beneficial for similar reasons, but there is again no evidence in favor or vitamin supplementation, and possibly some slight evidence to the contrary. A recent comprehensive epidemiologic study concluded that very high daily doses of vitamin A palmitate (15,000 U/day) slows the progress of RP by about 2% per year (Berson et al., 1993). However, some aspects of the study have been disputed, and this finding is controversial; the effects are also modest, and the use of such treatment must be weighed against the uncertain risk of long-term side effects from large chronic doses of vitamin A (Norton et al., 1993). Curiously, the study also found that high doses of vitamin E (400 U/day) were modestly deleterious, but the same questions and controversies exist about this finding (Berson et al., 1993).

Finally, there is a growing possibility of cellular transplantation to help patients with RP. It is technically feasible to transplant small patches of retinal or RPE tissue, or to inject cultured photoreceptor or RPE cells under the retina. Tissue transplantation could be beneficial in several ways. The presence of some normal tissue may exert humoral influences on more remote retinal areas that are degenerating (Silverman et al., 1994). To the extent that RPE damage or altered RPE metabolism may be at the root of some of the photoreceptor-degenerative changes, the insertion of healthy RPE cells may be beneficial.

Genetic and metabolic considerations. Within the last several years, a great deal has been learned about the molecular genetics of RP. The gene encoding rhodopsin was first cloned and mapped to Chromosome 3q in 1984 by Nathans and Hogness. Then in 1989, McWilliam and colleagues, using genetic linkage studies of a single large, autosomal-dominant RP family, mapped the diseased gene to the Chromosome 3q area. Then, using the candidate gene approach, Dryja and colleagues (1990) found the first mutations in the rhodopsin gene in autosomal-dominant RP. As of this writing (December 1995), over seventy different mutations have been found in the rhodopsin gene, which are thought to be associated and causative for the disease. It still remains unknown whether rhodopsin is expressed in the RPE, and how it is processed there. Even in autosomal-dominant RP, which is due to mutations

in rhodopsin, the cellular interaction resulting in cell death and bone spicule pigmentation is still unknown. Rhodopsin, a protein important in phototransduction of the rod outer segments, somehow causes cell death of the photoreceptors when modified by only one amino acid. It is suspected that the RPE is somehow important in the phagocytosis of these dying photoreceptors. With the increased rate of photoreceptor death, the RPE may become overwhelmed in RP. Additionally, there has been poor correlation between the genotype and the phenotype of RP. In single large families that have been extensively studied and found to have a rhodopsin mutation, there remains a great deal of phenotypic variability, expressed primarily in the variance of severity and onset of the disease. This suggests that additional environmental influences and/or other genes influence the expression (epistasis).

Rhodopsin mutations are also responsible for some autosomal-recessive RP cases. Rosenfeld and colleagues (1992) found a few autosomal recessive RP families with a particular rhodopsin mutation resulting in a functionally inactive protein. It is interesting to note that the heterozygote carriers of this mutation had reduced the ERGs with normal fundus findings.

Another protein, which was subsequently found to be mutated and a cause of autosomal-dominant RP, is the peripherin/rds gene (Travis et al., 1989). Using linkage analysis in an Irish family with autosomal-dominant RP, Farrar and colleagues (1991) and Jordan and colleagues (1992) found linkage to chromosome 6p and mutation in the peripherin/rds gene. Kajiwara and colleagues (1991), using a straight candidate gene analysis, also found mutations in peripherin causing autosomal-dominant RP. To make the situation even more confusing, mutations in the peripherin/rds gene have been found to be associated with Gass's adult foveal macular dystrophy, pattern dystrophy, and Stargardt's-like disease (Travis, 1993).

X-linked RP has been mapped to two or three loci on the short arm of the X chromosome known as RP-2 and RP-3. Recently RP-3 was cloned by Meindl and colleagues (1996) and is called the RPGR gene. The function of this gene is still being elucidated, but it appears to interact with GTP-ase and has an isoprenylation anchorage site.

An autosomal-recessive form of RP has been shown to be due to mutations in the gene encoding β-phosphodiesterase in a few families (McLaughlin et al., 1993). Beta-phosphodiesterase is important in the phototransduction cascade; its defect causes a decrease in phosphodiesterase activity, resulting in an increase in cyclic GMP levels within the rod photoreceptors. Mutations in the same gene in the mouse and in the Irish setter dog have been found to cause an outer segment retinal degeneration as well (Farber et al., 1992). One mutation in β-phosphodiesterase has been also found to cause CSNB-3 (congenital stationary night blindness) (Gal et al., 1994).

Several other loci of RP have been found, but the genes have not been cloned. Jordan and colleagues in 1993 mapped autosomal-dominant RP in a large Spanish family to chromosome 7q and Inglehearn and colleagues, also in 1993, mapped another family to chromosome 7p.

An extensive pedigree from the Netherlands with autosomal-recessive RP was studied by linkage analysis. It is interesting to note that a portion of one branch of this family had RP with para-arteriolar preservation of the RPE while other branches of the family did not. Analysis of five branches of the family yielded evidence of nonallelic genetic heterogeneity within this family corresponding to the observed clinical differences. A similar situation was found in an autosomal-recessive RP family reported by Leutelt and colleagues (1995), using a Pakistani family with consanguineous marriages. Two loci were linked, one to the 6 and one to 1q. Clear phenotypic differences were found between the matches of the family mapping to each locus.

A large South African kindred with autosomal-dominant RP (RP13) was mapped to chromosome 17p (Greenberg et al., 1994). Recoverin, which is a candidate gene in this region, was excluded as containing the mutation causing the disease (Weichmann et al., 1994).

Knowles and colleagues (1994) found, in a large Dominican autosomal-recessive RP family (RP14), linkage to Chromosome 6p. However, this locus is well away from the RDS region.

Recently, mutations have been found in the gene encoding cellular retinaldehyde-binding protein (CRALBP) in a family with autosomal recessive RP (Maw et al., 1997). This gene is not expressed in photoreceptors but is abundant in the RPE and Müller cells of the neuroretina. It is involved in the transport of 11-cis retinol and 11-cis retinaldehyde. Mutations in this gene prevent 11-cis retinol from acting as an efficient substrate for microsomal oxidation by 11-cis retinol dehydrogenase, and thus prevent the regeneration of rhodopsin.

Cone and Cone-Rod Dystrophies

Clinical review. These disorders, like the rod-cone dystrophies, represent a heterogeneous group of diseases, genetically and, presumably, metabolically. The cone or cone-rod dystrophies are characterized by poor visual acuity and poor color discrimination as early findings, although eventual involvement of rods, night vision, and peripheral vision is not infrequent (Szlyk et al.,

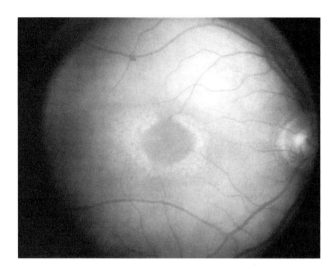

FIGURE 17-3. Cone/rod degeneration with bull's-eye maculopathy. This patient had an unrecordable cone ERG, while rod signals were near the lower limits of normal.

1993). The diagnosis is made in part by these clinical findings, but more definitively by the ERG, which shows severe and selective loss of cone function, with varying degrees of rod abnormality. The severe cone loss helps distinguish these diffuse dystrophic disorders from predominant macular diseases like Stargardt's disease or central choroidal dystrophy. The nature of RPE involvement in these diseases is presently unknown, but virtually all of the arguments by which RPE may be relevant to RP could apply to the cone and cone-rod dystrophies.

The reasons for certain patterns of RPE atrophy, such as bull's-eye maculopathy in some cone dystrophies (Fig. 17-3) have not been established. A different pattern of RPE disturbance, in the region of the vascular arcades, is seen in the enhanced S-cone syndrome (Fig. 17-4 and Plate 17-I) (Marmor et al., 1990). This disorder is characterized by an absence of rod function and enhanced activity of the short wavelength cone (S-cone) system. The degree of RPE and retinal degeneration is variable and this disorder may lie on a spectrum with the more severe Goldman-Favre disease.

Genetic and metabolic considerations. In a large kindred with autosomal-dominant cone rod dystrophy, Evans and colleagues (1994) demonstrated linkage to chromosome 19q13.1–q13.2. In this family, loss of visual acuity occurred early in life, during the first decade, with onset of night blindness occurring in the third decade (Evans et al., 1995). By the third decade of life, most individuals showed remarkable loss of cone and rod function. The gene has not yet been cloned.

Small and colleagues recently mapped an autosomal-dominant progressive cone degeneration to chromo-

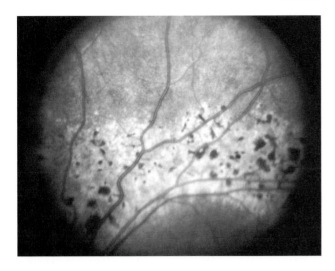

FIGURE 17-4. Enhanced S-cone syndrome. Pigmentary changes are most striking in the region of the vascular arcades. This syndrome can vary considerably among patients in the degree of pigmentary degeneration and ERG changes.

some 17p (Balciuniene et al., 1995; Small and Gehrs, 1996; Small et al., 1996). They ascertained a large family in eastern Tennessee with this disorder and screened the human genome in potential candidate regions until linkage was found to this region. There was a great deal of phenotypic variability within this single large family. Some affected individuals had relatively good central vision with impaired color vision and highly abnormal cone ERGs, while others had decreased central vision with only modestly decreased cone ERG and abnormal color vision. This family once again showed the value of having a single large family in order to be able to fully appreciate the extent of the phenotype.

This mapping was particularly important and interesting, because it mapped in the same region on chromosome 17p where the gene recoverin resides. Recoverin is thought to be highly expressed in cones and to play a significant role in allowing the phototransduction cascade to recover after stimulation (Murakami et al., 1992). A mutation of this gene could theoretically cause patients to have increased photophobia. That gene is currently being evaluated in this family. It may be relevant that the chick gene, visinin, has significant homology to recoverin and the chick retina is cone dominant.

MULTIPLE ORGAN SYSTEM DISORDERS

Leber's Congenital Amaurosis

There are a number of rare infantile syndromes that cause retinal degeneration in association with other systemic abnormalities. These include *Joubert's syndrome, neuronal ceroid lipofuscinosis, Alstrom's syndrome,*

and *Zellweger's syndrome.* These disorders overlap with *Leber's congenital amaurosis* (LCA), although the latter term should ideally be reserved for patients who lack systemic associations. Some of these conditions will be discussed later with respect to specific metabolic abnormalities.

Leber's congenital amaurosis, an autosomal-recessive retinal degeneration marked by profound visual impairment during childhood, was found to be responsible for 10% of blindness in Sweden (Alstrom, 1957). Keratoconus is sometimes associated with this disorder as well. No other systemic manifestations are known.

Camuzat and colleagues (1995), mapped Leber's congenital amaurosis (LCA1) to 17q using linkage analysis in 15 families. On a closer analysis of these 15 different families, they found that one group of five families of Maghrebian origin actually mapped to 17p instead of 17q. These researchers concluded that LCA1 in the North African families is located at 17p13. Linkage was not found to 17p in 10 families of French origin. There are several reasonable candidate genes in this area, including recoverin, beta-arrestin 2, retinal guanylate cyclase (GUC2D), and phosphotidylinositol transfer protein (PITPN). Of these, GUC2D most closely mapped to the LCA region. Most recently, using this information, Perrault and colleagues (1996) evaluated GUC2D in their families and found the mutations.

A different gene has recently been discovered to be abnormal in some families with Leber's amaurosis or early-onset autosomal recessive RP (Gu et al., 1997; Marlhens et al., 1997). This gene codes for a microsomal protein called RPE65, which is exclusively and abundantly expressed in the RPE and is important in retinoid metabolism. Marlhens and associates (1997) recently found mutations in this gene causing autosomal recessive Leber's congenital amaurosis as well as autosomal recessive childhood-onset severe retinal dystrophy.

Bardet-Biedl Complex of Diseases

Clinical review. The prototype of these disorders, the Bardet-Biedl syndrome, is an autosomal-recessive multisystem disease characterized by obesity, polydactily, hypogenitalism, mental retardation, and pigmentary retinopathy (Schachat and Maumenee, 1981). The retinal degeneration is quite severe (Fig. 17-5), with the ERG typically undetectable and both central and peripheral vision severely impaired. The fundus appearance, however, is generally atypical for RP, and is more characterized by granular pigment mottling and atrophy than by bone spicule deposits. This syndrome overlaps in some but not all features with a number of other entities such as the Lawrence-Moon syndrome (which includes spastic paresis and extensive choroidal atrophy

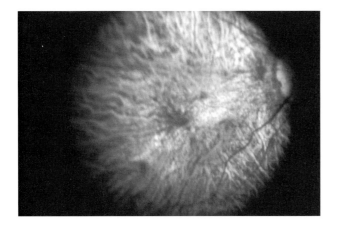

FIGURE 17-5. Bardet-Biedl syndrome. There is diffuse and severe retinal degeneration, but often with an atrophic or granular appearance rather than bone spicule figures.

but omits polydactily and obesity), and Alstrom disease (which adds deafness and diabetes mellitus to the list of abnormalities).

Genetic and molecular counseling. In a large, inbred Bedouin family from the Negev region of Israel, Kwitek-Black (1993) used linkage analysis to localize one of the genes of Bardet-Biedl syndrome (BBS) to chromosome 16q-21. Echocardiographic evaluation showed one-half of the affected individuals to demonstrate myocardial abnormalities, and renal ultrasonography was abnormal in half of the affected individuals (not necessarily the same ones). Leppert and colleagues (1994) found that there were some BBS families which did not map to chromosome 16. They performed a genome-wide search and found another locus on chromosome 11. Then, Sheffield and colleagues (1994) found a third locus on chromosome 3 in another Bedouin population. A fourth locus, on chromosome 15, was found in a separate inbred Bedouin family by Carmi and colleagues (1995). Therefore, it is apparent that BBS is genetically complex.

Usher's Syndrome (Retinal Dystrophy with Hearing Loss)

Clinical review. RP associated with sensory neural hearing loss has been termed *Usher's syndrome*. This is the most common cause of combined deafness and blindness in the United States, but it represents a heterogeneous group of autosomal-recessive disorders, and four types of Usher's syndrome have already been categorized (Fishman et al., 1983; Kimberling et al., 1994). The most prevalent type I patients have profound hearing loss, absent vestibular function, and

rather severe progressive retinal degeneration indistinguishable from RP. Type II patients have only moderate sensory neural loss, good vestibular responses, and somewhat milder RP.

Abnormalities in the ultrastructure of axonemes in cilia have been found in many Usher's patients (Hunter et al., 1986), which is intriguing since photoreceptors are modified cilia, and cilia are also the end organs for otologic function. Deafness may also be associated with disorders in which organ systems beyond the eye and ear are involved, such as Alstrom's syndrome, Bardet-Biedl syndrome, retinal renal syndromes, Refsum's disease, Leber's congenital amaurosis, mitochondrial myopathies, congenital rubella, and mucopolysaccharidoses.

Genetic and molecular counseling. Usher's syndrome type 1a, designated by the symbol Ush1a (French variety) was mapped to chromosome 14 (Kaplan et al., 1992). The Acadian variety was mapped to chromosome 11p, and Ush1b (non-Acadian variety) (Kimberling et al., 1992; Keats et al., 1994) was mapped to chromosome 11q (Weil et al., 1995). Ush1b accounts for about 75% of type 1 Usher's syndrome patients. A mutation in the gene encoding myosin VIIA was found to be responsible for the phenotype. Premature stop codon mutations have been demonstrated in five unrelated families. This mutation causes abnormalities in microtubules in the axoneme of the photoreceptor cells, nasal ciliary cells, and sperm cells; it also causes degeneration in the organ of Corti, resulting in deafness. Additionally, a mouse mutant known as "Shaker-1" (Sh1) was previously found to be homologous to human Usher's syndrome (Brown et al., 1992). The Sh1 homozygous mouse mutant demonstrates vestibular dysfunction and deafness. The olfactory protein (OMP) is linked to the mouse Sh1 chromosome on mouse chromosome 7. This was subsequently shown to be the gene encoding myosin VIIA. Therefore, Ush1b and "Shaker" are due to primary cytoskeleton protein defects. To date, three different mutations in the myosin VIIA have been demonstrated in humans to be responsible for Usher's syndrome. The myosin VIIA gene is expressed in the RPE and the cochlear hair cells but not in the neurosensory retina.

Of Usher's syndrome type 2 patients, approximately 5%–10% are known to link to chromosome 1q34–q41 (Kimberling et al., 1990). In this region is the "choroideremia-like gene," which may be a candidate for Ush2. A distinctive type of Usher's syndrome characterized by progressive hearing loss and vestibular dysfunction, was described by Karjalainen and colleagues (1985). This disease was additionally mapped by linkage by Sankila in 1995 to chromosome 3q12–q15. In

Finland, this accounts for 42% of Usher's syndrome, and is known as Usher's syndrome type 3 (Ush3).

Usher's syndrome type 1 (Acadian variety) was linked (Smith et al., 1992) to Chromosome 11p. A brain-derived neurotrophic factor also mapped to 11p13 and is a possible candidate gene. The mouse mutant characterized by deafness, known as "Twister," maps to the homologous region.

Neuromuscular Disorders

Retinal degeneration, most often associated with some degree of pigment epithelial change, is found in several diverse neuromuscular disorders. Some of the spinocerebellar degenerations such as Friedreich's ataxia and olivopontocerebellar degeneration are associated with pigmentary degeneration of the retina. In the latter group of disorders, some are inherited in an autosomal-dominant fashion, while mitochondrial DNA mutations have been found in others.

Myotonic dystrophy. In myotonic dystrophy, the fundus can show ill-defined and usually mild retinal degenerative changes, sometimes mimicking a pattern dystrophy (Fig. 17-6) (Kimizuka et al., 1993). The expression of this disease is highly variable and the retinal pathology is usually of little visual significance. However, the ERG can be mildly reduced, while the EOG is typically normal.

Myotonic dystrophy was the first demonstration of autosomal linkage in humans. This was suspected in 1954 by Mohr, who found linkage to the Lutheran blood group. Subsequently, Eiberg (1983) definitively linked myotonic dystrophy with the Lutheran blood group in a protein marker known as fibroblast C-3, which is located on Chromosome 19. Subsequently, tightly linked flanking markers were established, narrowing the genomic region of interest. Then, Harley and colleagues (1993) and Buxton and colleagues (1992) detected a DNA fragment which was much larger and more variable in size in affected persons than in the normal siblings. By using positional cloning strategies, Brook and colleagues (1992) established a CTG triplet repeat expansion which was larger in myotonic dystrophy patients than in unaffected individuals. This trinucleotide repeat expansion disrupted a protein kinase gene. Additionally, it was found that the larger the expansion the more severe the disease, in that as it passed from one generation to the next, the expansion increased. This was the first molecular evidence of "genetic anticipation." The role of the RPE in this remains unknown, as the expression of this protein kinase gene has not been determined in this tissue.

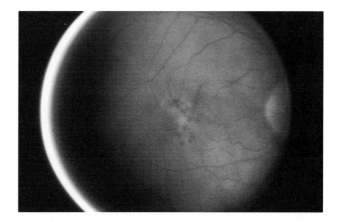

FIGURE 17-6. Myotonic dystrophy. Variable and patchy pigmentary changes are found, sometimes simulating a pattern dystrophy (as in this patient).

Duchenne's muscular dystrophy. Duchenne's muscular dystrophy, an X-linked disease, exhibits abnormal electroretinograms manifested primarily as a negative waveform on dark-adapted states (Sigesmund et al., 1994). This suggests abnormal panretinal neurotransmission. Interestingly, individuals with abnormal ERGs do not have nyctalopia and have normal dark adaptometry. Therefore, the significance of these ERG findings is unknown. Furthermore, the relationship to the RPE remains a mystery as well. The fundus in Duchenne's muscular dystrophy patients is typically normal.

The mutated protein known as *dystrophin* is ubiquitously present at basal levels in many cell types of these patients. Interestingly, the promoter for the dystrophin that is expressed in neural tissue is different than the dystrophin which is expressed in muscle tissue, as shown by Chelly and colleagues in 1990.

Friedreich's ataxia. Friedreich's ataxia was mapped by linkage (Chamberlain et al., 1988) to chromosome 9p22-cen. Other researchers subsequently showed that all Friedreich's ataxia families mapped to the same precise location, thus showing no evidence of genetic heterogeneity. French Canadian populations in Canada and in Louisiana were particularly helpful in narrowing the genetic region of interest. Recently another expanded triplet repeat of DNA in an intron was found to cause the disease (Campuzano et al., 1996). The gene, named frataxin, contains a potential mitochondrial targeting sequence. Thus, Friedreich's ataxia is a mitochondrial disease caused by mutations in the nuclear genome.

Olivopontocerebellar ataxia. Olivopontocerebellar ataxia (OPCA), an autosomal-dominant ataxia, was mapped by linkage to the HLA locus by Jackson and colleagues (1977). The reason this was mapped many years ago was the highly polymorphic nature of the HLA locus. Subsequently, OPCA-1 was partly renamed SCA-1 for spinal cerebellar atrophy type 1. The gene was subsequently found to be telomeric to the HLA complex and due to an expansion of a trinucleotide CAG repeat. Patients with early-onset and therefore more severe disease have a greater expansion of this trinucleotide repeat than patients with late-onset disease. This is similar to the mechanism of the mutations found in fragile X syndrome, myotonic dystrophy, Kennedy spinal and bulbar muscular atrophy, and in Huntington's disease. The mutated gene is called *ataxin-1*. The expression of this gene in the RPE has not been determined, but is highly expressed in cerebellar Purkinje cells, as demonstrated by Servadio and colleagues (1995).

Progressive cerebellar ataxia with pigmentary macular degeneration is called OPCA type 3. This gene was mapped to chromosome 3p21.1–p12 recently (Benomar et al., 1995). No genetic heterogeneity was found among Moroccan, Belgian, and French families studied.

Renal Disease

Several forms of congenital renal disease are associated with retinal degeneration.

Juvenile nephronothesis. Juvenile nephronothesis or renal-retinal dysplasia, is an autosomal-recessive disorder with juvenile renal failure and retinal pigmentary degeneration which is sometimes sectorial. It is suspected that this disease is a primary disorder of collagen and basement membrane. The defect was recently found to be a deletion of the gene NPHP1 on chromosome 2q13 (Hildebrandt et al., 1997).

Alport's disease. Renal disease is also a component of Alstrom's syndrome, Alport's disease, and some of the Bardet-Biedl complex disorders. Alport's disease shows considerable heterogeneity being inherited as an X-linked-recessive, autosomal-recessive, and autosomal-dominant trait. All have in common the features of nephritis with progressive renal failure and deafness. Anterior lenticonus is a particularly interesting feature of Alport's, which supported the hypothesis of this being a collagen or basement membrane disease. Retinal findings consist of whitish-gray dots in the superficial layer of the retina and flecks in the macular area that are not detectable by fluorescein angiography (Polak and Hogwind, 1977; Zylberman et al., 1980).

One gene defective in some patients with this disorder is type 4 collagen alpha 5 chain (COL4a5), located

on the X chromosome (Antignac et al., 1992, 1994; Barker et al., 1990, 1996, 1997). Many cases of Alport's have subsequently been demonstrated to be X-linked dominant. The autosomal-recessive form was mapped to chromosome 2q35–q37, where type 4 collagen genes COL4a3 and COL4a4 are located and are involved in several different types of mutations (Lemmink et al., 1994, 1997).

METABOLIC DEFECTS

It is beyond our scope to consider all of the metabolic disorders that have some retinal manifestation (Bateman et al., 1994). Some of the congenital abnormalities such as albinism are considered elsewhere in this book. We will focus on a few conditions which seem particularly relevant to RPE metabolism.

Neuronal Ceroid Lipofuscinosis

Clinical review. The neuronal ceroid lipofuscinoses are a group of recessive lysosomal storage disorders characterized broadly by dementia, seizures, and pigmentary retinopathy with progressive visual loss in the early-onset cases (Brod et al., 1987; Traboulsi et al., 1987). These have been categorized clinically in relation to the age of onset and the temporal relation of visual loss to neurologic symptoms: the infantile form has its onset at 8 to 18 months of age; the late infantile form (Janssky-Bielshovsky) appears between 2 and 4 years of age; the juvenile form (Vogt-Spielmeier-Batten) at 4 to 8 years (Elze et al., 1978); and the adult form (Kufs) in adulthood. The infantile disease is characterized by optic atrophy, macular pigmentary changes with mottling of the periphery, and low or absent electrophysiologic findings (ERG and visual evoked response). In the infantile forms, the retinal changes can lead to confusion with Leber's amaurosis congenital. The later infantile and juvenile cases, however, show macular granularity or bull's-eye maculopathy more prominently, and the appearance can be mistaken for a primary retinal dystrophy such as Stargardt's disease. The adult forms of lipofuscinosis often do not have ophthalmological manifestations, but electrophysiologic changes indicative of inner and RPE damage have been observed (Dawson et al., 1985).

Infantile neuronal ceroid lipofuscinosis is a distinctive form found primarily in Finland (Bateman and Philippart, 1986). Typically, these patients are blind by the age of two, with optic atrophy and macular and retinal changes but without pigment aggregation.

Genetic and molecular counseling. Batten's disease was localized to chromosome 16p12.1–p11.2 by Eiberg (1989), who found linkage to haptoglobin. Additional markers in the area as well as additional families studied by others have confirmed this localization. The Batten's disease gene, denoted CLN3, was recently found to be disrupted by deletions in most affected subjects (International Batten Disease Consortium, 1995).

The infantile disease has been mapped by linkage to chromosome 1p35–p33 (Jarvela et al., 1991). The gene palmitoyl-protein thioesterase has been found to be mutated in all Finnish patients with this disease, as well as in several non-Finnish patients (Vesa et al., 1995). The expression of this gene in the RPE is unknown. This protein is thought to be involved in the catabolism of lipid modified proteins.

Abetalipoproteinemia

Abetalipoproteinemia is an autosomal-recessive disorder in which apolipoprotein B is not synthesized, leading to fat malabsorption, fat-soluble vitamin deficiencies, spinocerebellar degeneration, and retinal degeneration (Cogan et al., 1984). The red blood cells show acanthocytosis. High-dose therapy with the fat-soluble vitamins A and E can prevent or ameliorate the retinal degeneration.

In abetalipoproteinemia the mutated protein in this disease is microsomal triglyceride transfer protein (Wetterau et al., 1992; Shoulders et al., 1993). This protein catalyzes the transport of triglyceride and cholesteryl ester from phospholipid surfaces. Microsomal triglyceride transfer protein is present in the lumen of the microsomal fraction of liver and intestine. The role of this protein in the RPE is unknown.

Peroxisomal Disorders and Refsum's Disease

Clinical review. The peroxisomal disorders result from dysfunction or absence or peroxisomes or peroxisomal enzymes (Folz and Trobe, 1991). The hallmarks biochemically are defective oxidation and accumulation of very long chain fatty acids. Zellweger's syndrome is the prototype of these disorders, and is characterized by infantile retinal degeneration associated with hypotonia, psychomotor retardation, seizures, characteristic facies, renal cortical cysts, and hepatic interstitial fibrosis. Patients with neonatal adrenal leucodystrophy may present in infancy, but generally survive until seven to ten years of age. Less severe but similar findings are present in infantile Refsum's disease, so-called because serum phytanic acid is elevated, as it is in regular Refsum's disease. Classic Refsum's disease (phytanic acid storage disease), however, may not be a true peroxisomal disorder. It is often not diagnosed until adulthood, and it is characterized by cerebellar ataxia, polyneuropathy, pigmentary retinopathy, anosmia, deafness, ichthyosis, and cardiac myopathy with arrhythmias. Night blindness may be an early symptom.

Genetic and metabolic considerations. Zellweger's syndrome was mapped in 1994 by Masuno and colleagues to chromosome 8q21.2. The human gene is known as PAF-1 (peroxisome assembly factor-1) and at least nine different genes are involved in the assembly of peroxisomes (Shimozawa et al., 1992). There was found to be no obvious relationship between genotype and phenotype. A second form of Zellweger's syndrome was identified in peroxisomal membrane protein-70, which mapped to Chromosome 1, and another form to chromosome 7 by demonstration of chromosomal rearrangement in two cases (Naritomi et al., 1989).

A third disorder, known as pseudo-Zellweger's syndrome, has been mapped to chromosome 3 to the peroxisomal thiolase gene (Bout et al., 1989). The role these proteins play in the RPE remains elusive. Refsum's disease has been neither mapped nor cloned.

Primary Hyperoxaluria Type 1

Clinical review. Primary hyperoxaluria type 1 (oxalosis) is an autosomal-recessive trait marked by high urinary oxalate excretion with progressive urolithiasis and nephrocalcinosis with subsequent renal failure. Oxalosis, or deposition of oxalate crystals in tissue, can occur in the cardiac conduction system, causing heart block, and in the peripheral blood vessels causing vascular insufficiency, arteriolar occlusion, and gangrene. Additionally, there is extensive deposition of the crystals in bone, causing marked bony malformations and spontaneous fractures. Small and colleagues in 1990 examined 24 patients with primary hyperoxaluria and found eight to have a striking and distinctive crystalline retinopathy with marked RPE hyperplasia (Fig. 17-7). Histopathology of eyes from primary hyperoxaluria patients typically shows marked RPE hyperplasia surrounding embedded oxalate crystals in the RPE. It would seem that the oxalate crystal deposition in the RPE is likely due to a hyperconcentration of oxalate due to a pumping action of the RPE. The RPE reacts to the crystalline deposit in a proliferative fashion.

Genetic and molecular considerations. The enzyme defective in primary hyperoxaluria is alanine:glyoxylate aminotransferase, which is a peroxisomal enzyme. In humans, the enzyme's activity is largely confined to the

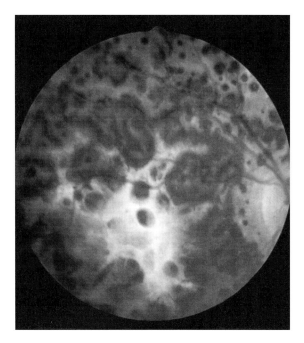

FIGURE 17-7. Primary hyperoxaluria, type I. (From Small, 1990.)

peroxisomes. In lower mammals, the enzyme has activity in the mitochondria as well (Danpure et al., 1986). The gene encoding alanine:glyoxylate aminotransferase was mapped by Purdue in 1990 to chromosome 2q36–q37. Six different point mutations within this gene have been shown to cause primary hyperoxaluria. Some of these mutations are associated with a peroxisome to mitochondrion mistargeting, also called *trafficking defects*.

Cystinosis

Cystinosis is an accumulation of intralysosomal cystine caused by a defect in its transportation out of lysosomes. Three types of cystinosis are recognized: nephropathic, late-onset (or intermediate), and benign. Cystine crystals accumulate in the cornea and conjunctiva in all three types, but only patients with nephropathic cystinosis develop retinopathy. These patients typically present as infants of 8 to 15 months of age with progressive renal failure, growth retardation, renal rickets, and hypothyroidism. Patchy areas of depigmented RPE are seen alternating with irregularly distributed clumps of pigment. Despite the fundus abnormalities, however, there is no significant disturbance of vision. Treatment with cystamine, which reacts with lysosomal cystine to form a mixed disulfide that can leave the lysosome, may be beneficial.

The Cystinosis Collaborative Research Group (Mc-Dowell et al., 1995) mapped cystinosis to the short arm of chromosome 17 by linkage analysis. All families analyzed had the infantile form of cystinosis. One juvenile cystinosis family was also consistent with linkage to this same region on 17p. The adult form has not been localized, nor the gene cloned.

Mitochondrial DNA Disorders

Clinical review. Mitochondrial myopathy is a result of defects in mitochondrial DNA, and can have a wide range of ocular manifestations (Brown et al., 1994). Progressive external ophthalmoplegia is most characteristic, and may be associated with pigmentary retinopathy, cardiomyopathy (the Kearns-Sayre syndrome) or other systemic abnormalities. The retina can show granular pigmentation, but the degree of retinopathy is quite variable (Fig. 17-8). In some patients, visual function is excellent and the ERG normal. But in others (especially those with full-blown Kearns-Sayre syndrome) the retinopathy and ERG loss can be severe. There is also a syndrome (NARP) of neurogenic muscle weakness, ataxia, and retinitis pigmentosa.

Genetic and molecular consideration. Deletions in muscle mitochondrial DNA were found by Moraes and colleagues (1991) in 32 of 123 patients with various mitochondrial myopathies and encephalopathies. All of these patients had progressive external ophthalmoplegia. The deletions varied in size. Large-scale deletions in muscle mitochondrial DNA in seven patients with Kearns-Sayre syndrome were found by Zeviani and colleagues in 1988. The proportion of mutated chromosomes in each Kearns-Sayre patient ranged from 45%

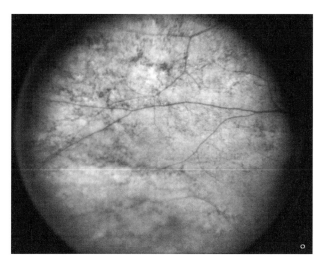

FIGURE 17-8. Kearns-Sayre syndrome (mitochondrial myopathy). There may be a granular pigmentary retinopathy, but the degree of involvement is variable and visual function often remains good.

to 75% of the total mitochondrial DNA. Partially deleted and normal mitochondrial DNA have been demonstrated in all tissues, but in very different proportions, indicating that the mutation originated before the primary cells diverged (Johns et al., 1989). The role of the mitochondrial deletions on the RPE has not been studied.

ACKNOWLEDGMENTS

This work is supported in part by The Foundation Fighting Blindness (KWS), National Eye Institute NIH/NEI RO1-EY12039 (KWS) and The McCone Endowment (KWS)

REFERENCES

Alstrom CH. 1957. Heredo-retinopathia congenitalis monohybrida recessiva autosomalis: a genetical-statistical study in clinical collaboration with Olof Olson. Hereditas 43:1–178.

Antignac C, Zhou J, Sanak M, Cochat P, Roussel B, Deschenes G, Gros F, Knebelmann B, Hors-Cayla M-C, Tryggvason K, Gubler M-C. 1992. Alport syndrome and diffuse leiomyomatosis: deletions in the 5-prime end of the COL4A5 collagen gene. Kidney Int 42:1178–1183.

Antignac C, Knebelmann B, Drouot L, Gros F, Deschenes G, Hors-Cayla M-C, Zhou J, Tryggvason K, Grunfeld J-P, Broyer M, Gubler M-C. 1994. Deletions in the COL4A5 collagen gene in X-linked Alport syndrome: characterization of the pathological transcripts in nonrenal cells and correlation with diseaseexpression. J Clin Invest 93:1195–1207.

Balciuniene J, Johansson K, Sandgren O, Wachtmeister L, Holmgren G, Forsman K. 1995. A gene for autosomal dominant progressive cone dystrophy (CORD5) maps to chromosome 17p12–p13. Genomics 30:281–286.

Barker DF, Hostikka SL, Zhou J, Chow LT, Oliphant AR, Gerken SC, Gregory MC, Skolnick MH, Atkin CL, Tryggvason K. 1990. Identification of mutations in the COL4A5 collagen gene in Alport syndrome. Science 248:1224–1227.

Barker DF, Pruchno CJ, Jiang X, Atkin CL, Stone EM, Denison JC, Fain PR, Gregory MC. 1996. A mutation causing Alport syndrome with tardive hearing loss is common in the western United States. Am J Hum Genet 58:1157–1165.

Barker DF, Denison JC, Atkin CL, Gregory MC. 1997. Common ancestry of three Ashkenazi-American families with Alport syndrome and COL4A5 R1677Q. Hum Genet 99:681–684.

Bateman JB, Lang GE, Maumenee IH. 1994. Multisystem genetic disorders associated with retinal dystrophies. In: Ryan SJ, ed., Retina, 2nd ed. St. Louis: Mosby, 467–491.

Bateman JB, Philippart M. 1986. Ocular features of the Hagberg-Santavuori syndrome. Am J Ophthalmol 102:262–271.

Benomar A, Krols L, Stevanin G, Cancel G, LeGuern E, David G, Ouhabi H, Martin J-J, Durr A, Zaim A, et al. 1995. The gene for autosomal dominant cerebellar ataxia with pigmentary macular dystrophy maps to chromosome 3p12–p21.1. Nature Genet 10:84–88.

Berson EL. 1994. Hereditary retinal diseases. In: Albert DM, Jakobies FA, eds., Principles and Practice of Ophthalmology. Philadelphia: Saunders, 1181–1262.

Berson EL, Rosner B, Sandberg MA, Hayes KC, Nicholson BW, Weigel-DiFranco C, Willett W. 1993. A randomized trial of vitamin A and vitamin E supplementation for retinitis pigmentosa. Arch Ophthalmol 111:761–772.

Brod RD, Packer AJ, Van Dyk HJL. 1987. Diagnosis of neuronal ceroid lipofuscinosis by ultrastructural examination of peripral blood lymphocytes. Arch Ophthalmol 105:1388–1393.

Bout A, Hoovers JMN, Bakker E, Mannens MMAM, Geurts van Kessel A, Westerveld A, Tager JM, Benne R. 1989. Assignment of the gene coding for human peroxisomal 3-oxoacyl-CoA thiolase (ACAA) to chromosome region 3p22–p23. Cytogenet Cell Genet 52:147–150.

Brook JD, McCurrach ME, Harley HG, Buckler AJ, Church D, Aburatani H, Hunter K, Stanton VP, Thirion J-P, Hudson T, et al. 1992. Molecular basis of myotonic dystrophy: expansion of a trinucleotide (CTG) repeat at the 3-prime end of a transcript encoding a protein kinase family member. Cell 68:799–808.

Brown KA, Sutcliffe MJ, Steel KP, Brown SDM. 1992. Close linkage of the olfactory marker protein gene to the mouse deafness mutation shaker-1. Genomics 13:189–193.

Brown MD, Lott MR, Wallace DC. 1994. Mitochondrial DNA Mutations and the Eye. In: Wright AF, Jay B, eds, Molecular Genetics of Inherited Eye Disorders. Chur (Switzerland): Harwood, 469–490.

Buxton J, Shelbourne P, Davies J, Jones C, Van Tongeren T, Aslanidis C, de Jong P, Jansen G, Anvret M, Riley B, et al. 1992. Detection of an unstable fragment of DNA specific to individuals with myotonic dystrophy. Nature 355:547–548.

Campuzano V, Montermini L, Molto MD, Pianese L, Cossee M, Cavalcanti F, Monros E, Rodius F, Duclos F, Monticelli A, Zara F, Canizares J, Koutnikova H, Bidichandani SI, Gellera C, Brice A, Trouillas P, De Michele G, Filla A, De Frutos R, Palau F, Patel PI, Di Donato S, Mandel J-L, Cocozza S, Koenig M, Pandolfo M. 1996. Friedreich's ataxia: autosomal recessive disease caused by an intronic GAA triplet repeat expansion. Science 271:1423–1427.

Camuzat A, Dollfus H, Rozet J-M, Gerber S, Bonneau D, Bonnemaison M, Briard M-L, Dufier J-L, Ghazi I, Leowski C, et al. 1995. A gene for Leber's congenital amaurosis maps to chromosome 17p. Hum Molec Genet 4:1447–1452.

Carmi R, Rokhlina T, Kwitek-Black AE, Elbedour K, Nishimura D, Stone EM, Sheffield VC. 1995. Use of a DNA pooling strategy to identify a human obesity syndrome locus on chromosome 15. Hum Molec Genet 4:9–13.

Chamberlain S, Shaw J, Rowland A, Wallis J, South S, Nakamura Y, von Gabain A, Farrall M, Williamson R. 1988. Mapping of mutation causing Friedreich's ataxia to human chromosome 9. Nature 334:248–250.

Chelly J, Kaplan J-C, Maire P, Gautron S, Kahn A. 1988. Transcription of the dystrophin gene in human muscle and non-muscle tissues. Nature 333:858–860.

Clayton PT, Patel E, Lawson AM, Carruthers RA, Collins, J. 1990. Bile acid profiles in peroxisomal 3-oxoacyl-coenzyme A thiolase deficiency. J Clin Invest 85:1267–1273.

Cogan DG, Rodrigues M, Chu FC, Schaeffer EJ. 1984. Ocular abnormalities in abetalipoproteinemia: a clinicopathologic correlation. Ophthalmology 91:991–998.

Danpure CJ, Jennings PR. 1986. Peroxisomal alanine:glyoxylate aminotransferase deficiency in primary hyperoxaluria type I. FEBS Lett 201:20–24.

Dawson WW, Armstrong D, Greer M, Maida TM, Samuelson DA. 1985. Disease-specific electrophysiological findings in adult ceroid-lipofuscinosis (KuPs disease). Doc Ophthalmol 60:163–171.

Dryja TP, McGee TL, Reichel E, Hahn LB, Cowley GS, Yandell DW, Sandberg MA, Berson EL. 1990. A point mutation of the rhodopsin gene in one form of retinitis pigmentosa. Nature 343:364–366.

Eiberg H, Mohr J, Nielsen LS, Simonsen N. 1983. Genetics and linkage relationships of the C3 polymorphism: discovery of C3-Selinkage and assignment of LES-C3-DM-Se-PEPD-Lu synteny to chromosome 19. Clin Genet 24:159–170.

Eiberg H, Gardiner RM, Mohr J. Batten disease (Spielmeyer-Sjogren disease) and haptoglobins (HP): indication of linkage and assignment to chromosome 16. Clin Genet 36:217–218.

Elze K-L, Koepp P, Lagenstein I, Steinhausen H-C, Colmant HJ, Schwendemann G. 1978. Juvenile type of generalized ceroid-lipofuscinosis (Spielmeyer-Sjogren syndrome). Neuropadiatrie 9:3–27.

Evans K, Fryer A, Inglehearn C, Duvall-Young J, Whittaker JL, Gregory CY, Butler R, Ebenezer N, Hunt DM, Bhattacharya S. 1994. Genetic linkage of cone-rod retinal dystrophy to chromosome 19q and evidence for segregation distortion. Nature Genet 6:210–213.

Evans K, Duvall-Young J, Fitzke FW, Arden GB, Bhattacharya SS, Bird AC. 1995. Chromosome 19q cone-rod retinal dystrophy: ocular phenotype. Arch Ophthalmol 113:195–201.

Farber DB, Danciger JS, Aguirre G. 1992. The beta subunit of cyclic GMP phosphodiesterase mRNA is deficient in canine rod-cone dysplasia 1. Neuron 9:349–356.

Farrar GJ, Kenna P, Jordan SA, Kumar-Singh R, Humphries MM, Sharp EM, Sheils DM, Humphries P. 1991. A three-base-pair deletion in the peripherin-RDS gene in one form of retinitis pigmentosa. Nature 354:478–480.

Fishman GA, Kumar A, Joseph ME, Torok N, Anderson RJ. 1983. Usher's syndrome. Arch Ophthalmol 101:1367–1374.

Fishman GA, Gilbert LD, Fiscella RG, Kimura AE, Jampol LM. 1989. Acetazolamide for treatment of chronic macular edema in retinitis pigmentosa. Arch Ophthalmol 107:1445–1452.

Fishman GA, Gilbert LD, Anderson RJ, Marmor MF, Weleber RG, Viana MAG. 1994. Effect of methazolamide on chronic macular edema in patients with retinitis pigmentosa. Ophthalmology 101:687–693.

Folz SJ, Trobe JD. 1991. The peroxisome and the eye. Surv Ophthalmol 35:353–368.

Gal A, Xu S, Piczenik Y, Eiberg H, Duvigneau C, Schwinger E, Rosenberg T. 1994. Gene for autosomal dominant congenital stationary night blindness maps to the same region as the gene for the beta-subunit of the rod photoreceptor cGMP phosphodiesterase (PDEB) in chromosome 4p16.3. Hum Molec Genet 3:323–325.

Gawande AA, Donovan WJ, Ginsburg AP, Marmor MF. 1989. Photoaversion in retinitis pigmentosa. Br J Ophthalmol 73:115–120.

Greenberg J, Goliath R, Beighton P, Ramesar R. 1994. A new locus for autosomal dominant retinitis pigmentosa on the short arm of chromosome 17. Hum Molec Genet 3:915–918.

Gu S, Thompson DA, Srikumari CRS, Lorenz B, Finckh U, Nicoletti A, Murthy KR, Rathmann M, Kumaramanickavel G, Denton MJ, Gal A. 1997. Mutations in RPE65 cause autosomal recessive childhood-onset severe retinal dystrophy. Nature Genet 17:194–197.

Harley HG, Rundle SA, MacMillan JC, Myring J, Brook JD, Crow S, Reardon W, Fenton I, Shaw DJ, Harper PS. 1993. Size of the unstable CTG repeat sequence in relation to phenotype and parental transmission in myotonic dystrophy. Am J Hum Genet 52:1164–1174.

Hildebrandt F, Otto E, Rensing C, Nothwang HG, Vollmer M, Adolphs J, Hanusch H, Brandis M. 1997. Novel gene encoding an SH3 domain protein is mutated in nephronophthisis type 1. Nature Genet 17:149–153.

Hunter DG, Fishman GA, Mehta RS, Kretzer FL. 1986. Abnormal sperm and photoreceptor axonemes in Usher's syndrome. Arch Ophthalmol 104:385–389.

Inglehearn CF, et al. 1993. A new locus for autosomal dominant retinitis pigmentosa on chromosome 7p. Nature Genet 4:51–53.

International Batten Disease Consortium. 1995. Isolation of a novel gene underlying Batten disease, CLN3. Cell 82:949–957.

Jackson JF, Currier RD, Terasaki PI, Morton NE. 1977. Spinocere-

bellar ataxia and HLA linkage: risk prediction by HLA typing. New Eng J Med 296:1138–1141.

Jarvela I, Schleutker J, Haataja L, Santavuori P, Puhakka L, Manninen T, Palotie A, Sandkuijl, LA, Renlund M, White R, et al. 1991. Infantile form of neuronal ceroid lipofuscinosis (CLN1) maps to the short arm of chromosome 1. Genomics 9:170–173.

Johns DR, Rutledge SL, Stine OC, Hurko O. 1989. Directly repeated sequences associated with pathogenic mitochondrial DNA deletions. Proc Nat Acad Sci 86:8059–8062.

Jordan SA, Farrar GJ, Kumar-Singh R, Kenna P, Humphries MM, Allamand V, Sharp EM, Humphries P. 1992. Autosomal dominant retinitis pigmentosa (adRP; RP6): cosegregation of RP6 and the peripherin-RDS locus in a late-onset family of Irish origin. Am J Hum Genet 50:634–639.

Jordan SA, Farrar GJ, Kenna P, Humphries MM, Sheils DM, Kumar-Singh R, Sharp EM, Soriano N, Ayuso C, Benitez J, Humphries P. 1993. Localization of an autosomal dominant retinitis pigmentosa gene to chromosome 7q. Nature Genet 4:54–58.

Kajiwara K, Hahn LB, Mukai S, Travis GH, Berson EL, Dryja TP. 1991. Mutations in the human retinal degeneration slow gene in autosomal dominant retinitis pigmentosa. Nature 354:480–483.

Kaplan J, Gerber S, Bonneau D, Rozet JM, Delrieu O, Briard ML, Dollfus H, Ghazi I, Dufier JL, Frezal J, Munnich A. 1992. A gene for Usher syndrome type I (USH1A) maps to chromosome 14q. Genomics 14:979–987.

Karjalainen S, Vartiainen E, Terasvirta M, Karja J, Kaariainen H. 1985. An unusual otological manifestation of Usher's syndrome in 4 siblings. Adv Audiol 3:32–40.

Keats BJB, Nouri N, Pelias MZ, Deininger PL, Litt M. 1994. Tightly linked flanking microsatellite markers for the Usher syndrome type I locus on the short arm of chromosome 11. Am J Hum Genet 54:681–686.

Kimberling WJ, Weston MD, Moller C, Davenport SLH, Shugart YY, Priluck IA, Martini A, Milani M, Smith RJ. 1990. Localization of Usher syndrome type II to chromosome 1q. Genomics 7:245–249.

Kimberling WJ, Moller CG, Davenport S, Priluck IA, Beighton PH, Greenberg J, Reardon W, Weston MD, Kenyon JB, Grunkemeyer JA, et al. 1992. Linkage of Usher syndrome type I gene (USH1B) to the long arm of chromosome 11. Genomics 14:988–994.

Kimberling WJ, Weston M, Moller C. 1994. Clinical and genetic heterogeneity of Usher syndrome. In: Wright AF, Jay B, eds, Molecular Genetics of Inherited Eye Disorders. Chur (Switzerland): Harwood, 359–382.

Kimizuka Y, Koyosawa M, Tamai M, Takase S. 1993. Retinal changes in myotonic dystrophy. Retina 13:129–135.

Kimura AE, Drack AV, Stone EM. 1995. Retinitis pigmentosa and associated disorders. In: Wright K, ed, Pediatric Ophthalmology and Strabismus. St. Louis: Mosby.

Knowles JA, Shugart Y, Banerjee P, Gilliam TC, Lewis CA, Jacobson SG, Ott J. 1994. Identification of a locus, distinct from RDS-peripherin, for autosomal recessive retinitis pigmentosa on chromosome 6p. Hum Molec Genet 3:1401–1403.

Kwitek-Black AE, Carmi R, Duyk GM, Buetow KH, Elbedour K, Parvari R, Yandava CN, Stone EM, Sheffield VC. 1993. Linkage of Bardet-Biedl syndrome to chromosome 16q and evidence for nonallelic genetic heterogeneity. Nature Genet 5:392–396.

Lemmink HH, Mochizuki T, van den Heuvel LPWJ, Schroder CH, Barrientos A, Monnens LAH, van Oost BA, Brunner HG, Reeders ST, Smeets HJM. 1994. Mutations in the type IV collagen alpha-3 (COL4A3) gene in autosomal recessive Alport syndrome. Hum Molec Genet 3:1269–1273.

Lemmink HH, Schroder CH, Monners LAH, Smeets HJM. 1997. The clinical spectrum of type IV collagen mutations. Hum Mutat 9:477–499.

Leppert M, Baird L, Anderson KL, Otterud B, Lupski JR, Lewis RA. 1994. Bardet-Biedl syndrome is linked to DNA markers on chromosome 11q and is genetically heterogeneous. Nature Genet 7: 108–112.

Leutelt J, Oehlmann R, Younus F, van den Born LI, Weber JL, Denton MJ, Mehdi SQ, Gal A. 1995. Autosomal recessive retinitis pigmentosa locus maps on chromosome 1q in a large consanguineous family from Pakistan. Clin Genet 47:122–124.

Marlhens F, Bareil C, Griffoin JM, Zrenner E, Amalric P, Eliaou C, Liu S-Y, Harris E, Redmond TM, Arnaud B, Claustres M, Hamel CP. 1997. Mutations in RPE65 cause Leber's congenital amaurosis. Nature Genet 17:139–141.

Marmor MF. 1979. The electroretionogram in retinitis pigmentosa. Arch Ophthalmol 97:1300–1304.

Marmor MF. 1986. Contrast sensitivity versus visual acuity in retinal disease. Br J Ophthalmol 70:553–559.

Marmor MF. 1990. Hypothesis concerning carbonic anhydrase treatment of cystoid macular edema: example with epiretinal membrane. Arch Ophthalmol 108:1524–1525.

Marmor MF, Jacobson, SG, Foerster MH, Kellner U, Weleber RG. 1990. Diagnostic clinical findings of a new syndrome with night blindness, maculopathy, and enhanced S cone sensitivity. Am J Ophthalmol 110:124–134.

Massof RW, Finkelstein D. 1981. Two forms of autosomal dominant primary retinitis pigmentosa. Doc Ophthalmol 51:289–346.

Masuno M, Shimozawa N, Suzuki Y, Kondo N, Orii T, Tsukamoto T, Osumi T, Fujiki Y, Imaizumi K, Kuroki Y. 1994. Assignment of the human peroxisome assembly factor-1 gene (PXMP3) responsible for Zellweger syndrome to chromosome 8q21.1 by fluorescence in situ hybridization. Genomics 20:141–142.

Maw MA, Kennedy B, Knight A, Bridges R, Roth KE, Mani EJ, Mukkadan JK, Nancarrow D, Crabb JW, Denton MJ. 1997. Mutation of the gene encoding cellular retinaldehyde-binding protein in autosomal recessive retinitis pigmentosa. Nature Genet 17:198–200.

McLaughlin ME, Sandberg MA, Berson EL, Dryja TP. 1993. Recessive mutations in the gene encoding the beta-subunit of rod phosphodiesterase in patients with retinitis pigmentosa. Nature Genet 4:130–134.

McDowell GA, Gahl WA, Stephenson LA, Schneider JA, Weissenbach J, Polymeropoulos MH, Town MM, van't Hoff W, Farrall M, Mathew CG. 1995. Linkage of the gene for cystinosis to markers on the short arm of chromosome 17. Nature Genet 10:246–248.

McWilliam P, Farrar GJ, Kenna P, Bradley DG, Humphries MM, Sharp EM, McConnell DJ, Lawler M, Sheils D, Ryan C, et al. 1989. Autosomal dominant retinitis pigmentosa (ADRP): localization of an ADRP gene to the long arm of chromosome 3. Genomics 5:619–622.

Meindl A, Dry K, Herrmann K, Manson F, Ciccodicola A, Edgar A, Carvalho MRS, Achatz H, Hellebrand H, Lennon A, Migliaccio C, Porter K, Zrenner E, Bird A, Jay M, Lorenz B, Wittwer B, D'Urso M, Meitinger T, Wright A. 1996. A gene (RPGR) with homology to the RCC1 guanine nucleotide exchange factor is mutated in X-linked retinitis pigmentosa (RP3). Nature Genet 13:35–42.

Mohr J. 1954. A Study of Linkage in Man. Copenhagen: Munksgaard.

Moraes CT, Shanske S, Tritschler H-J, Aprille JR, Andreetta F, Bonilla E, Schon EA, DiMauro S. 1991. mtDNA depletion with variable tissue expression: a novel genetic abnormality in mitochondrial diseases. Am J Hum Genet 48:492–501.

Murakami A, Yajima T, Inana G. 1992. Isolation of human retinal genes: recoverin cDNA and gene. Biochem Biophys Res Commun 187:234–244.

Naritomi K, Izumikawa Y, Ohshiro S, Yoshida K, Shimozawa N,

Suzuki Y, Orii T, Hirayama K. 1989. Gene assignment of Zellweger syndrome to 7q11.23: report of the second case associated with a pericentric inversion of chromosome 7. Hum Genet 84:79–80.

Nathans J, Hogness DS. 1984. Isolation and nucleotide sequence of the gene encoding human rhodopsin. Proc Nat Acad Sci USA 81:4851–4855.

Norton EWD, Marmor MF, Clowes DD, Gamel JW, Fielder AR (letters). 1993. A randomized trial of vitamin A and vitamin E supplementation for retinitis pigmentosa. Arch Ophthalmol 111:1460–1463.

Perrault I, Rozet JM, Calvas P, Gerber S, Camuzat A, Dollfus H, Chatelin S, Souied E, Ghazi I, Leowski C, Bonnemaison M, Le Paslier D, Frezal J, Dufier J-L, Pittler S, Munnich A, Kaplan J. 1996. Retinal-specific guanylate cyclase gene mutations in Leber's congenital amaurosis. Nature Genet 14:461–464.

Polak BCP, Hogwind BL. 1977. Macular lesions in Alport's syndrome. Am J Ophthalmol 84:532–535.

Purdue PE, Takada Y, Danpure CJ. 1990. Identification of mutations associated with peroxisome-to-mitochondrion mistargeting of alanine/glyoxylate aminotransferase in primary hyperoxaluria type 1. J Cell Biol 111:2341–2351.

Rosenfeld PJ, Cowley GS, Hahn LB, Sandberg MA, Berson EL, Dryja TP. 1992. A null mutation within the rhodopsin gene in a family with autosomal recessive retinitis pigmentosa. Invest Ophthal Vis Sci 33:1397 (Abstract).

Sankila E-M, Pakarinen L, Kaariainen H, Aittomaki K, Karjalainen S, Sistonen P, de la Chapelle A. 1995. Assignment of an Usher syndrome type III (USH3) gene to chromosome 3q. Hum Molec Genet 4:93–98.

Schachat AP, Maumenee IH. 1981. Bardet-Biedl syndrome and related disorders. Arch Ophthalmol 100:285–288.

Servadio A, Koshy B, Armstrong D, Antalffy B, Orr HT, Zoghbi HY. 1995. Expression analysis of the ataxin-1 protein in tissues from normal and spinocerebellar ataxia type 1 individuals. Nature Genet 10:94–98.

Sheffield V, Carmi R, Kwitek-Black A, Rokhlina T, Nishimura D, Duyk GM, Elbedour K, Sunden SL, Stone E. 1994. Identification of a Bardet-Biedl syndrome locus on chromosome 3 and evaluation of an efficient approach to homozygosity mapping. Hum Molec Genet 3:1331–1335.

Shimozawa N, Tsukamoto T, Suzuki Y, Orii T, Shirayoshi Y, Mori T, Fujiki Y. 1992. A human gene responsible for Zellweger syndrome that affects peroxisome assembly. Science 255:1132–1134.

Shoulders CC, Brett DJ, Bayliss JD, Narcisi TME, Jarmuz A, Grantham TT, Leoni PRD, Bhattacharya S, Pease RJ, Cullen PM, et al. 1993. Abetalipoproteinemia is caused by defects of the gene encoding the 97 kDa subunit of a microsomal triglyceride transfer protein. Hum Molec Genet 2:2109–2116.

Siegsmund DA, Weleber RG, Pillers D-AM, Westall CA, Panton CM, Powell BR, Heon E, Murphey WH, Musarella MA, Ray PN. 1994. Characterization of the ocular phenotype of Duchenne and Becker muscular dystrophy. Ophthalmology 101:856–865.

Silverman MS, Ogilvie JM, Lett J, Fang HJ, Wu M, Wang X, Landgraf M. 1994. Photoreceptor transplantation: potential for recovery of visual function. In: Christen Y, Doly M, Droy-Lefaix MT, eds, Retine, vieillissement et transplantation. Paris: Elsevier, 43–59.

Small KW, Letson R, Scheinman J. 1990. Ocular findings in primary hyperoxaluria. Arch Ophthalmol 108:89–93.

Small KW, Gehrs K. 1996. Clinical study of a large family with autosomal dominant progressive cone degeneration. Am J Ophthalmol 121:1–12.

Small KW, Syrquin M, Mullen L, Gehrs K. 1996. Mapping autosomal dominant cone degeneration to chromosome 17p. Am J Ophthalmol 121:13–18.

Smith RJH, Lee EC, Kimberling WJ, Daiger SP, Pelias MZ, Keats BJB, Jay M, Bird A, Reardon W, Guest M, et al. 1992. Localization of two genes for Usher syndrome type I to chromosome 11. Genomics 14:995–1002.

Szlyk JP, Fishman GA, Alexander KR, Peachey NS, Derlacki D. 1993. Clinical subtypes of cone-rod dystrophy. Arch Ophthalmol 111: 781–788.

Traboulsi EI, Green WR, Luckenbach MW, de la Cruz ZC. 1987. Neuronal ceroid lipofuscinosis: ocular histopathologic and electron microscopic studies in the late infantile, juvenile, and adult forms. Graefes Arch Clin Exp Ophthalmol 225:391–402.

Travis GH, Hepler JE. 1993. A medley of retinal dystrophies. Nature Genet 3:191–192.

Travis GH, Brennan MB, Danielson PE, Kozak CA, Sutcliffe JG. 1989. Identification of a photoreceptor-specific mRNA encoded by the gene responsible for retinal degeneration slow (rds). Nature 338:70–73.

Vesa J, Hellsten E, Verkruyse LA, Camp LA, Rapola J, Santavuori P, Hofmann SL, Peltonen L. 1995. Mutations in the palmitoyl protein thioesterase gene causing infantile neuronal ceroid lipofuscinosis. Nature 376:584–588.

Weil D, Blanchard S, Kaplan J, Guilford P, Gibson F, Walsh J, Mburu P, Varela A, Levilliers J, Weston MD, et al. 1995. Defective myosin VIIA gene responsible for Usher syndrome type 1B. Nature 374:60–61.

Weleber RG. 1994. Retinitis pigmentosa and allied disorders. In: Ryan SJ, ed, Retina, 2nd ed. St Louis: Mosby, 335–466.

Wetterau JR, Aggerbeck LP, Bouma M-E, Eisenberg C, Munck A, Hermier M, Schmitz J, Gay G, Rader DJ, Gregg RE. 1992. Absence of microsomal triglyceride transfer protein in individuals with abetalipoproteinemia. Science 258:999–1001.

Wiechmann AF, Haro KC, Bowden DW. 1994. Three microsatellite polymorphisms at the recoverin locus on chromosome 17. Hum Molec Genet 3:1028.

Zeviani M, Moraes CT, DiMauro S, Nakase H, Bonilla E, Schon EA, Rowland LP. 1988. Deletions of mitochondrial DNA in Kearns-Sayre syndrome. Neurology 38:1339–1346.

Zylberman R, Silverstone BZ, Brandes E, Drukker A. 1980. Retinal lesions in Alport's syndrome. Ped Ophthalmol 17:255–260.

V | DETACHMENT AND ADHESION

18. Biology of the interphotoreceptor matrix–retinal pigment epithelium–retina interface

GREGORY S. HAGEMAN AND MARKUS H. KUEHN

One important function of the retinal pigment epithelium (RPE) is to support photoreceptor cell integrity through exchange of catabolites and catabolic by-products (Adler and Southwick, 1992; Lin et al., 1994), degradation of shed photoreceptor outer segments, regulation of the ionic milieu within the subretinal space (Perry and McNaughton, 1993; Bialek and Miller, 1994; Hodson et al., 1994), and maintenance of retinal adhesion (Hollyfield et al., 1989; Yao et al., 1990; Hageman et al., 1995). The basal surface of the RPE is exposed to Bruch's membrane—an acellular connective tissue composed primarily of collagen and elastin—and its apical surface abuts the interphotoreceptor matrix (IPM). These two extracellular environments are uniquely distinct from one another in composition, structure, and function. The IPM fills the subretinal space, which is delineated by the apices of Müller, photoreceptor, and RPE cells (Fig. 18-1). The IPM is not an extracellular matrix *per se* but is more analogous to epithelial glycocalyces. Based on its strategic location, there is general consensus that the IPM mediates biochemical and physical interactions between the neural retina and RPE (Anderson et al., 1986; Hewitt and Adler, 1989; Kaplan et al., 1990; Bok et al., 1993).

The focus of this chapter is devoted to advances that have been made over the past several years related to our understanding of the biology of the IPM and the molecular constituents that comprise it. A number of significant advances and intriguing observations have been made during this time. Techniques for the enrichment of the IPM have been perfected. A variety of molecules have been identified as inhabitants of the IPM in normal and pathological retinas. Significant progress has been made toward isolating, cloning, and characterizing a few unique IPM constituents. Although a role in retinal adhesion for the IPM has been suspected, based largely on its location, recent studies from various laboratories have provided compelling evidence that specific IPM glycoconjugates, most likely proteoglycans, participate in maintaining a normal RPE–retina interface and are especially important in mediating retinal adhesion. Other observations, especially from studies of retinal devel-

opment and degeneration, have suggested a role for the IPM in the maintenance of photoreceptor cell viability. Elegant studies have demonstrated light-evoked changes in the distribution and/or conformation of some IPM constituents. Several investigators have identified previously undetected "domains" within the IPM that vary not only between species, but topographically within the same species. For example, recent studies suggest that the composition of cone photoreceptor–associated IPM glycoconjugates in the primate fovea appears to differ significantly from that of the extrafoveal retina. Similarly, the quantities of specific glycoconjugates associated with different classes of cone photoreceptors appear to vary in some species. Insoluble IPM has been identified in the vitreous of patients with rhegmatogenous retinal detachments and may be responsible for Shafer's sign, a clinical indication of retinal detachment. These same IPM components exhibit distinct compositional changes that are correlated with macular drusen, extracellular deposits in Bruch's membrane known to be a risk factor for the development of age-related macular degeneration (AMD) in humans.

Every effort has been made to include information pertaining to established relationships between the RPE and IPM in this chapter. Readers are referred to a number of previous reviews for a historical perspective and detailed information pertaining to the IPM and its relationship to RPE and photoreceptor cells prior to 1990 (Hewitt and Adler, 1989; Berman, 1991; Hageman and Johnson, 1991; Mieziewska, 1993).

COMPOSITION OF THE IPM

The IPM is comprised of an elaborate array of diffusible molecules that are distributed within an intricate, relatively insoluble network of proteoglycans and glycoconjugates that surround rod and cone photoreceptor cells (see Table 18-1). IPM components have been loosely classified *aqueous soluble* or *aqueous insoluble*. Perhaps because the aqueous-soluble IPM constituents are readily isolated (Berman and Bach, 1968; Bach and

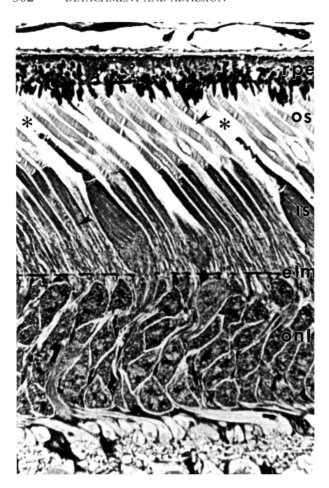

FIGURE 18-1. Silver-stained section of central monkey retina. The IPM surrounds the photoreceptor inner segments (is) and outer segments (os) and ellipsoids of both cone *(asterisks)* and rod *(arrowheads)* photoreceptors lying between the apical surface of the RPE (rpe) and the external limiting membrane (elm). (onl) = outer nuclear layer.

the apical surfaces of these tissues with various buffers to remove the soluble components (Berman and Bach, 1968; Bach and Berman, 1970; Adler and Serverin, 1981a; 1981b; Adler and Klucznik, 1982; Berman, 1982; Liou et al., 1986). While this approach facilitated the identification of a number of IPM constituents, these preparations can be contaminated with molecules from the surrounding tissues, including the choroid, vitreous, retina, and vasculature. To avoid these problems, Pfeffer and colleagues (1983) developed a method for cannulating the interphotoreceptor space in situ and subsequently collecting the aqueous-soluble IPM constituents, following buffer lavage.

Early biochemical studies indicated that the "aqueous-extractable" components of the IPM are predominantly proteins and glycoproteins, with some glycosaminoglycans (GAGs), including chondroitin sulfates and hyaluronic acid (Wortman and Freeman, 1962; Bach and Berman, 1971a; 1971b; Feeney 1973; Adler and Serverin, 1981a). The major soluble glycoprotein of the IPM is the interphotoreceptor retinoid-binding protein (IRBP) a retinoid-binding protein which has been purified and characterized from a number of species (Chader, 1989). Other soluble IPM constituents include a variety of glycosaminoglycans, enzymes, enzyme inhibitors, mucins, complex carbohydrates, growth and neurotrophic factors, survival-promoting factor(s), glucose, lactate, and miscellaneous proteins (see Table 18-1) (Bach and Berman, 1971a; 1971b; Adler and Martin, 1983; Adler, 1989; Hewitt and Adler, 1989; Azuma et al., 1990; Hewitt et al., 1990; Hageman et al., 1991; Hageman and Johnson, 1991; Adler and Southwick, 1992; Hunter et al., 1992; Plantner, 1992a; 1992b; Li et al., 1995; Ying et al., 1995).

Aqueous-Insoluble IPM

Techniques for isolating the aqueous-insoluble IPM constituents have been developed recently (Hageman et al., 1989; Hollyfield et al., 1989; 1990a; Johnson and Hageman, 1991; Hageman et al., submitted). These techniques, which elicit delamination of the insoluble IPM as large "sheets" from the neural retina following separation from the RPE, have facilitated subsequent studies directed toward the structural, compositional, and molecular characterization of these unique extracellular matrix domains. The ability to enrich insoluble IPM molecules has aided investigators in their subsequent characterization. For example, these preparations have helped to confirm that the glycoconjugates labeled by the lectin peanut agglutinin (PNA) and antibodies directed against chondroitin 6-sulfate (AC6S) are components of the aqueous-insoluble IPM (Hollyfield et al.,

Berman, 1970; Adler and Serverin, 1981a; 1981b; Adler and Klucznik, 1982; Berman, 1982; Pfeffer et al., 1983; Liou et al., 1986), they have been more completely characterized. More recently, techniques have been developed for enriching the aqueous-insoluble IPM; these preparations have been used to examine not only its molecular composition, but have also revealed insight into the elaborate substructure of the IPM (Hollyfield et al., 1990; Hageman and Johnson, 1991; Johnson and Hageman, 1991).

Aqueous-Soluble IPM

A variety of techniques for isolating aqueous-soluble constituents of the IPM have been used for many years to isolate and characterize these molecules (see Table 18-1). The most common technique that has been employed is to separate the retina from the RPE and rinse

TABLE 18-1. *IPM constituents*

Molecule	Species	Reference
Proteins/glycoproteins		
α2-Macroglobulin	Human	Hageman*
bFGF	Monkey, human	Hageman et al., 1991; Gao, 1995
GP147	Human	Tien et al., 1992
IGF-1	Human	Waldbillig et al., 1991
IgG and IgA	Human	Hageman, 1985
Inhibin	Bovine	Ying et al., 1995
IRBP	Various	Adler et al., 1982
Mucin(s)	Bovine	Plantner, 1992a; Adler et al., 1982
Neurotrophic Activity	Monkey, bovine	Tombran-Tink et al., 1992
PEDF	Human	Tombran-Tink et al., 1995
PSPA	Bovine	Hewitt et al., 1990
Purpurin	Chicken	Schubert, 1985
Serum albumin	Various	Adler et al., 1988
S-Antigen	Various	Wacker et al., 1977
S-Laminin	Skate, rat, rabbit	Hunter et al., 1992
Vitronectin	Monkey, human	Hageman and Anderson*
Enzymes		
Acid hydrolases	Bovine, human	Adler, 1989; Hayasaka et al., 1981
Arylsulfatase	Human	Hayasaka et al., 1981
Cathepsin D	Bovine, human	Hayasaka et al., 1981; Adler, 1989
cGMP-Phosphodiesterase	Monkey, cow	Barbehenn et al., 1985
Metalloproteinase inhib.	Bovine	Plantner, 1992
MMP-2	Bovine, human	Jones et al., 1994
NAcGAL-Aminylphosphotransferase	Monkey, chicken, frog	Sweatt et al., 1991
Neuron-specific enolase	Human, cow	Li et al., 1995
Neutral proteases (MMPs)	Bovine	Plantner, 1992
TIMP-1	Bovine, human	Jones et al., 1994
Glycosaminoglycans/proteoglycans		
Decorin	Human	Mullins*
Chondroitin-sulfate proteoglycans	Human	Hageman et al., 1987
Hyaluronan	Rabbit, human	Tate et al., 1993; Korte et al., 1994; Adler et al., 1981
IPM 150/IPM 200	Various	Hageman et al., 1991
Miscellaneous		
Fatty acids	Monkey	Bazan et al., 1985
Glucose	Bovine	Adler et al., 1992
Lactate	Bovine	Adler et al., 1992
Serum albumin	Monkey, human	Adler*
Vitamin A (retinol)	Bovine	Adler et al., 1982
Uncharacterized components		
Anti-HNK-binding glycoprotein	Human	Hageman*
MAB 7-H11 binding protein	Mouse, chicken	Lemmon, 1988
MAB F-22 binding protein (250 kDa)	Mouse, dog	Mieziewska et al., 1994
Major proteins	Various	Adler et al., 1981
Various lectin binding proteins	Various	Hageman*

*Unpublished

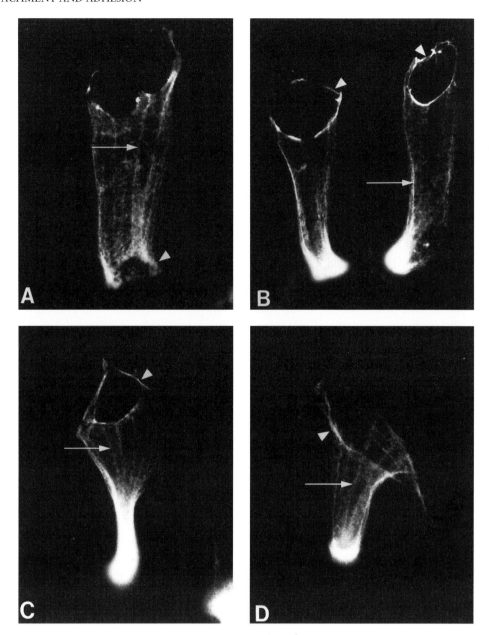

FIGURE 18-2. Fluorescence light micrographs of isolated bovine cone matrix sheaths in calcium-free media sheaths stained with PNA-FITC. Longitudinal filaments *(arrows)* extend between apical and basal rings *(arrowheads)* and appear to be interconnected by a finer anastomosing network of filamentous material. (Reprinted from Johnson and Hageman, 1991.)

1989; 1990a; Hageman et al., 1991; Johnson and Hageman, 1991). Isolated insoluble IPM preparations have also provided insight into the organization of this matrix (Johnson and Hageman, 1991). Upon exposure of isolated IPM "sheets" to calcium-free media, cone matrix sheaths (CMS)—compositionally distinct domains of the IPM surrounding cone photoreceptors—swell to two to three times their normal size, facilitating visual-

ization of their substructural organization. These preparations have revealed that longitudinally-oriented filaments extend the entire length of the CMS and terminate in filamentous rings at their apical and basal ends. These longitudinal filaments are interconnected by finer, anastomosing filamentous networks (Fig. 18-2).

The "aqueous-insoluble" constituents of the IPM constitute a significant proportion of the IPM in higher vertebrate species (Blanks and Johnson, 1984; Fariss et al., 1990; Hollyfield et al., 1990a; Hageman and Johnson, 1991; Landers et al., 1991; Iwasaki et al., 1992a; 1992b; Lazarus and Hageman, 1992; Bishop et al., 1993; Lazarus et al., 1993). Only a few insoluble IPM constituents have been identified and/or partially characterized. These include: (1) two proteoglycans, designated IPM 150 and IPM 200; (2) a WGA-binding glycoprotein, designated GP147 (Tien et al., 1992); (3) a high-molecular-weight mucin (Plantner, 1992a); and (4) a variety of uncharacterized glycoproteins (see Table 18-1) (Uehara et al., 1986; Shuster et al., 1987).

CHARACTERIZATION OF IPM CONSTITUENTS

Since complete descriptions of many components of the IPM are available in a variety of excellent reviews (Berman, 1985; Hewitt and Adler, 1989; Hageman and Johnson, 1991), only recently characterized IPM constituents are reviewed herein.

Proteoglycans/Glycosaminoglycans

Significant progress has been made toward characterizing IPM proteoglycans, two of which appear to be unique to the IPM. In addition, a number of studies have confirmed earlier biochemical observations showing that hyaluronic acid is present in the IPM.

IPM 150 and IPM 200. Western blot analyses of chondroitinase-treated IPM preparations from pig, monkey, and human retinas demonstrate bands of approximately 150 kDa and 200 kDa (and minor bands of 180 kDa and 220 kDa in pig and monkey, respectively) that are labeled by AC6S antibody and PNA (Hageman and Johnson, 1991; Hageman et al., 1992; Kuehn et al., 1993). These two proteoglycans have been designated IPM 150 and IPM 200. The 150 kDa band appears to contain two glycoproteins. One (designated IPM 150) binds both PNA and AC6S antibody and migrates to a lower-molecular-weight doublet of 55–58 kDa following exposure to neuraminidase and O-glycanase. Following complete deglycosylation of IPM 150 and IPM 200, AC6S antibody binds to a doublet of approximately 55–58 kDa.

The second 150 kDa constituent is neuraminidase insensitive, does not bind AC6S, and binds the lectin Phaseolus vulgaris agglutinin type IV (PHA-L). PHA-L intensely labels the IPM associated with the apical RPE in vitro. Furthermore, a 150 kDa PHA-L-binding glycoprotein has also been identified on Western blots of protein extracts derived from cultured RPE cells. Col-

lectively, these studies indicate that at least two distinct proteoglycans containing chondroitin 6-sulfate are associated with CMS, and that a distinct 150 kDa glycoprotein is associated with the apical RPE.

In order to identify the core proteins of IPM 150 and IPM 200, monkey eyes have been injected intravitreally with ^{35}S-methionine, ^{3}H-serine, or ^{35}SO$_4$ (Hageman and Johnson, 1986b; Rotramel et al., 1992). At 1, 3, 5, 8, 11, and 16 days following injections, the insoluble, radiolabeled IPM was isolated, digested with chondroitinase, and separated by SDS-polyacrylamide gel electrophoresis. Following deglycosylation of IPM 200, a doublet of approximately 55–58 kDa was resolved, whereas IPM 150 resolved as a doublet of 57–58 kDa and a band of 105 kDa. These results provide evidence that IPM 150 and IPM 200 have core proteins of similar molecular weights, but that each may be comprised of two distinct proteins. The relationship of the 105 kDa IPM glycoprotein to IPM 200 is unclear at this time.

Amino-terminal amino acid sequences of IPM 150 and IPM 200 from human, monkey, and pig IPM have been determined (Hageman et al., 1992; Kuehn et al., 1993; 1995). The sequences show that (1) the core proteins of the IPM 150 and IPM 200 share strongly conserved N-termini, (2) these proteins are conserved among higher mammalian species, and (3) the amino acid sequences are unique. Specific conservative amino acid substitutions are observed, however, at both the intraspecies and interspecies levels. Several internal peptides derived from pig and human IPM 150 and IPM 200 following trypsin digestion have been sequenced. None of these sequences exhibit homology with other proteins, although a few oligopeptides obtained from different species exhibit homology with one another. Based on N-terminal and internal amino acid sequences of IPM 150 and IPM 200, several cDNA clones have been isolated; these clones are novel based on comparison with existing databases. The deduced amino acid sequence of one of these clones features two possible N-glycosylation sites, numerous potential O-glycosylation sites, four cysteine residues, and two hyaluronate-binding motifs.

F22 epitope. A 250 kDa constituent of mouse IPM, recognized by a monoclonal antibody designated F22, appears to be a chondroitin sulfate proteoglycan that is distinguishable from chondroitin 4- and 6-sulfate proteoglycans that are also present. The F22-recognized epitope does not codistribute with antibodies that bind chondroitin 4- and 6-sulfates in the developing mouse eye (for more information on F22-detectable proteoglycan see "IPM in Retinal Development," below).

Decorin. Decorin is a member of the family of small chondroitin/dermatan sulfate proteoglycans; it is relatively abundant in bone, tendon, skin, and vessels and in the sclera and cornea (Hay, 1991). Decorin binds to specific types of collagen, appears to inhibit collagen fibrillogenesis, and neutralizes the biological activity of transforming growth factor beta. Recently, reactivity of antidecorin antibodies to cone matrix sheaths has been detected on sections of human retinas (Mullins and Hageman, unpublished). Additional studies will be required to confirm the presence of this proteoglycan as a constituent of the IPM.

Hyaluronic acid. Approximately 75% of the carbohydrates in the aqueous-soluble IPM are hyaluronidase sensitive and contain uronic acid. A portion of the glycosaminoglycans in this fraction appear to be hyaluronate (Berman and Bach, 1968; Berman, 1969; Bach and Berman, 1971a; 1971b).

A few recent histochemical studies have provided additional evidence that the IPM may contain hyaluronate. The distribution of hyaluronate in a rabbit model of RPE regeneration has been examined immunohistochemically. A mouse monoclonal antibody, ND OG1, generated against human trophoblast membrane and thought to react with hyaluronate (Korte et al., 1994), reacts with material (most likely IPM) that is closely apposed to photoreceptor cell outer segments in normal and sodium-iodate-treated rabbits (Fig. 18-13). Similar reaction of ND OG1 with adult human and monkey IPM has been observed (Hageman, unpublished). In another study, the IPM of adult human eyes was shown to bind biotinylated hyaluronic-acid-binding protein, although no controls were depicted (Tate et al., 1993). This result is in contrast to that obtained in a recent study of developing human retinas, in which Alcian Blue–positive staining of the IPM could not be removed by *Streptomyces* hyaluronidase pretreatment (Azuma et al., 1990).

Glycoproteins/Miscellaneous Proteins

GP147. A 147 kDa WGA-binding glycoprotein, termed GP147, has been identified on Western blots of reduced, insoluble IPM prepared from human retinas (Hollyfield et al., 1992; Tien et al., 1992). Following neuraminidase treatment, this band exhibits decreased binding of WGA and a concomitant binding of PNA, suggesting that GP147 may be a rod-associated IPM constituent which exhibits similar lectin-binding properties on sections of human retinas. However, a polyclonal antiserum generated against purified GP147 reacts with IPM associated with both rod and cone photoreceptors. As such, and since the epitope recognized by the antiserum has not

been determined, the precise distribution of GP147 within the IPM remains conjectural. GP147 is reduced in molecular weight and migrates to an approximate molecular weight of 105 kDa following exposure to N-glycopeptidase F; a neuraminidase-resistant protein of similar molecular weight has been identified fluorographically following deglycosylation of IPM 150 (Lazarus et al., 1991; Hageman et al., 1992; Rotramel et al., 1992). A 16-amino-acid N-terminal sequence of GP147 (NH_2—EQPGRQAGGKLDPDNL—COOH) has been determined (Tien et al., 1993); this sequence shares 83% homology with the hevein domain of a plant-derived protein that binds chitin.

Vitronectin. Reaction of antivitronectin antibodies with the IPM has been observed recently (Hageman, Anderson, and Johnson, unpublished). This observation has not been confirmed biochemically, although vitronectin mRNA is present in the neural retina. Significantly, the vitronectin receptor (V_nR), an integrin, has recently been identified in association with photoreceptor cell inner and outer segments and RPE apical microvilli (Anderson et al., 1995).

S-laminin. S-laminin, a homolog of laminin B1, is a novel laminin isoform that is concentrated in synaptic regions of muscle fiber and kidney glomerular basal laminae. S-laminin also possesses a site with which motor neurons bind. Hunter and colleagues have identified s-laminin immunoreactivity within the IPM of skate, rabbit, and rat retinas, using a variety of monoclonal and polyclonal antibodies (Hunter et al., 1992). A 190 kDa s-laminin immunoreactive band was observed on retinal extracts from all three species; sequential extraction of rabbit retinas suggested that this 190 kDa s-laminin was associated with the retinal extracellular matrix. Based on the observation that photoreceptor cells adhered to s-laminin and that its expression paralleled rod photoreceptor cell differentiation, the investigators proposed that s-laminin plays a role in retinal differentiation.

Cell surface glycosyltransferase. Glycosyltransferases are a diverse family of enzymes involved in oligosaccharide biosynthesis and mediation of cell–cell and cell–matrix adhesion (Lopez et al., 1985; Paietta et al., 1987; Ellies et al., 1994; Huang et al., 1995). N-acetyl galactosaminylphosphotransferase (GalNAcPTase) has been identified on the surfaces of rod photoreceptor cells and within the IPM of adult mice, frogs, cows, and monkeys. Western blot analyses demonstrate that the soluble IPM fraction contains a protein which reacts with antibodies to GalNAcPTase and which possesses

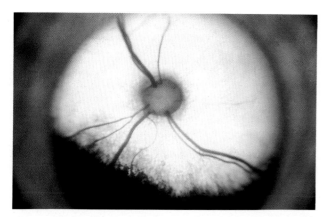

PLATE 2-I. Fundus of the cat. The tapetal area *(upper portion of the fundus)* is brilliantly reflective and the overlying RPE is devoid of pigment. The nontapetal RPE *(lower area)* is heavily pigmented. See also Plates 14-I and 14-V.

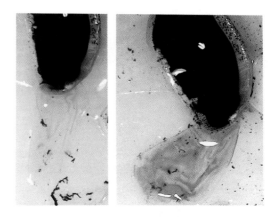

PLATE 2-II. Visual pigment regeneration in the frog. Peeled retina and eyecup from *Rana pipiens. Left:* Retina, light-adapted for 15 minutes. *Right:* Same retina after laying it back over the RPE for 3 hours in the dark.

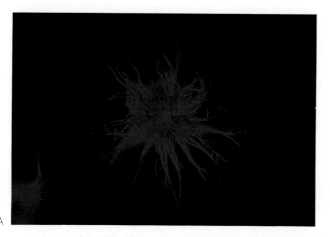

A

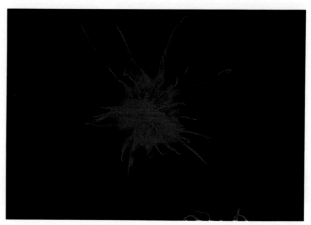

B

PLATE 3-I. Sunfish RPE cells in culture. (A) Tubulin staining. (B) Rhodamine-phalloidin labeling of actin. These images correspond to Figure 3-6c and d (see caption).

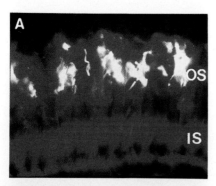

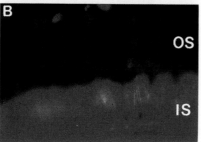

PLATE 8-I. Fluorescent images of vibratome slices of *Xenopus laevis* retinas labeled with the actin filament probe, rhodamine-phalloidin. Retinas were isolated from eyecups as in Figure 8-10 after treatment with 12 mM L-glutamate (A) or normal medium (B). (IS) and (OS) indicate the inner and outer segment layers, respectively. The inner segments in both images stain intensively with the f-actin probe. After L-glutamate treatment and retinal isolation f-actin containing processes *(stained intensively)* are associated with outer segments. In both images the outer segments are invisible. Approximate magnification ×600.

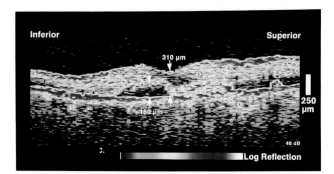

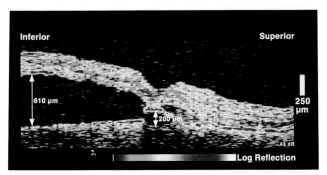

PLATE 12-I. False color vertical OCT of AMD/occult choroidal neo-vascularization. There is thickening and disruption of the reflective band corresponding to the RPE/choriocapillaris subfoveally and extending superiorly, consistent with a well-defined CNV. Inferior to the membrane, subretinal fluid is noted (180 μm).

PLATE 12-II. False color vertical OCT of central serous chorioretinopathy. There is a subfoveal pigment epithelial detachment and a neurosensory retina detachment inferiorly (610 μm). An RPE break is noted, allowing fluid leakage from the RPE detachment into the subretinal space.

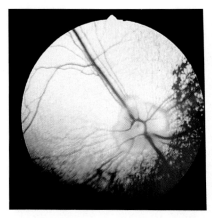

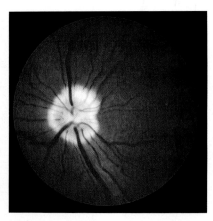

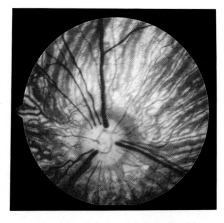

PLATE 14-I. Normal dog fundus illustrating the green color of the tapetal zone. The RPE in this region is not pigmented. The dark zone below the optic disc is the nontapetal zone in which the RPE is pigmented.

PLATE 14-II. Hereditary tapetal degeneration in the beagle dog. The fundus has a uniform red appearance.

PLATE 14-III. Albinotic fundus of a blue-merle Shetland sheepdog. The tapetal layer is absent, and there is lack of pigmentation in the RPE and choroid. The underlying white sclera is visible.

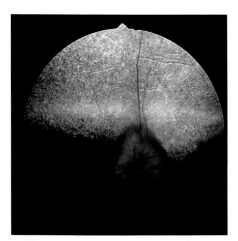

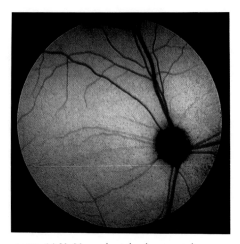

PLATE 14-IV. Advanced progressive retinal atrophy (PRA) in the dog. The fundus shows a marked loss of retinal vessels, and increased reflectivity of the tapetal layer (note that the light intensity used for this figure is 10 times less than for Plate 14-I).

PLATE 14-V. Normal cat fundus, tapetal zone.

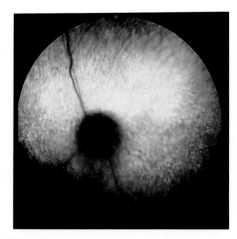

PLATE 14-VI. Early onset progressive retinal atrophy in a 16-week-old Persian cat. In the advanced stage of the disease, the fundus shows a marked loss of retinal vessels, and increased reflectivity of the tapetal layer (note that the light intensity used for this figure is 10 times less than for Plate 14-V).

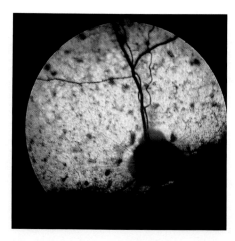

PLATE 14-VII. Retinal pigment epithelial dystrophy (RPED) in an adult dog. In the intermediate stages of the disease, there is accumulation of irregular foci of light brown pigment in the tapetal zone. Retinal thinning is indicated by the increased reflectivity of the tapetal layer, but there is preservation of the major retinal vessels.

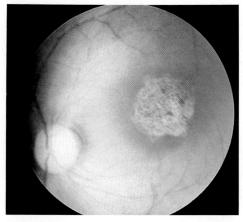

PLATE 14-VIII. Advanced macular degeneration associated with widespread outer retinal disease in a Guinea baboon. The macula appears honeycombed and atrophic. (Courtesy of Dr. S. Vainisi).

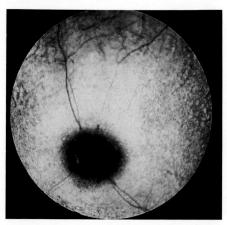

PLATE 14-IX. Gyrate atrophy of the choroid and retina in a cat. Deficiency of ornithine-δ-amino transferase (OAT) activity results in advanced retinal atrophy (loss of retinal vessels and increased reflectivity of the tapetal layer). Note that the scalloped, atrophic lesions characteristic of the human disease are not present in the cat.

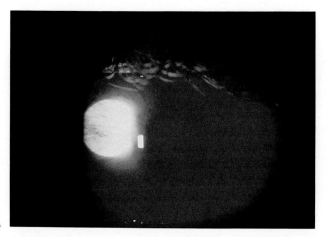

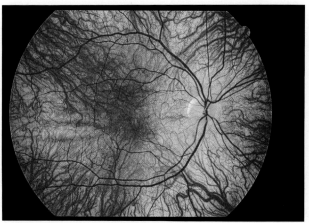

PLATE 15-I. Albinism. (A) Diffuse transillumination of the iris by retroillumination. (B) Hypopigmentation of the fundus.

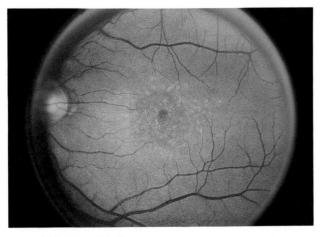

PLATE 16-I. Stargardt's disease.

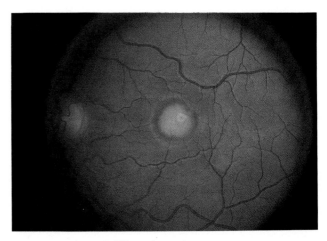

PLATE 16-II. Best's vitelliform dystrophy.

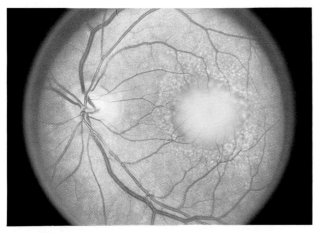

PLATE 16-III. Adult vitelliform degeneration in a patient with diffuse cuticular drusen.

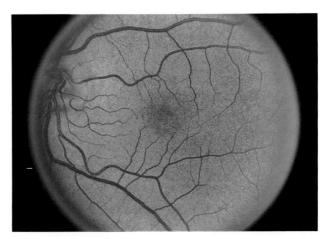

PLATE 16-IV. *Peau d'orange* pigmentary stippling (a prelude to angioid streaks).

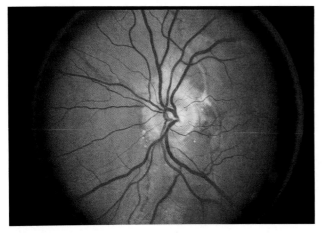

PLATE 16-V. Angioid streaks. The Bruch's membrane abnormalities mimic vessels.

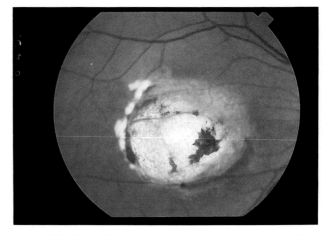

PLATE 16-VI. North Carolina macular dystrophy. (From Small, 1996.)

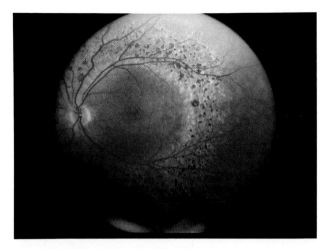

PLATE 17-I. Enhanced S-cone syndrome.

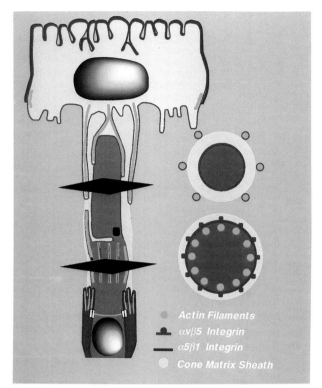

Actin Filaments
αvβ5 Integrin
α5β1 Integrin
Cone Matrix Sheath

PLATE 18-I. Schematic illustration of the putative location of VnR and FnR integrins at the photoreceptor–RPE interface, and their distribution in relation to the actin cytoskeleton. A cone photoreceptor is depicted in a plane parallel to its longitudinal axis *(left)*, as well as in two cross-sectional views, one at the level of the cone outer segment *(top, right)* and one at the level of the cone inner segment ellipsoid *(bottom, right)*. The distribution of VnR on the cell surface of the cone corresponds closely to the distribution of CMS and to actin filaments located in the cone ellipsoids and myoids. A transcellular linkage between components of the CMS, VnR integrins on the surfaces of photoreceptor and RPE cells, and their actin cytoskeletons has been suggested to function as a molecular mechanism for maintaining retinal adhesion. (Reprinted from Anderson et al., 1995.)

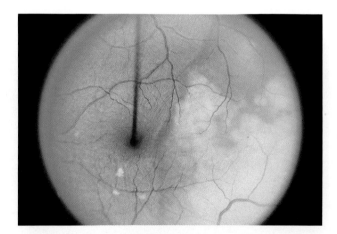

PLATE 22-I. Thrombotic thrombocytopenic purpura with serous detachment overlying a yellow placoid region of RPE abnormality. There are cotton-wool spots inferior to the fovea.

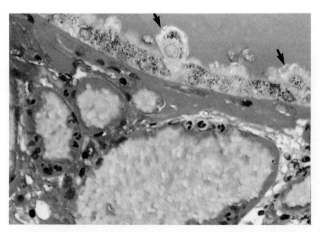

PLATE 24-I. Chorioretinal interface in an eye with retinal detachment. Some RPE cells show signs of detaching from their normal monolayer *(arrows)*. Light micrograph; magnification ×500.

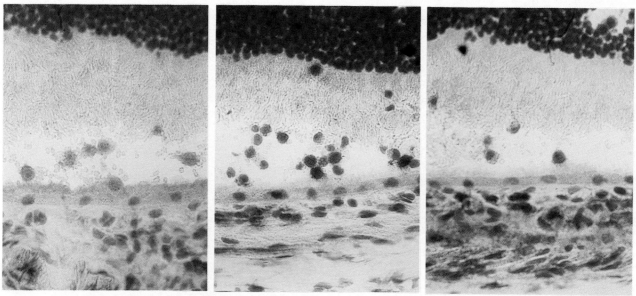

PLATE 26-I. Complement regulatory protein CD59 (MAC inhibitor) expression during experimental autoimmune uveoretinitis. Staining is selective for *(left)* antibody to CD59, *(middle)* for CD2+ve T-lymphocytes, and *(right)* for ED1+ve monocyte/macrophages. See legend to Figure 26-3.

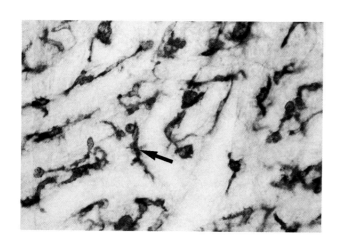

PLATE 26-II. Antigen-presenting cells within the choroid. Choroidal whole mount (rat), dual-stained for MHC class II antigen using alkaline phosphatase-conjugated OX6 antibody *(red)* and ED2 antibody bound to peroxidase via biotin-streptavidin *(blue)*, which is specific for tissue resident macrophages *(blue)*. Two separate populations of potential antigen-presenting cells are present within the choroid beneath the RPE layer and lining the vessel walls; these are highly MHC class II positive dendritic cells *(red)* and MHC class II negative tissue macrophages *(blue)*. Only the occasional macrophage also expresses MHC class II antigen and is double stained *(purple; arrowed)*. Original magnification ×120. (Courtesy of Dr. P. G. McMenamin, Department of Anatomy and Human Biology, University of Western Australia, Perth.)

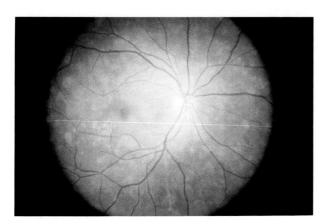

PLATE 28-I. Multiple evanescent white dot syndrome.

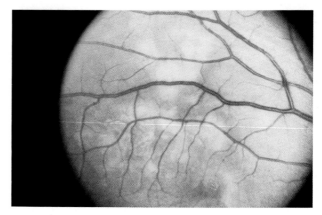

PLATE 28-II. Acute multifocal placoid pigment epitheliopathy (APMPPE). (Courtesy of Everett Ai, M.D.)

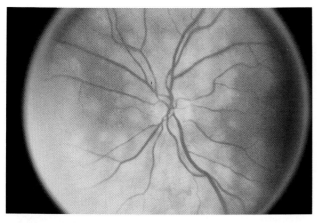

PLATE 28-III. Bird shot retinopathy.

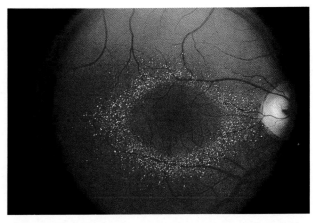

PLATE 32-I. Canthaxanthin retinopathy. (Courtesy of Michael F. Marmor, M.D.)

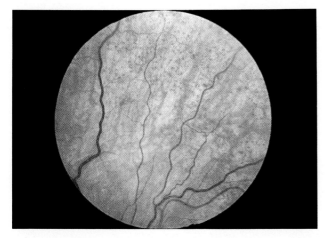

PLATE 32-II. Early thioridazine retinopathy, showing coarse pigment stippling. (Courtesy of Michael F. Marmor, M.D.)

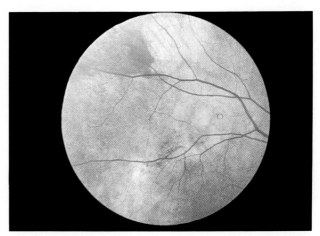

PLATE 32-III. Late thioridazine retinopathy, showing nummular areas of atrophy and hyperpigmentation. (Courtesy of Michael F. Marmor, M.D.)

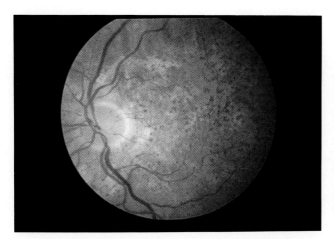

PLATE 32-IV. Desferrioxamine retinopathy. (From Lakhanpal et al., 1985)

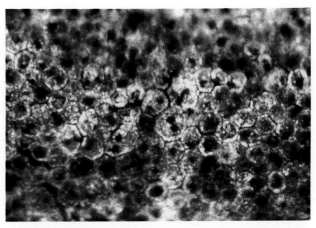

PLATE 33-I. Flat mount of human RPE from a 67-year-old subject. The cells are packed with brownish lipofuscin.

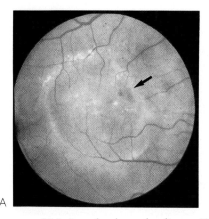 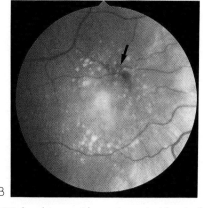 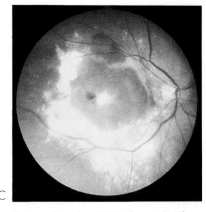

PLATE 35-I. Age-related macular disease. (A) RPE detachment with neovascular notch *(arrows)*. (B) Choroidal neovascular membrane *(arrow)* with retinal hemorrhage and exudate. (C) End-stage disciform lesion with massive subretinal exudate.

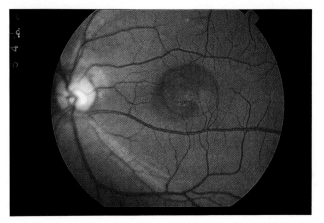

PLATE 36-I. Pigment epithelial detachment in a darkly pigmented fundus.

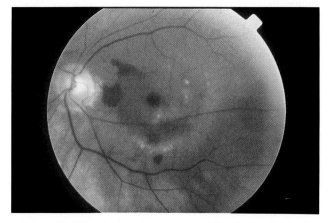

PLATE 36-II. Hemorrhagic pigment epithelial detachment.

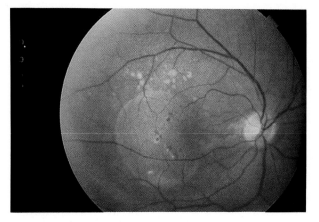

PLATE 36-III. Pigment epithelial detachment associated with atrophic change.

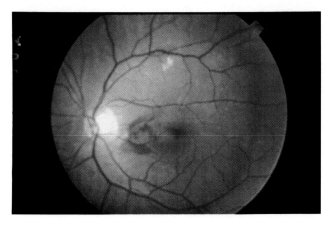

PLATE 36-IV. Hemorrhagic pigment epithelial detachment.

transferase activity toward itself and a few other large proteins, which may be proteoglycans (Sweatt et al., 1991; 1995). The ligands of the GalNAcPTase in the embryonic chicken retina have been identified as endogenous IPM proteoglycans possessing core proteins with a molecular weight of 250 kDa. Amino acid sequence analyses of these core proteins indicates that they may share sequence homology to neurocan, phosphocan, and aggrecan (Balsamo et al., 1995). It has been proposed that GalNAcPTase may act as a lectinlike adhesion molecule between the photoreceptor outer segments and the IPM (Balsamo and Lilien, 1990).

Miscellaneous glycoconjugates. A number of insoluble nonproteoglycan glycoconjugates have been identified in our laboratory as components of the aqueous-insoluble IPM in human and monkey IPM. These include: (1) a PHA-L-binding glycoprotein of 150 kDa, that is also synthesized by fetal and adult human cultured RPE cells; (2) a 140 kDa PNA-binding glycoprotein that is prevalent on Western blots of insoluble IPM preparations that are not exposed to chondroitinase prior to electrophoresis; (3) distinct IPM proteins of 120 kDa, 105 kDa, and 80 kDa that react strongly with monoclonal and/or polyclonal antibodies that were generated against insoluble human and monkey IPM; and (4) high-molecular-weight constituents of approximately 800–900 kDa peak that have been resolved by HPLC size exclusion chromatography (Hageman et al., 1990; Lazarus et al., 1991; Hageman et al., 1992; Rotramel et al., 1992).

Mucins

Early evidence for the presence of mucins in the IPM was provided by Adler and Klucznik (1982). A large-molecular-weight mucinlike glycoprotein (in excess of 10^7 kDa), has recently been isolated from bovine IPM and characterized (Plantner, 1992a). Exposure of this molecule to SDS or GuHCl does not alter its elution on filtration gels. However, treatment with reducing agents, such as β-mercaptoethanol, cause it to elute at an apparently lower molecular weight (100–200 kDa), suggesting that it exists in the IPM as disulfide-linked polymers. The core protein of this mucin is decorated with both O- and N-glycosidically linked oligosaccharides; it is bound by the lectins PNA, JAC, WGA, RCA I, and GS I, but not by SBA, GS II, UEA I, DBA, or BPA. It does not appear to contain glycosaminoglycan, as it is resistant to digestion with chondroitinase ABC, heparinase, and hyaluronidase. In addition, its density on cesium chloride/guanidine hydrochloride gradients is much lower than that typical for proteoglycans. In vivo

labeling studies have provided evidence that this mucinlike glycoprotein may be synthesized by the neural retina.

Metalloproteinases/TIMPs

Metalloproteinases and their endogenous inhibitors (TIMPs) have been demonstrated as components of the IPM. Data gathered in vitro indicate that both the retina (Sheffield and Graff, 1991) and the RPE (Alexander et al., 1990) may participate in the secretion of these proteins. Planter has demonstrated the presence of a high-molecular-weight proteolytic compound within bovine IPM which could be inactivated by metalloproteinase inhibitors (Plantner, 1992b). This proteolytic activity could also be blocked by an uncharacterized endogenous compound of lower molecular weight. More recent studies, employing both enzymatic and immunohistochemical methods, demonstrate the presence of proteinases which are recognized by an antibody to MMP-2, and of a protein which is labeled by an antibody generated against TIMP-1 (Jones et al., 1994). Earlier in vitro studies suggest that these molecules are synthesized by the RPE (Alexander et al., 1990). Interestingly, the metalloproteinases within the IPM appear to be present in a latent form in vivo, requiring activation before they can be detected by enzymatic methods.

Recently, a third member of the TIMP family, TIMP-3, which appears to be very similar to TIMP-1 and TIMP-2 in size and activity, has been cloned and characterized (Apte et al., 1994; 1995). Mutations in the gene encoding TIMP-3 have been linked to the etiology of Sorsby's fundus dystrophy in several families (Weber et al., 1994). The presence of TIMP-3 in the IPM has not yet been demonstrated in normal or diseased retinas. However, a recent in situ hybridization study has demonstrated the presence of TIMP-3 transcripts within photoreceptor cells of retinas from donors with simplex retinitis pigmentosa, but not in controls (Jones et al., 1994; Jomary et al., 1995).

Growth and Trophic Factors

A number of growth, survival, and neurotrophic factors have been identified as residents of the RPE–photoreceptor cell interface in normal and pathological retinas.

Basic fibroblast growth factor. It has been suggested that the RPE may provide basic fibroblast growth factor (bFGF) to the photoreceptor cells (Faktorovich et al., 1990) and that the IPM may serve as a depot for bFGF in normal adult retinas (Hageman et al., 1991). bFGF, or a protein that is immunologically and biochemically similar to it, has been identified immunochemically and biochemically within the IPM in adult monkeys (Hageman et al., 1991), humans (Hanneken and Baird, 1992), and mice (Gao and Hollyfield, 1992; 1995), using a variety of polyclonal and monoclonal antibodies directed against native bFGF and various peptide sequences derived from it. bFGF-immunoreactive IPM has not been detected in normal or Royal College of Surgeon (RCS) rats (Connolly et al., 1992) or in cows (Hanneken et al., 1989).

Hageman and colleagues have shown that the same antibodies that react with primate IPM also bind bands of 16.5–17.5 kDa on Western blots of insoluble monkey IPM proteins (Hageman et al., 1991). Sequences obtained by amino acid sequence analyses of these bands are homologous to those reported for native bFGF (Hageman, unpublished). It should be pointed out that remarkably diverse immunohistochemical results have been obtained, even in the same species, when various fixation, embedding, and antibody conditions are employed (Hageman et al., 1991; Hanneken and Baird, 1992), making it difficult to draw comparisons between studies that do not utilize identical conditions.

Although the role of IPM-sequestered bFGF has not been elucidated, it may be pertinent that (1) photoreceptor degeneration in RCS rats is delayed following subretinal injections of bFGF (Faktorovich et al., 1990); (2) photoreceptors are rescued in light-damaged rat retinas following subretinal injection of bFGF (Faktorovich et al., 1992); and (3) elevated expression of bFGF in degenerating photoreceptor cells is observed, prior to cell death, in *rd* mice (Gao and Hollyfield, 1995).

Pigment-epithelium-derived factor. A 50 kDa doublet on SDS-polyacrylamide gels, termed *pigment-epithelium-derived factor* (PEDF), has been isolated from the media of cultured fetal human RPE cells using ion exchange and size exclusion HPLC (Tombran-Tink et al., 1991). This factor, which induces neuronal differentiation of Y79 retinoblastoma cells in vitro (Steele et al., 1993), appears to be an IPM constituent based on immunohistochemical analyses (Tombran-Tink et al., 1995).

Insulinlike growth factor. The presence of IGF-I within the IPM has been established by Immunohistochemical and biochemical methods (Waldbillig et al., 1991). Interestingly, whereas both photoreceptor and RPE cells possess IGF receptors, the receptors on RPE cells have a slightly higher molecular weight (referred to as the *peripheral type*) than those associated with photoreceptor cells (*brain type*). The cellular source and function of

IPM-sequestered IGF is unknown. However, RPE cells synthesize IGF in vitro; IGF mRNA has also been detected within the neural retina (Hansson et al., 1989).

Neuron-specific enolase. Neuron-specific enolase (NSE), an enzyme that participates in glycolysis and has been implicated as an potential neuronal survival factor in the central nervous system, has been isolated from bovine IPM (Li et al., 1995). The amino acid sequence of a 46 kDa band purified from IPM exhibited homology with human NSE. The authors conclude from immunohistochemical analyses that immunoreactive NSE is present in the basal domain of the IPM between photoreceptor cell ellipsoids, although upon close examination of the micrographs depicted, it appears that NSE immunoreactivity may be associated with photoreceptor inner/outer segments. Nonetheless, it seems certain that NSE is associated with the photoreceptor–IPM interface, where it has been postulated to function as a neurotrophic factor for retinal neurons.

"Photoreceptor-survival-promoting activity." Crude extracts of chick "and bovine IPM have been shown to increase embryonic chick photoreceptor cell survival by a factor of three to four times in vitro (Hewitt et al., 1990). An IPM photoreceptor-survival-promoting activity (PSPA) has been eluted from Sepharose columns in two regions—400–450 kDa and 33 kDa. Although the PSPA binds to heparin affinity columns, it elutes at a salt concentration much lower than that required to elute growth factors such as bFGF, indicating that PSPA is an unrelated protein.

"Y79 neurotrophic activity." A potent neurotrophic activity has been demonstrated within adult bovine and monkey IPM (Tombran-Tink et al., 1992). This activity induces morphological differentiation of Y79 cell aggregates in vitro. In addition, this factor increases the expression of neuron-specific enolase by these cells. Although the molecule responsible for this activity has not been identified, it does not appear to be nerve growth factor, fibroblast growth factor, epidermal growth factor, transforming growth factor beta, or platelet-derived growth factor (Tombran-Tink et al., 1991).

Inhibin. A recent report has demonstrated the presence of inhibin, a member of the transforming growth factor beta superfamily, in the IPM of the bovine retina (Ying et al., 1995). The investigators employed a single polyclonal antibody, generated against an amino-terminal peptide of the inhibin alpha subunit, in their immunohistochemical study.

Miscellaneous Components

Based on the hypothesis that gradients of nutrients and waste products should be present across the IPM if indeed the IPM mediates neural retina nutrition, Adler and colleagues characterized the concentrations of glucose and lactate associated with the IPM adjacent to the retina and to the RPE (Adler and Southwick, 1992). Both constituents were present at levels approximating those found in serum in the IPM near the RPE. In contrast, glucose was nearly undetectable and lactate present in high concentrations in the IPM nearest the neural retina. The investigators point out that such levels are consistent with the hypothesis that nutrients are transported from the choroid to the photoreceptors via the IPM.

DISTRIBUTION OF IPM CONSTITUENTS

Although relatively little is known about the molecular nature, origin, and/or precise functions of most IPM molecules, it is clear that some of the constituents of the subretinal space are compartmentalized. Research in a number of laboratories has been directed toward determining the biochemical and molecular bases for these patterns of heterogeneity (Hageman and Johnson, 1986a; Uehara et al., 1986; Hageman and Johnson, 1987; Landers et al., 1991; Tien et al., 1992).

Patterns of IPM Heterogeneity

Immunohistochemical and lectin histochemical studies have revealed that the distributions of some IPM glycoconjugates are complex; numerous patterns of molecular heterogeneity have been described within the same species, as well as between species. To date, three basic patterns of distribution have been documented. These include IPM molecules that are associated specifically with rod or cone photoreceptor cells, are localized in apical–basal distributions, or are distributed homogeneously (Fig. 18-3). To complicate this situation, the distributions of some IPM molecules appear to fluctuate both temporally and regionally.

The most well-characterized IPM glycoconjugates to date are those that display photoreceptor cell type-specific distributions. *Arachis hypogaea* (PNA), *Bauhinia purpurea* (BPA), and perhaps *Wisteria floribunda* (WFA) agglutinins bind to glycoconjugates that are specifically associated with "cone matrix sheaths" (CMS), distinct compartments of the IPM that surround cone photoreceptor cells, in all mammalian species that

have been investigated (Uehara et al., 1983; Sameshima et al., 1984; Johnson et al., 1985; Hageman and Johnson, 1986a; Johnson et al., 1986; Porrello and LaVail, 1986; Hageman and Johnson, 1987; Hewitt and Adler, 1989; Fariss et al., 1990; Hollyfield et al., 1990a; Yao et al., 1990; Hageman and Johnson, 1991; Hageman et al., 1991; Johnson and Hageman, 1991; Mieziewska et al., 1991; Takumi and Uehara, 1991; Uehara et al., 1991b; Lazarus and Hageman, 1992; Yao et al., 1992; Bishop et al., 1993; Lazarus et al., 1993; Mieziewska et al., 1993b; Szel et al., 1993; Marmor et al., 1994; Yao et al., 1994; Hageman et al., 1995). These highly organized cylindrical subdomains of the IPM have also been identified in human retinas using the cationic copper phthalocyanin dyes Cuprolinic and Cupromeronic Blue, stains that selectively label for sulfated polyanions such as proteoglycans (Hollyfield et al., 1989; 1990). PNA also labels the basalmost aspect of the IPM between rod photoreceptor ellipsoids in some species; this binding is most apparent in isolated insoluble IPM preparations placed into calcium-free solutions (Johnson and Hageman, 1991; Mieziewska et al., 1991). Immunohistochemical studies have demonstrated that anti-chondroitin 6-sulfate antibody (AC6S) and PNA colocalize to CMS in higher mammalian species, including pigs, monkeys, and humans. Since all of these species possess distinctly tapered cone photoreceptor cells, it is possible that the presence of PNA-binding molecules may serve to maintain the correct orientation of outer segments by filling the spaces created by their distinct morphology (Hageman and Johnson, 1987; 1991; Carter-Dawson and Burroughs, 1992; Lazarus and Hageman, 1992).

Rod-photoreceptor-cell-associated IPM is bound intensely by *Triticum vulgaris* (WGA), *Maackia amurensis* (MAA), and *Limax flavus* (LFA) agglutinins (Fariss et al., 1990; Hollyfield et al., 1990a; Mieziewska et al., 1991; Iwasaki et al., 1992a; Tien et al., 1992; Bishop et al., 1993; Yao et al., 1994). LFA and WGA also bind to cone matrix sheaths, albeit less intensely (Fariss et al., 1990; Hollyfield et al., 1990; Mieziewska et al., 1993b).

Other constituents of the insoluble IPM are selectively distributed near the apical surface of the RPE; this domain has been identified by *Phaseolus vulgaris* type IV agglutinin (PHA-L) and MO-225 (an antibody directed against a chondroitin sulfate proteoglycan) in higher mammals. A similar domain is labeled by AC6S antibody and copper phthalocyanin dyes in rodents (Hageman and Johnson, 1991; Lazarus et al., 1991; Iwasaki et al., 1992a; 1992b; Bishop et al., 1993; Lazarus et al., 1993). It has been shown that a marked rearrangement of a subclass of the apical proteoglycans in the mouse retina occurs following detachment of the retina from

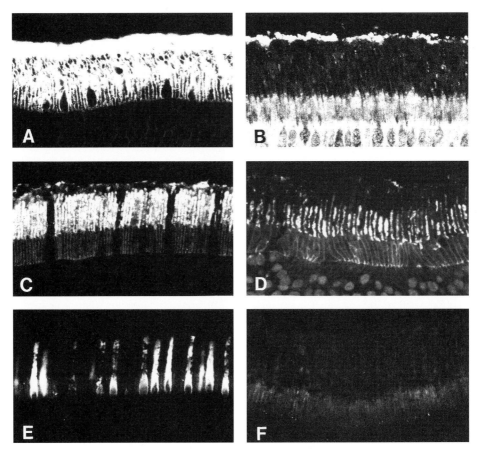

FIGURE 18-3. Light micrographs of sections of human retinas stained with a variety of lectins and antibodies. Distinct patterns of heterogeneity are observed within the IPM. Probes such as JAC label the entire IPM (A). Other IPM constituents are distributed along the apical surface of the RPE, as detected by PHA-L (B). Rod- but not cone-associated IPM is bound by WGA (C), yet WGA binds intensely to foveal cones and/or IPM (D). In contrast, AC6S reacts strongly with CMS in the central retina (E), but not the fovea (F).

the RPE (Iwasaki et al., 1992b). These authors speculate that a close apposition of the retina to the RPE may be required for maintaining the normal distribution of apically distributed proteoglycans in this species.

In contrast, other IPM components, such as those bound by *Helix aspersa* (HAA), *Pisum sativum* (PSA), *Lens culinaris* (LCA), and *Phaseolus vulgaris* type III (PHA-E) agglutinins, and perhaps anti-chondroitin 4-sulfate antibody, are distributed homogeneously within the IPM.

One must consider that at least some of the heterogeneity observed within the IPM may be due to differential glycosylation of the same, or nearly identical, proteins. It is conceivable that the various cell types (rod photoreceptor, cone photoreceptor, RPE, and Müller cells) apposed to the IPM might decorate similar core proteins with different oligosaccharides. For example, it appears that the amino acid sequences of the IPM 150

and IPM 200 core proteins are similar. As such, one explanation for the difference in their molecular weights is that it is due largely to their carbohydrate composition. Further characterization of specific IPM constituents and their associated saccharides will be required to test this theory.

Nonetheless, it is likely that the saccharides associated with IPM glycoconjugates are important to the functional properties of these molecules. An initial characterization of IPM glycoconjugates, using lectin-based histochemistry, has been published by Bishop and colleagues (1993). A group of lectins that specifically bind to N-glycans (ConA, PSA, LCA, and PHA-E), showed widespread labeling of the IPM, suggesting the presence of complex bisected and nonbisected biantennary and/or triantennary N-glycans. A number of lectins that bind specifically to O-glycans were shown to bind intensely to the IPM; PNA and BPA bound specifically to cone matrix sheaths. Based on these studies, four putative glycan outer sequences appear to be associated with IPM glycoconjugates. These include sialylated glycans with subterminal GalNAcα1,3GalNAc, sialylated glycans with subterminal N-acetyl-lactosamine residues, except in the cone matrix sheath, and GalNAcα1,6Galβ1 residues substituted in part with sialic acid.

More recently, it has become apparent that an already complex pattern of IPM heterogeneity is complicated by observations that show marked differences in the distribution of specific IPM glycoconjugates between lower and higher mammals (Porrello and LaVail, 1986; Porrello et al., 1986; Hageman et al., submitted), major light-evoked shifts in the distribution and/or molecular conformation of some constituents (Uehara et al., 1990a; 1991a; Huang and Karwoski, 1992), and topographical differences (e.g. foveal versus extrafoveal IPM) in the distribution of specific glycoconjugates within the same species.

Interspecies Heterogeneity

Little is known about interspecies variation in the molecular composition and/or distribution of insoluble IPM constituents, or of the relationship between PNA- and AC6S-binding glycoconjugates. Biochemical analyses of IPM preparations from pig, monkey, and human retinas have demonstrated that the IPM contains proteoglycans of approximately 150 kDa and 200 kDa that are bound by both PNA and anti-chondroitin 6-sulfate (AC6S) antibody (Hageman and Johnson, 1991). In contrast to these higher mammalian species, chondroitin 6-sulfate immunoreactive proteoglycan does not colocalize with PNA in the IPM of the mouse and rat, species which possess cylindrical cone photoreceptor cell outer segments (Porrello and LaVail, 1986; Hageman and Johnson, 1991). In these species, PNA-binding glycoconjugates are associated solely with cone matrix sheaths, whereas C6S-containing molecules are distributed throughout the IPM and are most prominent in its apical and basal regions.

The volume of cone matrix sheaths varies among mammals as a consequence of cone photoreceptor cell morphology. Biochemical studies have been conducted to characterize those IPM glycoconjugates bound by PNA and AC6S antibody in a variety of mammals possessing either "tapered" or "cylindrical" cone photoreceptors. Both PNA and AC6S antibody bind to bands of approximately 150 kDa and 200 kDa derived from human, monkey, pig, cow, and goat IPM. In dogs and cats, PNA binds bands of 150 kDa and 200 kDa, whereas AC6S antibody binds only a single band of approximately 230 kDa. In IPM isolated from rabbit retinas,

neither PNA nor AC6S antibody label any high-molecular-weight glycoconjugates. Rat interphotoreceptor matrix contains AC6S antibody-binding bands of approximately 150 kDa, 200 kDa, and 230 kDa; PNA does not bind any of these bands, but does label lower molecular weight bands.

These studies indicate that there is species-specific molecular heterogeneity in PNA- and AC6S antibody-binding glycoconjugates that appears to be correlated with cone photoreceptor cell morphology. Proteoglycans of 150 kDa and 200 kDa are present in species, such as primates, that possess tapered cone photoreceptor cells, but are not observed in species, such as rats and rabbits, that possess cylindrical cone photoreceptors. It has been suggested that these larger proteoglycans may provide structural support in these species, thereby maintaining the orientation of adjacent rod photoreceptor outer segments.

Developmental Heterogeneity

Changes in the distributions of various IPM constituents have been observed during ocular development in some species. These are described in more detail in the section on IPM and development.

Topographical Heterogeneity

Two patterns of topographical heterogeneity of specific IPM molecules have been reported.

Foveal IPM-associated molecules. The IPM associated with foveal cone photoreceptor cells in humans and monkeys is markedly different than that associated with extrafoveal cones. The foveal IPM is bound intensely by PNA, but AC6S antibody immunoreactivity is not observed. AC6S antibody reactivity is observed, however, in these same eyes in regions peripheral to the capillary-free zone of the macula. In addition, WGA binds intensely to foveal cones or cone-associated IPM, in contrast to extrafoveal cone matrix sheaths. Most strikingly, elderberry bark lectin (EBL) binds intensely and specifically to the IPM between cone photoreceptor inner segment ellipsoids in the foveola, a region that occupies the central floor of the fovea (Fig. 18-3).

The significance of this observation it not apparent at this time. The absence of chondroitin 6-sulfate (C6S) and, conversely, the presence of EBL-reactive glycoconjugates, may reflect potentially unique molecular, structural, and/or physiological features of foveal cone photoreceptors. It is also possible that the absence of AC6S antibody immunoreactivity in foveal cone matrix sheaths is related to the morphology of the foveal cones.

These cones, which are not fully differentiated until 3–5 years after birth, are structurally distinct from extrafoveal cones in that they more closely resemble rod photoreceptors. Since they are cylindrical and, thus, more rodlike, the presence of a "space-filling" proteoglycan may not be required for functions such as the maintenance of outer segment alignment in this region.

Based on our understanding that the viability and functions of cells are dependent upon their interactions with the extracellular matrix, the foveal IPM may be important to the function and homeostasis of these specialized cones. It is conceivable that disruption of the synthesis and/or maintenance of these IPM constituents could result in degenerative changes that occur within the macula, such as those in patients with various macular degenerations.

Cone photoreceptor class heterogeneity. A recent report provides compelling evidence that subtle differences in glycoconjugate composition may be associated with different classes of cone photoreceptors. In the cone-dominant ground squirrel, *Spermophilus tridecemlineatus*, the cone matrix sheaths of short-wavelength-sensitive cone photoreceptor cells (S-cones) exhibit an extreme affinity for PNA. In contrast, the cone matrix sheaths of the middle-wavelength-sensitive cone photoreceptors (M-cones), which constitute the majority of photoreceptors in this retina, are bound by PNA less intensely than the S-cones. This observation suggests that PNA-binding glycoconjugates associated with various cone photoreceptor populations may be compositionally or quantitatively different.

Light-Evoked Heterogeneity

Signal transduction by rod and cone photoreceptor cells is accompanied by substantially increased metabolism, production of waste products, and establishment of ionic concentration gradients. During the past few years, significant progress has been made toward understanding light/dark-induced changes that occur in the extracellular milieu of the IPM. These include fluctuations in extracellular K^+ (Bialek and Miller, 1994), Na^+ (Perry and McNaughton, 1993; Hodson et al., 1994), Ca^{2+} (Steinberg et al., 1980; Oakley and Steinberg, 1982; Frishman et al., 1992) and pH (Yamamoto et al., 1992). These processes appear to be accompanied by a light-evoked increase of IPM volume. Huang and Karwoski (1992) measured the concentration differences of an extracellular tracer molecule in dark- and light-adapted IPM of frogs and estimated that the subretinal space increases by 7% following illumination. Similar observations have been made in chick (Li et al., 1994a) and cat

(Li et al., 1994b) retinas. The latter observations, based on in vivo experiments, indicated that the volume of the IPM increases as much as 60%–90%. It has been suggested that the swelling of the IPM is accompanied by a reciprocal decrease of RPE cell volume due to movement of salts and water out of the RPE. It has been proposed that this may decrease the magnitude of ionic concentration fluctuations induced by altered conditions of illumination (Huang and Karwoski, 1992; Bialek and Miller, 1994; Li et al., 1994b).

Fluctuations in IPM volume are likely to precipitate alterations in the structural organization of this molecular constituents. Several recent reports indicate that the organization of IPM glycoconjugates may be influenced by light conditions (Uehara et al., 1990a; 1991a). In the subretinal space of normal, light-adapted rats, colloidal iron (a stain for polyanionic glycoconjugates) intensely stains the apical surface of the RPE and the ellipsoids of photoreceptor cells. The central portion of the IPM—that associated with the photoreceptor cell outer segments—is only weakly labeled (Fig. 18-4). In dark-adapted eyes, the pattern of colloidal iron staining is altered radically. The most intense staining is observed throughout the IPM. In contrast to the light-adapted pattern, virtually no staining is observed between photoreceptor cell inner segments. An antibody directed against chondroitin 6-sulfate reacts in a similar pattern, indicating that much of the colloidal iron staining may be due to chondroitin 6-sulfate proteoglycan (Uehara et al., 1990a). A similar light-adapted pattern is observed with the lectin WGA. Some of the WGA staining has been attributed to IRBP, since IRBP binds WGA, and nearly identical patterns are obtained with an antibody directed against IRBP (Uehara et al., 1990a).

Not all IPM constituents exhibit a light/dark-dependent reorganization. No difference in the distribution or intensity of IPM glycoconjugates bound by PNA are observed between light- or dark-adapted eyes (Uehara et al., 1991c). Such observations suggest that some IPM molecules may provide for its structural integrity.

The molecular mechanisms responsible for light-evoked changes in the distribution of various IPM constituents have not been elucidated, although evidence has been provided that illumination itself, and not circadian mechanisms or systemic factors, triggers the changes (Uehara et al., 1990a; 1991a; 1991c). The transition between the dark-adapted and the light-adapted patterns occurs quite rapidly, the altered distribution is clearly discernible within five minutes of light-onset. This is in stark contrast to the time required to reestablish the "dark" pattern (1–2 hours). This time period is significantly longer than those required to establish light-induced pH, ion or volume changes within the

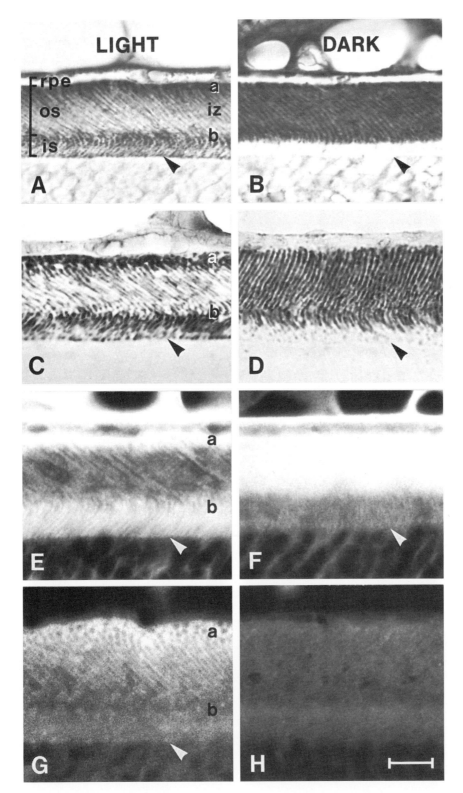

FIGURE 18-4. Light-evoked changes in the IPM of albino rat eyes. Retinal sections of eyes taken either during the light *(left column)* or dark period *(right column)* were labeled either with colloidal iron (A and B), AC6S (C and D), WGA (E and F), or an antibody directed against IRBP (G and H). The retinal pigment epithelium (rpe), the photoreceptor outer segments (os) and inner segments (is), the interstitial zone (iz), and the apical (a) and basal (b) IPM are indicated in (A). The arrowhead marks the outer limiting membrane. All probes display a markedly different distribution pattern in the light and dark adapted retina. (Reprinted from Uehara et al., 1990.)

IPM (Steinberg et al., 1980; Frishman et al., 1992; Yamamoto et al., 1992; Li et al., 1994a; 1994b). It is possible that both IPM volume variations and changes in ion concentrations affect the spatial reconfiguration of IPM glycoconjugates, leading to masking or unmasking of PNA- or WGA-binding epitopes. Studies employing sheets of isolated IPM in vitro have demonstrated that the IPM is extremely sensitive to the ionic concentration. In the absence of Ca^+, CMSs swell substantially and often enlarge to two- to three times their normal size. It is interesting to note that not all CMSs expand at the same rate and that it may take up to an hour for all CMSs to enlarge (Johnson and Hageman, 1991).

CELLULAR ORIGIN AND TURNOVER OF IPM CONSTITUENTS

Based largely on morphological and histochemical observations, many investigators have speculated upon the cellular source(s) of IPM components (Hewitt and Adler, 1989; Hageman and Johnson, 1991). Few of these studies, however, have provided information pertaining to the cellular source(s) of specific IPM constituents (Porrello et al., 1986; Landers et al., 1991). As such, our understanding of the synthesis, turnover, and degradation of IPM constituents is extremely limited.

An electron microscopic study of mouse IPM (detected by Cupromeronic Blue) has provided evidence that the RPE is the primary source of IPM-associated chondroitin sulfate proteoglycans (Tawara et al., 1989). However, subsequent autoradiographic and biochemical studies from the same laboratory (Landers et al., 1991; Landers and Hollyfield, 1992) have indicated that photoreceptor cells are also involved in the synthesis of IPM-associated chondroitin sulfates. More recently, Northern blot analyses have shown that transcripts encoding the IPM proteoglycan IPM 150 core protein are expressed in neural retina, but not RPE. Some antibodies directed against IPM 150 bind to Golgi within photoreceptor inner segments, which suggests that these cells synthesize this proteoglycan (Hageman, unpublished).

Based on autoradiographic and electron microscopic analyses, it has been shown that rod and cone photoreceptor cells are the primary cells involved in the synthesis of IRBP (Hollyfield et al., 1985; Rodrigues et al., 1987); this observation has been confirmed using molecular biological techniques (Liou et al., 1991; Porello et al., 1991). In vitro biosynthetic studies have provided evidence that the neural retina synthesizes the high-molecular-weight mucinlike glycoprotein characterized by Plantner (1992a). In the mouse retina, bFGF mRNA

has been localized mainly to the photoreceptor cells from P10 to the adult (Gao and Hollyfield, 1995). IGF mRNA has also been detected within the neural retina (Hansson et al., 1989).

Some indirect information pertaining to the putative sources of IPM constituents has been obtained from analyses of molecules synthesized and/or secreted by cultures of RPE and neural retina cells. Such studies have demonstrated that these cell types are capable of synthesizing and secreting an array of glycosaminoglycans, including hyaluronate, and proteoglycans (Adler and Serverin, 1981b; Edwards, 1982; Morris et al., 1987; Hewitt and Newsome, 1988; Needham et al., 1988; Landers et al., 1991; Murillo-Lopez et al., 1991; Stramm et al., 1991). Glia-free cultures of mouse retinal multipolar neurons and photoreceptors actively synthesize proteoglycans; chondroitin/dermatan sulfate proteoglycans are detected in the media from these cultures (Murillo-Lopez et al., 1991). Cultured RPE cells synthesize IGF (Hansson et al., 1989), PEDF (Tombran-Tink et al., 1991), and the 150 kDa PHA-L-binding glycoprotein. They do not secrete IPM 150 or IPM 200 (Pfeffer et al., 1991), which suggests either that these proteoglycans are synthesized by the neural retina, or that their synthesis by RPE cells is downregulated in culture. The latter is consistent with the results obtained from Northern analyses.

Even less is known about the turnover and degradation of IPM constituents. Autoradiographic and fluorographic studies have suggested that the IPM proteoglycans IPM 150 and IPM 200 have a half-life of approximately ten days, although nothing is known about the mechanisms involved in their turnover. The presence of acid hydrolases and metalloproteinases and their inhibitors in the IPM indicates that proteolytic and/or glycolytic processing of various IPM constituents may occur within the subretinal space, although this has not been documented.

It is anticipated that future in situ hybridization and Northern blot analyses will allow us to characterize more fully the distribution of IPM constituents and their transcripts, to determine their cellular sources, and to investigate changes in the expression of IPM-specific molecules in normal, developing, aging, and pathologic retinas.

IPM IN RETINAL DEVELOPMENT

A few studies have provided insight regarding the developmental expression of some IPM constituents, especially the proteoglycans. Electron microscopic studies have demonstrated that chondroitin-sulfate-containing proteoglycans, identified by Cupromeronic Blue, are first detectable in the mouse IPM a few days prior to the elaboration of photoreceptor cell outer segments. Organization of these molecules into elaborate, photoreceptor-associated networks occurs subsequently during outer segment elongation (Landers and Hollyfield, 1992).

Uehara and colleagues (1990b) have shown a dramatic increase of wheat germ agglutinin (WGA)-binding glycoconjugates in the IPM between P14 and P16 in rats. Similar changes of other IPM-associated molecules, such as chondroitin 6-sulfate proteoglycan, have not been detected (Chu et al., 1992). The increased expression of WGA-binding glycoconjugate(s) occurs concomitantly with a significant decrease in RCA-binding glycoconjugates. One explanation for this phenomenon is that sialic acid residues are added to the termini of IPM-associated glycoconjugates between P14 and P16, and thereby mask β-galactose residues and decrease RCA binding. In situ hybridization studies of rat retinas between P12 and P42 show specific labeling of photoreceptor cells by a probe for β-galactoside α2,6-sialyltransferase, beginning at P14. The investigators have suggested that this enzyme is responsible for sialyating the N-linked Galβ1,4GlcNAc residues of IPM glycoconjugates beginning at P14.

Interestingly, this "redistribution" of PNA- and WGA-binding IPM glycoconjugates does not appear to occur during ocular development in the mouse or dog, suggesting that these domains remain stable throughout development (Mieziewska, 1993; Mieziewska et al., 1993a; 1994). However, a 250 kDa constituent of the mouse IPM, recognized by a monoclonal antibody designated F22, shows a striking redistribution in the later stages of postnatal photoreceptor cell development (Mieziewska et al., 1993a; 1994). F22 is initially detected within the subretinal space at P3, concomitant with the early stage of outer segment genesis. It is distributed homogeneously within the IPM until P16–17, at which time rod-photoreceptor-cell-associated F22 epitope begins to disappear. By P20, F22-detectable antigen is associated solely with cone matrix sheaths. In the dog the distribution of F22-reactive IPM molecules does not exhibit these developmental changes. Although its developmental expression has been examined only in the dog and mouse, the F22-reactive molecule is present in cow, rat, cat, and monkey IPM, suggesting that it is a conserved component of this matrix. The authors provide evidence that the molecule recognized by F22 is probably not one of the chondroitin 4- or 6-sulfate proteoglycans that are also present in the IPM of the developing mouse eye.

Very little information is available regarding the developmental expression of IPM constituents in primates, with the exception of a single study of IRBP ex-

pression in the developing human retina (Johnson et al., 1985). Preliminary studies of the expression of cone-matrix-sheath-associated molecules during human retinal development have been initiated in our laboratory to monitor the expression of IPM-specific molecules in developing human retinas and to define critical developmental periods when various IPM domains are established (Fig. 18-5) (Anderson et al., 1989; Blanks et al., 1989; Hageman and Johnson, 1991). Rudimentary cone photoreceptor cell outer segments begin to differentiate at approximately 20 weeks. At this time, cone photoreceptors are well polarized, and enlarged domes of IPM are associated with them. Concentrated accumulations of PNA-binding constituents are observed at 17 to 18 weeks. Chondroitin 6-sulfate, a major component of cone matrix sheaths, is first detected in the IPM between 20 and 23 weeks and is solely associated with cone outer segments. At birth, AC6S antibodies bind specifically to cone matrix sheaths. In contrast, however, PNA binds homogeneously throughout the IPM; only after five years of age, PNA-binding IPM glycoconjugates are solely associated with cone matrix sheaths. These studies suggest that there is a staggered expression of PNA- and C6S-containing IPM constituents, and that cone matrix sheaths may be involved in the differentiation and survival of outer segments, as well in the maintenance of their polarity.

This contention is supported further by observations that photoreceptors exhibit some degree of polarity, but are unable to maintain differentiated outer segments in vitro (Adler, 1987) and that RPE-conditioned medium causes a significant increase in the number of embryonic chick photoreceptor cells forming outer-segment-like structures in vitro (Spoerri et al., 1988) and stimulates their survival and differentiation (Liu et al., 1990; Gaur et al., 1992).

IPM IN RETINAL PATHOLOGY

A number of studies have produced evidence suggesting that the IPM may play a significant role in the etiology of photoreceptor cell degeneration in a variety of species. The fate of IPM constituents has been reported for a number of animal models exhibiting inherited and induced degenerations, as well as humans with various diseases; these included *rd* and *rds* mice, RCS and taurine-deficient rats, humans with retinitis pigmentosa and mucopolysaccharidoses (Hewitt and Adler, 1989; Berman, 1991; Hageman and Johnson, 1991; Mieziewska, 1993). In the past few years, new information pertaining to the IPM in retinal pathologies has been forthcoming; these studies are outlined below.

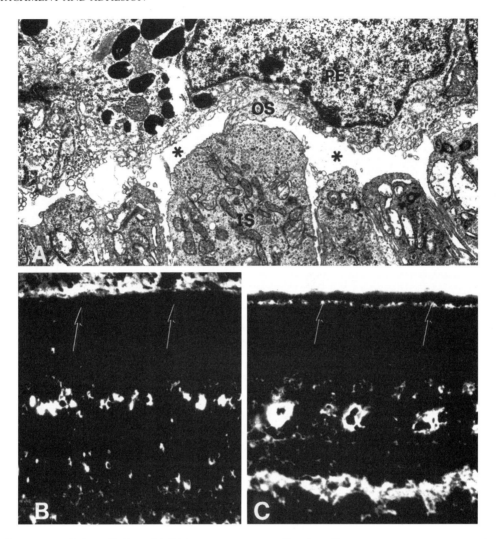

FIGURE 18-5. In humans, morphologically detectable IPM appears at 16–18 weeks gestation; flocculent material begins to accumulate within the subretinal space (A) *(asterisks)*. While cone photoreceptors can first be distinguished at 13 weeks, AC6S immunoreactive material sur-

rounding the rudimentary outer segments can not be detected at that point (B) *(arrows)*. However, at 18 weeks AC6S can readily be detected, paralleling the establishment of the extracellular compartment (C) *(arrows)*. (Reprinted from Hageman and Johnson, 1991.)

RCS Rat

A dramatic example of the deleterious effects that abnormal RPE function can have on IPM composition is exhibited by the Royal College of Surgeons (RCS) rat. This strain carries a hereditary defect in the ability of its RPE cells to phagocytose shed photoreceptor cell outer segments. Despite extensive studies on these animals, the molecular basis for the defect remains an enigma. Histochemical investigations have demonstrated that photoreceptor cells develop normally until about two postnatal weeks. After this time whorls of outer segment membranes accumulate in the subretinal space, concomitant with photoreceptor cell degeneration (Mullen and LaVail, 1976). Eventually the few surviving pho-

toreceptor cells are restricted to the peripheral retina (Sheedlo et al., 1989).

Abnormal changes in the distribution of IPM glycoconjugates occur immediately following the onset of photoreceptor disc shedding, well before the photoreceptor cells begin to degenerate (Fig. 18-6). In unaffected rat retinas, negatively charged glycosaminoglycans—identified with cationic dyes—are concentrated at the apical surface of the pigment epithelium; less intense staining is observed between the outer segments. In the IPM of the RCS rat, this band of glycoconjugates is not observed focally. As membranous debris accumulates within the subretinal space, IPM staining is almost obliterated along the pigment epithelial cell surface and in the debris zone. In contrast, the IPM surrounding the

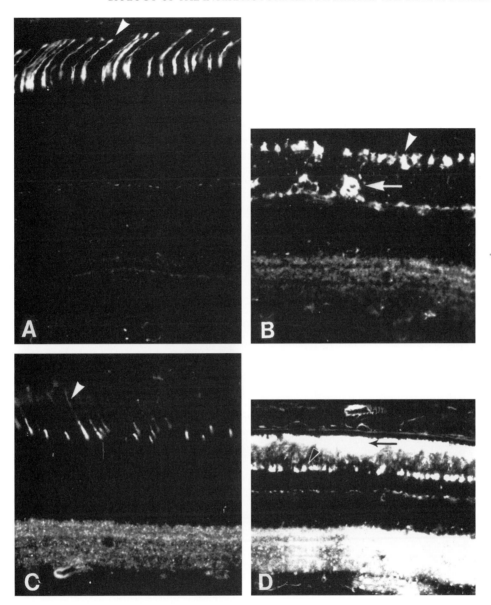

FIGURE 18-6. Retinal sections from normal (A) and *rd* mutant (B) mice at postnatal day 14, and from normal (C) and RCS mutant (D) rats at postnatal day 55, labeled with the lectin PNA. Arrowheads indicate CMS in control retinae and remnants of CMS associated with degenerating photoreceptors in mutant retinae. CMS remain present until late in the degenerative process in both *rd* mice and RCS rats. Degenerating photoreceptor cells are also labeled by PNA in the *rd* retina (D) *(arrow)*. Autoflourescent material accumulates in the interphotoreceptor matrix of the RCS retina (D) *(arrow)*. (Reprinted from Hageman and Johnson, 1991.)

photoreceptor outer segments is stained more intensely than in unaffected animals (LaVail et al., 1981). More recent studies indicate that much of the debris consists of chondroitin 6-sulfate glycosaminoglycans (Porrello et al., 1989; Chu et al., 1992). Contrary to early suggestions that the increased amounts of C6S around the outer segments in RCS rats might be due to a build up of glycoconjugates within the IPM because of an inability of RPE cells to remove them, more recent evidence suggests that chondroitin sulfate and/or heparan sulfate proteoglycans might actually be synthesized at a higher rate by the retinas of RCS rats (Landers et al., 1994).

rds Mouse

The photoreceptors of mutant mice with the hereditary disorder retinal degeneration slow *(rds)* fail to express peripherin, a glycoprotein implicated in the organization of photoreceptor outer segment discs (Connell et al., 1991). Photoreceptor cells fail to form outer segments and begin to degenerate around two weeks postnatally. By one year of age, essentially all photoreceptor cells are degenerated and the subretinal space is reduced to a narrow cleft (Sanyal et al., 1980). During the active stage of the degeneration, the subretinal space is filled with many photoreceptor-cell-derived membranous vesicles.

Transmission electron microscopic studies using dyes for polyanionic molecules, such as proteoglycans, indicate that the IPM develops normally in these animals. However, the absence of outer segments eventually results in the establishment of an irregular distribution of these IPM constituents, since they are normally localized along the photoreceptor outer segments. Eventually, as the subretinal space collapses, only scant staining remains on the apical surface of the RPE, which is now devoid of its apical microvilli (Tawara and Hollyfield, 1990).

Mucopolysaccharidoses

The mucopolysaccharidoses (MPS) are a family of lysosomal storage disorders resulting from the partial to complete absence of enzymes involved in the degradation of sulfated mucopolysaccharides, including dermatan, keratan, heparan, and chondroitin sulfates. These congenital afflictions are manifested by mental retardation, skeletal abnormalities, corneal opacities, and, in some syndromes, retinal degenerations. Since the degradation of shed photoreceptor cell outer segment membranes and, most likely, various IPM components is afforded, at least in part, by RPE cells, it has been suggested that the absence of lysosomal enzymes in individuals with mucopolysaccharidoses results in abnormal function of the IPM–RPE interface.

Over the past several years, animal models of various mucopolysaccharidoses have become available, providing the opportunity to test these hypotheses. MPS VII is characterized by the lack of β-glucuronidase—an enzyme that degrades chondroitin sulfate and other β-glucuronide-containing glycosaminoglycans (Heinegard and Paulsson, 1984). An accumulation of partially degraded glycosaminoglycans within extended lysosomes of RPE cells has been reported in a mouse model of MPS VII (Birkenmeier et al., 1989). Photoreceptor cell outer segments progressively shorten and degenerate during postnatal months one to eight, concomitant with a reduction in the thickness of the IPM. Whereas chondroitin sulfate in control mice is restricted to domains of IPM that abut the apical RPE surface and the spaces between the photoreceptor inner segments, it becomes

distributed more or less homogeneously throughout the IPM in MPS VII mice during the first seven postnatal months (Lazarus et al., 1993). By six to eight months, the RPE thickens to twice that of control animals and numerous membrane-bounded vesicles are noted within the cells (Fig. 18-7). It has been suggested that the accumulation of the abnormal degradation products within the MPS VII mouse IPM may lead to photoreceptor degeneration due to a disruption of photoreceptor support by the RPE cells (Lazarus et al., 1993).

RPE hypertrophy in itself, however, does not always lead to photoreceptor degeneration. For example, massive RPE atrophy occurs in the MPS VI cat, but photoreceptor degeneration does not occur (Aguirre et al., 1986). It is also pointed out that the morphological and biochemical manifestations of murine MPS VII differ significantly from those observed previously in canines (Long et al., 1989). Factors that might influence the pathology of MPS in the retina are the degree of enzyme deficiency and the differential glycosylation of IPM constituents between species. This may explain why no RPE or photoreceptor abnormalities were observed in an eye obtained from a human MPS VII donor, even though intracellular inclusions typical of this disease were observed (Hageman and Sly, unpublished).

Irish Setter (rcd-1)

The autosomal-recessive retinal degeneration rod-cone dysplasia 1 (rcd-1) is caused by insufficient activity of the enzyme cGMP-phosphodiesterase which leads to photoreceptor cell death and retinal degeneration over a period of months. Histochemical observations indicate that the retina and the IPM in these animals develop and differentiate normally until about three postnatal weeks (Aguirre et al., 1982), after which the photoreceptor cell outer segments shorten, become disorganized, and eventually die. The WGA- and PNA-binding components of the IPM appear to remain closely associated with the outer segments throughout this process (Mieziewska et al., 1993b). As photoreceptor cell loss continues, the extracellular space is virtually obliterated and neither PNA- nor WGA-binding in the IPM is observed.

Miniature Poodle (prcd)

In contrast to the rcd-1 Irish setter, progressive rod-cone degeneration in the miniature poodle (prcd) is characterized by a slow progression of visual loss over a period of five to seven years. Much like the rcd-1 retina, PNA- and WGA-binding IPM molecules in prcd-afflicted dogs persist within the subretinal space in a more or less organized state until photoreceptor cell outer and

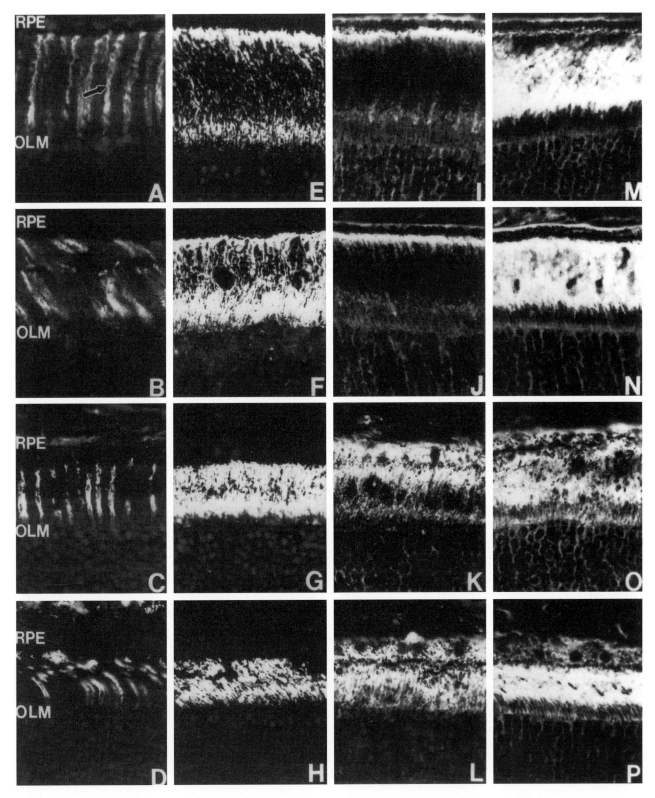

FIGURE 18-7. Sections of retinas from normal mice *(first row)* and MPS VII–affected animals at 1 *(second row)*, 4 *(third row)*, and 7.5 postnatal months *(fourth row)*. Sections were labeled with PNA *(first column)*, AC6S *(second column)*, PHA-L *(third column)*, and WGA *(fourth column)*. PNA specifically labels "cone matrix sheaths" *(arrow)*, which shorten progressively in MPS VII–afflicted animals. AC6S and PHA-L binding glycoconjugates are restricted to distinct re-

gions in the apical and basal IPM in healthy animals, yet in MPS VII mice they become uniformly distributed throughout the entire sub-retinal space as the disease advances. Note the progressive accumulation of PHA-L and WGA binding glycoconjugates within the RPE of affected retinas, as well as the disappearance of PHA-L and WGA binding to Burch's membrane at later ages in MPS VII mice. (Reprinted from Lazarus et al., 1993.)

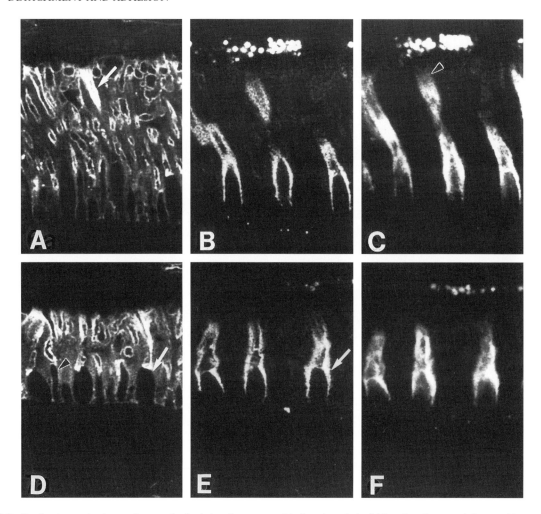

FIGURE 18-8. Confocal scanning laser micrographs depicting the central (A–C) and peripheral (D–F) retina of a poodle with advanced stage progressive rod-cone degeneration *(prcd)*. WGA labeling is prominent around the surviving photoreceptor outer segments (A) *(arrow)*, and diffuse in the remaining IPM. In contrast, PNA binding to the CMS is diminished in these animals (B and E), although the PNA binding domain is thicker than in normal dogs and is not identical to the domain occupied by WGA binding molecules (compare arrows in D and E). (C) and (F) represent composites of several images taken at different focus planes to give a more accurate representation of the cone domain, since only a fraction of it could be displayed in a single section. (Reprinted from Mieziewska et al., 1993b.)

inner segments have degenerated (Fig. 18-8) (Mieziewska et al., 1993a).

Alaskan Malamute (cd).

A hereditary cone degeneration has been described in Alaskan malamutes *(cd)* (Long et al., 1991). The adult retinas of these animals is characterized by a complete absence of cone function due to an unknown genetic defect. Rod photoreceptors appear completely normal both functionally and morphologically. Whereas a few cone photoreceptors do survive in older animals, they often lack outer segments. Nonetheless, these severely degenerated cones are typically surrounded by IPM that

binds PNA, suggesting that at least some components of cone matrix sheaths may be synthesized by the *cd* retina.

Retinitis Pigmentosa

During the course of the last decade tremendous advances have been made in the understanding of the genetic defects underlying retinitis pigmentosa (RP); defects in several genes, including rhodopsin, peripherin, and the beta subunit of phosphodiesterase have been identified in RP families (for reviews see Berson, 1993; Bird, 1995). The early stages of the disease are characterized by a progressive shortening of the photoreceptor outer segments and a concomitant reduction in the vol-

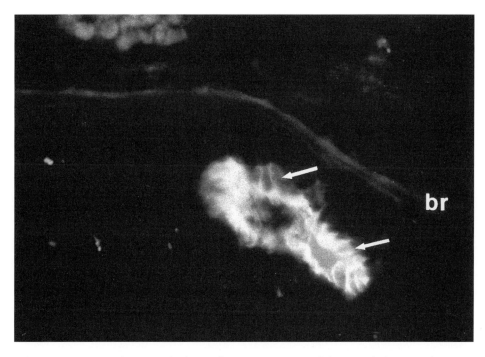

FIGURE 18-9. Section depicting a rosette in the retina of a donor who had retinitis pigmentosa. Cone photoreceptors line rosettes; remnants of their outer segments are oriented toward the lumen. The lumens of rosettes are bound by PNA-FITC, suggesting that some of the normal components of the IPM which surround cone outer segments are retained and may promote cone photoreceptor survival *(arrows)*. (br) = Bruch's membrane. (Reprinted from Milam and Jacobson, 1990.)

ume of the IPM. Later in the disease process, as RPE cells migrate to the inner retina and Müller cell processes can be observed even in Bruch's membrane, the subretinal space is completely lost (Milam et al., 1995). Rod photoreceptor cell death often precedes the degeneration of cone photoreceptors in RP retinas; histological observations have revealed the presence of cone photoreceptor "rosettes" in some donor RP retinas (Milam and Jacobson, 1990). These structures are formed in the remnants of the outer nuclear layer by cone photoreceptors, with their outer segments located within a newly formed extracellular space. The outer segments within the rosettes are surrounded by matrix material which reacts with PNA (Fig. 18-9), suggesting retention and/or synthesis of some normal IPM constituents by rosette-associated cells (Milam and Jacobson, 1990). These observations provide support for the contention that some IPM constituents participate in the maintenance of photoreceptor cell viability.

Aged Human Eyes with Drusen

A number of studies suggest a correlation between changes in IPM composition and the etiology of photoreceptor degeneration in some retinal/photoreceptor degenerations (LaVail et al., 1981; Porrello et al., 1986; Hageman and Johnson, 1991; Lazarus and Hageman, 1992; Lazarus et al., 1993). Recently, an abnormality of the rod-associated IPM has been identified in human retinas (Hollyfield et al., 1990a; Hageman et al., 1992; Iwasaki et al., 1992a). The IPM surrounding some rod photoreceptor cells (termed *PNA-binding rod photoreceptors*) was noted to bind the lectin PNA, a lectin that normally does not react with the rod-associated IPM (Fig. 18-10). Definitive identification of these cells as rod photoreceptors was achieved by double-labeling with PNA and a rod-specific antibody directed against the C-terminus of rhodopsin. The density of "PNA-binding rods" has been shown to increase in correlation with increasing quantities of macular drusen, extracellular deposits in Bruch's membrane associated with AMD (Hageman and Lazarus, 1992a; 1992b). Preliminary analyses of neutral and amino sugars from the IPM of retinas with and without significant numbers of these PNA-binding rods show a decrease in IPM sialic acid concentration. These studies provide the first direct evidence that changes in IPM proteoglycan composition are associated with drusen; we propose that these changes may be related to photoreceptor dysfunction and visual loss that occurs in individuals with AMD.

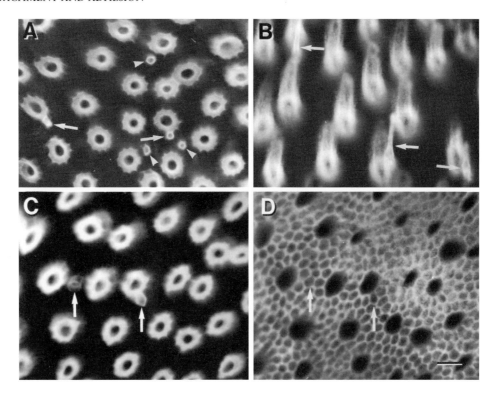

FIGURE 18-10. Cross-sectional (A, C and D) and longitudinal (B) views of human photoreceptors labeled with PNA-FITC and WGA-rhodamine. PNA binds to IPM associated with all cone photoreceptors and some rod photoreceptors located either directly adjacent (A) *(arrows)* or apart from cones (A) *(arrowheads)*. PNA-binding molecules appear to be present throughout the entire rod-associated IPM (B) *(arrows)*. Double labeling with PNA and WGA demonstrates that rods which bind PNA also bind WGA (C and D) *(arrows)*. (Reprinted from Iwasaki et al., 1992a.)

Understanding the molecular basis for the relationship between compositional changes in the IPM and photoreceptor cell degeneration in humans, especially in foveal cones, may provide valuable information pertinent to our understanding of the etiology of photoreceptor cell degeneration during aging and in diseases such as AMD and cone-rod dystrophies/degenerations. The PNA-bound molecules associated with PNA-binding rods have not been characterized. These IPM constituents could arise from de novo expression of an aberrant rod-associated IPM molecule. Alternatively, they might be abnormally glycosylated variants of normal rod sheath components that lack terminal sialic acid residues. This contention is supported by the observation that rod photoreceptor cells are bound by PNA after exposure to neuraminidase (Tien et al., 1992). Until it becomes clear which molecular defects underlie the compositional alterations in rod-associated IPM, theories on the connection between the increase in PNA-binding rod density and the pathogenesis of photoreceptor dysfunction and visual loss in AMD remain highly speculative.

Rhegmatogenous Retinal Detachment

The development of macular epiretinal membranes is a common complication of surgery for rhegmatogenous retinal detachments. The factors that precipitate the genesis of these membranes are not known, although a number of paradigms have been postulated. Based on a report that intravitreally injected chondroitin sulfate elicits epiretinal membrane formation in rabbits (Russell and Hageman, 1992), we conducted studies to determine whether insoluble IPM is present in the vitreous of human eyes following retinal detachment. Vitreous collected from patients during retinal reattachment surgery or membrane peeling for retinal-detachment-related macular epiretinal membranes was analyzed for the presence of IPM (Russell et al., 1997). Based on their unique morphology and ability to bind PNA and an

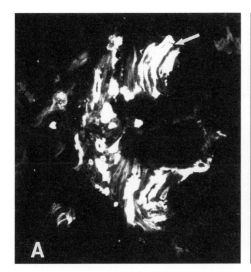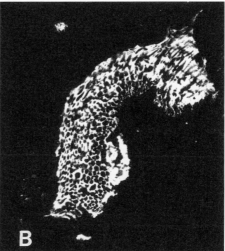

FIGURE 18-11. Serial sections of vitreous removed during a vitrectomy procedure from a patient with proliferative vitreoretinopathy. Insoluble IPM material detected by PNA (A) and a polyclonal antibody specific to IPM material, (B) are present. Both images document the smaller domains surrounding rod photoreceptors and the larger cone matrix sheaths (A) *(arrow)*.

IPM-specific antiserum, insoluble IPM domains were identified in the vitreous samples collected from 11 of 12 patients (Fig. 18-11). These patients also exhibited Shafer's sign (pigmented material, also referred to as tobacco dust, often associated with rhegmatogenous detachment) clinically. These results demonstrate that insoluble IPM constituents gain access to the vitreous cavity following RD, coincide with Shafer's sign, and may remain incompletely degraded for several months following RD. It is proposed that IPM liberated into the vitreous following a retinal tear may be a significant stimulus for the development of macular epiretinal membranes.

Central Serous Chorioretinopathy

Orzalesi and colleagues have speculated that cone matrix sheaths may play a role in the pathogenesis of central serous chorioretinopathy (Orzalesi et al., 1990). They suggest a number of mechanisms by which this might occur, but provide no data to support their contention. We are unaware of any studies that have been directed toward testing their hypothesis.

Retinal and RPE Transplants

A recent study (Juliusson et al., 1994) evaluated the ability of the transplanted retina to synthesize and secrete four major components of the IPM: chondroitin 6-sul-

fate, IRBP, PNA-binding proteins, and the F22 antigen (Mieziewska et al., 1994). The investigators transferred rabbit embryonic retinal cells into the retinas of normal adult rabbits. Transplanted cells organized into rosettes within the host retina. Photoreceptor inner and outer segments projected into the lumens of rosettes and were surrounded by extracellular matrix. Histochemical analyses indicated that PNA-binding molecules, chondroitin-6-sulfate-containing proteoglycans, and F22-reactive antigen were present within the rosette lumens. IRBP could not be detected within the rosettes, even though it was abundant in the host IPM.

Transplantation of healthy RPE cells into the subretinal space of the RCS rat retina appears to prevent photoreceptor cell death (LaVail et al., 1992). It also leads to the establishment of a phenotypically normal IPM, as the IPM assumed a normal appearance and distribution in areas where photoreceptor cell rescue was complete.

IPM AND RETINAL ADHESION

The molecular mechanisms involved in the establishment and maintenance of the attachment between the neural retina and the RPE remain poorly understood (Marmor, 1992). Physiologically, retina–RPE adhesion is maintained by a variety of interacting mechanisms, including active fluid transport, osmotic pressure gradients, intraocular pressure, physical interaction between

RPE and photoreceptor outer segments, and microenvironmental conditions. Based on their distribution and composition, it has been proposed that IPM glycoconjugates are also likely candidates for mediation of the molecular attachment between the neural retina and RPE. A number of recent studies, which are described below, have provided compelling evidence for such a role of IPM constituents in retinal adhesion. It now appears that specific components of the IPM act as major adhesive elements bridging the RPE–retina interface.

Xyloside-Induced IPM Perturbation

Intravitreal injections of β-D-xylopyranoside, a specific inhibitor of chondroitin sulfate proteoglycan synthesis, have been administered to micropigs in order to examine the potential role of CMS-associated proteoglycans in retinal adhesion (Lazarus and Hageman, 1992). The IPM was selectively affected by this treatment; at early stages, disorganization of AC6S- and PNA-binding glycoconjugates, alterations of cone outer segment plasma membranes, and/or transverse splitting of CMS was observed. Clinically, peripheral retinal detachments were sometimes detected. Cone, but not rod, outer segments degenerate subsequent to the initial loss of AC6S immunoreactivity. These observations suggest that intravitreal administration of β-D-xylopyranoside elicits disruption of CMS-associated proteoglycan synthesis and retinal detachment, supporting the hypothesis that RPE–outer segment attachment is dependent on continuous synthesis of CMS-associated proteoglycans.

Enzymatic Perturbation of Retinal Adhesion

The role of IPM constituents in mediating retinal adhesion has been investigated following subretinal or intravitreal injections of various enzymes into rabbit eyes and examination of the consequent morphological, biochemical, and physiological changes in retinal structure and function (Yao et al., 1990). Chondroitinase ABC, neuraminidase, and testicular hyaluronidase, three enzymes that degrade oligosaccharides known to be constituents of the IPM, caused diffuse loss of adhesion associated with changes in PNA-binding to CMS, without affecting photoreceptor function (based on ERG recordings). Retinal adhesion, which recovers steadily between 5 and 20 days following exposure to chondroitinase and neuraminidase, correlates closely with the reestablishment of the normal distribution of PNA-binding glycoconjugates in the IPM. These studies suggest that IPM constituents are involved in retinal adhesion, and that their adhesive properties can be modified in vivo.

Retinal Adhesion in Monkeys and Humans

The mechanisms of retinal adhesion in humans and monkeys have been studied in vitro and in vivo (Yao et al., 1992; Marmor et al., 1994; Yao et al., 1994; Hageman et al., 1995). These studies have demonstrated that the rate of postmortem failure of adhesiveness in the monkey is sensitive to temperature, pH, and calcium concentrations. Subretinal injections of neuraminidase weaken retinal adhesiveness and result in changes in the organization of PNA-binding glycoconjugates.

Additional studies have been performed in which monkey and human eyes were removed immediately following euthanasia or optic cross-clamp, respectively, and the retinas partially "peeled" from the RPE. CMS remained firmly attached to both the apical RPE and neural retina and elongated four to six times their normal length in eyes peeled within 45 seconds of enucleation (Fig. 18-12) (Hageman et al., 1995). Additional peeling separation results in separation of the entire RPE from Bruch's membrane, or splitting of the CMS. Another study has shown that remnants of IPM material, specifically cone matrix sheaths, adhere to the microvilli of the RPE when the neural retina is manually removed from the RPE cell layer (Hollyfield et al., 1989). Collectively, these investigations suggest that adhesion between CMS constituents and the RPE or photoreceptors is stronger than the integrity of CMS themselves and, as such, provide evidence that CMS have characteristics consistent with their participation in the establishment and maintenance of retinal attachment.

Vitronectin Receptor and CD44: A Proposed Model for Retinal Adhesion

Integrins constitute a family of ubiquitous extracellular matrix receptor molecules. They are heterodimeric transmembrane glycoproteins composed from two noncovalently linked subunits (α and β). Integrin binding often is mediated through the presence of an Arg-Gly-Asp (RGD) tripeptide within the ligand, but molecules lacking this tripeptide may still bind to integrins in a conformation-dependent manner. Integrins have been found to play important roles in nearly all tissues of the body and in such diverse processes as inflammation, development, gene regulation, thrombosis, and homeostasis.

The presence of integrins in the neural retina and the RPE has been established in the recent years (Philp and Nachmias, 1987; Fisher and Anderson, 1989; Anderson et al., 1991; Rizzolo and Heiges, 1991). Immunohistochemical investigations indicate that during the early

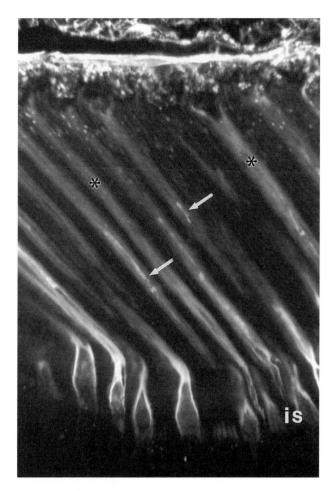

FIGURE 18-12. Photomicrographs of elongated cone matrix sheaths stained with PNA-FITC following manual separation of the retina from the RPE. Note the extreme elongation of CMS *(asterisks),* fragmented cone outer segments *(arrows)* and continued attachment of CMS to the apical RPE surface. is = inner segments (Reprinted from Hageman et al. 1995.)

stages of embryogenesis in chicken, β_1 and α_6 integrin subunits are present on all domains of the RPE plasma membrane. Later, both become localized to the basal surface of the epithelium. In contrast, α_3 and α_v subunits remain confined to the basolateral and apical surfaces, respectively, of the RPE throughout development (Rizzolo et al., 1994). More recently, it has been demonstrated that an integrin, the $\alpha_v\beta_{3/5}$ vitronectin receptor (VnR), is associated with apical RPE and cone photoreceptor outer and inner segment plasma membranes (Fig. 18-13). VnR colocalizes with structural components of apposed cone matrix sheaths, and cytoplasmically, with actin cables within apical RPE microvilli and cone photoreceptor inner segments (Anderson et al., 1995). Based on the known functions of VnR, it is likely that its interaction with IPM ligands might modulate other

cellular activities, such as translation of external cues into signals that affect cytoskeletal organization or modification of other IPM ligands (Juliano and Haskill, 1993).

Based on these observations, we have proposed a model for integrin-mediated retinal adhesion to the RPE (Anderson et al., 1995). It assumes that the integrins of the RPE microvilli and photoreceptor outer segment cell surfaces are linked to one other through unidentified IPM ligand(s). Intracellularly, the integrins are bound to the actin cytoskeleton, providing not only tensile support, but also an opportunity to transduce intracellular conditions to the exterior and vice versa. The IPM ligand(s) capable of mediating this interaction have not yet been identified. However, a number of potential candidates can be proposed; these include IPM 150/200, hyaluronate, and/or vitronectin.

IPM 150 and IPM 200. Some experimental evidence suggests that the chondroitin sulfate IPM proteoglycans, specifically IPM 150 and IPM 200, may be involved in maintaining retinal adhesion (Hollyfield et al., 1989; Hageman et al., 1995). Based on studies that implicate RGD-containing proteoglycans in cell matrix adhesion in other cellular systems (Hay, 1991), IPM 150 and/or IPM 200 have been considered potential candidates for mediating retinal adhesion. Elucidation of their complete amino acid sequences will reveal whether they possess RGD consensus sequences that would allow them to bind to photoreceptor and RPE VnR. To date, no deduced RGD sequences have been identified within the clones encoding IPM 150 or IPM 200. Interestingly, however, polyclonal antisera generated against RGD-containing peptides do react with the IPM on sections of human retina, suggesting the presence of an RGD-containing protein in the IPM.

Hyaluronate. Biochemical studies have indicated that hyaluronic acid is present as a component of the IPM (Fig. 18-13) (Bach and Berman, 1971a; 1971b; Kaneko, 1987; Tate et al., 1993; Korte et al., 1994). In the developing eye, hyaluronan is synthesized by the RPE and deposited both apically and basally; as RPE cells mature, hyaluronan deposition is restricted to their apical surface (Tate et al., 1993). It has been established that hyaluronan binds to chondroitin sulfate glycosaminoglycans in other systems. Based on the observations that IPM 150 core protein possesses potential hyaluronan-binding motifs and that hyaluronidase degrades cone matrix sheaths in vitro (Johnson and Hageman, 1987) and weakens retinal adhesion in vivo (Yao et al., 1990), we speculate that hyaluronan may stabilize the IPM

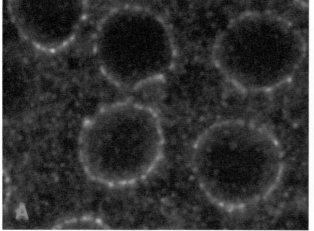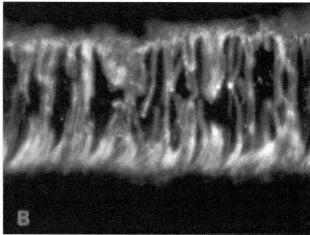

FIGURE 18-13. (A) Transverse sections of the adult monkey retina perpendicular to the longitudinal axis of the photoreceptors at the level of the cone photoreceptor inner segment, labeled with an antibody to the vitronectin receptor (VnR) integrin. Immunoreactivity is evident at the cell surface of each ellipsoid. (B) Section of rabbit IPM stained with a monoclonal antibody directed against hyaluronate. The antibody reacts with material associated with photoreceptor inner and outer segments extending to the apical surface of the RPE. ([A] reprinted from Anderson et al., 1995; [B] courtesy of GE. Korte.)

through interactions with IPM 150, IPM 200, and perhaps other insoluble IPM constituents.

CD44. This hyaluronan meshwork could be anchored directly to the neural retina by CD44, a cell surface glycoprotein capable of binding hyaluronan extracellularly (Wight et al., 1992) and actin filaments cytoplasmically (Lacy and Underhill, 1987). Interaction between CD44 and hyaluronan has been shown to be important in cell matrix adhesion in other systems (Aruffo et al., 1990; Toole, 1991). Recent studies have demonstrated that CD44 is associated with mouse and human Müller cell apical microvilli (Chaitin et al., 1994; Hageman et al., 1995). The distribution and molecular weight of retinal CD44 appears to be identical to that of a glycoprotein identified previously with an antibody designated 22/G9 (Korte et al., 1992).

Indirect anchorage of a hyaluronan network to the RPE and/or photoreceptors could conceivably be mediated by IPM proteoglycans, either through interactions with the chondroitin sulfate glycosaminoglycans (Turley and Roth, 1980) or through linkages to the proteoglycan core proteins. Alternatively, the close apposition between the RPE cell layer and hyaluronan could be mediated through a hyaluronan-binding protein distinct from CD44 (Hardwick et al., 1992; Jaworski et al., 1994).

In summary, we hypothesize that VnR and CD44 may mediate the linkage of photoreceptor, Müller, and RPE cell cytoskeletons (Vaughan and Fisher, 1987; Spencer et al., 1991) to as-yet-unidentified IPM ligands (Plate 18-I). Such a system would provide a framework for a molecular model of retinal adhesion, whereby IPM molecules, such as insoluble CMS-associated proteoglycans, bind to the extracellular domains of VnR and CD44. These, in turn, might be stabilized by other IPM constituents, such as hyaluronan. Additional studies will be required to test this theory.

REFERENCES

Adler AJ. 1989. Selective presence of acid hydrolases in the interphotoreceptor matrix. Exp Eye Res 49(6):1067–1077.

Adler AJ, Klucznik KM. 1982. Some functional characteristics of purified bovine interphotoreceptore retinol binding protein. Invest Ophthalmol Vis Sci 26:273–282.

Adler AJ, Martin KJ. 1982. Retinol-binding in the interphotoreceptor matrix. Biochem Biophys Res Comm 108:1601–1608.

Adler AJ, Martin KJ. 1983. Lysosomal enzymes in the interphotoreceptor matrix: acid protease. Curr Eye Res 2:359–366.

Adler AJ, Serverin KM. 1981a. Proteins of the bovine interphotoreceptor matrix. Doc Ophthalmol Proc Ser 25:25–40.

Adler AJ, Severin KM. 1981b. Proteins of the bovine interphotoreceptor matrix: tissues of origin. Exp Eye Res 32:755–769.

Adler AJ, Southwick RE. 1992. Distribution of glucose and lactate in the interphotoreceptor matrix. Ophthalmic Res 24(2):243–252.

Adler AJ, Spencer SA, Heth CA, Schmidt SY. 1988. Comparison of proteins in the interphotoreceptor matrix of vertebrates. Ophthalmic Res 20(5):275–285.

Adler R. 1987. The differentiation of retinal photoreceptor and neurons in vitro. In: Osborne N, Chader G., eds., Progress in Retinal Research, Oxford: Pergamon Press, 1–27.

Aguirre G, Farber D, Lolley R, O'Brian P, Alligood J, Fletcher RT, Chader G. 1982. Retinal degenerations in the dog: III abnormal cyclic nucleotide metabolism in rod-cone dysplasia. Exp Eye Res 35:625–642.

Aguirre GD, Stramm LE, Haskins M, Jezyk P. 1986. Animal models of metabolic eye disease. In: Goldberg MF, ed, Genetics and Metabolic Eye Disease. Boston: Little, Brown, 146–152.

Alexander JP, Bradley JMB, Gabourel JD, Acott TS. 1990. Expression of matrix metalloproteinases and inhibitor by the human retinal pigment epithelium. Invest Ophthalmol Vis Sci 31(12):2520–2528.

Anderson DH, Guerin CJ, Erikson PA, Stern WH, Fisher SK. 1986. Morphological recovery in the reattached retina. Invest Ophthalmol Vis Sci 27:168–183.

Anderson DH, Guerin CJ, Matsumoto B, Pfeffer BA. 1991. Identification and localization of a beta-1 receptor from the integrin family in mammalian retinal pigment epithelial cells. Invest Ophthalmol Vis Sci 31:81–93.

Anderson DH, Johnson LV, Hageman GS. 1995. Vitronectin receptor expression and distribution at the photoreceptor-retinal pigment epithelium interface. J Comp Neurol 360:1–16.

Anderson K, Hageman GS, Banks JC, Spee C. 1989. Developmental expression of human cone matrix sheath-specific molecules. Invest Ophthalmol Vis Sci 30(suppl):490.

Apte SS, Mattei MG, Olsen BR. 1994. Cloning of the cDNA encoding human tissue inhibitor of metalloproteinases-3 (TIMP-3) and mapping of the TIMP-3 gene to chromosome 22. Genomics 19: 86–90.

Apte SS, Olsen BR, Murphy G. 1995. The gene structure of tissue inhibitor of metalloproteinases (TIMP)-3 and its inhibitory activities define the distinct TIMP gene family. J Biol Chem 270:14313–14318.

Aruffo A, Stamenkovic I, Melnick M, Underhill CB, Seed B. 1990. CD44 is the principal cell surface receptor for hyaluronate. Cell 61:1303–1313.

Azuma N, Hida T, Akiya S, Uemura Y, Kohsaka S, Tsukada Y. 1990. Histochemical studies on hyaluronic acid in the developing human retina. Graefes Arch Clin Exp Ophthalmol 228:158–160.

Bach G, Berman ER. 1970. Characterization of a sialoprotein isolated from cattle retina. Ophthalmol Res 1:257–272.

Bach G, Berman ER. 1971a. Amino sugar-containing compounds of the retina. I. Isolation and characterization. Biochim Biophys Acta 252:453–461.

Bach G, Berman ER. 1971b. Amino sugar-containing compounds of the retina. II. Structural studies. Biochim Biophys Acta 252:462–471.

Balsamo J, Lilien J. 1990. N-cadherin is stably associated with and is an acceptor for a cell surface N-acetylgalactosaminylphosphotransferase. J Biol Chem 265(5):2923–2928.

Balsamo J, Ernst H, Zanin MKB, Hoffman S, Lilien J. 1995. The interaction of the retina cell surface N-acetylgalactosaminylphosphotransferase with an endogenous proteoglycan ligand results in inhibition of cadherin-mediated adhesion. J Cell Biol 129(5):1391–1401.

Barbehenn EK, Wiggert B, Lee L, Kapoor CL, Zonnenberg BA, Redmond TM, Passonneau JV, Chader GJ. 1985. Extracellular cGMP phosphodiesterase related to the rod outer segment phosphodiesterase isolated from bovine and monkey retinas. Biochemistry 24:1309–1316.

Bazan NG, Reddy TS, Redmont TM, Wiggert B, Chader GJ. 1985. Endogenous fatty acids are covalently and non-covalently bound to interphotoreceptor retinoid-binding proteinin the monkey retina. J Biol Chem 260:13677–13680.

Berman ER. 1969. Mucopolysaccharides (glycosaminoglycans) of the retina: identification, distribution and possible biological role. Biblio Ophthalmologica 79:5–31.

Berman ER. 1982. Isolation and characterization of the interphotoreceptor matrix. Meth Enzymol 81:77–85.

Berman ER. 1985. An overview of the biochemistry of the interphotoreceptor matrix. In: Bridges CD, Adler AJ, eds, The Interphotoreceptor matrix in health and disease. New York: Liss, 47–64.

Berman ER. 1991. Biochemistry of the eye. New York: Plenum Press.

Berman ER, Bach G. 1968. The acid mucopolysaccharides of cattle retina. Biochem J 108:75–88.

Berson EL. 1993. Retinitis pigmentosa: the Friedenwald lecture. Invest Ophthalmol Vis Sci 34:1659–1676.

Bialek S, Miller SS. 1994. K+ and Cl− transport mechanisms in bovine pigment epithelium that could modulate subretinal space volume and composition. J Physiology 475(3):401–417.

Bird AC. 1995. Retinal photoreceptor dystrophies. Am J Ophthalmol 119(5):543–562.

Birkenmeier EH, Davisson MT, Beamer WG, Ganschow RE, Vogler CA, Gwynn B, Lyford KA, Maltais LM, Wawrzynick CJ. 1989. Murine mucopolysaccaridosis type VII: characterization of a mouse with β-glucoronidase deficiency. J Clin Invest 83:1258–1266.

Bishop PN, Boulton M, McLeod D, Stoddart RW. 1993. Glycan localization within the human interphotoreceptor matrix and photoreceptor inner and outer segments. Glycobiology 3:403–412.

Blanks JC, Johnson LV. 1984. Specific binding of peanut lectin to a class of retinal photoreceptor cells: a species comparison. Invest Ophthalmol Vis Sci 25:546–557.

Blanks JC, Anderson K, Spee C, Hageman GS. 1989. Developmental expression of human cone matrix sheath-specific molecules. Soc Neurosci 15:494.

Bok D, Hageman GS, Steinberg RH. 1993. Repair and replacement to restore sight. Report from the panel on Photoreceptor/Retinal Pigment Epithelium. Arch Ophthalmol 111:463–471.

Carter-Dawson L, Burroughs M. 1992. Interphotoreceptor retinoid-binding protein in the Golgi apparatus of monkey foveal cones. Electron microscopic immunocytochemical localization. Invest Ophthalmol Vis Sci 33:1589–1594.

Chader GJ. 1989. Interphotoreceptor retinoid-binding protein (IRBP): a model protein for molecular biological and clinically relevant studies. Invest Ophthalmol Vis Sci 30:7–22.

Chaitin MH, Wortham HS, Brun-Zinkernagel AM. 1994. Immunocytochemical localization of CD44 in the mouse retina. Exp Eye Res 58(3):359–365.

Chu Y, Walker LN, Vijayasekaran SL, Cooper RL, Porrello KV, Constable IJ. 1992. Developmental study of chondroitin-6-sulphate in normal and dystrophic rat retina. Graefes Arch Clin Exp Ophthalmol 230(5):476–482.

Connell G, Bascom R, Molday L, Reid D, McInnes RR, Molday RS. 1991. Photoreceptor peripherin is the normal product of the gene responsible for retinal degeneration in the rds mouse. Proc Natl Acad Sci USA 88:723–726.

Connolly SE, Hjelmeland LM, LaVail MM. 1992. Immunohistochemical localization of basic fibroblast growth factor in mature and developing retinas of normal and RCS rats. Curr Eye Res 11:1005–1017.

Edwards RB. 1982. Glycosaminoglycan synthesis by cultured human retinal pigmented epithelium from normal postmortem donors and a postmortem donor with retinitis pigmentosa. Invest Ophthalmol Vis Sci 23:435–446.

Ellies LG, Jones AT, Williams MJ, Ziltener HJ. 1994. Differential regulation of CD43 glycoforms on CD4+ and CD8+ T lymphocytes in graft-versus-host disease. Glycobiology 4(6):885–893.

Faktorovich EG, Steinberg RH, Yasumura D, Matthes MT, LaVail MM. 1990. Photoreceptor degeneration in inherited retinal dystrophy delayed by the basic fibroblast growth factor. Nature 347:83–86.

Faktorovich EG, Steinberg RH, Yasumura D, Matthes MT, LaVail

MM. 1992. Basic fibroblast growth factor and local injury protect photoreceptors from light damage in the retina. J Neurosci 12:3554–3567.

Fariss RN, Anderson DH, Fisher SK. 1990. Comparison of photoreceptor-specific matrix domains in the cat and monkey. Exp Eye Res 51:473–485.

Feeney L. 1973. The interphotoreceptor space. II. Histochemistry of the matrix. Dev Biol 32:115–128.

Fisher SK, Anderson DH. 1989. Cellular effects of detachment on the neural retina and the retinal pigment epithelium. In: Ryan S, ed, Retinal Diseases. St Louis: Mosby, 165–189.

Frishman LJ, Yamamoto JF, Bogucka J, Steinberg RH. 1992. Light evoked changes in [K+] in proximal portion of light-adapted cat retina. J Neurophys 67(5):1201–1212.

Gao H, Hollyfield JG. 1992. Basic fibroblast growth factor (bFGF) immunolocalization in the reodent outer retina demonstrated with an anti-rodent bFGF antibody. Brain Res 585:355–360.

Gao H, Hollyfield JG. 1995. Basic fibroblast growth factor in retinal development: differential levels of bFGF expression and content in normal and retinal degeneration (rd) mutant mice. Dev Biol 169(1):168–184.

Gaur VP, Liu Y, Turner JE. 1992. RPE conditioned medium stimulates photoreceptor cell survival, neurite outgrowth, and differentiation in vitro. Exp Eye Res 54:645–659.

Hageman GS, Johnson LV. 1985. Distribution of IgA and IgG within the interphotoreceptor matrix: selective association with cone photoreceptors. Invest Ophthalmol Vis Sci 26(suppl):239.

Hageman GS, Johnson LV. 1986a. Biochemical characterization of the major peanut-agglutinin-binding glycoproteins in vertebrate retinae. J Comp Neurol 249:499–510.

Hageman GS, Johnson LV. 1986b. Further characterization of cone-associated interphotoreceptor matrix domains. Proc Int Soc Eye Res 4:22.

Hageman GS, Johnson LV. 1987. Chondroitin 6-sulfate glycosaminoglycan is a major constituent of primate cone photoreceptor matrix sheaths. Curr Eye Res 6:639–646.

Hageman GS, Johnson LV. 1991. Structure, composition and function of the retinal interphotoreceptor matrix. In: Osborne N, Chader J, eds, Progress in Retinal Research, vol 10, Oxford: Pergamon Press, 207–249.

Hageman GS, Lazarus HS. 1992a. An altered composition of rod photoreceptor-associated with macular degeneration. Ophthalmol Vis Sci 33(suppl):803.

Hageman GS, Lazarus HS. 1992b. Compositional changes in human interphotoreceptor matrix proteoglycans associated with macular drusen. Exp Eye Res 55(suppl):237.

Hageman GS, Hewitt AT, Kirchoff M, Johnson LV. 1989. Selective extraction and characterization of cone matrix sheath-specific molecules. Invest Ophthalmol Vis Sci 30(suppl):489.

Hageman GS, Kirchoff MA, Anderson DH. 1990. Biochemical characterization and distribution of retinal interphotoreceptor matrix glycoconjugates. Glycoconjugate J 7(5):129.

Hageman GS, Kirchoff-Rempe MA, Lewis GP, Fisher SK, Anderson DH. 1991. Sequestration of basic fibroblast growth factor in the primate retinal interphotoreceptor matrix. Proc Natl Acad Sci USA 88:6706–6710.

Hageman GS, Kirchoff-Rempe MA, Rotramel JR, Kuehn MH. 1992. Molecular and compositional characterization of interphotoreceptor matrix proteoglycans. Proc Int Soc Eye Res 7:33.

Hageman GS, Marmor MF, Yao XY, Johnson LV. 1995. The interphotoreceptor matrix mediates primate retinal adhesion. Arch Ophthalmol 113:655–660.

Hageman GS, Kim CK, Mullins RF. Submitted. Interspecies biochem-

ical heterogeneity of cone matrix sheath-associated proteoglycans. J Comp Neurol.

Hanneken A, Baird A. 1992. Immunolocalization of basic fibroblast growth factor: dependence on antibody type and tissue fixation. Exp Eye Res 54:1011–1014.

Hanneken A, Lutty GA, McLeod DS, Robey F, Harvey AK, Hjelmeland LM. 1989. Localization of basic fibroblast growth factor in the developing capillaries of the bovine retina. J Cell Physiol 138:115–120.

Hansson HA, Holmgren A, Norstedt G, Rozell G. 1989. Changes in the distribution of insulin-like growth factor I, thioredoxin, thioredoxin reductase and ribonucleotide reductase during the development of the retina. Exp Eye Res 48:411–420.

Hardwick C, et al. 1992. Molecular cloning of a novel hyaluronan receptor that mediates tumor cell motility. J Cell Biol 117(6):1343–1350.

Hay E, ed. 1991. Cell Biology of Extracellular Matrix. New York: Plenum Press.

Hayasaka S, Shiono T, Hara S, Mizuno K. 1981. Regional distribution of lysosomal enzymes in the retina and choroid of human eyes. Graefes Arch Clin Exp Ophthalmol 216:269–273.

Heinegard D, Paulsson M. 1984. Structure and metabolism of proteoglycans. In: Piez K, Reddi A, eds, Cell Biology of the Extracellular Matrix. New York: Elsevier, 277–328.

Hewitt AT, Adler R. 1989. The retinal pigment epithelium and interphotoreceptor matrix: structure and specialized function. In: Ogden TE, ed, Retina. St Louis: Mosby, 57–64.

Hewitt AT, Newsome DA. 1988. Altered proteoglycans in cultured human retinitis pigmentosa retinal pigment epithelium. Invest Ophthalmol Vis Sci 29:720–726.

Hewitt AT, Lindsey JD, Carbott D, Adler R. 1990. Photoreceptor survival-promoting activity in interphotoreceptor matrix preparations: characterization and partial purification. Exp Eye Res 50(1):79–88.

Hodson S, Armstrong I, Wigham C. 1994. Regulation of the retinal interphotoreceptor matrix Na by the retinal pigment epithelium during the light response. Experientia 50(5):438–441.

Hollyfield JG, Fliesler SJ, Rayborn ME, Fong SL, Landers RA, Bridges CD. 1985. Synthesis and secretion of interstitial retinol-binding protein by the human retina. Invest Ophthalmol Vis Sci 26:58–67.

Hollyfield JG, Varner HH, Rayborn ME, Osterfeld AM. 1989. Retinal attachment to the pigment epithelium. Retina 9:59–68.

Hollyfield J, Rayborn ME, Landers RA, Myers KM. 1990a. Insoluble interphotoreceptor matrix domains surround rod photoreceptors in the human retina. Exp Eye Res 51(1):107–110.

Hollyfield JG, Varner HH, Rayborn ME. 1990b. Regional variation within the interphotoreceptor matrix from fovea to the retinal periphery. Eye 4:333–339.

Hollyfield JG, Rayborn ME, Tien L, Iwasaki M, Landers RA. 1992. Characterization, distribution and origin of the insoluble components of the IPM. Proc Int Soc Eye Res 7:814.

Huang B, Karwoski CJ. 1992. Light-evoked expansion of subretinal space volume in the retina of the frog. J Neuroscience 12(11):4243–4252.

Huang Q, Shur BD, Begovac PC. 1995. Overexpressing cell surface beta 1,4-galactosyltransferase in PC12 cells increases neurite outgrowth on laminin. J Cell Sci 108:839–847.

Hunter DD, Murphy MD, Olsson CV, Brunken WJ. 1992. S-Laminin expression in adult and developing retinae: a potential cue for photoreceptor morphogenesis. Neuron 8:399–413.

Iwasaki M, Myers KM, Rayborn ME, Hollyfield JG. 1992a. Interphotoreceptor matrix in the human retina: cone-like domains surround a small population of rod photoreceptors. J Comp Neurol 319(2):277–284.

Iwasaki M, Rayborn ME, Tawara A, Hollyfield JG. 1992b. Proteoglycans in the mouse interphotoreceptor matrix. V. Distribution at the apical surface of the pigment epithelium before and after retinal separation. Exp Eye Res 54:415–432.

Jaworski DM, Kelly GM, Hockfield S. 1994. BEHAB, a new member of the proteoglycan tandem repeat family of hyaluronan-binding proteins that is restricted to the brain. J Cell Biol 125(2):495–509.

Johnson AT, Kretzer FL, Hittner HM, Glazebrook PA, Bridges CD, Lam DM. 1985. Development of the subretinal space in the preterm human eye: ultrastructural and immunocytochemical studies. J Comp Neurol 233:497–505.

Johnson LV, Hageman GS. 1987. Enzymatic characterization of peanut agglutinin-binding components in the retinal interphotoreceptor matrix. Exp Eye Res 44:553–565.

Johnson LV, Hageman GS. 1991. Structural and compositional analyses of isolated cone matrix sheaths. Invest Ophthalmol Vis Sci 32(7):1951–1957.

Johnson LV, Hageman GS, Blanks JC. 1985. Restricted extracellular matrix domains ensheath cone photoreceptors in vertebrate retinae. In: Bridges CDB, Adler AJ, eds, The Interphotoreceptor Matrix in Health and Disease. New York: Liss, 36–46.

Johnson LV, Hageman GS, Blanks JC. 1986. Interphotoreceptor matrix domains ensheath vertebrate cone photoreceptor cells. Invest Ophthalmol Vis Sci 27:129–135.

Jomary C, Neal MJ, Jones SE. 1995. Increased expression of retinal TIMP3 mRNA in simplex retinitis pigmentosa is localized to photoreceptor-retaining regions. J Neurochem 64(5):2370–2373.

Jones BE, Moshyed P, Gallo S, Tombran-Tink J, Arand G, Reid DA, Thompson EW, Chader GJ, Waldbillig RJ. 1994. Characterization and novel activation of 72-kDa metalloproteinase in retinal interphotoreceptor matrix and Y-79 cell culture medium. Exp Eye Res 59:257–269.

Jones SE, Jomary C, Neal MJ. 1994. Expression of TIMP-3 mRNA is elevated in retinas affected by simplex retinitis pigmentosa. FEBS Lett 352:171–174.

Juliano RL, Haskill S. 1993. Signal transduction from the extracellular matrix. J Cell Biol 120:577–585.

Juliusson B, Mieziewska K, Bergstrom A, Wilke K, van Veen T, Ehinger B. 1994. Interphotoreceptor matrix components in retinal cell transplants. Exp Eye Res 58:615–622.

Kaneko M. 1987. Interphotoreceptor matrix glycosaminoglycans in bovine eye. Ophthalmic Res 19:330–337.

Kaplan MW, Iwata RT, Sterrett CB. 1990. Retinal detachment prevents normal assembly of disk membranes in vitro. Invest Ophthalmol Vis Sci 31:1–8.

Korte GE, Hageman GS, Pratt DV, Glusman S, Marko M, Ophir A. 1992. Changes in Muller cell plasma membrane specializations during subretinal scar formation in the rabbit. Exp Eye Res 55:155–162.

Korte GE, Moskowitz L, Mrowiec E, Hamou D. 1994. Hyaluronate distribution in the regenerating retinal pigment epithelium of the rabbit: a study using confocal laser scanning microscopy. Microscopy Res Tech 29:34–349.

Kuehn MH, Hageman GS. 1995. Characterization of a cDNA encoding IPM 150, a novel human interphotoreceptor matrix chondroitin 6-sulfate proteoglycan. Invest Ophthalmol Vis Sci Suppl 36:510.

Kuehn MH, Mullins RF, Hageman GS. 1993. Retinal interphotoreceptor matrix proteoglycan core protein sequences are unique and highly conserved. Invest Ophthamol Vis Sci 34(suppl):1201.

Lacy BE, Underhill CB. 1987. The hyaluronate receptor is associated with actin filaments. J Cell Biol 105:1395–1404.

Landers RA, Hollyfield JG. 1992. Proteoglycans in the mouse interphotoreceptor matrix. VI. Evidence for photoreceptor synthesis of chondroitin sulfate proteoglycan using genetically fractionated retinas. Exp Eye Res 55:345–356.

Landers RA, Tawara A, Varner HH, Hollyfield JG. 1991. Proteoglycans in the mouse interphotoreceptor matrix. IV. Retinal synthesis of chondroitin sulfate proteoglycan. Exp Eye Res 52:65–74.

Landers RA, Rayborn ME, Myers KM, Hollyfield JG. 1994. Increased retinal synthesis of heparan sulfate proteoglycan and HNK-1 glycoproteins following photoreceptor degeneration. J Neurochem 63(2):737–750.

LaVail MM, Pinto LH, Yasumura D. 1981. The interphotoreceptor matrix in rats with inherited retinal dystrophy. Invest Ophthalmol Vis Sci 21:658–668.

LaVail MM, Li L, Turner JE, Yasumura D. 1992. Retinal pigment epithelial cell transplantation in RCS rats: normal metabolism in rescued photoreceptors. Exp Eye Res 55(4):555–562.

Lazarus HS, Hageman GS. 1992. Xyloside-induced disruption of interphotoreceptor matrix proteoglycans results in retinal detachment. Invest Ophthalmol Vis Sci 33:364–376.

Lazarus HS, Kirchoff-Rempe MA, Hageman GS. 1991. Characterization of apically-distributed interphotoreceptor glycoconjugates in the primate retina. Invest Ophthalmol Vis Sci 32(suppl):1216.

Lazarus HS, Sly WS, Kyle JW, Hageman GS. 1993. Photoreceptor degeneration and altered distribution of interphotoreceptor matrix proteoglycans in the mucopolysaccharidosis VII mouse. Exp Eye Res 56:531–541.

Lemmon V. 1988. A monoclonal antibody that binds to the surface of photoreceptors. Dev Brain Res 39:117–123.

Li JD, Gallemore RP, Dmitriev A, Steinberg RH. 1994a. Light-dependent hydration of the space surrounding photoreceptors in chick retina. Invest Ophthalmol Vis Sci 35(6):2700–2711.

Li JD, Govardovskii VI, Steinberg RH. 1994b. Light-dependent hydration of the space surrounding photoreceptors in the cat retina. Visual Neurosci 11(4):743–752.

Li A, Lane WS, Johnson LV, Chader GJ, Tombran-Tink J. 1995. Neuron-specific enolase: a neuronal survival factor in the retinal extracellular matrix? J Neurosci 15(1):385–393.

Lin H, la Cour M, Andersen MV, Miller SS. 1994. Proton-lactate cotransport in the apical membrane of frog retinal pigment epithelium. Exp Eye Res 59:679–688.

Liou GI, et al. 1986. Bovine interstitial retinol-binding protein (IRBP): isolation and sequence analysis of cDNA clones, characterization and in vitro translation of mRNA. Vision Res 26:1645–1653.

Liou GI, Geng L, Baehr W. 1991. Interphotoreceptor retinoid-binding protein: biochemistry and molecular biology. Prog Clin Biol Res 362:115–137.

Liu H, Gaur VP, Turner JE. 1990. Photoreceptor cell survival and differentiation stimulated by rat retinal pigment epithelium in tissue culture. Invest Ophthalmol Vis Sci 31:75.

Long K, Haskins M, Aguirre G. 1989. Photoreceptor interface in β-glucuronidase deficiency: An anatomical and immunocytochemical study. Invest Ophthalmol Vis Sci 30(suppl):488.

Long KO, Aguirre GD. 1991. The cone matrix sheath in the normal and diseased retina: Cytochemical and biochemical studies of peanut agglutinin-binding proteins in cone and rod-cone degeneration. Exp Eye Res 52:699–713.

Lopez LC, Bayna EM, Litoff D, Shaper NL, Shaper JH, Shur BD. 1985. Receptor function of mouse sperm surface galactosyltransferase during fertilization. J Cell Biol 101:1501–1510.

Marmor MF. 1992. Mechanisms of retinal adhesion. Prog Ret Res 12:179–204.

Marmor MF, Yao XY, Hageman GS. 1994. Retinal adhesiveness in surgically enucleated human eyes. Retina 14:181–186.

Mieziewska K. 1993. The interphotoreceptor matrix: a study of structure and composition in normal and degenerating retinas. Doctoral dissertation, University of Göteborg.

Mieziewska K, Szel A, van Veen T, Aguirre GD, Philp N. 1994. Redistribution of insoluble interphotoreceptor matrix components during photoreceptor differentiation in the mouse retina. J Comp Neurol 345(1):115–124.

Mieziewska K, van Veen T, Aguirre GD. 1993a. Development and fate of interphotoreceptor matrix components during dysplastic photoreceptor differentiation: a lectin cytochemical study of rod-cone dysplasia 1. Exp Eye Res 56(4):429–441.

Mieziewska K, van Veen T, Aguirre GD. 1993b. Structural changes of the interphotoreceptor matrix in an inherited retinal degeneration: a lectin cytochemical study of progressive rod-cone degeneration. Invest Ophthalmol Vis Sci 34(11):3056–3067.

Mieziewska KE, van Veen T, Murray JM, Aguirre GD. 1991. Rod and cone specific domains in the interphotoreceptor matrix. J Comp Neurol 308(3):371–380.

Milam AH, Jacobson SG. 1990. Photoreceptor rosettes with blue cone opsin immunoreactivity in retinitis pigmentosa. Ophthalmology 97:1620–1631.

Milam AH, Zong YL. 1995. Retinal pathology in retinitis pigmentosa. In: Anderson RE, ed, Degenerative Diseases of the Retina. New York: Plenum Press, 275–284.

Morris JE, Yanagishita M, Hascall VP. 1987. Proteoglycans synthesized by embryonic chicken retina in culture: composition and compartmentalization. Arch Biochem Biophys 258:206–218.

Mullen RJ, LaVail MM. 1976. Inherited retinal dystrophy: primary effect in pigment epithelium determined with experimental rat chimeras. Science 192:799–801.

Murillo-Lopez F, Politi L, Adler R, Hewitt AT. 1991. Proteoglycan synthesis in cultures of murine retinal neurons and photoreceptors. Cell Molec Neurobiol 11(6):579–591.

Needham LK, Adler R, Hewitt AT. 1988. Proteoglycan synthesis in flat cell-free cultures of chick embryo retinal neurons and photoreceptors. Dev Biol 126:304–314.

Oakley B II, Steinberg RH. 1982. Effects of maintained illumination upon [K+] in the subretinal space of frog retina. Vision Res 22:767–773.

Orzalesi N, Bottoni F, Staurenghi G. 1990. Is there a role for cone interphotoreceptor matrix in the pathogenesis of central serous chorioretinopathy? Ophthalmologica 201:49–51.

Paietta E, Hubbard AL, Wiernik PD, Diehl V, Stockert RJ. 1987. Hodgkin's cell lectin: an ectosialyltransferase and lymphocyte agglutinant related to the hepatic asialoglycoprotein receptor. Cancer Res 47:2461–2467.

Perry RJ, McNaughton PA. 1993. The mechanism of ion transport by the Na(+)−Ca2+,K+ exchange in rods isolated from the salamander retina. J Physiol 466:443–480.

Pfeffer B, Wiggert B, Lee L, Zonnenberg B, Newsome D, Chader G. 1983. The presence of a soluble interphotoreceptor retinol-binding protein (IRBP) in the retinal interphotoreceptor space. J Cell Physiol 117:333–341.

Pfeffer BA, Kirchoff-Rempe MA, Guerin CJ, Matsumoto B, Anderson DH, Hageman GS. 1991. RPE contribution to primate interphotoreceptor matrix, assessed by analysis of proteins biosynthetically labelled in situ and in vivo. Invest Ophthalmol Vis Sci 32(suppl):1217.

Philp NJ, Nachmias VT. 1987. Polarized distribution of integrin and fibronectin in retinal pigment epithelium. Invest Ophthalmol Vis Sci 28:939–949.

Plantner JJ. 1992a. High molecular weight mucin-like glycoproteins of the bovine interphotoreceptor matrix. Exp Eye Res 54:113–125.

Plantner JJ. 1992b. The presence of neutral metalloproteolytic activity and metalloproteinase inhibitors in the interphotoreceptor matrix. Curr Eye Res 11(1):91–101.

Porrello K, LaVail MM. 1986. Immunocytochemical localization of chondroitin sulfates in the interphotoreceptor matrix of the normal and dystrophic rat retina. Curr Eye Res 5:981–993.

Porrello K, Yasumura D, LaVail MM. 1986. The interphotoreceptor matrix in RCS rats: histochemical analysis and correlation with the rate of retinal degeneration. Exp Eye Res 43:413–429.

Porrello K, Yasumura D, LaVail MM. 1989. Immunogold localization of chondroitin 6-sulfate in the interphotoreceptor matrix of normal and RCS rats. Invest Ophthalmol Vis Sci 30(4):638-651.

Porello K, Bhat SP, Bok D. 1991. Detection of interphotoreceptor retinoid binding protein (IRBP) mRNA in human and cone-dominant squirrel retinas by in situ hybridization. J Histochem Cytochem 39:171–176.

Rizzolo LJ, Heiges M. 1991. The polarity of the retinal pigmented epithelium is developmentally regulated. Exp Eye Res 53:549–553.

Rizzola LJ, Zhou S, Li Z-Q. 1994. The neural retina maintains integrins in the apical membrane of the RPE early in development. Invest Ophthalmol Vis Sci 35(5):2567–2576.

Rodrigues M, Hackett, J, Wiggert B, Gery I, Speigel A, Krishna G, Stein P, Chader G. 1987. Immunoelectron microscopic localization of photoreceptor-specific markers in the monkey retina. Curr Eye Res 6:369–380.

Rotramel JR, Kirchoff-Rempe, MA, Hageman GS. 1992. Identification of core proteins from primate interphotoreceptor matrix chondroitin sulfate proteoglycans. Invest Ophthalmol Vis Sci 33(suppl):815.

Russell SR, Hageman GS. 1992. Chondroitin-sulfate induced generation of epiretinal membranes. Arch Ophthalmol 110:1000–1006.

Russell SR, Hageman GS. 1997. Insoluble interphotoreceptor matrix in human vitreous after rhegmatogenous retinal detachment. Am J Ophthalmol 123:386–391.

Sameshima M, Ohba N, Euhara F, Kawano KF. 1984. Binding sites of peanut agglutinin in mammalian retina. Jpn J Ophthalmol 28:205–214.

Sanyal S, de Ruiter A, Hawkins RK. 1980. Development and degeneration of retina in rds mutant mice: light microscopy. J Comp Neurol 194:193–207.

Schubert D, LaCorbiere M. 1985. Isolation of an adhesion-mediating protein from the chick neural retina adherons. J Cell Biol 101:1071–1077.

Sheedlo HJ, Li L, Turner JE. 1989. (Na+ + K+)−ATPase and opsin in retinas of RCS dystrophic rats: time course study. Curr Eye Res 8:741–750.

Sheffield JB, Graff D. 1991. Extracellular proteases in developing chick neural retina. Exp Eye Res 52:733–741.

Shuster TA, Walter AE, Williams DS, Farber DB. 1987. Identification of a peanut agglutinin-binding protein from human retina. Exp Eye Res 45(5):685–694.

Spencer M, Moon RT, Milam AH. 1991. Membrane skeleton protein 4.1 in inner segments of retinal cones. Invest Ophthalmol Vis Sci 32:1–7.

Spoerri PE, Ulshafer RJ, Ludwig HC, Allen CB, Kelley KC. 1988. Photoreceptor cell development in vitro: influence of pigment epithelium conditioned medium on outer segment differentiation. Eur J Cell Biol 46:362–367.

Steele FR, Chader GJ, Johnson LV, Tombran-Tink J. 1993. Pigment epithelium-derived factor: neurotrophic activity and identification as a member of the serine protease inhibitor gene family. Proc Natl Acad Sci USA 90(4):1526–1530.

Steinberg RH, Oakley BI, Neimeyer G. 1980. Light evoked changes in [K+] in retina of the intact cat eye. J Neurophys 44:897–921.

Stramm L, Li W, Haskins M, Aguirre G. 1991. Glycosaminoglycan and collagen metabolism in arylsulfatase B-deficient retinal pigment epithelium in vitro. Invest Ophthalmol Vis Sci 32:2034–2041.

Sweatt AJ, Balsamo J, Lilien J. 1991. Immunolocalization of N-acetyl-galactosaminylphosphotransferase in the adult retina and subretinal space. Exp Eye Res 53(4):479–487.

Sweatt AJ, Balsamo J, Lilien J. 1995. Rod outer segment-associated N-acetylgalactosaminylphosphotransferase. Invest Ophthalmol Vis Sci 36(1):163–173.

Szel A, von Schantz M, Rohlich P, Farber DB, van Veen T. 1993. Difference in PNA label intensity between short- and long-wavelength sensitive cones in the ground squirrel retina. Invest Ophthalmol Vis Sci 34:3641–3645.

Takumi K, Uehara F. 1991. In vivo lectin-binding of photoreceptors and interphotoreceptor matrix in rat. Jpn J Ophthalmol 35:16–22.

Tate DJ, Oliver PO, Miceli MV, Stern D, Shuster S, Newsome DA. 1993. Age-dependent change in the hyaluronic acid content of the human chorioretinal complex. Arch Ophthalmol 111:963–967.

Tawara A, Hollyfield JG. 1990. Proteoglycans in the mouse interphotoreceptor matrix. III. Changes during photoreceptor development and degeneration in the rds mutant. Exp Eye Res 51(3):301–315.

Tawara A, Varner HH, Hollyfield JG. 1989. Proteoglycans in the mouse interphotoreceptor matrix. II. Origin and development of proteoglycans. Exp Eye Res 48:815–839.

Tien L, Rayborn ME, Hollyfield JG. 1992. Characterization of the interphotoreceptor matrix surrounding rod photoreceptors in the human retina. Exp Eye Res 55(2):297–306.

Tien L, Rayborn ME, Hollyfield JG. 1993. Characterization of GP147, a major WGA-binding glycoprotein in the IPM of human retina. Invest Ophthalmol Vis Sci 34(suppl):1204.

Tombran-Tink J, Chader GG, Johnson LV. 1991. PEDF: a pigment epithelium derived factor with potent neuronal differentiative activity. Exp Eye Res 53:411–414.

Tombran-Tink J, Li A, Johnson MA, Johnson LV, Chader GJ. 1992. Neurotrophic activity of interphotoreceptor matrix on human Y79 retinoblastoma cells. J Comparative Neurol 317:175–186.

Tombran-Tink J, Shivaram SM, Chader GJ, Johnson LV, Bok D. 1995. Expression, secretion and age-related down regulation of pigment epithelium-derived factor, a serpin with neurothropic activity. J Neurosci 15:4992–5003.

Toole B. 1991. Proteoglycans and hyaluronan in morphogenesis and differentiation. In: Hay E, ed, Cell Biology of Extracellular Matrix. New York: Plenum Press, 305–341.

Turley EA, Roth S. 1980. Interactions between the carbohydrate chains of hyaluronan and chondroitin sulfate. Nature 283:268–271.

Uehara F, Sameshima M, Muramatsu T, Ohba N. 1983. Localization of fluorescence-labeled lectin binding sites on photoreceptor cells of the monkey retina. Exp Eye Res 36:113–123.

Uehara F, Muramatsu T, Ohba N. 1986. Two-dimensional gel electrophoretic analysis of lectin receptors in the bovine interphotoreceptor matrix. Exp Eye Res 43(2):227–234.

Uehara F, Matthes MT, Yasumura D, LaVail MM. 1990a. Light-evoked changes in the interphotoreceptor matrix. Science 248(4963):1633–1636.

Uehara F, Yasumura D, LaVail MM. 1990b. Lectin binding of the interphotoreceptor matrix during retinal development in normal and RCS rats. Curr Eye Res 9:687–695.

Uehara F, Yasumura D, LaVail MM. 1991a. Development of light-evoked changes of the interphotoreceptor matrix in normal and RCS rats with inherited retinal dystrophy. Exp Eye Res 53(1):55–60.

Uehara F, Yasumura D, LaVail MM. 1991b. Rod- and cone-associated interphotoreceptor matrix in the rat retina. Invest Ophthalmol Vis Sci 32(2):285–292.

Uehara F, Yasumura D, Matthes MT, LaVail MM. 1991c. Light-induced changes in the interphotoreceptor matrix: implications for inherited retinal degenerations and normal photoreceptor physiology. In: Anderson RE, Hollyfield JG, LaVail MM, eds, Retinal Degenerations. Boca Raton, FL: CRC Press, 227–241.

Vaughan DK, Fisher SK. 1987. The disruption of F-actin in cells isolated from vertebrate retinas. Exp Eye Res 44:393.

Wacker WB, Donoso LA, Kalsow CM, Yankeelow JA, Organischiak DT. 1977. Experimental allergic uveitis: isolation, characterization and localization of a soluble uveitopathogenic antigen from the bovine retina. J Immunol 119:1499.

Waldbillig RJ, Pfeffer BA, Schoen TJ, Adler AA, Shen-Orr Z, Scavo L, LeRoith D, Chader GJ. 1991. Evidence for an insulin-like growth factor autocrine-paracrine system in the retinal photoreceptor-pigment epithelial cell complex. J Neurochem 57(5):1522–1533.

Weber BH, Vogt G, Pruett RC, Stohr H, Felbor U. 1994. Mutations in the tissue inhibitor of metalloproteinases-3 (TIMP3) in patients with Sorsby's fundus dystrophy. Nature Genetics 8(4):352–356.

Wight TN, Kinsellaa MG, Qwarnstrom EE. 1992. The role of proteoglycans in cell adhesion, migration and proliferation. Curr Opin Cell Biol 4:793–801.

Wortman B, Freeman M. 1962. Resolution of bovine mucopolysaccharides by anion-exchange chromatography. Fed Proc 21:483.

Yamamoto F, Borgula GA, Steinberg RH. 1992. Effects of light and darkness on pH outside rod photoreceptors in the cat retina. Exp Eye Res 54(5):685–697.

Yao XY, Hageman GS, Marmor MF. 1990. Retinal adhesiveness is weakened by enzymatic modification of the interphotoreceptor matrix in vivo. Invest Ophthalmol Vis Sci 31(10):2051–2058.

Yao XY, Hageman GS, Marmor MF. 1992. Recovery of retinal adhesion after enzymatic perturbation of the interphotoreceptor matrix. Invest Ophthalmol Vis Sci 33:498–503.

Yao XY, Hageman GS, Marmor MF. 1994. Retinal adhesiveness in the monkey. Invest Ophthalmol Vis Sci 35(2):744–748.

Ying SY, Li S, Ishikawa M, Johnson LV. 1995. Immunohistochemical localization of inhibin in the retinal interphotoreceptor matrix. Exp Eye Res 60:585–590.

19. Mechanisms of retinal adhesiveness

MICHAEL F. MARMOR

The primary role of the retinal pigment epithelium (RPE) in the eye is to support retinal function. This is accomplished in a variety of ways, including the absorption of scattered light which might degrade visual images, the provision of a cellular barrier to prevent unwanted proteins from entering the neural domain, active transport to bring nutrients to the retina and dispose of undesirable material, the storage and processing of visual pigments to sustain the visual cycle, the phagocytosis and digestion of waste material from outer segment metabolism and regeneration, and the control of subretinal fluid to keep the subretinal space tight and dry (which facilitates many of the other support functions). None of these would be effective, however, without another RPE function, the maintenance of retinal adhesion. The subretinal space is the remnant of the embryonic cavity within the optic vesicle that forms as a bud off the developing brain. This vesicle collapses into a cup, which forms neural retina from its inner surface and RPE from the outer. The space between is never bridged by tissue (Steinberg and Wood, 1974), and yet the retina remains rather firmly attached to RPE throughout life (barring the intervention of pathology). This adhesion is vital to the retina, since a detached retina can no longer register focused images, and detached photoreceptors eventually degenerate for lack of nutrients or other factors from the RPE.

The mechanisms of retinal adhesiveness are complex and multifactorial, because a variety of physical and physiological forces impinge upon the subretinal space and the matrix which fills it. The earliest studies on retinal adhesion, more than twenty years ago, by Berman (1969) and Zauberman and Berman (1969), recognized a viscous tension between the layers, as if there was a physiologic glue keeping them together. Work in the ensuing 10–15 years demonstrated that retinal adhesiveness also depended upon metabolism (Zauberman and deGuillebon, 1972; Marmor et al., 1980a) and it seemed like active processes rather than a passive matrix (Adler and Klucznik, 1982a) were the keys to understanding why retina adheres. In the most recent decade, we have learned more about the structure and composition of the interphotoreceptor matrix (IPM), and how it binds across the subretinal space. The pen-

dulum of opinion has settled back in the middle, insofar as the IPM appears to provide the primary bond between retina and RPE, but the strength of this bond is dependent upon RPE metabolic activity and fluid transport.

Two reviews on mechanisms of adhesion have been published recently, which covered much of the literature on retinal adhesive force including techniques of measurement (Marmor, 1993; 1994). This chapter will concentrate on recent work that frames our current understanding of the process.

MEASUREMENT OF RETINAL ADHESION: NORMAL VALUES

It is difficult to measure retinal adhesive force because of limited access to the tissue in the living eye and the problem of rapid failure of adhesive strength (within minutes) in excised tissue. Most experimenters have used excised tissue, prepared as rapidly as possible. The retina has been pulled (Zauberman et al., 1972; Owczarek et al., 1975; Böse et al., 1981) or peeled (Lincoff et al., 1970; deGuillebon et al., 1971; Marmor et al., 1980a) from the RPE while measuring the force required, or secondary effects at the retina–RPE interface (such as the adherence of RPE pigment to peeled retina [Endo et al., 1988]) have been monitored. The first accurate in vivo measurements of adhesive force were made by Kita and colleagues, 1990, who measured the pressure required to expand experimental detachments within the living eye. Small detachments were made by injecting fluid into the subretinal space through a micropipette, after which a second micropipette was inserted into the detachment cavity to measure fluid pressure. Pressure measurements (Fig. 19-1) were converted mathematically by LaPlace's law into values for adhesive force at the margin of the detachment where retinal separation was taking place.

Using this technique, the adhesive force in the rabbit was found to be 100 to 180 dynes/cm (Kita and Marmor, 1992a; Kita et al., 1990). The adhesive force was roughly 80% stronger in cats and 40% stronger in monkeys.

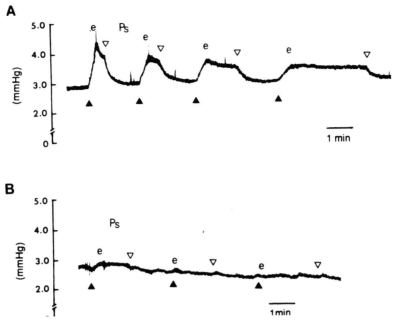

FIGURE 19-1. Recordings of subretinal pressure in the living rabbit eye from within blisterlike experimental detachments. The magnitude of pressure that causes the detachment to expand is dependent on the retinal adhesive force. (A) Normal eye (detachments filled with Hanks' solution). As fluid was injected into the subretinal space (▲), the pressure rose until the retinal adhesive force was overcome and the detachment began to expand (e); expansion continued until the injection was stopped (∇). (B) Detachments filled with Ca^{2+}-free EDTA solution. Adhesive force was low and detachments expanded after only minimal elevation of pressure. (Modified from Kita, Negi and Marmor, 1992.)

MODULATION OF ADHESIVENESS: MODIFYING FACTORS AND REVERSIBILITY

Ionic Environment

Retinal adhesiveness is sensitive to calcium and magnesium concentration, and to pH. Removal of calcium and magnesium from the subretinal space in vivo (Fig. 19-1) weakens retinal adhesion in rabbits to about 30% of normal (Kita et al., 1992). Calcium and magnesium removal also hastens postmortem adhesive failure in rabbit, primate, and human tissue, as does lowering the pH to 6.0 (Marmor et al., 1994; Yao et al., 1994). Changes in potassium, sulfate, and phosphate did not alter retinal adhesiveness in rabbit experiments (Marmor and Maack, 1982b). The effects of calcium changes in rabbits can be observed within seconds, suggesting that this ion plays an important and active role in regulating some aspect of the adhesive mechanism. The calcium and pH effects are also reversible: in both rabbit (Yao et al., 1989) and human tissue (Marmor et al., 1994), after postmortem adhesive failure has begun in a low-calcium bath, adhesiveness will recover to control levels within a few minutes after restoring a normal ionic en-

vironment (Fig. 19-2). It has been argued that postmortem adhesive failure is a result of proteolytic destruction of the IPM, since proteolytic enzymes (Adler and Martin, 1983) can be activated at low calcium levels (Kain and Libondi, 1986). However, this explanation is difficult to reconcile with the fact that adhesiveness recovers very quickly upon restoring normal calcium, since this would be unlikely had the adhesive IPM been enzymatically destroyed.

Temperature

Cooling has a powerful effect upon retinal adhesion— or at least upon the rate of postmortem degradation (Endo et al., 1988; Marmor et al., 1994; Marmor and Yao, 1989; 1990; Yao et al., 1994; 1989; Yoon and Marmor, 1988a). In eye tissue kept at body temperature (37 °C) after enucleation, retinal adhesiveness fails almost completely within 5 minutes in the rabbit, and within 40 to 50 minutes in human or primate tissue. These changes are slowed severalfold by cooling to 16 to 20 °C (Fig. 19-3), and adhesive force can be maintained at control levels for hours in tissue that is cooled to 4 °C. Adhesive strength that has been lost through

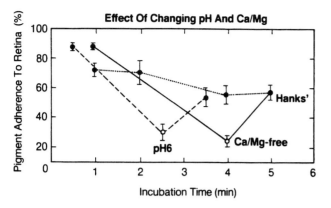

FIGURE 19-2. Reversibility of low-pH or low-Ca/Mg effects on retinal adhesiveness. In this experiment, the residual adherence of pigment (as retina was peeled from the RPE) was used as an index of adhesiveness. Control tissue maintained in Hanks' solution *(closed circles)* showed a stable retinal adhesive force. Tissue changed from pH 7.4 to 6.0 *(dashed line, open circle)* lost adhesiveness, but recovered it on restoration of pH 7.4. Similarly, exposure to Ca/Mg-free solution *(solid line, open circle)* caused a loss of adhesiveness that was recovered on restoring normal Ca/Mg levels. (From Marmor, 1993.)

postmortem incubation at 37 °C will recover to a large degree after cooling to 4 °C.

The mechanism of these temperature effects on retinal adhesiveness is still obscure. Temperature modulates metabolic activity, which is a factor in the maintenance of adhesion (see "Mechanisms of Retinal Adhesion," below). However, active RPE metabolism supports adhesion, while the effect of cold (which shuts down metabolism) is to strengthen rather than weaken adhesive force. Some of the adhesion-enhancing effects of cold may result from inhibition of the sodium pump and secondary tissue swelling, which makes interdigitated outer segments and RPE microvilli harder to separate (Marmor et al., 1980a; Marmor and Yao, 1989). Cold may also modify the binding and elastic properties of the IPM in ways that makes separation more difficult. Whatever their mechanism, the effects of cold are powerful; they block or mask the adhesive-weakening effects of low pH and low calcium.

Oxidative Metabolism

The rapid failure of retinal adhesion postmortem or in excised tissue can be prevented to a large degree by improving the oxygenation of the excised tissue (Kim et al., 1993; Marmor and Yao, 1992). Strips of monkey eyecup kept at 37 °C in a balanced salt solution in an open petri dish (oxygen pressure, $pO_2 = 205$ mm Hg) lose most of their retinal adhesive strength in about 30 minutes. If the tissue is bathed in a hypoxic nitrogen-bubbled solution ($pO_2 = 101$), the adhesive strength is lost in only 10 minutes (Fig. 19-4). However, circulating

oxygenated balanced salt solution ($pO_2 = 500$) over the tissue preserves adhesive strength well beyond an hour. The effect of oxygen is not simply the result of delaying a degradative process. Tissue that had lost adhesiveness while incubated in nitrogen-circulated solution regained adhesive strength back to control levels upon restoration of an oxygenated medium. In other words, the level of oxygenation reversibly modulates adhesive strength. These effects depend upon oxidative rather than anaerobic metabolism, since adhesive strength was unaffected (at least within the time frame of these experiments) by replacement of glucose in the bath with sucrose (which does not readily cross cell membranes). As might be expected, cyanide placed in the bath reduced adhesiveness.

The results from in vivo experiments are also supportive of an oxidative metabolic requirement for retinal adhesiveness (Marmor and Yao, 1992; Marmor and Takeuchi, 1996). When rabbit eyes were made ischemic (by raising intraocular pressure) for just two minutes, the strength of retinal adhesion (measured either in vivo or in vitro after rapidly enucleating the eye) was reduced to very low levels. Subretinal injection of the metabolic inhibitor dinitrophenol also reduces adhesive force (measured in vivo) to an unrecordable level. This ischemic adhesive failure was reversible either by restoring the ocular circulation or by placing excised tissue in a circulating oxygen-bubbled bath. However, the longer the duration of in vivo ischemia, the longer the duration of reperfusion required to restore normal adhesive strength. After one minute of ischemia, in vivo adhesive

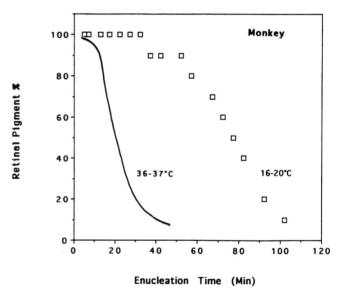

FIGURE 19-3. Effect of cooling on the rate at which retinal adhesiveness fails in the monkey after enucleation. Adhesive failure was delayed at a cooler temperature. (Data from Yao et al., 1994.)

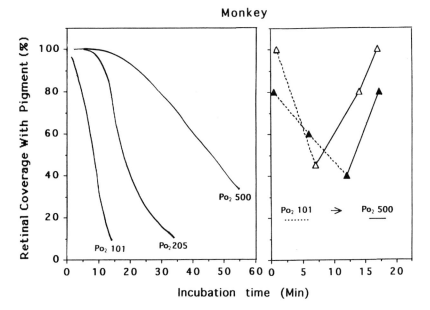

FIGURE 19-4. Effects of oxygenation on the maintenance of retinal adhesive strength in excised primate retina. *Left:* Tissue at pO_2 = 205 lost most of its adhesiveness within 30 minutes. The loss was even faster at pO_2 = 101, but tissue at pO_2 = 500 maintained high levels for more than one hour. *Right:* Restoring oxygen to poorly oxygenated tissue (that had lost adhesiveness) restored normal adhesive force. (Data from Marmor and Yao, 1995.)

strength returned to near normal values within 15 minutes of reperfusion; after 10 minutes of ischemia, more than one hour of reperfusion was required (Fig. 19-5).

Transport Inhibitors

Acetazolamide was found many years ago in rabbit experiments in vitro to strengthen retinal adhesiveness and enhance the rate of outward fluid transport across the RPE (Marmor et al., 1980a; Marmor and Maack, 1982a). This result has since been confirmed by in vivo experiments in both rabbits and monkeys (Fig. 19-6) (Kita and Marmor, 1992a). Acetazolamide is effective only when given systemically, and it does not enhance adhesion if placed in the subretinal space (Kita and Marmor, 1992b) or in an experimental bath (Marmor et al., 1980a; Marmor and Maack, 1982a). Thus, it appears to act primarily on the basal RPE membrane. Acetazolamide is a carbonic anhydrase inhibitor, but the mechanism by which it enhances either fluid transport or adhesiveness remains obscure. There is a rapid acidification of the subretinal space after acetazolamide administration to the basal RPE (Yamamoto and Steinberg, 1991), and this acidification may well be responsible for the enhanced transport and secondarily the enhanced adhesiveness. However, it is not yet clear how the drug causes this rapid apical change.

In contrast, furosemide and amiloride do act within

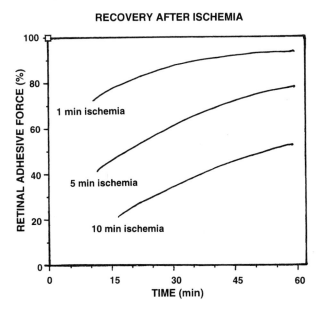

FIGURE 19-5. Effects of ocular ischemia (from elevated intraocular pressure) on retinal adhesive force, measured within the living eye. Adhesive force was reduced by as little as 1 minute's interruption of the ocular circulation, but recovery was very rapid upon restoring the circulation. Interrupting the circulation for 5 to 10 minutue caused a greater loss of adhesive force and slower recovery (still incomplete one hour after reperfusion). (Data from Marmor and Takeuchi, 1996.)

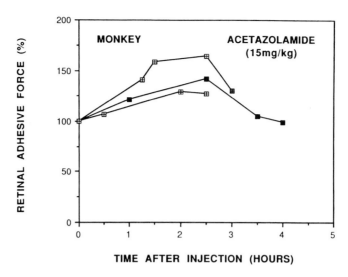

FIGURE 19-6. Enhancement of retinal adhesive force in the living primate eye by intravenous acetazo-lamide (15 mg/Kg). (From Kita and Marmor, 1992a.)

the subretinal space (Fig. 19-7), causing a small decrease in retinal force (Kita and Marmor, 1992b). They are known to reduce apical-to-basal fluid transport in epithelial systems (Frambach and Misfeldt, 1983; Tsuboi

and Pederson, 1986). Cyclic AMP is even more effective as an inhibitor of RPE fluid transport and an inhibitor of retinal adhesive force, measured either in vitro or in vivo (Kita and Marmor, 1992b; Yoon and Marmor,

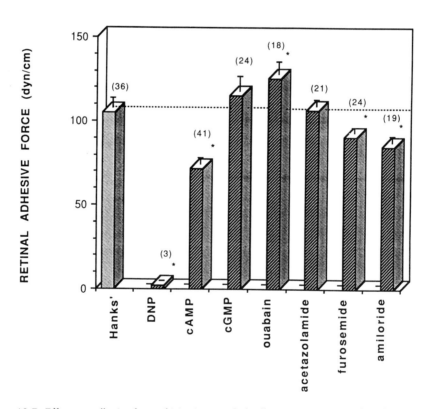

FIGURE 19-7. Effects on adhesive force of injecting metabolically active agents into the subretinal space of rabbits. The columns show mean value; the bars show standard error; the numbers of experiments are in parentheses; data with an asterisk differed significantly from control Hanks' solution (p ≤ 0.05). (From Kita and Marmor, 1992b.)

1988a). Measurements within the living eye showed a drop in adhesive force of 31% after subretinal cAMP administration. Cyclic GMP has an opposite effect upon RPE fluid transport, but no clear effect on retinal adhesiveness (Kawano and Marmor, 1988; Marmor and Negi, 1986).

The actions of the electrogenic sodium pump inhibitor ouabain are more complicated (Kita and Marmor, 1992b; Marmor et al., 1980a; Marmor and Yao, 1989). When applied to excised eyecup tissue, or to the subretinal space in vivo, its effect is to strengthen retinal adhesiveness. In the short term this may reflect loss of Na transport (and thus lower water movement) *into* the subretinal space. However, the alteration in Na gradients eventually interferes with *outward* fluid transport, and thus should in theory hydrate the subretinal space and diminish adhesiveness. Ouabain-poisoned retina rapidly becomes edematous, from accumulated intracellular sodium, and the apparent rise in adhesive strength may be a result of cellular swelling in the region of the photoreceptor outer segments and RPE microvilli (Marmor and Yao, 1989). The outer segments are firmly interdigitated between the microvillous processes, and tissue swelling tightens this mechanical interdigitation and acts to resist forces of separation.

Hydrostatic and Osmotic Pressure

Intraocular pressure contributes to retinal adhesion by moving water against the flow resistance of the retina (Fatt and Shantinath, 1971). Conversely, the placement of a hyperosmotic solution into the vitreous draws fluid in the opposite direction and produces rapid detachment of the retina (Marmor, 1979; Marmor et al., 1980b). Intravitreal injection of just 50 microliters of a 500 mOsm solution was sufficient in rabbits to produce low detachments, and massive separation occurred with solutions over 1000 mOsm. These data suggest that fluid pressure against the retina is relevant to adhesion, but they also indicate the need for caution in administering or evaluating intravitreal drugs (particularly those of low molecular weight) which have relatively high osmolarity.

Consistent with these results, the intravenous injection of mannitol, which raises choroidal osmolarity, increases retinal adhesiveness in both monkeys (Fig. 19-8) and rabbits (Kita and Marmor, 1991; Kita and Marmor, 1992a; Yao et al., 1991). The effects of a 2g/Kg mannitol injection last for roughly two hours, with retinal adhesive force rising to values 50% above normal. It remains to be determined whether this transient strengthening of adhesion might be useful in clinical circumstances where there is imminent danger of detachment (or of the spread of a detachment).

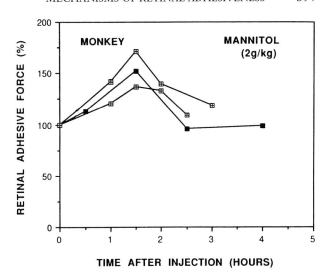

FIGURE 19-8. Enhancement of retinal adhesive force in the living primate eye by intravenous mannitol (2.0 g/Kg). (Modified from Kita and Marmor, 1992a.)

Enzymatic and Structural Modifications

Enzymes that degrade specific components of the IPM include chondroitinase ABC (which degrades chondroitin sulfate) (Yamada, 1974) and neuraminidase (which breaks down sialic acid bonds) (Uehara et al., 1985). When injected into the vitreous, or into the subretinal space of rabbits, these enzymes cause a marked reduction in retinal adhesive strength that correlates with cytochemical evidence of damage to the IPM (Fig. 19-9) (Yao et al., 1990; 1994). This IPM damage, and the loss of adhesive strength, are both reversible within about three weeks (Yao et al., 1992). It is perhaps relevant that while adhesive loss after enzyme administration correlates with the morphology of peanut or wheat germ agglutinin binding, there are no changes in lectin-binding characteristics during the first few minutes after death, when postmortem adhesive loss occurs (Hageman et al., 1995). Disrupting matrix proteoglycans with xyloside also weakens adhesion (Lazarus and Hageman, 1992).

Cytochalasin D polymerizes actin microfilaments and disrupts cytoskeletal networks, both of which affect microvilli and thus might be postulated to affect the RPE and retinal adhesion. Retinal adhesive force, measured in vivo, drops within 30 minutes of injecting cytochalasin into the vitreous of rabbit eyes (Fig. 19-10) (Chiang et al., 1995). This loss of adhesion is accompanied by changes of the surface morphology of the RPE, which showed swelling of the cone sheaths, the appearance of unusual bulletlike microvilli, and disappearance of the normal filamentous microvilli (Immel et al., 1986; Chi-

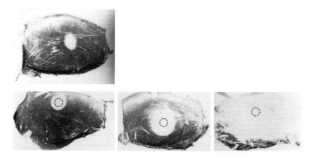

FIGURE 19-9. Effects of degradative enzymes on retinal adhesiveness. These illustrations show rabbit retinal whole-mounts that were peeled from the RPE immediately after enucleation. Where adhesion was strong, fragments of apical RPE pigment remained stuck to the retina; where it was weak, the retinal surface was clean. *Top row:* Hanks' solution was injected into the subretinal space. Only the injected locus was free of pigment 3 days later. *Bottom row:* Testicular hyaluronidase was injected subretinally into the small region shown by dotted lines, and the eyes were enucleated 1, 2, and 3 days later, respectively. Adhesive force was severely weakened over almost the entire retina by day 3. Similar effects were observed after chondroitenase and neuraminidase. (From Yao et al., 1990.)

ang et al., 1995). These anatomical changes gradually disappeared over 72 hours, concomitant with a recovery of retinal adhesive strength. Actin filaments are involved in more than microvillous morphology (Burnside and Laties, 1976) in mammalian epithelial cells; they have been implicated in sodium channel activity and in the binding of cellular adhesion molecules (Cantiello et al., 1991; Fredriksen and Leyssac, 1977; Chaitin et al., 1994). Thus, although these results suggest that actin systems are involved in retinal adhesion, they do not indicate how the microvilli participate.

Hemicholinium-3 (HC-3) interferes with choline transport, and when injected into the rabbit vitreous it causes photoreceptor outer segment and RPE degeneration within a few days (Pu and Masland, 1984; Yoon and Marmor, 1993). The photoreceptor degeneration is presumed to be a result of faulty synthesis of new membrane material, but the mechanism of the RPE damage is unclear. Retinal adhesive force fell markedly by three days after HC-3 injection, in conjunction with these anatomic changes (Negi, et al., 1993; Yoon and Marmor, 1993). However, in the first day after HC-3 injection, attempts to peel retina from the RPE often resulted in tissue separation at the level of Bruch's membrane instead of the subretinal space (Fig. 19-11). In other words, RPE rather than retinal detachment occurred. Similar results were observed within the first few minutes after intravenous injection of sodium iodate, a potent RPE toxin (Ashburn et al., 1980; Takeuchi et al., 1991; Yoon and Marmor, 1993).

MECHANISMS OF RETINAL ADHESION

Forces outside the Subretinal Space

Both the retina and RPE offer a substantial resistance to water movement (Fatt and Shantinath, 1971; Tsuboi, 1987). A side effect of the retinal resistance to flow is that the outward movement of fluid (in response to either intraocular pressure or oncotic pressure from the choroid) acts to push the retina against the RPE. Under normal conditions, there is relatively little posterior fluid flow in the eye (see Chapter 21), but Fatt and Shantinath (1971) calculated that only a minute pressure difference (less than 10^{-3} mm Hg) across the retina would generate a force sufficient to keep retina firmly positioned against the wall of the eye. In further support

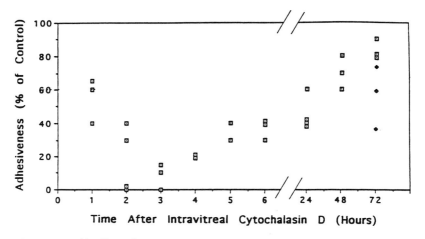

FIGURE 19-10. Reversible effects of intravitreal cytochalasin D on retinal adhesiveness in the rabbit (measured by the amount of adherent apical RPE pigment, as shown in Fig. 19-9). Adhesiveness is lost within hours of the injection, but recovers over the next 3 days. (Modified from Chiang et al., 1995.)

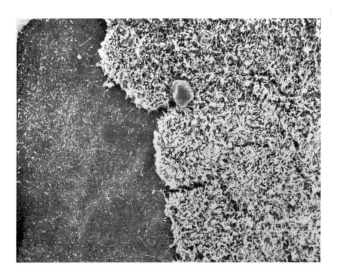

FIGURE 19-11. Scanning electron micrograph of the rabbit RPE surface after peeling the retina, 13 hours following intravitreal hemicholinium-3 injection. In large areas full-thickness RPE remained adherent to the retina and detached from Bruch's membrane (which is bare in left half of the figure). Magnification bar = 10 μm. (From Yoon and Marmor, 1993.)

of an adhesive role for hydrostatic and osmotic pressure is the evidence noted earlier (Marmor, 1979) that raising the osmotic pressure of the vitreous can cause retinal detachment. Increasing the choroidal osmotic pressure with intravenous mannitol strengthens retinal adhesion, although this effect may reflect modification of the viscosity and binding properties of the IPM as well as a movement of water (Kita and Marmor, 1991; 1992a; Yao et al., 1991).

Another possible adhesive factor, external to the subretinal space, is the vitreous gel which may physically impede retinal separation and which may serve to seal or tamponade small holes (Foulds, 1975; Osterlin, 1977). Experimentally, it is surprisingly difficult to produce or maintain experimental rhegmatogenous detachments in mammals as long as the vitreous body remains intact (Foulds, 1963; Machemer and Norton, 1968). Liquid vitreous must have access to the subretinal space in order to produce long-lasting experimental detachments.

Although hydrostatic and osmotic pressure do represent adhesive forces, they are probably not the most important adhesive forces under normal conditions. If they were, for example, one would expect retinal detachment to be a frequent finding under conditions of hypotony (which it is not). One also might expect to see many more rhegmatogenous detachments, since peripheral holes are present in roughly 10% of autopsy eyes (Rutnin and Schepens, 1978) (even granting that many of these holes not functionally open because of surround-

ing pigmentation or because of tamponade by vitreous gel). More critical, however, is the fact that there are other powerful mechanisms of adhesion (as discussed in the following sections) which seem dominant in most situations.

Mechanisms within the Subretinal Space

Anatomic relationships. The RPE microvilli wrap closely around the tips of the outer segments, an interdigitation that facilitates the daily phagocytosis of outer segment material as the photoreceptors renew their discs (Anderson and Fisher, 1986; Steinberg and Wood, 1974; Young, 1976). One might predict that retinal adhesion would be higher about the time of peak of disc shedding (in the morning for rods, and possibly late in the day for cones), as the microvilli indent the outer segments to ingest their tips. Such an effect has not been demonstrated experimentally (Marmor and Maack, 1982b), but there is evidence that retinal adhesion becomes stronger under conditions of cellular swelling (caused by cold temperature or ouabain) that would tighten the interdigitation between outer segments and RPE microvilli (Marmor and Yao, 1989).

Close ensheathment of outer segments by microvilli might also provide a frictional or electrostatic resistance to withdrawal (Gingell and Fornes, 1975). The magnitude of these effects is uncertain, but the cytoarchitecture of the RPE microvilli appears to be relevant to adhesion. As noted earlier, the disruption of actin filaments with cytochalasin-D severely weakens retinal adhesiveness (Moore et al., 1991; Chiang et al., 1995). This could be a result of loosening the villous ensheathment of the outer segments and/or a result of disrupting filamentous structures that contribute to bonding to cellular adhesion molecules in the IPM.

Interphotoreceptor matrix. The IPM is not merely a layer of viscous glue, but a highly complex material (Adler and Klucznik, 1982b; Porello and LaVail, 1986) with structural components that serve the rods and cones independently (Uehara et al., 1991; Hageman and Johnson, 1991) (see also Chapter 18). The cone matrix material can be recognized histochemically by the binding of peanut agglutin (PNA) (Hollyfield et al., 1989; Johnson et al., 1986) whereas the rod matrix material stains selectively with wheat germ agglutin (WGA) or other lectins (Hageman et al., 1990). Using these lectin stains, one can observe in fresh human and primate tissues that, as the retina is peeled from the RPE, the cone and rod matrix material stretches dramatically before breaking (Fig. 19-12) (Hageman et al., 1995; Marmor et al., 1994). The stretching indicates that the bond of IPM to

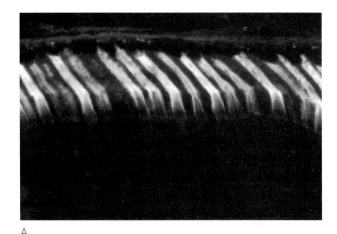

A

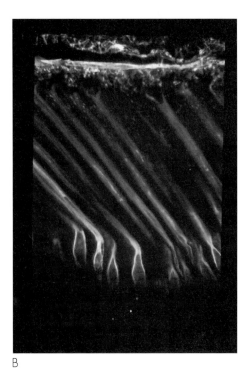

B

FIGURE 19-12. Photomicrographs of cone matrix sheaths stained with fluorescein-conjugated peanut agglutinin. In these pictures the RPE is above and neurosensory retina below. *Left:* Normal sheaths in attached retina. *Right:* Markedly elongated sheaths at the junction where retina is being peeled from the RPE. The stretching indicates that IPM had bonded across the subretinal space. Original magnification ×130. (From Hageman et al., 1995.)

retina and RPE is stronger than the elastic force of the elongated cone and rod sheaths. Within the first two minutes of death, the bond is so strong that cone matrix sheaths can stretch to more than double their normal length, and RPE cells are sometimes pulled intact off Bruch's membrane (Fig. 19-12). However, these bonds

are highly sensitive to postmortem change, and within just 4–5 min after death or enucleation, the IPM will separate without stretching. The attachment of IPM to outer segments and RPE is thought to occur with cellular adhesion molecules that have receptors at the cellular membranes. Receptors for fibronectin, integrins, and mannose have been found in outer segment or RPE membranes, but their functional importance for adhesion has not been determined (Hageman and Johnson, 1991; Kohno et al., 1987; Opas and Kalnins, 1985; Philp and Nachmias, 1987; Shirakawa et al., 1987). The localization of cellular adhesion molecules may depend upon neural retina–RPE contact (Gunderson et al., 1993) or access to ligands in the IPM structures that present to Müller cell or RPE microvilli (Chaitin et al., 1994). Similar factors may modulate adhesion of the RPE to Bruch's membrane (Ho and Del Priore, 1997).

Adhesive strength must also depend upon the viscosity and structural integrity of the matrix material itself, which is a complex mixture of proteins, glycoproteins, proteoglycans, and glycosaminoglycans. The properties of these large and intercolated molecules will be modified by hydration, ionic environment, and other factors that have been noted above to modulate retinal adhesive force. Of most direct relevance, of course, is the evidence that enzymatic degradation of chondroitin sulfate or sialic acid bonds in the IMP leads to a rapid loss of retinal adhesiveness (Yao et al., 1990; 1994).

The sum of current evidence suggests that the IPM physically bonds between retina and RPE, and that it is probably responsible for much of the retinal adhesive force under normal circumstances. However, the strength and viscosity of this bond is modulated by metabolic activity (which controls fluid movement and ionic environment), and also by forces outside the subretinal space that influence the movement and accumulation of fluid in the subretinal space.

Metabolic factors. Evidence has already been presented that retinal adhesiveness is highly sensitive to metabolic inhibitors and to the level of available oxygen. Changing the metabolic state rapidly and reversibly alters the strength of adhesion. The target cell for these effects is probably the RPE which, through active transport, controls the hydration and ionic homeostasis of the subretinal space (see Chapter 6). It is unlikely to be a coincidence that experimental factors and conditions which facilitate or inhibit the rate of fluid absorption across the RPE have a similar influence on retinal adhesion. The two are linked because the control of subretinal ions and fluid modulates the adhesive properties of the IPM. Conditions that dehydrate the subretinal space serve not only to keep the retina closely apposed, but also to keep the matrix viscous and the matrix molecules tightly interactive at ionic and receptor-binding sites.

Multifactorial issues. It is clear that different adhesive forces act upon the subretinal space simultaneously to keep retina in apposition against the RPE. The IPM is probably the major adhesive element, but its effectiveness depends critically upon the metabolic status of the RPE and the degree of hydration in the subretinal space, and it is backed up by physical forces such as hydrostatic and oncotic pressure. Retinal adhesiveness is markedly weakened by enzymatic damage to the IPM. However, it is also weakened by anoxia, metabolic inhibitors, and conditions such as vitreous hyperosmolarity which draw fluid into the subretinal space. Even under conditions where the IPM has been enzymatically damaged, the retina does not spontaneously detach. In fact, retinal detachments are rarely seen even after surgical procedures where the RPE and choroid have been totally removed (such as *en bloc* resection of a choroidal tumor). Why does the retina stay flat and attached under these circumstances where the retinal apposition cannot be a result of either IPM bonding or RPE metabolic activity? Attachment is probably a result of passive hydrostatic and osmotic forces that draw fluid through the relatively impermeable retina and push it against the wall of the eye. The actual strength of attachment may be very weak under these conditions, and retinal detachment would probably occur easily under adverse stress. Nonetheless, the detachment will still not take place unless there is such stress, such as traction on the retina and/or the development of holes. The bottom line is that retinas will not detach unless positive forces conspire to defeat the collective power of the normal mechanisms that hold retina in apposition—and this scenario fits clinical experience in which retinal detachment is, all considered, a rather rare event.

ENHANCEMENT AND REPAIR OF ADHESION

Pharmacologic Enhancement of Adhesion

It would be useful clinically to have agents that pharmacologically enhance retinal adhesive force. They could help to reduce the risk of retinal detachment in high-risk eyes. They might minimize the spread of existing detachments that are awaiting surgical repair. They could improve or hasten the healing process after surgical repair. To the extent that they act upon the absorption of subretinal fluid, they could also hasten the recovery of nonrhegmatogenous detachments, minimize the risk of their reformation, and perhaps enhance visual recovery. There are no agents presently in use for this purpose, but several strategies can be postulated.

Hyperosmotic agents such as mannitol cause a 50% increase in retinal adhesiveness in living primate eyes for a few hours after injection (see Fig. 19-8) (Kita and Marmor, 1992a). This effect will not be useful for the long-term management of recovery from detachments, but could be beneficial preoperatively or for short-term stabilization of a detachment that is threatening the macula.

Retinal adhesiveness has been increased experimentally by the pathologic conditions of cold temperature and sodium pump inhibition with ouabain. These agents block metabolic activity, and appear to increase adhesiveness by causing tissue edema rather than by enhancing the normal mechanisms of adhesion (Marmor and Yao, 1989). It is doubtful that such approaches would be useful for any long-term clinical applications, but there are special situations in which they could be valuable. For example, cooling the irrigating solution during vitrectomy might reduce the risk of a detachment developing or spreading during the manipulations of surgery.

Acetazolamide, which enhances the absorption of subretinal fluid and is in clinical use for some conditions with macular edema, increases retinal adhesiveness for several hours after intravenous injection (see Fig. 19-6) (Kita and Marmor, 1992a). The drug can be given orally, and it might theoretically be of benefit for strengthening adhesiveness over longer periods of time, although systemic side effects are sometimes troublesome. A membrane-limited carbonic anhydrase inhibitor, benzolamide, has similar effects on adhesiveness and may prove to cause fewer side effects (Wolfensberger et al., 1995). There is no direct evidence, however, as to whether the beneficial effects of these agents can be maintained beyond a few hours, or whether they are even large enough to be meaningful under clinical conditions. The effects of acetazolamide on RPE transport are relatively weak, and in clinical practice it seems to be most effective in clearing retinal edema under conditions where the RPE is relatively healthy—and thus responsive to the drug (Marmor, 1990). Possibly some other transport-enhancing agents will prove to be more effective in enhancing retinal adhesiveness. Adhesion would also be strengthened if drugs can be found that strengthen the physical or bonding properties of the IPM, or with agents that stabilize the structural interdigitation of RPE and outer segments.

The reparative process, after detached retina becomes

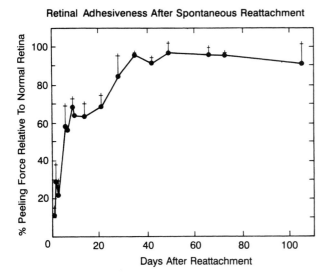

FIGURE 19-13. Recovery of retinal adhesive force after spontaneous reattachment of the retina. Small detachments were made in rabbit eyes by injecting a balanced salt solution into the subretinal space. The fluid absorbed within a few hours, but normal adhesive strength was not reached for almost 6 weeks. (Data from Yoon and Marmor, 1988b.)

reapposed, is another potential target for drug therapy. In rabbits, the fluid under an experimental detachment may absorb within a few hours, but normal adhesive strength does not return for several weeks (Kita et al., 1994; Yoon and Marmor, 1988b) (Fig. 19-13). This time is required, we may presume, for reconstructing the anatomic interdigitation between outer segments and RPE, and for resynthesizing the cone and rod matrix sheaths and their binding elements. It is not yet known which of these steps are rate limiting in this time course of 4–6 weeks, but such knowledge could lead to the design of therapy that would enhance healing after the repair of retinal detachments.

Finally, even if detachments are repaired, and adhesion restored, visual recovery may be compromised by degeneration of the photoreceptors while detached. Preventing such degeneration, and facilitating recovery after reattachment, is not strictly an enhancement of adhesiveness—but neither adhesion without visual function, nor visual function without adhesion is a satisfactory long-term result. Therapeutic strategies that strengthen adhesion before and after detachment will minimize photoreceptor degeneration and facilitate natural recovery mechanisms. Conversely, retinal degeneration can be minimized, and recovery enhanced, by agents that ameliorate mechanisms of neuronal injury and final common pathways of cellular death. The neuronal injury cascade involves membrane damage, free-

radical activity, ionic decompensation, and, eventually, terminal events such as apoptosis (programmed cell death). Modulation of these processes with agents such as antioxidants, calcium channel blockers, excitotoxin antagonists, growth factors, and apoptosis inhibitors is being investigated for the treatment of strokes and neurodegenerative disorders, and drugs that prove effective for these disorders will very likely help in retinal disorders, including detachment.

Recovery from Detachment and Retinopexy

Visual recovery from retinal detachment is dependent on a variety of factors including reapposition, recovery of adhesion, restoration of anatomic relationships between RPE and photoreceptors (Anderson et al., 1986; Kroll and Machemer, 1969), and restoration of the functional capacity of the visual cells. Some of these processes are considered elsewhere in this book (see Chapter 20), and our concern here is with the recovery of adhesive force. We made measurements of the in vitro and in vivo adhesive force in rabbits after injecting saline fluid into the subretinal space and letting it absorb (which takes place within a few hours). Even though the retina settled back upon the RPE within hours, normal levels of adhesive force were not reached for 5–6 weeks (Fig. 19-13) (Kita et al., 1994; Yoon and Marmor, 1988b). This time frame may, if anything, be optimistic for clinical conditions where the detachment has persisted for longer periods and serous fluid had been present in the subretinal space. These data are consistent with clinical reports that retinal detachments can be repaired without retinopexy (Chignell and Markham, 1981; Machemer, 1984; Zauberman and Rosell, 1975), but they also show why results without retinopexy are not as reliable: the recovery process is slow, and will be subverted if any adverse mechanical forces such as vitreous traction persist.

Retinopexy increases the strength of retinal adhesion, but the time frame varies for different methods of scarification (Fig. 19-14) (Kita et al., 1991; Kwon and Kim, 1995; Yoon and Marmor, 1988b). Measurement of adhesive force in vivo in rabbits showed that both laser treatment and diathermy increased adhesiveness to roughly 125% of normal within 24 hours of application. Adhesive force was nearly double normal values by 2–4 weeks after the applications, and increased even further over the next several months. Similar results were obtained from in vitro measurements of adhesion. Cryopexy ultimately had similar beneficial effects, but for the first few days after application adhesiveness was weakened, perhaps as a result of local inflammation or

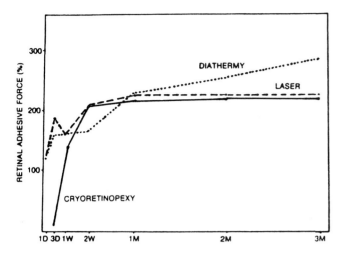

FIGURE 19-14. Changes in retinal adhesive force within living rabbit eyes, at different times after retinal scarification. Both laser *(dashes)* and diathermy *(dots)* produced enhanced adhesiveness within 1 day of application, while cryopexy *(solid line)* left adhesion very weak for the first 3 days. However, all three techniques ultimately produced bonds with at least twice normal adhesive strength. (Data from Kita et al., 1991.)

edema. Normal or enhanced adhesiveness was not reliably recorded until several days to one week after cryopexy, but thereafter the adhesive strength matched the results with laser or diathermy. All forms of retinopexy will ultimately form strong bonds through scar formation, but laser and diathermy are preferable if rapid bonding is clinically important.

CONCLUSIONS

The eye is designed with multiple systems to keep retina in place, so that retina prefers to adhere rather than to detach. Passive hydrostatic forces, interdigitation of outer segments and RPE microvilli, active transport of subretinal fluid, and the complex structure and binding properties of the IPM—all work together to keep retina apposed to the wall of the eye. Detachment does not occur simply because there is a hole in the retina or a leak in the RPE; there must be positive traction pulling on the retina or a positive force pushing fluid into the subretinal space. Retinal detachment is not simply a disease of physical separation but is the result of a vital battle between pathologic influences and the mechanisms that work routinely to maintain attachment. Through better physiologic knowledge of these mechanisms of adhesion, and better understanding of the metabolic role of the RPE in the adhesive process, better strategies may be devised in the future to manage disorders of detachment.

REFERENCES

Adler AJ, Klucznik KM. 1982a. Interaction of bovine pigment epithelium cells, photoreceptor outer segments, and interphotoreceptor matrix: a model for retinal adhesion. Curr Eye Res 1:579–589.

Adler AJ, Klucznik KM. 1982b. Proteins and glycoproteins of the bovine interphotoreceptor matrix: composition and fractionation. Exp Eye Res 34:423–434.

Adler AJ, Martin KJ. 1983. Lysosomal enzymes in the interphotoreceptor matrix: acid protease. Curr Eye Res 2:359–366.

Anderson DH, Fisher SK. 1986. The relationship of primate foveal cones to the pigment epithelium. J Ultrastruc Res 67:23–32.

Anderson DH, Guerin CJ, Erickson PA, Stern WH, Fisher SK. 1986. Morphological recovery in the reattached retina. Invest Ophthalmol Vis Sci 227:168–183.

Ashburn FS Jr, Pilkerton A, Rao NA, Marak GE. 1980. The effects of iodate and iodoacetate on the retinal adhesion. Invest Ophthalmol Vis Sci 19:1427–1432.

Berman ER. 1969. Mucopolysaccharides (glycosaminoglycans) of the retina: identification, distribution and possible biological role. Mod Probl Ophthalmol 8:5–31.

Böse M, Rassow B, Willie M. 1981. Zur Festigkeit retinaler Narben nach Argon- und Xenonkoagulation und Kryopexie. Graefes Arch Klin Exp Ophthalmol 216:291–299.

Burnside B, Laties AM. 1976. Actin filaments in apical projections of the primate pigmented epithelial cell. Invest Ophthalmol 15:570–575.

Cantiello HF, Stow JL, Prat AG, Ausiello DA. 1991. Actin filaments regulate epithelial Na+ channel activity. Am J Physiol 261:882–888.

Chaitin M, Wortham H, Brun-Zinkernagel AM. 1994. Immunocytochemical localization of CD 44 in the mouse retina. Exp Eye Res 58:359–365.

Chiang RK, Yao X-Y, Takeuchi A, Dalal R, Marmor MF. 1995. Cytochalasin D reversibly weakens retinal adhesiveness. Curr Eye Res 14:1109–1113.

Chignell AH, Markham RHC. 1981. Retinal detachment surgery without cryotherapy. Br J Ophthalmol 65:371–373.

deGuillebon H, de la Tribonniere MM, Pomerantzeff O. 1971. Adhesion between retina and pigment epithelium. Arch Ophthalmol 86:679–684.

Endo EG, Yao X-Y, Marmor MF. 1988. Pigment adherence as a measure of retinal adhesion: dependence on temperature. Invest Ophthalmol Vis Sci 29:1390–1396.

Fatt I, Shantinath K. 1971. Flow conductivity of retina and its role in retinal adhesion. Exp Eye Res 12:218–226.

Foulds WS. 1963. Experimental retinal detachment. Trans Ophthalmol Soc UK 83:153–170.

Foulds WS. 1975. The vitreous in retinal detachment. Trans Ophthalmol Soc UK 95:412–416.

Frambach DA, Misfeldt DS. 1983. Furosemide-sensitive Cl transport in embryonic chicken retinal pigment epithelium. Am J Physiol 244:F679–F685.

Frederikson O, Leyssac PP. 1977. Effects of cytochalasin B and dymethylsulfoxide on isosmotic fluid transport by rabbit gall-bladder in vitro. J Physiol 265:103–118.

Gingell D, Fornes JA. 1975. Demonstration of intermolecular forces in cell adhesion using a new electrochemical technique. Nature 256:210–211.

Gunderson D, Powell SK, Rodriguez-Boulan E. 1993. Apical polarization of N-CAM in retinal pigment epithelium is dependent on contact with the neural retina, J Cell Biol 121:335–343.

Hageman GS, Johnson LV. 1991. Structure, composition and function of the retinal interphotoreceptor matrix. In Osborne N, Chader J, eds, Progress in Retinal Research. Oxford: Pergamon Press, 207–249.

Hageman GS, Kirchoff MA, Anderson DH. 1990. Biochemical characterization and distribution of retinal interphotoreceptor matrix glycoconjugates. Glycoconjugate J 7:512.

Hageman GS, Marmor MF, Yao X-Y, Johnson LV. 1995. The interphotoreceptor matrix mediates primate retinal adhesion. Arch Ophthalmol 113:655–660.

Ho T-C, Del Priore LV. 1997. Reattachment of cultured human retinal pigment epithelium to extracellular matrix and human Bruch's membrane. Invest Ophthalmol Vis Sci 38:1110–1118.

Hollyfield JG, Varner H, Rayborn ME, Osterfeld AM. 1989. Retinal attachment to the pigment epithelium. Retina 9:59.

Immel J, Negi A, Marmor MF. 1986. Acute changes in RPE apical morphology after retinal detachment in rabbit: a SEM study. Invest Ophthalmol Vis Sci 27:1770–1776.

Johnson LV, Hageman GS, Blanks MC. 1986. Interphotoreceptor matrix domains ensheath vertebrate cone photoreceptor cells, Invest Ophthalmol Vis Sci 27:129–135.

Kain HL, Libondi T. 1986. Experimentelle Netzhautablöaung—Untersuchungen zum Pathomechanismus. Fortschr Ophthalmol 83:590–596.

Kawano S-I, Marmor MF. 1988. Metabolic influences on the absorption of serous subretinal fluid. Invest Ophthalmol Vis Sci 29:1255–1257.

Kim RY, Yao X-Y, Marmor MF. 1993. Oxygen dependency of retinal adhesion. Invest Ophthalmol Vis Sci 34:2074–2078.

Kita M, Marmor MF. 1991. Systemic mannitol increases the retinal adhesive force in vivo. Arch Ophthalmol 109:1449–1450.

Kita M, Marmor MF. 1992a. Retinal adhesive force in living rabbit, cat and monkey eyes: normative data and enhancement by mannitol and acetazolamide. Invest Ophthalmol Vis Sci 33:1879–1882.

Kita M, Marmor MF. 1992b. Effects on retinal adhesive force in vivo of metabolically active agents in the subretinal space. Invest Ophthalmol Vis Sci 33:1883–1887.

Kita M, Negi A, Kawano S-I, Honda Y, Maegawa S. 1990. Measurement of retinal adhesive force in the in vivo rabbit eye. Invest Ophthalmol Vis Sci 31:624–628.

Kita M, Negi A, Kawano S-I, Honda Y. 1991. Photothermal, cryogenic, and diathermic effects on retinal adhesive force in vivo. Retina 11:441–444.

Kita M, Negi A, Marmor MF. 1992. Lowering the calcium concentration in the subretinal space in vivo loosens retinal adhesion. Invest Ophthalmol Vis Sci 33:23–29.

Kita M, Negi A, Honda Y, Marmor MF. 1994. The recovery of retinal adhesion and subretinal fluid absorption after experimental retinal detachment. Invest Ophthalmol Vis Sci 35(suppl):1903.

Kohno T, Sorgente N, Ishibashi T, Goodnight R, Ryan SJ. 1987. Immunofluorescent studies of fibronectin and laminin in the human eye. Invest Ophthalmol Vis Sci 28:506–514.

Kroll AJ, Machemer R. 1969. Experimental retinal detachment in the owl monkey. V. Electron microscopy of the reattached retina. Am J Ophthalmol 67:117–130.

Kwon O-W, Kim S-Y. 1995. Changes in adhesive force between the retina and the retinal pigment epithelium by laser photocoagulation in rabbits. Yonsei Med J 36:243–250.

Lazarus HS, Hageman GS. 1992. Xyloside-induced disruption of interphotoreceptor matrix proteoglycans results in retinal detachment. Invest Ophthalmol Vis Sci 33:364–376.

Lincoff H, O'Connor P, Bloch D, Nadel A, Kreissig I, Grinberg M. 1970. The cryosurgical adhesion, part II. Trans Am Acad Ophthalmol Otolaryngol 74:98–107.

Machemer R. 1984. The importance of fluid absorption, traction, intraocular currents, and chorioretinal scars in the therapy of rhegmatogenous retinal detachments. Am J Ophthalmol 98:681–693.

Machemer R, Norton EWD. 1968. Experimental retinal detachment in the owl monkey. I. Methods of production and clinical picture. Am J Ophthalmol 66:388–396.

Marmor MF. 1979. Retinal detachment from hyperosmotic intravitreal injection. Invest Ophthalmol Vis Sci 18:1237–1244.

Marmor MF. 1990. Hypothesis concerning carbonic anhydrase treatment of CME: example with epiretinal membrane. Arch Ophthalmol 108:1524–1525.

Marmor MF. 1993. Mechanisms of retinal adhesion. In: Osborne NN, Chader GJ, eds, Progress in Retinal Research. Oxford: Pergamon Press, 179–204.

Marmor, MF. 1994. Mechanisms of normal retinal adhesion. In: Ryan SJ, Glaser BM, eds, Retina, 2nd ed. St Louis: Mosby-Year Book. 1931–1953.

Marmor MF, Maack T. 1982a. Enhancement of retinal adhesion and subretinal fluid resorption by acetazolamide. Invest Ophthalmol Vis Sci 23:121–124.

Marmor MF, Maack T. 1982b. Local environmental factors and retinal adhesion in the rabbit. Exp Eye Res 34:727–733.

Marmor MF, Negi A. 1986. Pharmacologic modification of subretinal fluid absorption in the rabbit eye. Arch Ophthalmol 104:1674–1677.

Marmor MF, Takeuchi A. 1996. Effects of choroidal ischemia on retinal adhesion in vivo. Invest Ophthalmol Vis Sci 37(suppl):S963.

Marmor MF, Yao X-Y. 1989. The enhancement of retinal adhesiveness by ouabain appears to involve cellular edema. Invest Ophthalmol Vis Sci 30:1511–1514.

Marmor MF, Yao X-Y. 1995. The metabolic dependency of retinal adhesion in rabbit and primate. Arch Ophthalmol 113:232–238.

Marmor MF, Abdul-Rahim AS, Cohen DS. 1980a. The effect of metabolic inhibitors on retinal adhesion and subretinal fluid resorption. Invest Ophthalmol Vis Sci 19:893–903.

Marmor MF, Martin LJ, Tharpe S. 1980b. Osmotically induced retinal detachment in the rabbit and primate. Invest Ophthalmol Vis Sci 19:1016–1029.

Marmor MF, Yao X-Y, Hageman GS. 1994. Retinal adhesiveness in surgically enucleated human eyes. Retina 14:181–186.

Negi, A, White MP, Marmor MF. 1993. Effects of hemi-cholinium-3, a photoreceptor and pigment epithelial toxin, on retinal adhesiveness and subretinal fluid absorption. Doc Ophthalmol 83:331–336.

Opas M, Kalnins VI. 1985. Distribution of spectrin and lectin-binding materials in surface lamina of RPE cells. Invest Ophthalmol Vis Sci 26:621–627.

Osterlin S. 1977. On the molecular biology of the vitreous in the aphakic eye. Acta Ophthalmol 55:353–361.

Owczarek FR, Marak GE, Pilkerton AR. 1975. Retinal adhesion in light- and dark-adapted rabbits. Invest Ophthalmol 14:353–358.

Philp NJ, Nachmias VT. 1987. Polarized distribution of integrin and fibronectin in retinal pigment epithelium. Invest Ophthalmol Vis Sci 28:1275–1280.

Porello K, LaVail MM. 1986. Histochemical demonstration of spatial heterogeneity in the interphotoreceptor matrix of the rat retina. Invest Ophthalmol Vis Sci 27:1577–1586.

Rutnin U, Schepens CL. 1978. Fundus appearance in normal eyes. IV. Retinal breaks and other findings. Am J Ophthalmol 64:1063–1078.

Shirakawa H, Ishiguro S-I, Itoh Y, Plantner JJ, Kean EL. 1987. Are sugars involved in the binding of rhodopsin-membranes by the retinal pigment epithelium? Invest Ophthalmol Vis Sci 28:628–632.

Steinberg RH, Wood I. 1974. Pigment epithelial cell ensheathment of cone outer segments in the retina of the domestic cat. Proc Royal Soc Lond B 187:461–478.

Takeuchi A, Negi A, Yamamoto F, Sakaue H, Honda Y. 1991. Effects of sodium iodate on retinal adhesive force in vivo. Invest Ophthalmol Vis Sci 32(suppl):667.

Tsuboi S. 1987. Measurement of the volume flow and hydraulic conductivity across the isolated dog retinal pigment epithelium. Invest Ophthalmol Vis Sci 28:1776–1782.

Tsuboi S, Pederson JE. 1986. Experimental retinal detachment. XI. Furosemide-inhibitable fluid absorption across retinal pigment epithelium in vivo. Arch Ophthalmol 104:602–603.

Uehara F, Muramatsu T, Sameshima M, Kawano K, Kode H, Ohba N. 1985. Effects of neuraminidase on lectin binding sites in photoreceptor cells of monkey retina. Jpn J Ophthalmol 29:54.

Uehara F, Yasumura D, LaVail MM. 1991. Rod- and cone-associated interphotoreceptor matrix in the rat retina. Invest Ophthalmol Vis Sci 32:285–292.

Wolfensberger TJ, Chiang R, Takeuchi A, Marmor MF. 1995. Inhibition of membrane-bound arbonic anhydrase enhances subretinal fluid absorption and retinal adhesiveness. Invest Ophthalmol Vis Sci 36:S921.

Yamada K. 1974. The effect of digestion with chondroitinases upon certain histochemical reactions of mucosaccharide-containing tissues. J Histochem Cytochem 22:266.

Yamamoto F, Steinberg RH. 1991. Effects of intravenous acetazolamide on retinal pH in the cat. Exp Eye Res 54:711–718.

Yao, X-Y, Endo EG, Marmor MF. 1989. Reversibility of retinal adhesion in the rabbit. Invest Ophthalmol Vis Sci 30:220–224.

Yao X-Y, Hageman GS, Marmor MF. 1990. Retinal adhesiveness is weakened by enzymatic modification of the interphotoreceptor matrix in vivo. Invest Ophthalmol Vis Sci 31:2051–2058.

Yao X-Y, Moore KT, Marmor MF. 1991. Systemic mannitol increases retinal adhesiveness measured in vitro. Arch Ophthalmol 109:275–277.

Yao X-Y, Hageman GS, Marmor MF. 1992. Recovery of retinal adhesion after enzymatic purturbation of the interphotoreceptor matrix. Invest Ophthalmol Vis Sci 33:498–503.

Yao X-Y, Hageman GS, Marmor MF. 1994. Retinal adhesiveness in the monkey. Invest Ophthalmol Vis Sci 35:744–748.

Yoon YH, Marmor MF. 1988a. Effects on retinal adhesion of temperature, cyclic AMP, cytochalasin B, and enzymes. Invest Ophthalmol Vis Sci 29:910–914.

Yoon YH, Marmor MF. 1988b. Rapid enhancement of retinal adhesion by laser photocoagulation. Ophthalmology 95:1385–1388.

Yoon YH, Marmor MF. 1993. Retinal pigment epithelium adhesion to Bruch's membrane is weakened by hemicholinium-3 and sodium iodate. Ophthalmic Res 25:386–392.

Young RW. 1976. Visual cells and the concept of renewal. Invest Ophthalmol 15:700–725.

Zauberman H, Berman ER. 1969. Measurement of adhesive forces between the sensory retina and the pigment epithelium. Exp Eye Res 8:276–283.

Zauberman H, deGuillebon H. 1972. Retinal traction in vivo and postmortem. Arch Ophthalmol 87:549–554.

Zauberman H, Rosell FG. 1975. Treatment of retinal detachment without inducing chorioretinal lesions. Trans Am Acad Ophthalmol Otolaryngol 79:835–844.

Zauberman H, deGuillebon H, Holly FJ. 1972. Retinal traction in vitro: biophysical aspects. Invest Ophthalmol 11:46–55.

20. Cellular responses of the retinal pigment epithelium to retinal detachment and reattachment

STEVEN K. FISHER AND DON H. ANDERSON

Our understanding of the responses of the retinal pigment epithelium (RPE) to retinal detachment is based primarily on studies of animal models in which detachments are created experimentally. Most of this data is derived from experimental detachments and/or reattachments in the retinas of domestic cats, rabbits, or, in a few cases, primates. To date, it seems fair to state that the responsiveness of the RPE has not received the same degree of attention as the neural retina, where detachment triggers numerous changes including, among others, photoreceptor outer segment degeneration (Machemer, 1968; Kroll and Machemer, 1968; see Fisher and Anderson, 1994 for a review), synaptic terminal degeneration (Erickson et al., 1983), changes in gene expression in Müller cells (Lewis et al., 1989; 1994), apoptotic photoreceptor cell death (Cook et al., 1995), and proliferation of all nonneuronal retinal cell types (Fisher et al., 1991). It is likely that the RPE plays a major role in the neural retina's reactions to detachment and reattachment, because of the diversity of interactions that occur between these two layers. These range from the exchange of molecules critical for retinal function (e.g. vitamin A and oxygen) to the phagocytosis of disk packets that have been shed from the tips of rods and cones (see Anderson et al., 1978; Bok, 1982; 1985 for reviews). It is also well established that RPE cells which migrate from the monolayer can participate in the complications that arise from detachment/reattachment, such as subretinal fibrosis and proliferative vitreoretinopathy (Machemer & Laqua, 1975).

In this chapter we will review the changes in the RPE that are induced by detachment, and some of the consequences of these specific changes that may affect chances for successful retinal reattachment and visual recovery.

THE RPE–PHOTORECEPTOR INTERFACE

The normal interface between the RPE and photoreceptors is similar in all three species of animals that have been used to study detachment experimentally, although the apical processes that ensheath the cone outer segments of the cat and rabbit retinas are organized into much more complex structures than their counterparts in primate retina (Figs. 20-1, 20-2A; also see Steinberg and Wood, 1974; Anderson et al., 1978; Anderson and Fisher, 1979; Fisher and Steinberg, 1982. It is important to note that the apical processes elaborated by the RPE consist of *both* cylindrical-shaped microvilli and more flattened, sheetlike structures that envelop the rod and cone photoreceptor outer segments (Fig. 20-2A). Both types of processes contain a core of actin filaments (Burnside and Laties, 1976; Anderson and Fisher, 1979), and both participate in the engulfment of phagosomes shed from the tips of outer segments (see Bok, 1985).

The most rapid morphological response of RPE cells to detachment that has been identified to date is the dedifferentiation of the apical surface. The highly specialized apical processes disappear rapidly, and are replaced by a carpet of greatly shortened microvilli that uniformly decorate the apical surface (Fig. 20-2B, 20-2D), or, in some instances, by a relatively smooth surface without large numbers of microvilli (Fig. 20-2C). In experimental rhegmatogenous detachments, the loss of these highly specialized apical processes occurs within 24 hours following detachment (Anderson et al., 1983). In non-rhegmatogenous "bleb" detachments, where a small quantity of isotonic fluid is microinjected into the subretinal space, such changes have been identified within one hour following detachment (Immel et al., 1986). Based upon these observations, it seems clear that the change(s) in extracellular milieu created by the separation of the neural retina from the RPE is sufficient to trigger a rapid dedifferentiation of the RPE apical surface. Conversely, this implies that the apposition of the photoreceptors and, perhaps, the appropriate interphotoreceptor matrix domains are required for induction and elaboration of the specialized ensheathing processes on the apical surface that occurs both developmentally and following reattachment (DeFoe and Easterling, 1994).

The RPE's capacity for such a rapid and dynamic

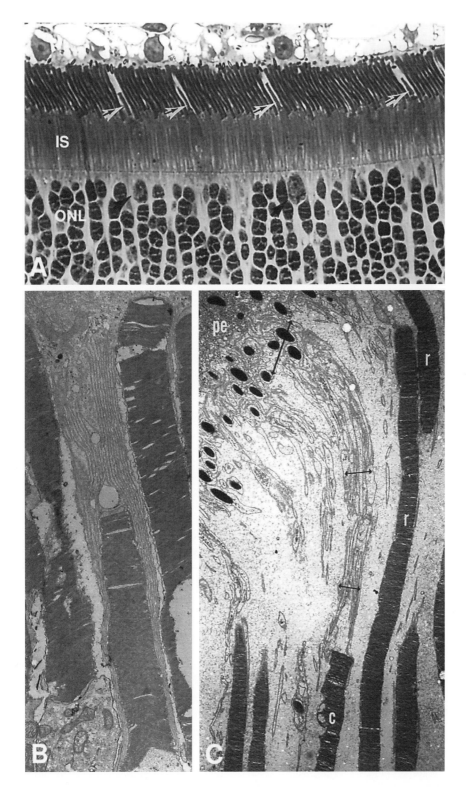

FIGURE 20-1. Micrographs showing the relationship between outer segments and the RPE in cat and primate retina. (A) Light micrograph of the interface between RPE and neural retina in the cat. The arrows indicate cone outer segments, which do not terminate at the RPE apical surface like rod outer segments, but are contacted by a highly organized array of ensheathing processes (see also Fig. 20-2A). (IS) = the layer of photoreceptor inner segments, (ONL) = outer nuclear layer. Magnification ×720. (Reprinted by permission from Anderson et al., 1983. (B) An electron micrograph illustrating the cone sheath in the cat retina. ×10,700. (Reprinted with permission from Fisher and Steinberg, 1982. (C) An electron micrograph showing the somewhat less elaborate array of apical processes *(arrows)* that contact extrafoveal cone outer segments in the primate *(Macaca mullata)* retina. (C) = cone outer segment, (r) = rod outer segments, (pe) = RPE. ×9000.

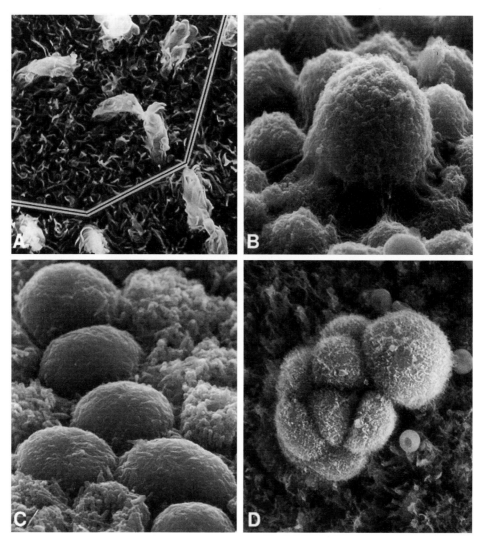

FIGURE 20-2. Scanning electron micrographs illustrating the apical surface of the RPE in: (A) Normal cat retina. The lines demarcate the border of one RPE cell. The apical surface has both short microvilli-like processes and sheetlike processes that interdigitate to form the cone sheaths. Magnification ×7500. (Reprinted with permission from Pfeffer and Fisher, 1981.) (B) Cat retina detached for 6 weeks, illustrating the loss of specialized apical processes and the mounding of the RPE cell bodies that occurs after detachment. ×4400. (Reprinted with permission from Fisher and Anderson, 1994.) (C) Rhesus monkey retina detached for 6 weeks, illustrating some cells that are highly mounded and with relatively smooth apical surfaces, while others are covered with microvilli-like processes. ×5000. (D) Rhesus monkey retina detached for 6 weeks, illustrating a mound of proliferated RPE cells attached to the original monolayer. These cells are covered with microvilli-like processes. ×4800.

transformation of its apical surface could be construed as highly advantageous for repair and recovery. When the retina–RPE interface is compromised through injury or disease, surgical or spontaneous reattachment does not result in exact realignment of photoreceptors to their original points of contact with the RPE apical surface. Since rods and cones are contacted by morphologically different RPE apical processes as well as by biochemically distinct extracellular matrix domains (Johnson et al., 1986; Hageman and Johnson, 1986), rapid dedifferentiation following separation may facilitate, rather than detract from, repair by providing for the specific induction of the appropriate apical processes and matrix components after reapposition, depending on whether the apical surface is contacted by a rod or cone.

Another prominent morphological change on the apical surface, and one that also occurs very rapidly, is a conversion of the apical surface from a relatively "flat" contour to one with a "mounded," more spherical contour from which the homogeneous "carpet" of microvilli extend (Fig. 20-2B–D) (Anderson et al., 1983; Immel et al., 1986). Like the loss of specialized processes, this change in cell shape has been shown to occur within minutes of producing a bleb-type experimental detachment (Immel et al., 1986). The nucleus of the RPE cell often migrates into the portion of the cell which protrudes into the expanded subretinal space. This morphology is highly similar to RPE cells when they are grown in primary culture. In fact, RPE cells in the detached state appear to exhibit many of the same characteristics as cultured RPE cells when they are grown to confluence on solid substrates composed of basement membrane components (Matsumoto et al., 1990). The cytoskeleton of flattened, undifferentiated RPE cells in primary culture assumes a pattern in which microtubules, intermediate filaments (e.g., vimentin), and actin filaments are distributed more or less randomly throughout the cytoplasm. However, as the cultured cells become confluent and begin to differentiate, the bulk of actin and vimentin filaments become concentrated in the basolateral cytoplasm in the form of a circumferential bundle that lines the perimeter of each cell (Burnside and Laties, 1986; Fisher and Steinberg, 1982). Under in vivo conditions normal RPE cells, as well as those in the detached state, also display a circumferential bundle composed of actin filaments. However, under normal in vivo conditions, vimentin is not usually expressed by primate and feline RPE cells, and the circumferential bundle does not contain vimentin filaments. In the detached state, however, vimentin filaments are found in the basal cytoplasm and in association with the circumferential bundle (Guérin et al., 1990). It appears that the "mounded" morphology, as well as other structural changes on the apical surface of RPE cells in the detached state, is just one manifestation of a general change in the cells' cytoskeletal organization that mimics the in vitro profile, and is inducible in vivo by various perturbations such as retinal detachment.

PROLIFERATION AND MIGRATION

Study of experimental detachments in primates (Machemer and Laqua, 1975) and later observations of histopathologic specimens of "periretinal membranes" from human patients (Clarkson et al., 1977; Machemer et al., 1978), led to the conclusion that RPE cells migrate away from the monolayer and then proliferate, under certain pathological conditions, in the subretinal space and in the vitreous cavity. As such, RPE cells were long regarded as a primary contributor to subretinal and vitreoretinal proliferative disorders, although retinal glia (i.e. Müller cells and astrocytes) are now regarded by some investigators as the principal cell types involved.

Subsequently, the proliferative response of RPE cells was quantified in experimental detachments in which retinal cells were labeled with either radiolabeled thymidine or an antibody to a nuclear antigen expressed only by dividing cells (Anderson et al., 1981; Geller et al., 1995). RPE cells in "normal" eyes are generally considered to be mitotically quiescent, or to turn over at an extremely low rate. Within 24 hours of producing an experimental detachment, however, RPE cells begin to proliferate, as demonstrated by ^{3}H-thymidine incorporation (see Fig. 20-3) or upregulation of a nuclear specific antigen, Ki-67 (Anderson et al., 1981, Geller et al., 1995). In these experiments, the proliferative response follows a time course similar to that of other nonneuronal cells in the retina (Fisher et al., 1991; Geller et al., 1995) and brain (Janeczko, 1989) where the response peaks at around 3 or 4 days following detachment, and then subsides within the next week to basal levels. Results from earlier studies suggest that at least some RPE proliferation continues to take place between 1 and 8 weeks following detachment (Machemer and Laqua, 1975).

The proliferative response of the RPE is responsible for significant alterations in the organization of the RPE–photoreceptor interface since the daughter cells assume a number of different configurations. These include long assemblies of cells that protrude into the subretinal space, mounds of cells that remain associated with the monolayer, discrete clumps of cells within the subretinal space, and/or multiple layers of cells adjacent to the original monolayer (Fig. 20-4A,B). In the latter case, these new layers can exhibit an altered polarity, such that their apical surface apposes the apical surface of the original monolayer and their basal surface faces the neural retina (Figs. 20-5, 20-6A) (Anderson et al., 1983). The presence of multiple layers of RPE appears to interfere with outer segment regrowth after successful reattachment, especially when the basal surface is presented to the neural retina (Anderson et al., 1986; Guérin et al., 1989). The fact that RPE proliferation is limited to the area of detachment provides some insight into the molecular event(s) that are involved in initiating the response (Anderson et al., 1981). Apposition of the RPE and neural retina is apparently sufficient to maintain mitotic quiescence. Their separation either triggers an intracellular response in some RPE cells that leads to entry into the cell cycle or, more likely, results in the local release of some regulatory factor that stimulates some detached RPE cells to begin proliferating. Understanding and identifying the mechanisms by which apposition inhibits proliferation and detachment stimulates proliferation may play a key role in developing therapeutics that prevent the proliferation of RPE

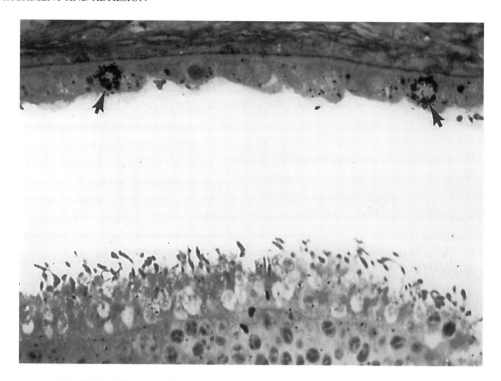

FIGURE 20-3. RPE proliferation in the cat retina 48 hours following experimental retinal detachment. Two radio-labeled RPE cell bodies are present in the field *(arrows)*. The concentrations of silver grains signify the incorporation of 3H-thymidine and DNA synthesis. Also note the degenerated layer of photoreceptor outer segments, and the absence of microvilli on the apical surfaces of the RPE cells. Magnification ×600.

and other nonneuronal cells, thereby decreasing the likelihood of epiretinal or subretinal membrane formation.

One potential molecular mediator of this response is basic fibroblast growth factor (bFGF or FGF-2) which is prevalent in various cellular and extracellular locations in the retina (Baird et al., 1985; Hageman et al., 1991; Hanneken et al., 1989; Hanneken and Baird, 1992). After injection of exogenous bFGF into the normal vitreous, the factor diffuses rapidly into the neural retina and the subretinal space (Lewis et al., 1996). Approximately 24 hours following injection, evidence of DNA synthesis and RPE cell division are first detected in an otherwise normal eye (De Juan et al., 1990; Lewis et al., 1992). bFGF is almost certainly not the only molecular species that could be involved. A number of other growth regulating factors including transforming growth factor beta (TGF-β) (Pfeffer et al., 1994; Anderson et al., 1995), insulin-like growth factor (IGF) (Waldbillig et al., 1991; Charkrabarti et al., 1991; Arnold et al., 1993), and FGF-5 (Kitaoka et al., 1993) are also expressed by the RPE, and could be involved in maintaining its mitotic quiescence. Nevertheless, bFGF

is the only factor thus far that has been shown to modulate RPE proliferation in vivo.

After detachment, RPE cells are occasionally observed in the process of migrating away from the monolayer. This phenomenon has been documented in several mammalian species following experimental detachment (Inahara, 1973; Johnson and Foulds, 1977; Clarkson et al., 1977) but is most clearly observed in the detached feline RPE. In electron micrographs, the process of "budding off" appears as a progressive reduction in the amount of basal surface area that is attached to basement membrane, coincident with severance of the junctional complexes at the cell's lateral borders (Anderson et al., 1983). After this process is complete and the cells enter the subretinal space, they often assume a macrophage-like appearance. Such cells often contain pigment granules, some of which are clearly melanin-like in appearance; this is not always the case, however, especially in species such as the cat, where nonpigmented RPE cells overlie the tapetum in the superior retina. Pigmented RPE cells may also lose pigmentation as they proliferate, whereas macrophages may acquire pigmentation by engulfment of pigment granules derived from

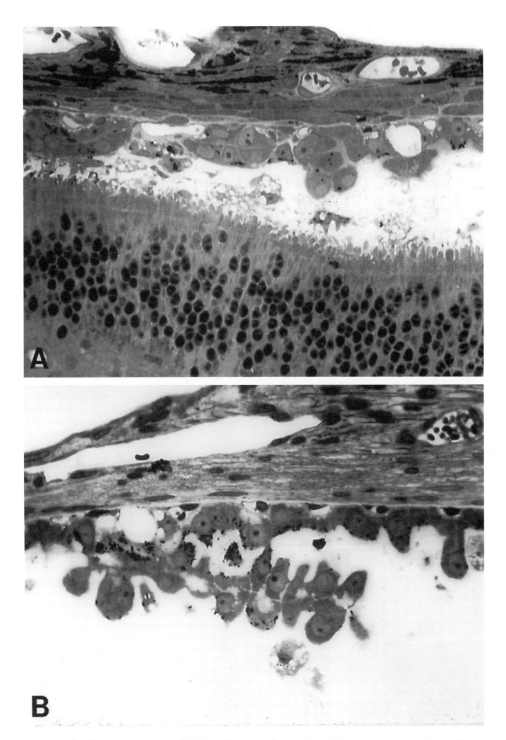

FIGURE 20-4. Light micrographs illustrating regions of RPE proliferation after experimental retinal detachment in the cat. (A) A transition zone between a detached area *(right)* and an adjacent attached region *(left)* in a retinal detachment of 13 days' duration. Outer segments are almost completely degenerated and clusters of proliferated RPE cells lie adjacent to the original RPE monolayer. A population of phagocytic cells is situated over the layer of inner segments. Magnification ×525. (B) A long assembly of RPE cells extends from the monolayer into the expanded subretinal space after 50 days of detachment. Note the overall contour of cells in the monolayer as well as the absence of specialized apical processes. ×600. (Reprinted with permission from Anderson et al., 1983.)

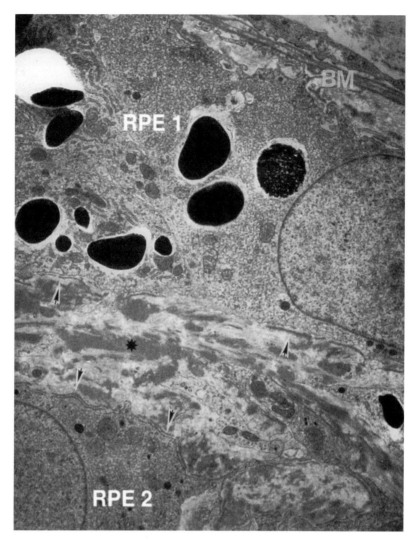

FIGURE 20-5. An electron micrograph showing the interface between the original RPE monolayer (RPE 1) and a second layer of RPE cells resulting from proliferation (RPE 2). Note that a basement membrane now occurs on the apical surface of the original monolayer and on the "basal" surface of the proliferated cell layer *(arrows)*. The intervening space is occupied by electron lucent extracellular matrix *(asterisk)* presumably synthesized and secreted by one or both cell layers. Magnification ×13,300.

necrotic cells. Thus, the identity of the macrophage-like cells is not always obvious based on morphological criteria alone. But, subretinal phagocytes of RPE origin can often be distinguished from cells of monocyte-macrophage lineage using an antibody to cellular retinaldehyde-binding protein (Fig. 20-7), a protein expressed only by RPE and Müller cells in the retina (Bunt-Milam et al., 1983). It is unlikely that the macrophage-like cells are of Müller cell origin since Müller cells assume a completely different morphology when they migrate into the subretinal space (Laqua and Machemer, 1975; Anderson et al., 1983; Hjelmeland

and Harvey, 1988). Macrophage-like RPE cells are typically situated next to the layer of truncated inner/outer segments to which they may adhere. It is not unusual for these cells to contain packets of engulfed outer segment disc membranes (Fig. 20-8), which is additional evidence for their phagocytic origin.

Local accumulations of RPE cells that occur as a result of both proliferation and migration almost certainly account for some of the fundoscopic signs of hyper- and hypopigmentation in the subretinal space that are associated with detachment and with other retinal pathologies involving the photoreceptor-RPE interface.

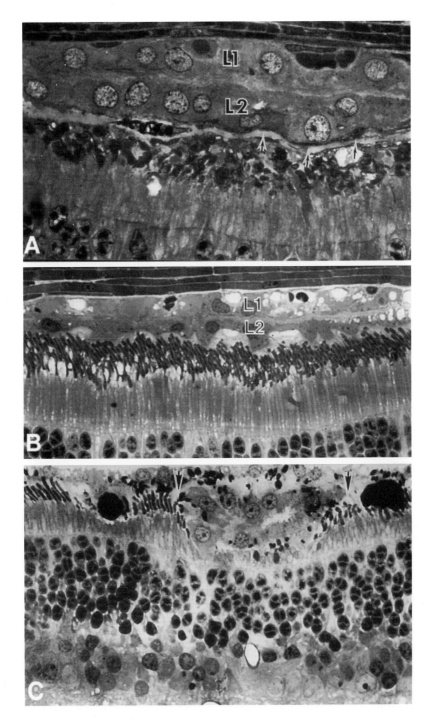

FIGURE 20-6. Light micrographs illustrating the effects of RPE proliferation on outer segment regeneration following experimental retinal reattachment in the cat. Note that the figures illustrate various configurations that occur and these do not necessarily correlate with the duration of detachment. (A) There are two monolayers of RPE (L1, L2) in this example. The second layer has its basal surface *(arrows)* apparently facing the neural retina. Note the poor regeneration of outer segments. Retina detached for 14 days, reattached for 30 days. Magnification ×1500. (B) In this example, the second layer of RPE cells has its apical surface facing the neural retina. Note the near normal appearance of the outer segment layer in this region. Retina detached for 30 days and reattached for 30 days. ×800. (C) Photoreceptors underlying the cluster of proliferated RPE cells *(arrows)* show essentially no outer segment regeneration while adjacent photoreceptors possess cylindrical, nearly normal appearing outer segments. Retina detached for 7 days and reattached for 10 days. ×1000. (B) and (C) (reprinted with permission from Anderson et al., 1986.)

413

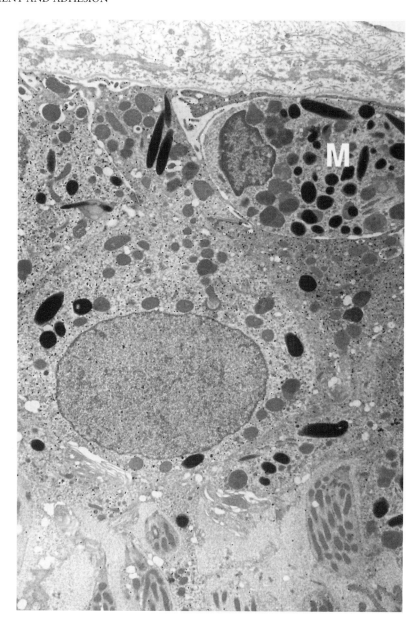

FIGURE 20-7. An electron micrograph from a primate retina detached for 7 days and reattached for 30 days. Tissue sections were probed with a polyclonal antibody to cellular retinaldehyde binding protein, and then a secondary antibody gold conjugate. The presence of electron-dense gold particles in the cytoplasm indicates that these cells are of RPE origin. Absence of gold particles over the cytoplasm of the cell in the upper right suggests that this cell is of monocyte/macrophage rather than RPE lineage. Such cells are frequently found in the sub-retinal space following retinal detachment. Magnification ×10,600.

These include the "demarcation lines" that often mark the boundary between attached and detached retina (Hilton et al., 1975). In experimentally detached cat retina, clusters of RPE cells often occur at the transition between detached and attached regions (Anderson et al., 1983).

CELL DEATH

Significant numbers of photoreceptor cells die after retinal detachment (Erickson et al., 1983; Wilson and Green, 1987) with a wave of apoptotic cell death occurring in the first few days after production of the de-

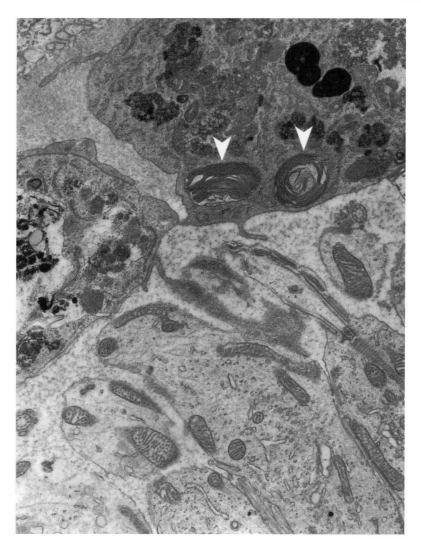

FIGURE 20-8. An electron micrograph showing a phagocytic cell overlying the layer of inner segments in the detached cat retina. Note the presence of lamellar bodies within the cell's cytoplasm *(white arrowheads)*, indicating that it has phagocytosed several packets of outer segment discs. These cells are most likely of RPE origin. Magnification ×13,500.

tachment (Cook et al., 1995). There is no evidence at present that RPE cells are similarly affected.

CHANGES IN GENE EXPRESSION

Compared with studies of the neural retina, changes in the expression of specific proteins by the RPE after perturbation or insult have been studied relatively infrequently in vivo. Potentially, this is an important area of investigation, because changes in the expression of such molecules as vitamin A binding proteins, vitamin A isomerases, membrane ion transporters, trophic factors,

cytokines, or adhesion molecules could have profound effects on the ability of the RPE to interact normally with the reattached neural retina. Based on observations in the neural retina (see Lewis et al., 1994), it is likely that significant changes in gene expression do occur in the RPE as well. It is known, for example, that the cytoskeletal protein vimentin is a component of the cytoskeleton in cultured mammalian RPE cells (Matsumoto et al., 1990). In contrast, it is not expressed by normal cat or primate RPE cells in situ; but it can be induced within two days following retinal detachment (Guerin et al., 1990). Intermediate filaments are generally thought to stabilize overall cell architecture, and the

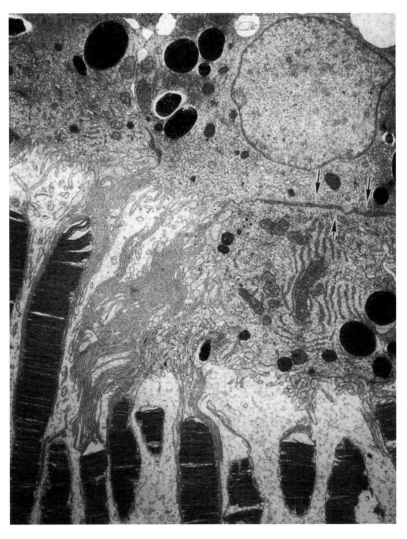

FIGURE 20-9. An electron micrograph of the RPE–photoreceptor interface from a cat retina detached for 3 days and reattached for 10 days. Note the dramatic remodeling of the apical surface (compare to Fig. 20-1B) that has taken place during this relatively short detach- ment interval. The arrows indicate the junctional complex between an RPE cell lying in the original monolayer and an adjacent cell with an abnormal bulging of its apical surface into the subretinal space. Magnification ×10,000.

induction of this protein may reflect the many changes in RPE morphology that occur around this same time after detachment.

There is some evidence that the profile of adhesion receptors on the apical surface of RPE cells undergoes a shift in response to detachment. Under normal conditions, β1 integrins are expressed primarily on the basal and basolateral surface of the adult RPE in vivo (Philp et al., 1987; Anderson et al., 1995). Under in vitro conditions they are also expressed on the apical surface, at least in cultured mammalian RPE cells (Anderson et al., 1991). Following detachment, however, this profile changes and there appears to be an upregulation of β1 integrins on the apical surface that is confined to the region of detachment (Philp and Anderson, unpublished data). Thus, it seems likely that the molecular profile of

proteins found on the apical surface of the RPE in the presence of the neural retina is somewhat different from the profile in the detached state. The latter profile may more closely correspond to cultured RPE cells, where the apical surface is exposed directly to the culture media. In large part, this is a relatively unexplored area of inquiry that may have important implications for the recovery process that ensues once the retina reattached.

RPE RESPONSE TO RETINAL REATTACHMENT

Reestablishment of the interface between RPE and neural retina is essential for significant visual recovery following detachment. There are several important factors that must be recognized in order to appreciate the complex nature of this repair process. In the human retina, as in that of most animals, rods and cones have different anatomical relationships to the RPE; moreover, foveal cones have a different structural relationship with the RPE than do peripheral cones. There are more cones per RPE cell in the fovea, and foveal cone outer segments terminate much closer to the apical surface than do their peripheral counterparts (Anderson and Fisher, 1979). In addition, the extracellular matrix that ensheaths the distal portion of rod and cones is somewhat different in biochemical composition (Hageman and Johnson, 1986; Sameshima et al., 1987; Fariss et al., 1990). Since dedifferentiation of the apical processes occurs very rapidly after detachment, each RPE cell retains its ability to redifferentiate its apical surface when the detached retina is reapposed to the RPE apical surface upon reattachment. Although it remains unclear the extent to which the recovery process recapitulates the developmental process, the capacity for recovery at the cellular and molecular levels must be an important determinant of recovery at the functional level. Outer segment regeneration, which must occur in order to have significant visual recovery, is a complex process involving the appropriate synthesis and delivery of molecular components from the inner segment to the outer segment of the photoreceptors (Young, 1968), and the assembly of these molecular components into an appropriate configuration (Steinberg et al., 1980). The photoreceptor–RPE interface in a normal retina has a remarkably uniform appearance in histological sections. This is not the case in feline and monkey retinas that are reattached following experimental retinal detachment, where there is considerable variability in morphology. After reattachment periods of up to one month, the retina–RPE interface is best described as a "patchwork" in which some areas show almost normal RPE and outer segment morphology while adjacent regions appear highly abnormal (Fig. 20-9) (Anderson et al., 1986; Guérin et al., 1989; Fisher and Anderson, 1994). RPE abnormalities range from subtle changes in the size, numbers, and configurations of the apical processes to highly abnormal regions where clusters or even multiple layers of RPE cells occur in the subretinal space. At these highly abnormal locations, photoreceptors almost always have abnormal outer segment configurations or none at all (Fig. 20-6). While this may be of minor significance in the peripheral retina, where small patches of missing or abnormal outer segments probably have little impact on overall vision, it may be highly significant within the fovea. For example, in primate maculas detached for 7 days and reattached for varying intervals (Guérin et al., 1989), the RPE–photoreceptor interface undergoes considerable remodeling and reorganization during the first week of reattach-

ment, including the apparent migration of RPE pigment granules toward the apical surface and the beginning of redifferentiation of the apical processes to ensheath the growing outer segments. At 7 days after reattachment, the process of disc shedding and phagosome engulfment by the RPE appears to resume. During the next week, specialized processes ensheathing cone outer segments are recognizable, although the tips of regenerated cone outer segments are not contacted by the typical 8–10 μm–long apical processes. Rather, regenerated cone outer segments tend to terminate at or very close to the RPE cell body. The impact of this morphological difference on retinal function is unknown. The results from this same study dramatically illustrate the effects of RPE proliferation within the fovea. In one animal with a 7-day detachment, 30-day reattachment interval, an area of significant RPE proliferation was identified adjacent to the foveal pit. There was no regeneration of cone outer segments underlying this area even though the neural retina was directly apposed to the RPE, whereas a nearby area free from intervening RPE proliferation showed the presence of rudimentary cone outer segments (Guérin et al., 1989).

The available experimental studies, as well as acuity measurements obtained from human detachment patients, strongly suggest that it is highly desirable to reattach the retina as soon as possible following detachment. The underlying assumption is that cellular repair, as well as visual recovery, is optimized by reestablishing the photoreceptor–RPE interface as quickly as possible. At this point, it seems reasonable to conclude that a better understanding of the cell–cell interactions between neural retina and RPE that induce the rod and cone specializations on the apical RPE surface will be an important step forward in defining the limits of repair and recovery following reattachment. Likewise, understanding how the RPE affects the differentiation, growth, and maintenance of the photoreceptors (or other cells in the neural retina) will not only help us to devise ways to optimize recovery after retinal reattachment, but may ultimately hold the key to treating other retinal degenerative diseases as well.

ACKNOWLEDGMENTS

The original research included in this report was supported by NEI grants R37-EY-00888 (SKF), and RO1-EY-02082(DHA). The authors would like to acknowledge those who contributed to the preparation of this manuscript: Ms. Maura Jess, Dr. Geoffrey P. Lewis, and Mr. Kenneth A. Linberg.

REFERENCES

Anderson DH, Fisher SK. 1979. The relationship of primate foveal cones to the pigment epithelium. J Ultrastruc Res 67:23–32.

Anderson DH, Fisher SK, Steinberg RH. 1978. Mammalian cones: disc shedding, phagocytosis, and renewal. Invest Ophthalmol Vis Sci 17:117–133.

Anderson DH, Stern WH, Fisher SK, Erickson PA, Borgula GA. 1981. The onset of pigment epithelial proliferation after retinal detachment. Invest Ophthalmol Vis Sci 21:10–16.

Anderson DH, Stern WH, Fisher SK, Erickson PA, Borgula GA. 1983. Retinal detachment in the cat: the pigment epithelial-photoreceptor interface. Invest Ophthalmol Vis Sci 24:906–926.

Anderson DH, Guerin CJ, Erickson PA, Stern WH, Fisher SK. 1986. Morphological recovery in the reattached retina. Invest Ophthalmol Vis Sci 27:168–183.

Anderson DH, Guerin CJ, Hageman GS, Pfeffer BA, Flanders KC. 1995. The distribution of TGF-β isoforms in the mammalian retina, retinal pigment epithelium, and choroid. J Neurosci Res 42:63–79.

Arnold DR, Moshayedi P, Shoen TJ, Jones BE, Chader GJ, Waldbillig RI. 1993. Distribution of IGF-I and -II, IGF binding proteins (IGFBPs) and IGFBP mRNA in ocular fluids and tissues: potential sites of synthesis of IGFBPs in aqueous and vitreous. Exp Eye Res 56:555–565.

Baird A, Esch F, Gospodarowica D, Guillemin R. 1985. Retina- and eye-derived endothelial growth factors: partial molecular characterization and identity with acidic and basic fibroblast growth factors. Biochemistry 24:7855–7860.

Bok D. 1982. Renewal of photoreceptor cells. Methods in Enzymology 81:763–772.

Bok D. 1985. Retinal photoreceptor–pigment epithelial interactions. Invest Ophthalmol Vis Sci 12:1659–1694.

Bunt-Milam AH, Saari JC, 1983. Immunocytochemical localization of two retinoid binding proteins in vertebrate retina. J Cell Biol 97:703–712.

Burnside MB, Laties AM. 1976. Actin filaments in apical projections of the primate pigmented epithelial cell. Invest Ophthalmol Vis Sci 15:570–578.

Charkrabarti S, Ghahary A, Murphy LJ, Sima AA. 1991. Insulin-like growth factor-I expression is not increased in the retina of diabetic BB/W-rats. Diabetes Research and Clinical Practice 14:91–97.

Clarkson JG, Green WR, Massof D. 1977. A histopathologic review of 168 cases of preretinal membrane. Am J Ophthalmol 84:1–17.

Cook B, Lewis GP, Fisher SK, Adler R. 1995. Apoptotic photoreceptor degeneration in experimental retinal detachment. Invest Ophthalmol Vis Sci 36:990–996.

Defoe DM, Easterling KC. 1994. Reattachment of retinas to cultured pigment epithelial monolayers from Xenopus laevis. Invest Ophthalmol Vis Sci 35:2466–2476.

deJuan E, Steffansson E, Ohira A. 1990. Basic fibroblast growth factor stimulates ³H-thymidine uptake in retinal venular and capillary endothelial cells in vivo. Invest Ophthalmol Vis Sci 31:1238–1244.

Erickson PA, Fisher SK, Anderson DH, Stern WH, Borgula GA. 1983. Retinal detachment in the cat: the outer nuclear and outer plexiform layers. Invest Ophthalmol Vis Sci 24:927–942.

Fariss RN, Anderson DH, Fisher SK. 1990. Comparison of photoreceptor–specific matrix domains in the cat and monkey retinas. Exp Eye Res 51: 473–485.

Fisher SK, Anderson DH. 1994. Cellular effects of detachment on the neural retina and retinal pigment epithelium. In: Ryan ST, ed, Retina, 2nd ed. Vol III, Glaser BM, ed, Surgical Retina. Mosby: St Louis, 2035–2061.

Fisher SK, Steinberg RH. 1982. Origin and organization of pigment epithelial apical projections to cones in the cat retina. J Comp Neurol 206:131–145.

Fisher SK, Erickson PA, Lewis GP, Anderson DH. 1991. Intraretinal proliferation induced by retinal detachment. Invest Ophthalmol Vis Sci 32:1739–1748.

Geller SF, Lewis GP, Anderson DH, Fisher SK. 1995. Use of the MIB-1 antibody for detecting proliferating cells in the retina. Invest Ophthalmol Vis Sci 36:737–744.

Guérin CJ, Anderson DH, Fariss RN, Fisher SK. 1989. Retinal reattachment of the primate macula. Invest Ophthalmol Vis Sci 30:1708–1725.

Guérin CJ, Anderson DH, Fisher SK. 1990. Changes in intermediate filament immunolabeling occur in response to retinal detachment and reattachment in primates. Invest Ophthalmol Vis Sci 31: 1474–1482.

Hageman GS, Johnson LV. 1986. Characterization of the major peanut agglutinin-binding glycoproteins in vertebrate retinae. J Comp Neurol 249:499–510.

Hageman GS, Johnson LV. 1991. Structure, composition and function of the retinal interphotoreceptor matrix. In: Osborne N, Chader G eds, Progress in Retinal Research, vol 10. Oxford: Pergamon Press, 207–249.

Hageman GS, Kirchoff-Rempe MA, Lewis GP, Fisher SK, Anderson DH. 1991. Sequestration of basic fibroblast growth factor in the primate retinal interphotoreceptor matrix. Proc Nat Acad Sci USA 88:6706–6710.

Hanneken A, Baird A. 1992. Immunolocalization of bFGF: dependence on antibody type and tissue fixation. Exp Eye Res 54: 1011–1014.

Hanneken A, Lutty GA, McCleod DS, Robey F, Harvey AK, Hjelmeland LM. 1989. Localization of basic fibroblast growth factor to the developing capillaries of the bovine retina. J Cell Physiol 138:115–120.

Hilton GF, McLean EB, Norton WWD. 1979. Retinal Detachment. Rochester, MN: Am Acad Ophthalmol, 35.

Hjelmeland LM, Harvey AK. 1988. Gliosis of the mammalian retina: migration and proliferation of retinal glia. In: Osborn N, Chader J, eds, Progress in Retinal Research, vol 7. Oxford: Pergamon 259–281.

Immel J, Negi A, Marmor MF. 1986. Acute changes in RPE apical morphology after retinal detachment in rabbit: a SEM study. Invest Ophthalmol Vis Sci 27:1770–1776.

Inahara M. Studies on the fine structure of experimental retinal detachment. Acta Soc Ophthalmol Jpn 77:1002.

Janeczko K. 1989. Spatiotemporal patterns of the astroglial proliferation in rat brain injured at the postmitotic stage of postnatal development: a combined immunocytochemical and autoradiographic study. Brain Res 485:236–243.

Johnson NF, Foulds WS. 1977. Observations on the retinal pigment epithelium and retinal macrophages in experimental retinal detachment. Br J Ophthalmol 61:564.

Johnson LV, Hageman GS, Blanks JC. 1986. Interphotoreceptor matrix domains ensheath vertebrate cone photoreceptor cells. Invest Ophthalmol Vis Sci 27:129–135.

Kitaoka T, Aotaki-Keen AE, Hjelmeland LM, 1993. Distribution of FGF-5 in the rhesus macaque retina. Invest Ophthalmol Vis Sci 35(8):3189–3198.

Kroll AJ, Machemer R. 1968. Experimental retinal detachment in the owl monkey. III. Electron microscopy of retina and pigment epithelium. Am J Ophthalmol 66:410–427.

Lewis GP, Erickson PA, Guérin CJ, Anderson DH, Fisher SK. 1989. Changes in the expression of specific Mueller cell proteins during long-term retinal detachment. Exp Eye Res 49:93–111.

Lewis GP, Erickson PA, Guérin CJ, Anderson DH, Fisher SK. 1992. Basic fibroblast growth factor: a potential regulator of proliferation and intermediate filament expression in the retina. J Neurosci 12: 3968–3978.

Lewis GP, Guérin CJ, Anderson DH, Matsumoto B, Fisher SK. 1994. Rapid changes in the expression of glial cell proteins caused by experimental retinal detachment. Am J Ophthalmol 118:368–376.

Lewis GP, Fisher SK, Anderson DH. 1996. Fate of biotinylated basic fibroblast growth factor in the retina following intravitreal injection. Exp Eye Res 62:309–324.

Machemer R. 1968. Experimental retinal detachment in the owl monkey. II. Histology of retina and pigment epithelium. Am J Ophthalmol 66:396–410.

Machemer R, Laqua H. 1975. Pigment epithelial proliferation in retinal detachment (massive periretinal proliferation). Am J Ophthalmol 80:1–23.

Machemer R, van Horn D, Aaberg TM. 1978. Pigment epithelial proliferation in human retinal detachment with massive periretinal proliferation. Am J Ophthalmol 85:181–191.

Matsumoto B, Guérin CJ, Anderson DH. 1990. Cytoskeletal redifferentiation of feline, monkey, and human RPE cells in culture. Invest Ophthalmol Vis Sci 31:879–889.

Philp NJ, Nachmias VT. 1987. Polarized distribution of integrin and fibronectin in retinal pigment epithelium. Investigative Ophthalmol Vis Sci 28:1275–1280.

Sameshima M, Uehara F, Ohba N. 1987. Specialization of the inter-photoreceptor matrices around cone and rod photoreceptor cells in the monkey retina as revealed by lectin cytochemistry. Exp Eye Res 45:845–863.

Steinberg RH. 1987. Monitoring communications between photoreceptors and pigment epithelial cells: effects of "mild" systemic hypoxia. Invest Ophthalmol Vis Sci 28:1888–1904.

Steinberg RH, Wood I. 1978. Pigment epithelial cell ensheathment of cone outer segments in the retina of the domestic cat. Proc Royal Soc Lond (Biol) 187:461–478.

Steinberg RH, Fisher SK, Anderson DH. 1980. Disc morphogenesis in vertebrate photoreceptors. J Comp Neurol 190:501–519.

Waldbillig RJ, Pfeffer BA, Schoen TJ, Adler AA, Shen-Orr Z, Scavo L, LeRoith D, Chader GJ. 1991. Evidence for an insulin-like growth factor autocrine-paracrine system in the retinal photoreceptor-pigment epithelial cell complex. J. of Neurochem 57:1522–33.

Wilson DJ, Green WR. 1987. Histopathologic study of the effect of retinal detachment surgery on 49 eyes obtained post mortem. Am J Ophthalmol 103:167–179.

Young RW., Droz, B. 1968. The renewal of protein in retinal rods and cones. J. Cell Biol. 39:169–183.

21. Control of subretinal fluid and mechanisms of serous detachment

MICHAEL F. MARMOR

The subretinal space (SRS) is normally compact with little appreciable free fluid or protein. The photoreceptors interdigitate tightly with the apical processes of the retinal pigment epithelium (RPE), and the intervening space is filled with a complex interphotoreceptor matrix (IPM), specialized to accommodate the architecture and chemistry of the rods and cones. This tight apposition serves a number of purposes. The optics of the eye depend on a fixed retinal plane, and both refractive error and image quality change when the retina is elevated by edema or subretinal fluid. The close apposition is also vital to the exchange of nutrients and oxygen from choroid to photoreceptors, and indeed for many of the interactive functions between retina and RPE that form the physiological and pathophysiological focus of this book. A variety of forces, both passive and active, work synergistically to keep fluid out of the SRS and maintain this tight apposition of retina to RPE. This chapter reviews the mechanisms that control fluid in the SRS, and considers the implication of these physiological systems for pathologic conditions such as serous retinal detachment. Some of the material but not its organization overlaps with other recent reviews (Marmor, 1993; Tsuboi, 1990; Marmor, 1994; Pederson, 1994).

FLUID BARRIERS AND TRANSPORT SYSTEMS AT THE SUBRETINAL SPACE

Flow Barriers

The anatomic boundaries of the SRS are, on one side, the outer segments and external limiting membrane; and on the other side, the apical microvilli of the RPE and the tight junctions (zonula occludens) between the RPE cells. There are also functional boundaries to the subretinal space. The SRS is a part of the neural environment of the retina which, like the brain, is protected from exposure to proteins and other substances that leak out of the general (non-CNS) vasculature. The "blood–brain barrier" for retina is maintained by the tight endothelial junctions of the intrinsic retinal capillaries, but choroidal vessels are inherently leaky and the barrier on the choroidal side is provided by the tight junctions of the RPE. The SRS is also protected from free entry of fluid because the RPE (with its tight junctions) and the retina (with tightly packed cells) are relatively impermeable to water flow. Fluid can cross the RPE by facilitated and active transport, but there is no easy passage for volume flow.

Measurements of the fluid permeability of the retina in the dog indicate values in the range of only 0.03 μl/min/mm Hg/cm^2 (Tsuboi, 1989). Permeability of the RPE is even less, at 0.01 μl/min/mm Hg/cm^2 in the dog, and half that in the monkey (Tsuboi, 1987; Tsuboi and Pederson, 1986; 1988a). Thus, both retina and RPE offer considerable resistance to fluid movements. Intraocular pressure is a driving force for vitreous-to-choroid flow, but the actual pressure drop across the retina is small, since the sclera provides ultimate containment of the hydrostatic pressure of the eye. Fatt and Shantinath (1971) calculated the transretinal pressure difference to be only 0.5×10^{-3} mm Hg, and while this difference is enough to push retina forward against the wall of the eye, it would be insufficient to move much fluid across the retina. On the other hand, it has been estimated that there is a 4 mm Hg drop between the vitreous and the suprachoroidal space in the monkey, which would translate into a volume flow of roughly 0.3 μl/min across the entire RPE (Emi et al., 1989). This represents about 10%–15% of aqueous secretion (Brubaker, 1991), an amount consistent with estimates that up to 20% of aqueous secretion is absorbed posteriorly, but well below the maximum capacity of the RPE to transport fluid (see below). The evidence above, and studies on tritiated water movement (Kirchhof and Ryan, 1993), indicate that the retinal resistance to water flow is rate limiting with respect to the SRS. There is a constant percolation of water (derived from aqueous secretion) through the retina, but it is an amount that can easily be removed by transport across the RPE and no fluid accumulates in the SRS.

Passive Fluid Movement

Because the retina and RPE are slightly permeable to water, hydrostatic pressure is one factor controlling the movement of fluid across normal and pathological eyes. The rate of fluid absorption from experimental detachments in the rabbit rises 39% when intraocular pressure changes from 0 to 38 mm Hg (Negi et al., 1987); in monkeys, there is a 32% decrease in the inward permeability of fluorescein across the blood–retinal barrier in response to a 20 mm Hg rise in intraocular pressure (Tsuboi and Pederson, 1988b).

Osmotic pressure can also draw fluid out from the eye and the subretinal space, because the protein concentration of the choroid is high (Toris et al., 1990). Elevating systemic osmotic pressure with mannitol increases the rate at which fluid leaves experimental detachments in rabbits (Negi and Marmor, 1984a). Conversely, injecting hyperosmolar solutions into the vitreous causes a reversal of the normal direction of flow and rapid detachment of the retina (Fig. 21-1) (Marmor, 1979; Marmor et al., 1980b). One might wonder whether the presence of protein within the subretinal space, under conditions of serous or rhegmatogenous detachment, might similarly modify or even reverse the direction of normal fluid movement. This does not appear to be the case for several reasons. Experiments in which fluid is introduced into the subretinal space show that the rate of fluid absorption across the RPE is only slightly slower when serum rather than saline is in the subretinal space (Negi and Marmor, 1983; 1984b; 1984c; Pederson and MacLellan, 1982). The transport mechanisms of normal RPE are capable of overcoming whatever osmotic differences exist, and even a serum-filled experimental detachment will absorb in the rabbit within a few hours' time. Second, and perhaps of greater consequence, is the fact that the osmotic pressure of the SRS equilibrates continuously and rapidly with the vitreous (Fig. 21-2) (Takeuchi et al., 1994; 1995). When Hanks' solution (289 mOsm/kg) was injected into the SRS, fluid withdrawn just one minute later had risen to vitreous osmolarity (293 mOsm/kg). Even if protein becomes concentrated in the SRS as water is absorbed across the RPE, fluid influx (and possibly ionic shifts) from the vitreous will keep the osmolarity similar. Thus, the oncotic difference between choroid and vitreous will tend to be maintained, and favor the removal of fluid from the subretinal space.

Active Fluid Transport

Measurements of fluid movement across the RPE have varied considerably, depending on the species studied and the experimental technique. Transport rates between 0.1 and 0.3 μl/mm^2/hr were recorded in experiments on the absorption of fluid from experimental detachments in cat and rabbit (Frambach and Marmor, 1982; Negi and Marmor, 1986b), but lower rates, in the range of 0.03–0.05 μl/mm^2/hr, were found across isolated tissue from frog, dog, or monkey (Hughes et al., 1984; Tsuboi, 1987; Tsuboi and Pederson, 1988a). Estimates in man, from clinical data in cases of RPE detachment, are consistent with these data, and suggest that the human RPE can probably transport fluid at about 0.1 μl/hr/mm^2, which extrapolates to roughly ?

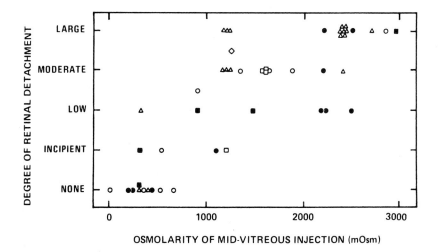

FIGURE 21-1. Effects of mid-vitreal injection of 0.05 ml of hyperosmolar solutions in the rabbit; ○ = NaCl; ● = Na aspartate; △ = penicillin; □ = mannitol; ■ = sucrose. The effects were graded approximately 15 minutes after injection. (Modified from Marmor, 1979.)

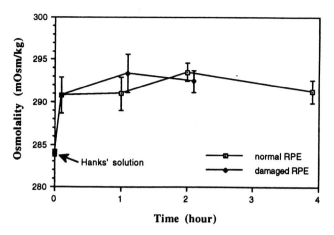

FIGURE 21-2. Rapid equilibration of vitreous with the subretinal space in the rabbit. When Hanks' solution at 284 mOsm/kg was injected into the subretinal space, the osmolality of subretinal fluid rose within one minute to 291 mOsm/kg (vitreous level). It remained in this range thereafter, regardless of whether the RPE barrier was intact or damaged with sodium iodate. (From Takeuchi et al., 1994.)

ml per 24 hours across the entire RPE. This represents a substantial percentage of the vitreous volume, and corresponds with clinical experience that most of the fluid under a large retinal detachment can absorb within 24 hours

after nondrainage surgery (Chihara and Nao-i, 1985). This estimate is apt to be low, if anything, considering that the RPE in experimental or clinical detachments, and certainly in isolated tissue, may well be damaged. As a point of reference, the human eye secretes roughly 5 ml of aqueous per day (Brubaker, 1991).

The high transport capacity of the RPE is dependent primarily on metabolic activity (Fig. 21-3), although hydrostatic and osmotic forces do contribute to fluid absorption. The rate of subretinal fluid absorption is reduced dramatically under conditions of anoxia (Fig. 21-3 *right*) or cold, which suppress oxidative metabolism, and the rate of fluid absorption is also depressed by exposure to toxins such as cyanide and dinitrophenol (Frambach and Marmor, 1982; Marmor et al., 1980b; Marmor and Negi, 1986). Furthermore, if an isosmolar solution of sucrose (which does not cross membrane ion channels) is placed into the subretinal space (Fig. 21-3 *left*), fluid absorption is halted almost completely until enough time has passed for ions to diffuse into the subretinal space and restore the ionic transport that carries water along with it osmotically (Frambach and Marmor, 1982). If the fluid absorption did not involve ionic transport, the sucrose solution would have been absorbed as quickly as normal saline. There are, in

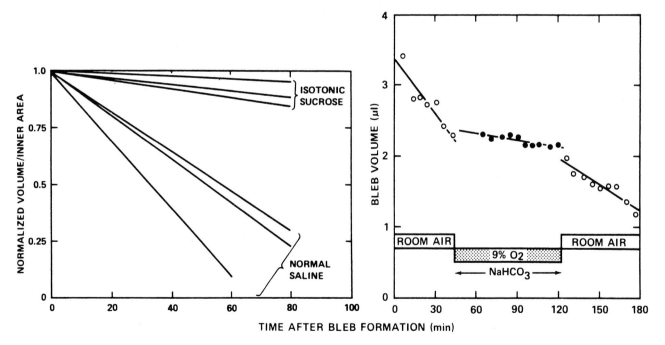

FIGURE 21-3. Evidence for active transport of fluid across the rabbit RPE. *Left:* Absorption of experimental detachments filled with isotonic sucrose or normal saline respectively. There was very little absorption of the sucrose solution, presumably because the sucrose is not transported actively. *Right:* Effect of hypoxia on the rate of fluid absorption. While monitoring the volume of an experimental detach-

ment (bleb), the animal was switched from room air to 9% O₂. Sodium bicarbonate was infused during this period of hypoxia to minimize acidosis. Fluid absorption slowed dramatically during the hypoxia, and then sped up upon restoration of room air. (From Frambach and Marmor, 1982.)

fact, quite a number of different ionic transport systems in the RPE membranes (Quinn and Miller, 1992; Joseph and Miller, 1991) (see Chapter 6), some inward and some outward, and it is only the *net* result from these diverse ionic movements that favors water transport in an apical-to-basal direction. In other words, there is no single water transport system, but rather a number of ionic pathways, the summation of which favors a net outward transport of water.

Since the RPE has such a large capacity for water transport, why doesn't most intraocular fluid (aqueous secretion) leave the eye posteriorly instead of anteriorly? Because, as noted earlier, the retina is a barrier to flow. The amount of water that can percolate through the retina under the normal pressure dynamics of the eye is well below the transport capacity of the RPE. However, if the retinal blockage to flow is removed (as by a retinal tear in a rhegmatogenous detachment), water can freely reach the SRS and the result is posterior drainage of aqueous and hypotony (Pederson and Cantrill, 1984).

CONTROL OF PROTEIN IN THE SUBRETINAL SPACE

The subretinal space normally contains little protein, except as a component of the IPM (Adler and Klucznik, 1982). There is a small amount of protein in the vitre-

ous fluid, and while the RPE tight junctions do not admit proteins, the retina itself has no anatomic or junctional barrier against protein diffusion. A recent series of experiments set out to measure protein movement in and out of the subretinal space, across RPE and retina, by measuring the protein content within small experimental detachments in the rabbit (Takeuchi et al., 1994; 1995). Albumin concentration was measured both by gel electrophoresis and by the use of fluorescein-labeled albumin and fluorophotometry. When the subretinal space was filled with saline, and protein entry monitored, there was virtually no entry from the serum (despite its very high protein concentration: 36.7 mg/ml). However, protein entered the subretinal space from the vitreous (Fig. 21-4 *left*) at a rate of 2%–3% of the vitreous concentration (0.24 mg/ml) per hour. Conversely, when native or fluorescein-labeled protein was injected into the subretinal space (Fig. 21-4 *right*), none of it could be measured in the serum, but the protein concentration of the vitreous rose at approximately 5% of the concentration gradient per hour. In other words, protein will cross the retina at a rate of 2%–5% per hour (relative to an existing concentration gradient) but passage across an intact RPE is unmeasurable within this time frame.

These results are generally consistent with clinical findings and results from previous physiological and

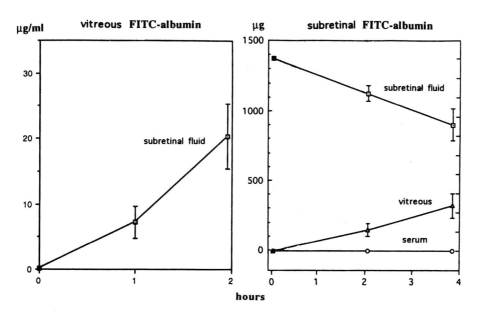

FIGURE 21-4. Diffusability of albumin across the retina. Small experimental detachments were made in rabbits by injecting fluid into the subretinal space. Fluorescein-labeled (FITC) albumin was injected either into the vitreous or the subretinal space, and the rate of its appearance in the other compartment was measured. *Left:* Injection of fluoresceinated albumin into the vitreous. Protein diffused into the subretinal space across the retina. (From Takeuchi et al., 1994.) *Right:* Injection of fluoresceinated albumin into the subretinal space. Labeled albumin appeared in the vitreous, as it disappeared from the subretinal space. Virtually none was measurable in the serum, indicating that diffusion occurred across the retina but not the intact RPE. (From Takeuchi et al., 1995.)

anatomical experiments. Fluorescein does not leak through a normal RPE on clinical angiography, but does diffuse into the vitreous whenever it reaches the retina. When fluorescein-labeled dextrans of various molecular weights were injected into the subretinal space, they diffused across the retina in proportion to their size, and large dextrans of molecular radius comparable to albumin entered the vitreous very slowly (Marmor et al., 1985). Some fluoresceinated material was still visible in the subretinal space three days after injection, even though the fluid had long since disappeared. The external limiting membrane has been reported to be the retinal structure most resistant to protein diffusion, and there is anatomical evidence that thorotrast (with an effective radius of 50 angstroms) does not penetrate the external limiting membrane (Smelser et al., 1965). Albumin has an effective radius of approximately 35 angstroms (Bellhorn et al., 1977) and may be expected to cross to some degree, consistent with the physiologic results.

These findings have several implications. They indicate that protein does not ordinarily enter the subretinal space to any great degree, although a small amount of diffusion might occur from the vitreous and require ongoing removal. On the other hand, if any protein accumulates in the subretinal space, it will tend to diffuse out into the vitreous in proportion to the concentration gradient that exists. If protein is to be maintained in high concentration under pathological conditions, there must be a continual influx to balance whatever diffuses out. It should also be emphasized that protein within the subretinal space does not block subretinal fluid absorption or cause its accumulation. One reason is that the retina is relatively permeable to water and ions, and the subretinal space is in osmotic equilibrium with the vitreous even when protein is present (Takeuchi et al., 1994, 1995). As noted earlier, even serum-filled detachments (Negi and Marmor, 1983; 1984c) or dextran-filled detachments (Marmor et al., 1985) absorb quickly as long as the RPE is undamaged. Nevertheless, as the fluorescein-labeled dextran experiments show, a certain amount of material may remain in the subretinal space for an extended period of time after all the fluid is absorbed. It is not clear whether this represents free protein concentration that may continue to diffuse out, or material that is now inspissated or bound in a fashion where it may persist until it can be removed by phagocytosis or digestion.

MODULATION OF THE BARRIERS AND TRANSPORT SYSTEMS

Actions on the RPE

Physical damage to the RPE barrier. One might think, given the high rate at which RPE transports water, that

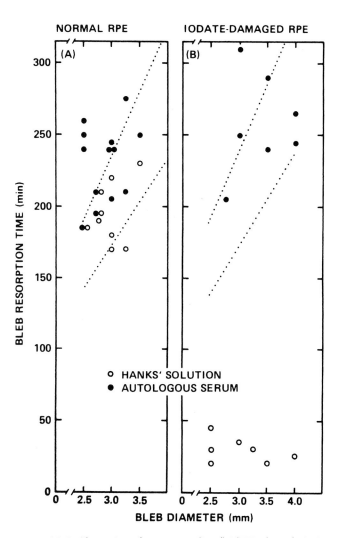

FIGURE 21-5. Absorption of serum or saline fluid (Hanks' solution) from the rabbit subretinal space. The solutions were injected into the subretinal space to create a small detachment (bleb), and the rate of its absorption was monitored. Over normal RPE, serum absorbed slightly more slowly than saline. Over a damaged RPE barrier (after sodium iodate administration), the saline fluid absorbed very much faster. (From Negi and Marmor, 1983.)

damage to the RPE would severely impair the rate at which fluid is removed from the subretinal space. In fact, quite the opposite occurs. When the RPE is damaged physically (with mechanical damage or laser burns) or chemically (with the toxin sodium iodate), the absorption of saline fluid from the subretinal space occurs very much *faster* (Fig. 21-5) (Negi and Marmor, 1983; 1984b; 1984c). All of these injuries destroy the RPE barrier to fluid movement, and allow subretinal fluid to move more freely into the choroid under the influence of choroidal oncotic and hydrostatic (intraocular) pressure. Experimental detachments in the rabbit of a size that requires three hours to absorb over intact RPE will collapse in less than 30 minutes when the RPE has been damaged. Even if the subretinal space is filled with serum instead of saline, the fluid will still be absorbed through damaged RPE at a rate similar to that over intact RPE (Fig. 21-5), which suggests that hydrostatic pressure (Negi and Marmor, 1987) plays a significant role under these circumstances, since the presence of serum greatly reduces the osmotic gradient.

From a functional standpoint, it appears that the eye has both active and passive systems available to remove subretinal fluid. The passive hydrostatic and osmotic mechanisms (Negi and Marmor, 1987; 1984a) are, in the absence of any flow barriers, quite powerful. However, in the normal eye, these pathways are largely blocked by the diffusion barrier of the RPE, and thus active transport is necessary in order to maintain subretinal space homeostasis.

As might be expected, damage to the RPE barrier also provides a conduit for protein to enter the subretinal space. Whereas virtually no protein enters over an intact RPE, RPE damage with sodium iodate allowed the prompt entry of albumin into the subretinal space (Takeuchi et al., 1994; 1995). Curiously, however, the rate at which protein diffused through sodium-iodate-damaged RPE was only about 2.5% of serum concentration per hour, similar to the rate of 2%–5% per hour at which proteins move down a concentration gradient across the retina. In other words, although iodate-damaged RPE is grossly leaky by fluorescein angiography and shows cellular disruption by histology, the impediment to protein diffusion is still comparable to, or even greater than, that of intact retina. Of course, the degree of RPE barrier damage and the potential rate of protein entry may vary considerably depending upon the nature of the pathology.

These observations have implications for the interpretation of fluorescein angiography. The entry of fluorescein through a "leak" may represent only a very small amount of material or a slow rate of entry—even small quantities of dye will be highly visible because of fluorescence and will spread in any available space by convection. The experimental work makes another important point (Fig. 21-6): no fluorescein leakage was observed in iodate-damaged rabbit eyes except into areas where experimental detachments had been made (Negi and Marmor, 1983). In other words, even though the RPE may be leaky, as long as the retina is tightly apposed there is no space into which proteinaceous fluid can move! The presence of "leakage" on angiography is itself proof that there is a reservoir (even if a small or subclinical one) of overlying subretinal fluid.

Metabolic and transport inhibitors. Whereas physical damage to the RPE barrier facilitates the passive egress of subretinal fluid, metabolic damage to the RPE (while the barrier remains intact) has exactly the opposite ef-

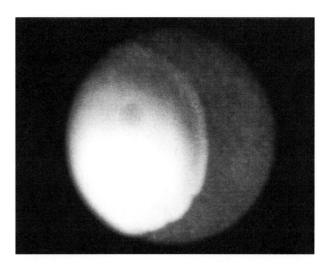

FIGURE 21-6. Fluorescein angiogram from a rabbit eye, after administration of intravenous sodium iodate to damage the RPE barrier, and formation of an experimental detachment by injecting Hanks' solution into the subretinal space. Fluorescein leakage is only observed into the region of retinal separation, even though the RPE barrier is damaged everywhere. (From Negi and Marmor, 1983.)

fect. Poisoning RPE metabolism with cyanide or dinitrophenol slows the absorption of subretinal fluid (Marmor et al., 1980; Negi and Marmor, 1986a), as would be predicted from inhibition of metabolic fluid transport systems while the RPE barrier remains intact to prevent the passive absorption of fluid. Cyclic AMP slows markedly the transport of fluid, measured both in vitro and in vivo, because it suppresses chloride transport which normally draws a component of the water across the RPE. (Hughes et al., 1984; Marmor and Negi, 1986; Miller and Farber, 1984; Kawano and Marmor, 1988). Furosemide, which blocks chloride transport, also reduces subretinal fluid absorption (Frambach and Misfeldt, 1983; Tsuboi and Pederson, 1986b), as does ouabain (Marmor et al., 1980a), which blocks the apical electrogenic sodium–potassium exchange pump. Since the apical sodium pump produces a net ionic movement *into* the subretinal space, it normally carries water inward rather than outward, and blockade might be expected to increase net water transport out of the subretinal space (Hughes et al., 1984). However, net ionic movement across the RPE is a balance of membrane mechanisms, and much of the driving force for the outward transport of water comes from the sodium gradient that is maintained by the electrogenic pump.

Fluid transport across the RPE can be enhanced to a slight degree by cyclic GMP (which tends to have membrane actions opposite to cyclic AMP) (Kawano and Marmor, 1988; Marmor and Negi, 1986), and to greater degree by carbonic anhydrase inhibitors such as acetazolamide (Fig. 21-7) (Marmor et al., 1980a; Marmor and Maack, 1982; Marmor and Negi, 1986; Tsu-

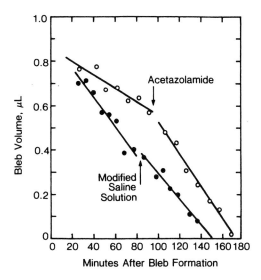

FIGURE 21-7. Absorption of fluid from an experimental detachment in the rabbit, comparing the effects of intravenous saline or acetazolamide (50 mg/kg). The rate of fluid absorption was unaffected by saline, but increased markedly after acetazolamide. The average rate of absorption (μl/mm²/hr) from these experiments was 0.09 before acetazolamide and 0.16 after. (From Marmor and Negi, 1986b.)

boi and Pederson, 1985; 1987a). The mechanism of acetazolamide action is unknown. It is only effective when applied to the basal side of the RPE in vitro, or through the systemic circulation in vivo. Its effects are not related to systemic acid/base shifts, but a rapid acidification of the subretinal space has been documented after acetazolamide administration (Yamamoto and Steinberg, 1991; Edelman et al., 1994). It appears that this hydrogen ion concentration increase facilitates ionic and water transport, although the means by which the drug at the basal surface affects apical pH so rapidly is unclear. The transport-enhancing effects of carbonic anhydrase inhibitors are modest, but the drugs can help to clear retinal edema in a number of clinical conditions (Cox et al., 1988; Fishman et al., 1989; Marmor, 1990)—although it seems most effective in disorders where the RPE is still relatively intact, and thus able to respond to the drug such as an epiretinal membrane (Fig. 21-8) (Marmor, 1990).

The transport-enhancing effects of acetazolamide may result from action upon membrane-bound rather than intracellular carbonic anhydrase. The former predominates in the RPE (Wolfensberger et al., 1994), and similar positive effects on both fluid transport and retinal adhesiveness can be obtained with benzolamide, a carbonic anhydrase inhibitor which is hydrophilic and does not penetrate beyond the cell membrane (Fig. 21-9) (Wolfensberger et al., 1995). Since the unpleasant systemic side effects of acetazolamide are thought to result primarily from intracellular carbonic anhydrase, the use

of a membrane-limited drug such as benzolamide may have clinical advantages.

Retinal Pathology

Retinal damage is not directly influential on the transport of fluid from the subretinal space, since both the passive and active mechanisms act across the RPE. The main concern is the degree to which retinal holes or tears modify fluid and protein access to or egress from the subretinal space. Retinal holes are found in roughly 10% of autopsy eyes (Rutnin and Schepens, 1978), but retinal detachment is a rare disease. Clearly, most of these holes are either not functional (as a result of surrounding scarring or tamponade by vitreous gel), or they are not of clinical significance because normal RPE surrounding the hole maintains retinal adhesion and

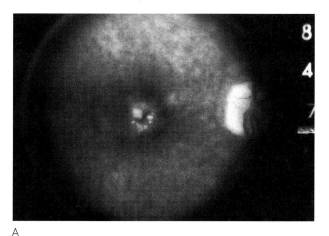

A

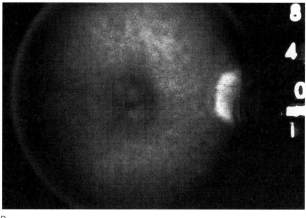

B

FIGURE 21-8. Late-phase angiograms from a 41-year-old man with epiretinal membrane and cystoid macular edema. (A) Right fovea before treatment; visual acuity 20/30. (B) Right fovea after 19 days of methazolamide therapy (50 mg bid); visual acuity 20/20. (From Marmor, 1990.)

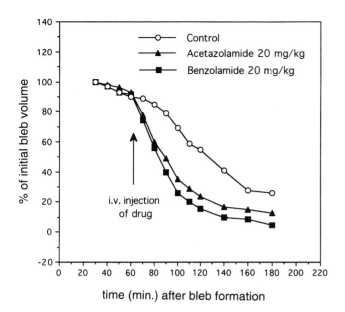

FIGURE 21-9. Comparison of the effects of acetazolamide and benzolamide on the absorption of subretinal fluid in the rabbit. The volume of small experimental detachments was monitored after intravenous injection of the drugs. Acetazolamide and benzolamide produced a marked increase in the rate of fluid absorption relative to control injections of saline solution.

prevents fluid from moving laterally within the subretinal space. However, when holes are large enough, and there is access to liquid vitreous, fluid can enter the subretinal space and lead to rhegmatogenous detachment. Vitreous fluid entering the subretinal space is different from serum and normal saline: it contains a small concentration of protein (roughly $\frac{1}{100}$ of the concentration in serum), as well as hyaluronic acid. Some questions about vitreous toxicity have been raised (Zhu et al., 1988a; 1988b), but experiments in rabbits show that subretinal liquid vitreous is absorbed at a normal rate for subretinal fluid (at least over a period of 4 hours) (Takeuchi et al., 1996b). As fluid is absorbed, the protein concentration of the subretinal space rises proportionally, which suggests that continuous fluid absorption as vitreous percolates into the subretinal space could be a mechanism by which the protein is concentrated in the subretinal fluid over time.

SUBRETINAL FLUID IN RHEGMATOGENOUS RETINAL DETACHMENT

As discussed in Chapter 19, normal mechanisms of retinal adhesion—of which fluid transport is one—are quite strong; multiple factors interact synergistically so that pathology of only one does not necessarily cause detachment (Marmor, 1993; 1994). There must either be

gross traction upon the retina to cause separation, or rather severe damage to the physiologic systems that maintain adhesion. The hallmark of rhegmatogenous detachment is the presence of a hole or tear in the retina which provides a conduit for liquid vitreous to enter the subretinal space. Once a detachment is started, this fluid seems able to gradually dissolve or damage the binding IPM and allow the detachment to spread. However, one may still ask why the fluid is not absorbed.

Eyes with rhegmatogenous detachment are typically hypotonous, which may have several causes (Pederson, 1994; 1982; Tsuboi, 1990). Some inflammation or uveitis is often present, and aqueous secretion is reduced, but some of the hypotony results from the posterior flow of aqueous. As noted earlier, the access of liquid vitreous to the subretinal space allows the RPE to transport a large volume of fluid per unit time, relative to normal (Chihara and Nao-i, 1985), and the only source of new fluid is a relative shift of aqueous movement from the anterior chamber to the vitreous cavity. Such movement is facilitated by the liquification of the vitreous, which not only allows fluid to enter through a retinal hole but also reduces the vitreous diffusion barrier to aqueous. Normal aqueous secretion occurs at a rate roughly comparable to the transport capability of normal RPE over the whole eye, but there could be some degree of RPE injury relative to water transport in cases of detachment. Fluorescein leakage has been noted during the earliest stages of detachment, which would suggest damage to the RPE barrier (Tsuboi and Pederson, 1987b); later on, this leakage stops—and of course once a buckle is placed subretinal fluid can be absorbed very rapidly. Furthermore, there must be water movement across the RPE in chronic detachments, insofar as a balance is reached between the rate of transport out and the rate of fluid entry into the subretinal space.

Hammer has shown that because of this continued RPE transport, a retinal hole does not have to be completely sealed in order for subretinal fluid to be absorbed (Hammer, 1981). In nondrainage procedures, just moving the wall of the eye closer to the hole modifies the pattern of flow and creates an effective suction that draws the retina closer to the buckle (and by narrowing the channel, reduces the rate at which fluid enters the subretinal space). As the balance is tipped in favor of RPE transport, the retina is further sucked against the buckle and the subretinal fluid removed.

Chronic subretinal fluid is highly proteinaceous (Akhmeteli et al., 1975; Himi, 1975; Chignell et al., 1971) and the origin of this fluid may involve both vitreous and serum sources. Experiments on the placement of liquid vitreous in the subretinal space (Fig. 21-10)

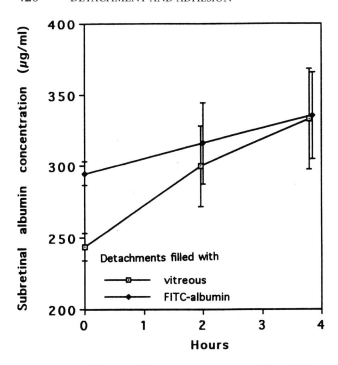

FIGURE 21-10. Changes in the protein concentration of liquefied vitreous within the subretinal space of rabbits. Liquefied vitreous was injected into the subretinal space of rabbits, and the protein concentration measured over time. The concentration rose steadily over 4 hours, presumably reflecting the absorption of fluid. The results were similar if fluoresceinated albumin rather than vitreous was injected, which suggests that vitreous is not toxic to the mechanisms of absorption within this time frame. (From Takeuchi et al., 1966.)

show that the protein concentration rises slowly as a result of fluid absorption (Takeuchi et al., 1996b). This mechanism could allow the chronic buildup of protein, as more vitreous (and new protein) enters the subretinal space while fluid continues to be actively transported out. Of course, a limit will be reached when the rate of protein entry is balanced by protein diffusion back across the retina into the vitreous. This finding of fluorescein leakage early in detachments (Tsuboi and Pederson, 1987b) suggests that some degree of RPE barrier damage is present, however, and this would allow an even more rapid entry of protein. This protein also would be further concentrated over time until a steady state is reached, in which protein entry balances protein diffusion across the retina into the vitreous.

RPE DETACHMENT

In some respects it is surprising that RPE detachments do not occur more frequently, since the fluid pressure for serous detachment comes from the choroid. Gass (1967) has argued that serous detachments in central serous

chorioretinopathy are preceded by local RPE detachment, and perhaps the reason that the RPE detachments are not more prominent or obvious is that the pathologic circumstances which favor RPE detachment, or the RPE detachment itself, may lead also to breaks in the RPE barrier that allows an overlying serous detachment to form and expand. We know little about the strength of attachment between the RPE and Bruch's membrane, which may be strong enough to provide resistance against RPE detachment under circumstances where the RPE cells or the RPE barrier break down under pathologic stress.

One mechanism by which RPE detachment may occur has been proposed by Bird (1991). There are increased lipid deposits in the aging Bruch's membrane, and thus a greater resistance to water flow (see Chapter 34). Since the RPE is normally in the business of actively transporting fluid in an apical-to-basal direction, a decrease in the permeability of Bruch's membrane could cause the RPE to effectively pump itself off. Indeed, RPE cells cultured on an impermeable barrier can form localized detachments by this exact mechanism (Pfeffer et al., 1987). For this to occur in vivo, one would require that Bruch's membrane become significantly impermeable while the overlying RPE retains sufficient health and transport capacity to create a separation.

RPE detachments may also occur in clinical circumstances where there is a rise in choroidal pressure or a focal source of choroidal exudation, but no breach of the RPE barrier that would form a conduit for serous detachment. These conditions occur in inflammatory conditions where there is prominent exudation without direct RPE damage, or in the presence of neovascularization and age-related macular degeneration, where a fibrovascular net leaks fluid extensively in an area where the RPE is still relatively intact. Many RPE detachments in aging eyes overlie occult neovascularization. The mix of conditions may be fairly delicate, since serous fluid is more often (or also) found subretinally. The mere presence of "leakage" from neovascularization, for example, is evidence for at least a local degree of retinal separation, since experimental studies show fluorescein will not leak into firmly apposed retina (Negi and Marmor, 1983). When fluorescein angiography is done after laser burns have been applied, one sees leakage at the margins of the burns. Histology of even very light burns in the monkey shows RPE cells to be vacuolated and disrupted just at the margin of the burn where the choriocapillaris is *still patent* (Marmor et al., 1996; Borges et al., 1987). In the burn core, the capillaries are occluded and there is no leakage, but at the edge the capillaries leak from subclinical injury and the RPE (presumably injured as well) cannot resist the fluid pressure. Detach-

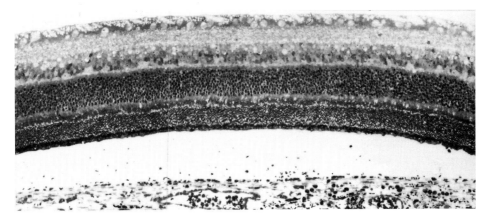

FIGURE 21-11. Light micrograph from a rabbit eye about 15 minutes after an intravitreal injection of n-ethylmaleimide. There is RPE detachment over a moderately edematous choroid. Original magnification ×20; Toluidine Blue stain. (From Chon et al., 1996.)

ment of the RPE is not seen because injury sufficient to cause vascular leakage is also likely to weaken the RPE barrier.

RPE detachments have rarely been produced experimentally. The adhesion of the RPE to Bruch's membrane may weaken acutely under the influence of toxins such as sodium iodate and hemicholinium-3 (see Fig. 19-11) (Yoon and Marmor, 1993). This suggests that metabolic systems may be involved in some way with the bond of RPE to Bruch's membrane, but the mechanisms by which this might occur are unknown. RPE detachments have been observed to develop acutely after intravitreal administration of a sulfhydryl alkylating agent, n-ethyl maleimide (Fig. 21-11) (Chon et al., 1996). This drug causes rapid and massive choroidal edema, resulting in RPE detachment and then later (as the RPE degenerates) in massive serous detachment.

SEROUS RETINAL DETACHMENT

Necessary Conditions for Serous Detachment

In some respects, the intriguing question about serous detachments—at least elevated and prominent ones—is not so much why they form, but why they form so rarely (Marmor, 1988). Considering that RPE defects are seen in many eyes, that the RPE barrier is often broken clinically with photocoagulation, and that subretinal neovascularization with subretinal exudation occurs with troubling frequency in age-related maculopathy and other conditions as well, it is intriguing that large or bullous serous detachments are relatively rare entities. One reason, of course, is that retina does not detach easily

(see Chapter 19), but more important is the fact that powerful mechanisms work to remove fluid from the subretinal space.

From a theoretical standpoint, serous detachment requires three conditions (Marmor and Yao, 1994): (1) There must be access of fluid to the subretinal space; (2) There must be a positive pressure gradient to move fluid into the subretinal space; (3) If the detachment is to spread beyond the source of leakage or persist, there must be an impediment to the absorption of the subretinal fluid. The first two conditions are obvious, but the latter may be the key to disorders such as central serous chorioretinopathy (CSC). It helps explain why a large rhegmatogenous detachment can lose its subretinal fluid within 24 hours after buckling, while a small serous detachment may persist for months and require 1–2 weeks to absorb even after the leak has been stopped with laser photocoagulation.

In some diseases of serous detachment, the area of exudation through damaged RPE is large, and the serous detachment covers little additional area beyond the leak. This is often the circumstance in diffuse uveitic conditions such as Harada's disease, where inflammation and damage to the overlying RPE can involve a large portion of the fundus, and fluorescein leakage occurs diffusely. Under these circumstances the first two conditions (access and leakage) are present, and the third condition is moot, since the fluid is accumulating directly over the area of leakage. A similar situation may occur in ischemic disorders such as disseminated intravascular coagulation (DIC) and preeclampsia, where serous detachment occurs over areas of choroidal ischemia. The situation is different, however, in CSC and other conditions where the site of leakage is quite small

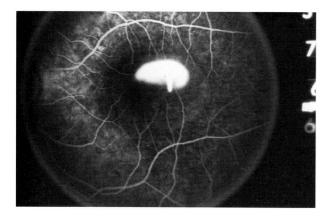

FIGURE 21-12. Fluorescein angiogram from a patient with central serous chorioretinopathy. Dye can be seen diffusing from a small site of focal leakage, and rising by convection to mushroom out within the area of serous detachment.

and focal (Fig. 21-12). It also may be different in the occasional case of age-related maculopathy where the neovascular source of leakage is relatively small but a serous detachment extends widely in the posterior pole. Under these circumstances one must ask how the focal leakage could possibly be so massive as to overwhelm the systems for removing fluid in the surrounding tissue; or conversely, whether there may also be unrecognized pathology of the fluid removal system (i.e., the RPE

and/or choroid) beyond the site of leakage (Fig. 21-13) (Marmor, 1988; Marmor and Yao, 1994; Marmor, 1997).

Idiopathic Central Serous Chorioretinopathy (CSC)

There is little evidence that leakage from a focal source can be so vigorous as to overwhelm the *normal* transport capabilities of the RPE. Neovascular nets are not uncommon, and typically produce only local edema and very limited serous detachment, which suggests that the rate of fluid entry can be handled by surrounding RPE. These active neovascular lesions seem likely to be exuding fluid at a greater rate than the small focal nonneovascular sources in CSC. Spitznas (1986) has suggested that CSC may result from reverse fluid transport through a focal region of RPE cells. The concept of reverse transport is quite reasonable, insofar as the RPE membranes contain a variety of ion transport systems that are simultaneously working in both directions. Exposing the RPE to cyclic AMP, for example, reduces RPE water transport by shifting the balance of transport systems (Miller and Farber, 1984). However, if the only region of backward transport were the small region of leakage seen on fluorescein angiography, it still remains unclear why the surrounding RPE cannot easily remove the fluid. Furthermore, the fact that fluorescein and indocya-

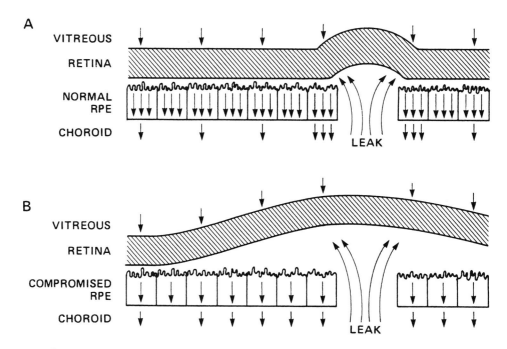

FIGURE 21-13. Diagram illustrating that active transport across healthy RPE (A) prevents the accumulation or persistence of overlying subretinal fluid. For serous detachment to persist, fluid absorption must be compromised (B) so that a balance is reached between the rate of entry through the leak and the absorption through surrounding RPE. The cause of compromised transport may be metabolic dysfunction within the RPE or pathology within the choroid. (From Marmor, 1988.)

nine green can pass through these leakage sites suggests that there is damage to the RPE barrier rather than aberrant transport alone.

The mechanism by which large serous detachments persist over a small focal site of leakage seems more likely to involve the diffuse compromise of fluid transport in the area surrounding the leakage site, with the additional proviso that the RPE barrier in the surrounding region must be fundamentally intact (Fig. 21-13). The intact barrier prevents the passive egress of fluid, while compromised transport prevents active clearance of a normal rate. The mechanisms for impaired fluid transport could involve either metabolic abnormality within the RPE or primary pathology within the choroid that alters fluid dynamics or secondarily compromises the RPE (Marmor, 1988; 1997). Serous detachments are often associated with disorders of choroidal ischemia (de Venecia and Jampol, 1984; Fastenberg and Ober, 1983; Hoines and Buettner, 1989; Cunningham et al., 1966). Recent ICG studies of CSC have shown diffuse areas of early choriocapillary hypoperfusion suggesting ischemia, and then late hyperpermeability, underlying the central retina (Hayashi et al., 1986; Scheider et al., 1993; Prünte and Flammer, 1996). This indicates that the pathology in CSC is not limited to the leakage site itself. Other authors have argued that the choroidal hyperperfusion and/or hyperpermeability rather than hypoperfusion is the primary disorder (Guyer et al., 1994; Piccolino and Borgia, 1994; Prünte and Flammer, 1996; Spaide et al., 1996a; 1996b). In either case, there is a driving force for the accumulation of subretinal fluid should breaks develop in the RPE barrier. There may well be many individuals in our stressful society who have such diffuse choroidal pathology; but only if the patient has the misfortune to develop a focal RPE break, which would allow fluid to enter the region of compromised transport, will serous detachment occur.

Idiopathic CSC in man has been associated with stress and Type A personality (Gelber and Schatz, 1987; Yannuzzi, 1987), and with systemic usage of corticosteroids (Wakakura and Ishkawa, 1984). Multifocal serous detachments can be produced in rabbits (Miki et al., 1982) and monkeys (Yoshioka et al., 1982; Yoshioka, 1991) by chronic administration of adrenalin (or adrenalin and steroids). Adrenalin undoubtedly affects the choroidal vasculature, but may also act directly upon RPE which has both α_1 and β receptors (Frambach et al., 1988; Tran, 1992). In the scheme we have been considering, one might postulate that chronic stress, along with adrenalin and steroid secretion, leads to choroidal vascular changes (possibly ischemic with resultant hyperpermeability and/or metabolic changes in the RPE) that create a condition of impaired RPE transport with

an underlying head of pressure from the hyperperfusing choriocapillaries. These individuals are then at risk for leakage with poor absorption should the RPE break down focally because of local capillary dropout or ischemia, infection, inflammation, or other pathology. This model would help explain why CSC is not purely a focal disease, but in fact is usually characterized by the finding of multifocal and often bilateral areas of RPE damage (Nadel et al., 1979). Furthermore, recurrences can occur even after laser treatment, suggesting that the underlying pathology is not relieved by curing a particular leak.

Why does laser treatment work at all? Because the disease still represents a balance of fluid entering and leaving the subretinal space. In the steady state, that is, when there is a stable serous detachment, the rate of fluid leakage must be exactly balanced by fluid absorption through the rest of the RPE in the area covered by the serous detachment. Histology of low intensity laser burns in animals has shown RPE cells are destroyed by the burn, but fresh RPE cells fill in the defect within a period of 1 to 2 weeks (Fig. 21-14) (Negi and Marmor, 1984c). This new RPE will seal the site of leakage, and possibly restore better fluid transport. The laser treatment also may destroy the underlying vessels that were exuding fluid. This allows the surrounding RPE and choroid to gradually absorb water from the subretinal space (even if at a slow or compromised rate) now that the entry of fluid has stopped. The ultimate resolution of the disease, however, will depend upon a reduction of stress, a reduction of the systemic chemical abnormality, or an eventual restoration of normal circulatory and RPE function.

Protein Content

Serous detachments by definition contain proteinaceous fluid, the source of which is probably serum. In experimental serous detachments, created by focal ischemia or the toxin n-ethylmaleimide, the protein concentration of the subretinal space was found to be roughly 70% of that in serum within 3 hours of formation of detachment (Fig. 21-15) (Takeuchi et al., 1996a; Chon et al., 1996). This suggests that the initial entry of fluid is partially filtered. The concentration rose closer to serum levels over the next 24 hours, suggesting a continued leakage of protein while fluid absorption was taking place. The ultimate concentration of albumin in serous detachments will be limited by diffusion across the retina into the vitreous. The steady state must represent a balance of the rates at which protein enters from the serum, fluid is absorbed across the RPE, and protein is lost by diffusion into the vitreous cavity.

LASER PHOTOCOAGULATION LESIONS IN RABBIT

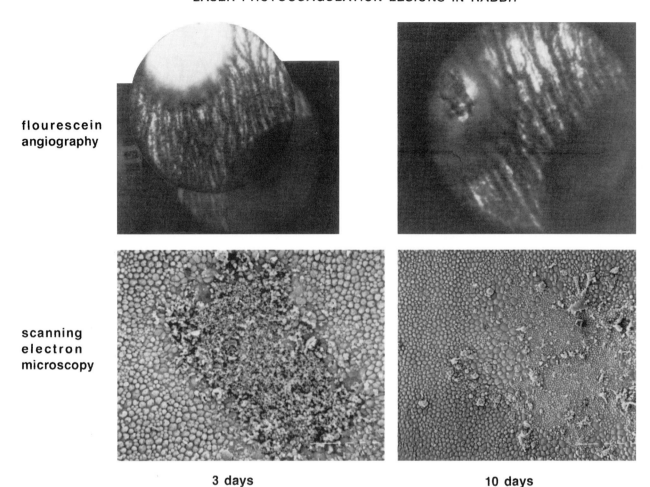

flourescein
angiography

scanning
electron
microscopy

3 days   10 days

FIGURE 21-14. Healing of laser photocoagulation lesions in the rabbit, with restoration of the RPE barrier. Each of the fluorescein angiograms (*top row*) shows two experimental detachments in the same eye: one over an area of photocoagulation burns (towards the upper left) and one over normal RPE (towards the lower right). Fluorescein leaks vigorously over 3-day-old laser burns, but there is very little leakage over 10-day-old burns and none over normal RPE. The scanning electron micrographs (magnification bar = 100 μm) show that at three days after photocoagulation lesions are filled with debris and devoid of RPE cells. By ten days after photocoagulation, lesions are filled with small, proliferating RPE cells that have reestablished a blood–retinal barrier. (From Negi and Marmor, 1984c.)

One might ask whether protein entry or the high protein content of serous detachments would account, on the basis of oncotic pressure, for the formation and persistence of subretinal fluid. Serous detachments have been occasionally observed in paraproteinemias (Cohen et al., 1996) where there is presumed to be excessive vascular leakage of protein. However, when albumin or even larger molecules are introduced into the SRS experimentally, subretinal water (although not all of the protein) absorbs within a few hours (Negi and Marmor, 1983, 1984b; Marmor et al., 1985). Furthermore, the retina is sufficiently permeable to ions and water that the osmotic pressure of subretinal fluid equilibrates very

rapidly and continuously with the vitreous to neutralize any gradients (Takeuchi et al., 1995). As noted earlier, albumin can cross the retina at a modest rate so that a high subretinal protein content can only be maintained if there is a continued entry of new protein (Takeuchi et al., 1994, 1995). Protein may be concentrated within the SRS as proteinaceous fluid leaks in, and water is pumped out, but the protein is not itself responsible for the presence of detachment. For a detachment to form there must be an influx of subretinal fluid that initially exceeds (and eventually balances) the capacity of the RPE and choroid to remove subretinal fluid (Marmor, 1997).

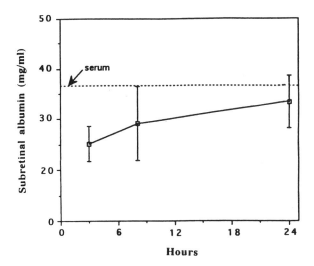

FIGURE 21-15. Protein entry into a self-forming serous detachment in the rabbit. A region of choroidal ischemia was produced by illumination from an operating microscope after sensitization with Rose Bengal dye. Subretinal fluid began to accumulate shortly after this photic injury, and after three hours the subretinal fluid had a protein concentration roughly 70% of serum. The concentration approached serum levels by 24 hours. (From Takeuchi et al., 1996.)

Experimental Models of Central Serous Chorioretinopathy

The complexity of these mechanisms for causing serous detachment may account for the fact that central serous choroidopathy (that is, serous detachment from a local leak) has been notoriously difficult to produce experimentally. Chronic systemic administration of adrenalin leads to multifocal detachments in rabbit and monkey (Yoshioka et al., 1982; Yoshioka, 1991), but it is hard to produce conditions acutely that cause an accumulation of subretinal fluid. Laser burns do not cause serous detachment, although they are leaky at the burn borders where injured RPE cells decompensate over patent choriocapillaries. This holds true even if an eye is made hypotonous to favor fluid movement toward the subretinal space or if subretinal fluid transport is impaired with cyclic AMP (Tsukhara and Marmor, 1991). Small serous detachments have been produced combining focal laser burns with choriocapillary ischemia (facilitated with rose bengal photosensitization), or when an area of retina surrounding a laser burn has been subjected to intense light exposure (which presumably produces a degree of RPE damage) (Marmor and Yao, 1994; Yao and Marmor, 1992). The amount of serous leakage was larger where the light damage had occurred than where it had not (Fig. 21-16), which strongly suggests that the spread or persistence of serous detachment is dependent more on the condition of surrounding RPE and choroid than on the leak itself. However, large

serous detachments have not been produced experimentally with focal leakage. Large serous detachments have been produced over regions of diffuse pathology, such as choroidal ischemia as a result of rose bengal-sensitized light damage (Wilson et al., 1991; Marmor and Yao, 1994; Yao and Marmor, 1992), microsphere blockage of vessels (Collier, 1967; Algvere, 1976), or induced severe hypertension. They have also been induced by drug toxicity as from n-ethylmaleimide (Chon et al., 1996). Ischemia may be a part of the mechanism by which systemic chronic administration of adrenalin produces multifocal detachments.

It may seem puzzling that serous detachments develop over areas of choroidal vascular occlusion, since nonperfused capillaries provide no source of fluid. However,

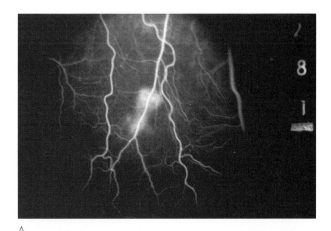

A

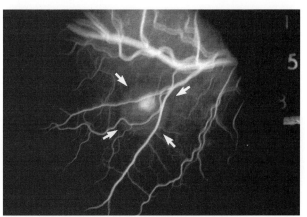

B

FIGURE 21-16. Effect of diffuse RPE damage on the ability of a focal leak to produce serous detachment in the cat. In both (A) and (B) a small cluster of laser burns was made after photosensitization with Rose Bengal to create a focal source of leakage through the RPE. However, the eye in (B) had also been pretreated with intense light exposure to injure RPE in a diffuse area surrounding the laser site. Fluorescein leakage extends much further beyond the laser burns in (B) than (A). (From Marmor and Yao, 1994.)

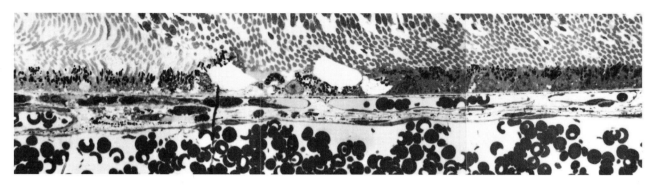

FIGURE 21-17. Light micrograph of the margin of a laser burn in the monkey. Gross disruption of the RPE cells occurred only at the junction of occluded choriocapillaris *(left)* and normal choriocapillaris *(right)*, but over the last bit of capillaries that were still patent. The RPE cells were not normal over the region of total capillary occlusion, but they were not disrupted. Disrupted RPE cells over patent capillaries are a conduit for leakage into the subretinal space. Original magnification ×100; Toluidine Blue stain. (From Marmor et al., 1996.)

the fluid leakage into ischemic detachments typically occurs at the margin of the ischemia where vessels are still patent and can produce fluid to leak through compromised RPE. Vascular leakage is evident angiographically around the edge of rose bengal-sensitized ischemic detachments, similar to the vascular leakage that is seen around the margin of clinical laser burns (Marmor and Yao, 1994; Yao and Marmor, 1992). Histology of laser burns in the monkey showed this pathophysiologic situation dramatically (Marmor et al., 1996; Borges et al., 1987). In the base of the laser burn, the RPE cells stained abnormally and showed some internal disorganization, but remained cuboidal in shape and attached to Bruch's membrane over the occluded choriocapillaris. At the margin of the burn, however, the RPE cells were massively vacuolated and disrupted just beyond the area of capillary occlusion (Fig. 21-17). In other words, the RPE disruption, which represents the conduit for fluid leakage, occurred over *intact* capillaries that are the source of fluid exudation. This disruption of RPE cells is similar to what is found in osmotic serous detachments, where fluid is drawn so forcefully through the RPE as to damage the cells.

Therapeutic Applications

Does this physiologic knowledge give us clues as to a therapy for serous detachment? First, the most critical message is to treat any underlying circulatory or metabolic disorder that is contributing to vascular damage or transport dysfunction. This may represent psychiatric treatment to reduce stress, specific blockers against adrenergic damage, or general membrane-stabilizing agents which can minimize vascular or RPE damage. Yoshioka found that the formation of adrenalin-related detachments in the rabbit could be blocked by pretreat-

ment with an α-adrenergic blocking agent (Yoshioka, 1991), but there is no clinical evidence to date as to whether α-antagonists would be therapeutic given after serous detachments had formed in human disease. The facilitating effect of steroids in some of Yoshioka's experiments raises concern about the role of steroids clinically. Steroid usage is now considered an association or possible cause of serous detachment (Gass and Little, 1995). Unless there is clear evidence for inflammation, steroids are probably contraindicated in CSC.

Agents to hasten the removal of fluid by improving RPE transport have so far not proven effective. Acetazolamide and other carbonic anhydrase inhibitors can help clear macular edema from a variety of causes, including retinitis pigmentosa and aphakia (Cox et al., 1988; Fishman et al., 1989). However, this effect seems to require a relatively intact RPE in order for the drug to have a substrate to work upon (see Fig. 21-8) (Marmor, 1990). This, of course, may not be available in CSC to the extent that the fundamental problem in the disorder is abnormal transport across the RPE (as discussed earlier). It has been noted that the acetazolamide-induced hyperpolarization of the standing potential (as well as the hyperosmolarity response and light response) are normal in patients with CSC (Gupta and Marmor, 1996). Anecdotally, acetazolamide has not made a major impact upon patients with CSC, and there is evidence that it is not as effective at absorbing serum as saline from the subretinal space (Kawano and Marmor, 1988). Acetazolamide systemic side effects are also a problem, although these might be minimized by use of carbonic anhydrase inhibitors such as benzolamide that act only on membrane-bound enzymes (Wolfensberger et al., 1995). There may be other more potent transport-enhancing agents available. Osmotic agents can theoretically help the removal of nonproteinaceous fluid

(Negi and Marmor, 1983; 1984a) but would be less able to reduce serous fluid (Kawano and Marmor, 1988). Their use would also be limited to acute situations, since they cannot be administered chronically.

Visual Effects of Serous Detachment

Finally, passing comment should be made about the surprising ability of visual function to persist in retina overlying serous detachment. Visual function is lost rather abruptly in rhegmatogenous retinal detachment. This may in part represent disruption of images optically, but physical degeneration of the photoreceptors begins within days and becomes severe within only a few weeks (Kroll and Machemer, 1968; Erickson et al., 1983). Presumably, the separation of retina from its source of nutrients and its environmental control is damaging and the retina is unable to survive. In serous detachments, however, visual function can remain surprisingly good for many months, even though the retina is moderately elevated. Contrast sensitivity is reduced and dark adaptation somewhat slowed, but dark adaptation still occurs (meaning that visual pigments can be regenerated and reach the retina) and the loss of central acuity can often be compensated for to a large degree by adding plus lenses (Mori et al., 1990; van Meel et al., 1984; Chuang et al., 1987; Miyake et al., 1988). These observations suggest that the RPE is still providing nutrients to the subretinal space, and their concentration is adequate because no washout is taking place. In a rhegmatogenous detachment there is a continual entry of liquid vitreous (Pederson and Cantrill, 1984), which will dilute and remove nutrient substances and visual pigment in the SRS along with vigorous RPE transport.

CONCLUSIONS

The subretinal space is normally dehydrated, as a result of active RPE mechanisms for transporting fluid. Hydrostatic and osmotic pressures also work to keep the subretinal space dehydrated, but probably are not major factors under normal circumstances since the RPE severely limits passive fluid movement. When the RPE barrier is injured, however, subretinal fluid may leave even more rapidly than normal because of these passive mechanisms. Serous detachments form and persist only when the area of leakage is large (and accounts for the detachment), or under circumstances where both passive and active fluid absorption are compromised in an area surrounding the site of fluid and protein entry. Although protein can accumulate in the subretinal space by entry from the choroid, and build up as water is ab-

sorbed, the protein concentration in a serous detachment (like the amount of fluid) represents a balance between continual entry and continual egress (for proteins by diffusion across the retina). The subretinal space is never a static environment, even in the presence of a "stable" detachment, but always represents a dynamic interplay of entry and egress of both fluid and protein.

REFERENCES

Adler AJ, Klucznik KM. 1982. Proteins and glycoproteins of the bovine interphotoreceptor matrix: composition and fractionation. Exp Eye Res 34:423–434.

Akhmeteli L, Kasavina D, Petropavlovskajaga G. 1975. Biochemical investigation of the subretinal fluid. Br J Ophthalmol 59:70–77.

Algvere P. 1991. Retinal detachment and pathology following experimental embolization of choroidal and retinal circulation. Graef Arch Ophthalmol 201:123–134.

Bellhorn MB, Bellhorn RW, Poll DS. 1977. Permeability of fluorescein-labeled dextrans in fundus fluorescein angiography of rats and birds. Exp Eye Res 24:595–605.

Bird AC. 1991. Pathogenesis of retinal pigment epithelial detachment in the elderly: the relevance of Bruch's membrane change. Eye 5:1–12.

Borges JM, Charles HC, Lee CM, Smith RT, Cunha-Vaz JG, Goldberg MF, Tso MOM. 1987. A clinicopathologic study of dye laser photocoagulation on primate retina. Retina 7:46–57.

Brubaker RF. 1991. Flow of aqueous humor in humans. Invest Ophthalmol Vis Sci 32:3145–3177.

Chignell A, Caruthers M, Rahi A. 1971. Clinical, biochemical, and immunoelectrophoretic study of subretinal fluid. Br J Ophthalmol 55:525–532.

Chihara E, Nao-i N. 1985. Resorption of subretinal fluid by transepithelial flow of the retinal pigment epithelium. Graefes Arch Klin Exp Ophthalmol 223:202–204.

Chon CH, Yao X-Y, Dalal R, Takeuchi A, Kim RY, Marmor MF. 1996. An experimental model of retinal pigment epithelial and serous detachment. Retina 16:139–144.

Chuang EI, Sharp DM, Fitzke FW, Kemp CM, Holden AL, Bird AC. 1987. Retinal dysfunction in central serous retinopathy. Eye 1:120–125.

Cohen SM, Kokame GT, Gass JDM. 1996. Paraproteinemias associated with serous detachments of the retinal pigment epithelium and neurosensory retina. Retina 16:467–473.

Collier RH. 1967. Experimental embolic ischemia of the choroid. Arch Ophthalmol 77:683–692.

Cox SN, Hay E, Bird AC. 1988. Treatment of chronic macular edema with acetazolamide. Arch Ophthalmol 106:1190–1195.

Cunningham ET, Alfred PR, Irvine AR. 1996. Central serous chorioretinopathy in patients with systemic lupus erythematosus. Ophthalmology 103:2081–2090.

de Venecia G, Jampol LM. 1984. The eye in accelerated hypertension. II. Localized serous detachments of the retina in patients. Arch Ophthalmol 102:68–73.

Edelman JL, Lin H, Miller SS. 1994. Acidification stimulates chloride and fluid absorption across frog retinal pigment epithelium. Am J Physiol 266:C946–C956.

Emi K, Pederson JE, Toris CB. 1989. Hydrostatic pressure of the suprachoroidal space. Invest Ophthalmol Vis Sci 30:233–238.

Erickson PA, Fisher SK, Anderson DH, Stern WH, Borgula GA. 1983. Retinal detachment in the cat: the outer nuclear and outer plexiform layers. Invest Ophthalmol Vis Sci 24:927–942.

Fastenberg DM, Ober RR. 1983. Central serous choroidopathy in pregnancy. Arch Ophthalmol 101:1055–1058.

Fatt I, Shantinath K. 1971. Flow conductivity of retina and its role in retinal adhesion. Exp Eye Res 12:218–226.

Fishman GA, Gilbert COT, Fiscella RG, Kimura AE, Jampol LM. 1989. Acetazolamide for treatment of chronic macular edema in retinitis pigmentosa. Arch Ophthalmol 107:1445–1452.

Frambach DA, Marmor MF. 1982. The rate and route of fluid resorption from the subretinal space of the rabbit. Invest Ophthalmol Vis Sci 22:292–302.

Frambach DA, Misfeldt DS. 1983. Furosemide-sensitive Cl transport in embryonic chicken retinal pigment epithelium. Am J Physiol 244:F679–F685.

Frambach DA, Valentine JL, Weiter JJ. 1988. Alpha-1 adrenergic receptors on rabbit retinal pigment epithelium. Invest Ophthalmol Vis Sci 29:737–741.

Gass JDM. 1967. Pathogenesis of disciform detachment of neuroepithelium. II. Idiopathic central serous choroidopathy. Am J Ophthalmol 63:587–615.

Gass JDM, Little H. 1995. Bilateral bullous exudative retinal detachment complicating idiopathic central serous chorioretinopathy during systemic corticosteroid therapy. Ophthalmology 1102:737–747.

Gelber GS, Schatz H. 1987. Loss of vision due to central serous chorioretinopathy following psychological stress. Am J Psychiatry 144:46–50.

Gupta LY, Marmor MF. 1996. Electrophysiology of the retinal pigment epithelium in central serous chorioretinopathy. Doc Ophthalmol 91:101–107.

Guyer DR, Yannuzzi LA, Slakter JS, Sorenson JA, Ho A, Orlock D. 1994. Digital indocyanine-green videoangiography of central serous chorioretinopathy. Arch Ophthalmol 112:1057–1062.

Hammer ME. 1981. Retinal re-attachment forces created by absorption of subretinal fluid. Doc Ophthalmol Proc Series 25:61–75.

Hayashi K, Hasegawa Y, Tokoro T. 1986. Indocyanine green angiography of central serous chorioretinopathy. Int Ophthalmol 9:37–41.

Himi T. 1975. Total protein concentration of subretinal fluid in rhegmatogenous detachment of the retina. Acta Soc Ophthalmol Jpn 79:1865–1878.

Hoines J, Buettner H. 1989. Ocular complications of disseminated intravascular coagulation (DIC) in abruptio placentae. Retina 9:105–109.

Hughes BA, Miller SS, Machen TE. 1984. Effects of cyclic AMP on fluid absorption and ion transport across frog retinal pigment epithelium: measurements in the open-circuit state. J Gen Physiol 83:875–899.

Joseph DP, Miller SS. 1991. Apical and basal membrane ion transport mechanisms in bovine retinal pigment epithelium. J Physiol 435:439–463.

Kawano S-I, Marmor MF. 1988. Metabolic influences on the absorption of serous subretinal fluid. Invest Ophthalmol Vis Sci 29:1255–1257.

Kirchhof B, Ryan SJ. 1993. Differential permeance of retina and retinal pigment epithelium to water: implications for retinal adhesion. Int Ophthalmol 17:19–22.

Korte GE. 1989. Choriocapillaries regeneration in the rabbit. Invest Ophthalmol Vis Sci 30:1938–1950.

Kroll AJ, Machemer R. 1968. Experimental retinal detachment in the owl monkey: III. Electron microscopy of retina and pigment epithelium. Am J Ophthalmol 66:410–427.

Marmor MF. 1979. Retinal detachment from hyperosmotic intravitreal injection. Invest Ophthalmol Vis Sci 18:1237–1244.

Marmor MF. 1988. New hypothesis on the pathogenesis and treatment of serous retinal detachment. Graefes Arch Clin Exp Ophthalmol 226:548–552.

Marmor MF. 1990. Hypothesis concerning carbonic anhydrase treatment of CME: example with epiretinal membrane. Arch Ophthalmol 108:1524–1525.

Marmor MF. 1993. Mechanisms of retinal adhesion. In: Osborne NN, Chader GJ, eds, Progress in Retinal Research, vol 12. Elmsford, NY: Pergamon Press, 179–204.

Marmor MF. 1994. Mechanisms of normal retinal adhesion. In: Ryan SJ, Glaser BM, eds, Retina, 2nd ed, vol 3. St. Louis: Mosby, 1931–1953.

Marmor MF. 1997. On the cause of serous detachments and acute central serous chorioretinopathy. Br J Ophthalomol 81:812–813.

Marmor MF, Maack T. 1982. Enhancement of retinal adhesion and subretinal fluid resorption by acetazolamide. Invest Ophthalmol Vis Sci 23:121–124.

Marmor MF, Negi A. 1986. Pharmacologic modification of subretinal fluid absorption in the rabbit eye. Arch Ophthalmol 104:1674–1677.

Marmor MF, Yao X-Y. 1994. Conditions necessary for the formation of serous detachment: experimental evidence from the cat. Arch Ophthalmol 112:830–838.

Marmor MF, Abdul-Rahim AS, Cohen DS. 1980a. The effect of metabolic inhibitors on retinal adhesion and subretinal fluid resorption. Invest Ophthalmol Vis Sci 1:893–903.

Marmor MF, Martin LF, Tharpe S. 1980b. Osmotically induced retinal detachment in the rabbit and primate. Invest Ophthalmol Vis Sci 19:1016–1029.

Marmor MF, Negi A, Maurice DM. 1985. Kinetics of macromolecules injected into the subretinal space. Exp Eye Res 40:687–696.

Marmor MF, Dalal R, Yao X-Y. 1996. Effects of visible, subclinical and photosensitized argon laser burns on monkey retinal pigment epithelium and choriocapallaris. Lasers and Light in Ophthalmol. 7:97–103.

Miki T, Sunada I, Higaki T. 1972. Studies on chorioretinitis induced in rabbits by stress (repeated administration of epinephrine). Acta Soc Ophthalmol Jap 76:1037–1045.

Miller S, Farber D. 1984. Cyclic AMP modulation of ion transport across frog retinal pigment epithelium: measurements in the short-circuit state. J Gen Physiol 83:853–874.

Miyake Y, Shiroyama S, Ota I, Horiguchi M. 1988. Local macular electroretinographic responses in idiopathic central serous chorioretinopathy. Am J Ophthalmol 106:546–550.

Mori T, Pepperberg DR, Marmor MF. 1990. Dark adaptation in locally detached retina. Invest Ophthalmol Vis Sci 31:1259–1263.

Nadel AJ, Turan MI, Coles RS. 1979. Central serous retinopathy. Mod Probl Ophthal 20:76–88.

Negi A, Marmor MF. 1983. The resorption of subretinal fluid after diffuse damage to the retinal pigment epithelium. Invest Ophthalmol Vis Sci 24:1475–1479.

Negi A, Marmor MF. 1984a. Effects of subretinal and systemic osmolality on the rate of subretinal fluid resorption. Invest Ophthalmol Vis Sci 25:616–620.

Negi A, Marmor MF. 1984b. Experimental serous retinal detachment and focal pigment epithelial damage. Arch Ophthalmol 102:445–449.

Negi A, Marmor MF. 1984c. Healing of photocoagulation lesions affects the rate of subretinal fluid resorption. Ophthalmology 91:1671–1683.

Negi, A, Marmor MF. 1986a. Mechanisms of subretinal fluid resorption in the cat eye. Invest Ophthalmol Vis Sci 27:1560–1563.

Negi A, Marmor MF. 1986b. Quantitative estimation of metabolic transport of subretinal fluid. Invest Ophthalmol Vis Sci 27:1564–1568.

Negi A, Kawano S-I, Marmor MF. 1987. Effects of intraocular pressure and other factors on subretinal fluid resorption. Invest Ophthalmol Vis Sci 28:2099–2102.

Pederson JE. 1982. Experimental retinal detachment. IV. Aqueous humor dynamics in rhegmatogenous detachments. Arch Ophthalmol 100:1814–1816.

Pederson JE. 1994. Fluid physiology of the subretinal space. In: Ryan SJ, Glaser BM, eds, Retina, 2nd ed, vol 3. St. Louis: Mosby, 1955–1967.

Pederson JE, Cantrill HL. 1984. Experimental retinal detachment. V. Fluid movement through the retinal hole. Arch Ophthalmol 102:136–139.

Pederson JE, MacLellan HM. 1982. Experimental retinal detachment. I. Effect of subretinal fluid composition on resorption rate and intraocular pressure. Arch Ophthalmol 100:1150–1154.

Pfeffer BA, Usukura J, Bok D. 1987. Ouabain and furosemide reversibly suppress domes in cultured human RPE. Invest Ophthalmol Vis Sci 28(suppl):374.

Piccolino FC, Borgia L. 1994. Central serous chorioretinopathy and indocyanine green angiography. Retina 14:231–242.

Prünte C, Flammer J. 1996. Choroidal capillary and venous congestion in central serous chorioretinopathy. Am J Ophthalmol 121:26–34.

Quinn RH, Miller SS. 1992. Ion transport mechanisms in native human retinal pigment epithelium. Invest Ophthalmol Vis Sci 33:3513–3527.

Rutnin U, Schepens CL. 1978. Fundus appearance in normal eyes. IV. Retinal breaks and other findings. Am J Ophthalmol 64:1063–1078.

Scheider A, Nasemann JE, Lund O-E. 1993. Fluorescein and indocyananine green angiographies of central serous choroidopathy by scanning laser ophthalmoscopy. Am J Ophthalmol 115:50–56.

Smelser GK, Ishikawa T, Pei YF. 1965. Electron microscopic studies of intraretinal spaces: diffusion of particulate materials. In: Rohen EW, ed, Structure of the Eye, vol 2. Stuttgart: Schattauer-Verlag, 109–120.

Spaide RF, Campeas L, Haas A, Yannuzzi LA, Fisher YL, Guyer DR, Slakter JS, Sorenson JA, Orlock DA. 1996a. Central serous chorioretinopathy in younger and older adults. Ophthalmology 103:2070–2080.

Spaide RF, Hall L, Haas A, Campeas L, Yannuzzi LA, Fisher YL, Guyer DR, Slakter JS, Sorenson JA, Orlock DA. 1996b. Indocyanine green videoangiography of older patients with central serous chorioretinopathy. Retina 16:203–213.

Spitznas M. 1986. Pathogenesis of central serous retinopathy: a new working hypothesis. Graefes Arch Clin Exp Ophthalmol 224:321–324.

Takeuchi A, Kricorian G, Yao X-Y, Kenny JW, Marmor MF. 1994. The rate and source of albumin entry into saline-filled experimental retinal detachments. Invest Ophthalmol Vis Sci 35:3792–3798.

Takeuchi A, Kricorian G, Marmor MF. 1995. Albumin movement out of the subretinal space after experimental retinal detachment. Invest Ophthalmol Vis Sci 36:1298–1305.

Takeuchi A, Kricorian G, Wolfensberger T, Marmor MF. 1996a. The source of fluid and protein in serous retinal detachments. Curr Eye Res 15:764–767.

Takeuchi A, Kricorian G, Marmor MF. 1996b. When vitreous enters the subretinal space: implications for subretinal fluid protein. Retina 16:426–430.

Toris CB, Pederson JE, Tsuboi S, Gregerson DS, Rice TJ. 1990. Extravascular albumin concentration of the uvea. Invest Ophthalmol Vis Sci 31:43–53.

Tran VT. 1992. Human retinal pigment epithelial cells possess beta-2 adrenergic receptors. Exp Eye Res 55:413–417.

Tsuboi S. 1987. Measurement of the volume flow and hydraulic conductivity across the isolated dog retinal pigment epithelium. Invest Ophthalmol Vis Sci 28:1776–1782.

Tsuboi S. 1990. Fluid movement across the blood-retinal barrier: a review of studies by vitreous fluorophotometry. Jpn J Ophthalmol 34:133–141.

Tsuboi S, Pederson JE. 1985. Experimental retinal detachment. X. Effect of acetazolamide on vitreous fluorescein disappearance. Arch Ophthalmol 103:1557–1558.

Tsuboi S, Pederson JE. 1986a. Fluid transport and its interaction with the diffusional movement of fluorescent tracers across the retinal pigment epithelium of the cynomolgus monkey. In: Iwata S, ed, Proceedings of the International Society for Eye Research, vol 4. New York: International Society for Eye Research.

Tsuboi S, Pederson JE. 1986b. Experimental retinal detachment. XI. Furosemide-inhibitable fluid absorption across retinal pigment epithelium in vivo. Arch Ophthalmol 104:602–603.

Tsuboi S, Pederson JE. 1987a. Acetazolamide effect on the inward permeability of the blood-retinal barrier to carboxyfluorescein. Invest Ophthalmol Vis Sci 28:92–95.

Tsuboi S, Pederson JE. 1987b. Permeability of the blood-retinal barrier to carboxyfluorescein in eyes with rhegmatogenous retinal detachment. Invest Ophthalmol Vis Sci 28:96–100.

Tsuboi S, Pederson JE. 1988a. Volume flow across the isolated retinal pigment epithelium of cynomolgus monkey eyes. Invest Ophthalmol Vis Sci 29:1652–1655.

Tsuboi S, Pederson JE. 1988b. Effect of plasma osmolality and intraocular pressure on fluid movement across the blood-retinal barrier. Invest Ophthalmol Vis Sci 29:1747–1749.

Tsukahara Y, Marmor MF. 1991. Experimental studies on the accumulation of subretinal fluid. Ophthalmologica 202:202–207.

van Meel GJ, Smith VC, Pokorny J, van Norren D. 1984. Foveal densitometry in central serous choroidopathy. Am J Ophthalmol 98:359–368.

Wakakura M, Ishikawa S. 1984. Central serous chorioretinopathy complicating systemic corticosteroid treatment. Br J Ophthalmol 68:329–331.

Wilson CA, Royster AJ, Tiedeman JS, Hatchell DL. 1991. Exudative retinal detachment after photodynamic injury. Arch Ophthalmol 109:125–134.

Wolfensberger TJ, Mahieu I, Jarvis-Evans J, Boulton M, Carter N, Nogradi A, Hollande E, Bird AC. 1994. Membrane-bound carbonic anhydrase in human retinal pigment epithelium. Invest Ophthalmol Vis Sci 35:3401–3407.

Wolfensberger TJ, Chiang R, Takeuchi A, Marmor MF. 1995. Inhibition of membrane-bound carbonic anhydrase enhances subretinal fluid absorption and retinal adhesiveness. Invest Ophthalmol Vis Sci 36:S921.

Yamamoto F, Steinberg RH. 1991. Effects of intravenous acetazolamide on retinal pH in the cat. Exp Eye Res 54:711–718.

Yannuzzi LA. 1987. Type-A behavior and central serous chorioretinopathy. Retina 7:111–130.

Yao X-Y, Marmor MF. 1992. Induction of serous retinal detachment in rabbit eyes by pigment epithelial and choriocapillary injury. Arch Ophthalmol 110:541–546.

Yoon YH, Marmor MF. 1993. Retinal pigment epithelium adhesion to Bruch's membrane is weakened by hemicholinium-3 and sodium iodate. Ophthalmic Res 25:386–392.

Yoshioka H. 1991. The etiology of central serous chorioretinopathy. Acta Soc Ophthalmol Jpn 95:1181–1195.

Yoshioka H, Katsume Y, Akune H. 1982. Experimental central serous chorioretinopathy in monkey eyes: fluorescein angiographic findings. Ophthalmologica 185:168–178.

Zhu Z, Goodnight R, Ishibashi T, Sorgente N, Ogden TE, Ryan SJ. 1988a. Breakdown of Bruch's membrane after subretinal injection of vitreous. Ophthalmology 95:925–929.

Zhu Z, Goodnight R, Sorgente N, Blanks JC, Orden TE, Ryan SJ. 1988b. Cellular proliferation induced by subretinal injection of vitreous in the rabbit. Arch Ophthalmol 106:406–411.

22. Manifestations and pathophysiology of serous detachment of the retinal pigment epithelium and retina

RICHARD F. SPAIDE AND LAWRENCE A. YANNUZZI

Good visual function depends on the proper apposition between the retina and the retinal pigment epithelium (RPE), and in turn, between the RPE and Bruch's membrane. This chapter examines the balance of forces that maintain apposition and proposes a framework to understand how the breakdown of these normal adhesive interactions can lead to serous detachment of the RPE, the retina, or both.

Forces Maintaining Attachment of the Retina

The main interactions between the retina and RPE, such as nutritional support, retinol metabolism, phagocytosis of the outer segments of the photoreceptors, and bidirectional trophic support through production of growth factors and other substances, depend on the apposition of the retina with the RPE. Ordinarily, cells attach themselves to other cells with structures such as desmosomes, zona adherens, and zona occludens. Because of the unique sequence in the embryologic development of the eye, the apical surface of the retina is in contact with the apical surface of the underlying RPE. The cells of these structures maintain an attachment, of sorts, to each other on the basis of both passive and active factors without direct cell-to-cell junctions.

Under normal circumstances there is a net flow of fluid from the vitreous cavity toward the choroid (Fig. 22-1). The impetuses for this bulk flow include osmotic, hydrostatic, and active transport mechanisms. The retina offers some resistance to the flow of fluid from the vitreous to the choroid, giving rise to a vector force driving the retina toward the RPE (Kirchof and Ryan, 1993). Evidence for this comes from laboratory data showing the retina to be relatively impermeable to the free flow of fluid (Kirchof and Ryan, 1993), and from clinical observations of patients with retinal detachment (Foulds, 1969; Chihara and Nao, 1985; Pederson and Cantrill, 1984). When a significant portion of the retina is detached, decreased intraocular pressure may ensue, because posterior absorption of aqueous occurs across

bare RPE. A large retinal detachment can resorb in a short period of time after closure of a retinal defect. Bare RPE is capable of pumping almost half of the intraocular volume per day (Chihara and Nao, 1985). On the other hand, when the retina is attached the amount of fluid passing posteriorly has been estimated to be only 0.3 cc per day because of the resistance to flow by the relatively impermeable retina (Pederson, 1994).

The RPE has a complex arrangement of apical processes that interdigitate between the photoreceptor outer segments (Fisher and Steinberg, 1982). The apical processes increase the surface area of the RPE apical plasma membrane about thirtyfold (Steinberg and Miller, 1979). The interstices between the interdigitated elements are occupied by interphotoreceptor matrix, an extracellular matrix that is composed of a number of different molecules, including proteoglycans such as glycosoaminoglycans, which are viscous and form structured sheaths about the cone and rod outer segments. The cone and rod matrix sheaths bond across the subretinal space, and can be seen to stretch dramatically as the retina is peeled from the RPE (Hageman, 1995). Interposition of a viscous material between the large surfaces of adjacent plasma membrane of retina and RPE may contribute to the cohesiveness between these layers (Berman, 1969; Adler and Kluznik, 1985). Evidence for the importance of the interphotoreceptor matrix in maintaining adhesion includes observations that injections of enzymes such as neuraminidase, chondroitinase, and hyaluronidase lead to diffuse loss of adhesiveness between the retina and RPE (Hageman et al., 1995; Yao et al., 1992). Subretinal administration of xyloside, a sugar that inhibits chondroitin synthesis, also causes decreased adhesiveness (Lazarus and Hageman, 1992). The adhesiveness caused by the proteoglycans may be enhanced by relative dehydration of the interphotoreceptor matrix and the maintainence of a proper ionic environment. Leakage of fluid into the subretinal space, such as through the RPE, may contribute to retinal detachment through hydrostatic effects and also to

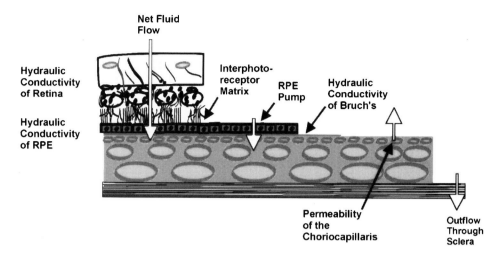

FIGURE 22-1. Overall schematic of forces maintaining attachment. The light downward arrows show the net movement of water from the vitreous to the choroid that occurs under normal circumstances . The permeability of the choriocapillaris may increase the hydrostatic pressure within the choroid to varying degrees. Increased hydrostatic pressure within the choroid may lead to leakage through the RPE originating from the choroid *(upward arrow)*.

anomalous hydration of the interphotoreceptor matrix, resulting in reduced cohesion.

Other components in the interphotoreceptor matrix may promote functional interactions between the retina and RPE, such as factors to promote neuronal survival such as neuron-specific enolase and pigment epithelium-derived factor (Gregory et al., 1990; Hageman, et al., 1991; Li et al., 1995; Tombran-Tink, et al., 1995). Loss of trophic factors may affect both outer segment morphology and integrity. Retinal detachment causes the RPE to lose their microvilli on their apical surface. Degradation of the bidirectional promotion of cell growth and differentiation may result in both less appositional surface area and altered interphotoreceptor matrix production, causing decreased adhesion between the retina and RPE.

Forces Maintaining Attachment of the RPE to Bruch's Membrane

Near the apical portion of the RPE cell are zonula occludens, manifested by membrane fusion between adjacent RPE cells. These are tight junctions which restrict the passage of molecules and ions, enabling the RPE to form the outer part of the blood–ocular barrier. In addition to zonula occludens, adjacent RPE cells also have zonula adherens (Hudspeth and Yee, 1973), which do not appear to participate in maintaining the blood–retinal barrier, but may enhance the structural adhesion between adjacent cells to retain the monolayer structure of the RPE.

The layer of RPE cells is positioned to act as a control over the flow of fluid between the retina and the choroid. However, experimental evidence shows that hydrostatic forces will drive fluid from the retina into the choroid in the absence of an intact RPE. Subretinal fluid in experimental detachments is absorbed more rapidly if the underlying RPE is damaged by chemical poisoning with sodium iodate or thermal injury from cryopexy or laser burns (Negi and Marmor, 1983; 1984). The RPE offers more resistance to the flow of fluid moving from the vitreous to the choroid than the retina (Kirchhof and Ryan, 1993). This suggests that the flow of fluid from the vitreous to the choroid may create a vector maintaining contact between the RPE and Bruch's membrane.

The RPE, while relatively impermeable to the free diffusion of fluid, has active mechanisms to transport water, ions, and larger molecules. In particular, there are several interrelated pathways controlling the movement of ions in the subretinal space including Na+-K+, Na+-K+-CL- cotransport, and Cl-bicarbonate pumps (Miller and Edelman, 1990; Joseph and Miller, 1991; la Cour, 1991; Adorante and Miller, 1990). The Na/K ATPase pumping capacity appears to decrease with age (Burke and McKay, 1993). Concomitant with the movement of ions, these pathways modulate pH and govern the movement of water from the subretinal space (Lin et al, 1992). The ability of the pigment epithelium to pump fluid is enhanced by carbonic anhydrase inhibitors (Marmor and Maack, 1982) and is decreased by hypoxia, cyanide, and dinitrophenol (Negi and Marmor, 1986; Marmor et al., 1980).

The RPE is proficient at phagocytic and autophagic

activities (Reme, 1977). Incomplete digestion of phagocytized material can lead to the formation of waste material such as lipofuscin (Gaillard et al., 1995; Bazan et al., 1990). The amount of lipofuscin in an RPE cell increases with age (Bazan et al., 1990). Accumulation of lipid moieties within the RPE cells may lead to the transport of these partially digested lipids through the basal surface of the RPE cell to Bruch's membrane (Holz et al., 1994; Starita et al., 1995). Because of the lack of transport mechanisms in Bruch's membrane, lipid moieties may accumulate there.

Bruch's membrane is traditionally considered to be formed of five layers. However, the innermost and outermost layers are actually the basement membranes of the RPE and capillary endothelial cells, respectively. The central portion of Bruch's membrane is formed by an elastic layer bounded on either side by layers of collagen fibers that have a random orientation. The RPE basement membrane merges into the structure of Bruch's membrane; cellular attachment of the RPE cell to its basement membrane is mediated with the help of laminin, collagen, and proteoglycans. It is possible that either exposure to toxins (Yoon and Marmor, 1993), senescence, or disease alteration in the chemical composition, proportion, or function of these molecules may alter the ability of the RPE cells or their basement membrane to maintain contact with Bruch's membrane.

Fluid Dynamics of the Choroid

On the external side of Bruch's membrane is the choroid, a densely packed vascular structure that has a very high blood flow. At one time it was assumed that the choroidal vessels were innervated with sympathetic fibers and that the choroidal vasculature does not have autoregulation (Ernest, 1994). Recent studies have shown that in addition to being innervated by sympathetic fibers, the choroidal vasculature is innervated by parasympathetic fibers (Nakanome et al., 1994; Shih et al., 1993). The Edinger-Westphal nucleus is involved in the parasympathetic control of blood flow in the choroid (Fitzgerald et al., 1990). Several different lines of investigation have established that the choroidal vasculature has a sophisticated autoregulation of blood flow (Kiel, 1994; Lopez-Costa et al., 1995; Mann et al., 1995). In addition to autonomic innervation and autoregulation, the choroidal vessels appear responsive to endogenous circulating vasoactive mediators such as epinephrine and angiotensin (Yoshioka and Katsume, 1982; Yoshioka et al., 1982).

Blood enters the eye at a fairly high pressure through the posterior ciliary arteries. This blood pressure must be reduced to the much lower level found in the choriocapillaris. Proper control of capillary pressure is established through sympathetic and parasympathetic nervous innervation, autoregulation, and endogenous vasoactive factors. The choriocapillaris is a tightly packed capillary system composed of relatively large diameter vessels with walls that are fenestrated and ordinarily allow the passage of water, ions, and smaller protein molecules (Pino, 1985). This is different than the retina, where the passage of even small molecules such as fluorescein (molecular weight 374) is ordinarily restricted.

Ordinarily, the interstitial fluid in the choroid can be expected to have a larger range of molecules than what is found within the vitreous or retina. The additional solutes in the interstitial fluid of the choroid creates a larger osmotic force, creating a net suction force toward the choroid. This creates a hydrostatic force that would drive fluid from the vitreous toward the choroid as well. The net fluid flow from the vitreous toward the choroid, then, depends on the hydrostatic and osmotic gradients that are intrinsic in normal ocular function.

Absorption of fluid and protein molecules within the choroid primarily occurs by free exchange through the fenestrated choriocapillaris. Unlike most other organ systems, the eye does not have a lymphatic system, which ordinarily functions to help drain excess fluid and protein from tissue. It is possible that fluid and protein generated in excess to what the choriocapillaris can resorb may partly escape from the eye through the sclera. This may explain, somewhat, the collection of fluid seen by ultrasonography within Tenon's space in patients with certain inflammatory conditions. Alterations in scleral permeability may lead to accumulation of abnormal amounts of fluid and protein, such as seen in nanophthalmia (Brockhurst, 1975) or in the uveal effusion syndrome (Gass, 1983). Nanophthalmic eyes have increased scleral thickness, abnormal collagen fibrillogenesis (Stewart et al., 1991), and increased deposition of fibronectin and glycosoaminoglycans (Yue et al., 1988; Ward et al., 1988; Kawamura et al., 1995), all which may make the sclera more impermeable.

Normal apposition of the retina, RPE, Bruch's membrane, and choroid relies on interconnected and interdependent function of several subsystems. There is a bulk flow of fluid from the vitreous cavity toward the choroid. This bulk flow depends on the hydrostatic and osmotic forces within the vitreous cavity and the choroid. The retina maintains apposition to the pigment epithelium through the effects of its limited hydraulic conductivity in the face of the bulk flow. The interphotoreceptor matrix acts as a mucilage of sorts, particularly when dehydrated by the pumping action of the RPE. The apical processes of the RPE interdigitate with the photoreceptors in a manner presaging Velcro. The

RPE has an active pump that contributes to the movement of fluid toward the choroid. The hydrostatic and osmotic milieu in the choroid is established by the blood pressure within and permeability of the choriocapillaris. The choroidal vasculature has mechanisms to maintain both a low hydrostatic pressure and a high flow rate, all the while restricting the passage of solutes into the choroidal interstium. The accumulation of fluid and protein in the choroidal interstitium may be affected by the permeability of the sclera.

Production of a pigment epithelial detachment (PED) would occur when the forces separating the RPE and its basement membrane from Bruch's membrane are greater than the forces keeping them opposed. If the integrity of the zona occludens, zona adherens, or the RPE cell structure is not violated by mechanical., inflammatory, or ischemic damage, fluid from under the PED will not go to the subretinal space. If fluid enters the subretinal space, it produces a force acting to elevate the retina. Production of a serous retinal detachment of the retina beyond the point of entry would occur if the forces generated by the fluid overcame both the mechanisms to remove fluid from the subretinal space and the forces maintaining retinal attachment to the RPE.

The clinical conditions examined in this paper appear to result from a breakdown in one or more of these subsystems, causing an accumulation of fluid under the retina, the RPE, or both. Four different classes of disorders will be examined, idiopathic, inflammatory, ischemic, and degenerative. Several attempts have been made in the past to explain the accumulation of fluid in these disorders by focusing only on particular physiologic aspects of a limited number of the subsystems. This has produced widely divergent theories about the same disease, particularly in the case of central serous chorioretinopathy.

IDIOPATHIC CHOROIDAL VASCULAR HYPERPERMEABILITY: CENTRAL SEROUS CHORIORETINOPATHY

Central serous chorioretinopathy (CSC) is characterized by a circumscribed serous retinal detachment that is usually confined to the posterior pole. Eyes with CSC do not have signs of intraocular inflammation, accelerated hypertension, infiltration or infarction of the choroid or RPE. The age group of patients most commonly affected in older studies was young adults 30 to 50 years of age (Cassel et al., 1984; Gilbert et al., 1984; Jalkh et al., 1984; Frederick, 1984; Spitznas and Huke, 1987; Castro-Correia et al., 1992). Male patients substantially outnumber female patients, with a ratio reported in older studies of at least 6:1 (Cassel et al., 1984;

Gilbert et al., 1984; Jalkh et al., 1984; Frederick, 1984; Spitznas and Huke, 1987; Castro-Correia et al., 1992). CSC seems notably severe in certain races, particularly in patients of Hispanic and Asian descent. On the other hand, CSC appears to be less common and less severe in African Americans. Patients with CSC are frequently hyperopic. Patients with CSC frequently have had a preceding stressful event (Gelber and Schatz, 1987) and are more likely to have a type A personality (Yannuzzi, 1987). Many patients with CSC are motivated, pressure themselves to succeed, and seem to internalize stress.

There are two main types of CSC (Gass, 1987; Spaide et al., 1996a; 1996b). The first, and more common type, is usually seen in younger patients and causes an acute, localized detachment of the retina with mild to moderate loss of visual acuity. There is usually one or a few obvious leaks at the level of the RPE during fluorescein angiography. The extent of the retinal detachment is generally limited to the immediate vicinity of the leaks. The source of the leak is usually not under the fovea, but the serous detachment of the retina almost always extends into the foveal region. Occasionally there is a descending track of fluid into the inferior periphery. The second principle presentation of CSC has widespread alteration of pigmentation of the RPE in the posterior pole related to the chronic presence of subretinal fluid, and this variant of CSC has been termed *diffuse retinal pigment epitheliopathy, decompensated RPE,* or *chronic CSC.* This form of CSC generally has a slowly progressive, chronic course, and the patients frequently have a more pronounced loss of visual acuity (Spaide et al., 1996b). The retinal detachment usually is not prominently elevated, but may involve a large area of the fundus. Descending tracks of fluid are common in patients with chronic CSC.

It is not uncommon for patients with CSC to have subretinal exudative deposits (Ie et al., 1993; Gass, 1991). Deposition of grayish translucent material on the undersurface of the retina is thought to represent fibrin (Ie et al., 1993; Gass, 1991; de Venecia, 1987). Histopathologic and histochemical study of one case of central serous chorioretinopathy has shown the presence of subretinal and sub-pigment epithelial fibrin (de Venecia, 1987). Subretinal fibrin deposition occurred in 12% of patients in one series (Gass, 1991) and 16.2% in another (Spaide et al., 1996b). Subretinal lipid may also occur, particularly in patients with chronic CSC (Spaide et al., 1996b).

Fluorescein Angiography

Fluorescein angiography in acute cases of CSC demonstrates one or several hyperfluorescent leaks at the level of the RPE (Spitznas and Huke, 1987) (Fig. 22-2A). In

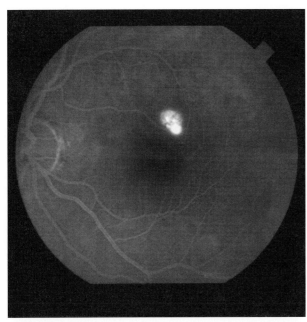

A

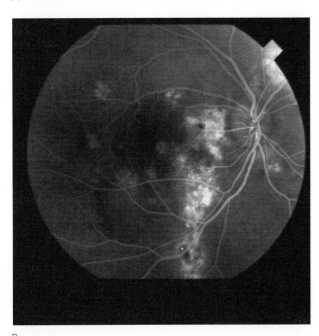

B

FIGURE 22-2. (A) Fluorescein of a patient with classic central serous chorioretinopathy demonstrating a PED and a leak from the level of the retinal pigment epithelium. (B) Fluorescein of a patient with chronic central serous chorioretinopathy demonstrating a granular hyperfluorescence and indistinct leaks.

a minority of cases (10%) the dye rises up under the neurosensory detachment as a "smokestack" leak. This pattern is thought to be related to the increased concentration of protein in the fluid accumulating in the detachment (Shimizu and Tobari, 1971). The new fluid

entering into the detachment has less protein and consequently a lower specific gravity. The newly entering fluid rises up and then spreads out when it reaches the dome of the detachment. A more commonly seen pattern of dye leakage is manifested as a small blotlike leak that increases in size during the angiographic evaluation (Spitznas and Huke, 1987). In the later phases of the angiogram the dye diffuses throughout the fluid and is seen to pool within the detachment. Patients with diffuse retinal pigment epitheliopathy (Fig. 22-2B) associated with chronic CSC have scattered areas of disturbance of the RPE that are best seen with fluorescein angiography. These areas have a granular hyperfluorescence due to relative atrophy of the involved RPE and also subtle, often indistinct, leaks.

Indocyanine Green Angiography

Patients with CSC may appear to have patchy filling of the choriocapillaris. However, proper analysis of the filling of the choroid in patients with CSC is limited by the almost complete lack of standardized knowledge of the filling characteristics of normal people. Later in the Indocyanine Green angiographic examination, patients with CSC demonstrate patchy areas of hyperfluorescence thought to represent choroidal vascular hyperpermeability (Spaide et al., 1996a; Hayashi et al., 1986; Scheider et al., 1993; Guyer et al., 1994; Piccolino and Borgia, 1994; Piccolino et al., 1995) (Fig. 22-3). These areas are best seen in the middle-phases of the angiogram, and appear localized in the inner choroid (Spaide et al., 1996a). With time the liver removes the Indocyanine Green from the circulation, and the dye that has leaked into the choroid appears to disperse somewhat, particularly into the deeper layers of the choroid. This produces a characteristic appearance of hyperfluorescent patches in the choroid with negative staining or silhouetting of the larger choroidal vessels in the later phases of the ICG angiographic evaluation (Spaide et al., 1996a). Some areas of choroidal vascular hyperpermeability may be seen during ICG angiography in patients with CSC that do not appear to be associated with active leaks (Spaide et al., 1996a). This does not imply, however, that these areas are clinically silent. The Indocyanine Green angiographic findings of multifocal choroidal hyperpermeability are the same in the classic and the chronic, more diffuse form of central serous retinopathy (Fig. 22-3) (Spaide, et al. 1996a, Spaide, et al. 1996b).

Proposed Pathophysiology

With the advent of fluorescein angiography, ophthalmologists had a more precise method of diagnosing and

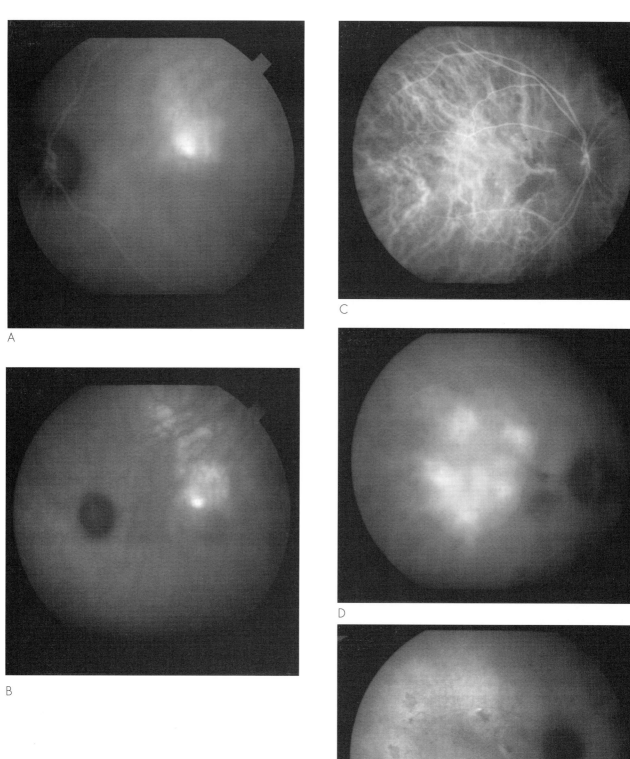

FIGURE 22-3. (A) Midphase ICG angiogram of case in Figure 22-2A showing multifocal areas of choroidal vascular hyperpermeability. (B) Somewhat later in the ICG angiogram, there is dispersion of the dye and silhouetting of the larger choroidal vessels. The area of the leak is still visible. (C) Early phase ICG angiogram corresponding to Figure 22-2B. (D) A midphase ICG angiogram of the patient shown in Figure 22-2B shows multifocal choroidal vascular hyperpermeability. (E) Late-phase ICG angiogram demonstrating dispersion of the dye in a fashion similar to that seen in the patient with classic central serous.

evaluating CSC. Fluorescein angiography demonstrates a site or sites of fluorescein leakage in cases of active CSC. With cessation of these leaks the detachment was seen to regress. This suggested, at least to some observers, that the leak seen during fluorescein angiography represented fluid coming from the choroid into the subretinal space through a defect in the continuity of the RPE (Matsunaga et al., 1994). The fluorescein, contained in the choroidal fluid, was brought into the subretinal space with the bulk fluid flow going from the choroid toward the retina.

Ordinarily, the balance of the tissue osmotic and hydrostatic pressures causes fluid flow from the retina toward the choroid. In experimental models, injury or destruction of the RPE was seen to speed the resorption of subretinal defect (Negi and Marmor, 1983; 1984). These findings suggested to some that a simple defect in the integrity of the RPE alone could not explain the findings seen in CSC (Marmor, 1988).

One theory suggested that a focus of RPE cells, losing their normal polarity, pumps water in a choroid-to-retina direction, causing a neurosensory detachment (Spitznas, 1986). This theory could not explain why the cells pumped in the wrong direction. It could not explain the presence of PEDs, as pigment epithelial cells pumping in the wrong direction should drive the pigment epithelium toward Bruch's membrane, not away from it. This theory could not explain why subretinal fibrin forms, as the passage of protein and water through the RPE occurs by way of different channels, or how a few RPE cells pumping in the wrong direction could overcome the pumping ability of legions of surrounding RPE cells.

Theories about the pathogenesis of central serous chorioretinopathy must address why protein, particularly fibrin, is found in the subretinal space, and how subretinal deposits of fibrin form. Fibrinogen, the monomeric precursor of fibrin, has a molecular weight of 345,000, a size ordinarily restricted to the intravascular space. For protein, and specifically fibrin, to be present in the subretinal space, a considerable alteration in the normal physiology of the choriocapillaris and the RPE must occur. To gain access into the subretinal space, large protein molecules must traverse first the choriocapillaris and then the barrier formed by the RPE. The fluorescein leak of the patients with subretinal fibrin almost always appears to be energetic, and the typical subretinal deposit of fibrin usually overlies the leak. This suggests that the subretinal exudation may be deposited secondary to protein laden fluid jetting toward the retina from the leakage site rather than passive diffusion of protein into the subretinal space.

Integration of the clinical findings of CSC with recent research into the ICG angiographic abnormalities of the choroidal circulation in patients with CSC has led to new theoretical considerations (Fig. 22-4). During ICG angiography the choroidal circulation appears to have multifocal areas of hyperpermeability (Spaide, 1996a). Excessive tissue hydrostatic pressure within the choroid from the vascular hyperpermeability may lead to PEDs, mechanical disruption of the RPE barrier, and abnormal egress of fluid under the retina (Spaide, 1996a; Guyer et al., 1994) (Fig. 22-4D). In past studies leaks demonstrable at the level of the RPE invariably are contiguous with areas of choroidal vascular hyperpermeability. On the other hand, most areas of hyperpermeability are not associated with actual leaks. This is not to say that areas of hyperpermeability without leaks are clinically silent; indeed, increased tissue hydrostatic pressure within the choroid may affect the ability of the overlying RPE to pump fluid from the retina to the choroid. This may affect the size, shape, and chronicity of the overlying neurosensory detachment.

The blood pressure in the short posterior ciliary vessels is about 70% of the systemic pressure. The branching structure, the tortuosity, and precapillary arteriole control of luminal diameter act in coordination to reduce the blood pressure by a factor of ten within the .25 millimeter thickness of the choroid. The blood flow within the choriocapillaris is quite pulsatile, and may have a duty cycle as low as 30% (Flower, 1995). It is possible that any alteration in the function of this system to reduce the blood pressure could result in increased pressure transmitted to the choriocapillaris. It is also possible that venous congestion in the choroid may also cause increased intravascular pressure in the choriocapillaris. This pressure overload may be the cause of the choroidal vascular hyperpermeability, which appears to require the presence of the choriocapillaris to occur (Spaide, et al., 1996a). Abnormal leakage from the choriocapillaris allows escape of both excessive amounts of fluid and large molecules such as fibrinogen. Mechanical breakdown of intercellular attachments in the RPE monolayer, possibly related to the increased hydrostatic pressure may provide a pathway for the fluid and protein molecules to gain access to the subretinal space.

The presence of subretinal and subpigment epithelial fluid depends on abnormal hyperpemeability of the choriocapillaris, a defect in the RPE barrier, and to a certain extext, a deficiency in the absorption of the subretinal fluid. Alterations in the degree of hyperpermeability, RPE barrier function, or resorption of subretinal fluid would change the size and morphology of the retinal detachment. Spontaneous resolution of the neurosensory detachment in CSC may occur with decreased choroidal vascular hyperpermeability, restoration of the

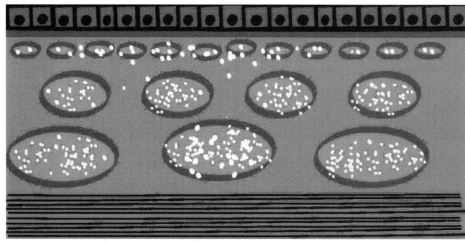

A

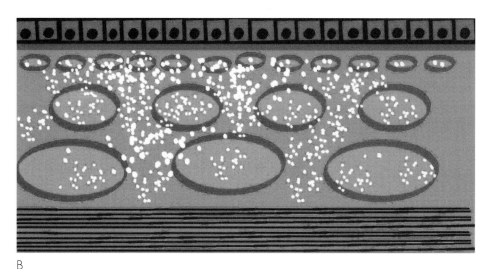

B

FIGURE 22-4. Drawings. (A) ICG early phase. Soon after injection, the dye *(gray dots)* is largely confined within the choroidal vessels. (B) Midphase of the ICG angiogram showing hyperpermeability from the choroidal vessels. (C) Late phase showing dispersion of the dye within the choroid and silhouetting of the larger choroidal vessels. (D) Cross-sectional drawing demonstrating formation of serous pigment epithelial and retinal detachment secondary to increased hydrostatic forces arising from the choroid. Note that the formation of the PED can not be explained by alterations in the pumping ability of the RPE. (from Spaide RF, et al. 1996a)

RPE barrier, or increased resorption of the subretinal fluid. The mechanisms by which laser photocoagulation work to cause a more rapid resolution of the leak are not known, but laser photocoagulation may affect the hyperpermeable vessels in the region of the leak or it may stimulate the RPE to either cover the defects at the site of the leak or to secrete factors that control choriocapillaris function (Sakamoto, 1995; Mancini, 1986; Morse, 1989; Goureau, 1994).

A curious aspect of CSC is that it develops primarily in patients who are hyperopic and almost never occurs in patients with pathologic myopia. Hyperopes have increased scleral thickness, which may decrease outflow of fluid through the posterior sclera. In light of the lack of lymphatic drainage from the choroid, relative impermeability by the sclera may accentuate any abnormal fluid dynamics caused by hyperpermeable choroidal vessels. If the sclera is relatively impermeable in patients with CSC, there might be an abnormal accumulation of protein within the choroid. This protein may stain during the ICG angiographic evaluation to produce the patchy areas of hyperfluorescence seen.

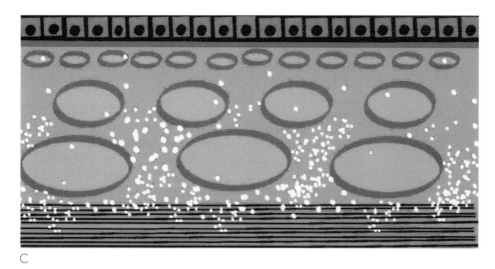

C

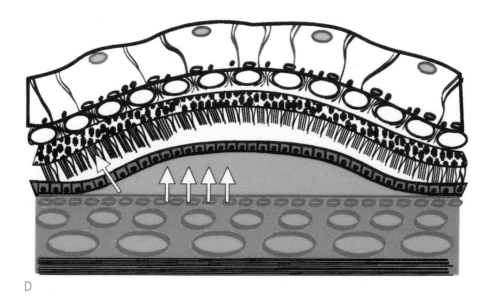

D

Abnormal vascular hyperpermeability must be involved in patients with CSC, however, because PEDs and leaks are seen to overlie areas of choroidal vascular hyperpermeability.

INFLAMMATORY: VOGT-KOYANAGI-HARADA SYNDROME

Eyes affected with Vogt-Koyanagi-Harada (VKH) syndrome have decreased visual acuity, show signs of iritis or vitritis, and have exudative detachments of the retina and RPE (Rao et al., 1995). Harada's disease most commonly occurs in young patients of both sexes. In the United States VKH is uncommon, but occurs most frequently in patients of Asian or American Indian descent (Davis et al., 1990). In Japan, VKH is a common form of uveitis (Murakami et al., 1994). VKH has occurred simultaneously in monozygotic twins (Rutzen et al., 1995), and it shows associations with certain HLA types (Islam et al., 1994), supporting the theory that there may be a genetic propensity for the disease. Indeed, patients with VKH vary in course of the disease in relation to the subtype of HLA-DRB1 that they have (Islam, 1994).

Patients with VKH have a variety of intraocular and systemic problems. Extraocular findings include fever, headache, and neck stiffness. The cerebral spinal fluid frequently demonstrates pleocytosis, but no organisms (Norose et al., 1990). Hearing problems are common and include high-frequency hearing loss, dysacusia, and tinnitus (Nussenblat, 1994). Changes of pigmentation are prevalent in VKH, including vitiligo, perilimbal vitiligo, and poliosis.

The intraocular findings are related to inflammation that appears to have a partiality for melanin pigment. In the anterior segment granulomatous iritis, shallowing of the anterior chamber, pupillary membranes, synechia, or cataract may occur. Vitritis and swelling of the optic disk are usually present. Bullous collections of fluid cause round or oval detachments of the retina. The fluid in the detachments may be clear, serous, or fluid, or may be slight turbid, presumably from increased protein content. The underlying RPE may have scattered yellow half-disk-diameter areas of yellow discoloration. Some patients have multiple PEDs. Later in the course of the disease, particularly in the periphery, well defined areas of atrophy appear and cause depigmentation of the RPE and choroid. These atrophic spots vary in size from pinpoint to medium-sized $\frac{1}{4}$ to $\frac{1}{2}$ disk diameter to larger areas caused by the confluence of smaller lesions. They may have a punched-out appearance similar to multifocal choroiditis and panuveitis. The patients may also have a more generalized depigmentation of the choroid in the later phases of the disease. Increased visibility of the choroidal vasculature accentuates the reddish orange hue of the fundus, and has been termed the "setting sun" fundus (Inomata and Sakamoto, 1990). Patients with VKH frequently show the ultrasonographic findings of thickening of the choroid and sclera (Forster et al., 1990).

Fluorescein Angiography

Immediately after injection, patients with VKH display patchy filling of the choroid. Shortly afterward, multiple pinpoint leaks are visible at the level of the RPE. Over the course of the study these leaks cause pooling of dye into the subretinal space. Multiple PEDs may be seen. Some of these are the typical round or oval dome-shaped elevations, while others have a more diffuse and flatter appearance. Patients may also have staining later in the angiographic evaluation, particularly in the areas of filling delays.

Indocyanine Green Angiography

Less is known about the ICG angiographic findings of VKH because of the limited number of examinations performed. Choroidal filling defects are seen during the early phases of ICG angiography (Matsunaga et al., 1994). Pinpoint leaks may be less visible than during fluorescein angiography, but are present. There is widespread leakage of dye from the choroidal vessels, partially obscuring the visibility of the larger vessels (Yuzawa et al., 1993). In the later phases of the ICG angiography areas involved with retinal detachment may be hypofluorescent, possibly because of blockage of fluorescence by the protein-laden subretinal fluid (Yuzawa et al., 1993).

Proposed Pathophysiology

Inflammation causes a breakdown in the blood–ocular barrier, increased permeability from vessels (Edamitsu et al., 1995; Green et al., 1990), and inflammation may also may lead to vascular occlusion within the eye (Sanders and Graham, 1988). VKH appears to show a predilection for melanin, and thereby, may have a profound effect on the choroid, a highly pigmented, vascular structure. Direct and indirect involvement of the choroidal vessels may lead to diffuse leakage. Indeed, the blood vessels throughout the choroid show diffuse hyperpermeability during ICG angiography. This pattern of hyperpermeability in VKH is different from the discrete zones of choriocapillaris hyperpermeability seen in CSC. In VKH, inflammatory and ischemic injury to the RPE cells and their intercellular connections may vitiate the integrity of the outer blood–ocular barrier, promoting leakage through the RPE. Turbidity of the subretinal fluid may arise from the egress of protein from the vascular hyperpermeability.

Treatment with corticosteroids generally causes a fairly rapid decrease in the extent of serous retinal detachment, number and size of PEDs, and the amount of clinically evident intraocular inflammation. Corticosteroids (Schleimer, 1993) modulate or reduce the production of a number of different inflammatory and proinflammatory mediators that potentially can affect the choroidal circulation, including prostaglandins, leukotrienes, bradykinin, cytokines, nitric oxide, free radicals, and platelet activating factor. Corticosteroids also reduce or inhibit cellular mediators of inflammation such as leukocytes. Reduction of the inflammation in the choroid appears to allow restoration of more normal vascular and blood–ocular barrier function allowing a resolution of the detachment of the RPE and retina.

Another inflammatory entity that may cause collection of fluid under the retina or pigment epithelium is posterior scleritis. Patients with posterior scleritis have multiple pinpoint leaks from the RPE. By ultrasonography patients have thickening of the choroid and sclera. It is possible that patients with posterior scleritis not only have widespread choroidal vascular leakage, but also have inflammatory-induced scleral outflow changes, leading to the abnormal accumulation of fluid.

ISCHEMIC: THROMBOTIC THROMBOCYTOPENIC PURPURA (TTP), DISSEMINATED INTRAVASCULAR COAGULATION (DIC), ECLAMPSIA, MALIGNANT HYPERTENSION

Although TTP, DIC, eclampsia, and malignant hypertension seemingly are a disparate group, they share some similarities in the manifestation of serous retinal detachment that often is associated with necrotic areas of RPE. TTP causes a classic pentad of findings: microangiopathic hemolytic anemia, thrombocytopenia, fever, and neurologic and renal dysfunction (Melton and Spaide, 1996). TTP may occur secondary to malignancies, connective tissue diseases, sepsis, and HIV infection. Patients with DIC have hemorrhage from multiple sites and ischemia from vasopasm and microthrombi. There are many possible causes for DIC, but the final pathway for end organ damage is intravascular activation of the coagulation cascade. Consumption of coagulation proteins as well as production of fibrin degradation products from fibrinolysis leads to widespread hemorrhage. The hallmarks of eclampsia are hypertension, proteinuria, consumptive coagulopathy, and seizures. Malignant hypertension causes profoundly elevated blood pressure with widespread organ damage from the combined effects of edema and ischemia. Malignant hypertension has been related to abnormalities in the renin-aldosterone-angiotensin system and endothelin-1 plasma levels in some patients.

Patients with any of these ischemic disorders present with decreased visual acuity related to serous detachments of the retina associated with yellow placoid discoloration of the RPE. (Fig. 22-5A and Plate 22-I). On occasion occlusion of larger choroidal vessels may be seen as streaks radiating in the fundus. In TTP and DIC there may be cotton-wool spots related to retinal microvascular occlusion. In addition to cotton-wool spots, patients with malignant hypertension and eclampsia often have retinal hemorrhages, intraretinal lipid (including star figures in the macula), and swelling of the nerve head. In all of these entities, the choroidal circulation

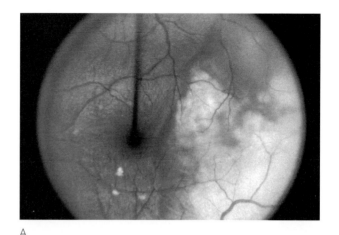

A

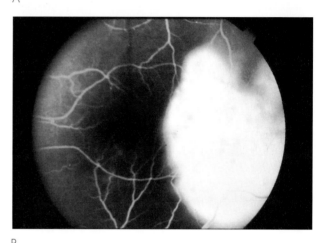

B

FIGURE 22-5. (A) The left eye of a patient with TTP demostrating a serous detachment of the retina overlying a yellowish geographic placoid region at the level of the RPE. Note the small cluster of cotton-wool spots inferior to the fovea. (B) Fluorescein angiography of the same region shows intense leakage from and staining of the yellow placoid area.

appears to be affected more than the retinal circulation. It is possible that because of the rapid deceleration of the blood flow and the larger volumetric flow within the choroid, platelet emboli may be more likely to become lodged there (Melton and Spaide, 1996; Cogan, 1975).

With resolution of these conditions the serous detachments abate as leakage from the RPE decreases. Infarcted areas of the RPE and choroid may lead to scattered hyperpigmented spots (Elschnig's spots), branching yellowish lines in the posterior pole (Siegrist's lines), triangular areas of RPE scarring with an apex pointing toward the posterior pole (Amalric's triangles), or, in patients with severe affectation, widespread pigmentary disturbance.

Fluorescein Angiography

Irregular filling of the choroid during fluorescein angiography is common. Multiple leaks from the level of the RPE associated with the yellowish patches are seen in patients with serous detachment of the retina. The yellow patches demonstrate late staining and diffuse leakage (Fig. 22-5B). Sometimes the leaks seem to be more common in areas of relatively normal perfusion adjacent to ischemic areas. Leakage from the retinal vessels may occur, and particularly in cases of malignant hypertension. Staining in the optic nerve head may be seen in all of the ischemic disorders.

With cessation of the inciting event, diminution of the serous detachment and resolution of the acute RPE injury occurs. Patients develop coarse granularity of the pigmentation with transmission defects seen in areas of infarcted RPE. If the RPE has been damaged but not infarcted, it may heal with varying degrees of pigmentation. Infarcted vessels in the choroid may show lack of substantive filling.

Indocyanine Green Angiography

Patients with ischemic disorders are usually incapacitated because of their serious illnesses and often can not participate in angiography of the eye. Because ICG angiography is not as available and the length of the angiographic examination is longer than fluorescein angiography, there is a relative paucity of published cases of any of these seriously ill patients.

Proposed Pathophysiology

Common to all of these disorders is damage to the formed elements of the blood and microvascular occlusion secondary to deposition of fibrin within small vessels. This leads to ischemia and necrosis. Damage to the vessel walls may lead to leakage if the vessel is not completely occluded. In the eye there is occlusion of the choroidal arterioles, choriocapillaris, and venules, necrosis of the RPE, and serous detachment of the retina.

Integration of the clinical, angiographic, and histopathologic findings points to widespread breakdown of the blood–ocular barrier. There is leakage from the retinal and choroidal vessels, leading to accumulation of fluid in the subretinal space through the RPE. PEDs are not common in this group of disorders. It is possible that the ischemic injury to the RPE damages the zona occludens and zona adherens allowing a relatively free flow of fluid from the choroid directly to the subretinal space. If the RPE offers ineffectual resistance to the passage of fluid because the cells in the monolayer have diapha-

nous interconnections, little force would be generated by choroidal vascular hyperpermeability to elevate the RPE to form a PED. With necrosis of the RPE some of the passive mechanisms to maintain retinal attachment, such as the integrity of the interdigitation of apical processes with the outer receptors and the adhesion due to the interphotoreceptor matrix, would suffer as well. Because of the breakdown of these factors, fluid generated in the choroid could directly elevate the retina, producing a serous detachment.

DEGENERATIVE: NONEXUDATIVE AGE-RELATED MACULAR DEGENERATION

The most common reason for visual loss in older patients is age-related macular degeneration (AMD) (Leibowitz et al., 1980). The exudative form accounts for the majority of blindness in patients with AMD. The nonexudative form, which generally precedes the exudative form, has as its hallmark drusen. The Beaver Dam Eye Study found that drusen were commonly found in patients over 43 years of age, with large and indistinct drusen being more prevalent in patients 75 years or older (Klein et al., 1992).

PEDs are commonly seen in association with drusen in nonexudative AMD (Bird and Marshall, 1986). The size of PEDs seen in nonexudative AMD usually ranges from $\frac{1}{4}$ to 2 disk diameters. Patients with PEDs may retain good visual acuity (Klein et al., 1980). PEDs may flatten spontaneously, many times leaving an area of atrophy at the level of the RPE. It is possible to flatten serous PEDs with laser photocoagulation, but often patients do not enjoy an improvement in visual acuity. Some patients have had tears of the RPE after laser treatment of PEDs. Laser photocoagulation of PEDs was examined in a one prospective study; however, a number of these eyes may have harbored occult choroidal neovascularization making any conclusions difficult (Moorfields Macular Study Group, 1982).

Fluorescein Angiography

PEDs in nonexudative AMD fill uniformly during the early stages of fluorescein angiography (Fig. 22-6). The fluorescence reaches a peak during the middle phases of the angiographic evaluation, and then recedes later in the study. Pigmentary figures appear as dark lines against the bright background of the PED. Fluorescein angiographic findings of irregular hyperfluorescence, hypofluorescence, notching, folds in the PED, and irregular elevation of the PED all suggest the presence of occult choroidal neovascularization (Gass, 1984; Schatz

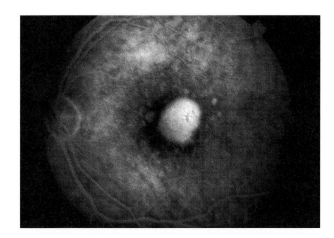

FIGURE 22-6. Fluorescein angiogram of serous PED in an older patient with age-related macular degeneration without choroidal neovascularization.

et al., 1990). With spontaneous flattening of a PED and resultant atrophy, a window defect may be seen.

Indocyanine Green Angiography

There has been limited published data on the ICG angiographic findings of serous PEDs without concurrent choroidal neovascularization (Yuzawa et al., 1995) (Fig.

22-7). ICG angiography has an important clinical utility in delineating areas of choroidal neovascularization underlying PEDs because the ability of ICG angiography to image the choroidal vasculature is greater that fluorescein angiography. In our experience, serous PEDs associated with nonexudative AMD do not show increased choroidal vascular hyperpermeability.

Proposed Pathophysiology

With age several important physiochemical changes occur in Bruch's membrane itself. Increases in collagen, thickening of the intercapillary pillars, accumulation of basal laminar deposit, diffuse accumulation of neutral lipids and phospholipids—all contribute to a generalized thickening of Bruch's membrane with aging (Marshall et al., 1994; Ramrattan et al., 1994). Because of the continued deposition of collagen and accumulation of lipid, the ability of water and other molecules to traverse Bruch's membrane decreases with the increasing age. The hydraulic conductivity of Bruch's membrane in the macular area decreases by half every decade, while the decrease in hydraulic conductivity in the periphery is less prominent (Moore et al., 1995). The RPE pumps fluid, but, with increasing resistance to water flow by an increasingly hydrophobic Bruch's membrane (Bird and

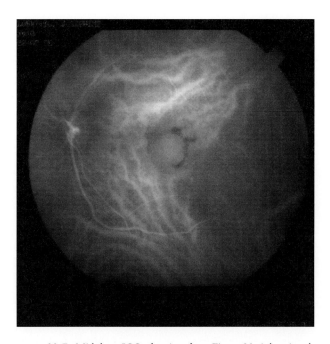

FIGURE 22-7. Midphase ICG of patient from Figure 22-6 showing the lack of underlying hyperpermeability. The serous PED is attributed to decreased permeability of Bruch's membrane to the movement of water.

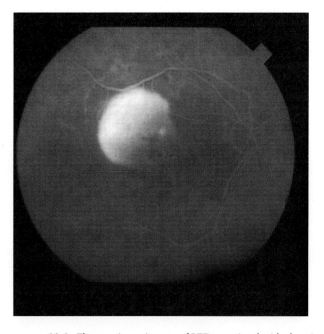

FIGURE 22-8. Fluorescein angiogram of PED associated with choroidal neovascularization showing diffuse hyperfluorescence. Note that the actual area of choroidal neovascularization is not well seen because of the prominent amount of overlying dye.

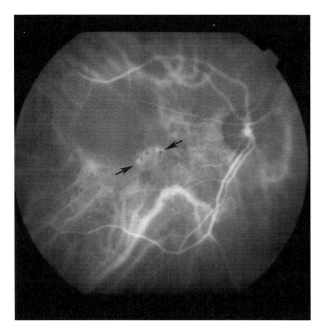

FIGURE 22-9. Midphase ICG angiogram demonstrating the area of choroidal neovascularization in the notch of the PED *(arrows)*.

Marshall, 1986), the fluid may accumulate between the RPE and Bruch's membrane.

The mechanism of spontaneous flattening of a PED is interesting, especially in light of the subsequent atrophy commonly seen in the wake of the PED. It is possible that the primary event in spontaneous flattening of a PED is RPE atrophy with a concomitant loss of pump function. Laser-induced PED flattening may arise from several possible mechanisms. The laser may induce atrophy of some RPE cells in the detachment, leading to less overall pumping in the area of detachment. It is also possible that thermal, photochemical, or inflammatory changes induced by the laser may increase the hydraulic conductivity of Bruch's membrane, improving the egress of fluid from under the elevated RPE.

Although it does not cause a purely serous detachment, and so is not strictly the focus of this manuscript, exudative AMD secondary to choroidal neovascularization may also cause detachment of the retina or RPE (Figs. 22-8 and 22-9). The new vessels growing in the inner portion of Bruch's membrane may lead to detachment of the RPE though hydrostatic forces caused by leakage from the new vessels (Fig. 22-10). The way the fluid enters the subretinal space is not known with certainty. In some cases the fluid may enter through a small rip in the RPE (Ie, 1992). In most cases the passage of fluid is not readily apparent, leading to the concept of leakage from an undetermined source, such as that seen in occult CNV. Bleeding, transudation of proteins, and the breakdown of blood and sequestered proteins may increase the osmotic pressure within the sub-RPE space, encouraging the accumulation and persistence of fluid within this space. Clearing of the blood and proteinaceous material appears to come, in part, from inflammatory and wound-healing mechanisms (Lopez et al., 1991). These may secondarily damage the RPE and Bruch's membrane, causing a further localized breakdown in the mechanisms favoring proper apposition of the retina, RPE, and Bruch's membrane. Relative im-

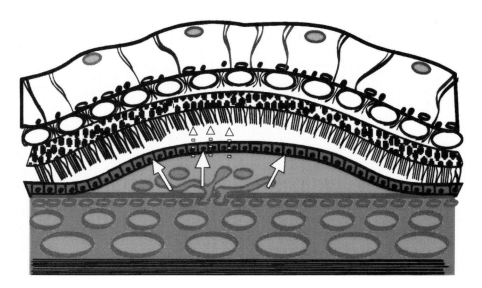

FIGURE 22-10. Cross-sectional drawing of PED and serous detachment of the retina related to the discrete, underlying source of leakage, namely the CNV. The mechanism by which the fluid enters the subretinal space is not known with certainty.

permeability of Bruch's membrane may play a role, as serous PEDs are common in CNV secondary to AMD, but much less common in patients with CNV associated with pathologic myopia, angioid streaks, and presumed ocular histoplasmosis syndrome.

SUMMARY

The close apposition of the retina, RPE, and Bruch's membrane is accomplished through the orchestrated action of several different mechanisms acting in the eye. Perturbation of any of these mechanisms could potentially lead to the formation of fluid under the retina, RPE, or both. This paper examined four different classes of abnormalities that may act as paradigms for these perturbations. Central serous chorioretinopathy may result from zones of increased choroidal vascular hyperpermeability. The cause of this hyperpermeability is not known, but may be related to chronically increased endogenous andrenergic or corticoid stimulation to the choroidal vessels. VKH may lead to detachment of the retina and RPE through diffuse choroidal vascular hyperpermeability combined with alteration in RPE function, both secondary to inflammation. Malignant hypertension may cause serous detachments from the combined effects of ischemia and hyperpermeability associated with placoid areas of RPE necrosis. Nonexudative AMD may lead to PEDs because of decreased hydraulic conductivity of Bruch's membrane.

This chapter has looked at the formation of serous detachment of the retina and RPE by examining the net pathophysiologic effect disease states have on all of the interrelated processes designed to maintain attachment. The assessment of the relative importance of each of these systems in the formation of detachment is based on available scientific data, which changes with time. Although knowledge of the physiology of each of the separate mechanisms will certainly increase, it will still be necessary to examine the aggregate effect of all interrelated systems affecting attachment.

REFERENCES

Adler AJ, Kluznik KM. 1985. Proteins and glycoproteins of the bovine interphotoreceptor matrix: composition and fractionation. Exp Eye Res 34:423–434.

Adorante JS, Miller SS. 1990. Potassium-dependent volume regulation in retinal pigment epithelium is mediated by Na,K,Cl cotransport. J Gen Physiol 96:1153–1176.

Bazan HE, Bazan NG, Feeney-Burns L, Berman ER. 1990. Lipids in human lipofuscin-enriched subcellular fractions of two age populations. comparison with rod outer segments and neural retina. Invest Ophthalmol Vis Sci 31:1433–1443.

Berman ER. 1969. Mucopolysaccharides (glycosaminoglycans) of the retina: indentification, distribution, and possible biological role. Mod Prob Ophthalmol 8:5–31.

Bird AC, Marshall J. 1986. Retinal pigment epithelial detachments in the elderly. Trans Ophthalmol Soc UK 105:674–682.

Brockhurst RJ. 1975. Nanophthalmos with uveal effusion: a new clinical entity. Arch Ophthalmol 93:1289.

Burke JM, McKay BS. 1993. In vitro aging of bovine and human retinal pigment epithelium: number and activity of the Na/K ATPase pump. Exp Eye Res 57:51–57.

Cassel GH, Brown GC, Annesley WH. 1984. Central serous chorioretinopathy: a seasonal variation? Br J Ophthalmol 68:724–726.

Castro-Correia J, Coutinho MF, Rosas V, Maia J. 1992. Long-term follow-up of central serous retinopathy in 150 patients. Documenta Ophthalmologica 81:379–386.

Chihara E, Nao-I N. 1985. Resorption of subretinal fluid by transepithelial flow of the retinal pigment epithelium. Graefes Arch Klin Exp Ophthalmol 223:202–204.

Cogan DG. 1975. Ocular involvement in disseminated intravascular coagulopathy. Arch Ophthalmol 93:1–8.

Davis JL, Mittal KK, Freidlin V, Mellow SR, Optican DC, Palestine AG, Nussenblatt RB. 1990. HLA associations and ancestry in Vogt-Koyanagi-Harada disease and sympathetic ophthalmia. Ophthalmology 97:1137–1142.

de Venecia G. 1987. Fluorescein angiographic smoke stack: case presentation at Verhoeff Society meeting, Washington, D.C., April 24–25, 1982. Quoted from Gass JDM, Stereoscopic Atlas of Macular Diseases. St Louis: Mosby, 56–57.

Edamitsu S, Matsukawa A, Ohkawara S, Takagi K, Nariuchi H, Yoshinaga M. 1995. Role of TNF alpha, IL-1, and IL-1ra in the mediation of leukocyte infiltration and increased vascular permeability in rabbits with LPS-induced pleurisy. Clin Immunol Immunopathol 75(1):68–74.

Ernest JT. 1994. Choroidal circulation. In: Ryan SJ, ed, Retina. St Louis: Mosby, 76–80.

Fisher SK, Steinberg RH. 1982. Origin and organization of pigment epithelial apical projections to cones in cat retina. J Cell Bio 206: 131–145.

Fitzgerald ME, Vana BA, Reiner A. 1990. Control of choroidal blood flow by the nucleus of Edinger-Westphal in pigeons: a laser Doppler study. Invest Ophthalmol Vis Sci 31(12):2483–2492.

Flower RW. 1995. Difficult Aspects of ICG choroidal angiography and future development of the technique. In: Update of Indocyanine Green Angiography. Proceedings of The Second International Symposium on Indocyanine Green Angiography, Nara, Japan. 38–45.

Forster DJ, Cano MR, Green RL, Rao NA. 1990. Echographic features of the Vogt-Koyanagi-Harada syndrome. Arch Ophthalmol 108(10):1421–1426.

Foulds WS. 1969. Experimental detachment of the retina and its effect on the intraocular fluid dynamics. Mod Probl Ophthalmol 8:51–63.

Frederick AR Jr. 1984. Multifocal and recurrent (serous) choroidopathy (MARC) syndrome: a new variety of idiopathic central serous choroidopathy. Documenta Ophthalmologica 56:203–235.

Gaillard ER, Atherton SJ, Eldred G, Dillon J. 1995. Photophysical studies on human retinal lipofuscin. Photochem Photobiol 61:448–453.

Gass JDM. 1983. Uveal effusion syndrome: a new hypothesis concerning pathogenesis and technique of surgical treatment. Trans Am Ophthalmol Soc 81:246.

Gass JDM. 1984. Serous retinal pigment epithelial detachment with a notch: a sign of occult choroidal neovascularization. Retina 4:205.

Gass JDM. 1987. Stereoscopic Atlas of Macular Disease. St Louis: Mosby, 46–59.

Gass JDM. 1991. Central serous chorioretinopathy and white sub-retinal exudation during pregnancy. Arch Ophthalmol 109:677–681.

Gelber GS, Schatz H. 1987. Loss of vision due to central serous chorioretinopathy following psychological stress. Am J Psych 144:46–50.

Gilbert CM, Owens SL, Smith PD, Fine SL. 1984. Long-term follow-up of central serous chorioretinopathy. Brit J Ophthalmol 68:815–820.

Goureau O, Hicks D, Courtois Y. 1994. Human retinal pigmented epithelial cells produce nitric oxide in response to cytokines. Biochem Biophys Res Comm 198(1):120–126.

Green K, Paterson CA, Cheeks L, Slagle T, Jay WM, Aziz MZ. 1990. Ocular blood flow and vascular permeability in endotoxin-induced inflammation. Ophthalmic Res 22(5):287–294.

Gregory CY, Converse CA, Foulds WS. 1990. Effect of glycoconjugates on rod outer segment phagocytosis by retinal pigment epithelial explants in vitro assessed by a specific double radioimmunoassay procedure. Curr Eye Res 9:65–77.

Guyer DR, Yannuzzi LA, Slakter JS, Sorenson JA, Ho A, Orlock D. 1994. Digital indocyanine green videoangiography of central serous chorioretinopathy. Arch Ophthalmol 112:1057–1062.

Hageman GS, Kirchoff-Rempe MA, Lewis GP, Fisher SK, Anderson DH. 1991. Sequestration of fibroblastic growth factor in the primate retinal interphotoreceptor matrix. Proc Nat Acad Sci USA 88:6706–6710.

Hageman GS, Marmor MF, Yao XY, Johnson LV. 1995. The interphotoreceptor matrix mediates primate retinal adhesion. Arch Ophthalmol 113:655–660.

Hayashi K, Hasegawa Y, Tokoro T. 1986. Indocyanine green angiography of central serous chorioretinopathy. Int Ophthalmol 9:37–41.

Holz FG, Sheraidah G, Pauleikhoff D, Bird AC. 1994. Analysis of lipid deposits extracted from human macular and peripheral Bruch's membrane. Arch Ophthalmol 112:402–406.

Hudspeth AJ, Yee AG. 1973. The intercellular junctional complexes of retinal pigment epithelia. Invest Ophthalmol Vis Sci 12:354–365.

Ie D, Yannuzzi LA, Spaide RF, Woodward K, Singerman LJ, Blumenkranz MS. 1992. Micro-rips of the retinal pigment epithelium. Arch Ophthalmol 110:1443–1449.

Ie D, Yannuzzi LA, Spaide RF, Rabb MF, Blair NP, Daily MJ. 1993. Subretinal exudative deposits in central serous chorioretinopathy. Br J Ophthalmol 77:349–353.

Inomata H, Sakamoto T. 1990. Immunohistochemical studies of Vogt-Koyanagi-Harada disease with sunset sky fundus. Curr Eye Res 9(suppl):35–40.

Islam SM, Numaga J, Matsuki K, Fujino Y, Maeda H, Masuda K. 1994. Influence of HLA-DRB1 gene variation on the clinical course of Vogt-Koyanagi-Harada disease. Invest Ophthalmol Vis Sci 35(2):752–756.

Jalkh AE, Jabbour N, Avila MP, Trempe CL, Schepens CL. 1984. Retinal pigment epithelium decompensation. I. Clinical features and natural course. Ophthalmology 91:1544–1548.

Joseph DP, Miller SS. 1991. Apical and basal membrane ion transport mechanisms in bovine retinal pigment epithelium. J Physiol (Lond) 435:439–463.

Kawamura M, Tajima S, Azuma N, Katsura H, Akiyama K. 1995. Biochemical studies of glycosaminoglycans in nanophthalmic sclera. Graefes Arch Clin Exp Ophthalmol 233:58–62.

Kiel JW. 1994. Choroidal myogenic autoregulation and intraocular pressure. Exp Eye Res 58(5):529–543.

Kirchhof B, Ryan SJ. 1993. Differential permeance of retina and retinal pigment epithelium to water: implications for retinal adhesion. Int Ophthalmol 17:19–22.

Klein ML, Obertynski H, Patz A, Fine SL, Kini M. 1980. Follow-up study of detachment of the retinal pigment epithelium. Br J Ophthalmol 64(6):412–416.

Klein R, Klein BEK, Moss SE. 1992. Prevalence of age-related maculopathy: The Beaver Dam Eye Study. Ophthalmology 99:1527–1534.

la Cour M. 1991. pH homeostasis in the frog retina: the role of $Na^+:HCO_3^-$ co-transport in the retinal pigment epithelium. Acta Ophthalmol (Copenh) 69:496–504.

Lazarus HS, Hageman GS. 1992. Xyloside-induced disruption of interphotoreceptor matrix proteoglycans results in retinal detachment. Invest Ophthalmol Vis Sci 33(2):364–376.

Leibowitz HM, et al. 1980. The Framingham Eye Study Monograph: an ophthalmological and epidemiological study of cataract, glaucoma, diabetic retinopathy, macular degeneration and visual acuity in a general population of 2631 adults. Surv Ophthalmol 24:335–610.

Li A, Lane WS, Johnson LV, Chader GJ, Tombran-Tink J. Neuron-specific enolase: a neuronal survival factor in the retinal extracellular matrix? J Neurosci 385–393.

Lin H, Kenyon E, Miller SS. 1992. Na-dependent pH regulatory mechanisms in native human retinal pigment epithelium. Invest Ophthalmol Vis Sci 33:3528–3538.

Lopez PF, Grossniklaus HE, Lambert HM, Aaberg TM, Capone A Jr, Sternberg P Jr, L'Hernault N. 1991. Pathologic features of surgically excised subretinal neovascular membranes in age-related macular degeneration. Am J Ophthalmol 112:647–656.

Lopez-Costa JJ, Goldstein J, Mallo G, Saavedra JP. 1995. NADPH-diaphorase distribution in the choroid after continuous illumination. Neuroreport 6:361–364.

Mancini MA, Frank RN, Keirn RJ, Kennedy A, Khoury JK. 1986. Does the retinal pigment epithelium polarize the choriocapillaris? Invest Ophthalmol Vis Sci 27:336–345.

Mann RM, Riva CE, Stone RA, Barnes GE, Cranstoun SD. 1995. Nitric oxide and choroidal blood flow regulation. Invest Ophthalmol Vis Sci 36:925–930.

Marmor MF. 1988. New hypotheses on the pathogenesis and treatment of serous retinal detachment. Graefes Arch Clin Exp Ophthalmol 226:548–552.

Marmor MF, Maack T. 1982. Enhancement of retinal adhesion and subretinal fluid resorption by acetazolamide. Invest Ophthalmol Vis Sci 23:121–124.

Marmor MF, Abdul-Rahim AS, Cohen DS. 1980. The effect of metabolic inhibitors on retinal adhesion and subretinal fluid resorption. Invest Ophthalmol Vis Sci 19:893–903.

Marshall GE, Konstas AG, Reid GG, Edwards JG, Lee WR. 1994. Collagens in the aged human macula. Graefes Arch Clin Exp Ophthalmol 232:133–140.

Matsunaga H, Matsubara T, Fukushima I, Uyama M. 1994. Indocyanine green fluorescence agiography in Harada disease. Nippon Ganka Gakkai Zasshi 98:852–857.

Melton RC, Spaide RF. 1996. Visual problems as a presenting sign for thrombotic thrombocytopenic purpura. Retina 16:78–80.

Miller SS, Edelman JL. 1990. Active ion transport pathways in the bovine retinal pigment epithelium. J Physiol (Lond) 24:283–300.

Moore DJ, Hussain AA, Marshall J. 1995. Age-related variation in the hydraulic conductivity of Bruch's membrane. Invest Ophthalmol Vis Sci 36:1290–1297.

Moorfields Macular Study Group. 1982. Retinal pigment epithelial detachments in the elderly: a controlled trial of argon laser photocoagulation. Br J Ophthalmol 66(1):1–16.

Morse LS, Terrell J, Sidikaro Y. 1989. Bovine retinal pigment epithelium promotes proliferation of choroidal endothelium in vitro. Arch Ophthalmol 107:1659–1663.

Murakami S, Inaba Y, Mochizuki M, Nakajima A, Urayama A. 1994. A nationwide survey on the occurrence of Vogt-Koyanagi-Harada disease in Japan. Jpn J Ophthalmol 38(2):208–213.

Nakanome Y, Karita K, Izumi H, Tamai M, Okabe H, Abe S. 1994. Experimental research on choroidal circulation. 2. Choroidal blood flow increase elicited by electrical stimulation of parasympathetic nerve behind the eyeball in the cat. Nippon Ganka Gakkai Zasshi 98:962–967.

Negi A, Marmor MF. 1983. The resorption of subretinal fluid after diffuse damage to the retinal pigment epithelium. Invest Ophthalmol Vis Sci 24:1475–1479.

Negi A, Marmor MF. 1984. Experimental serous retinal detachment and focal pigment epithelial damage. Arch Ophthalmol 102:445–449.

Negi A, Marmor MF. 1986. Quantitative estimation of metabolic transport of subretinal fluid. Invest Ophthalmol Vis Sci 27:1564–1568.

Norose K, Yano A, Aosai F, Segawa K. 1990. Immunologic analysis of cerebrospinal fluid lymphocytes in Vogt-Koyanagi-Harada disease. Invest Ophthalmol Vis Sci 31(7):1210–1216.

Nussenblat RB, Palestine AG. 1994. The Vogt-Koyanagi-Harada syndrome (uveomeningitic syndrome). In Ryan SJ, ed, Retina, 2nd ed. St Louis: Mosby, 1737–1743.

Pederson JE, Cantrill HL. 1984. Experimental retinal detachment. V. Fluid movement through the retinal hole. Arch Ophthalmol 102:136–139.

Pederson JE. 1994. Fluid physiology of the subretinal space. In: Ryan SJ, ed, Retina, St Louis: Mosby, 1955–1967.

Piccolino FC, Borgia L. 1994. Central serous chorioretinopathy and indocyanine green angiography. Retina 14:231–242.

Piccolino FC, Borgia L, Zinicola E, Zingirian M. 1995. Indocyanine green angiographic findings in central serous chorioretinopathy. Eye 9(3):324–332.

Pino RM. 1985. Restriction to endogenous plasma proteins by a fenestrated capillary endothelium: an ultrastructural immunocytochemical study of the choriocapillary endothelium. Am J Anat 172:279.

Ramrattan RS, van der Schaft TL, Mooy CM, de Bruijn WC, Mulder PG, de Jong PT. 1994. Morphometric analysis of Bruch's membrane, the choriocapillaris, and the choroid in aging. Invest Ophthalmol Vis Sci 35:2857–2864.

Rao NA, Moorthy RS, Inomata H. 1995. Vogt-Koyanagi-Harada syndrome. Int Ophthalmol Clin 35(2):69–86.

Reme CE. 1977. Autophagy in visual cells and pigment epithelium. Invest Ophthalmol Vis Sci 16:807–814.

Rutzen AR, Ortega-Larrocea G, Schwab IR, Rao NA. 1995. Simultaneous onset of Vogt-Koyanagi-Harada syndrome in monozygotic twins. Am J Ophthalmol 119:239–240.

Sakamoto T, Sakamoto H, Murphy TL, Spee C, Soriano D, Ishibashi T, Hinton DR, Ryan SJ. 1995. Vessel modulation by choroidal endothelial cells in vitro is modulated by retinal pigment epithelial cells. Arch Ophthalmol 113:512–520.

Sanders MD, Graham EM. 1988. Retinal vasculitis. Postgrad Med J 64:488–496.

Schatz H, McDonald HR, Johnson RN. 1990. Retinal pigment epithelial folds associated with retinal pigment epithelial detachment in macular degeneration. Ophthalmology 97(5):658–665.

Scheider A, Nasemann JE, Lund OE. 1993. Fluorescein and indocyanine green angiographies of central serous choroidopathy by scanning laser ophthalmoscopy. Am J Ophthalmol 115:50–56.

Schleimer RP. 1993. An overview of glucocorticoid anti-inflammatory actions. Eur J Clin Pharmacol 45(suppl 1):S3–7.

Shih YF, Fitzgerald ME, Reiner A. 1993. Effect of choroidal and ciliary nerve transection on choroidal blood flow, retinal health, and ocular enlargement. Vis Neurosci 10:969–979.

Shimizu K, Tobari I. 1971. Central serous retinopathy dynamics of subretinal fluid. Mod. Prob. Ophthalmol 9:152.

Smith RS, Rudt LA. 1975. Ocular vascular and epithelial barrier to microperoxidase. Invest Ophthalmol Vis Sci 14:556.

Spaide RF, Hall L, Haas A, Campeas L, Yannuzzi LA, Guyer DR, Slakter JS, Sorenson JA. 1996a. Indocyanine green videoangiography of central serous chorioretinopathy in older adults. Retina 16:203–213.

Spaide RF, Campeas L, Haas A, Yannuzzi LA, Fisher Y, Guyer DR, Slakter JS, Sorenson JA, Orlock DA. 1996b. Central serous chorioretinopathy in younger and older adults. Ophthalmology. 103:2070–2080.

Spitznas M. 1986. Pathogenesis of central serous retinopathy: a new working hypothesis. Graefes Arch Clin Exp Ophthalmol 224:321–324.

Spitznas M, Huke J. 1987. Number, shape, and topography of leakage points in acute type I central serous retinopathy. Graefes Arch Clin Exp Ophthalmol 438–440.

Starita C, Hussain AA, Marshall J. 1995. Decreasing hydraulic conductivity of Bruch's membrane: relevance to photoreceptor survival and lipofuscinoses. Am J Med Genet 57(2):235–237.

Stewart DH III, Streeten BW, Brockhurst RJ, Anderson DR, Hirose T, Gass DM. 1991. Abnormal scleral collagen in nanophthalmos: an ultrastructural study. Arch Ophthalmol 109:1017–1025.

Tombran-Tink J, Shivaram SM, Chader GJ, Johnson LV, Bok D. 1995. Expression, secretion, and age-related downregulation of pigment epithelium-derived factor, a serpin with neurotrophic activity. J Neurosci 15:4992–5003.

Toris CB, Pederson JE. 1984. Experimental retinal detachment. VII. Intravenous horseradish peroxidase diffusion across the blood-retinal barrier. 102:752.

Ward RC, Gragoudas ES, Pon DM, Albert DM. 1988. Abnormal scleral findings in uveal effusion syndrome. Am J Ophthalmol 106:139–146.

Yannuzzi LA. 1987. Type-A behavior and central serous chorioretinopathy. Retina 7:111.

Yao XY, Hageman GS, Marmor MF. 1992. Recovery of retinal adhesion after enzymatic perturbation of the interphotoreceptor matrix. Invest Ophthalmol Vis Sci 33:498–503.

Yoon YH, Marmor MF. 1993. Retinal pigment epithelium adhesion to Bruch's membrane is weakened by hemicholinium-3 and sodium iodate. Ophthalmic Res 25(6):386–392.

Yoshioka H, Katsume Y. 1982. Experimental central serous chorioretinopathy. III: ultrastructural findings. Jpn J Ophthalmol 26:397–409.

Yoshioka-H, Katsume-Y, Akune-H. 1982. Experimental central serous chorioretinopathy in monkey eyes: fluorescein angiographic findings. Ophthalmologica 185:168–178.

Yue BY, Kurosawa A, Duvall J, Goldberg MF, Tso MO, Sugar J. 1988. Nanophthalmic sclera. Fibronectin studies. Ophthalmology 95:56–60.

Yuzawa M, Kawamura A, Matsui M. 1993. Indocyanine green videoangiographic findings in Harada's disease. Japanese Journal of Ophthalmology 37:456–466.

Yuzawa M, Kawamura A, Yamaguchi C, Shouda M, Shimoji M, Matsui M. 1995. Indocyanine green videoangiographic findings in detachment of the retinal pigment epithelium. Ophthalmology 102(4):622–629.

VI | CELLULAR GROWTH AND TRANSPLANTATION

23. Growth factors in the retinal pigment epithelium and retina

PETER A. CAMPOCHIARO

The structure and functions of cells are modulated by many signals derived from their extracellular matrix, from neighboring cells, and from distant cells. Growth factors are one of the major types of such signals; they are proteins that bind to cell surface receptors and influence a number of intracellular parameters. The retinal pigmented epithelium (RPE) is located between the neural retina and the vascular choroid and influences the structure and function of cells in both. Many of these interactions are likely to be mediated by growth factors. This chapter reviews the growth factors that have been demonstrated to be produced by the RPE and retina, those to which the RPE responds, and the possible roles of these growth factors in retinal physiology and pathophysiology.

BASIC RESEARCH

It has been known for several years that cultured RPE cells secrete growth-promoting activity for themselves and for other cells (Bryan and Campochiaro, 1986). Several types of cultured cells produce growth-stimulating activity, but RPE cells produce more than some other types of nontransformed cells (Bryan and Campochiaro, 1986). This is not surprising in view of the subsequent demonstration that cultured RPE cells produce many growth factors (Tables 23-1 and 23-2). Some of these growth factors have been demonstrated only in cultured RPE and while such demonstrations are likely to have significance, their relevance to the situation in vivo is uncertain, because growth factor production can be induced in cultured cells (Terracio et al., 1988). Therefore, in vitro findings indicating growth factor production or responsiveness should be followed up by in vivo studies to explore physiologic significance. This chapter focuses on five growth factor families for which there is information regarding expression in vitro and in vivo: platelet-derived growth factor, vascular endothelial growth factor, fibroblast growth factor, transforming growth factor-β, and insulin-like growth factors; it

also deals briefly with the epidermal growth factor family and several cytokines.

The Platelet-Derived Growth Factor Family

Platelet-derived growth factor (PDGF) was first identified as a mitogen for smooth-muscle cells that is released by platelets into serum (Ross et al., 1974). The name is somewhat misleading, because PDGF is now known to be produced by several cell types and stimulates proliferation and chemotaxis of several cell types (for review, see Heldin and Westermark, 1990). PDGF is actually a family of three polypeptides which are disulfide-bonded homodimers or heterodimers of two homologous (60% sequence identity) gene products, PDGF A chain (PDGF-A) and PDGF B chain (PDGF-B). The three isoforms of PDGF exert their effects on target cells by binding to two structurally related tyrosine kinase receptors designated PDGF α-receptor and PDGF β-receptor (for review, see Hart and Bowen-Pope, 1990). The extracellular portion of each receptor consists of five immunoglobulin-like domains with 30% sequence homology and the intracellular portion contains two tyrosine kinase domains separated by a kinase insert domain. PDGF-A binds to either α- or β- receptors, while PDGF-B binds only to β-receptors. Ligand binding induces receptor dimerization, which results in receptor autophosphorylation and is necessary for signal transduction.

PDGF is involved in regulation of cell growth and differentiation during development (Mercola et al., 1990; Rappolee et al., 1988). In the eye, it has been implicated in differentiation of oligodendrocytes and type 2 astrocytes of the optic nerve (for review, see Barres and Raff, 1994). Both of these cell types originate from a common precursor cell, the oligodendrocyte-type 2 astrocyte (O-2A) progenitor cell, which has PDGF α-receptors. PDGF promotes the proliferation of O-2A progenitor cells and prevents their premature differentiation. There is no direct evidence indicating that PDGF stimulates the migration of glial progenitor cells from

TABLE 23-1. *Growth factors produced by RPE cells*

Growth factor	From cultured RPE	From RPE in situ	
		Constitutive	Wound repair
PDGF family	Campochiaro et al., 1989		
PDGF-A	Yoshida et al., 1992; Campochiaro et al., 1994	Mudhar et al., 1993	Campochiaro et al., 1994; Robbins et al., 1994; Vinores et al., 1995a
PDGF-B	Yoshida et al., 1992; Campochiaro et al., 1992		Campochiaro et al., 1994; Robbins et al., 1994; Vinores et al., 1995
VEGF famliy	Adamis et al., 1993; Shima et al., 1994; Guerrin et al., 1995; Chen et al., 1997		Dastgeib et al., 1995; Vinores et al., 1995b; Vinores et al., 1997
FGF Famliy			
aFGF	Kitaoka et al., 1993	Jacquemin et al., 1990; Noji et al., 1990	Baudoin et al., 1990; Fredj-Reygrobelet et al., 1991; Malecaze et al., 1994; Amin et al., 1994
bFGF	Schweigerer et al., 1987; Sternfeld et al., 1989; Bost et al., 1992; 1993; 1994; Campochiro et al., 1993; Hackett et al., 1997	Fayein et al., 1990; Connolly et al., 1992; Gao and Hollyfield, 1992; Rakoczy et al., 1993	Amin et al., 1994
FGF-5	Bost et al., 1992	Kitaoka et al., 1994	
TGF-β family			
Activan	Jaffe et al., 1992		
TGF-β_1	Tanihara et al., 1993; Kvanta, 1994		
TGF-β_2	Tanihara et al., 1993; Kvanta, 1994; Matsumoto et al., 1994	Pfeffer et al., 1994; Anderson et al., 1995	
TGF-β_3	Tanihara et al., 1994; Kvanta, 1994		
Insulin Family			
IGF-I	Martin et al., 1992; Moriarty et al., 1994; Waldbilling et al., 1991a; 1991b; Takagi et al., 1994		
IGF-II	Takagi et al., 1994; Martin et al., 1992		

the optic nerve into the retina, but it is interesting that this occurs soon after retinal ganglion cells begin to express PDGF-A. Transgenic mice that express PDGF-A in the lens under control of the αA-crystallin promoter exhibit a marked increase in GFAP-positive cells (probably astrocytes) along the inner surface of the retina (Reneker and Overbeek, 1996); PDGF-A clearly stimulates the proliferation and migration of these glial cells. PDGF-A promotes the survival of oligodendrocytes and it may do the same for retinal astrocytes; in adult animals, astrocytes reside adjacent to ganglion cells and

surrounding retinal blood vessels, two sources of PDGF-A (Mudhar et al., 1994; Campochiaro et al., 1994). PDGF has also been demonstrated to have neurotrophic effects (Smits et al., 1991).

In adult animals, it has been hypothesized that PDGF may function as a wound hormone, because it is present in high amounts in platelets and stimulates chemotaxis, proliferation, and matrix production of connective tissue cells (Heldin and Westermark, 1990). This hypothesis is supported by experimental data that demonstrate that PDGF promotes the formation of granulation tis-

TABLE 23-2. *Cytokines produced by RPE cells*

Cytokine	From cultured RPE
Interleukin family	
IL-1α	Jaffe et al., 1992a
IL-1β	Jaffe et al., 1992a; Planck et al., 1993
IL-6	Benson et al., 1992; Elner et al., 1992; Kuppner et al., 1995; Planck et al., 1992
IL-8	Kuppner et al., 1995
Macrophage colony stimulating factor	Planck et al., 1993; Jaffe et al., 1992b
MGSA/gro	Jaffe et al., 1993; Shettuck et al., 1994
TNF-α	Tanihara et al., 1992

sue (Sprugel et al., 1987), shortens the time required for healing (Pierce et al., 1991), and increases wound strength (Pierce et al., 1989). Altered expression of PDGF and PDGF receptors has been implicated in repair of traumatic skin injury (Antonaides et al., 1991), synovitis (Rubin and Terracio, 1988), and vascular injury (Majesky et al., 1990). There is also ample evidence implicating altered expression of PDGF and its receptors in several diseases in which there is exaggerated wound repair resulting in scarring, including atherosclerosis (Wilcox et al., 1988; Ross et al., 1990), rheumatoid arthritis (Reuterdaul et al., 1991; Remmers et al., 1991), scleroderma (Gay et al., 1989), and pulmonary fibrosis (Martinet et al., 1987). PDGF-B is virtually identical to p28^{sis}, the transforming protein of simian sarcoma virus (Waterfield et al., 1983; Doolittle et al., 1983), and altered expression of PDGF and PDGF receptors has been demonstrated in several human malignancies (Coltrera et al., 1995; Gunha et al., 1995). Therefore, PDGF plays an important role in normal and excessive wound repair throughout the body.

Cultured RPE cells express PDGF-A, PDGF-B, PDGF α-receptor, and PDGF β-receptor (Campochiaro et al., 1989; 1994; Yoshida et al., 1992). Exogenous PDGF stimulates the proliferation (Leschey et al., 1990; Campochiaro et al., 1994) and migration (Campochiaro and Glaser, 1985) of RPE cells. RPE-derived PDGF also stimulates the growth of RPE cells; PDGF accounts for a substantial amount of the growth-promoting activity in RPE-conditioned medium (Campochiaro et al., 1989) and antibodies to PDGF partially inhibit RPE growth in serum-free medium (Campochiaro et al., 1994). This indicates the presence of a PDGF autocrine loop in cultured RPE. In an in vitro model of wound repair in which a scrape is made in a monolayer culture of RPE cells in serum-free medium, cells along the edge of the defect show increased expression of PDGF and PDGF

receptor and increased labeling with proliferating cell nuclear antigen, indicating that upregulation of PDGF and its receptors occurs in cells that are proliferating to fill in the defect. Cells in subconfluent areas of the culture also show increased expression of PDGF and its receptors suggesting that the PDGF autocrine loop may be regulated in part by cell–cell contact.

Immunohistochemistry and in situ hybridization in adult mouse or rat retina demonstrate PDGF-A expression in ganglion cells and RPE, while PDGF-B is expressed in cells of blood vessels (Mudhar et al., 1993; Campochiaro et al., 1994). After laser, there is an increase in PDGF-A expression in proliferating RPE cells adjacent to laser burns and after retinal detachment, PDGF-A is increased in RPE beneath detached retina (Campochiaro et al., 1994). This indicates that like RPE in vitro, RPE cells in situ have increased PDGF-A expression when participating in normal wound repair. There is also an increase in PDGF-A expression in RPE participating in abnormal wound repair; RPE cells in epiretinal membranes express high levels of PDGF-A and both types of PDGF receptors (Campochiaro et al., 1994; Vinores et al., 1995a; Robbins et al., 1994). Therefore, upregulation of the PDGF autocrine loop in RPE may play a role in epiretinal membrane formation and provides a good target for therapeutic intervention.

Vascular Endothelial Growth Factor

Vascular endothelial growth factor (VEGF) was first discovered as a tumor-secreted protein that increases the permeability of microvessels to circulating macromolecules and was originally named vascular permeability factor (VPF) because of this property (Senger et al., 1983). It is one of the most potent vascular permeability agents known, acting at concentrations below 1 nM. It was independently isolated based on its ability to stimulate vascular endothelial cell proliferation (Ferrara et al., 1989; Gospodarowicz et al., 1989) and is often referred to as VEGF/VPF or more simply VEGF.

There are four isoforms of VEGF due to alternative splicing of mRNA resulting in polypeptides of 206, 189, 165, and 121 amino acids. Each of the polypeptides form disulfide-bonded dimeric glycoproteins with Mr ranging from 34 to 45 kd. In this respect VEGF is similar to PDGF, and in fact VEGF shares low but significant sequence homology with PDGF. Each of the four VEGF isoforms have similar biological activity, but the two smaller isoforms are secreted, while the two larger isoforms remain largely cell-associated (Park et al., 1993). Two receptors for VEGF have been identified and are referred to as fms-like tyrosine kinase-1 (Flt-1—DeVries et al., 1992) and fetal liver kinase-1 (Flk-1—

Quinn et al., 1993; Terman et al., 1992). While it has been suggested that these receptors are expressed predominantly, if not exclusively on vascular endothelium, they are also expressed on RPE cells (Guerrin et al., 1995; Chen et al., 1997).

Recently, VEGF has been the focus of a great deal of interest, because it stimulates angiogenesis in vivo (Connolly et al., 1989; Leung et al., 1989) and its expression is increased by hypoxia (Shweiki et al., 1992; Plate et al., 1992); high levels of expression in hypoxic regions of tumors has lead to speculation that it may act as a tumor angiogenesis agent. VEGF may also participate in ocular neovascularization. There are increased levels of VEGF in the vitreous cavity (Adamis et al., 1994; Aiello et al., 1994; Malcaze et al., 1995) and increased expression of VEGF in the retina (Pe'er et al., 1995) of patients with ischemic retinopathy and ocular neovascularization. Increased expression of VEGF has also been demonstrated in primate (Miller et al., 1994), mouse (Pierce et al., 1995), and rat (Vinores et al., 1997) models of ischemic retinopathy. In the primate and mouse models, immunohistochemical staining for VEGF was identified in cells of the inner nuclear layer, felt to be Müller cells. In the rat ischemia retinopathy model, immunostaining for VEGF was demonstrated in ganglion cells (Vinores et al., 1997). Staining for VEGF has also been demonstrated in ganglion cells and other retinal neurons in rats with experimental autoimmune uveoretinitis (EAU) and in eyes from patients with diabetes, ischemic retinopathies, pseudophakic macular edema, inflammatory eye disease, macular degeneration, or intraocular tumors (Vinores et al., 1995b; 1997; Pe'er et al., 1995; Dastgheib et al., 1995). VEGF staining was seen in the RPE in patients with choroidal melanoma (Vinores et al., 1995b) and in patients and rats with diabetes (Vinores et al., 1997); VEGF is also expressed in cultured RPE (Adamis et al., 1993; Shima et al., 1995). These findings support a role for VEGF as a mediator of ocular neovascularization in ischemic retinopathies, but several of the above listed ocular disorders are not associated with ischemia or with neovascularization. Inflammation, however, is present in each of these disorders. Since cytokines have been demonstrated to increase expression of VEGF (Li et al., 1995; Harada et al., 1994), production of cytokines by inflammatory cells, or in some cases tumor cells, may be responsible for the increased VEGF seen in these conditions. Interestingly, severe and prolonged intraocular inflammation can be associated with retinal or iris neovascularization that resolves when the inflammation is treated.

These findings also indicate that VEGF immunoreactivity can be increased in the retina and RPE without associated neovascularization. The stimulus for increased production of VEGF may be important in this regard. Hypoxia increases the expression of VEGF receptors (Shweiki et al., 1992), while this has not been demonstrated for cytokines. Perhaps simultaneous increased expression of VEGF and its receptors is required for the development of retinal neovascularization, unless the increase in VEGF expression is large.

In transgenic mice in which VEGF expression is driven by a rhodopsin promoter, there is sustained high expression of VEGF in photoreceptors and these mice develop intraretinal and subretinal neovascularization (Okamoto et al., 1997). These data indicate that increased expression of VEGF alone under the right circumstances is sufficient to cause neovascularization in the retina. This and demonstrations that VEGF antagonists partially inhibit ocular neovascularization (Aiello et al., 1995; Robinson et al., 1996; Adamis et al., 1996) indicate that VEGF plays a central role, but they do not rule out the possibility that upregulating of VEGF receptors and production of other growth factors also contribute to the development of retinal neovascularization in ischemic retinopathies. In fact, a recent study suggests that growth hormone working through IGF-I also contributes to retinal neovascularization in ischemic retinopathies (Smith et al., 1997).

In addition to its role in neovascularization, VEGF may have other effects in the retina. Breakdown of the blood retinal barrier occurs in each of the conditions in which VEGF is increased and in eyes with ocular melanoma, VEGF immunoreactivity colocalizes with sites of blood retinal barrier breakdown (Vinores et al., 1995b). Therefore, VEGF may contribute to macular edema, as well as ocular neovascularization.

While evidence suggesting these pathologic effects of VEGF is mounting, the physiologic role of VEGF in the retina is unknown. It may be one of the stimuli for normal development of the retinal vasculature (Stone et al., 1995) and in adults could serve as a trophic factor for vascular endothelial cells. The latter may be the reason for VEGF production by RPE cells. The reason for VEGF receptor expression by RPE in vitro is unknown, but like PDGF, VEGF is an autocrine growth stimulator in cultured RPE (Guerrin et al., 1995). If there is expression of VEGF receptors by RPE in situ, there may be an as yet uncharacterized function of VEGF in RPE.

The Fibroblast Growth Factor Family

The fibroblast growth factor family is known to have many members (for review, see Baird and Klagsburn, 1991). Basic fibroblast growth factor (bFGF) was the first to be identified and was named for its mitogenic effect on fibroblasts (Gospodarowicz et al., 1986). It is now recognized that the FGFs have numerous target cells and several activities in vitro including stimulation of chemotaxis, proliferation, and production of proteolytic enzymes by vascular endothelial cells (Gospodarowicz et al., 1986), and induction of neuronal differentiation (Wagner and D'Amore, 1986; Walicke et al., 1986). FGFs play a critical role in development (Herbert et al., 1990; Amaya et al., 1991), and mice with FGF receptor deficiency have multiple developmental abnormalities resulting in embryonic death (Yamaguchi et al., 1994; Deng et al., 1994). Other in vivo activities include stimulation of angiogenesis (Gospodarowicz et al., 1986), keratinocyte differentiation (Werner et al., 1993), epithelial differentiation and branching morphogenesis in lungs (Peters et al., 1994), and promotion of neuronal survival after several types of insults (Anderson et al., 1988; Freese et al., 1992).

The actions of FGFs are mediated through a family of tyrosine kinase receptors (for review, see Johnson and Williams, 1993). Four distinct FGF receptor (FGFR) genes have been identified and in the case of FGFR 1 and FGFR 2, alternative splicing results in multiple mRNA transcripts. There are three extracellular immunoglobulin-like domains; alternative splicing in the third domain is important for determining ligand binding specificities. As is true for PDGF and VEGF receptors, ligand binding results in FGFR dimerization and is necessary for signal transduction.

Cultured RPE cells produce at least three members of the FGF family, bFGF (Schweigerer et al., 1987; Sternfield et al., 1989), acidic FGF (Kitaoka et al., 1993), and FGF-5 (Bost et al., 1992). The expression of bFGF by cultured RPE cells is modulated by cell density, cell adhesion, extracellular matrix components, stress, and cytokines (Bost et al., 1993; 1994; Hackett et al., 1997). Localization of FGFs in situ is complicated by species differences and technical problems that have contributed to differences in reported localization in the retina (Hanneken and Baird, 1992; Hanneken et al., 1991; Kitaoka et al., 1994; Gao and Hollyfield, 1992; Connolly et al., 1992; Baudouin et al., 1990; Raymond et al., 1992; Consigli et al., 1993; Caruelle et al., 1989; Noji et al., 1992; Bugara et al., 1993; Ishigooka et al., 1993; Jacquemin et al., 1990; 1993). However, based upon both immunohistochemistry and in situ hybridization, it can be concluded that the RPE and essentially all retinal neurons are capable of expression of bFGF, acidic FGF, and FGF-5, although the relative level of expression determined among cell types varies based upon developmental stage and differences in technical aspects of reported studies. Several studies have also demonstrated bFGF around retinal blood vessels (Hanneken et al., 1989; 1991; Ishigooka et al., 1993; Connolly et al.,

1992), and one study has suggested that it may be present in interphotoreceptor matrix (Hageman et al., 1991). RPE and photoreceptors also express FGF receptors (Plouet et al., 1988; Fugiwara, 1994; Mascarelli et al., 1989; Fayein et al., 1990); FGFR-1 and FGFR-2 have been localized to RPE and photoreceptors by immunohistochemistry (Tcheng et al., 1994; Ohachi et al., 1994). The response of RPE in organ culture or cell culture to FGFs is dependent on the species and to some extent on culture conditions. In human RPE, bFGF stimulates proliferation on a plastic substratum (Leschey et al., 1990), but can promote expression of markers of differentiation in cells grown on basement membrane components (Campochiaro et al., 1993). Addition of bFGF or aFGF to embryonic chick eyecups causes regeneration of neural retina from the RPE (Park and Hollenberg, 1989; 1993). Transdifferentiation also occurs in embryonic chick RPE cultures, but is dependent on the physical configuration of cells (Pittack et al., 1991) or the substratum (Opas and Dziak, 1994). In cultures of retinal neurons, FGFs promote survival and stimulate opsin expression, a marker of differentiation (Tcheng, 1994; Hicks and Courtois 1988; 1992a; 1992b).

Since FGFs have angiogenic activity, their demonstration in the retina caused speculation that they might provide the stimulus for the development of retinal and/or choroidal neovascularization. Such a role is supported by studies that suggest that FGFs are increased in the vitreous of patients with ischemic retinopathies, in vascularized epiretinal membranes, and in choroidal neovascular membranes (Amin et al., 1994; Sivalingam et al., 1990; Baudouin et al., 1990; Fredj-Reygrobellent; 1991). However, some studies have demonstrated FGFs in avascular epiretinal membranes (Baudouin et al., 1990; Fredj-Reygrobellet et al., 1991; Malecaze et al., 1991), and one study failed to demonstrate basic FGF in fibrovascular epiretinal tissue (Hanneken et al., 1991). At this time, the role of FGFs in ocular neovascularization is uncertain (for review, see D'Amore, 1994).

Recently, attention has focused on the neurotrophic effects of the FGFs. Acidic and basic FGF promote photoreceptor survival in Royal College of Surgeons rats with an inherited retinal dystrophy (Faktorovich et al., 1990) and rats exposed to constant light (LaVail et al., 1992). Basic FGF also protects inner retinal neurons from ischemic damage (Zhang et al., 1994). If endogenous FGFs have a neuroprotective effect in the retina, it would be expected that their expression would be increased by various insults in an attempt to limit retinal damage. This is the case, as basic FGF expression is increased in the retina following optic nerve transection (Kostyk et al., 1994), exposure to constant light (Steinberg et al., 1995), or penetrating trauma (Wen et al., 1995). Intense light exposure and oxidizing agents also increase basic FGF expression in cultured RPE (Hackett et al., 1997). After transection of the optic nerve, photoreceptors show increased basic FGF immunoreactivity (Kostyk et al., 1994) and are more resistant to the damaging effects of constant light (Sievers et al., 1987). Recently, it has been demonstrated that transgenic mice with photoreceptor-specific expression of dominant-negative FGF receptor mutants (mutants that specifically disrupt FGF signaling in photoreceptors) undergo photoreceptor degeneration (Campochiaro et al., 1995). This strongly suggests that one or more FGF acts as a survival factor in the outer retina.

Both photoreceptors and RPE produce FGFs and both contain FGF receptors. Perhaps FGFs act as neuroprotective agents independently in an autocrine fashion in photoreceptors and RPE, but they may also mediate trophic interactions between RPE and photoreceptors. For the latter to be true, FGFs must have some way of getting outside cells, and both acidic and basic FGF lack signal sequences and are not secreted through the endoplasmic reticulum-Golgi pathway. However, FGF-5 is a secreted protein and may mediate paracrine functions of the FGFs in the retina while acidic and basic FGF act in an autocrine manner (Kitaoka et al., 1994). Alternatively, basic and acidic FGF may gain access to the extracellular space through novel pathways (Mignatti et al., 1992).

Why do FGFs have neuroprotective activity as well as mitogenic and angiogenic activity? The answer to this question is not known, but it may be that acidic and basic FGF function primarily as autocrine neuroprotective agents, but serve secondarily as wound repair hormones when widespread cell damage causes them to leak into the extracellular space. Alternatively, if acidic and basic FGF normally have paracrine neuroprotective functions, their mitogenic and angiogenic activities may be limited by other mechanisms, such as soluble receptors, that act as sponges and prevent activation of wound repair functions until critical extracellular levels are reached (Hanneken and Baird, 1995). In any case, it may not be possible to use FGFs as pharmacologic agents for neuroprotection, unless their neuroprotective and mitogenic activities can be dissociated.

The Transforming Growth Factor-β Family

The transforming growth factor-β (TGF-β) superfamily consists of a large number of structurally related proteins including five isoforms of TGF-β (three of which occur in mammals), activins and inhibins, bone morphogenic proteins, Müllerian inhibitory substances, and the product of the decapentaplegic gene complex in *Drosophila* (for review, see Roberts and Sporn, 1990). The three mammalian isoforms of TGF-β, TGF-β_1, -β_2, and β_3, are coded by separate genes, but the mature proteins share 70%–80% amino acid identity, bind to the same receptors, and induce similar responses. The active molecules are 25 kd homodimers derived from inactive precursors by proteolytic cleavage of the amino terminal ends of the chains. In most cells and tissues, TGF-β is found in latent form in which the residue of the precursor remains noncovalently attached and prevents interaction with TGF-β receptors. Latent TGF-β is produced by almost all cells and therefore its activation represents an important control mechanism. In cocultures of endothelial cells and pericytes (or smooth muscle cells), activation of TGF-β requires cell–cell contact and is mediated by surface-bound plasmin (Antonelli-Orlidge et al., 1989; Rifkin et al., 1993). Addition of bFGF to endothelial cell cultures results in activation of latent TGF-β and may constitute a negative feedback loop, since TGF-β inhibits endothelial cell proliferation (Rifkin et al., 1993). Unlike most other cell types, bovine hyalocytes secrete TGF-β in active form (Lazarus et al., 1993).

Regulation of TGF-β activity is also achieved through binding proteins, some of which are located on cell surfaces (for review, see Sporn and Roberts, 1992). The type III TGF-β receptor, betaglycan, and a related cell surface molecule, endoglin, do not have signaling capabilities themselves, but may modulate TGF-β activity by enhancing its presentation to the signaling receptors. Other proteins in extracellular matrix or serum, including α_2-macroglobulin and decorin, bind and sequester TGF-β which limits its activity, while thrombospondin-bound TGF-β is active.

There are two signaling receptors for TGF-β, the type I and type II receptors, which are present on essentially all nontransformed cells (for review, see Massagué, 1992). The type II receptor belongs to a family of serine/threonine kinases which also includes two activin receptors. Cooperativity between type II and type I receptors may be needed for signaling.

TGF-β inhibits the growth of endothelial cells and epithelial cells, including RPE cells, in which it blocks the mitogenic effects of other growth factors (Leschey et al., 1990). It stimulates the growth of some cells by activating an autocrine loop (Battegay et al., 1990). TGF-β is a potent stimulator of extracellular matrix production, it promotes differentiation of some cells, and it has neuroprotective effects, possibly by acting indirectly through glial cells (Roberts and Sporn, 1990; Sporn and Roberts, 1992). TGF-β is an important regulator of inflammation and immune function and an excess or a deficiency can cause problems. Mice deficient in TGF-β_1 and those overexpressing TGF-β_1 show leukocyte infiltration of several organs and a high rate of perinatal death indicating that regulated expression is needed for normal development and survival (McCartney-Francis and Wahl, 1994).

Cultured RPE cells express all three isoforms of TGF-β, but TGF-β_2 is predominant (Kvanta, 1994; Pfeffer et al., 1994). TGF-β_2, but not TGF-β_1, accumulates in the media of RPE cells (Pfeffer et al., 1994) and is increased by laser photocoagulation (Matsumoto et al., 1994). Most of the TGF-β secreted by RPE cells is in latent form (Matsumoto et al., 1994), which is consistent with previous observations that RPE-conditioned media stimulate proliferation of RPE and endothelial cells (Leschey et al., 1990; Wong et al., 1988; Morse et al., 1989). In contrast, hyalocytes secrete active TGF-β and hyalocyte-conditioned media inhibit proliferation of RPE and endothelial cells (Lazarus et al., 1996).

Immunohistochemical studies have localized TGF-β_1 to choroidal endothelium (Lutty et al., 1991; 1993), photoreceptor outer segments (Lutty et al., 1993; Anderson et al., 1995), and Müller cells (Anderson et al., 1995). TGF-β_2 has been localized to the stroma of the choroid (Lutty et al., 1993), the RPE (Pfeffer et al., 1994; Anderson et al., 1995), photoreceptor outer segments (Lutty et al., 1993; Pfeffer et al., 1994; Anderson et al., 1995), and hyalocytes (Lutty et al., 1993). TGF-β_3 has been localized to photoreceptor inner segments (Anderson et al., 1995), Müller cells (Anderson et al., 1995), ganglion cells (Anderson et al., 1995), and hyalocytes (Lutty et al., 1993; Anderson et al., 1995). Sandwich enzyme-linked immunosorbent assays on freshly isolated tissues from monkey eyes demonstrated that TGF-β_2 is the predominant isoform present in RPE/choroid, neural retina, and vitreous (Pfeffer et al., 1994).

The function of TGF-β in the retina and the choroid is unknown. It is likely to modulate inflammation and immune response since this appears to be a general function of TGF-β and there is evidence to suggest that it plays such a role in the anterior segment of the eye (Cousins et al., 1991; de Boer et al., 1994). This hypothesis is supported by an in vitro study demonstrating that TGF-β_1 and β_2 inhibit interferon-γ-induced upregulation of class III histocompatibility antigens on human RPE cells (Gabrielian et al., 1994). Another possible function of TGF-β is neuroprotection. TGF-β increases the survival of telencephalic neurons exposed to metabolic inhibitors or excitotoxic agents (Prehn et al., 1993). In support of this hypothesis, it has been demonstrated that TGF-β increases the expression of heme oxidase in cultured RPE (Kutty et al., 1994). Avascular

tissues have high levels of TGF-β and this has led to speculation that TGF-β may help to prevent vascular invasion (Eisenstein and Grant-Bertacchini, 1991). TGF-β in the vitreous and the outer retina may contribute to a biochemical barrier to neovascularization, a concept supported by in vitro studies. TGF-β may also participate in normal and excessive wound repair (Conner et al., 1989), and exogenous TGF-β may enhance the rate of sealing of macular holes treated by vitrectomy and fluid–gas exchange (Lansing et al., 1993). Finally, TGF-β may serve to modulate the effects of other growth factors, particularly bFGF. A feedback loop involving TGF-β and bFGF has been implicated in regulation of endothelial cell growth (Rifkin et al., 1993). A similar loop may be involved in regulation of scleral growth (Seko et al., 1995; Roher and Stell, 1994). A link between neuronal signaling in the retina and scleral growth has been established in form-deprivation myopia; the RPE, a source of both FGFs and TGF-β, may be the effector cell that makes the link possible. In vivo studies are needed to test all of the above hypotheses.

Insulin and Insulin-like Growth Factors

The insulin-like growth factors, IGF-I and IGF-II, are growth-promoting peptides that are structurally related to insulin. They were first described as *sulfation factor,* based upon an ability to stimulate cartilage sulfation (Salmon and Daughaday, 1957), but because sulfation factor was found to have numerous other activities including stimulation of DNA, protein, and proteoglycan synthesis, it was proposed to be a circulating factor mediating the effect of growth hormone and was renamed somatomedin (Daughaday et al., 1972). At the same time, it was noted that serum contains factors that have insulin-like activity that cannot be blocked by anti-insulin antibody; this was called *nonsuppressible insulin-like activity* (Froesch et al., 1966). It was subsequently demonstrated that two proteins were responsible for all of the above activities, and they were named IGF-I and IGF-II (Rinderknecht and Humbel, 1978a; 1978b; Svoboda et al., 1980).

There are two receptors that specifically recognize the IGFs, the type I and type II IGF receptors (for review, see Jones and Clemmons, 1995). Most of the cellular effects of both IGF-I and IGF-II occur through the type I receptor which is a tyrosine kinase. The type II receptor is identical to the mannose-6-phosphate receptor and may sequester the IGFs, but has not been shown to mediate IGF signaling. The type I receptor has 50%–60% overall sequence identity with the insulin receptor and 84% homology in tyrosine kinase domains. IGFs bind to the insulin receptor with 100 times less affinity than insulin and insulin binds to the IGF receptors with 100 to 1000-fold lower affinity than the IGFs. Both the type I IGF and the insulin receptor are formed from disulfide-bonded half receptors consisting of extracellular (α) and intracellular (β) subunits that are also disulfide bonded. As is true for the other tyrosine kinase receptors discussed above, dimer formation is critical for signaling, but in this case, occurs prior to ligand binding; ligand binding stimulates transphosphorylation of the two β subunits. Hybrid receptors form in cells that express both insulin and IGF type I receptors. IGFs also bind to a family of binding proteins (IGFBPs) that modulate IGF activity directly by modulating interaction with receptors, and indirectly by serving as transport proteins that prolong half-life and may provide a means for tissue- and cell-specific localization.

IGF-I receptors are expressed on numerous cell types and, therefore, IGFs have widespread effects (Jones and Clemmons, 1995). Their best-characterized action is stimulation of cell proliferation, but in some cell types they inhibit apoptosis and in others they stimulate differentiated functions. Mice with null mutations of the IGFs and/or IGF receptors demonstrate that both IGFs play a critical role in development that is independent of growth hormone (Behringer et al., 1988; Liu et al., 1993), while transgenic mice that overexpress growth hormone and/or IGF-I demonstrate that most of the growth-promoting activity of growth hormone (GH) occurs through IGF-I (Palmiter et al., 1983; Mathews et al., 1988a; 1988b).

Several studies have demonstrated insulin and IGF receptors in the retina (Waldbillig et al., 1987a; 1987b; 1988a; Im et al., 1986; Rosenzweig, 1993; Rosenzweig et al., 1990; Zetterstrom et al., 1991; 1992). In a detailed study of the outer retina–RPE complex, Waldbillig and colleagues (1991b) demonstrated IGF-I and IGFBPs in IPM and IGF receptors on photoreceptors and RPE. It was postulated that the RPE is the source of IGF-I in IPM because cultured RPE produces IGF-I. It has subsequently been shown that cultured RPE also expresses IGF-II, IGFBPs, type I and type II IGF receptors and insulin receptors (Waldbillig et al., 1991b; 1992; Martin et al., 1992; Takagi et al., 1994; Feldman and Randolph, 1994; Moriarty et al., 1994). Both insulin and IGFs stimulate RPE proliferation (Leschey et al., 1990; Grant et al., 1990), and therefore IGFs, like PDGF and VEGF, may act as autocrine growth stimulators in RPE. At high concentrations, insulin also stimulates retinal ester synthetase activity, melanin formation, and phagocytosis (Kurtz and Edwards, 1991; Edwards et al., 1992; Miceli and Newsome, 1994); the significance of these findings is unknown.

The IGFs may play a role in retinal development. IGF binding and expression of mRNA for IGF type I receptor, insulin receptor, IGF-I, and insulin are developmentally regulated in embryonic chick retina (Waldbillig et al., 1991a; de la Rosa et al., 1994). Teleost fish retinas continue to add neurons throughout life and insulin and IGF-I stimulate the proliferation of fish neural progenitor cells in vitro which give rise to rod photoreceptors (Mack and Fernald, 1993). In situ hybridization demonstrates IGF mRNA in cone receptors, which produce progenitor cells, consistent with the hypothesis that IGFs play a role in regulating production of new neurons in teleost retina (Mack et al., 1994) and they may have a similar role in mammalian retina during development.

The observations that hypophysectomy and other conditions of GH deficiency have an ameliorative effect on proliferative diabetic retinopathy (PDR), has implicated GH in the pathogenesis of PDR. Since IGF-I mediates most of the proliferative effects of GH, there is good reason to suspect that IGF-I could play a role. Although this hypothesis remains unproven, it is supported by several studies. Patients with rapidly progressive PDR have higher levels of IGF-I in serum (Merimee et al., 1983) and vitreous (Grant et al., 1986) than diabetics with quiescent disease. IGF-I stimulates migration and proliferation of vascular endothelial cells (Grant et al., 1987) and intravitreous injection of IGF-I stimulates disc neovascularization in pigs with branch retinal vein occlusion (Davis et al., 1994). Specific binding of radiolabeled IGF-I has been demonstrated in human diabetic epiretinal membranes (Ulbig et al., 1995).

In a murine model of ischemic retinopathy, mice expressing a GH antagonist gene or mice given an inhibitor of GH secretion had partial inhibition of retinal neovascularization (Smith et al., 1997). Inhibition was reversed by administration of exogenous IGF-I. Therefore, it is likely that IGF-I collaborates with VEGF in the development of retinal neovascularization.

There are several other growth factors that have been demonstrated to be produced by cultured RPE and/or to influence retinal cells. Evidence relating to epidermal growth factor and interleukins and other cytokines will be briefly summarized.

Epidermal Growth Factor

Epidermal growth factor is present in serum and could potentially influence retinal cells. It stimulates proliferation of neural progenitor cells (Anchan et al., 1991) including fetal human retinal cells (Kelley et al., 1995), cultured RPE (Leschey et al., 1990; Arrindell et al., 1992), and retinal glia (Sagar et al., 1991; Roque et al., 1992). There is weak immunoreactive staining for EGF and EGF receptor in normal human retina and moderate staining for TNF-α, which is very closely related to EGF, both structurally and functionally; each is increased in diabetic retinas and is present in surgically removed diabetic epiretinal membranes (Patel et al., 1994). Therefore, EGF/TGF-α may play a role in retinal development and could contribute to the proliferative stimuli that influence epiretinal membrane formation.

Interleukins and Other Cytokines

Although many growth factors have effects on cells of erythroid and myeloid lineage, some have very prominent effects and are therefore strongly associated with inflammatory and immune responses; they are often referred to as cytokines. Numerous cytokines are produced by cultured RPE cells, either unstimulated or stimulated by other cytokines. They include IL-1α (Jaffe et al., 1992a), IL-1β (Jaffe et al., 1992a; Planck et al., 1993), IL-6 (Benson et al., 1992; Elner et al., 1992; Kuppner et al., 1995; Planck et al., 1992), IL-8 (Kuppner et al., 1995), macrophage colony stimulating factor, and TNF-α (Tanihara et al., 1993). RPE cells also present antigen and therefore appear likely to play an important role in the inflammatory response in the eye.

CLINICAL IMPLICATIONS

The physiologic role of constitutive production of growth factors in the RPE and retina is unknown, but based on experimental evidence, much of which has been cited above, certain speculations can reasonably be made. It has been known for some time that many neurons require constant exposure to one or more soluble factors to maintain viability; however, there is mounting evidence to suggest that nonneuronal cells may have similar requirements (Desmouliere et al., 1995). This survival-promoting function of growth factors is called their *trophic function*; factors that promote survival, but not growth, are referred to as *trophic factors*. There appears to be considerable redundancy in trophic interactions, such that one of several soluble factors or extracellular matrix components may suffice to maintain the viability of a particular cell. Extracellular matrix components may activate intracellular signaling pathways through growth factor receptors or through receptors that are also used for cell adhesion (e.g., integrin receptors). The withdrawal of trophic support leads to cell death by apoptosis, a default cell death program (Majno and Joris, 1995). Since growth factors stimulate proliferation, constitutive production for trophic support must be at very low concentrations that are insuf-

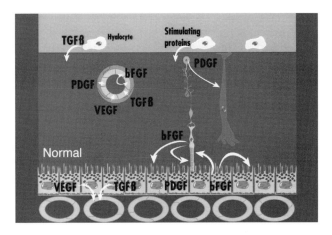

FIGURE 23-1. Schematic representation of constitutive production of growth factors in the retina and RPE and potential targets. Platelet-derived growth factor (PDGF) is produced by the RPE, vascular endothelial cells, and ganglion cells and its potential targets are the RPE, pericytes, smooth-muscle cells, and retinal glia. Vascular endothelial growth factor (VEGF) is produced by the RPE, pericytes, smooth muscle cells, and retinal glia *(not shown)* and may target retinal and choroidal vascular endothelial cells and the RPE. Basic fibroblast growth factor (bFGF) is produced by the RPE, retinal neurons *(only photoreceptors shown)*, and vascular endothelial cells, and its potential targets are the RPE, retinal neurons, and vascular endothelial cells. Transforming growth factor-β (TGF-β) is produced by pericytes and smooth-muscle cells, hyalocytes, the RPE, and cells in the choroid *(not shown)*, and its potential targets are retinal and choroidal vascular endothelial cells, the RPE, retinal glia, and retinal neurons. This schematic representation is incomplete, as there are likely to be many more stimulatory and inhibitory proteins that are produced. For example, hyalocytes are a likely source of some growth stimulators that are balanced by TGF-β production under basal conditions.

ficient for growth stimulation, or it must be balanced by inhibitory stimuli.

Figure 23-1 shows a schematic representation of how constitutive production of stimulatory and inhibitory growth factors might occur to achieve trophic support and normal growth regulation in the retina and RPE. The best experimental evidence for such a trophic function exists for the FGF family (Campochiaro et al., 1995), represented by bFGF in Figure 23-1. The RPE, retinal neurons, and cells of retinal vessels (probably endothelial cells) constitutively produce bFGF, and since its production is so widespread and it lacks a signal sequence, it may act primarily as an autocrine trophic factor. Increased levels of FGFs may help retinal cells survive noxious stimuli such as excessive exposure to light and its production may be modulated by soluble factors that travel between cells or by transcription factors induced by the noxious stimuli. However, FGFs are deposited in extracellular matrix by an unknown mechanism and from that site may affect the cell of origin and adjacent cells. TGF-β blocks the proliferative effects of FGFs (but not necessarily the trophic effects) and the constitutive production of TGF-β by RPE, photoreceptors, cells of the retinal vessels (probably pericytes), and hyalocytes may block the proliferative effects of FGFs on retinal cells.

PDGF-A is produced by RPE, in which it may have autocrine trophic effects, and retinal ganglion cells which may target retinal glia. PDGF-B is produced by endothelial cells and may act on pericytes, smooth-muscle cells, and glia. It is not yet known if VEGF is constitutively produced in the retina and RPE; if it is, it may provide trophic support for retinal and choroidal endothelial cells.

Age-Related Macular Degeneration

Abnormal extracellular matrix may decrease access of matrix-bound FGFs to cells and prevent activation of FGF receptors by other matrix components (Kinoshita et al., 1995). Diffuse thickening of Bruch's membrane and drusen may act in this way to cause or contribute to RPE dysfunction and death in patients with atrophic age-related macular degeneration. Loss of RPE leads to atrophy of photoreceptors and choriocapillaris (Del Priore et al., 1995), possibly due to loss of RPE-derived trophic support, including FGFs. This does not rule out primary defects in photoreceptors as a cause of AMD; they may secondarily cause thickening of Bruch's membrane and RPE dysfunction. Dysfunctional RPE could release increased amounts of FGFs and VEGF, and decreased amounts of TGF-β, which could contribute to growth of choroidal neovascularization (CNV), along with angiogenic factors produced by macrophages (Fig. 23-2).

Endothelial cells of CNV are likely to produce PDGF-A and PDGF-B; this may be why CNV becomes surrounded by RPE cells, which proliferate and form large scars (Fig. 23-2). Substitution of soluble trophic factors for those normally provided by the ECM could provide a new approach to therapy in patients with atrophic AMD. With respect to CNV, several agents that block angiogenesis have been identified and one or more are likely to be used in the future to treat and/or prevent CNV. PDGF antagonists may help to limit disciform scarring.

Wound Repair

When the RPE monolayer is disrupted by laser, cryopexy, or mechanical debridement, as shown in Figure 23-3, there is upregulation of PDGF and PDGF receptors. This contributes to the proliferation and migration of RPE cells, which results in repair of the defect; however, there may be other factors that also contribute that

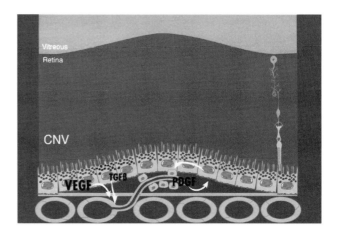

FIGURE 23-2. Schematic representation of modulation of growth factor production that could contribute to choroidal neovascularization (CNV). Due to alterations in the RPE, there may be increased production of vascular endothelial growth factor (VEGF) and fibroblast growth factors (*not shown*) and decreased production of transforming growth factor-β. Production of these same growth factors by macrophages is not shown. Once CNV invades the sub-RPE space, the production of platelet-derived growth factor by vascular endothelial cells is likely to contribute to recruitment and proliferation of RPE.

are not represented in Figure 23-3. FGFs are probably released from injured cells and could contribute, as could autocrine loops for VEGF and IGFs. However, PDGF is a strong stimulator of RPE migration (Campochiaro and Glaser, 1985), which plays a prominent role in would repair of this type. Another important factor is the ECM; RPE defects are not repaired if Bruch's membrane is severely damaged (Del Priore et al., 1995).

Mechanical removal of the RPE commonly occurs

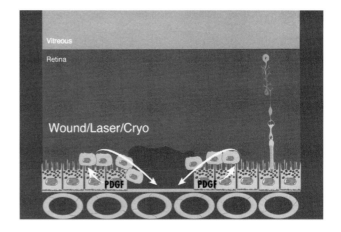

FIGURE 23-3. Schematic representation of possible growth factor modulation during normal RPE wound repair. A defect in the RPE monolayer results in upregulation of autocrine loops in RPE. One autocrine loop involves PDGF, but there is also a vascular endothelial growth factor autocrine loop and possible loops for fibroblast growth factor and insulin-like growth factor that may contribute (*not shown*).

during surgical removal of submacular CNV. In young patients the defect is often repaired and good vision can result, but in patients with AMD, the defect is rarely repaired and return of central vision is unusual. The PDGF autocrine loop, as well as other autocrine loops, may be abnormal in the RPE of patients with AMD and could, along with abnormalities in Bruch's membrane, contribute to poor repair after mechanical removal of the RPE. It would be useful to determine if RPE repair can be augmented by GF administration in animal models of RPE debridement to determine if such an approach could be considered in patients. It would be reasonable to include TGF-β as part of a GF cocktail, since it has already been demonstrated to enhance repair of macular holes with no identifiable toxicity (Lansing et al., 1993) and could potentially stimulate ECM production and help prevent excessive cellular proliferation. The use of TGF-β and other GF in the treatment of macular holes may be limited by the high rate of hole closure without adjunctive therapy. However, as noted above, the magnitude of the wound repair problem is much greater in patients with AMD who have undergone CNV removal, and, therefore, such patients provide an important potential application of GF therapy to augment wound repair.

Posterior Vitreous Detachment and Idiopathic Epiretinal Membranes

In a series of 101 patients with idiopathic epiretinal membranes (ERMs) reviewed by Smiddy et al. (1990), all of the patients were felt to have a posterior vitreous detachment (PVD) preoperatively. The high association of PVD with ERM formation has never been adequately explained. We often tell patients that when the vitreous separates, it may create defects in the internal limiting membrane, allowing cells to migrate onto the surface of the retina. However, defects in the ILM are often created at the time of surgery for ERMs, and yet ERMs rarely recur. Also, retinotomies to remove submacular CNV rarely result in ERM formation. Therefore, it is likely that PVD does more than create defects in the ILM; it is likely that it alters the balance of stimulatory and inhibitory factors at the retinal surface (Fig. 23-4). Hyalocytes are located in the cortical vitreous and constitutively produce all three types of TGF-β, which could provide tonic inhibition of cell migration and proliferation at the retinal surface. PVD results in separation of hyalocytes from the retinal surface and is likely to cause them to be relatively hypoxic; this could result in decreased production of TGF-β and increased production of stimulatory factors. Another situation in which hyalocytes are hypoxic is in ischemic retino-

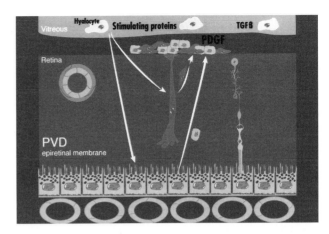

FIGURE 23-4. Schematic representation of possible modulation of growth factor production and its consequences after posterior vitreous detachment (PVD). Separation of the vitreous from the retinal surface increases the distance between hyalocytes and their supply of oxygen, resulting in relative hypoxia. This may result in decreased production of TGF-β and increased production of stimulating proteins. If RPE and glia are activated by an unknown mechanism (e.g., up-regulation of receptors by a bout of inflammation), the imbalance of stimulatory and inhibitory factors from hyalocytes may result in recruitment of RPE and glia to the retinal surface to form epiretinal membranes.

pathies in which the vitreous, from which inhibitors of NV can normally be extracted (Jacobson et al., 1983), becomes a scaffold for NV. As noted above, production of stimulatory growth factors in the lens has been demonstrated to cause migration of cells through the retina and cell proliferation on the retinal surface (Reneker et al., 1996). Therefore, production of stimulatory factors by hyalocytes in the vitreous cavity is also likely to be capable of stimulating migration of cells onto the retinal surface. A bout of inflammation or another insult might cause upregulation of necessary receptors on RPE or glia. Requirement for the latter might explain why all patients with PVD do not get ERMs. Further work is needed to explore the effect of hypoxia on hyalocytes and its potential impact on ERM formation.

Retinal Detachment and PVR

Retinal detachment results in increased expression of PDGF in RPE. It is accompanied by cell proliferation, resulting in multilayered colonies of RPE cells beneath the detached retina. PDGF may also stimulate Müller cells (Fig. 23-5), which send processes that migrate along the outer surface of the retina.

Retinal reattachment results in reversal of these processes, although they are not always reversible and their persistence in the macula may be a cause of poor

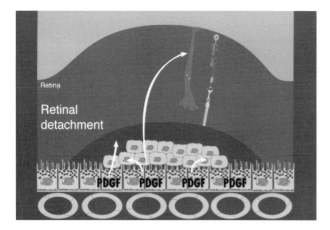

FIGURE 23-5. Schematic representation of possible modulation of growth factor production and its consequences after retinal detachment. Retinal detachment results in upregulation of the PDGF autocrine loop in RPE that may contribute to proliferation and migration of RPE and retinal glia. Other autocrine loops, including those for vascular endothelial growth factor, basic fibroblast growth factor, and insulin-like growth factor, may also contribute *(not shown)*.

recovery of visual acuity after retinal reattachment. If there is persistent inflammation, either from surgery or from other causes, the migration and proliferation of RPE and glia may continue; once these cells are established on the retinal surface and/or in the vitreous, they may provide another source of stimulatory factors (Fig. 23-6). For simplicity, only PDGF is listed in Figure 23-6, but it is likely that many GFs and cytokines participate, and, therefore, specific antagonism of any one GF

may not be sufficient for treatment of PVR. For this reason, agents that antagonize several GFs may hold more promise than specific antagonists for drug therapy of PVR (Campochiaro et al., 1991).

Diabetes and Retinal NV

Experiments using cultured cells, as summarized above (see "The Transforming Growth Factor-β Family"), have led to the hypothesis that pericyte-derived TGF-β provides a tonic inhibitory influence on endothelial cells of retinal vessels. After several years of diabetes, pericytes begin to drop out and make endothelial cells more responsive to stimulatory factors. Retinal hypoxia results in increased expression of VEGF by Müller cells and possibly by other cells. VEGF in collaboration with other factors, such as IGF-1, stimulates retinal neovascularization (Fig. 23-7). Endothelial cells of retinal NV produce PDGF, which may contribute to recruitment of RPE and glia into neovascular tissue on the surface of the retina (Fig. 23-8). It is not known if FGFs or other angiogenic factors contribute, but antagonism of VEGF partially inhibits retinal NV in a murine model (Aiello et al., 1995). Therefore, VEGF antagonists and/or other angiogenesis inhibitors may be useful adjuncts for the treatment of retinal NV. However, because PRP is very effective, it is unlikely that drug therapy will completely replace PRP.

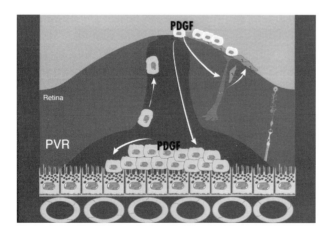

FIGURE 23-6. Schematic representation of possible modulation of growth factor production and its consequences after proliferative vitreoretinopathy (PVR). Once established, RPE and glia in epiretinal membranes produce PDGF, vascular endothelial growth factor, and other growth factors *(not shown)*, which recruit other RPE and glia, making the process self-sustaining. In this figure migration is shown in the area of a retinal break, but it can occur through intact retina.

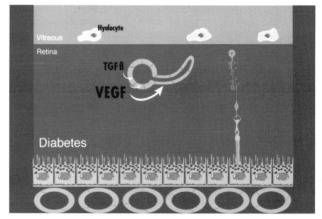

FIGURE 23-7. Schematic representation of modulation of growth factor production that could contribute to early retinal neovascularization in diabetes and other ischemic retinopathies. Retinal ischemia results in increased production of VEGF by Müller cells and retinal neurons. VEGF targets vascular endothelial cells made more responsive by decreased production of TGF-β after pericyte dropout and alteration of VEGF receptors. Other factors, including insulin-like growth factors and fibroblast growth factors, may also contribute *(not shown)*.

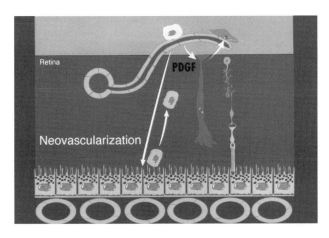

FIGURE 23-8. Schematic presentation of modulation of growth factor production that could contribute to fibrovascular epiretinal membrane production in the presence of retinal neovascularization. Once established, endothelial cells in retinal neovascularization produce PDGF and vascular endothelial growth factor *(not shown)*, which contribute to recruitment of RPE and glia that also produce these and other growth factors. This provides a self-sustaining feature, as seen in proliferative vitreoretinopathy.

CONCLUSIONS

Studies over the past ten years have demonstrated that the RPE is essentially a factory for many growth factors. It also responds to several growth factors, and there are at least three that act as autocrine stimulators of RPE growth in vitro. A bigger challenge is to define the role(s) of these growth factors in retinal physiology and pathophysiology. Although some progress has been made in this area, as indicated in the previous section, it is really just beginning. Over the next few years, targeted expression of growth factors and mutated growth factor receptors should provide many new insights. These insights could serve as the basis for new therapeutic approaches for a host of retinal diseases, ranging from retinal degenerations to ocular neovascularization.

ACKNOWLEDGMENTS

This work was supported by PHS grant EY05951 and core grant P30EY01765 from the National Eye Institute, Bethesda, Md., and by a Lew R. Wasserman Merit Award and an unrestricted grant from Research to Prevent Blindness, Inc., New York, N.Y.

REFERENCES

Adamis AP, Shima DT, Yeo K-T, Yeo T-K, Brown LF, Berse B, D'Amore PA, Folkman J. 1993. Synthesis and secretion of vascular permeability factor/vascular endothelial growth factor by human retinal pigment epithelial cells. Biochem Biophys Res Comm 93:631–638.

Adamis AP, Miller JS, Bernal MT, D'Amico DJ, Folkman J, Yeo TK, Yeo KT. 1994. Increased vascular endothelial growth factor levels in the vitreous of eyes with proliferative diabetic retinopathy. Am J Ophthalmol 118:445–450.

Adamis AP, Shima DT, Tolentino MJ, Gragoudas ES, Ferrara N, Folkman J, D'Amore PA, Miller JW. 1996. Inhibition of vascular endothelial growth factor prevents retinal ischemia-associated iris neovascularization. Arch Ophthalmol 114:66–71.

Aiello LP, Avery RL, Arrigg PG, Keyt BA, Jampel HD, Shah ST, Pasquale LR, Thieme H, Iwamoto MA, Park JE, et al. 1994. Vascular endothelial growth factor in ocular fluid of patients with diabetic retinopathy and other retinal disorders. N Eng J Med 331: 1480–1487.

Aiello LP, Pierce EA, Foley ED, Takagi H, Chen H, Riddle L, Ferrara N, King GL, Smith LEH. 1995. Suppression of retinal neovascularization in vivo by inhibition of vascular endothelial growth factor (VEGF) using soluble VEGF-receptor chimeric proteins. Proc Nat Acad Sci USA 92:10457–10461.

Amaya E, Musci TJ, Kirschner MW. 1991. Expression of a dominant negative mutant of the FGF receptor disrupts mesoderm formation in Xenopus embryos. Cell 66:257–270.

Amin R, Puklin JE, Frank RN. 1994. Growth factor localization in choroidal neovascular membranes of age-related macular degeneration. Invest Ophthalmol Vis Sci 35:3178–3188.

Anchan RM, Reh TA, Angello J, Balliet A, Walker M. 1991. EGF and TGF-α stimulate retinal neuroepithelial cell proliferation in vitro. Neuron 6:923–936.

Anderson KJ, Dam D, Lee S, Cotman CW. 1988. Basic fibroblast growth factor prevents death of lesioned cholinergic neurons in vivo. Nature 332:360–361.

Anderson DH, Guerin CJ, Hageman GS, Pfeffer BA, Flanders KC. 1995. Distribution of transforming growth factor-β isoforms in the mammalian retina. J Neurosci Res 42:63–79.

Antonaides HN, Galanopoulous T, Neville-Golden J, Diritsy CP, Lynch SE. 1991. Injury induces an in vivo expression of platelet-derived growth factor (PDGF) and PDGF receptor mRNAs in skin epithelial cells and PDGF mRNA in connective tissue fibroblasts. Proc Nat Acad Sci USA 88:565–569.

Antonelli-Orlidge A, Saunders KB, Smith SR, D'Armore PA. 1989. An activated form of transforming growth factor is produced by cultures of endothelial cells and pericytes. Proc Nat Acad Sci USA 86:4544–4548.

Arrindell EL, McKay BS, Jaffe GJ, Burke JM. 1992. Modulation of potassium transport in cultured retinal pigment epithelium and retinal glial cells by serum and epidermal growth factor. Exp Cell Res 203:192–197.

Baird A, Klagsburn M. 1991. The fibroblast growth factor family. Cancer Cells 3:239–243.

Barres BA, Raff MC. 1994. Control of oligodendrocyte number in the developing rat optic nerve. Neuron 12:935–942.

Battegay EJ, Raines EW, Seifert RA, Bowen-Pope DF, Ross R. 1990. TGF-β induces bimodal proliferation of connective tissue cells via complex control of an autocrine PDGF loop. Cell 63:515–524.

Baudouin C, Fredj-Reygrobellet D, Caruelle JP, Barritault D, Gastaud P, Lapalus P. 1990. Acidic fibroblast growth factor distribution in normal human eye and possible implications in ocular pathogenesis. Ophthalmic Res 22:733–781.

Behringer RR, Mathews LS, Palmiter RD, Brinster RL. 1988. Dwarf mice produced by genetic ablation of growth hormone-expressing cells. Genes Dev 2:453–461.

Benson MT, Shepherd L, Rees RC, Rennie IG. 1992. Production of interleukin-6 by human retinal pigment epithelium in vitro and its regulation by other cytokines. Curr Eye Res 11:173–179.

Bost LM, Aotaki-Keen AE, Hjelmeland LM. 1992. Coexpression of FGF-5 and bFGF by the retinal pigment epithelium in vitro. Exp Eye Res 55:727–734.

Bost LM, Hjelmeland LM. 1993. Cell density regulates differential production of bFGF transcripts. Growth Factors 9:195–203.

Bost LM, Aotaki-Keen AE, Hjelmeland LM. 1994. Cellular adhesion regulates bFGF gene expression in human retinal pigment epithelial cells. Exp Eye Res 58:545–552.

Bryan JA, Campochiaro PA. 1986. A retinal pigment epithelial cell-derived growth factor(s). Arch Ophthalmol 104:422–425.

Bugra K, Oliver L, Jacquemin E, Laurent M, Courtois Y, Hicks D. 1993. Acidic fibroblast growth factor is expressed abundantly by photoreceptors with the developing and mature rat retina. European J Neurosci 5:1586–1595.

Campochiaro PA, Glaser BM. 1985. Platelet-derived growth factor is chemotactic for human retinal pigment epithelial cells. Arch Ophthalmol 104:1685–1687.

Campochiaro PA, Hackett SF. 1993. Corneal endothelial cell matrix promotes expression of differentiated features of retinal pigmented epithelial cells: implication of laminin and basic fibroblast growth factor as active components. Exp Eye Res 57:539–547.

Campochiaro PA, Sugg R, Grotendorst G, Hjelmeland LM. 1989. Retinal pigment epithelial cells produce PDGF-like proteins and secrete them into their media. Exp Eye Res 49:217–227.

Campochiaro PA, Hackett SF, Conway BP. 1991. Retinoic acid promotes density-dependent growth arrest in retinal pigment epithelial cells. Invest Ophthalmol Vis Sci 32:65–72.

Campochiaro PA, Hackett SF, Vinores SA, Freund J, Csaky C, LaRochelle W, Henderer J, Johnson M, Rodriguez IR, Friedman Z, et al. 1994. Platelet-derived growth factor is an autocrine growth stimulator in retinal pigmented epithelial cells. J Cell Sci 107:2459–2469.

Campochiaro PA, Chang M, Osato M, Vinores SA, Nie Z, Hjelmeland L, Mansukhani A, Basilico C, Zack DJ. 1995. Photoreceptor degeneration in transgenic mice with PR-specific expression of a dominant negative fibroblast growth factor receptor. Invest Ophthalmol Vis Sci 36:5424.

Caruelle D, Groux-Muscatelli B, Gaudric A, Sestier C, Coscas G, Caruelle JP, Barritault D. 1989. Immunological study of acidic fibroblast growth factor (aFGF) distribution in the eye. J Cell Biochem 39:117–128.

Chen Y-S, Hackett SF, Schoenfeld C-L, Vinores MA, Vinores SA, Campochiaro PA. 1997. Localization of vascular endothelial growth factor and its receptors to cells of vascular and avascular epiretinal membranes. Br J Ophthalmol, 81:919–926.

Coltrera MD, Wang J, Porter PL, Gown AM. 1995. Expression of platelet-derived growth factor B-chain and the platelet-derived growth factor beta receptor subunit in human breast tissue and breast carcinoma. Canc Res 55:2703–2708.

Connolly DT, Heuvelman DM, Nelson R, Olander JV, Eppley BL, Delfino JJ, Siegel NR, Leimgruber RM, Feder J. 1989. Tumor vascular permeability factor stimulates endothelial cell growth and angiogenesis. J Clin Invest 84:1470–1478.

Connolly SE, Hjelmeland LM, LaVail MM. 1992. Immunohistochemical localization of basic fibroblast growth factor in mature and developing retinas of normal and RCS rats. Curr Eye Res 11:1005–1017.

Connor TB, Roberts AB, Sparn MB, Dart LL, Michels RG, de Bustros S, et al. 1989. Correlation of fibrosis and transforming growth factor-β type 2 leves in the eye. J Clin Invest 83:1661–1666.

Consigli SA, Lyser KM, Joseph-Silverstein J. 1993. The temporal and spatial expression of basic fibroblast growth factor during ocular development in the chicken. Invest Ophthalmol Vis Sci 34:559–566.

Cousins SW, Trattler WB, Streilein JW. 1991. Immune privilege and suppression of immunogenic inflammation in the anterior chamber of the eye. Curr Eye Res 10:287–297.

D'Amore PA. 1994. Mechanisms of retinal and choroidal neovascularization. Invest Ophthalmol Vis Sci 35:3974–3979.

Danis RP, Grant M, Bingaman D, Ladd B. 1994. Intravitreal IGF-1 enhances preretinal neovascularization induced by ischemia in pigs. Invest Ophthalmol Vis Sci 35:1996.

Dastgheib K, Li Q, Chan C-C, Roberge FG, Csaky K, Green WR. 1995. Vascular endothelial growth factor (VEGF) in neovascular age-related macular degeneration. Invest Ophthalmol Vis Sci 36: S102.

Daughaday WH, Hall K, Raben MS, Salmon WD, van den Brande JL, Van Wyck JJ. 1972. Somatomedin: proposed designation for sulfation factor. Nature 234:107–108.

de Boer JH, Limpens J, Orengo-Nania S, de Jong PTVM, LaHeij E, Kijlstra A. 1994. Low mature TGF-β₂ levels in aqueous humor during uveitis. Invest Ophthalmol Vis Sci 35:3702–3710.

de la Rosa EJ, Bondy CA, Hernandezsanchez C, Wu X, Zhou J, Lopezcarranza A, Scavo LM, Depablo F. 1994. Insulin and insulin-like growth factor system components gene expression in the chicken retina from early neurogenesis until late development and their effect on neuroepithelial cells. Eur J Neurosci 6:1801–1810.

de Vries C, Escobedo JA, Ueno H, Houck K, Ferrara N, Williams LT. 1992. The fms-like tyrosine kinase, a receptor for vascular endothelial growth factor. Science 255:989–991.

Del Priore LV, Hornbeck R, Kaplan HJ, Jones Z, Valentino TL, Mosinger-Ogilvie J, Swinn M. 1995. Debridement of the pig retinal pigment epithelium in vivo. Arch Ophthalmol 113:939–944.

Deng C-X, Wynshaw BA, Shen MM, Daugherty C, Ornitz DM, Leder P. 1994. Murine FGFR-1 is required for early postimplantation growth and axial organization. Genes Develop 8:3045–3057.

Desmoulière A, Redard M, Darby I, Gabbiani G. 1995. Apoptosis mediates the decrease in cellularity during transition between granulation tissue and scar. Am J Pathol 146:56–66.

Doolittle RF, Hunkapiller MW, Hood LE, Devare SG, Robbins KC, Aaronson SA, Antoniades HN. 1983. Simian sarcoma virus oncogene, v-sis, is derived from the gene (or genes) encoding a platelet-derived growth factor. Science 221:275–277.

Edwards RB, Adler AJ, Claycomb RC. 1992. Requirement of insulin of IGF-1 for the maintenance of retinyl ester synthetase activity by cultured retinal pigment epithelial cells. Exp Eye Res 52:51–57.

Eisenstein R, Grant-Bertacchini. 1991. Growth inhibitory activities in avascular tissues are recognized by anti-transforming growth factor-β antibodies. Curr Eye Res 10:157–162.

Elner VM, Strieter RM, Elner SG, Baggiolini M, Lindley I, Kunkel S. 1990. Neutrophil chemotactic factor (IL-8) gene expression by cytokine-treated retinal pigment epithelial cells. Am J Pathol 136:745–750.

Elner VM, Scales W, Elner SG, Danforth J, Kunkel SL, Strieter RM. 1992. Interleukin-6 (IL-6) gene expression and secretion by cytokine-stimulated human retinal pigment epithelial cells. Exp Eye Res 54:361–368.

Faktorovich EG, Steinberg RH, Yasumura D, Matthes MT, LaVail MM. 1990. Photoreceptor degeneration in inherited retinal dystrophy delayed by basic fibroblast growth factor. Nature 347:83–86.

Fayein NH, Courtois Y, Jeanny JC. 1990. Ontogeny of basic fibroblast growth factor binding sites in mouse ocular tissues. Exp Cell Res 188:75–88.

Feldman EL, Randolph AE. 1994. Regulation of insulin-like growth factor binding protein synthesis and secretion in human retinal pigment epithelial cells. J Cell Physiol 158:198–204.

Ferrara N, Henzel WJ. 1989. Pituitary follicular cells secrete a novel heparin-binding growth factor specific for vascular endothelial cells. Biochem Biophys Res Commun 161:851–858.

Fredj-Reygrobellet D, Baudouin C, Negre F, Caruelle JP, Gastaud P, Lapalus P. 1991. Acidic FGF and other growth factors in preretinal membranes from patients with diabetic retinopathy and proliferative vitreoretinopathy. Ophthalmic Res 23:154–161.

Freese A, Finklestein SP, DiFiglia M. 1992. Basic fibroblast growth factor protects striatal neurons in vitro from NMDA-receptor mediated excitotoxicity. Brain Res 575:351–355.

Freund J, Hackett S, Dooner J, DiStefano P, Gottsch J, Campochiaro PA. 1994. Modulation of bFGF mRNA in the RPE by stress neurotrophins, and cytokines. Invest Ophthalmol Vis Sci 35:1760.

Froesch ER, Muller WA, Burgi H. 1966. Nonsuppressible insulin-like activity of human serum. II. Biological properties of plasma extracts with nonsuppressible insulin-like activity. Biochim Biophys Acta 121:360–375.

Fujiwara M. 1994. Analysis of fibroblast growth factor receptor genes expressed in the retinal pigment epithelium of chick embryos by reverse transcription polymerase chain reaction. Acta Soc Ophthalmol Jpn 98:625–629.

Gabrielian K, Osusky R, Sippy BD, Ryan SJ, Hinton K. 1994. Effect of TGF-β on interferon-γ-induced HLA-DR expression in human retinal pigment epithelial cells. Invest Ophthalmol Vis Sci 35:4253–4259.

Gao H, Hollyfield JG. 1992. Basic fibroblast growth factor (bFGF) immunolocalization in the rodent outer retina demonstrated with an anti-rodent bFGF antibody. Brain Res 585:355–360.

Gay S, Jones RE, Huang G, Gay RE. 1989. Immunohistological demonstration of platelet-derived growth factor and sis-oncogene expression in scleroderma. J Invest Dermatol 92:301–303.

Gospodarowicz D, Neufeld G, Schweigerer L. 1986. Molecular and biological characterization of fibroblast growth factor, an angiogenic factor which also controls the proliferation and differentiation of mesoderm and neuroectoderm derived cells. Cell Differ 19:1–17.

Gospodarowicz D, Abraham JA, Schilling J. 1989. Isolation and characterization of a vascular endothelial cell mitogen produced by pituitary-derived folliculo stellate cells. Proc Nat Acad Sci USA 86:7311–7315.

Grant M, Russell B, Fitzgerald, Merimee J. 1986. Insulin-like growth factors in the vitreous studies in central and diabetic subjects with neovascularization. Diabetes 35:416–420.

Grant M, Jerdan J, Merimee TJ. 1987. Insulin-like growth factor I modulates endothelial cell chemotaxis. J Clin Endocrinol Metab 65:370–371.

Grant MB, Guay C, Marsh R. 1990. Insulin-like growth factor I stimulates proliferation, migration, and plasminogen activator release by human retinal pigment epithelial cells. Curr Eye Res 9:323–335.

Guerrin M, Moukadiri H, Chollet P, Moro F, Datt K, Melecaze F, Plouet J. 1995. Vasculotropin/vascular endothelial growth factor is an autocrine growth factor for human retinal pigment epithelial cells cultured in vitro. J Cell Physiol 164:385–394.

Guha A, Dashner K, Black PM, Wagner JA, Stiles CD. 1995. Expression of PDGF and PDGF receptors in human astrocytoma operation specimens supports the existence of an autocrine loop. Int J Canc 60:168–173.

Hackett SF, Schoenfeld C-L, Freund J, Gottsch JD, Bhargave S, Campochiaro PA. 1997. Neurotrophic factors, cytokines and stress in-

crease expression of basic fibroblast growth factor in retinal pigmented epithelial cells. Exp Eye Res 64:865–873.

Hageman GS, Kirchoff-Rempe MA, Lewis GP, Fisher SK, Anderson DH. 1991. Sequestration of basic fibroblast growth factor in the primate retinal interphotoreceptor matrix. Proc Nat Acad Sci USA 88:6706–6710.

Hanneken A, Baird A. 1992. Immunolocalization of basic fibroblast growth factor: dependence on antibody type and tissue fixation. Exp Eye Res 54:1011–1014.

Hanneken A, Baird A. 1995. Soluble forms of the high-affinity fibroblast growth factor receptor in human vitreous fluid. Invest Ophthalmol Vis Sci 36:1192–1196.

Hanneken A, Lutty GA, McLeod DS, Robey F, Harvey AK, Hjelmeland LM. 1989. Localization of basic fibroblast growth factor to the developing capillaries of bovine retina. J Cell Physiol 138:115–120.

Hanneken A, deJuan E, Lutty GA, Fox GM, Schiffer S, Hjelmeland LM. 1991. Altered distribution of basic fibroblast growth factor in diabetic retinopathy. Arch Ophthalmol 109:1005–1011.

Harada S, Nagy JA, Sullivan KA, Thomas KA, Endo N, Rodan GA, Rodan SB. 1994. Induction of vascular endothelial growth factor expression by prostaglandin E$_2$ and E$_1$ in osteoblasts. J Clin Invest 93:2490–2496.

Hart CE, Bowen-Pope DF. 1990. Platelet-derived growth factor receptor: current views of the two subunit model. J Invest Dermatol 94:535–575.

Heldin C-H, Westermark B. 1990. Platelet-derived growth factor: mechanism of action and possible in vivo function. Cell Reg 8:555–566.

Herbert JM, Basilico C, Goldfarb M, Haub O, Martin GR. 1990. Isolation of cDNAs encoding four mouse FGF family members and characterization of their expression pattern during embryogenesis. Dev Biol 138:454–463.

Hicks D, Courtois Y. 1988. Acidic fibroblast growth factor stimulates opsin levels in retinal photoreceptor cells in vitro. FEBS Lett 234:475–479.

Hicks D, Courtois Y. 1992a. Basic fibroblast growth factor stimulates photoreceptor differentiation in vitro. Devel Biol 134:201–205.

Hicks D, Courtois Y. 1992b. Fibroblast growth factor stimulates photoreceptor differentiation in vitro. J Neurosci 12:2022–2033.

Im JH, Pillon DJ, Meezan E. 1986. Comparison of insulin receptors from bovine retinal blood vessels and nonvascular retinal tissue. Invest Ophthalmol Vis Sci 27:1681–1690.

Ishigooka H, Kitaoka T, Boutilier SB, Bost LM, Aotaki-Keen A, Tablin F, Hjelmeland LM. 1993. Developmental expression of bFGF in the bovine retina. Invest Ophthalmol Vis Sci 34:2813–2823.

Jacquemin E, Halley C, Alterio J, Laurent M, Courtois Y, Jeanny JC. 1990. Localization of acidic fibroblast growth factor (aFGF) mRNA in mouse and bovine retina by in situ hybridization. Neurosci Lett 116:23–28.

Jacquemin E, Jonet L, Oliver L, Bugra K, Laurent M, Courtois Y, Jeanny JC. 1993. Developmental regulation of acidic fibroblast growth factor (aFGF) expression in bovine retina. Int J Dev Biol 37:417–423.

Jacobson B, Sullivan D, Raymard L, Basu PK, Hasany SM. 1983. Further studies on a vitreous inhibitor of endothelial proliferation. Exp Eye Res 36:447–450.

Jaffe GJ, Van Le L, Valea F, Haskill S, Roberts W, Arend WP, Stuart A, Peters WP. 1992a. Expression of interleukin-1α, interleukin-1β, and an interleukin receptor-1 antagonist in human retinal pigment epithelial cells. Exp Eye Res 55:325–335.

Jaffe GJ, Peters WP, Roberts W, Kurtzberg J, Stuart A, Wang AM,

Stoudemire JB. 1992b. Modulation of macrophage colony stimulating factor in cultured human retinal pigment epithelial cells. Exp Eye Res 54:595–603.

Jaffe GJ, Richmond A, Van Le L, Shattuck RL, Cheng QC, Wong F, Roberts W. 1993. Expressions of three forms of melanoma growth stimulating activity (MSGA)/gro in human retinal pigment epithelial cells. Invest Ophthalmol Vis Sci 34:2776–2785.

Jaffe GJ, Roberts WL, Hong HL, Yurochko AD, Cianciolo GJ. 1995. Monocyte-induced cytokine expression in cultured human retinal pigment epithelial cells. Exp Eye Res 60:533–543.

Johnson DE, Williams LT. 1993. Structural and functional diversity in the FGF receptor multigene family. Adv Canc Res 60:1–41.

Jones JI, Clemmons DR. 1995. Insulin-like growth factors and their binding proteins: biological actions. Endocrine Rev 16:3–34.

Kelley MW, Turner JK, Reh TA. 1995. Regulation of proliferation and photoreceptor differentiation in fetal human retinal cell cultures. Invest Ophthalmol Vis Sci 36:1280–1289.

Kinoshita N, Minshull J, Kirschner MW. 1995. The identification of two novel ligands of the FGF receptor by a yeast screening method and their activity in xenopus development. Cell 83:621–630.

Kitaoka T, Bost LM, Ishigooka H, Aotaki-Keen AE, Hjelmeland LM. 1993. Increasing cell density down-regulates the expression of acidic FGF by human RPE cells in vitro. Curr Eye Res 12:993–999.

Kitaoka T, Aotaki-Keen AE, Hjelmeland LM. 1994. Distribution of FGF-5 in the rhesus macaque retina. Invest Ophthalmol Vis Sci 35:3189–3198.

Kohner EM, Hamilton AM, Joplin GF. 1953. Florid diabetic retinopathy and its response to treatment by photocoagulation or pituitary ablation. Diabetes 25:104–110.

Kostyk SK, D'Amore PA, Herman IM, Wagner JA. 1994. Optic nerve injury alters basic fibroblast growth factor localization in retina and optic tract. J Neurosci 14:1441–1449.

Kuppner MC, McKillop-Smith S, Forrester JV. 1995. TGF-beta and IL-1 beta act in synergy to enhance IL-6 and IL-8 mRNA levels and IL-6 production by human retinal pigment epithelial cells. Immunology 84:265–271.

Kurtz MJ, Edward RB. 1991. Influence of bicarbonate and insulin on pigment synthesis by cultured adult human retinal pigment epithelial cells. Exp Eye Res 53:681–684.

Kutty RK, Nagineni CN, Kutty G, Hooks JJ, Chader GJ, Wiggert B. 1994. Increased expression of heme oxygenase-1 in human retinal pigment epithelial cells by transforming growth factor-beta. J Cell Physiol 159:371–378.

Kvanta A. 1994. Expression and secretion of transforming growth factor-beta in transformed and nontransformed retinal pigment epithelial cells. Ophthalmic Res 26:361–367.

Lansing MB, Glaser MD, Liss H, Hanham A, Thompson JT, Sjaarda RN, Gordon AJ. 1993. The effect of pars plana vitrectomy and transforming growth factor-beta 2 without epiretinal membrane peeling on full-thickness macular holes. Ophthalmology 100:868–872.

Lazarus HS, Schoenfeld C-L, Fekrat S, Cohen S, Carol H, Hageman GS, Hackett SF, Chen Y-S, Vinores SA, Campochiaro PA. 1996. Hyalocytes synthesize and secrete inhibitors of retinal pigment epithelial cell proliferation in vitro. Arch Ophthalmol 114:731–736.

LaVail MM, Unoki K, Yasumura D, Matthes MT, Yancopoulos GD, Steinburg RH. 1992. Multiple growth factors, cytokines, and neurotrophins rescue photoreceptors from the damaging effects of constant light. Proc Nat Acad Sci USA 89:11249–11253.

Leschey KH, Hackett SF, Singer JH, Campochiaro PA. 1990. Growth factor responsiveness of human retinal pigment epithelial cells. Invest Ophthalmol Vis Sci 31:839–846.

Leung DW, Cachianes G, Kuang W-J, Goeddel DV, Ferrara N. 1989. Vascular endothelial growth factor is a secreted angiogenic mitogen. Science 246:1306–1309.

Li J, Perrella MA, Tsai J-C, Yet S-F, Hsieh C-M, Yoshizumi M, Patterson C, Endege WO, Zhou F, Lee M-E. 1995. Induction of vascular endothelial growth factor gene expression by interleukin-1β in rat aortic smooth muscle cells. J Bio Chem 279:308–312.

Liu J-P, Fitzgibbon F, Nash M, Osborne NN. 1992. Epidermal growth factor potentiates the transmitter-induced stimulation of C-AMP and inositol phosphates in human pigment epithelial cells in culture. Exp Eye Res 55:489–497.

Liu J-P, Baker J, Perkins AS, Robertson EJ, Efstratiadis A. 1993. Mice carrying null mutations of the genes encoding insulin-like growth factor I (Igf-1) and type 1 IGF receptor (Igf1r). Cell 75:73–82.

Lutty G, Ikeda K, Chandler C, McLeod DS. 1991. Immunohistochemical localization of transforming growth factor-β in human photoreceptors. Curr Eye Res 10:61–74.

Lutty GA, Merges C, Threlkelt AB, Crone S, McLeod DS. 1993. Heterogeneity in localization of isoforms of TGF-β in human, retina, vitreous and choroid. Invest Ophthalmol Vis Sci 34:477–487.

Mack AF, Fernald RD. 1993. Regulation of cell division and rod differentiation in the teleost retina. Dev Brain Res 76:183–187.

Mack AF, Balt SL, Fernald RD. 1995. Localization and expression of insulin-like growth factor in the teleost retina. Vis Neurosci 12:457–461.

Majesky MW, Reidy MA, Bowen-Pope DF, Hart CE, Wilcox, JN, Schwartz SM. 1990. PDGF ligand and receptor gene expression during repair of arterial injury. J Cell Biol 111:2149–2158.

Majno G, Joris I. 1995. Apoptosis, oncosis and necrosis. An overview of cell death. Am J Pathol 146:3–15.

Malecaze F, Mathis A, Arne JL, Raulais D, Courtois Y, Hicks D. 1991. Localization of acidic fibroblast growth factor in proliferative vitreoretinopathy membranes. Curr Eye Res 10:719–729.

Malecaze F, Mascarelli F, Bugra K, Fuhrmann G, Courtois Y, Hicks D. 1993. Fibroblast growth factor receptor deficiency in dystrophic retinal pigmented epithelium. J Cell Physiol 154:631–642.

Malecaze F, Clamens S, Simorre-Pinatel V, Mathis A, Chollet P, Favard C, Bayard F, Plouet J. 1994. Detection of vascular endothelial growth factor messenger RNA and vascular endothelial growth factor-like activity in proliferative diabetic retinopathy. Arch Ophthalmol 112:1476–1482.

Martin DM, Yee D, Feldman EL. 1992. Gene expression of the insulin-like growth factors and their receptors in cultured human retinal pigment epithelial cells. Brain Res Mol Brain Res 12:181–186.

Martinet Y, Rom WN, Rom WN, Grotendorst GR, Martin GR, Crystal RG. 1987. Exaggerated spontaneous release of plate-derived growth factor by alveolar macrophages from patients with idiopathic pulmonary fibrosis. N Eng J Med 317:202–209.

Masagué J. 1992. Receptors for the TGF-β family. Cell 69:1067–1070.

Mascarelli F, Raulais D, Courtois Y. 1989. Fibroblast growth factor phosphorylation and receptors in rod outer segments. EMBO J 8:2265–2273.

Mathews LS, Hammer RE, Brinster RL, Palmiter RD. 1988a. Expression of insulin-like growth factor I in transgenic mice with elevated levels of growth hormone is correlated with growth. Endocrinology 123:433–437.

Mathews LS, Hammer RE, Behringer RR, D'Ercole AJ, Bell GI, Brinster RL, Palmiter RD. 1988b. Growth enhancement of transgenic mice expressing human insulin-like growth factor-I. Endocrinology 123:2827–2833.

Matsumoto M, Yoshimura N, Honda Y. 1994. Increased production of transforming growth factor-β_2 from cultured human retinal pigment epithelial cells by photocoagulation. Invest Ophthalmol Vis Sci 35:4245–4252.

McCartney-Francis NL, Wahl SM. 1994. Transforming growth factor β: a matter of life and death. J Leukoc Biol 55:401–409.

Mercola M, Wang C, Kelly J, Brownlee C, Jackson-Grusby L, Stiles C, Bowen-Pope D. 1990. Selective expression of PDGF and its receptor during early mouse embryogenesis. Dev Biol 138:114–122.

Merimee TJ, Zapf J, Froesch ER. 1983. Insulin-like growth factors: studies in diabetics with and without retinopathy. N Eng J Med 309:527–530.

Miceli MV, Newsome DA. 1994. Insulin stimulation of retinal outer segment uptakes by cultured human retinal pigmented epithelial cells determined by a flow cytometric method. Exp Eye Res 59:271–280.

Mignatti P, Morimoto T, Rifkin DB. 1992. Basic fibroblast growth factor, a protein devoid of secretory signal sequence, is released by cells via a pathway independent of the endoplasmic reticulum–Golgi complex. J Cell Physiol 151:81–93.

Miller JW, Adamis AP, Shima DT, D'Amore PA, Molton RS, O'Reilly MS, Folkman J, Dvorak HF, Brown LF, Berse B, et al. 1994. Vascular endothelial growth factor/vascular permeability factor is temporally and spatially correlated with ocular angiogenesis in a primate model. Am J Path 145:574–584.

Moriarty P, Boulton M, Dickson A, McLeod D. 1994. Production of IGF-I and IGF binding proteins by retinal cells in vitro. Br J Ophthalmol 78:638–642.

Morse L, Terrell J, Sidikaro Y. 1989. Bovine retinal pigment epithelium promotes proliferation of choroidal endothelium in vitro. Arch Ophthalmol 107:1659–1663.

Mudhar HS, Pollock RA, Wang C, Stile CD, Richardson WD. 1993. PDGF and its receptors in the developing rodent retina and optic nerve. Development 118:539–552.

Noji S, Matsuo T, Koyama E, Yamaai T, Nohno T, Matsuo N, Tanaguchi S. 1990. Expression pattern of acidic and basic fibroblast growth factor genes in adult rat eyes. Biochem Biophys Res Commun 168:343–349.

Ohuchi H, Koyama E, Myokai F, Nohno T, Shiraga F, Matsuo T, Matsuo N, Taniguchi S, Noji S. 1994. Expression patterns of two fibroblast growth factor receptor genes during early chick eye development. Exp Eye Res 58:649–658.

Okamoto N, Tobe T, Hackett SF, Ozaki H, Vinores MA, LaRochelle W, Zack DJ, Campochiaro PA. 1997. Transgenic mice with increased expression of vascular endothelial growth factor in the retina. A new model of intraretinal and subretinal neovascularization. Amer J Pathol 151:281–291.

Opas M, Dziak E. 1994. bFGF-induced transdifferentiation of RPE to neuronal progenitors is regulated by the mechanical properties of the substratum. Dev Biol 161:440–454.

Palmiter RD, Norstedt RE, Gelinas RE, Hammer RE, Brinster RL. 1983. Metallothionein-human GH fusion genes stimulate growth of mice. Science 222:809–814.

Park CM, Hollenberg MJ. 1989. Basic fibroblast growth factor induces retinal regeneration in vivo. Dev Biol 134:201–205.

Park CM, Hollenberg MJ. 1993. Growth factor-induced retinal regeneration in vivo. Int Rev Cytol 146:49–74.

Park J, Keller G-A, Ferrera N. 1993. The vascular endothelial growth factor (VEGF) isoforms: differential deposition into the subepithelial extracellular matrix and bioactivity of extracellular matrix-bound VEGF. Mol Biol Cell 4:1317–1326.

Patel B, Hiscott P, Charteris D, Mather J, McLeod D, Boulton M. 1994. Retinal and preretinal localization of epidermal growth factor, transforming growth factor alpha, and their receptor in proliferative diabetic retinopathy. Br J Ophthalmol 78:714–718.

Pe'er J, Shweiki D, Itin A, Heme I, Gnessin H, Keshet E. 1995. Hypoxia-induced expression of vascular endothelial growth factor by retinal cells is a common factor in neovascularizing ocular diseases. Lab Invest 72:638–645.

Peters K, Werner S, Liao X, Wert S, Whitsett J, Williams L. 1994. Targeted expression of a dominant negative FGF receptor blocks branching morphogenesis and epithelial differentiation of the mouse lung. EMBO J 13:3296–3301.

Pfeffer BA, Flanders KC, Guerin CJ, Danielpour D, Anderson DH. 1994. Transforming growth factor-β_2 is the predominant isoform in the neural retina, retinal pigment epithelium-choroids and vitreous of the monkey eyes. Exp Eye Res 59:323–333.

Phren JHM, Peruche B, Unsicker K, Krieglstein J. 1993. Isoform-specific effects of growth factor-β on degeneration of primary neuronal cultures induced by cytotoxic hypoxia or glutamate. J Neurochem 60:1165–1672.

Pierce EA, Avery RL, Foley ED, Aiello LP, Smith LEH. 1995. Vascular endothelial growth factor/vascular permeability factor expression in a mouse model of retinal neovascularization. Proc Nat Acad Sci USA 92:905–909.

Pierce GF, Mustoe TA, Lingelbach J, Masakowski VR, Griffin GL, Senior RM, Deuel TF. 1989. Platelet-derived growth factor and transforming growth factor-β enhance tissue repair activities by unique mechanisms. J Cell Biol 109:429–440.

Pierce GF, Mustoe TA, Altrock BW, Deuel TF, Thomason A. 1991. Role of platelet-derived growth factor in wound healing. J Cell Biochem 45:319–326.

Pittack C, Jones M, Reh TA. 1991. Basic fibroblast growth factor induces retinal pigment epithelium to generate neural retina in vitro. Development 113:577–578.

Planck SR, Dang TT, Graves D, Tara D, Ansel JC, Rosenbaum JT. 1992. Retinal pigment epithelial cells secrete interleukin-6 in response to interleukin-I. Invest Ophthalmol Vis Sci 33:78–82.

Planck SR, Huang XN, Robertson JE, Rosenbaum JT. 1993. Retinal pigment epithelial cells produce interleukin-1 β and granulocyte-macrophage colony-stimulating factor in response to interleukin-1 alpha. Curr Eye Res 12:205–212.

Plate KH, Breier G, Welch HA, Risau W. 1992. Vascular endothelial growth factor is a potential tumor angiogenesis factor in human gliomas in vivo. Nature 359:845–848.

Plouet J, Mascarelli F, Loret MD, Faure JP, Courtois Y. 1988. Regulation of eye derived growth factor binding to membranes by light, ATP or GTP in photoreceptor outer segments. EMBO J 7:373–376.

Poulson JE. 1953. The Houssay phenomenon in man: recovery from retinopathy in a case of diabetes with Simmond's disease. Diabetes 2:7–12.

Quinn TP, Peters KG, DeVries C, Ferrara N, Williams LT. 1993. Fetal-liver kinase 1 is a receptor for vascular endothelial growth factor and is selectively expressed in endothelium. Proc Nat Acad Sci USA 90:7533–7557.

Randolph A, Yee D, Feldman EL. 1993. Insulin-like growth factor binding protein expression in human retinal pigment epithelial cells. Ann NY Acad Sci 692:265–267.

Rappolee DA, Brenner CA, Schultz R, Mark D, Werb Z. 1988. Developmental expression of PDGF, TGF-α and TGF-β genes in preimplantation mouse embryos. Science 241:1823–1825.

Raymond PA, Barthel LK, Rounsifer ME. 1992. Immunolocalization of basic fibroblast growth factor and its receptor in adult goldfish retina. Exp Neurol 115:73–78.

Reneker LW, Overbeek PA. 1996. PDGF induces abnormal development of both lens epithelium and retinal astrocytes in transgenic eyes. Invest Ophthalmol Vis Sci 37:2455–2466.

Remmers EF, Sano H, Lafyatis R, Case JP, Kumkumian GK, Hla T, Maciag T, Wilder RL. 1991. Production of platelet-derived growth factor B-chain mRNA and immunoreactive PDGF B-like polypeptide by rheumatoid synovium: co-expression with heparin binding acidic fibroblast growth factor-1. J Rheumatol 18:7–13.

Reuterdahl C, Tingstrom A, Terracio L, Funa K, Heldin CH, Rubin K. 1992. Characterization of platelet-derived growth factor-β receptor expressing cells in the vasculature of human rheumatoid synovium. Lab Invest 64:321–329.

Rifkin DB, Kojima S, Abe M, Harpel JG. 1993. TGF-β: structure, function, formation. Thrombosis and Haemostasis 70:177–179.

Rinderknecht E, Humbel RE. 1978a. The amino acid sequence of human insulin-like growth factor I and its structural homology with proinsulin. J Biol Chem 253:2769–2776.

Rinderknecht E, Humbel RE. 1978b. Primary structure of human insulin-like growth factor II. FEBS Lett 89:283–286.

Robbins SG, Mixon RN, Wilson DJ, Hart CE, Robertson JE, Westra I, Planck SR, Rosenbaum JT. 1994. Platelet-derived growth factor ligands and receptors immunolocalized in proliferative retinal diseases. Invest Ophthalmol Vis Sci 35:3649–3663.

Roberts AB, Sporn MB. 1990. Transforming growth factor β. Adv Canc Res 51:107–145.

Robinson GS, Pierce EA, Rook SL, Foley E, Webb R, Smith LES. 1996. Oligodeoxynucleotides inhibit retinal neovascularization in a murine model of proliferative retinopathy. Proc Nat Acad Sci USA 93:4851–4856.

Rohrer B, Stell WK. 1994. Basic fibroblast growth factor (bFGF) and transforming growth factor beta (TGF-β) act as stop and go signals to modulate postnatal ocular growth in the chick. Exp Eye Res 58:553–562.

Roque RS, Caldwell RB, Behzadian MA. 1992. Cultured Müller cells have high levels of epidermal growth factor receptors. Invest Ophthalmol Vis Sci 33:2587–2595.

Rosenzweig SA. 1993. Retinal insulin receptors. Meth Neurosci 11:294–316.

Rosenzweig SA, Zetterström C, Benjamin A. 1990. Identification of retinal insulin receptors using site-specific antibodies to a carbonyl-terminal peptide of the human insulin receptor α-subunit. Up-regulation of neuronal insulin receptors in diabetes. J Biol Chem 265:18030–18034.

Ross R, Glomset JA, Kariya B, Harker L. 1974. A platelet-dependent serum factor that stimulates the proliferation of arterial smooth muscle cells in vitro. Proc Nat Acad Sci USA 71:1207–1210.

Ross R, Masuda J, Raines E, Gown AM, Katsuda S, Sashara M, Malden LT, Masuko H, Sato H. 1990. Localization of PDGF-B protein in all phases of atherogenesis. Science 248:1009–1012.

Rubin K, Terracio L. 1988. Expression of platelet-derived growth factor receptors is induced on connective tissue cells during chronic synovial inflammation. Scand J Immunol 27:285–294.

Sagar SM, Edwards RH, Sharp FR. 1991. Epidermal growth factor and transforming growth factor alpha induce c-fos gene expression in retinal Müller cells in vivo. J Neurosci Res 29:549–559.

Salmon Jr WD, Daughaday WH. 1957. A hormonally controlled serum factor which stimulates sulfate incorporation by cartilage in vitro. J Lab Clin Med 49:825–836.

Schweigerer L, Malerstein B, Neufeld G, Gospodarowicz D. 1987. Basic fibroblast growth factor is synthesized in cultured retinal pigment epithelial cells. Biochem Biophys Res Comm 143:934–940.

Seko Y, Shimokawa H, Tokoro T. 1995. Expression of bFGF and TGF-Beta-2 in experimental myopia in chicks. Invest Ophthalmol Vis Sci 36:1183–1187.

Senger DR, Galli SJ, Dvorak AM, Perruzzi CA, Harvey VS, Dvorak HF. 1983. Tumor cells secrete a vascular permeability factor that promotes accumulation of ascites fluid. Science 219:983–985.

Shima DT, Adamis AP, Ferrara M, Yeo K-T, Yeo T-K, Allende R, Folkman J, D'Amore PA. 1985. Hypoxic induction of endothelial growth factors in retinal cells—identification and characterization of vascular endothelial growth factor (VEGF) as the mitogen. Molec Med 1:182–193.

Shweiki D, Itin A, Soffer D, Keshet E. 1992. Vascular endothelial growth factor induced by hypoxia may mediate hypoxia-initiated angiogenesis. Nature 359:843–845.

Sievers J, Hausmann B, Unsicker K, Berry M. 1987. Fibroblast growth factors promote the survival of adult rat retinal ganglion cells after transection of the optic nerve. Neurosci Lett 76:157–162.

Sivalingam A, Kenney J, Brown GC, Benson WE, Donoso L. 1990. Basic fibroblast factor levels in the vitreous of patients with proliferative diabetic retinopathy. Arch Ophthalmol 108:869–872.

Smiddy WE, Michels RG, Green WR. 1990. Morphology, pathology, and surgery of idiopathic vitreoretinal macula disorders: a review. Retina 10:288–296.

Smith LEH, Kopchick JJ, Chen W, Knapp J, Kinose F, Daley D, Foley E, Smith RG, Schaeffer JM. 1997. Essential role of growth hormone in ischemia-induced retinal neovascularization. Science 276:1706–1709.

Smits A, Kato M, Westermark B, Nister M, Helden CH, Funa K. 1991. Neurotrophic activity of platelet-derived growth factor (PDGF): rat neuronal cells possess functional PDGF beta-type receptors and respond to PDGF. Proc Nat Acad Sci USA 88:8159–8163.

Sporn MB, Roberts AB. 1992. Transforming growth factor-β: Recent progress and new challenges. J Cell Biol 119:1017–1021.

Sprugel KH, McPherson JM, Clowes AW, Ross R. 1987. Effects of growth factors in vivo. I. Cell ingrowth into porous subcutaneous chambers. Am J Pathol 129:601–613.

Steinberg RH, Song Y, Cheng T, Mathes MT, Yasumura D, LaVail MM, Wen R. 1995. Exposure to constant light upregulates the expression of bFGF, CNTF, FGFR-1 and GFAP mRNA in the rat retina. Invest Ophthalmol Vis Sci 36:5637.

Sternfield MD, Robertson JE, Shipley GD, Tsai J, Rosenbaum JT. 1989. Cultured human retinal pigment epithelial cells express basic fibroblast growth factor and its receptor. Curr Eye Res 8:1029–1037.

Stone J, Itin A, Alon T, Pe'er J, Ghessin H, Chen-Ling T, Keshet E. 1995. Development of retinal vasculature is mediated by hypoxia-induced vascular endothelial growth factor (VEGF) expression by neuroglia. J Neurosci 15:4738–4747.

Svoboda ME, Van Wyck JJ, Klapper DG, Fellows RE, Grissom FE, Schlueter RJ. 1989. Purification of somatomedin-C from human plasma: chemical and biological properties, partial sequence analysis and relationship to other somatomedins. Biochemistry 19:790–797.

Takagi H, Yoshimura N, Tanihara H, Honda Y. 1994. Insulin-like growth factor-related genes, receptors, and binding proteins in cultured human retinal pigment epithelial cells. Invest Ophthalmol Vis Sci 35:916–923.

Tanihara H, Yoshida M, Matsumoto M, Yoshimura N. 1993. Identification of transforming growth factor-β expressed in cultured human retinal pigment epithelial cells. Invest Ophthalmol Vis Sci 34:413–419.

Taniwaki T, Becerra SP, Chader GJ, Schwartz JP. 1995. Pigment epithelium-derived factor is a survival factor for cerebellar granule cells in culture. J Neurochem 65:2509–2517.

Tcheng M, Fuhrman G, Hartmann M-P, Courtois Y, Jeanny J-C. 1994. Spatial and temporal expression patterns of FGF receptor genes type 1 and type 2 in the developing chick retina. Exp Eye Res 58:351–358.

Tcheng M, Oliver L, Courtois Y, Jeanny J-C. 1994. Effects of exogenous FGFs on growth, differentiation, and survival of chick neural retina cells. Exp Cell Res 212:30–35.

Terman BI, Dougher-Vermazen M, Carrion ME, Dimitrov D, Armellino DC, Gospodarowicz D, Böhlen P. 1992. Identification of the KDR tyrosine kinase as a receptor for vascular endothelial growth factor. Biochem Biophys Res Comm 187:1579–1586.

Terracio L, Ronnstrand L, Tingstrom A, Rubin K, Claesson-Welsh L, Funa K, Heldin C-H. 1988. Induction of platelet-derived growth factor expression in smooth muscle cells and fibroblasts upon tissue culturing. J Cell Biol 107:1947–1957.

Ulbig MW, Wolfensberger TJ, Hiscott P, Ationu A, Carter ND, Gregor ZJ. 1995. German J Ophthalmol 4:264–268.

Vinores SA, Henderer JD, Mahlow J, Chiu C, Derevjanik NL, LaRochelle W, Csaky C, Campochiaro PA. 1995a. Isoforms of platelet-derived growth factor and its receptors in epiretinal membranes: immunolocalization to retinal pigmented epithelial cells. Exp Eye Res 60:607–619.

Vinores SA, Küchle M, Mahlow J, Chiu C, Green WR, Campochiaro PA. 1995b. Blood-ocular barrier breakdown in eyes with ocular melanoma: a potential role for vascular endothelial growth factor/vascular permeability factor. Am J Pathol 147:1289–1297.

Vinores SA, Youssri AI, Luna JD, Chen YS, Bhargave S, Vinores MA, Schoenfeld C-L, Peng B, Chan C-C, LaRochelle W, et al. 1997. Upregulation of vascular endothelial growth factor in ischemic and non-ischemic human and experimental retinal disease. Histol Histopathol 12:99–109.

Waldbillig RJ, Fletcher RT, Chader GJ, Rajagopalan S, Rodrigues M, LeRoth D. 1987a. Retinal insulin receptors. 1. Structural heterogeneity and functional characterization. Exp Eye Res 45:823–835.

Waldbillig RJ, Fletcher RT, Chader GJ, Rajagopalan S, Rogrigues M, LeRoth D. 1987b. Retinal insulin receptors. 2. Characterization and insulin-induced tyrosine kinase activity in bovine rod outer segments. Exp Eye Res 45:837–844.

Waldbillig RJ, Fletcher RT, Somers RL, Chader GJ. 1988. IGF-I receptors in the bovine neural retina: structure, kinase activity and comparison with retinal insulin receptors. Exp Eye Res 47:587–607.

Waldbillig RJ, Arnold DR, Fletcher RT, Chader GJ. 1991a. Insulin and IGF-I binding in developing chick neural retina and pigment epithelium: a characterization of binding and structural differences. Exp Eye Res 53:13–22.

Waldbillig RJ, Pfeffer BA, Schoen TJ, Adler AA, Shen-Orr Z, Scavo L, LeRoith D, Chader GJ. 1991b. Evidence for an insulin-like growth factor autocrine-paracrine system in the retinal photoreceptor-pigment epithelial cell complex. J Neurochem 57:1522–1533.

Waldbillig RJ, Schoen TJ, Chader GJ, Pfeffer BA. 1992. Monkey retinal pigment epithelial cells in vitro synthesize, secrete, and degrade insulin-like growth factor binding proteins. J Cell Physiol 150:76–83.

Waterfield MD, Scrace T, Whittle N, Stroobant P, Johnson A, Wasteson A, Westermark B, Heldin C-H, Huang JS, Deuel TF. 1983. Platelet-derived growth factor is related to the putative transforming protein p28[sis] of simian sarcoma virus. Nature 304:35–39.

Wen R, Song Y, Chen T, Mathes MT, Yasumura D, LaVail MM, Steinberg RH. 1995. Increase in expression of survival factors in rat retina induced by mechanical injury. Invest Ophthalmol Vis Sci 36:5637.

Werner S, Weinberg W, Liao X, Peters KG, Blassing M, Yuspa SH, Weiner RL, Williams LT. 1993. Targeted expression of dominant-negative FGF receptor mutant in the epidermis of transgenic mice reveals a role of FGF in keratinocyte organization and differentiation. EMBO J 12:2635–2643.

Wilcox JN, Smith KM, Williams LT, Schwartz SM, Gordon D. 1988. Platelet-derived growth factor mRNA detection in human atherosclerotic plaques by in situ hybridization. J Clin Invest 82:1134–1143.

Wong HC, Boulton M, McLeod D, Bayly M, Clark P, Marshall J. 1988. Retinal pigment epithelial cells in culture produce retinal vascular mitogens. Arch Ophthalmol 106:1439–1443.

Yamaguchi TP, Harpal K, Henkemeyer M, Rossant J. 1994. FGFR-1 is required for embryonic growth and mesodermal patterning during mouse gastrulation. Genes Develop 8:3032–3044.

Yoshida M, Tanihara H, Yoshimura N. 1992. Platelet-derived growth factor gene expression in cultured human retinal pigment epithelial cells. Biochem Biophys Res Comm 189:66–71.

Youssri AI, Luna J, Vinores S, Campochiaro PA. 1995. Immunohistochemical localization of vascular endothelial growth factor in retinas with oxygen-induced ischemic retinopathy and non-ischemic retinas. Invest Ophthalmol Vis Sci 36:5401.

Zetterström C, Fang C, Benjamin A, Rosenzweig SA. 1991. Characterization of a novel receptor in toad retina with dual specificity for insulin and insulin-like growth factor I. J Neurochem 57:1332–1339.

Zetterström C, Benjamin A, Rosenzweig SA. 1992. Differential expression of retinal insulin receptors in STZ-induced diabetic rats. Diabetes 41:818–825.

Zhang C, Takahaski K, Lam TT, Tso MOM. 1992. Effects of basic fibroblast growth factor in retinal ischemia. Invest Ophthalmol Vis Sci 33:722.

24. The retinal pigment epithelium, epiretinal membrane formation, and proliferative vitreoretinopathy

PAUL HISCOTT AND CARL M. SHERIDAN

Cellular, fibrocellular, or fibrovascular proliferations may form at several locations within the vitreous cavity, but most frequently and importantly they are situated on the inner retinal surface. The proliferations on the inner retina are called epiretinal membranes. Many epiretinal membranes do not produce symptoms; Foos (1974) called such asymptomatic membranes *simple epiretinal membranes*. Conversely, epiretinal membranes that produce symptoms are regarded as *complex epiretinal membranes* (Foos, 1978). Simple epiretinal membranes occasionally progress to complex membranes (Foos, 1978; Kampik et al., 1980; 1981). There is good evidence that both complex and, less commonly, simple epiretinal membranes may involve retinal pigment epithelium (RPE) cells. In particular, RPE cells are a major component of the epiretinal membranes of proliferative vitreoretinopathy (PVR), a condition which complicates rhegmatogenous retinal detachment (see below).

SIMPLE EPIRETINAL MEMBRANES AND RETINAL PIGMENT EPITHELIAL CELLS

Simple epiretinal membranes typically have a simple histological appearance, usually consisting of thin layers of cells or cell processes on undistorted retina (Fig. 24-1). Although the first investigators generally considered that simple epiretinal membranes were derived from endothelial cells (see Parsons, 1905 for a review), subsequent electron microscopic and immunohistochemical investigations demonstrated that most simple epiretinal membranes were composed of glial cells (Foos, 1974; Hiscott et al., 1984a). However, Kurz and Zimmerman (1962) showed that in the presence of a retinal defect the RPE can extend as a thin layer over the retina. Such thin RPE epiretinal membranes have also been designated "simple" (Wallow and Miller, 1978).

COMPLEX EPIRETINAL MEMBRANES AND RETINAL PIGMENT EPITHELIAL CELLS

Epiretinal membranes most often cause symptoms by virtue of a tendency to contract. Membrane contraction may cause partial- or full-thickness folding of the subjacent retina (Fig. 24-2—Kleinert, 1954), or even retinal hole formation with subsequent rhegmatogenous retinal detachment (Wadsworth, 1952; Klien, 1955). In addition, opaque membranes may impede the passage of light to the retina.

Symptomatic epiretinal membranes typically have a complicated histopathological appearance. It has long been recognized that what would now be considered complex epiretinal membranes contain connective tissue (fibrous) and cellular components (Parsons, 1905—Fig. 24-2). However, the origins of the cells in complex membranes has been the subject of debate (Gloor, 1976; Machemer, 1978). RPE are implicated in complex-membrane formation on account of the presence of epithelial cells in the vitreous of eyes with a retinal detachment (Gonin, 1930) and melanin in some of the related membranes (Smith, 1960).

THE PROBLEMS OF IDENTIFYING RETINAL PIGMENT EPITHELIAL CELLS IN EPIRETINAL MEMBRANES

Although RPE cells are virtually stationary and exhibit a low proliferation rate in the normal adult eye, it is well established that the cells retain the ability to migrate and divide in response to a wide range of pathological insults (reviewed by Grierson et al., 1994). This reparative response is associated with a dramatic phenotypic transformation. The cells detach from their polarized simple epithelial monolayer and become isolated (Fig. 24-3 and Plate 24-I). The sequestrated cells are highly mobile and

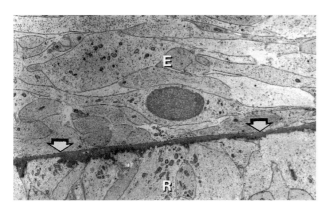

FIGURE 24-1. Transmission electron micrograph of an epiretinal membrane (E) overlying the retina (R). The inner limiting lamina *(arrows)* is undistorted, indicating that the membrane is "simple" in nature. The membrane consists chiefly of glial cell processes. Magnification ×4500.

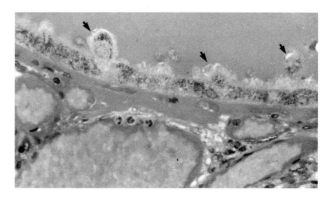

FIGURE 24-3. Light micrograph of the chorioretinal interface in an eye with a retinal detachment. Retinal pigment epithelial cells show signs of detaching from their location *(arrow)* in the normal retinal pigment epithelial monolayer. Magnification ×500.

usually adopt either a macrophage-like or a fibroblast-like appearance (Machemer and Laqua, 1975; Mandelcorn et al., 1975; Muller-Jensen et al., 1975; Vidaurri-Leal et al., 1984; Machemer et al., 1978). Moreover, as the cells undergo these changes (which have been called *metaplasia, dedifferentiation,* and *transdifferentiation*) they may release melanin. The free melanin can then be phagocytosed by other cells such as mononuclear phagocyte system (MPS) and glia (Friedenwald and Chan, 1932).

MPS macrophages and glia, together with fibroblasts

from a variety of potential sources (e.g., perivascular cells), are among the major cellular components implicated in the formation of complex epiretinal membranes. In some membranes ectopic RPE cells keep or regain their tertiary differentiation characteristics (e.g., by forming monolayers of polarized cells—Fig. 24-4) to the extent that their origins can be determined with reasonable confidence (Machemer et al., 1978; Green et al., 1979; Kampik et al., 1981; Trese et al., 1983). On the other hand, in many membranes RPE cells remain dedifferentiated and, even at the electron microscopic level, are difficult to distinguish from glia or other cell types (Green et al., 1979; Kampik et al., 1981; Trese et al., 1983).

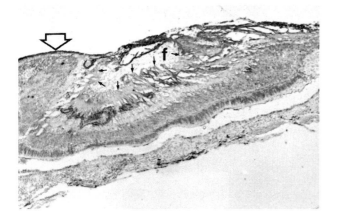

FIGURE 24-2. Light micrograph of a section through the retina with an overlying epiretinal membrane. The section was stained with hematoxylin and immunoperoxidase for the glial marker glial fibrillary acidic protein (to delineate the neuroretina). Note that the retinal surface *(small closed arrows)* is grossly distorted with folding of adjacent neuroretina *(large open arrow)*. The complex epiretinal membrane has a substantial fibrous component (f) and a glial element. Magnification ×35.

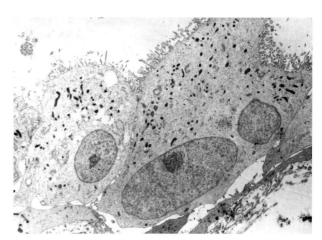

FIGURE 24-4. Transmission electron micrograph of a surgically resected epiretinal membrane. The tissue contains a layer of polarized pigmented cells. The morphology of these cells is consistent with a retinal pigment epithelial origin. Magnification ×6000.

METHODS OF DETECTING RETINAL PIGMENT EPITHELIAL CELLS IN EPIRETINAL MEMBRANES

Histological and Ultrastructural Methods

Because histological and ultrastructural methods have proved inadequate for detecting the origins of ectopic and metaplastic epiretinal cells (see above), attempts have been made to identify transformed epiretinal RPE cells by other methods.

In Vitro Techniques

Evidence that RPE cells contribute to complex epiretinal membranes was provided by studying the morphology (Newsome et al., 1981) and locomotory characteristics (Hiscott et al., 1983) of cellular outgrowths from epiretinal membranes in tissue culture. Further testimony that cultured monolayers from complex membranes include epithelial cells was provided by immunofluorescent studies of the cytoskeletal components of the cultured cells (Hiscott et al., 1983; 1984a; 1984b—Fig. 24-5). However, in vitro methods do not give information about the distribution or proportion of RPE cells in epiretinal membranes.

Immunohistochemistry

The distribution and proportion of cells in a tissue may be evaluated using immunohistochemical techniques: methods which depend on antibody recognition of specific proteins in tissue sections.

Light microscopic immunohistochemistry. Light microscopic immunohistochemistry was first conducted on epi-

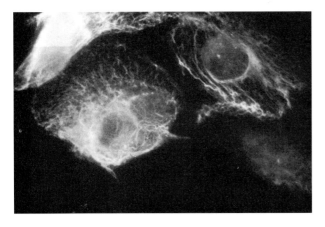

FIGURE 24-5. Cells grown in tissue culture from a surgically excised epiretinal membrane and stained with the immunofluorescent technique for cytokeratins. The cells exhibit strong immunoreactivity for cytokeratins within the cytoskeleton, indicating an epithelial origin. Magnification ×1400.

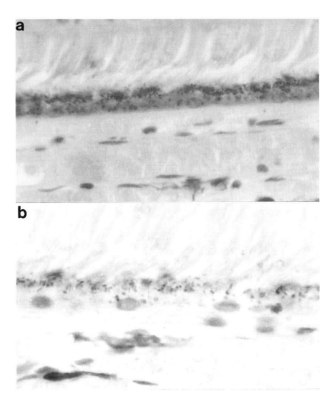

FIGURE 24-6. (a) Normal retinal pigment epithelium stained with the immunoperoxidase method for cytokeratins and counterstained with haematoxylin. (b) As in (a), but following omission of primary antibody during the staining procedure. Note in (a) that the retinal pigment epithelium is immunoreactive for cytokeratins. Magnification ×1000.

retinal membranes by Rodrigues and colleagues (1981). In their study, the authors identified glial cells in the tissue using antibodies to glial intermediate filament proteins (Rodrigues et al., 1981). This method is based on the concept that tissue-specific intermediate filament proteins are retained when cells undergo phenotypic transformation (Lazarides, 1980). A similar approach was applied by Hiscott and colleagues to investigate the RPE cell content of epiretinal membranes, this time using cytokeratins (a family of intermediate filament proteins found in epithelia) as a marker of RPE cells (Hiscott et al., 1984b). These authors found that normal RPE was weakly immunoreactive for cytokeratins (Fig. 24-6), but that as RPE cells became transdifferentiated their cytokeratin staining became more prominent.

There has been controversy, however, concerning the nature of RPE intermediate filaments and thus debate concerning the value of cytokeratins as a marker for RPE cells in epiretinal membranes (Weller et al., 1989). Some researchers reported that the cytoskeleton of RPE cells contained vimentin (Docherty et al., 1984; Philp and Nachmias, 1985; White et al., 1989), while others found cytokeratins (Hiscott et al., 1983; 1984b; Aronson, 1983). The controversy was resolved by McKechnie and colleagues and Owaribe and colleagues, who showed that avian RPE contains only vimentin whereas mammalian (including human) and amphibian RPE cells express several members of the cytokeratin family with or without vimentin (McKechnie et al., 1988; Owaribe et al., 1988; Owaribe, 1988). These findings have largely been confirmed by others (Turksen et al., 1989; Fuchs et al., 1991; Robey et al., 1992; McKay and Burke, 1994) (see also Chapter 3 on retinal pigment epithelial cytoskeleton).

Cytokeratins are a better marker for RPE cells than vimentin; vimentin is expressed by most cell types, whereas cytokeratins are thought to be specific for epithelia. It is important to use antibodies which recognize a range of cytokeratins, as mammalian RPE cells can express a broad spectrum of cytokeratins. Studies with such "wide-screening" antibodies on epiretinal membranes have provided further evidence that (1) RPE cells may be involved in the tissue; (2) at least some of the fibroblast-like and macrophage-like cells in the tissue are derived from RPE cells (Fig. 24-7) and (3) RPE cells may be the major cell type in epiretinal membranes, especially in membranes arising in the presence of a retinal hole (Hiscott et al., 1984b; Shirakawa et al., 1987; Jerdan et al., 1989; Morino et al., 1990; Weller et al., 1991). On the other hand, many of the cells in complex epiretinal membranes do not label with wide-screening cytokeratin antibodies.

Electron microscopic immunohistochemistry.

Electron microscopic immunohistochemistry permits the combination of both immunohistochemical and ultrastructural analysis, although light microscopic immunohistochemistry on multiple sections of epiretinal membranes allows more representative tissue sampling for analysis than electron microscopic techniques. Nevertheless, immunogold studies have provided further proof that RPE cells may play a prominent role in epiretinal membrane formation (Vinores et al., 1990). However, coexpression of glial and epithelial markers has been found in occasional cells in epiretinal membranes examined with ultrastructural immunohistochemistry (Vinores et al., 1992), albeit similar "double-labeled" cells have not yet been observed at the light microscopic level (Hiscott et al., 1994). In addition, the immunogold approach demonstrated that many epiretinal cells do not label with a "cocktail" of monoclonal antibodies to cytokeratins (Vinores et al., 1990).

The observation that many cells in epiretinal membranes are not immunoreactive for a range of cytokeratins can be explained in several ways. One possibility

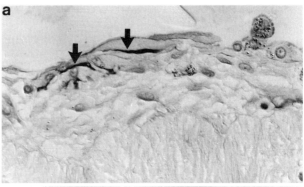

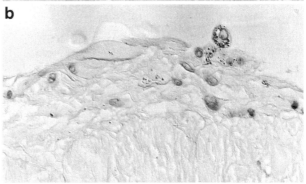

FIGURE 24-7. Differential interference contrast micrographs of sections through the retinal surface and an overlying complex epiretinal membrane. (a) Stained with the immunoperoxidase method for cytokeratins. Note the membrane contains fibroblast-like retinal pigment epithelial cells *(arrows)*. (b) As in (a), but following substitution of the anticytokeratin antibody with an inappropriate antibody as a control. Magnification ×700.

is that the cytokeratin-negative cells are not of RPE origin. Alternatively, RPE cells in the tissue may express cytokeratins or even epitopes of individual cytokeratins not recognized by the antibodies employed in immunohistochemistry. Since the cytokeratins expressed by RPE cells vary with cell behavior and differentiation state (McKechnie et al., 1988; Robey et al., 1992; Grisante and Guidry, 1995), there is a chance of "false-negative" staining in membranes where the cells are engaged in a diversity of activities (see Activities of RPE Cells in Epiretinal Membranes). False-negative cytokeratin staining also would occur if some retinal pigment epithelial cells lose their cytokeratins completely during transformation.

Attempts have been made to resolve the potential problem of false-negative cell staining in epiretinal membranes by employing a battery or "panel" of antibodies in immunohistochemical studies. For example, MPS macrophages can be differentiated from macrophage-like RPE cells not only by their lack of cytokeratin immunoreactivity, but also by their positive staining with macrophage markers such as M718, Leu M3, OKM1, CD68, and MAC 387 (Weller et al., 1988; Jerdan et al., 1989; Baudouin et al., 1990; Charteris et al., 1992).

Lectin Histochemistry

Lectin histochemistry provides an alternative to the immunohistochemical detection of cells and is based on the ability of lectins (sugar-binding proteins or glycoproteins of nonimmune origin) to bind to complex carbohydrate structures (reviewed by Ponder, 1983). Carbohydrate components of cell membrane proteins and glycoproteins may be useful markers of cell type. Bopp and colleagues have determined that normal RPE cells have receptors for concavalin A (Con A), wheat germ agglutinin (WGA), peanut agglutinin (PNA) and *rhicinus communis* agglutinin (RCA 1) (Bopp et al., 1989) and that the binding of these four lectins is chiefly in the apical region of the cells. Reactive RPE cells also stain with Con A, WGA, PNA, and RCA 1, but, apart from photoreceptor cells which express addition lectins, other retinal elements do not bind the lectins (Bopp et al., 1989; 1990). In addition, macrophage-like RPE cells exhibit receptors to soybean agglutinin (SBA) (Bopp et al., 1992). Cells binding Con A, WGA, PNA, and RCA 1 with or without SBA binding are found in epiretinal membranes and are thought to be retinal pigment epithelial in origin (Bopp et al., 1992).

The evidence from light and electron microscopic, in vitro, immunohistochemical, and lectin histochemical studies argues cogently that RPE cells are frequently present in complex epiretinal membranes and that the cells may play a major role in the development of the tissue.

WHICH MEMBRANES CONTAIN RETINAL PIGMENT EPITHELIAL CELLS?

Epiretinal Membranes in the Absence of a Retinal Hole

There are several reports of RPE cells in epiretinal membranes arising in the apparent absence of a retinal hole, including idiopathic and developmental membranes and membranes complicating intraocular inflammation and ocular trauma without clinically detectable retinal hole formation (Michels, 1982; Hiscott et al., 1984b; Smiddy et al., 1989).

The fibrovascular epiretinal membranes of proliferative diabetic retinopathy (PDR) may contain RPE cells (Fig. 24-8; Smith et al., 1976; Hamilton et al., 1982; Weller et al., 1991). Hamilton and colleagues observed cells with the morphological characteristics of RPE cells in PDR epiretinal membranes from eyes with previous

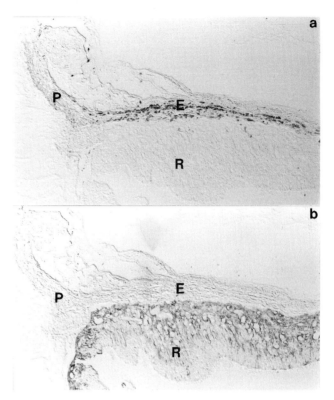

FIGURE 24-8. Differential interference contrast micrographs of the retina (R), epiretinal (E), and posterior hyaloid membranes (P) in sections through an eye with proliferative diabetic retinopathy (PDR). (a) Labeled with the immunoperoxidase method for cytokeratins (no counterstain). Numerous retinal pigment epithelial cells can be seen in the PDR membranes. (b) Control section, stained as in (a), but following substitution of the antikeratin antibodies with antiglial fibrillary acidic protein antibodies (a glial marker). The retinal glia are highlighted but no reaction is seen in the membranes. Magnification ×80.

retinal detachment (Hamilton et al., 1982). A subsequent investigation of surgically removed PDR membranes demonstrated that most of the specimens containing retinal pigment epithelial cells occurred in eyes with a retinal hole (Hiscott et al., 1994). Nevertheless, retinal pigment epithelial cell-containing PDR membranes occasionally are observed in eyes devoid of detectable retinal holes (Hiscott et al., 1994). However, PDR membranes generally do not contain such a high proportion of RPE cells as the epiretinal membranes of proliferative vitreoretinopathy (Hiscott et al., 1994).

Epiretinal Membranes of Proliferative Vitreoretinopathy (PVR)

PVR is strictly defined as a complication of rhegmatogenous retinal detachment characterized by the formation of membranes on both surfaces of the detached retina and on the posterior surface of the detached vit-

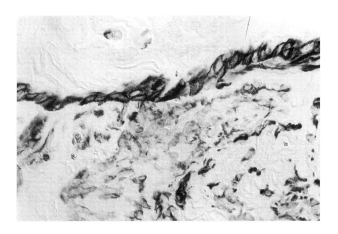

FIGURE 24-9. Differential interference contrast micrograph of a section through a surgically excised PVR epiretinal membrane. The section has been stained with the immunoperoxidase method for cytokeratins (no counterstain). The vast majority of the cells are of retinal pigment epithelial origin, including a prominent layer of cells. Magnification ×700.

reous gel (Retina Society Terminology Committee, 1983; Machemer et al., 1991). Usually, the posterior hyaloid membranes are continuous with epiretinal membranes and thus have a similar composition.

Clinicopathological studies indicate that RPE cells are present in the vast majority of the epiretinal membranes of proliferative vitreoretinopathy (PVR) (Clarkson et al., 1977; Machemer et al., 1978; Kampik et al., 1981; Hiscott et al., 1984b; Jerdan et al., 1989; Morino et al., 1990; Heidenkummer and Kampik, 1991). Moreover, RPE cells are the vast majority of cells in some of the membranes (Fig. 24-9). In these membranes, it is logical to assume that RPE cells are responsible for events such as cell recruitment, membrane contraction, and extracellular matrix synthesis during the development of the tissue (see below).

Anterior PVR

RPE cells are thought to be a major component of anterior PVR membranes: membranes on the peripheral retina which can extend as far forward as the pupillary margin in PVR (Elner et al., 1988).

Subretinal Membranes of PVR

In PVR, problematic membranes beneath the neuroretina (subretinal membranes) are not as common as complex epiretinal membranes (Sternberg and Machemer, 1984). Nevertheless, subretinal membranes are responsible for preventing retinal reattachment in 13% of all cases of PVR (Lewis et al., 1989). In PVR, subretinal membranes may commence as sheets of replicating cells

which condense into fibrocellular strands or bands as the membranes begin to contract (Sternberg and Machemer, 1984; Federman et al., 1983). The taut bands require surgical removal if they impede retinal reattachment and the excised specimens have been the subject of several morphological investigations (Federman et al., 1983; Trese et al., 1985; Matsumura et al., 1986; 1987; Morino et al., 1987; Schwartz et al., 1988; Hiscott et al., 1989). The evidence from these studies, together with studies of PVR subretinal membranes in enucleated eyes (Wilkes et al., 1987), shows that RPE cells are a major component of the tissue. Indeed, semiquantitative immunohistochemical evaluation of PVR subretinal membranes indicates that the RPE cell content is generally higher, and the glial element less, than in PVR epiretinal membranes (Hiscott et al., 1989; Garcia-Arumi et al., 1992). Thus retinal pigment epithelial cells, embracing transdifferentiated forms, are probably responsible for the tension in the bands and the resulting clinical problems.

Non-PVR Subretinal Membranes

Retinal pigment epithelial cells also are thought to be involved in non-PVR subretinal membranes, including membranes complicating penetrating ocular trauma and corneoscleral rupture (Winthrop et al., 1980; Daicker, 1985), Coats's disease (Manschot and Bruijn, 1967), and intraocular inflammation (Palestine et al., 1984; 1985). In subretinal neovascularization, there is experimental evidence that RPE cells proliferate on the surface of the new vessels and eventually may cause involution of the lesion (Miller et al., 1986—see also macular degeneration chapter).

HOW DO RETINAL PIGMENT EPITHELIAL CELLS GET INTO EPIRETINAL MEMBRANES?

It is not surprising that RPE cells are the principle component of subretinal membranes since the membranes form adjacent to the pigment epithelial layer. Conversely, the retinal pigment epithelial monolayer is relatively remote from the vitreous surface of the retina where epiretinal membranes form.

Migratory retinal pigment epithelial cells can traverse the neuroretina and become incorporated in epiretinal tissue during the development of experimental epiretinal membranes (Hitchins and Grierson, 1988). This mechanism may account for the retinal pigment epithelial cell component of human epiretinal membranes which arise in the absence of a defect in the neuroretina. Trans-retinal-pigment-epithelial cell migration is presumably facilitated by damage to the neuroretina, as occurs, for example, following photocoagulation (Gloor and Daicker, 1975).

Although trans-RPE migration might be involved in the development of PVR epiretinal membranes, the current data suggest that the cells arrive at the retinal surface via a different route. In PVR, the retinal pigment epithelial cells are believed to gain access to the inner retinal surface via the retinal holes. After a retinal tear has formed fluid components of the vitreous pass through the hole. The resulting retinal detachment is associated with a breakdown in the blood–retina barrier and exudation of plasma proteins into the vitreous, including the fluid vitreous beneath the retina (the subretinal fluid). The subretinal fluid thus becomes rich in plasma derivatives, some of which are chemoattractants for retinal pigment epithelial cells and may induce the cells to detach from Bruch's membrane (Fig. 24-3—Campochiaro et al., 1984; 1985). The detached cells (which resemble macrophages—see above) accumulate in the subretinal space (Machemer, 1978). It is postulated that some of the retinal pigment epithelial macrophages either migrate, or are swept, through the retinal hole into the vitreous cavity where they are visible biomicroscopically as "tobacco dust" (Hamilton and Taylor, 1972; Machemer, 1978). Once in the vitreous cavity the cells can settle on the inner retinal surface.

THE ACTIVITIES OF RETINAL PIGMENT EPITHELIAL CELLS IN EPIRETINAL MEMBRANES

Epiretinal pigment epithelial cells are thought to be involved in a variety of cellular activities, some of which are akin to the behavior of cells in healing wounds. In fact, epiretinal membranes have been likened to the scars of wound repair elsewhere in the body (Constable et al., 1974).

Cell Recruitment

On the retinal surface, the retinal pigment epithelial cells can both synthesize and be influenced by biologically active substances such as peptide growth factors and glycoproteins. These factors are thought to induce further proliferation and migration of retinal pigment epithelia, glia, and fibroblasts (see reviews by Burke, 1989; Weidemann, 1992; and Charteris, 1995) and thus increase the cell mass of the developing epiretinal membrane.

Interactions between growth factors and pigment epithelial cells are discussed in detail in Chapter 23. However, it is worth noting that a plethora of growth factors

have been implicated in epiretinal membrane formation (Burke, 1989; Wiedemann, 1992; Charteris, 1995). The evidence for the involvement of some peptides is derived from both experimental and human studies. For example, immunohistochemical studies of human epiretinal membranes show colocalization of both platelet-derived growth factor (PDGF) ligands and PDGF receptors on cells of retinal pigment epithelial origin (Robbins et al., 1994a). In addition, retinal pigment epithelial cells in vitro produce PDGF, a chemotactic agent for several cell types including retinal pigment epithelial cells themselves (Campochiaro and Glaser, 1985; Campochiaro et al., 1989). Thus PDGF produced locally by retinal pigment epithelial cells may recruit more cells to the retinal surface in an autocrine- or paracrine-like way.

Although diverse growth factors are present in the plasma, Burke has pointed out that peptides of hematogenous origin are unlikely to reach chemotactic concentrations for retinal cells at the site of membrane formation (Burke, 1989). Conversely, chemotactic levels of glycoproteins (e.g., fibronectin) probably are derived from plasma following breakdown of the blood–retina barrier and may well influence retinal pigment epithelial migration in the early stages of membrane formation (Campochiaro et al., 1984; 1985). Nevertheless, in situ hybridization and immunohistochemical studies of human epiretinal membranes demonstrate that epiretinal cells, including pigment epithelial cells, also produce fibronectin (Figs. 24-10 and 24-11—Hiscott et al., 1992a). Moreover, migratory retinal pigment epithelial cells (detected by immunoreactivity for a migration-related epitope of cytokeratin 18—Robey et al., 1992) are often codistributed with fibronectin-producing cells in both epiretinal and subretinal membranes (Fig. 24-12; Hiscott et al., 1992a; Grierson et al., 1994). Therefore, cellular fibronectin of retinal pigment epithelial origin also may have paracrine- and autocrine-like effects in developing epiretinal membranes. Recently, we have observed a more consistent association between the extracellular matrix glycoprotein thrombospondin 1 and migratory RPE (Fig. 24-13), and to a less extent between osteonectin (another glycoprotein, also known as SPARC) and migratory RPE (Magee, Sheridan, Hiscott, and Grierson, unpublished observations).

Epiretinal Membrane Contraction and Retinal Pigment Epithelial Cells

In addition to their chemotactic and mitogenic properties, glycoproteins play a role in cell-to-cell and cell-to-substrate adhesion (Yamada et al., 1975; D'Ardenne and McGee, 1984). For example, cellular fibronectin secreted by the cells in wounds can bind to other early extracellular matrix components, such as the glycoprotein thrombospondin, and thus may produce a provisional matrix (see Lawler, 1986 for a review). Both thrombospondin and cellular fibronectin occur in epiretinal membranes (Figs. 24-11 and 24-13—Hiscott et al., 1985; Esser et al., 1991; Hiscott et al., 1992b). The data suggest that epiretinal pigment epithelial cells produce both fibronectin and thrombospondin (Hiscott et al., 1992a; Larkin et al., 1994), which together might form an early extracellular matrix. Such a matrix may be important in linking contractile elements in the membranes into a "contractile cohesive unit" (Hiscott et al., 1985).

From the clinical point of view, epiretinal membrane contraction is a prominent event and there is little doubt that it is mediated by the membrane cells (Grierson and Rahi, 1981). Since retinal pigment epithelial cells are the principal cells in some membranes, these cells are presumably responsible for the forces generated. Indeed,

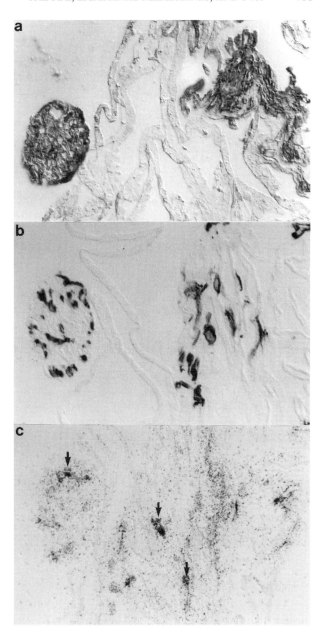

FIGURE 24-11. Sections from a surgically excised epiretinal membrane stained with the immunoperoxidase method without counterstain (a, b) or by in situ hybridization (c). (a) Staining for fibronectin reveals the glycoprotein in relation to cellular components of the membrane. (b) Cytokeratin staining demonstrates that most of the cells in the tissue are of retinal pigment epithelial origin. (c) A section labeled with an antisense ssRNA probe for fibronectin mRNA, employing the in situ hybridization technique. Many of the cells, including some retinal pigment epithelial cells, contain fibronectin mRNA *(arrows)*. Differential contrast micrographs; magnification ×600.

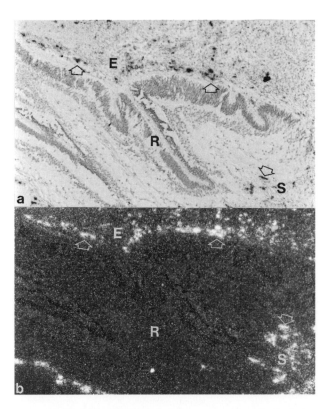

FIGURE 24-10. Differential interference contrast (a) and epipolarization (b) micrographs of a section through detached, folded retina (R) in an enucleated eye. Epiretinal (E) and subretinal (S) membranes of PVR are present. The section has been labeled with an antisense single-stranded RNA (ssRNA) probe for fibronectin mRNA, employing the in situ hybridization technique. Cells within the epi- and subretinal membranes are replete with fibronectin mRNA *(arrows)*, whereas cells in the retina show only background labeling. Magnification ×50.

retinal pigment epithelial cells cause contraction in a collagen matrix model of PVR. In this model, retinal pigment epithelial cells are more efficient constrictors of the matrix than retinal glia but do not execute matrix

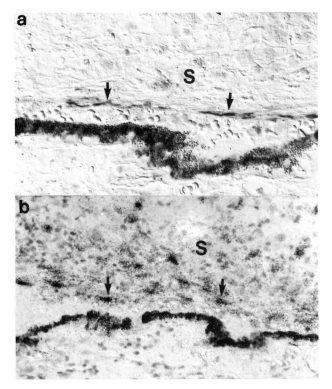

FIGURE 24-12. (a) Section through a subretinal membrane (S) of PVR with subjacent retinal pigment epithelium and choroid. The section has been stained with the immunoperoxidase method for cytokeratin 18 (CK18). CK18-positive cells are present in the membrane *(arrows)* (differential contrast micrograph; magnification ×500). (b) Another section through the membrane has been labeled with an antisense ssRNA probe for fibronectin mRNA, employing the in situ hybridization technique. Cells containing fibronectin mRNA *(arrows)* are codistributed with CK18-positive cells. Bright field; magnification ×400.

contraction as well as fibroblasts (Mazure and Grierson, 1992).

The precise mechanism by which cells contract scar tissue—and hence epiretinal membranes—is still controversial (Rudolph et al., 1991). Wound contraction was thought of as a result of synchronized contraction by a syncytium of fibroblasts with musclelike features. These cells are called *myofibroblasts* (Gabbiani et al., 1971; 1972). Myofibroblast-like cells have been described in epiretinal membranes (Constable et al., 1974), as have cells immunoreactive for the contractile protein actin (Rodrigues et al., 1985). However, an actin content is not an index of cellular contraction; more recent in vitro research suggests that human retinal pigment epithelial cells do not behave like muscle cells (Glaser et al., 1987). Moreover, the myofibroblast may be a product rather than a cause of contraction in wounds (reviewed by Grierson et al., 1988; Ehrlich, 1988).

Cultured human RPE cells have been shown to interact with single strands of collagen and pull or reel in the fibers toward themselves (Glaser et al., 1987). Interactions with the extracellular matrix also occur during cell locomotion (Fig. 24-14; Grierson et al., 1988; Rudolph et al., 1991), and it has been suggested that tractional forces in the membranes are mediated by interactions between matrix and individual cells. Cell–matrix associations are dependent on cell surface receptors, including integrins (a group of transmembrane heterodimeric receptors, each consisting of one α and one β subunit). Various integrins have been detected on retinal pigment epithelial cells in situ and in epiretinal membranes (Anderson et al., 1990; Robbins et al., 1994b). However, it is not yet clear which integrins are expressed by epiretinal retinal pigment epithelial cells. Robbins and colleagues found variable immunohistochemical staining for α subunits 2 through 6 and V, and β subunits 1, 2, and 3 on pigment-epithelium-like epiretinal cells (Robbins et al., 1994b). We have found inconsistent expres-

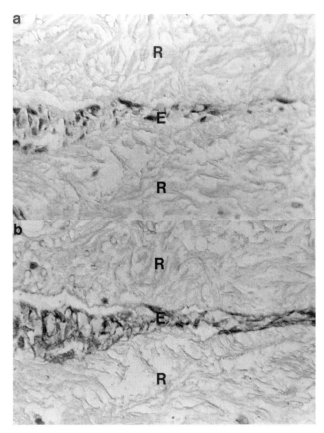

FIGURE 24-13. Differential interference contrast micrographs of sections through a complex epiretinal membrane (E) between folds of detached retina (R) in PVR. The sections have been stained with the immunoperoxidase method for (a) CK18 and (b) thrombospondin 1. CK18-positive cells colocalize with thrombospondin 1 in the membrane. Hematoxylin counterstained; magnification ×400.

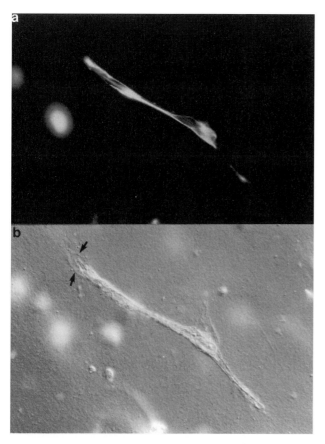

FIGURE 24-14. Retinal pigment epithelial cell in a collagen type I matrix seen by (a) immunofluorescent staining for cytokeratins and (b) phase contrast microscopy. Evidence of cell–matrix interaction is seen in the form of collagen raveling *(arrows)*. Magnification ×1200.

sion of α5, αV, β1, and β3 subunits by epiretinal pigment epithelia (unpublished observations).

Cell-matrix interactions may also involve remodeling of the extracellular matrix surrounding the cell, and enzymes such as the matrix metalloproteinases play a key role in this process. RPE cells are capable of matrix metalloproteinase synthesis (Hunt et al., 1993; Padgett et al., 1997) although initial studies suggest that these enzymes are not important in contraction in vitro (Hunt et al., 1993).

Synthesis of Extracellular Matrix by Epiretinal Pigment Epithelial Cells

Apart from glycoproteins, several other extracellular matrix components are found in complex epiretinal membranes, such as collagen and members of the elastic family.

Several collagen subtypes, including types I to V, may be present in epiretinal membranes (Sheiffarth et al.,

1988; 1989; Jerdan et al., 1989; Morino et al., 1990) and collagen is associated with retinal pigment epithelial cells in membranes (Machemer et al., 1978; Morino et al., 1990). The colocalization of epiretinal pigment epithelial cells and collagen does not indicate that the epithelial cells produced the collagen, since it is possible that the cells migrated into preformed matrix. However, there is evidence in vivo (Mueller-Jensen et al., 1975; Laqua, 1981) and in vitro (Campochiaro et al., 1986; Newsome et al., 1988) that retinal pigment epithelial cells produce collagens. Moreover, in epiretinal membranes composed chiefly of retinal pigment epithelial cells it is difficult to envisage where else the collagen, particularly interstitial collagen types I and III, may originate. Nevertheless, there has been some controversy regarding the ability of retinal pigment epithelial cells to synthesize type II collagen (Newsome et al., 1988) and the possibility that type II collagen in epiretinal membranes represents incarcerated vitreous collagen (Scheiffarth et al., 1989).

PVR membranes contain precursors (oxytalan) of elastic fibers and, since subretinal as well as epiretinal membranes contain oxytalan, it is postulated that these fibers are produced by retinal pigment epithelium (Alexander et al., 1992).

Extracellular matrix components like oxytalan and collagen build up in epiretinal membranes with time, as do matrix elements in the scars of healing wounds. In healing wounds, the deposition of extracellular matrix is reflected by a time-dependent decrease in wound cellularity. The proportion of retinal pigment epithelial cells (together with other cell types) in epiretinal membranes also declines with the clinical duration of the tissue (Hiscott et al., 1985; Morino et al., 1990). This decline in epiretinal pigment epithelial cell numbers may result from progressive entombment of the cells in their own collagen (Hiscott et al., 1985). However, in contrast to cells in healing skin wounds, the activities of epiretinal pigment epithelial cells appear protracted and disorganized (Hiscott et al., 1985).

FUTURE RESEARCH: EPIRETINAL PIGMENT EPITHELIAL CELLS AS THERAPEUTIC TARGETS

The clinical problems caused by complex epiretinal membranes have been a stimulus in the search for therapeutic agents which can control retinal pigment epithelial behavior. Pharmacology and the retinal pigment epithelium is discussed in detail in Chapter 31. Suffice it to point out here that, so far, drug prevention of complex epiretinal membrane formation has been based on antiproliferative and antiinflammatory agents and the results of such treatment have been disappointing (reviewed by Weidemann, 1989). There is a need for nontoxic agents which will block the activities of retinal pigment epithelial (and other) cells in membranes without damaging the subjacent retina. One approach is to target cell surface molecules such as the integrins (see above). Indeed, Kupper and Ferguson (1993) showed that the contraction of vitreous and collagen type II gels in vitro by human retinal pigment epithelium can be blocked by antibodies and peptides that antagonize the function of α2β1 integrin. However, the success of such an approach is likely to depend on identifying cell surface molecules specific to the cells involved in membrane formation. Normal retinal pigment epithelial cells also express β1 integrins (Anderson et al., 1990; Chu and Granwald, 1991). Indeed, β1 integrins have been shown to play a role in RPE attachment to Bruch's membrane (Ho and Del Priore, 1997) and it remains to be seen whether targeting β1 integrins will benefit patients.

ACKNOWLEDGMENTS

Support is provided by the Guide Dogs for the Blind Association, The Foundation for the Prevention of Blindness and the Research and Development Fund of the University of Liverpool.

REFERENCES

Alexander RA, Hiscott P, McGalliard J, Grierson I. 1992. Oxytalan fibres in proliferative vitreoretinopathy. Ger J Ophthalmol 1:382–387.

Anderson DH, Guerin JC, Matsumoto B, Pfeffer BA. 1990. Identification and localisation of a β1-receptor from the integrin family in mammalian retinal pigment epithelial cells. Invest Ophthalmol Vis Sci 31:81–85.

Aronson JF. 1983. Human retinal pigment cell culture. In Vitro 19:642–650.

Baudouin C, Fredj-Reygrobellet D, Gordon WC, et al. 1990. Immunohistologic study of epiretinal membranes in proliferative vitreoretinopathy. Am J Ophthalmol 110:593–598.

Bopp S, el Hifnawi ES, Laqua H. 1989. Localization of lectin-binding sites on retinal pigment epithelium and photoreceptor cells of the human eye. Fortschr Ophthalmol 86:515–518.

Bopp S, el Hifnawa ES, Laqua H. 1990. Lectin histochemical investigations on the retinal pigment epithelium after photocoagulation. Fortschr Ophthalmol 87:351–354.

Bopp S, el Hifnawi ES, Laqua H. 1992. Lectin binding pattern in human retinal pigment epithelium. Anat Anz 174:279–285.

Burke JM. 1989. Cell interactions in proliferative vitreoretinopathy: do growth factors play a role? In: Heimann K, Wiedemann P, eds. Proliferative Vitreoretinopathy. Heidelberg: Kaden, 80–87.

Campochiaro PA, Jerdan JA, Glaser BM. 1984. Serum contains chemo-attractants for human retinal pigment epithelial cells. Arch Ophthalmol 102:1830–1833.

Campochiaro PA, Glaser BM. 1985a. Platelet-derived growth factor is chemotactic for human retinal pigment epithelial cells. Arch Ophthalmol 103:576–579.

Campochiaro PA, Jerdan JA, Glaser BM, Cardin AC, Michels, RG. 1985b. Vitreous aspirates from patients with proliferative vitreo-

retinopathy stimulate retinal pigment epithelial cell migration. Arch Ophthalmol 103:1403–1405.

Campochiaro PA, Jerdan JA, Glaser BM. 1986. The extracellular matrix of human retinal pigment epithelial cells in vivo and its synthesis in vitro. Invest Ophthalmol Vis Sci 27:1615–1621.

Campochiaro PA, Sen HA, Robertson TJ, Conway BP. 1989. The role of the breakdown of the blood-retinal barrier in proliferative vitreoretinopathy. In: Heimann K, Wiedemann P, eds, Proliferative Vitreoretinopathy. Heidelberg: Kaden, 45–49.

Charteris DG. 1995. Proliferative vitreoretinopathy: pathobiology, surgical management, and adjunctie treatment. Br J Ophthalmol 79:953–960.

Charteris DG, Hiscott P, Grierson I, Lightman SL. 1992. Proliferative vitreoretinopathy: lymphocytes in epiretinal membranes. Ophthalmology 100:43–46.

Chu PG, Grunwald GB. 1991. Functional inhibition of retinal pigment epithelial cell-substrate adhesion with a monoclonal antibody against the beta 1 subunit of integrin. Invest Ophthalmol Vis Sci 32:1763–1769.

Clarkson JG, Green WR, Massof D. 1977. A histopathologic review of 168 cases of preretinal membrane. Am J Ophthalmol 84:1–17.

Constable IJ, Tolentino FI, Donovan RH, Schepens CL. 1974. Clinico-pathologic correlation of vitreous membranes. In: Pruett RD, Regan DJ, eds, Retinal Congress. New York: Appleton-Century-Crofts, 254–257.

D'Ardenne AJ, McGree JO. 1984. Fibronectin and disease. J Pathol 142:235–251.

Daiker, B. 1985. Constricting retroretinal membranes associated with traumatic retinal detachments. Graefes Arch Clin Exp Ophthalmol 222:147–153.

Docherty RJ, Edwards JG, Garrod DR, Mattey DL. 1984. Chick embryonic pigmented retina is one of the group of epithelioid tissues that lack cytokeratins and desmosomes and have intermediate filaments composed of vimentin. J Cell Sci 71:61–74.

Ehrlich HP. 1988. Wound closure: evidence of cooperation between fibroblast and collagen matrix. Eye 2:149–157.

Elner SG, Elner VM, Diaz-Rohena R, Freeman HM, Tolentino FI, Albert DM. 1988. Anterior proliferative vitreoretinopathy; clinical, light microscopic, and ultrastructural findings. Ophthalmology 95:1349–1357.

Esser P, Weller M, Heimann K, Wiedemann P. 1991. Thrombospondin and its importance in proliferative retinal diseases. Fortschr Ophthalmol 88:337–340.

Federman JL, Foldberg R, Ridley M, Arbizo VA. 1983. Subretinal cellular bands. Trans Am Ophthalmol Soc 81:172–179.

Foos, RY. 1974. Vitreoretinal juncture—simple epiretinal membranes. Graefes Arch Clin Exp Ophthal 189:231–250.

Foos RY. 1978. Nonvascular proliferative extraretinal retinopathies. Am J Ophthalmol 86:723–725.

Friedenwald JS, Chan E. 1932. Pathogenesis of retinitis pigmentosa. Arch Ophthalmol 8:173–181.

Fuchs U, Kivela T, Tarkkanen A. 1991. Cytoskeleton in normal and reactive human retinal pigment epithelial cells. Invest Ophthalmol Vis Sci 32:3178–3186.

Gabbiani G, Ryan GB, Majno G. 1971. Presence of modified fibroblasts in granulation tissue and their possible role in wound contraction. Experientia 27:549–550.

Gabbiani G, Hirschel BJ, Ryan GB, Statkov PR, Majno G. 1972. Granulation tissue as a contractile organ. J Exp Med 135:719–734.

Garcia Arumi J, Corcostegui B, Tallada N. 1992. Subretinal membranes in proliferative vitreoretinopathy: an immunohistochemical study. Retina 12:S55–S59.

Glaser BM, Cardin A, Biscoe B. 1987. Proliferative vitreoretinopathy:

the mechanism of development of vitreoretinal traction. Ophthalmology 94:327–332.

Gloor BP. 1976. Macular fibrosis and massive preretinal retraction. Doc Ophthalmol 7:105–112.

Gloor BP, Daicker BC. 1975. Pathology of the vitreo-retinal border structures. Trans Ophthalmol Soc UK 95:387–390.

Gonin J. 1930. Detachment of the retina and its treatment. Trans Ophthalmol Soc UK 50:531–551.

Green WR, Kenyon KR, Michels RG, Gilbert HD, de la Cruz ZC. 1979. Ultrastructure of epiretinal membranes causing macular pucker after retinal re-attachment surgery. Trans Ophthalmol Soc UK 99:65–77.

Grierson I, Rahi AHS. 1981. Structural basis of contraction in vitreal fibrous membranes. Br J Ophthalmol 65:737–749.

Grierson I, Joseph J, Miller M, Day JE. 1988. Wound repair: the fibroblast and the inhibition of scar formation. Eye 2:135–148.

Grierson I, Hiscott P, Hogg P, Robey H, Mazure A, Larkin G. 1994. Development, repair and regeneration of the retinal pigment epithelium. Eye 8:255–262.

Grisante S, Guidry C. 1995. Transdifferentiation of retinal pigment epithelial cells from epithelial to mesenchymal phenotype. Invest Ophthalmol Vis Sci 36:391–405.

Hamilton AM, Taylor W. 1972. Significance of pigment granules in the vitreous. Br J Ophthalmol 56:700–702.

Hamilton CW, Chandler D, Klintworth GK, Machemer R. 1982. A transmission and scanning electron microscopic study of surgically excised preretinal membrane proliferations in diabetes mellitus. Am J Ophthalmol 94:479–488.

Heidenkummer H, Kampik A. 1991. Comparative immunohistochemical investigations of epiretinal membranes in proliferative vitreoretinal disorders. Fortschr Ophthalmol 38:219–224.

Hiscott P, Grierson I, Hitchins CA, Rahi AHS, McLeod D. 1983. Epiretinal membranes in vitro. Trans Ophthalmol Soc UK 103:89–102.

Hiscott P, Grierson I, Trombetta CJ, Rahi AHS, Marshall J, McLeod D. 1984a. Retinal and epiretinal glia—an immunohistochemical study. Br J Ophthalmol 68:698–707.

Hiscott P, Grierson I, McLeod D. 1984b. Retinal pigment epithelial cells in epiretinal membranes: an immunohistochemical study. Br J Ophthalmol 68:708–715.

Hiscott P, Grierson I, McLeod D. 1985. Natural history of fibrocellular epiretinal membranes: a quantitative, autoradiographic and immunohistochemical study. Br J Ophthalmol 69:810–823.

Hiscott P, Morino I, Alexander R, Grierson I, Gregor Z. 1989. Cellular components of subretinal membranes in proliferative vitreoretinopathy. Eye 3:606–610.

Hiscott P, Waller HA, Butler MG, Grierson I, Scott DL. 1992a. Local production of fibronectin by ectopic human retinal cells. Cell Tissue Res 267:185–192.

Hiscott P, Larkin G, Robey HL, Orr G, Grierson I. 1992b. Thrombospondin as a component of the extracellular matrix of epiretinal membranes: comparisons with cellular fibronectin. Eye 6:566–569.

Hiscott P, Gray R, Grierson I, Gregor Z. 1994. Cytokeratin-containing cells in proliferative diabetic retinopathy membranes. Br J Ophthalmol 78:219–222.

Hitchins CA, Grierson I. 1988. Intravitreal injection of fibroblasts: the pathological effects on the ocular tissues of the rabbit following an intravitreal injection of autologous skin fibroblasts. Br J Ophthalmol 72:498–510.

Ho TC, Del Priore LV. 1997. Reattachment of cultured human retinal pigment epithelium to extracellular matrix and human Bruch's membrane. Invest Ophthalmol Vis Sci 38:1110–1118.

Hunt RC, Fox A, Al Pakalnis V, Sigel MM, Kosnosky W, Choudhury

P, Black EP. 1993. Cytokines cause cultured retinal pigment epithelial cells to secrete metalloproteinases and to contract collagen gels. Invest Ophthalmol Vis Sci 34:3179–3186.

Jerdan JA, Pepose JS, Michels RG, et al. 1989. Proliferative vitreoretinopathy membranes an immunohistochemical study. Ophthalmology 96:801–810.

Kampik A, Green WR, Michels RG, Nase PK. 1980. Ultrastructural features of progressive idiopathic epiretinal membrane removed by vitreous surgery. Am J Ophthalmol 90:797–809.

Kampik A, Kenyon KR, Michels RG, Green WR, de la Cruz ZC. 1981. Epiretinal and vitreous membranes. Comparative study of 56 cases. Arch Ophthalmol 99:1445–1454.

Kleinert H. 1954. Primäre Netzhautfältelung im Maculabereich. Graefes Arch Ophthalmol 155:350–358.

Klien BA. 1955. Concerning the pathogenesis of retinal holes. Am J Ophthalmol 40:515–522.

Kupper TS, Ferguson TA. 1993. A potential pathophysiologic role for alpha 2 beta 1 integrin in human eye diseases involving vitreoretinal traction. FASEB J 7:1401–1406.

Kurz GH, Zimmerman LE. 1962. Vagaries of the retinal pigment epithelium. In: Zimmerman LE, ed, Tumors of the Eye and Adnexa. Boston: Little, Brown, 441–464.

Laqua H. 1981. Collagen formation by periretinal cellular membranes. Dev Ophthalmol 2:396–406.

Larkin G, Hiscott P, Sheraidah G, Occleston NL, Khaw PT, Grierson I. 1994. The production of thrombospondin and fibronectin by retinal pigment epithelial cells. Invest Ophthalmol Vis Sci 35(suppl): S2039.

Lawler J. 1986. The structural and functional properties of thrombospondin. Blood 67:1197–1209.

Lazarides E. 1980. Intermediate filaments as mechanical integrators of cellular space. Nature 283:249–256.

Lewis H, Aaberg TM, Abrams GW, McDonald HR, Williams GA, Mieler WF. 1989. Subretinal membranes in proliferative vitreoretinopathy. Ophthalmology 96:1403–1415.

Machemer R. 1978. Pathogenesis and classification of massive periretinal proliferation. Br J Ophthalmol 62:737–747.

Machemer R, Laqua H. 1975. Pigment epithelial proliferation in retinal detachment (massive periretinal proliferation). Am J Ophthalmol 80:1–23.

Machemer R, van Horn D, Aaberg TM. 1978. Pigment epithelial proliferation in human retinal detachment with massive periretinal proliferation. Am J Ophthalmol 85:181–191.

Machemer R, Aaberg TM, Freeman HM, Irvine AR, Lean JS, Michels RM. 1991. An updated classification of retinal detachment with proliferative vitreoretinopathy. Am J Ophthalmol 112:159–165.

Mandelcorn MS, Machemer R, Fineberg E, Hersch SB. 1975. Proliferation and metaplasia of intravitreal retinal pigment epithelium cell autotransplants. Am J Ophthalmol 80:227–237.

Manschot WA, de Bruijn WC. 1967. Coats's disease: definition and pathogenesis. Br J Ophthalmol 51:145–157.

Matsumura M, Yamakawa R, Yoshimura N. et al. 1986. Subretinal strands: tissue culture and histological studies of subretinal strands. Acta Soc Ophthalmol Jpn 90:441–446.

Matsumura M, Yamakawa R, Yoshimura N, Shirakawa H, Okada M, Ogina N. 1987. Subretinal strands: tissue culture and histological study. Graefes Arch Clin Exp Ophthalmol 225:341–345.

Mazure A, Grierson G. 1992. In vitro studies of the contractility of cell types involved in proliferative vitreoretinopathy. Invest Ophthalmol Vis Sci 33:3407–3416.

McKay BS, Burke JM. 1994. Separation of phenotypically distinct subpopulations of cultured human retinal pigment epithelial cells. Exp Cell Res 213:85–92.

McKechnie NM, Boulton M, Robey HL, Savage FJ, Grierson I. 1988. The cytoskeletal elements of human retinal pigment epithelium in vitro and in vivo. J Cell Sci 91:303–312.

Michels RG. 1982. A clinical and histopathological study of epiretinal membranes affecting the macular and removed by vitreous surgery. Trans Am Ophthalmol Soc 80:580–656.

Miller H, Miller B, Ryan SJ. 1986. The role of retinal pigment epithelium in the involution of subretinal neovascularization. Invest Ophthalmol Vis Sci 27:1644–1652.

Morino I, Kazusa R, Yamanaka A. 1987. Glial cells in subretinal strand. J New Ophthalmol (Atarashii Ganka) 4:279–282.

Morino I, Hiscott P, McKechnie N, Grierson I. 1990. Variation in epiretinal membrane components with clinical duration of the proliferative tissue. Br J Ophthalmol 74:393–399.

Mueller-Jensen K, Machemer R, Azarnia R. 1975. Autotransplantation of retinal pigment epithelial cells in intravitreal diffusion chamber. Am J Ophthalmol 80:530–537.

Newsome DA, Rodrigues MM, Machemer R. 1981. Human massive periretinal proliferation: in vitro characteristics of cellular components. Arch Ophthalmol 99:873–880.

Newsome DA, Pfeffer BA, Hewitt AT, Robey PG, Hassell JR. 1988. Detection of extracellular matrix molecules synthesized in vitro by monkey and human retinal pigment epithelium: influence of donor age and multiple passages. Exp Eye Res 46:305–321.

Owaribe K. 1988. The cytoskeleton of retinal pigment epithelial cells. In: Osborne NN, Chader GJ, eds, Progress in Retinal Research. Oxford: Pergamon Press, 23–49.

Owaribe K, Kartenbeck J, Rungger-Brandle E, Franke WW. 1988. Cytoskeletons of retinal pigment epithelial cells: interspecies differences of expression patterns indicate independence of cell function from the specific complement of cytoskeletal proteins. Cell Tissue Res 254:301–315.

Padgett LC, Lui GM, Werb Z, LaVail MM. 1997. Matrix metalloproteinase-2 and tissue inhibitor of metalloproteinase-1 in the retinal pigment epithelium and interphotoreceptor matrix: Vectorial secretion and regulation. Exp Eye Res 64:927–938.

Palestine AG, Nussenblatt RB, Parver LM, Knox DL. 1984. Progressive subretinal fibrosis and uveitis. Br J Ophthalmol 68:667–673.

Palestine AG, Nussenblatt RB, Chan C, Hooks JJ, Friedman L, Kuwabara T. 1985. Histopathology of the subretinal fibrosis and uveitis syndrome. Ophthalmol 92:838–844.

Parsons JH. 1905. The Pathology of the Eye. Vol 2. London: Hodder and Stoughton, 542–600.

Philp NJ, Nachmias VT. 1985. Components of the cytoskeleton in the retinal pigment epithelium of the chick. J Cell Biol 101:358–362.

Ponder BAJ. 1983. Lectin histochemistry. In: Polak JM, Noorden SV, eds, Immunocytochemistry: Practical Application in Pathology and Biology. Bristol: John Wright and Sons, 129–142.

Retina Society Terminology Committee. 1983. The classification of retinal detachment with proliferative vitreoretinopathy. Ophthalmology 90:121–125.

Robbins SG, Mixon RN, Wilson DJ, et al. 1994a. Platelet-derived growth factor ligands and receptors immunolocalized in proliferative retinal diseases. Invest Ophthalmol Vis Sci 35:3649–3663.

Robbins SG, Brem RB, Wilson DJ, et al. 1994b. Immunolocalization of integrins in proliferative retinal membranes. Invest Ophthalmol Vis Sci 35:3475–3485.

Robey HL, Hiscott P, Grierson I. 1992. Cytokeratins and retinal epithelial cell behaviour. J Cell Sci 102:329–340.

Rodrigues MM, Newsome DA, Machemer R. 1981. Further characterisation of epiretinal membranes in human massive periretinal proliferation. Curr Eye Res 1:311–315.

Rudolph R, Vande Berg J, Pierce GF. 1991. Changing concepts in myofibroblast function and control. In: Janssen H, Rooman R, Robertson JIS, eds, Wound Healing. Petersfield (UK): Wrightson Biomedical Publishing 103–115.

Scheiffarth OF, Kampik A, Günther H, v d Mark K. 1988. Proteins of the extracellular matrix in vitreoretinal membranes. Graefes Arch Clin Exp Ophthalmol 226:357–361.

Scheiffarth OF, Kampik A, Guenther-Koszka H, v d Mark K. 1989. Collagens, fibronectin and laminin in proliferative vitreoretinopathy. In: Heimann K, Wiedemann P, eds, Proliferative Vitreoretinopathy. Heidelberg: Kaden, 134–138.

Schwartz D, de la Cruz ZC, Green WR, Michels RG. 1988. Proliferative vitreoretinopathy Ultrastructural study of 20 retroretinal membranes removed by vitreous surgery. Retina 8:275–281.

Shirakawa H, Yoshimura N, Yamakawa R, et al. 1987. Cell components in proliferative vitreoretinopathy: immunofluorescent double staining of cultured cells from proliferative tissues. Ophthalmologica 194:56–62.

Smiddy WE, Maguire AM, Green WR, et al. 1989. Idiopathic epiretinal membranes: ultrastructural characteristics and clinicopathologic correlation. Ophthalmology 96:811–821.

Smith RS, van Heuven WAJ, Streeten B. 1976. Vitreous membranes: a light and electron microscopic study. Arch Ophthalmol 94:1556–1560.

Smith TR. 1960. Pathologic findings after retina surgery. In: Schepens CL, ed, Importance of the Vitreous Body in Retina Surgery with Special Emphasis on Reoperations. St Louis: Mosby, 61–93.

Sternberg P, Machemer R. 1984. Subretinal proliferation. Am J Ophthalmol 98:456–462.

Trese MT, Chandler DB, Machemer R. 1983. Macular pucker. II Ultrastructure. Graefes Arch Clin Exp Ophthalmol 221:16–26.

Trese MT, Chandler DB, Machemer R. 1985. Subretinal strands: ultrastructural features. Graefes Arch Clin Exp Ophthalmol 223:35–40.

Turksen K, Opas M, Kalnins VI. 1989. Cytoskeleton, adhesion, and extracellular matrix of fetal human retinal pigmented epithelial cells in culture. Ophthalmic Res 21:56–66.

Vidaurri-Leal J, Hohman R, Glaser BM. 1984. Effect of vitreous on morphologic characteristics of retinal pigment epithelial cells: a new approach to the study of proliferative vitreoretinopathy. Arch Ophthalmol 102:1220–1223.

Vinores SA, Campochiaro PA, Conway BP. 1990. Ultrastructural and electron-immunocytochemical characterisation of cells in epiretinal membranes. Invest Ophthalmol Vis Sci 31:14–28.

Vinores SA, Van Niel E, Kim HJ. Campochiaro PA. 1992. Simultaneous expression of keratin and glial fibrillary acidic protein by the same cells in epiretinal membranes. Invest Ophthalmol Vis Sci 33:3361–3366.

Wadsworth JAC. 1952. Retinal detachment; etiology and pathology. Trans Am Acad Ophthalmol Otolaryngol 56:370–397.

Wallow IHL, Miller SA. 1978. Preretinal membrane by retinal pigment epithelium. Arch Ophthalmol 96:1643–1646.

Weller M, Heimann K, Wiedemann P. 1988. Immunochemical studies of epiretinal membranes using APAAP complexes: evidence for macrophage involvement in traumatic proliferative vitreoretinopathy. Int Ophthalmol 11:181–186.

Weller M, Heimann K, Wiedemann P. 1989. Immunochemical analysis of periretinal membranes; review and outlook. In: Straub W, ed, Developments in Ophthalmology, vol 16. Basel: Karger, 54–74.

Weller M, Esser P, Heimann K, Wiedemann P. 1991. Retinal microglia: a new cell in idiopathic proliferative vitreoretinopathy? Exp Eye Res 53:275–281.

White MF, Feist RM, Morris R, Douglas Witherspoon C, Couchman JR. 1989. A cytoskeletal characterization of human retinal pigment epithelial cells. In: Heimann K, Wiedemann P, eds, Proliferative Vitreoretinopathy. Heidelberg: Kaden, 98–103.

Wiedemann P. 1989. Medical treatment of proliferative vitreoretinopathy: the selection of drugs for clinical trials. In: Heimann K, Wiedemann P, eds, Proliferative Vitreoretinopathy. Heidelberg: Kaden, 248–250.

Wiedemann P. 1992. Growth factors in retinal disease: proliferative vitreoretinopathy, proliferative diabetic retinopathy, and retinal degeneration. Surv Ophthalmol 36:373–384.

Wilkes SR, Mansour AM, Green WR. 1987. Proliferative vitreoretinopathy histopathology of retroretinal membranes. Retina 7: 94–101.

Winthrop SR, Cleary PE, Minckler DS, Ryan SJ. 1980. Penetrating eye injuries: a histopathological review. Br J Ophthalmol 64:809–817.

Yamada KM, Yamada SS, Pastan I. 1975. The major cell surface glycoprotein of chick embryo fibroblasts is an agglutinin. Proc Nat Acad Sci USA 72:3158–3162.

25. Transplantation of retinal pigment epithelium

PETER GOURAS

The retinal pigment epithelium (RPE) layer is a logical starting point in any attempt to repair or reconstruct the retina by transplantation. This monolayer is self-contained, performing its functions by merely contacting the photoreceptors at its apical side and the choriocapillaris at its basal side. Even its apical/basal polarity appears to be modifiable (Al-Awqati, 1996; Cao et al., 1994). The other neural layers of the retina have a fixed polarity and are complexly interconnected, making transplantation a much greater challenge. The RPE layer is situated within a potential space, the subretinal space, that can be reversibly enlarged providing relatively easy access to the tissue and the surgery can be performed under direct vision through the pupil of the eye.

There is in addition an animal model, the Royal College of Surgeons (RCS) rat, in which a known defect of the RPE layer which leads to blindness has been shown to be correctable by RPE transplantation (Gouras et al., 1988; 1989; Li and Turner, 1988a; 1991; Lopez et al., 1989; Sheedlo et al., 1991b), and this is functional for the life of the animal. Therefore, transplantation can be therapeutic if the problem causing the retinal degeneration is due to a primary defect in the RPE layer. There are three retinal degenerations in man, which appear to be due to defects unique to the RPE, Sorsby's fundus dystrophy (Della et al., 1996) and two forms of autosomal recessive retinitis pigmentosa (Denton et al., 1997; Gu et al., 1997). In addition there are two more generalized retinal degenerations, Usher's syndrome (type 1B) (Hasson et al., 1995; Weil et al., 1995) and sex-linked retinitis pigmentosa (RP3) (Dryja et al., 1996), in which the defective gene is expressed strongly in the RPE but also weakly in the neural retina. We suspect that some forms of macular degeneration, such as vitelliform macular degeneration (Best's disease), and Malattia leventinese (dominant drusen) may also be due to primary defects in the RPE layer because of their clinical appearance and histopathology. Age related macular degeneration (AMD) and Stargardt's disease also appear to affect the RPE layer early in their courses, but the gene defect in some forms of these degenerations appears to involve the rods (Allikmets et al., 1997); this rod defect nevertheless has its most deleterious affect on the RPE layer of the macula. There are also certain generalized genetic defects that produce blindness by their early impact on the RPE layer, such as chorioderemia and gyrate atrophy, which might also be treatable by RPE transplantation. Molecular genetics and protein chemistry will ultimately clarify which degenerations are in fact primary to the RPE layer and what are the result of defects in other cell layers of the neural retina or choroid.

RPE transplantation is continuously evolving. There are many variables that can determine success or failure with this technique. Advances must come essentially by trial-and-error experimentation. It is well established that transplanted RPE survives and works in the subretinal space sufficiently to sustain photoreceptor function. Applying this technique, however, to the human retina and especially the macula, requires more than simply placing such transplants into the subretinal space without regard for their precise geometry and the potential trauma that is associated with the surgery. In addition, there is the question of host/graft rejection. Of these two problems, rejection seems less important because it can be prevented by immunosuppressive agents, perhaps even at a local level and therefore less toxically to the recipient. The problem of surgical technique, however, is a much greater challenge. Moving single cells into and within the subretinal and submacular space precisely and atraumatically requires methods even more refined than those currently employed in retinal surgery. This is an area with great potential, however, given the continuous developments in optics, microinstrumentation, and robotics.

This chapter covers the history of RPE transplantation, the current methodology, its application to human AMD, the question of host/graft rejection, and the possible future role of RPE transplantation. It supplements earlier reviews (Blair et al., 1990; Gouras and Lopez, 1989; Grierson et al., 1994; Sheedlo et al., 1991a, 1992; Turner et al., 1988).

HISTORY

The concept of RPE transplantation evolved from the successful culturing of RPE, especially human RPE from donor eyes (Flood et al., 1980). The fact that such tissue could be easily removed from Bruch's membrane by enzymatic dissection and maintained indefinitely in vitro was impressive. In vitro, the tissue is relatively well differentiated, maintaining an epitheloid appearance with an apical/basal polarity (see Chapter 5). It is capable of mediating the vitamin A cycle of vision (Das et al., 1990) and phagocytizing foreign outer segment material (Gouras et al., 1984), which are expressions of several of its major roles in vivo.

Therefore, it was logical to ask whether such RPE could be reimplanted into the retina and whether such transplants would continue to work effectively. Cultured RPE transplants were found to quickly attach to Bruch's membrane and survive in a foreign host retina (Gouras et al., 1984; 1985). Proving this was facilitated by culturing, because RPE cells routinely divide in vitro, making them susceptible to ^{3}H thymidine labeling. This is an ideal label for cell transplantation experiments, because it is virtually impossible to produce any false-positive labeling. A false-positive label would require high, maintained levels of the isotope in the subretinal space as well as host RPE cell division. Neither of these conditions occur to any significant extent. The amount of ^{3}H thymidine introduced in a transplant is miniscule even if all the transplanted tissue disintegrated. The intense labeling of the nuclei of transplanted cultured RPE left no doubt that it attached rapidly to Bruch's membrane and survived well in a foreign retina. It is also possible to label dividing RPE in vitro with the Lac Z reporter gene, chromosomally transfected with a retrovirus vector (Dunaief et al., 1995), which is a good marker at both the light and electron microscopic level (Du et al., 1992).

In order to demonstrate that the transplanted RPE could function in a foreign retina, we had to improve our surgical technique for delivering RPE to the subretinal space in order to facilitate reattachment of the neural retina. A closed-eye (Lopez et al., 1987) method to perform such surgery was obviously preferable to the more radical "open-sky" technique used initially. Today, a decade later, surgical technique still remains the foremost challenge in this field.

In the closed-eye approach, the retina is visualized through the pupil and access to the subretinal space is optimized by producing a "bleb" detachment (Marmor et al., 1980). Such detachments either spontaneously reattach or can be artificially reattached by the use of intravitreal gases or silicone oil. Under optimal conditions

transient neural retinal detachments are also not too harmful to the photoreceptors (Guerin et al., 1993).

A handicap of working under a bleb detachment, however, is that one cannot easily remove the host RPE layer before attempting to place an RPE transplant on Bruch's membrane. It is uncertain whether such a debridement is necessary for treating RPE dysfunction, as for example in the RCS rat, where layering healthy RPE over the host RPE layer can be therapeutically effective.

One strategy was to try to dislodge the host RPE from Bruch's membrane by the jet stream force required to produce the bleb detachment (Lopez et al., 1987). This approach is unpredictable and uncorrectable if coupled quasi-simultaneously with the injection of a suspension of dissociated RPE cells. Improvements with this technique—such as using a two-stage procedure in which the transplanted RPE is only introduced after the host RPE debridement is completed—should be possible. To a certain extent this occurs when neovascular membranes are removed (Algvere et al., 1994).

Nevertheless, the approach through a bleb detachment is successful in rapidly bringing the host photoreceptor outer segments in close contact with transplanted RPE shortly after surgery. This, combined with radiolabeling, proved that transplanted RPE was fully capable of phagocytizing host outer segments (Gouras et al., 1986). This immediately suggested that a therapeutic potential of RPE transplantation was possible in the RCS rat model if the method could be scaled down to an infant rat eye (Reppucci et al., 1988).

RPE ALLOGRAFTS IN THE RCS RAT

This is the only animal model of an hereditary disease in which RPE dysfunction is known to be responsible for a retinal degeneration that leads to blindness (see Chapter 13). Although the gene defect is not yet known, the pathogenesis of the disease at the cellular level is understood conceptually. The defective RPE is incapable of phagocytizing the growing outer segments of the photoreceptors (Bok and Hall, 1971; Dowling and Sidman, 1962; Herron et al., 1969; Mullin and LaVail, 1976). Therefore, the outer segments pile up in the subretinal space, which secondarily causes the photoreceptor cells to degenerate.

Introducing a suspension of RPE cells into the subretinal space of an infant rat (2–3 weeks old) is more difficult to do than it is in a much larger adult rabbit or monkey eye. In addition, the relatively large size of the rat lens makes a pars plana approach even more difficult. We used a more posterior, transretinal rather than a pars plana route to gain sufficient access to the vitre-

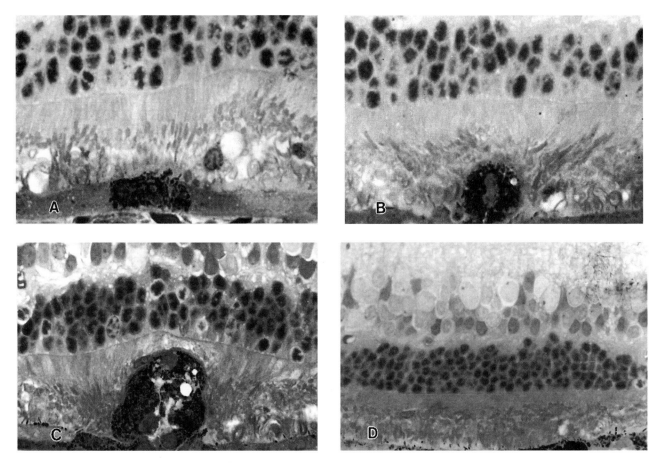

FIGURE 25-1. Light micrographs of 3- to 4-month-old RCS rat retina showing photoreceptor rescue from RPE transplants. In (A), (B), and (D) the pigmented transplants have insinuated into the albinotic host epithelial layer. In (B) and (C) the transplanted RPE forms a ball of cells, which also rescues receptors; these sections show the tendency for outer segments to orient toward the transplants.

al cavity in the rat eye (Reppucci et al., 1988). Turner's group modified a posterior approach they had been using to introduce neural grafts into rat retina (Turner et al., 1988) to also begin RPE transplantation in the RCS rat (Li and Turner, 1988a; 1991; Gaur et al., 1992). The posterior route is easier than the transvitreal one, but offers less feedback for visualizing the bleb detachment of the neural retina and the precise placement of the suspension of RPE cells.

Both groups quasi-independently (Johnson, 1992) discovered that the introduction of healthy RPE cells into the subretinal space of young RCS rats stopped the photoreceptors from degenerating. Figure 25-1 shows the rescue of photoreceptors in the RCS rat retina by RPE transplantation. The transplants are clumps of pigmented cells sitting on the host epithelial layer. Note how the preserved outer segments appear to orient

themselves toward the transplants. Figure 25-2 compares short with longer term photoreceptor rescue by RPE transplants and demonstrates in Fig. 25-2D the total loss of the photoreceptor layer in a control retina that has not received any transplant. Electron micrographs (Fig. 25-3) show a healthy appearance of such rescued outer segments. This was the first demonstration that a progressive neuronal degeneration in the central nervous system could be prevented by cell transplantation. It provided hope that RPE transplantation might also be able to prevent some forms of human retinal degenerations.

This rescue of photoreceptors can last for the life of the rat and is accompanied by a preservation of visual function from the photoreceptors to the output layers of the retina (LaVail et al., 1992; Sheedlo et al., 1993; Yamamoto et al., 1993; Jiang and Hamasaki, 1994b). Be-

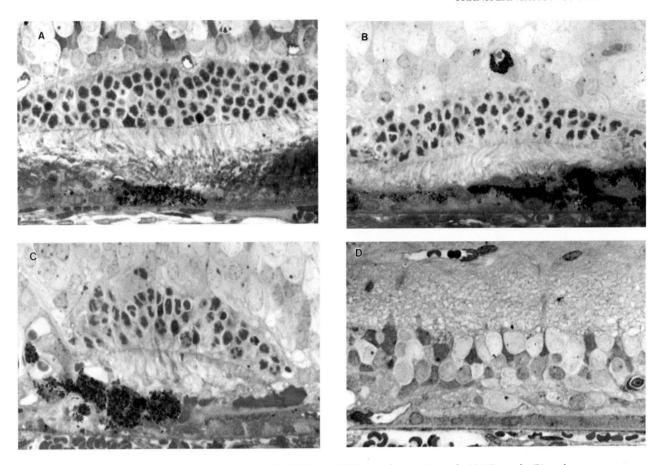

FIGURE 25-2. Photoreceptor rescue in the RCS rat by RPE transplants at 2 months (A), 7 months (B), and 10 months (C) after surgery. The retina of a 4-month-old RCS rat is shown in (D) as a control. In (B) and (C), microelectrode recording caused a small recent hemorrhage.

havioral experiments in RCS rats have also shown that RPE transplantation leads to a preservation of visual function (Whiteley et al., 1995). Transplantation also normalizes the retinal vascular changes accompanying this retinal dystrophy (Seaton and Turner, 1992; Seaton et al., 1994; Seregard et al., 1994) and also influences other retinal cells (Li et al., 1993a). It is ineffective in degenerations not due to an RPE defect (Li et al., 1993b) or at late stages of degeneration in the RCS rat (Sheedlo et al., 1991b). There can be no doubt about the efficacy of RPE transplantation in this well-established animal model of a hereditary retinal degeneration. It can, in fact, be used as a test of RPE transplant competence (Little et al., 1995).

A question that still exists is how the RPE transplants stop the photoreceptors from degenerating. The simplest explanation is that it is due to the reestablishment of outer segment phagocytosis which the host RPE is incapable of performing. Evidence for this viewpoint is the following: The rescue of the photoreceptors occurs only in the regions where there are RPE transplants and is closely related to the local number of transplanted RPE (Fig. 25-4). As soon as the RPE transplants reach the subretinal space, they appear to engorge themselves with the large pile-up of effete outer segment material in these developing retinas (Lopez et al., 1989); this phenomenon is shown quantitatively in Figure 25-5. By electron microscopy one can detect very fine processes from the transplanted RPE which extend over relatively long distances to engulf outer segment material. This can mimic a diffusion mediated effect if these ultrafine processes are not visualized by microscopy.

There is evidence that a diffusible factor is playing a role, although it appears to be a minor one compared with the physical presence of phagocytically competent RPE. A diffusible factor was suggested by experiments with chimeric rats where photoreceptors near but not directly over normal RPE patches failed to degenerate (Mullen and LaVail, 1976). This phenomenon could also be explained by fine processes of normal RPE ex-

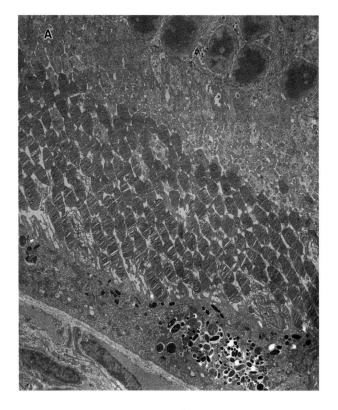

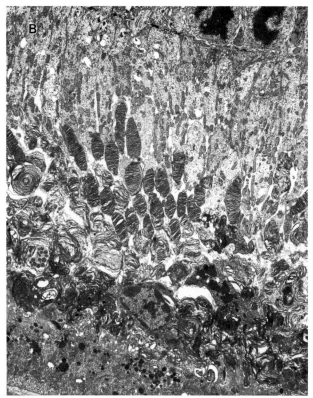

FIGURE 25-3. Electron micrographs of photoreceptor outer segments rescued by RPE transplantation in the RCS rat at 3 months after surgery. Phagosomes can be seen in the RPE in (B).

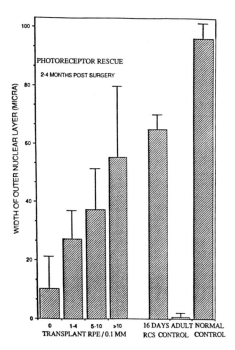

FIGURE 25-4. Histogram showing the relationship between outer nuclear layer thickness in the RCS rat and the concentration of RPE transplants (number/0.1 mm) in each local area at 2–4 months after surgery for five animals. On the right are results for RCS control retinas at 16 days and 4 months of age compared to a normal adult rat. The vertical lines show standard deviations.

tending into areas subserved by defective RPE. Stronger evidence came from sham surgery without RPE transplantation, which produces a small, transient retardation of the photoreceptor degeneration (Silverman and Hughes, 1990). More informative evidence came from intravitreal administration of basic fibroblastic growth factor (bFGF), which also leads to photoreceptor rescue in the RCS rat (Faktorovich et al., 1990; Perry et al., 1995). This is also a relatively smaller, more transient phenomenon than RPE transplantation. bFGF produces several effects in the retina such as neovascularization and the redistribution of retinal macrophages (Perry et al., 1995), both of which could influence the rate of photoreceptor degeneration in the RCS rat. These trophic effects do not appear to correct the basic defect, incompetent RPE phagocytosis, although some evidence for such a hypothesis exists (McLaren et al., 1992). Trophic factors could influence processes that lead secondarily to the degeneration of the photoreceptors. For example, neovascularization may promote a faster removal of a toxic material, such as retinol, building up from pileup of outer segments. Macrophages may also hasten the photoreceptor degeneration, and their removal by bFGF could delay this. The triggering of photoreceptor apoptosis could also be altered by trophic factors.

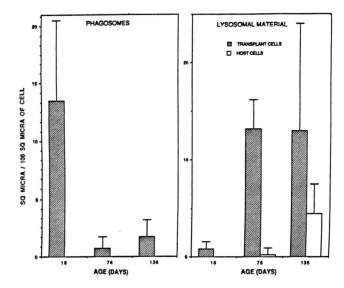

FIGURE 25-5. Histogram *(left)* showing the square microns of phago-some/square microns of cytoplasm found in transplanted *(hatched squares)* and host *(open squares)* RPE at 18, 76, and 136 days after surgery. The histogram *(right)* shows the amount of lysosomal material in these cells. The results indicate the enormous phagocytosis of outer segment material that the transplanted RPE must consume shortly after these cells are introduced into the subretinal space. The vertical lines show standard deviation.

RPE ALLOGRAFTS IN RABBITS

Because of the possibility that RPE transplantation could also have therapeutic potential in man, a number of laboratories have been exploring this technique in eyes that are larger and therefore more comparable to the human eye. Most of this research has been done in rabbits, transplanting pigmented RPE into albinotic retinas (Bhatt et al., 1993; 1994; El Dirini et al., 1992; Gouras et al., 1992; Lopez et al., 1987; Yamaguchi et al., 1992; Li and Wu, 1995); some has also been done in pigs (Lane et al., 1988; 1989; Lane and Boulton, 1988). The strategy of using pigmented cells as markers for transplants in albinotic retinas is reasonable but must be used with caution because albinotic host epithelium can phagocytize melanin released by degenerating or even viable RPE transplants. Usually this can be distinguished because it involves only small amounts of melanin, which makes such cells much less intensely pigmented than the transplants. If there is any question, it behooves the investigators to use more reliable markers (Ye et al., 1993).

Most of this research has involved the standard pars plana route to the retina. One study compared this with a posterior transchoroidal approach (Wongpichedchai et al., 1992). It concluded that a greater number of transplanted RPE could be delivered to Bruch's membrane by the posterior approach, but this had the disadvantage of being less precise in targeting the cells due to poorer visibility. This is similar to what occurs in RPE transplants to rat retina. Nevertheless, there is room for further experimentation with the posterior approach.

Most of the allografts in rabbit retina were suspensions of RPE cells that were injected into a bleb detachment of the neural retina. All of these studies have demonstrated that such RPE transplants survive and intermingle intimately with the host epithelium and the neural retina. Junctional complexes form between the previously dissociated transplants, as well as between host and transplanted epithelium (Gouras et al., 1992), implying considerable functional compatibility between these foreign epithelia.

In general, suspensions of dissociated cells do not lead to the reestablishment of a complete epithelial monolayer which replaces the host layer. First of all it is difficult to remove the host RPE layer working within a bleb detachment of the neural retina. Second, the suspension of RPE cells spreads over the host epithelial layer in an unpredictable way, producing clusters of cells resting within and between the host epithelium and the photoreceptors. Nevertheless such transplants, which form a double or even a triple layer of RPE, support reasonably healthy looking photoreceptors; quantitative measurements on this point are shown in Figure 25-9.

The creation of a bleb detachment of the neural retina can rip off the apical processes of RPE cells in rabbits (Lopez et al., 1955; Sheng et al., 1995a) and monkeys (Berglin et al., 1997). Such explosive detachments may be more deleterious in the fovea where cone outer segments are especially delicate. Methods that facilitate a more gentle separation of the neural retina from the RPE layer may improve the impact of RPE transplantation on visual function.

Several laboratories have been trying to improve the method for debriding the host RPE layer from Bruch's membrane working within the confines of a bleb detachment. One method uses Ca^{2+} chelating agents, EDTA, combined with gentle brushing of the host RPE layer off Bruch's membrane with a soft-tip silicone catheter (Del Priore et al., 1995). Others have used a silicone brush needle alone (Ozaka et al., 1995) or a subretinal forceps (Valentino et al., 1995). Another employs a microjet stream to dislodge the host RPE (Parolini et al., 1995). Displaced RPE cells are aspirated from the subretinal space. So far, no one has attempted to collect and measure the numbers removed by these methods, feedback that could be important at the time of surgery. Such an approach might be different in the macula of subjects with RPE degenerations, where cells may be removable much more easily than is the case in healthy young animal retinas.

There have also been attempts to use organized RPE monolayers (Castillo et al., 1995) rather than cell suspensions as transplants. Several teams have used artificial supports to maintain the RPE as a rigid monolayer, either growing the cells in vitro on collagen (Bhatt et al., 1994; Organesian et al., 1995) or biodegradable membranes (Moritera et al., 1993; Thomson et al., 1995) or embedding them in dissolvable gelatin (Liu et al., 1992; Fang et al., 1993; Yang et al., 1995). We have taken advantage of fetal human RPE's resiliency which makes them culturable and transplantable as monolayer patches (Gouras et al., 1994a). Ho and colleagues (1995) have reported similar results for porcine RPE. Without a rigid support such RPE patches can be folded and thereby transplanted within a relatively small pipette (Algvere et al., 1994; Sheng et al., 1995a). This requires a smaller retinotomy than those in which a rigid monolayer is introduced into the subretinal space. The method of folding an RPE monolayer within a pipette is not totally successful, because the monolayer does not completely unfold after ejection. A method that could unfold, spread and flatten such a monolayer patch within the subretinal space without damaging the adjacent photoreceptors would be advantageous.

RPE ALLOGRAFTS IN AMD

The development of surgical techniques to remove subfoveal neovascular membranes in both the presumed ocular histoplasmosis syndrome and in "wet" forms of AMD (Thomas and Kaplan, 1991; Thomas, 1994) offered a new approach to this serious complication. The results in histoplasmosis have been more promising than those in the older patients with AMD (Berger and Kaplan, 1992; deJuan and Machemer, 1988; Thomas, 1994). One hypothesis that could explain this difference is that the surgical removal of these neovascular membranes invariably removes some or even much of the subfoveal RPE layer together with the interwoven scar tissue (Algvere et al., 1994; Bynoe et al., 1994; Lopez et al., 1991; Seregard et al., 1994). In younger patients the vitality of the neighboring RPE layer may lead to the growth of RPE cells that covers the deficit. In older patients, whose RPE is not only more aged but also degenerate from the inherent AMD, there may be less potential for the adjacent RPE to reepithelialize the subfoveal retina. There is also less potential for mitosis (Flood et al., 1980). This lack of reepithelialization of the subfovea may be responsible for the poorer visual outcome in AMD patients.

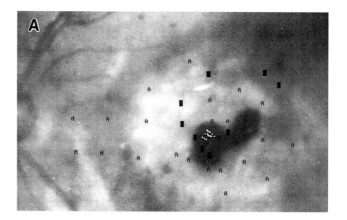
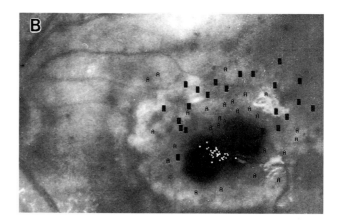
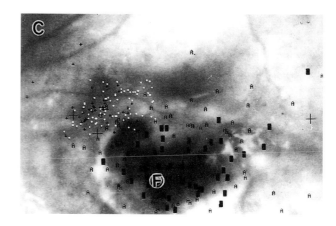

FIGURE 25-6. SLO perimetry of a human subject at 2 days (A), 1 month (B), and 3 months (C) after RPE transplantation surgery. The small white dots indicate the position of fixation during the detection of each test stimulus. The position of the test stimuli detected are illustrated as a naked "A"; those not detected as a black rectangle. At 2 days and 1 month, fixation is at the fovea and over the transplant; at 3 months it has become eccentric and less precise. Light detection occurs over the transplant, but only along its nasal edge at 3 months after transplantation. The foveal area is marked by (F). (Modified from Algvere et al., 1994.)

We attempted to compensate for this potential RPE deficit in five patients who were candidates for the surgical removal of subfoveal neovascular membranes secondary to AMD. When their subfoveal neovascular membranes were removed, a patch of previously cultured human fetal RPE was transplanted into the subretinal space to cover the subfoveal area (Algvere et al., 1994). Each RPE patch was folded within a glass micropipette, having a tip diameter of 0.2–0.3 mm, and injected into the submacular space over the fovea. After surgery four of the five patients who had had foveal fixation before surgery retained this function after surgery. Figure 25-6A shows an example of such a patient examined by a scanning laser ophthalmoscope (SLO). The SLO allows local light detection to be determined but also provides a monitor on the position of fixation. At one week after surgery the patient was detecting light and foveally fixating over the heavily pigmented fetal RPE allograft. This remained stable at one month after transplantation (Fig. 25-6B). But at three months after surgery and concomitant with chronic fluorescein leakage over the transplant, visibility and fixation over the transplant was lost (Fig. 25-6C). A similar pattern was seen in the other patients. Only one patient has maintained foveal fixation, but this was the only case where the transplant was not placed directly in the fovea.

At more than one year after surgery the transplants are still apparent as discrete patches darker than the adjacent retinal areas. They have also spread to cover a larger area, implying growth along their perimeter. The neural retina over the transplants is less transparent and local visual function has been lost. Most of the patients have had a mild loss of visual acuity compared to their preoperative level. The one patient who retains foveal fixation still has virtually the same acuity as she had before surgery (20/200). Such transplants are capable of supporting local visual function including foveal fixation for at least several months after transplantation, but they seem to encounter what must be chronic host/graft rejection that slowly compromises function and damages the contiguous neural retina.

Another group (Peyman et al., 1991) has also reported two cases of RPE transplants after the removal of subfoveal neovascular membranes in AMD. They used more radical surgery, folding a 250 degree pedicle flap of neural retina off the macula to remove the membranes. In one case they covered the fovea with a flap of autologous RPE from an adjacent area. This patient was reported to be fixating over the graft with an acuity of 20/400 at 14 months after surgery. The problem with using homologous RPE is that it increases the retinal surgery considerably and leaves the patient with what may be a degenerate RPE layer. In the second case they transplanted an allograft of RPE together with Bruch's membrane and the choriocapillaris dissected from an adult donor eye. Choroidal tissue was included to keep the RPE layer intact, a technically difficult feat. This graft failed to support vision and became encapsulated, probably due to rejection.

None of these patients had been immunosuppressed. It is now our impression that such transplants are more vulnerable to rejection because they are directly exposed to the choroid rather than immunologically isolated within a subretinal space. In addition, the presence and subsequent removal of the new vessel growth further increases the immunological provocation of such transplants.

We have tested this hypothesis by transplanting human fetal RPE into the submacular space of four patients with advanced but "dry" forms of AMD. In these cases, although there are widespread window defects in the macula, there is no leakage of fluorescein at angiography. We therefore assume that the blood–retinal barrier is intact. In order to minimize possible rejection, we reduced the size of the transplant to a circular patch, 0.6 mm in diameter. We also placed each transplant in nonfoveal areas of the macula where rejection, if it occurred, would have a minimal influence on visual function. All of these patients had acuities of 20/200 and three of four had foveal fixation, as determined by SLO microperimetry. At present, more than a year after surgery, none of these transplants have disturbed local visual function. One of the transplants, located very close to the retinotomy site has degenerated; this may be related to inflammation around the retinotomy site, which could have provoked rejection of this transplant. The other three transplants can be visualized continuously over this a two year period. One of these, lying over an intact host RPE layer, has remained unchanged during this entire time. The other two, which are lying over areas devoid of an RPE layer show evidence of growth along their edges, which appeared to stop at 3–6 months after transplantation surgery. Since a similar growth was also seen around the edges of transplants placed over areas from which neovascular membranes including much of the host RPE had been removed, it is tempting to suggest that RPE transplant growth will occur in vivo if there is no contact inhibition from neighboring RPE. This is, of course, what happens to RPE in vitro. The survival of these transplants for such a long period of time supports the hypothesis that if the blood-retinal barrier remains intact RPE allogafts are less likely to be rejected (Algvere et al., 1996).

These previous four patch transplants covered a very small and nonfoveal area of the macula. In order to try to cover a larger area including the fovea as gently as possible, we used a suspension of concentrated dissociated fetal human RPE rather than a patch transplant in seven subsequent cases of advanced but dry AMD. These cases have been followed for more than a year. Transplants of cell suspensions are more difficult to visualize if their concentrations are less than about 50,000 or less cells but become more apparent with suspensions containing 100,000 or more cells. These transplants also are showing evidence of host-graft rejection though they were also introduced into a subretinal space where the blood-retinal barrier appears to be intact.

The evidence for rejection is the development of fluorescein staining and leakage. This develops at about 8–12 months in transplants containing 50,000 cells (3 cases) and in about 3 months in transplants containing 500,000 cells (2 cases). One case receiving cell suspensions of 2,000 and another receiving 20,000 cells have shown no evidence of rejection at one year.

These results have led us to conclude that rejection of human fetal RPE allografts is common but not inevitable. The probability of rejection is high if there are a large number of cells in the transplant and/or the transplant is near a site of possible inflammation, i.e. a retinotomy.

RPE ALLOGRAFT REJECTION IN ANIMALS

The question of subretinal RPE allograft rejection remains a significant issue, which will probably be controversial for a long time. We argued above that it may not occur in human subjects, at least not in subjects with small RPE patch transplants when the blood–retinal barrier is intact. In these cases there is no histological evidence to confirm this conclusion, which is based on the absence of fluorescein leakage and the maintenance of visual function over the transplants at six months after surgery.

A review of the evidence on this point in animal experimentation where histological examination is routinely available is somewhat inconsistent. We have found no rejection of RPE allografts in the RCS rat where evidence for functional integrity of rescued photoreceptors was found at almost one year after transplantation (Yamamoto et al., 1993), and this is supported by reports of other laboratories (LaVail et al., 1992; Sheedlo et al., 1993; Jiang and Hamasaki, 1994). There is also evidence that RPE allografts are well tolerated in the subretinal space of rabbit retina (El Dirini et al., 1992).

Recently Bok and associates (unpublished results) have found a certain degree of rejection that also occurs in RPE allografts to the RCS rat. Jiang et al. (1995) have also reported that subretinal murine allografts are rejected in 35 days with a cellular form of rejection. We

have found that murine photoreceptor allografts survive for at least nine months in the subretinal space of *rd* mutant mice (Gouras et al., 1994b), but comparing photoreceptors with RPE allografts may not be appropriate because photoreceptors may be less immunogenic than RPE (Kaplan et al., 1995).

More research is necessary to resolve these contradictions. The subretinal space, like the anterior chamber of the eye, is an immunologically privileged site (Streilein, 1987; Jiang et al., 1993; see Chapter 26). This privileged status appears to depend completely or in part on an active process that promotes tolerance. In the anterior chamber the active process has been called *anterior chamber immune deviation* (ACAID); in this case antigen-specific suppressor T cells form and prevent a delayed hypersensitivity to a foreign antigen. Recently, the presence of Fas ligand, a member of the TNFa family of cytokines, which induces apoptosis in cells expressing the Fas receptor, has been found in RPE and photoreceptors (Griffth et al., 1995). This kills T cells, which express the Fas receptor, when they enter the retina to attack foreign protein. Fas ligand-induced apoptosis appears to be required to induce ACAID (Ferguson, 1997). In addition, the subretinal space is relatively isolated from the immune system, as is the rest of the central nervous system, making transplants less prone to immune surveillance and detection. Recognition of a foreign protein depends upon antigen-presenting APC cells incorporating the antigen and presenting to their MHC Class II surface antigens a peptide fragment, which then interacts with CD-4 positive T cells (Adorini, 1989; Stinman, 1991) (Fig. 25-7). The latter amplify and communicate this signal to the immune system. APC cells have been found in the choroid (Forrester et al., 1994) and are the most likely candidates for alerting the immune system to subretinal RPE allografts. In order for them to do this, foreign proteins or peptides from the allografts must reach the choroidal cells, perhaps by exocytosis and diffusion. It is also possible that either the RPE allografts or the host RPE can act as antigen-presenting cells since RPE can express MHC Class II antigens (Silbert et al., 1995; Liversidge et al., 1988; Zhang et al., 1995). When the blood–retinal barrier is broken, more direct access of APC and/or CD-4 T cells becomes possible (Fig. 25-7). All of these phenomena may occur, making RPE allograft rejection a response that depends upon both the unique circumstances within the retina and the surgical technique used in transplantation.

HUMAN RPE XENOGRAFTS

In an attempt to gain more experience in transplanting human fetal RPE we performed a series of xenograft ex-

HOST - GRAFT REJECTION

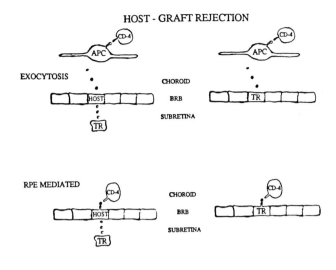

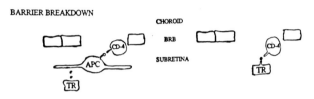

In similar xenografts to monkey retina the results are different; rejection is relatively uncommon even at six months after transplantation, our longest time point. Only 7 out of 21 (33%) of these transplants were rejected. Five of the transplants were placed in or near the fovea and 4 of 5 (80%) of these were rejected by six months. Such xenografts in the fovea appear to be more vulnerable to rejection. Again, rejection is most apparent histologically by cellular disruption of the transplant and damage to the overlying photoreceptors. Fluorescein leakage and depigmentation of the transplants are also apparent. In the perimacular or along the vascular arcades, rejection of such subretinal RPE xenografts was uncommon, only 3 of 16 (19%) rejected. Figure 25-8 illustrates the appearance of photoreceptors, both rods and cones, in intimate association with a nonrejected perimacular fetal human RPE patch transplant

FIGURE 25-7. A scheme indicating the potential factors that may contribute to host/graft rejection in the subretinal space. By exocytosis *(above)* of foreign protein antigens, antigen-presenting cells (APC) in the choroid can incorporate such antigens and present them to CD-4 lymphocytes. The exocytosis could proceed from transplant to host RPE or directly from transplants insinuated into the host RPE layer; by the host *(left)* or transplant *(RPE middle)* acting as the antigen-presenting cells. By blood–retinal barrier breakdown *(below)* in which both choroidal APC cells and/or CD-4 lymphocytes have more direct access to these transplants.

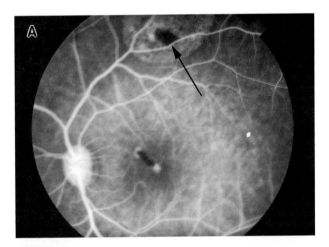

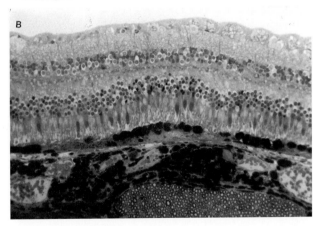

FIGURE 25-8. (A) Human fetal RPE patch transplant to macaque retina at 6 months after surgery as viewed in a late-stage fluorescein angiogram. One transplant *(arrow)* is located along the superior arcade; another transplant is located in the foveal area. There is no evidence of leakage. (B) Light micrograph showing the central area of the transplant, arrowed in (A). The heavily pigmented transplant is sitting on the host RPE layer, making contact with the outer segments of both rods and cones.

periments in rabbits and monkeys, some of which have been reported (Sheng et al., 1995b). Others are currently in press (Gouras et al., 1996; Berglin et al., 1997). In the subretinal space of rabbits, cultured human fetal RPE patch transplants will survive well for at least one week and preserve relatively good looking photoreceptors in association with the transplant, but at one month virtually all of the transplants are rejected. Others (Li et al., 1992) have examined rat-to-rabbit RPE xenografts and obtained similar results. Rejection is apparent funduscopically by a disruption and depigmentation of the transplant, angiographically by fluorescein leakage around and over the transplant, and histologically by infiltration of the transplant by monocytes together with destruction of the neighboring photoreceptors. This rejection response is extremely local, leaving the adjacent retina on either side of the transplant unscathed (Gabrielien et al., 1995; Sheng et al., 1995a). All of this can be prevented by postsurgical cyclosporine administration (Sheng et al., 1995b).

PERIPHERAL TRANSPLANT (6 MONTHS)

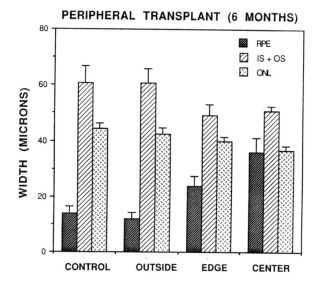

FIGURE 25-9. A histogram showing the width of the RPE layer (and the transplant when relevant), the outer nuclear layer (ONL), and the combined inner and outer segment (IS + OS) in undetached (control) retina, in detached retina that is not receiving the patch transplant (outside), and at the edge and the center of the transplant. The vertical lines show standard deviations.

for six months. On electron microscopy the transplanted fetal human RPE appeared to be more macrophagic than the host RPE (Gouras et al., 1996). The vulnerability of the foveal area to rejection may reflect its greater vascularity and/or a greater surgical trauma in producing a bleb detachment.

In order to obtain quantitative measurements of the effect of such human fetal patch transplants on the host retina, we measured the width of the outer nuclear layer, the inner segment, and the outer segment of the photoreceptors over the transplant and compared these measurements with those over the detached retina which did not receive any transplant, as well as with undetached retina in an adjacent region of the retina. We also included the width of the host RPE and that of the transplant combined with the host RPE. In general, these transplants are sitting on top of the host RPE layer, which makes a double layer and in some cases where there is folding of the transplant, a triple layer.

Figure 25-9 shows an example of such measurements from a transplant which was not rejected in the perimacular area. The results show several interesting points. First there is some slight damage due to the retinal detachment alone. There is reduction of the outer nuclear layer width and outer and inner segment length over the transplant, but it is not striking. Interestingly, the differences between a very thick (i.e. multilayered) transplant and a relatively thin one (i.e. at the edge of the transplant) are comparatively small. Photoreceptors

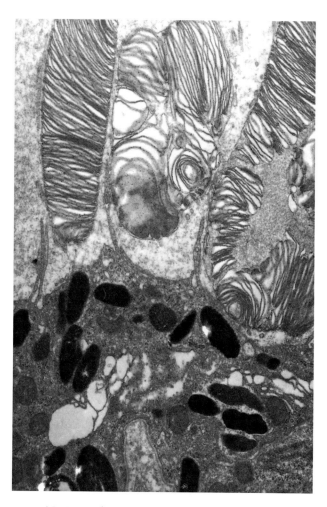

FIGURE 25-10. Monkey rod outer segment in intimate contact with the apical processes of a human fetal RPE transplant at 6 months after surgery.

including their outer segments are capable of surviving relatively well over a multilayered RPE transplant (Fig. 25-10).

Iris Pigment Epithelium (IPE)

An interesting strategy to eliminate rejection has been to use autografts of biopsied IPE to replace defective RPE (Gelanze et al., 1993; Gelanze et al., 1997; Lai et al., 1997; Mashhour and Renard, 1997). Several investigators have demonstrated the ability of IPE to phagocytize outer segments (Thurmann and Heimann, 1997; Bisantis et al., 1997). The question of vision specific retinoid metabolism has not been examined. Recently it has been shown that IPE transplants can delay the photoreceptor degeneration in the RCS rat with (Takeka et al., 1997) or without (Resai et al., 1997) bFGF-cDNA. In the RCS model the host RPE may be satisfying the unique retinoid metabolism of the photoreceptors but this may not occur if the host RPE is degenerate or completely absent.

THE FUTURE OR RPE TRANSPLANTATION

The future of RPE transplantation depends on whether it is capable of producing some therapeutic effect in man. The first attempt was to help repair the RPE layer after removal of neovascular membranes in AMD. This has not been successful yet, mainly because such transplants appear to be prone to rejection. Perhaps here immunosuppression using the standard triple-drug regimen of cyclosporine, azathioprine, and methylprednisone will prevent rejection. In addition, tissue typing as well as assessment of antibody titers in the recipients could serve to tailor the appropriate immunosuppression.

Rejection may be less of a problem if the blood–retinal barrier is intact. This is suggested by the current results in human subjects with dry forms of AMD as well as by the successful use of RPE allografts in rats. Again, the final answer has not been reached on rejection but, regardless of the answer, RPE transplantation could be performed with immunosuppression. This has become a very important consideration since several forms of retinal degeneration, especially Sorsby's fundus dystrophy, appear to be due to primary RPE defects and could therefore be treatable using methods that are known to be effective in the RCS rat model.

The question of technique also becomes relevant. Will suspension of RPE cells be as useful as organized monolayers? Intuitively it seems better to reconstruct a pristine new RPE monolayer that completely replaces the degenerate or defective host layer. This will require much greater sophistication in subretinal microsurgery and improvement in the delivery of the transplant monolayer. This, of course, may not be necessary to gain a beneficial effect in some degenerative diseases, but it remains the ultimate goal in attempting to repair the RPE layer.

The problems increase in the foveal area, which is exceedingly delicate and known to be less tolerant of retinal detachment. It may also be more prone to host/graft rejection and to cystoid macular edema. It is the foveal area, however, that holds most of the benefits to vision that patients with retinal degenerations seek. Therefore the future impact of RPE transplantation, if it proves in any way therapeutic, will depend on how well it can be applied to the fovea.

At present the technique has been used only in advanced stages of AMD, both the "wet" and more recently the "dry" forms. These are situations where the least can be gained because there must already be considerable photoreceptor degeneration present, much of it irreversible. If RPE transplantation can be performed without causing any untoward effects on a patient, we may be able to approach the early stages of degeneration, where more function can be preserved and possibly regained.

How far retinal cell transplantation can go in the future is difficult to predict, but success would seem to be inevitable given the improvements which should evolve in the microtechnology required to operate within the subretinal space. There are many additional possibilities that can be imagined. For example, photoreceptor allografts including both rods and cones can survive indefinitely in mouse (Gouras et al., 1994b), rat (Aramant and Seiler, in press), and rabbit (Adolph et al., 1994) retinas. The only question is whether they are capable of synaptically interacting with host neurons. Most certainly ways will be found to expedite such interactions since they have been demonstrated elsewhere in the central nervous system (Lund and Coffey, 1994). Under these circumstances it may become possible to transplant both RPE and photoreceptors either together or in stages. This would, of course, allow vision to be restored after it has been lost.

In addition, the possibility of gene therapy is on the horizon. The very same techniques used to transplant retinal cells can be used to introduce viral vectors, with either photoreceptor or RPE-specific gene promoters, directly adjacent to the cells they must transfect in order to be therapeutic (Bennett et al., 1996). Combinations of genetic engineering and cell transplantation can be used in innovative ways. For example, RPE cells in culture can be transfected with a retrovirus which can put unique new genes into chromosomal DNA, and these transgenic cells can be transplanted back into the retina (Dunaief et al., 1995; Lai et al., 1998). Ophthalmology and retinal surgery therefore has a great opportunity in advancing the frontier of cellular and molecular repair of the central nervous system.

REFERENCES

Adolph AR, Zucker CL, Ehinger B, Bergstrom A. 1994. Function and structure in retinal transplants. J Neural Transpl Plasticity 5:147–161.

Adorini L. 1989. The presentation of antigen by MHC class I molecular. Year Immunol 6:21–37.

Al-Awqati Q. 1996. Plasticity in the epithelial polarity of renal intercalated cells: targeting of the HRATpase and band 3. Am J Gen Physiol 270:C1571–1580.

Algvere PV, Berglin L, Gouras P, Sheng Y. 1994. Transplantation of fetal retinal pigment epithelium in age-related macular degeneration with subfoveal neovascularization. Graefes Arch Clin Exp Ophthalmol 232:707–716.

Algvere PV, Berglin L, Gouras P, Sheng Y. 1997. Human fetal RPE transplants in age related macular degeneration (ARMD). Graefes Arch Clin Eye Ophthalmol 235:149–158.

Allikmets R, Shroyer NF, Singh N, Seddon JM, Lewis RA, Bernstein PS, Peiffer A, Zabriskie NA, Li Y, Hutchinson A, Dean M, Lupski JR, Leppert M. 1997. Mutation of the Stargardt Disease gene (ABCR) in age-related macular degeneration. Science 277:1805–1807.

Aramant R, Seiler M. 1995. Fiber and synaptic connections between embryonic retinal transplants and host retina. Exper Neurol 133:244–255.

Bennett J, Tanabe T, Sun D, Zeng Y, Kjeldbye H, Gouras P, Maguire AM. 1996. Photoreceptor cell rescue in retinal degeneration (rd) mice by in vivo gene therapy. 2:649–654.

Berger AS, Kaplan HJ. 1992. Clinical experience with the surgical removal of subfoveal neovascular membranes: short-term postoperative results. Ophthalmol 99(6):969–975.

Berglin L, Gouras P, Sheng Y, Lavid J, Lin PK, Cao H, Kjeldbye H. 1997. Tolerance of human fetal RPE xenografts in monkey retina. Graefes Arch Clin Exp Ophthalmol 235:103–110.

Bhatt NS, Oliver PD, French T, et al. 1993. Transplantation of human retinal pigment epithelial cells into rabbits. Invest Ophthalmol Vis Sci 34:1093.

Bhatt NS, Newsome DA, French T, et al. 1994. Experimental transplantation of human retinal pigment epithelial cells on collagen substrates. Am J Ophthalmol 117:214–221.

Bisantis F, Fregona I, Mancini A, Dalla Pozza G, Bisantis C. 1997. Is phagocytosis in iris pigmented epithelium (IPE) cultures by human iridectomies a self-limited and dose-dependent mechanism? Invest Ophthalmol Vis Sci 38(4):S330.

Blair JR, Gaur V, Laedtke TW, Li L, Liu Y, Sheedlo H, Yamaguchi K, Yamaguchi K, Turner JE. 1990. Oculotransplantation studies involving the neural retina and its pigment epithelium. Prog Retinal Res 10:69–88.

Bok D, Hall MO. 1971. The role of the pigment epithelium in the etiology of inherited retinal dystrophy in the rat. J Cell Biol 49:664–682.

Bynoe LA, Chang TS, Funata M, Del Priore LV, Kaplan HJ, Green WR. 1994. Histopathologic examination of vascular patterns in subfoveal neovascular membranes. Ophthalmol 101(6):1112–1117.

Cao H, Sheng Y, Gouras P, Kjeldbye H, Tanabe T. 1994. Patch culturing and polarity independence of human fetal RPE. Invest Ophthalmol Vis Sci 35(suppl):1761.

Castillo BV Jr, Little CW, del Cerro C, del Cerro M. 1995. An improved method of isolating human fetal RPE. Invest Ophthalmol Vis Sci 36(4):S251.

Das SR, Bhardwaj N, Gouras P. 1990. Synthesis of retinoids by human retinal epithelium and transfer to rod outer segments. Biochem J 268:201–206.

DeJuan E Jr, Machemer R. 1988. Vitreous surgery for hemorrhagic and fibrous complications of age-related macular degeneration. Am J Ophthalmol 105:25–29.

Della NF, Campochiaro PA, Zack DJ. 1996. Localization of TIMP-3 mRNA expression to the retinal pigment epithelium. Invest Ophthalmol Vis Sci 37(3):S227.

Del Priore LV, Hornbeck R, Kaplan HJ, Jones Z, Silverman MS, Mosinger-Ogilvie J, Swinn M. 1995. Debridement of the pig retinal pigment epithelium in vivo. Arch Ophthalmol 113:939–944.

Dowling JE, Sidman RL. 1962. Inherited retinal dystrophy in the rat. J Cell Biol 14:73–109.

Dry KL, Manson FDC, Edgar AJ, Lennon AA, Porter KE, Bird AC, D'Urso M, Wright AF. 1996. Identification and characterization of the gene for X-linked retinitis pigmentosa. Am J Human Genetics 59(suppl):A256.

Du J, Gouras P, Kjeldbye H, Kwun R, Lopez R. 1992. Monitoring photoreceptor transplants with macular and cytoplasmic markers. Exper Neurol 115:79–86.

Dunaief JL, Kwun RC, Bhardwaj N, Lopez R, Gouras P, Goff SP. 1995. Retroviral gene transfer into retinal pigment epithelial cells followed by transplantation into rat retina. Human Gene Therapy 6:1225–1229.

El Dirini AA, Wang H, Ogden TE, Ryan SJ. 1992. Retinal pigment epithelium implantation in the rabbit: technique and morphology. Graefes Arch Clin Exp Ophthalmol 230:292–300.

Faktorovich EG, Steinberg RH, Tasumura D, Matthes MT, LaVail MM. 1990. Photoreceptor degeneration in inherited retinal dystrophy delayed by basic fibroblast growth factor. Nature 347:83–86.

Fang SR, Kaplan HJ, Del Priore LV, et al. 1993. Development of a surgical procedure and instrument for transplantation of extended gelatin sheets to the subretinal space. Invest Ophthalmol Vis Sci 34:1093.

Ferguson TA, Gao Y, Herndon JM, Griffith TS. 1997. Apoptotic cell death on IL-10 production in the eye are essential for the induction of immune deviation. Invest Ophthalmol Vis Sci 38:S492.

Flood MT, Gouras P, Kjeldbye H. 1980. Growth characteristics and ultrastructure of human retinal pigment epithelium in vitro. Invest Ophthalmol Vis Sci 19:1309–1320.

Forrester JV, McMenamin PG, Holthouse I, Lumsden L, Liversidge J. 1994. Localization and characterization of major histocompatibility complex class II-positive cells in the posterior segment of the eye: implications for induction of autoimmune uveoretinitis. Invest Ophthalmol Vis Sci 35:64–77.

Gabrielian K, Oganesian A, Patel SC, Nucci P, Ernest JT. 1995. Cellular response in rabbit eyes after subretinal injection of human fetal RPE cells. Invest Ophthalmol Vis Sci 36(4):5249.

Gaur V, Agarwal N, Li L, Turner JE. 1992. Maintenance of opsin and S-antigen gene expression in RCS dystrophic rats following RPE transplantation. Exp Eye Res 54(1):91–101.

Gelanze M, Breipohl W, Wiedemann P, Naib-majani W, Heimann K. 1993. First experimental iris pigment epithelial cell transplantation in subretinal space of RCS rats. Invest Ophthalmol Vis Sci 34(suppl):1097.

Gelanze M, Meneses P, Rosenfeld MR, Duvoisin RM, Coleman DJ. 1997. Long-term results of autologous transplantation of iris pigmented epithelial cells into the subretinal space. Invest Ophthalmol Vis Sci 38(4):S334.

Gouras P, Lopez R. 1989. Transplantation of retinal epithelial cells. Invest Ophthalmol Vis Sci 30:1681–1683.

Gouras P, Flood MT, Eggers HM, Kjeldbye H. 1984. Transplantation of cultured human retinal cells to monkey retina. An Acad Brasil, Ciencias 56(3):431–443.

Gouras P, Flood MT, Kjeldbye H, Bilek MK, Eggers H. 1985. Transplantation of cultured human retinal epithelium to Bruch's membrane of the owl monkey's eye. Curr Eye Res 4:253–265.

Gouras P, Lopez R, Brittis M, Kjeldbye H, Fasano MK. 1986. Transplantation of cultured retinal epithelium. In: Agardh E, Ehinger B, eds, Retinal Signals System, Degenerations and Transplants. Amsterdam: Elsevier, 271–286.

Gouras P, Lopez R, Brittis M, Kjeldbye H, Sullivan B. 1988. The experimental route to curing a rat retinal dystrophy by transplantation. In: Favilla I, ed, Proc. 5th International RP Congress. Melbourne: Australian RP Foundation, 267–276.

Gouras P, Lopez R, Kjeldbye H, Sullivan B, Brittis M. 1989. Transplantation of retinal epithelium prevents photoreceptor degeneration in the RCS rat. In: Progress in Clinical and Biological Research, vol 314. Inherited and Environmentally Induced Retinal Degenerations. New York: Liss, 659–671.

Gouras P, Lopez R, Du J, Gelanze M, Kwun R, Kjeldbye H. 1990.

Transplantation of retinal cells. Neuro-Ophthalmology 10:165–176.

Gouras P, Lopez R, Brittis M, Kjeldbye H. 1992. The ultrastructure of transplanted rabbit retinal epithelium. Graefes Arch Clin Exp Ophthalmol 230:468–475.

Gouras P, Cao H, Sheng Y, Tanabe T, Efremova Y, Kjeldbye H. 1994a. Patch culturing and transfer of human fetal retinal epithelium. Graefes Arch Clin Exp Ophthalmol 232:599–607.

Gouras P, Du J, Kjeldbye H, Yamamoto S, Zack DJ. 1994b. Long-term photoreceptor transplants in dystrophic and normal mouse retina. Invest Ophthalmol Vis Sci 35:3145–3153.

Gouras P, Berglin L, Sheng Y, Cao H, Lavid J, Lin PK, Bergman L, Kjeldbye H. 1995. Long term human RPE transplants in monkey retina. Invest Ophthalmol Vis Sci 36(4):S211.

Gouras P, Berglin L, Sheng Y. 1996. Human fetal RPE xenografts in monkey retina. Invest Ophthalmol Vis Sci 37(3):S95.

Grierson I, Hiscott P, Hogg P, Robey H, Mazure A, Larken G. 1994. Development, repair, and regeneration of the retinal pigment epithelium. Eye 8:255–262.

Griffith TS, Brunner T, Flectcher SM, Green DR, Ferguson TA. 1995. Fas-Ligand-induced apoptosis as a mechanism of immune priviledge. Science 270:1189.

Gus S-M, Thompson DA, Srisailapathy Srikumari CR, Lorenz B, Finckh U, Nicoletti A, Murphy KR, Rathmann M, Kumaramanickavel G, Denton MJ, Gal A. 1997. Mutations in RPE65 cause autosomal recessive childhood-onset severe retinal dystrophy. Nature Genetics 17:194-197.

Guerin G, Lewis P, Fisher SK, Anderson DH. 1993. Recovery of photoreceptor outer segment length and analysis of membrane assembly rates in regenerating primate photoreceptor outer segments. Invest Ophthalmol Vis Sci 34:175–183.

Hasson T, Heintzelman MB, Santos-Sacchi J, Corey DP, Mooseker MS. 1995. Expression in cochlea and retina of myosin VII, the gene product defective in Usher's syndrome type 1B. Proc Nat Acad Sci USA 92:9815–9819.

Herron WL, Riegel BW, Myers OE, Rubin ML. 1969. Retinal dystrophy in the rat: a pigment epithelial disease. Invest Ophthal 8:595–604.

Ho TC, Del Priore LV, Tezel TH, Hornbeck R, Kaplan HJ. 1995. Viability of retinal pigment epithelial cells harvested as a monolayer from tissue culture and freshly enucleated eyes by an improved method. Invest Ophthalmol Vis Sci 36(4):S251.

Ishioka M, Streilein JW, Jiang LQ. 1995. Effects of cyclosporine A on the intraocular retinal grafts. Invest Ophthalmol Vis Sci 36(4):S252.

Jiang LQ, Hamasaki D. 1994a. The immunological barrier to successful rescue of visual function in RCS rats. Invest Ophthalmol Vis Sci 35:1525.

Jiang LQ, Hamasaki D. 1994b. Corneal electroretinographic function rescued by normal retinal pigment epithelial grafts in retinal degenerative Royal College of Surgeons rats. Invest Ophthalmol Vis Sci 35:4300–4309.

Jiang LQ, Jorquera M, Streilein JW. 1993. Subretinal space and vitreous cavity as immunologically privileged sites for retinal allografts. Invest Ophthalmol Vis Sci 34:3347–3354.

Jiang LQ, Jorquera M, Malek TW. 1995. The neurobiological role of interleukin-2 expressed during rejection of intraocular RPE allografts. Invest Ophthalmol Vis Sci 36(4):S212.

Johnson J. 1992. Transplanted retinal cells may give sight to sore eyes. J NIH Res 4(3):48–52.

Kaplan HJ, Yu X-H, Zhang H, Wang X, Gao E-K. 1995. Antigen specific CTL fail to recognize neoretinal antigen in vivo. Invest Ophthalmol Vis Sci 36(4):S201.

Lai C, Pawliuk R, Gouras P, Tsang S, Lu F, Doi K, Goff S, Leboulch P. 1998. Genetically engineered human RPE transplants express green fluorescent protein in the subretinal space. Invest Ophthalmol Vis Sci 39(4) in press.

Lai W, Rezaei KA, Farrokh-Siar L, Pearlmann J, Shu J, Patel SC, Ernest JT. 1997. A new method of culturing and transferring iris pigment epithelium. Invest Ophthalmol Vis Sci 38(4):S335.

Lane CM, Boulton ME. 1988. Retinal pigment epithelial transplantation: technique and possible applications. In: Brunsmann F, Gyzicki R, eds, Advances in the Biosciences: Patient Case of Retinitis Pigmentosa. Oxford: Pergamon Press, 125.

Lane CM, Boulton ME, Bridgman A, Marshall J. 1988. Transplantation of retinal epithelium in the miniature pig. Invest Ophthalmol Vis Sci 29(suppl):405.

Lane C, Boulton M, Marshall J. 1989. Transplantation of retinal pigment epithelium using a pars plana approach. Eye 3:27–32.

LaVail MM, Li L, Turner JE, Yasumura D. 1992. Retinal pigment epithelial cell transplantation in RCS rats: normal metabolism in rescued photoreceptors. Exp Eye Res 55:555–562.

Li GH, Wu LZ. 1995. The study of retinal pigment epithelial transplantation. Invest Ophthalmol Vis Sci 36(4):S250.

Li L, Turner JE. 1988a. Inherited retinal dystrophy in the RCS rat: prevention of photoreceptor degeneration by pigment epithelial cell transplantation. Exp Eye Res 47:911–947.

Li LX, Turner JE. 1988b. Transplantation of retinal pigment epithelial cells to immature and adult rat hosts: short and long-term survival characteristics. Exp Eye Res 47:771–785.

Li L, Turner JE. 1991. Optimal conditions for long-term photoreceptor cell rescue in RCS rats: the necessity for healthy RPE transplants. Exp Eye Res 52(6):669–679.

Li L, Sheedlo HJ, Turner JE. 1993a. Muller cell expression of glial fibrilary acidic protein (GFAP) in RPE-cell transplanted retinas of RCS dystrophic rats. Curr Eye Res 12(9):841–849.

Li L, Sheedlo HJ, Turner JE. 1993b. Retinal pigment epithelial cell transplants in retinal degeneration slow mice do not rescue photoreceptor cells. Invest Ophthalmol Vis Sci 34(6):2141–2145.

Li ZT, Chu H, Stepkowski SM, Garcia CA. 1992. A model of xenogenic retinal pigment epithelial cell (RPEC) transplantation. Invest Ophthalmol Vis Sci 33(4):1071.

Little CW, Castillo BV, DiLoreto DA, del Cerro C, Cox C, del Cerro M. 1995. Experimental photoreceptor rescue by human fetal retinal pigment epithelial cells. Invest Ophthalmol Vis Sci 36(4):S212.

Liu Y, Silverman MS, Berger AS, Kaplan HJ. 1992. Transplantation of confluent sheets of adult human RPE. Invest Ophthalmol Vis Sci 33:1128.

Liversidge J, Sewell HF, Forrester JV. 1988. Human retinal pigment epithelial cells differentially express MHC class II (HLA DP, DR, DQ) antigens in response to in vitro stimulation with lymphokine or purified IFN-gamma. Clin Exp Immunol 73:489–494.

Lopez PF, Grossniklaus HE, Lambert M, Aaberg TM, Capone A Jr, Sternberg P Jr, L'Hernault N. 1991. Pathological features of surgically excised subretinal neovascular membranes in age-related macular degeneration. Am J Ophthalmol 112:647–656.

Lopez PF, Yan Q, Kohen L, et al. 1995. Retinal pigment epithelial wound healing in vivo. Arch Ophthalmol 113:1437–1446.

Lopez R, Gouras P, Brittis M, Kjeldbye H. 1987. Transplantation of cultured rabbit retinal opithelium to rabbit retina using a closed eye method. Invest Ophthal Vis Sci 28:1131–1137.

Lopez R, et al. 1989. Transplanted retinal pigment epithelium modifies the retinal degeneration in the RCS rat. Invest Ophthalmol Vis Sci 30:586–588.

Lund RD, Coffey PJ. 1994. Visual information processing by intracerebral retinal transplants in rats. Eye 8:263–268.

Mashhour B, Renard G. 1997. Iris pigment epithelium autotransplantation in exudative ARMD. Invest Ophthalmol Vis Sci 38(4):S657.

Marmor MF, Abdul-Rahim AS, Cohen DS. 1980. The effect of metabolic inhibitors on retinal adhesion and subretinal fluid absorption. Invest Ophthal Vis Sci 19:893–903.

Maw MA, Kennedy B, Knight A, Bridges R, Roth KE, Mani EJ, Mukkadan JK, Nancarrow D, Crabb JW, Denton MJ. 1997. Mutation of the gene encoding cellular retinaldehyde-binding protein in autosomal recessive retinitis pigmentosa. Nature Genetics 17: 198–200.

McLaren MJ, Holderby M, Brown ME, Inana G. 1992. Kinetics of ROS binding and ingestion by cultured RCS rat RPE cells: modulation by conditioned media and bFGF. Invest Ophthal Vis Sci 33(suppl):1027.

Moritera T, Peyman GA, Rahimy MH, Luo Q, Wafapoor H, Gebhardt BM. 1993. Transplants of monolayer retinal pigment epithelium grown on biodegradable membrane in rabbits. Invest Ophthalmol Vis Sci 34:1093.

Mullin RJ, LaVail MM. 1976. Inherited retinal dystrophy: primary defect in pigment epithelium determined with rat chimeras. Science 192:799–801.

Organesian A, Gabrielian K, Patel SC, Ernest JT, Khadem J. 1995. Growth of human fetal RPE patches on different biologic matrices. Invest Ophthalmol Vis Sci 36(4):S251.

Ozaki S, Yamana T, Kita M, Negi A, Honda Y. 1995. The reorganization process of the retinal pigment epithelium-photoreceptor interface for 6 months observation after RPE removal. Invest Ophthalmol Vis Sci 36(4):S252.

Parolini B, Sugino IK, Gordon E, Zarbin MA. 1995. A new method to debride RPE cells from Bruch's membrane. Invest Ophthalmol Vis Sci 36(4):S252.

Perry J, Du J, Kjeldbye H, Gouras P. 1995. The effects of bFGF on RCS rat eyes. Curr Eye Res 14:585–592.

Peyman GA, Blinder KJ, Paris CL, Alturki W, Nelson NC, Desai U. 1991. A technique for retinal pigment epithelium transplantation for age-related macular degeneration secondary to extensive subfoveal scarring. Ophthalmic Surg 22:102–108.

Reppucci V, Goluboff E, Wapner F, Syniuta L, Brittis M, Sullivan B, Gouras P. 1988. Retinal pigment epithelium transplantation in the RCS rat. Invest Ophthalmol Vis Sci 29(suppl):144.

Rezai KA, Kohen L, Wiedemann P, Heimann K. 1997. Iris pigment epithelium transplantation. Graefes Arch Clin Exp Ophthalmol 235: 588–562.

Seaton AD, Turner JE. 1992. RPE transplants stabilize retinal vasculature and prevent neovascularization in the RCS rat. Invest Ophthalmol Vis Sci 33(1):83–91.

Seaton AD, Sheedlo HJ, Turner JE. 1994. A primary role for RPE transplants in the inhibition and regression of neovascularization in the RCS rat. Invest Ophthalmol Vis Sci 35(1):162–169.

Seregard S, Algvere PV, Berglin L. 1994. Immunohistochemical characterization of surgically removed subfoveal fibrovascular membranes. Graefes Arch Clin Exp Ophthalmol 232:325–329.

Sheedlo HJ, Gaur V, Li LX, Seaton AD, Turner JE. 1991a. Transplantation to the diseased and damaged retina. Trends in Neurosci 14(8):347–350.

Sheedlo HJ, Li L, Turner JE. 1991b. Photoreceptor cell rescue at early and late RPE-cell transplantation periods during retinal disease in RCS dystrophic rats. J Neural Transplant and Plast 2(1):55–63.

Sheedlo HJ, Li L, Gaur VP, Young RW, Seaton AD, Stovall SV, Joynes CD, Turner JE. 1992. Photoreceptor rescue in the dystrophic retina by transplantation of retinal pigment epithelium. Int Rev Cytol 138:1–49.

Sheedlo HJ, Li L, Barnstable CJ, Turner JE. 1993. Synaptic and photoreceptor components in retinal pigment epithelial cell transplanted retinas of Royal College of Surgeons dystrophic rats. J Neurosci Res 36(4):423–431.

Sheng Y, Gouras P, Cao H, Berglin L, Kjeldbye H, Lopez R, Rosskothen H. 1995a. Patch transplants of human fetal retinal pigment epithelium in rabbit and monkey retina. Invest Ophthalmol Vis Sci 36:381–390.

Sheng Y, Li W, Cao H, Lin P-K, Lavid J, Saeki M, Gouras P. 1995b. Intravitreal cyclosporine prevents RPE xenograft rejection in rabbit retina. Invest Ophthalmol Vis Sci 36(4):S250.

Silbert JE, Gao E-K, Yu X-H, Kaplan HJ. 1994. Adult murine retinal pigment epithelium is immunogenic. Invest Ophthal Vis Sci 35(4): 1525.

Silbert JE, Gao E-K, Yu X-H, Kaplan HJ. 1995. Peptide specific T-cell recognition of adult murine RPE. Invest Ophthal Vis Sci 36(4): S549.

Silverman MS, Hughes SE. 1990. Photoreceptor rescue in the RCS rat without pigment epithelium transplantation. Curr Eye Res 9:183–191.

Stinman RM. 1991. The dendritic cell system and its role in immunogenicity. Ann Rev Immunol 9:271–296.

Streilein JW. 1987. Immune regulation and the eye: a dangerous compromise. FASEB J 75:199–208.

Takeda Y, Yamada K, Tomita H, Abe T, Kojima S, Ishiguor S-I, Tamai M. 1997. bFGF-cDNA transfected iris pigment epithelium cells rescue photoreceptor cell degeneration in RCS rats. Invest Ophthalmol Vis Sci 38(4):S337.

Thomas MA. 1994. The management of subfoveal choroidal neovascularization with vitreoretinal surgery. In: Lewis H, Ryan SJ, eds, Medical and Surgical Retina. St Louis: Mosby, 63–81.

Thomas MA, Kaplan HJ. 1991. Surgical removal of subfoveal neovascularization in the presumed ocular histoplasmosis syndrome. J Ophthalmol 111(1):1–7.

Thomson RC, Collier JH, Mikos AG, Garcia CA, Giordano GG. 1995. Physical characteristics of biodegradable polymer substrates for RPE cells. Invest Ophthalmol Vis Sci 36(4):S251.

Thurmann G, Heimann K, Schraermeyer U. 1997. Quantitative phagocytosis of rod outer segments by human and porcine iris pigment epithelial cells in vitro. Invest Ophthalmol Vis Sci 38(4):S330.

Turner JE, Blair JR, Seiler M, Aramant R, Laedtke TW, Chappell ET, Clarkson L. 1988. Retinal transplants and optic nerve bridges: possible strategies for visual recovery as a result of trauma or disease. Int Rev Neurobiol 29:281–308.

Valentino A, Kaplan HJ, Del Priore LV, Fang J, Berger A, Silverman JS. 1995. Retinal pigment epithelium repopulation and photoreceptor repair after submacular surgery. Arch Ophthalmol 113:932–938.

Weil D, et al. 1995. Defective myosin VIIa gene responsible for Usher's syndrome Type IB. Nature 374:60–61.

Whiteley SJ, Lichfield TM, Tyers P, Lund RD. 1995. Retinal pigment epithelium transplanted to the subretinal space improves the pupillary light reflex in RCS rats. Invest Ophthalmol Vis Sci 36(4):S212.

Wongpichedchai S, Weiter J, Weber P, Dorey CK. 1992. Comparison of external and internal approaches for transplantation of autologous retinal pigment epithelium. Invest Ophthalmol Vis Sci 33: 3341–3352.

Yamaguchi K, Yamaguchi K, Young RW, Gaur VP, Greven CM. 1992. Vitreoretinal surgical technique for transplanting retinal pigment epithelium in rabbit retina. Jpn J Ophthalmol 36(2):142–150.

Yamaguchi K, Yamaguchi K, Gaur VP, Turner JE. 1993a. Effect of neonatal retinal pigment cell transplantation on aged retinas. Nippon Ganka Gakkai Zasshi—Acta Soc Ophthal Jpn 97(1):36–42.

Yamaguchi K, Yamaguchi K, Gaur VP, Turner JE. 1993b. Retinal pigment epithelial cell transplantation into aging retina: a possible approach to delay age-related cell death. Jpn J Ophthalmol 37(1):16–27.

Yamamoto S, Du J, Gouras P, Kjeldbye H. 1993. Retinal pigment epithelial transplants and retinal function in RCS rats. Invest Ophthalmol Vis Sci 34:3068–3075.

Yang D, Peyman GA, Luo Q, Liang C. 1995. Partially cross-linked gelatin membranes for RPE cell transplantation and retinal tissue regeneration. Invest Ophthalmol Vis Sci 36(4):S249.

Ye J, Wang HM, Ogden TE, Ryan SJ. 1993. Allotransplantation of rabbit retinal pigment epithelial cells double-labelled with 5-bromodeoxyuridine (BrdU) and natural pigment. Curr Eye Res 12: 629–639.

Zhang XY, Ohmen JD, Bok D. 1995. Antigen presenting cell function of human retinal pigment epithelial cells in superantigens induced T cell activation. Invest Ophthal Vis Sci 36(4):S549.

VII | INFLAMMATION AND CHOROIDAL DISEASE

26. Regulation of immune responses by the retinal pigment epithelium

JANET LIVERSIDGE AND JOHN V. FORRESTER

Inflammation of the choroid, retina, and vitreous is an important pathogenic feature of a wide spectrum of inflammatory diseases of the eye, leucocytic infiltration representing the coordinated response of the immune system to infection or injury. The immune system has a number of different mechanisms to protect the individual. These may be separated into two forms; *natural or inate immunity,* which provides immediate protection but is broad spectrum, and *acquired immunity,* which is highly specific for the invading pathogen. Acquired immunity is initially slow (1–2 weeks) but is rapidly reactivated and amplified with each reexposure to the pathogen. Both systems utilize circulating molecules and cells which secrete mediators which activate other cells. In natural immunity, complement provides the circulating factor, with natural killer cells and phagocytes such as macrophages and neutrophils providing the cellular component. These cells secrete the soluble mediators (cytokines), which bring other inflammatory cells to the site, allowing specific immunity to be acquired or reactivated. The specificity of the acquired response is generated by specialized antigen-presenting cells (APCs) such as dendritic cells (DC), which have the ability to activate naive T helper lymphocytes, which in turn activate the B lymphocyte response and specific antibody secretion.

Physicochemical barriers such as the skin and mucosal surfaces are also important in both forms of immunity. The retinal pigment epithelium (RPE) and the underlying Bruch's membrane form the outermost layer of the retina and constitute one-half of the blood–retina barrier and can therefore also act as an immunological barrier. Strategically placed to interact with cells of both the choroid and retina, the RPE can regulate the traffic of both cells and cell products, and by influencing the microenvironment of the adjacent choroidal tissue to which circulating leucocytes have free access, the RPE will act as a component of the immune system.

RPE cells have been extensively studied in order to understand how they may participate in the pathogenesis of ocular inflammation associated with proliferative disorders or autoimmunity. Although considered to be a terminally differentiated cell, under certain pathological conditions such as inflammation the RPE cell undergoes activation and may become multilayered (Forrester et al., 1985), and under the influence of cytokines such as interferon-γ (IFN-γ), which is a product mainly of natural killer (NK) cells and T cells, cultured RPE cells undergo morphological changes involving the actin cytoskeleton and acquire a migratory phenotype (Martini et al., 1991) (Fig 26-1a & 26-1b). Such changes suggest that the barrier function of the RPE would be disrupted early in inflammation, allowing unimpeded access to the retina for inflammatory cells from the choroid. However, in vivo the barrier appears to remain largely intact with physical breakdown and RPE necrosis delayed until the later stages of acute inflammations such as experimental autoimmune uveoretinitis (EAU) (Dua et al., 1991; Greenwood et al., 1994) (Fig 26-2). Indeed a large body of research, largely in the animal model, would suggest that the RPE is actively immunosuppressive during inflammations (reviewed, Forrester et al., 1995). Conversely, selective chemical disruption of the RPE in Lewis rats by the administration of sodium iodate has been shown to inhibit the development (EAU) (Konda et al., 1994). This implies, in the animal model at least, that the RPE also has a physiological role in the induction and/or perpetuation of autoimmune uveoretinitis. Such conflicting data underline the complexity of the RPE and its role in maintaining a balance between assisting with the elimination of infectious organisms while protecting the retina from the potentially damaging consequences of cytotoxic immune mediators.

In this chapter we will review various aspects of RPE cell function in relation to its immunoregulatory role in ocular inflammation and where possible, compare in vitro data with in vivo observations from rat models and human tissue. The potential of the RPE to participate actively in regulating ocular inflammation, by secreting various pro- and antiinflammatory cytokines while interacting directly with infiltrating leucocytes via cell surface activation and accessory molecules, will be discussed in the context of the hypothesis that immunological homeostasis in the eye is the result of active immunosuppression by ocular cells such as the RPE.

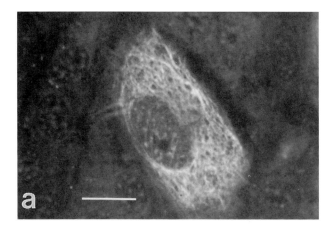 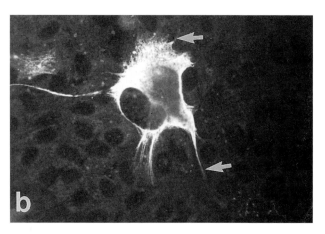

FIGURE 26-1. Actin cytoskeleton in RPE cells. Confocal scanning laser microscope images of human RPE cells labeled with an antibody to the filamentous form of actin and indirectly stained with fluorocein. Cells cultured in (a) medium alone, showing a regular, loose distribution of the filaments; (b) stimulated with 200 u/ml IFN-γ for 4 days, cell migrating beneath monolayer showing rearrangement of the filaments, the cell adopting a stellate morphology, with long cytoplasmic protrusions and bundles of actin fibers extending to adhesion foci (arrowed). Bar = 15 μm. (J. Liversidge.)

IMMUNOREGULATION AT THE BLOOD–RETINA INTERFACE; THE EYE AS A SITE OF IMMUNE PRIVILEGE

The blood–retina barrier, which effectively isolates the retina and the posterior segment of the eye from the circulation, creates a microenvironment in which normal immune responses to foreign antigens are modulated (Forrester et al., 1995). A similar situation exists in the brain, which is separated from the normal circulation by the blood–brain barrier (Thomsett, 1990), the absence of lymphatic drainage coupled with a previously assumed lack of acknowledged immunocompetent anti-

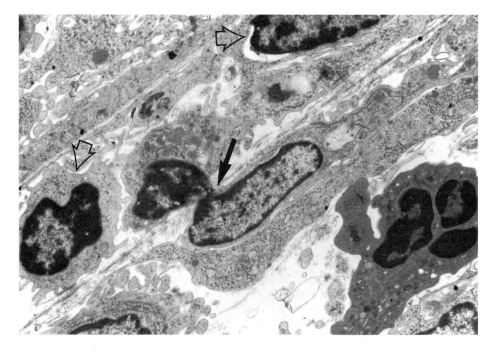

FIGURE 26-2. Inflammatory cells migrating across the RPE. Bruch's membrane is intact, but separated with the inner cuticular layer at the RPE and the outer collagenous layer at the choriocapilaris where a leucocyte can be seen migrating through a pore (black arrow). Other leucocytes (open arrows) are lying between the RPE cells and the layers of Bruch's membrane. (Dua et al., 1991.)

gen-presenting cells in both tissues creating the concept of sites of immune privilege. The purpose of these barriers has been assumed to be a mechanism for protecting these vulnerable sites from inflammation and cytotoxic damage. However, differences between the two sites exist, as one half of the barrier in the retina comprises neuroectodermal RPE cells, and unlike the brain, the immunosuppressive environment in the eye is not restricted to tissue behind the barrier. For instance, Hara and colleagues (1992) suppressed the development of posterior chamber EAU in mice by placing the retinal autoantigen IRBP in the anterior segment of the eye. This phenomenon has been extensively studied and is described as *anterior-chamber associated immune deviation* (ACAID) (Ferguson et al., 1987; Neiderkorn et al., 1990; Streilein et al., 1992a).

ACAID has been attributed to the secretion of immunosuppressive cytokines such as transforming growth factor (TGF)-β and tumor necrosis factor (TNF)-α (Cousins et al., 1991; Strielein et al., 1992b; Ferguson et al., 1994) and the presence of various neuropeptides such as melanocyte-stimulating hormone and vasointestinal active peptide (Taylor et al., 1992; 1994). As similar responses have been demonstrated with antigens placed within the vitreous cavity and subretinal space (Jiang et al., 1993), the immunosuppression observed within the posterior chamber is presumed to be an active process governed by the cells of the retina, rather than merely the effect of a physical barrier. APCs must also be involved in the ACAID response, since the immune suppression observed requires an intact spleen and involves an antigen-specific systemic response, which depresses cell-mediated immune responses such as delayed type hypersensitivity (DTH) reactions to the antigen at sites distant from the eye (Willbanks and Streilein, 1991; Streilein et al., 1992a; Ferguson and Herndon, 1994).

Dendritic cells (DC) present within the iris have been implicated in ACAID, but the APCs responsible for posterior chamber immune deviation are less readily identified. Antigens in the vitreous cavity could be available for processing and presentation by DCs in the ciliary body. Since ciliary body DCs have the same life history as DCs within the iris, migrating forward through the anterior chamber and being exposed to aqueous fluids before exiting the eye via the angle structures into the circulation (McMenamin and Holthouse 1992), ACAID-like responses to vitreous antigens could be induced. However, the vitreous also contains inhibitory factors (Young & Lutty 1987; Connor et al., 1989), so immunosuppression could also be induced by cells located in the posterior chamber such as the RPE, which is not only strategically positioned to interact with circulating lymphocytes, but also secretes the soluble mediators that have been shown to influence immune responses in the eye and beyond. In particular the RPE can produce both TGF-β and TGF-β-binding protein (Tanihara et al., 1993) which regulates TGF-β activity in vivo, and secrete both prostaglandin E$_2$ (PGE$_2$) and nitric oxide (NO), which inhibit lymphocyte proliferation (Liversidge et al., 1993a; 1994a; 1994b) (see below). Therefore the RPE, together with ciliary body cells (Helbig et al., 1990) and Müller cells (Caspi et al., 1987), which have also been shown to have immunosuppressive effects on lymphocyte activation, contributes to the predominantly immunosuppressive environment within the eye. All are important regulators of immunological homeostasis throughout the retina and posterior chamber of the eye.

RPE CELL EXPRESSION OF REGULATORY MOLECULES ASSOCIATED WITH NATURAL IMMUNE FUNCTION

A major function of the RPE is phagocytosis of the continually regenerating and diurnally shed photoreceptor outer segments. This process requires recognition, attachment, and ingestion, each event requiring cell surface receptors and ligands in a process similar to macrophage phagocytosis (Gordon, 1986). The RPE is derived from neural ectoderm and expresses simple cytokeratins, confirming that it is a true epithelium. However, RPE cells also express other antigens which are more usually associated with monocytic cells derived from the bone marrow. Expression of these monocyte/macrophage-like features may be linked to the principal phagocytic and degradative function of the cell, but also provides the RPE with additional, vital scavenging functions to minimize damage to the delicate retina in the event of inflammation or infection. For instance, Rao and colleagues (1996) have recently identified a novel, protective protein, secreted only by RPE cells which can inhibit superoxide generation by neutrophils and macrophages. This protein can be detected at a low level in normal rabbit eyes and is marked upregulated in both endotoxin-induced uveitis and EAU. In addition, CD68 is an intracytoplasmic molecule associated with lysosomes and is believed to be important in intracellular degradation of phagocytic material. This antigen is widely distributed in mononuclear phagocytes including monocytes and fully differentiated macrophages, but it is also constitutively expressed by up to 10% of human RPE in vivo (Liversidge and Forrester, 1991) and is upregulated in cultured cells (Elner et al., 1992a).

The primary function of mononuclear phagocytes is to function both as accessory and effector cells in the immune response, playing a role in the cognitive, activation, and effector phases of specific immunity. In the effector phase of the immune response, foreign antigens such as microbes become coated by antibody molecules and complement proteins. These opsonized particles can then be efficiently bound and phagocytosed by cells expressing specific receptors. Complement proteins therefore form an important part of the initial, natural immune response. The complement cascade is regulated at two critical steps. First, the formation and degradation of C3b and, second, at the formation and function of the terminal cytolytic membrane attack complex (MAC). Several receptors for these proteins have been found on RPE cells and probably reflect additional vital functions for the RPE in protecting the eye during an inflammation. For instance, receptors for the Fc portion of IgG immunoglobulin (CD16) have been found on freshly isolated but not cultured RPE cells, which would enable the ingestion and disposal of immune complexes (Elner et al., 1981; Dutt et al., 1986; Eckert and Hafeman, 1986), and in addition, Elner and colleagues (1981) have also demonstrated the complement receptor C3b (CD35) and the C3Bi complement receptor (CD11b/CD18) on freshly isolated RPE.

Complement-regulatory proteins are required to control the complement cascade and protect host tissue from damage. These are membrane-bound cofactor proteins including (MCP, CD46), decay accelerating factor (DAF, CD55), and membrane attack complex inhibiting protein (CD59). These proteins are differentially expressed by various tissues within the eye (Bora et al., 1993). In the retina, MCP and DAF are expressed at a low level within the photoreceptor cell layer layer but CD59, the MAC inhibitor, is strongly expressed throughout the retina, including in the RPE, providing evidence that a regulatory system exists to protect these cells from complement damage (Fig. 26-3a and Plate 26-I). These molecules may also have other functions which remain to be determined. CD59 for instance also regulates complement activation of platelets and moreover may interact with CD2 on T lymphocytes. A role for CD59 in the activation of T cells is controversial, but recent in vitro evidence has shown that CD59 expressed by RPE cells can activate T cells polyclonally, inducing IL-2 driven T cell growth (Liversidge et al., 1996).

Other monocytic immunoregulatory receptors identified on the RPE include CD11c and CD14 (Elner, 1989; Liversidge and Forrester 1991). The CD11/CD18 family of integrin molecules have previously been thought to be restricted to hematopoetic cells (Springer, 1990). Controversy over the presence of these receptors on RPE cells has stemmed from the failure to find expression on cultured cells; however, these receptors are rapidly shed in short-term culture, and their restoration depends upon a mature, differentiated phenotype being r-established (Limb et al., 1988).

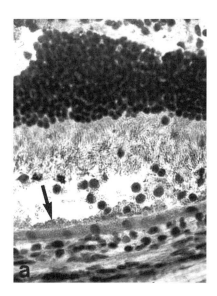 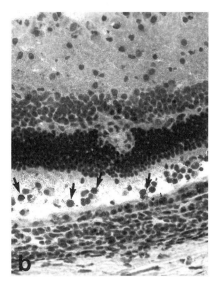 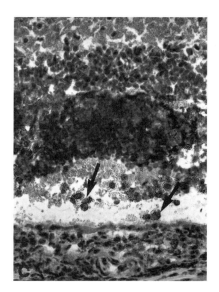

FIGURE 26-3. Complement regulatory protein CD59 (MAC inhibitor) expression during EAU. Photomicrographs of Lewis rat retina during early stages of retinal antigen induced EAU. The choroid is filled with inflammatory cells, and leucocytes can be seen in the rod photoreceptor outer segments of the retina in close apposition to the RPE. The inner and outer nuclear layers of the retina contain some inflammatory cells but are still relatively intact. The choroid is thickened and also contains lymphocytes and monocytes. (a) APAAP staining with a monoclonal antibody to rat CD59 showing strong staining on the apical surface of the RPE (arrowed) as well as on infiltrating inflammatory cells. Adjacent sections from the same eye indicate that the inflammatory cells are; (b) CD2+ve T-lymphocytes and (c) ED1+ve monocyte/macrophages. (J. Liversidge and S. Hoey.)

Interaction between receptors and their ligands usually transmit intracellular signals in the cells involved, resulting in further activation and functional changes. The major function of CD11b is to bind the complement component iC3b with induction of phagocytosis (Keizer et al., 1987) and to control the adhesion and degranulation of neutrophils (Shleiffenbaum et al., 1989). Possession of all these receptors by the RPE in combination with mannose 6-phosphate receptors (McLaughlin et al., 1987) and other scavenging receptors (Hayes et al., 1989) provides the RPE with the ability to eliminate foreign antigens and underlines their role as a first line of defense against infection in the absence of professional macrophages. In addition, expression of CD14, which is the lipopolysaccharide (LPS) receptor, assists with the clearance of gram-negative bacteria and specifically induces the synthesis of the cytokine TNF-α, one of the earliest mediators of an immune response.

RPE CELLS AS SOURCES OF REGULATORY INFLAMMATORY CYTOKINES

Cytokines are soluble mediators that are secreted by many cell types and control inflammation by inducing chemotaxis and activation of inflammatory cells, the combination of cytokines influencing the selection of leucocytes to the site. It is clear that cytokines have a major influence on the pathogenesis of various intraocular inflammations; several cytokines, including TNF, IL-1, IL-6, IL-8 and IFN-γ, have been shown to possess uveitogenic properties when inoculated into experimental animals (reviewed de Vos et al., 1992; 1994). In addition, various therapeutic strategies to inhibit certain cytokines can also exacerbate (de Vos et al., 1995) or ameliorate experimental ocular inflammations.

It might be expected that cytokines secreted by the initial leucocyte infiltrate would be proinflammatory while cytokines released by tissue cells would be antiinflammatory, with the aim of limiting tissue destruction. However cytokine gene expression is complex and human RPE cells have been shown to express mRNA and gene product for a wide variety of pro- inflammatory cytokines as well as other anti-inflammatory cytokines under various culture conditions, both in response to stimulation with exogenous cytokines or in response to endogenously generated signals during coculture with activated T lymphocytes (Fig. 26-4) (Liversidge et al., 1994a; 1994b). It is therefore important to consider the effects of cytokines produced by T cells present within the infiltrate on RPE cells. For instance, human sympathetic ophthalmitis has many characteristics typical of a delayed type hypersensitivity (DTH) reaction (Liver-

sidge, 1993b). DTH reactions are initiated by T helper 1 type lymphocytes which secrete IFN-γ, followed by granuloma formation under the influence of T helper 2 type lymphocytes which secrete IL-4 and are associated with downregulation of immune responses (Powrie et al., 1993).

IL-1-β and TNF-α are mediators of the host inflammatory response in natural immunity and are therefore among the first mediators produced in the cytokine cascade, and blockade of their action reduces structural damage to the retina in experimental autoimmune uveoretinitis (EAU). Jaffe and colleagues (1995) using supernatants from activated monocytes found that IL-1β and TNF-α were the principal activating cytokines stimulating RPE cytokine gene expression, and these cytokines, alone or in combination with others have been extensively used to stimulate RPE cells in vitro. RPE can themselves produce TNF-α in response to bacterial LPS or IFN-γ (de Kozak et al., 1994) but although human RPE cells synthesise IL-1β, the secreted form of the protein has not yet been detected (Jaffe et al., 1992; Planck et al., 1993). However, within the eye, Müller cells are known to secrete both IL-1β and TNFα (Roberge et al., 1988), which in turn induce RPE cells to secrete IL-6 (Benson et al., 1992; Plank et al., 1992; Forrester et al., 1995) and the neutrophil chemotactic factors IL-8 and MCP-1 (Elner et al., 1990; 1996).

Interleukin-6 secretion, in response to IL-1β and TNF-α, has been shown to be further increased by interaction with the cytokines IL-4, IL-13, and IFN-γ (Forrester et al., 1995). Both IL-6 and IL-8 are also involved in lymphocyte activation and chemotaxis, and induce an inflammatory response when injected intravitrally (Hoekzema et al., 1990; Ferrick et al., 1991). Moreover, Kuppner and colleagues (1995) found that the effect of IL-1β on IL-6 and IL-8 mRNA expression by RPE cells was synergistically enhanced by the addition of TGF-β, which is also present within the eye (Pasquale et al., 1993) and which can be secreted in an active form by RPE cells. TGF-β is thought to be primarily involved in the maintainance of the immunosuppressive ocular environment (Cousins et al., 1991), but it can also have transient proinflammatory properties (Wahl et al., 1989). For instance, TGF-β synergizes with IL-1β to enhance RPE cell expression of both IL-6 and IL-8 mRNA, however different transcriptional and translational mechanisms are involved since only IL-6 secretion is increased (Kuppner et al., 1995), further underlining the complexity of cytokine interactions during inflammation. Other cytokines expressed by RPE include basic fibroblast growth factor (bFGF), nerve growth factor (NGF) (Dicou et al., 1994), and the melanoma-growth-stimulating chemokine GROα and γ

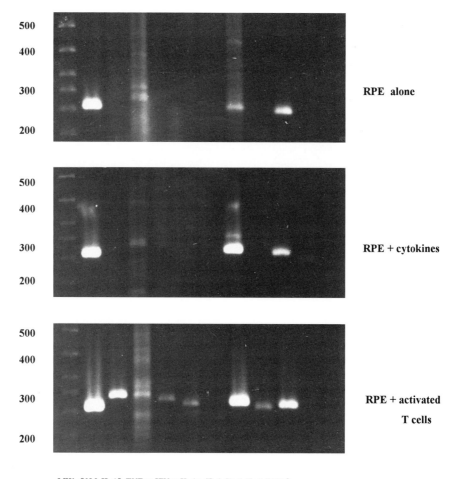

MW β2M IL-1β TNF-α IFN-γ IL-1α IL-2 IL-6 IL-8 TGF-β

FIGURE 26-4. Cytokine gene expression by human RPE cells co-cultured with activated T cells. mRNAs for specific cytokines were detected by RT-PCR of total RNA from unstimulated human RPE cells, cytokine-stimulated (IFN-γ, TNF-α, and LPS for 72 hours) and activated T-cells (5 μg/ml Con-A for 4 hours) cocultured with human RPE cells for 72 hours. (Liversidge et al., 1994b.)

(growth-regulated oncogene). GROα and β are pleiotropic modulators of cell proliferation and inflammation, secretion being increased by IL-1β (Shattuck et al., 1994; Jaffe et al., 1995). Conversely, increased fibronectin release by RPE cells as part of the healing response, although stimulated by TGF-β, is reduced by IL-1β and IFN-γ (Osusky et al., 1994).

Proinflammatory IL-1β and TNF-α also stimulate RPE cultures to secrete high levels of RANTES, which is a specific chemoattractant for CD4 memory T lymphocytes and monocytes, cells which may be initiators of ocular autoimmunity. RANTES production by RPE cells was in turn found to be regulated by T cell cytokines. IL-1β induction was increased by IFN-γ, while, in contrast, TNF-α induction was reduced by IL-4, even in the presence of IFN-γ. This indicates that RANTES production, and therefore continued T cell chemoat-traction, is differentially regulated by a network of cytokine interactions in which the RPE must participate (Kuppner et al., 1996b). TNF-α also synergizes with IL-1β in the stimulation of RPE secretion of granulocyte-macrophage colony-stimulating factor (GM-CSF), which stimulates hematopoietic progenitor cells to proliferate and differentiate into mature granulocytes and macrophages at the site of inflammation (Crane et al., 1998). TGF-β has a similar synergistic effect with IL-1β, and the three cytokines together result in a sixfold increase in GM-CSF production by RPE cells compared with levels induced by IL-1β alone. The Th1 cytokine IFN-γ, in contrast to its effects on RANTES production, reduces IL-1β-induced RPE production of GM-CSF and of GM-CSF mRNA levels. Thus, early effects of the cytokine cascade will encourage granulocyte and macrophage maturation at the site of inflammation as part of the natural immune response. In the presence of IFN-γ this response will be regulated by IFN-γ, which in turn stimulates RANTES secretion and attraction of T cells to the site and development of the antigen-specific response. Recently, IL-15 expression by transformed human fetal RPE has been detected (Kumaki et al., 1996). As IL-15 has similar T cell growth-stimulating properties to IL-2, these cells have the additional potential for regulating growth of infiltrating T cells.

The synergistic effects of cytokine combinations revealed by many of the in vitro experiments mentioned here are important, and indicate that leucocyte activation and chemotaxis in vivo may occur even when only very small amounts of the individual proinflammatory cytokines are present, allowing physiological levels of cytokines to be reached very early in injury or infection and rapid responses to be made by the immune system.

Leucocyte migration in response to chemokines such as RANTES, IL-8 (T lymphocytes and neutrophils), MIP-1α (monocytes/macrophages, T lymphocytes, and neutrophils), MCP-1 (monocyte chemotactic protein-1), and MCAF (monocyte attraction and activation factor) (Murphy, 1994) depends upon physical as well as soluble signals, involving interactions between adhesion molecules expressed by the leucocytes and the endothelium or RPE. Cytokines, which provide the soluble signals, also influence the expression of adhesion molecules by tissue cells, including the RPE cells which provide the physical signals, and these changes allow increased migration into the site, resulting in chronic inflammation and progressive tissue damage.

THE BLOOD–RETINA BARRIER AND TRANSEPITHELIAL MIGRATION OF LEUCOCYTES

The mechanisms by which inflammatory cells leave the circulation and cross the tight junctions of the blood–retina barrier to enter the retina have been studied mostly at the level of the endothelium, and although lymphocytes are known to migrate through endothelial cells (Greenwood et al., 1994) interactions with RPE cells are less well characterized. Since inflammatory cells must cross both the choroidal endothelium and the RPE to reach target autoantigens in the rod outer segment (ROS) of the retina, it has been proposed that the initial breakdown of the blood–retina barrier occurs at the retinal endothelium. However, Konda and colleageus (1994) have shown that the RPE is required for induction of retinal autoimmunity and that retinal antigen-specific T cells are also likely to be recruited via the choroidal circulation due to the proximity of the target antigens and the ease of diapedesis across fenestrated

endothelium. Other observations in chronic or mild disease such as cell transfer models of EAU (Forrester et al., 1992; Dick et al., 1995) suggest that a thickening of the choroid by inflammatory cells precedes retinal inflammation, and the earliest infiltrates appear to be CD4[+]ve T cells and macrophages within the ROS coincident with development of retinal vasculitis, indicating that breakdown of the barrier at the RPE can be an early event in autoimmune uveoretinitis (Fig. 26-5).

Cell–cell and cell–substratum interactions are mediated through several different families of receptors. In addition to targeting cell adhesion to specific extracellular matrix proteins and ligands on adjacent cells, adhesion molecules influence many diverse processes, including cellular growth, differentiation, junction formation, and polarity. Activation of adhesion molecules and their ligands is crucial for effective immune surveillance and aggregation at the site of infection, whereas abnormal expression of such molecules, for instance on RPE cells, is involved in pathological conditions such as proliferative vitreoretinopathy (Robbins et al., 1994). Cells of the immune system normally circulate as nonadherent cells in the blood and lymph, but rapid transition between nonadherent and adherent states occurs in response to soluble mediators and other changes in the tissue. Three families of molecules have been implicated in the interactions that culminate in firm leucocyte adherence and transendothelial or transepithelial migration: the selectins, the integrins (LFA-1, VLA-α), and the immunoglobulin (Ig) superfamily (ICAM-1 and ICAM-2, VCAM-1) (Albeda and Buck, 1990).

Receptors for many leucocyte adhesion molecules are more strongly expressed on RPE with intraocular inflammatory diseases such as sympathetic ophthalmia than with normal eye tissue, with the enhanced and sometimes de novo expression of adhesion molecules such as ICAM-1, VCAM-1, and ELAM-1, together with the "homing receptor" CD 44, which also controls lymphocyte trafficking (Duguid et al., 1991; Whitcup et al., 1992). Increased mRNA expression of these immune adhesion molecules can be induced by IL-1 and TNF-α, cytokines which, together with NK-cell-derived IFN-γ, are expressed early in the immune response to infections, and which also initiate the cytokine cascade (see above) (Elner SG et al., 1992b; Platts et al., 1995). These molecules regulate the migration of leucocytes into inflammatory sites (Oppenheimer-Marks et al., 1991; Bird et al., 1993) Kuppner and colleagues (1993), compared adhesion molecule expression in acute and fibrotic sympathetic ophthalmia with normal eyes. Expression of several integrins of the VLA family which form receptors for various extracellular matrix proteins were found to be expressed by the RPE. However, VLA-

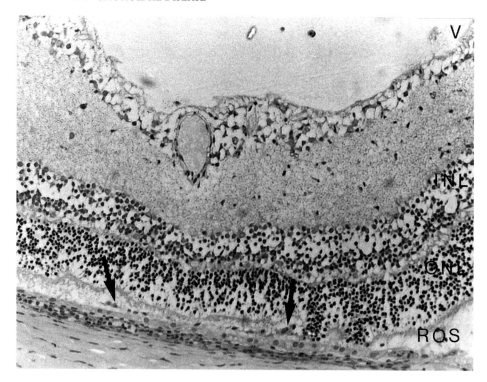

FIGURE 26-5. EAU induced by retinal-antigen-specific T-cell transfer. Transfer of 5×10^6 retinal-antigen-specific CD4+ve T-cells to naive rats induces retinal disease by day 5. The T-cells observed in the ROS *(arrowed)* can be identified as originating from the donor retinal-anti-gen-specific T-cell lines by immunocytochemical techniques. (V), vitreous; (INL), inner nuclear layer; (ONL), outer nuclear layer; (ROS), rod outer segments; (RPE), retinal pigment epithelium; (C), choroid. (Dick et al., 1996.)

4, (the ligand for VCAM-1 and fibronectin), VLA-5 (fibronectin), and VLA-6 (laminin), which were increased in acute and sympathetic eyes were not upregulated on RPE cells. In contrast, ICAM-1 and CD44 expression were greatly enhanced.

Cellular adhesion via integrins and Ig superfamily receptors are stable and of high avidity, enabling RPE–T cell interactions to be analyzed in vitro. RPE cells have been shown to retain many of their in vivo characteristic in vitro, secreting components of the extracellular matrix (Campochiario et al., 1986) and expressing endogenous cadherin which form adherens junctions and a tight monolayer (Marrs et al., 1995). Thus, RPE cells are useful for studies on leucocyte diapedesis. Using an adhesion assay, in which individual receptors are blocked physiologically or by specific antibodies, it was found that constitutive expression of ICAM-1 by human RPE cells is upregulated by cytokines, and that T cell binding to RPE cells is predominantly via the ICAM-1 receptor—although another important adhesion pathway used by endothelial cells, in which LFA-3 (CD58) binds T cell CD2, was not found (Liversidge et al., 1990). The lack of CD58 expression by an epithelium is very unusual, and may account for the poor co-stimulatory activity of RPE cells in antigen presentation assays (see below). Further work, carried out using rat RPE cells by Mesri and colleagues (1994a; 1996), has indicated that activation of the LFA-1 molecule on the T cell is crucial for adhesion to and subsequent migration across the monolayers to occur, and Devine and colleagues (1996) have shown that migration across RPE cells by antigen-specific T cells can be blocked by antibodies to both LFA-1 and VCAM-1. In addition, although endothelial cells preferentially bind CD4+ve T cells, RPE cells also bind significant numbers of CD8+ve T cells, suggesting that the RPE cells may have an additional adhesion receptor not expressed by endothelium (G. Neill, unpublished observation). The importance of these particular cell adhesion molecules in directing antigen-specific activated T cell to the target tissue is underlined by in vivo studies demonstating the inhibitory effects of antibodies to ICAM-1 and LFA-1 on the development of EAU (Whitcup et al., 1992; 1993).

Additional differences between the retinal endothelium and the RPE appear to be in the manner in which leucocytes cross the barrier that they represent. Dua and colleagues (1991) showed that inflammatory cell movement through Bruch's membrane involved separation of its constituent layers, migration through the pores in the membrane, and crossing between the RPE cells without causing significant disruption of the RPE cell layer (Fig. 26-2). Retinal vascular endothelium diapedesis, however, involved changes in the vessels to high endothelial venule morphology, indicating endothelial cell activation (Dua et al., 1991; McMenamin et al., 1992). Leucocyte migration appears to be intracellular rather than intercellular at the tight junctions (Greenwood et al., 1994; 1995).

Adhesion molecules also have costimulatory function during antigen presentation, and it has been proposed that T cells migrating across endothelium or epithelium may also be receiving activation signals, which would affect their function. This is particularly relevant to the RPE and the induction of retinal autoimmunity, since the candidate autoantigens are located at the RPE–photoreceptor interface. It has been hypothesized that free antigen from the retina, perhaps as a result of a retinal detachment, could pass across the RPE into the choroid (Foulds, 1976). In the choroid it would be available for processing and presentation to circulating T cells by choroidal APC (Forrester et al., 1994). Alternatively, antigen could be processed and presented by the RPE cells themselves.

RPE CELLS AS ANTIGEN-PRESENTING CELLS FOR ACQUIRED IMMUNITY AND AS POTENTIAL INDUCERS OF AUTOIMMUNITY

Although the primary immunoregulatory function of the RPE is believed to be suppression of immune reactivity (Forrester et al., 1995), RPE cells, as a result of their macrophage-like features, may also be able to act as antigen-presenting cells and be involved in the activation of an immune response. Indeed the in vitro observation that under certain culture conditions T lymphocytes cocultured with RPE cells produce IL-2 and can undergo non-antigen-specific proliferation, indicate that RPE cells are capable of providing the activating signal, perhaps via the CD2/CD59 receptor cross-linking that T cells require to cross the blood–retina barrier (Liversidge and Forrester, 1992; Liversidge, 1996).

Autoimmune disease might arise following an initial tissue injury such as viral or bacterial infection with release of partially degraded autoantigens which are subsequently presented to autoreactive T cells (Opendakker and van Damme, 1994). Retinal injury almost invariably is accompanied by photoreceptor outer segment damage, thereby releasing retinal autoantigens for presentation (McMenamin et al., 1992). Since the retina is considered not to contain "professional" antigen-pre-

senting cells such as DCs or macrophages, it has been suggested that resident retinal cells might act as APCs in this situation. An obvious candidate is the RPE cell, since its primary function is to engage in photoreceptor protein uptake and proteolysis.

During thymic education, immature T cells that are cross-reactive with self-antigens expressed within the thymus are deleted. However, not all tissue antigens are expressed within the thymus, and the immune system has developed mechanisms of controlling autoreactivity. T cells that recognize specific antigen on tissue cells in the periphery, but do not receive appropriate co-stimulation, may be deleted or rendered unresponsive (anergic). Cells that are rendered tolerant in this way cannot normally be activated by specific antigen. This mechanism is known to operate for abundant autoantigens, but self antigens expressed at very low levels may evade detection and T cells specific for these antigens retain the ability to respond. The blood–retina barrier prevents recirculation of naive lymphocytes and therefore circulating T lymphocytes autoreactive with many retinal antigens are not deleted. The rod outer segments (ROS) alone contain a number of well-defined autoantigens (Faure, 1980; Gery et al., 1986) including S-antigen, interphotoreceptor retinol binding protein, phosducin (Dua et al., 1992), recoverin (Polans et al., 1993; Gery et al., 1994), and rhodopsin (Broekhuyse et al., 1991). When injected with adjuvant into susceptible animals, these antigens induce an EAU and associated pinealitis (EAP) (Wacker et al., 1991; Forrester et al., 1992).

A number of antigens specific to the RPE which can also elicit an autoimmune response have also been described, but whether these antigens are normally sequestered from circulating lymphocytes and unavailable for T cell tolerization is uncertain. The generation of autoantibodies specific to the RPE has been demonstrated both in spontaneous (Caffe et al., 1993) and virally induced murine retinal dystrophies (Hooks et al., 1993). In both cases the RPE- associated pathology appears to be secondary to the development of tumors or vasculitis. Broekhuyse and colleagues (1991; 1992a; 1992b; 1993) have identified uveitogenic antigens in both insoluble and soluble preparations of purified bovine RPE cells. The insoluble uveitogenic peptide PEP-X initiated a T–cell dependent mononuclear cell infiltrate in the anterior chamber of rats. This antigen, which was found to be melanin bound, also induced a severe iridocyclitis and choroiditis. Within the soluble fraction of the RPE cell a 65 kD antigen (PEP-65) was isolated which induced a posterior EAU characterized by a choroiditis accompanied by epitheliod or monocyte accumulations adjacent to the RPE on either side of Bruch's membrane resembling Dalen Fuch's nodules (Broekhuyse et al., 1992b). In this model, despite the development of vitreous cell infiltrates, retinal vasculitis is rare and the photoreceptors remain largely intact. These endogenous antigens would be most unlikely to be presented via class II antigens expressed by the RPE, therefore phagocytosis and degradation of damaged RPE by other APCs would be required for autoimmunity to these antigens to arise.

Retinal autoimmunity may also arise as a result of cross-reactivity between parasite antigens and components of eye tissue. For instance, antiretinal antibodies in sera from onchocerciasis patients cross react with antigens on the surface and within the nucleoli of RPE and neural retinal cells (Braun et al., 1991, Zhou et al., 1994). Braun and colleagues (1995) have characterized a clone (hr44) isolated from a cDNA library of human retina which is recognized by an antibody to an *Onchocerca* derived antigen. This antigen is located in the optic nerve, neural retina, and RPE, as well as in the epithelial layers of the ciliary body and iris. Sequence analysis of hr44 did not reveal extensive homology with other known retinal antigens, but a short sequence was found to have identity with an octopeptide from rhodopsin. In such cases it may be presumed that the normal immunosuppressive environment generated by the RPE and other ocular cells has failed, and the barrier to inflammatory cell migration presented by the RPE has broken down.

Autoimmune uveal inflammation induced by retinal antigens requires APC to endocytose, process, and present those antigens to CD4[+]ve autoreactive T cells. The majority of these autoantigens are located at the photoreceptor–RPE interface and are in the unusual position of undergoing endocytosis, and proteolysis in a diurnal cyclical fashion (Young, 1974). This is particularly true of retinal S-antigen (Reid et al., 1987), one of the most abundant soluble outer segment proteins, and most potent autoantigen (Shinohara et al., 1988) (Fig. 26-6). Presentation of antigen to CD4[+]ve T cells occurs in a highly restricted, antigen-specific manner, involving the expression of the processed peptide bound in the groove of an MHC class II molecule on an APC and recognition of that peptide by the specific T cell. The

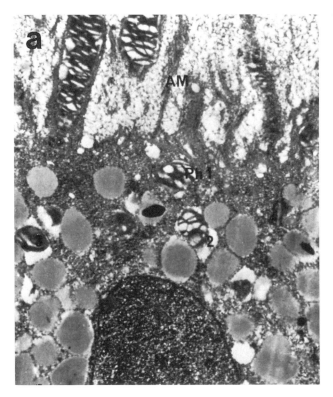
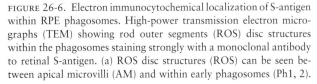
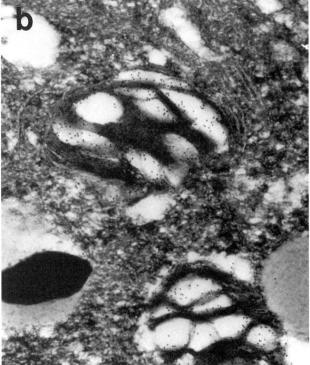

FIGURE 26-6. Electron immunocytochemical localization of S-antigen within RPE phagosomes. High-power transmission electron micrographs (TEM) showing rod outer segments (ROS) disc structures within the phagosomes staining strongly with a monoclonal antibody to retinal S-antigen. (a) ROS disc structures (ROS) can be seen between apical microvilli (AM) and within early phagosomes (Ph1, 2). Magnification ×7900; LR white. (b) High-power TEM of phagosomes Ph1 and Ph2. ROS structures showing immunogold labeling of the S-antigen epitope within the phagosomes. No staining was seen in the nucleus or cytoplasm, or within the electron-dense lysosomes. ×29,100; LR white. (Reid et al. 1987.)

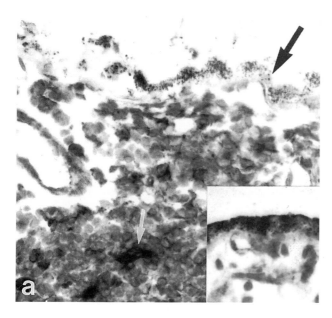
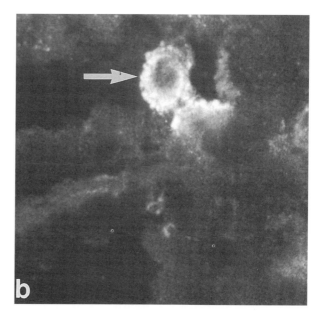

FIGURE 26-7. MHC class II antigen expression by RPE cells. (a) Acute sympathetic ophthalmia: cryostat section of human choroid stained for HLA-DR antigen, note intense staining of vascular endothelium and leucocytes including large dendritiform cells *(white arrow)*. The RPE, identified by the presence of melanin granules, was negative *(black arrow)*. In contrast, the RPE stains intensely for the ICAM-1 adhesion molecule *(inset)*. Magnification ×330. (b) Confocal image of retina and choroid from Lewis rat uveitic lesion (S-antigen-induced EAU) stained for MHC class II antigen (OX6 monoclonal antibody). The lymphocyte *(arrowed)* and central RPE cell are intensely fluorescent, with high membrane expression present on the RPE cell; note the close apposition of this RPE cell and the lymphocyte. Neighboring RPE cells show only faint staining indicating the local nature of aberrant high MHC class II expression by the RPE. ([a] J. Liversidge.)

MHC class II molecule is usually only expressed on professional APCs such as DCs, B lymphocytes, and macrophages. However, its expression can be induced on other tissue cells such as endothelial and epithelial cells by interferon-γ (IFN-γ), a proinflammatory cytokine released by activated T helper 1–type CD4[+]ve lymphocytes (Th1) or natural killer cells (NKs) as a result of viral infection or inflammation.

The hypothesis that local aberrant expression of MHC class II antigens by epithelial cells might enable these cells to present autoantigen on their surfaces to T lymphocytes as a primary event in autoimmunity was first proposed by Bottazzo and colleagues (1983). Both rat and human RPE express high levels of MHC class II antigens in vitro after exposure to IFN-γ (Liversidge et al., 1988a; 1988b) and RPE cells during experimental and clinical uveoretinitis have also been reported to express MHC class II (Chan et al., 1986a; 1986b). However expression in vivo is usually only in patchy or focal (Liversidge et al., 1993a), and morphologically normal RPE cells may fail to express MHC class II even in severe inflammation (Liversidge and Forrester, 1990; Liversidge et al., 1993b) (Fig. 26-7a and 26-7b).

Several attempts have been made to show that RPE cells can present antigen, including retinal antigens, to T cells in vitro. IFN-γ-treated rat RPE cells were found to be able to present antigen and induce IL-2 secretion, although the proliferation was not marked (Liversidge and Forrester, 1990; Percopo et al., 1990). This poor level of proliferation was found to be due to the secretion of prostaglandin E₂ (PGE₂); more efficient presentation of retinal antigen was found when indomethacin was added to the cultures and a membrane inhibitory factor removed by trypsin pretreatment (Liversidge et al., 1993a). In fact, RPE cells were found to inhibit lymphocyte proliferation induced by antigen or mitogen, even in the presence of other, immunocompetent antigen-presenting cells, a finding which reinforced the concept of immunosuppression as the primary immunological function of the RPE (see below).

RPE CELLS AS SUPPRESSORS OF LYMPHOCYTE ACTIVATION THROUGH ACTIVATION OF THE CYCLO-OXYGENASE AND INDUCIBLE NITRIC OXIDE SYNTHASE PATHWAYS

Many of the experiments which led to the concept of RPE cells as potential activators of T lymphocytes involved the addition of exogenously applied T cell cytokines in various combinations and at various concentrations which may not reflect physiological concentrations found in vivo. This is particularly evident in the general failure of RPE in vivo to express the high levels of MHC class II antigens observed in vitro. In order to mimic the in vivo situation as closely as possible, a coculture system in which T lymphocytes are cultured on monolayers of RPE cells without the addition of any exogenous cytokines has been developed (Liversidge et al., 1993a; 1994a). Using this experimental system, it was found that RPE cells were not only poor presenters of antigen to sensitized T lymphocytes but that lymphocyte proliferation to antigen even in the presence of additional, "professional" antigen-presenting cells was profoundly suppressed. Even the addition of the T cell mitogen concanavalin-A to the RPE/T cell cultures failed to induce T cell proliferation. These results were initially attributed to the secretion of high levels of PGE_2 by the RPE, but as addition of IL-2 to the cultures did not restore full T cell responsiveness, additional inhibitory factors were assumed to be present.

Similar immunosuppressive effects on T cell proliferation by macrophages have been described and have been attributed to reactive nitrogen intermediates, in particular nitric oxide (NO) (Mills, 1990) in combination with activation of the cyclooxygenase pathway and PGE_2 (Albina et al., 1991). Nitric oxide is a highly soluble free radical whose diverse roles include signal transduction and the regulation of vascular resistance, and cytostatic and cytotoxic effector roles in tumor cell killing, antimicrobial activity, and the killing of a variety of intracellular parasites (Moncada et al., 1991). Recently, in addition to these actions as an immune defense molecule, a role for NO as an immunoregulator in inflammation has been proposed. In particular the cytostatic effects of l-arginine metabolism by macrophages has been shown to regulate the immune system by reducing or suppressing allogeneic activation and mitogen-induced proliferation of lymphocytes. The wide range of activity attributed to this molecule is due to the existence of different isoforms of the nitric oxide synthase (NOS) family of enzymes which are the products of separate genes.

The cytokines identified as appearing early in inflammation (IL-1β, TNF-α, and IFN-γ with or without additional mitogenic stimulation by bacterial LPS) have been shown to be potential inducers of the NOS gene in many cell types including the RPE (Moncada et al., 1991; Nathan, 1992; Goureau et al., 1992; 1994). To identify the NOS species expressed by rat RPE cells, degenerate oligonucleotide primers were designed based on the known sequences of the various NOS genes. These primers recognized nucleotide motifs conserved between the published sequences for both constitutive and inducible forms of the enzyme. From the stimulat-

ed RPE cells a cDNA product was amplified and cloned which when sequenced showed identity with the rat vascular smooth muscle inducible NOS sequence, confirming that the inducible, cytotoxic/cytostatic form of the enzyme (iNOS) rather than the constitutive endothelial or neuronal form (i.e. the physiological form) was involved. Northern blot analysis of total RNA extracted from rat RPE before and after cytokine treatment showed a fivefold induction of the iNOS gene (Liversidge et al., 1994a).

The expression of iNOS and the secretion of cytotoxic or cytostatic levels of NO has been well documented in the murine system, but evidence that inducible NO might have an important role in the etiology of human disease has been scarce. It has been suggested that limited expression of iNOS by human cells reflects the lack of certain cofactors in some human cells or that other genetic variables are involved. High- and low-iNOS-expressing strains of rats and mice have been described, which correlate with variations in susceptibility to parasitic infections and induction of EAU (Fu and Blankenhorn, 1992). However, human RPE can secrete high levels of NO when cocultured with activated T lymphocytes. RT-PCR analysis of mRNA for endogenously generated cytokines in the cocultured cells revealed the presence of IFN-γ, IL-1α, IL-β, and TNFα, together with GM-CSF and IL-6, which is endogenously expressed by the cultured RPE (Liversidge et al., 1994b) (Fig. 26-7). In addition, Goureau and colleagues (1994b) also induced cultured human RPE cells to secrete NO in response to exogenous IFN-γ and IL-1β, and showed that induction was inhibited by TGF-β.

Excessive production of NO would have destructive effects, particularly in tissues such as the retina where high levels of cGMP cause destruction of photoreceptors, therefore iNOS expression is likely to be under tight control. For instance TGF-β is a major modulator of iNOS, and is reciprocally expressed in a number of pathological conditions (Vodovotz et al., 1993; Goureau et al., 1994b), and in RPE cells, both acidic and basic fibroblast growth factors which are required for the normal functioning of the photoreceptors, inhibit the induction of iNOS (Goureau et al., 1993). Although expression of iNOS by cultured rat RPE cells is very strong, little if any expression can be detected in the RPE in vivo. Hoey and colleagues (1997) have found that iNOS expression in the rat model of EAU is highly restricted, being found almost exclusively in monocyte/macrophages infiltrating the ROS during the early stages (days 12–14) of retinal antigen-induced EAU (Fig. 26-8). Although mRNA for iNOS can be detected in the eye at all stages of disease, during later stages the enzyme itself is only weakly expressed in the tissues and

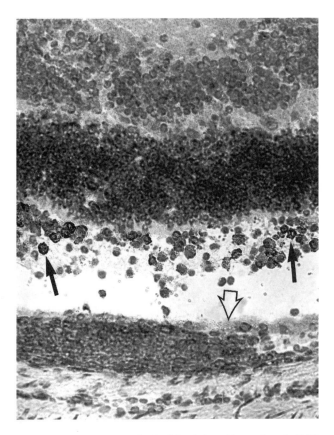

FIGURE 26-8. Expression of inducible nitric oxide synthase in EAU. Retinal antigen induced EAU: cryostat section of rat retina at day 12 labeled with an antibody to the inducible form of nitric oxide synthase. Many large mononuclear inflammatory cells within the subretinal exudate, where the autoantigen is located, are positively stained *(black arrows)*, but the retinal pigment epithelial cells are negative *(white arrow)*. (Hoey et al., 1997.)

has disappeared by day 18, indicating that translation of the gene is under separate control.

Whether inducible NO exerts an immunosuppressive effect in EAU by inhibiting T cell proliferation, as suggested by the in vitro experiments, or has cytotoxic effects which increase severity of disease is controversial. The cytotoxic properties are known to be beneficial for combating bacterial and parasitic infections, and may play a vital role as a first line of defense against such pathogens before a specific immune response can take effect. Phagocytosis of ROS is decreased by NO (Goureau et al., 1994), which could lead to photoreceptor degeration. On the other hand, NO inhibits RPE proliferation, which could also be beneficial (Goureau et al., 1993). In vivo experiments in rat EAU models suggest that excessive NO produced within the eye is destructive (Hoey et al., 1995; Goureau et al., 1995a). Whether RPE cell NO production is significant in vivo in human uveoretinitis is presently unknown. The rat model of

EAU is hyperacute, and failure to detect iNOS in rat RPE in the model could reflect a rapid induction of TGF-β in the RPE that may not occur uniformly in human uveoretinitis; or, FGF, which is present within the normal retina, may be sufficient to prevent induction of the iNOS gene.

Both iNOS and iCOX pathways are induced by IL-1β. Vasodilation, induced by arachidonic acid is inhibited by either indomethacin, which inhibits PGE_2, or L-NAME, the competitive inhibitor of the l-arginine pathway. Endogenous PGE_2 production is known to increase NO synthesis, and inhibition of the inducible cyclooxygenase pathway (iCOX) in RPE cells significantly reduces NO secretion (Liversidge et al., 1994a). Equally, inhibition of iNOS reduces PGE_2 production, suggesting that either a synergy between prostaglandins and NO exists, or that their release is linked (Corbett et al., 1993). The major regulatory effect of PGE_2 on T cell immune responses is through the increase of intracellular cAMP. This inhibits cell proliferation and IFN-γ and IL-2 production by Th_1 cells but not IL-4 synthesis by Th_2 cells. In addition, PGE_2 also exerts an immunosuppressive effect upon accessory cells, inhibiting production of IL-1 and TNF post transcriptionally and decreasing cytokine-induced MHC class II expression. Secretion of PGE_2 can therefore modulate the immune response by several mechanisms: by reducing expression of the proinflammatory cytokines IL-1 and TNF; by reducing the activity of APC; by promoting downregulatory Th_2- type responses, which provide the cytokines for B cell development and antibody secretion; and by synergizing with NO, providing powerful cytotoxic and cytostatic effects.

CONCLUSION

The inflammatory infiltrate of leucocytes which marks the response of the immune system to infection or injury involves the orderly recruitment of immunocompetent cells to the site in response to physical as well as soluble signals sent out by local cells. It is evident that the RPE is not merely a passive barrier in this situation, but functions as an active component of the immune system in the eye, providing not only scavenging and phagocytic activity but also expressing many of the surface receptors and soluble mediators required to coordinate the immune response. RPE cells also provide homeostatic mechanisms which operate to control inflammatory responses.

Whether the RPE exerts a proinflammatory or antiinflammatory effect will depend on the microenvironment of the cells, the presence or absence of a particular cytokine, or the expression of a control mechanism such as cytokine receptor antagonists. These factors may be genetically determined. For instance, variable secretion of NO, TNF-α, and NGF by RPE from different strains of rat correlates with susceptibility to inflammation such as EAU. Much of the data discussed in this chapter have been obtained from cultured cells, and how the RPE functions in vivo during inflammation is not well understood although the induction of cytokine mRNA expression by RPE cells in coculture with activated T lymphocytes indicates that endogenous cytokine levels generated during an inflammation would be sufficient to trigger RPE cell activation. The failure of RPE cells to express MHC class II molecules and iNOS in vivo during retinal antigen-induced EAU, despite high expression by other inflammatory cells in the vicinity, indicates that regulatory mechanisms are operating expressly within the RPE. For example, failure to express the iNOS enzyme in vivo may reflect the predominant expression of TGF-β and/or FGF by the RPE in the cytokine milieu of the acute EAU lesion, and induction of the iCOX pathway would restrict MHC class II expression. In addition, modulation of cytokine activity is achieved by natural inhibitors, such as receptor antagonists and soluble receptors, expressed by the RPE, which provides further evidence for an immunosuppressive function for the RPE. For example, IL-1 is a pivotal cytokine in the initiation of inflammation, and although the RPE can be induced to express the gene and make the protein in vitro, the secreted form of the protein has never been detected. RPE cells respond to exogenous IL-1 stimulation via the IL-1 receptor, but expression of the IL-1 receptor antagonist by RPE suggests that the effect of the cytokine may be limited (Jaffe et al., 1992; de Vos et al., 1994b), particularly if physiological levels in vivo are low.

If the RPE is mainly immunosuppressive, how does inflammation, such as uveoretinitis occur? Focal, patchy MHC class II expression by RPE cells in vivo during EAU (Fig. 26-7) indicates that proinflammatory events can occur locally at the RPE, but the limited nature of the expression confirms the predominantly suppressive microenvironment. The significance of this for disease is uncertain. The choroid contains a network of bone-marrow-derived antigen-presenting cells (Plate 26-II), including macrophages and dendritic cells, the latter often being found in very close proximity to Bruch's membrane and having the ability to initiate T cell responses to retinal antigens (Forrester et al., 1994). The interactions of these cells with the RPE are probably central to the induction of immune responses within the eye, inflammation occuring when homeostatic mechanisms break down as a result of infection or injury.

REFERENCES

Albeda SM, Buck CA. 1990. Integrins and other cell adhesion molecules. FASEB J 4:2868–2880.

Albina JE, Abate JA, Henry EA. 1991. Nitric oxide is required for murine resident peritoneal macrophages to suppress mitogen-stimulated T cell proliferation. J Immunol 147:144–148.

Benson MT, Sheperd L, Rees RC, Rennie IG. 1992. Production of IL-6 by human retinal pigment epithelium in vitro and its regulation by other cells. Curr Eye Res 11(suppl):173–179.

Bequet F, Courtois Y, Goureau O. 1994. Nitric oxide decreases in vitro phagocytosis of photoreceptor outer segments by bovine retinal pigmented epithelial cells. J Cell Physiol 159:256–262.

Bird IN, Spragg JH, Ager A, Matthews N. 1993. Studies of lymphocyte transendothelial migration: analysis of migrated cell phenotypes with regard to CD31(PECAM-1), CD45RA and CD45RO. Immunol 88:553–560.

Bora NS, Gobleman CS, Atkinson JP, Pepose JS, Kaplan HJ. 1993. Differential expression of the complement regulatory proteins in the human eye. Invest Ophthalmol Vis Sci 34:3579–3584.

Bottazzo GF, Pujol-Borel R, Hanafusa T, Feldman M. 1983. Role of aberrant HLA-DR expression and antigen presentation in induction of endocrine autoimmunity. Lancet 2:1115–1119.

Braun G, McKechnie NM, Connor V, Gilbert CE, Engelbrecht F, Whitworth JA, Taylor DW. 1991. Immunological cross reactivity in the pathogenesis of ocular onchocerciasis. J Exp Med 174:169–177.

Braun G, McKechnie N, Gürr W. 1995. Molecular and immunological characterisation of hr44, a human ocular component immunologically cross reactive with antigen Ov39 of Onchocerca volvulus. J Exp Med 182:1121–1131.

Broekhuyse GF, Winkens HJ, Kuhlmann ED, Vugt AHM. 1984. Opsin-induced experimental autoimmune retinitis in rats. Curr Eye Res 3:1405–1412.

Broekhuyse GF, Kuhlmann ED, Winkens HJ, Vugt AHM. 1991. Experimental autoimmune anterior uveitis (EAAU), a new form of experimental uveitis.1. Induction by a detergent insoluble, intrinsic protein fraction of the retinal pigment epithelium. Exp Eye Res 52:465–474.

Broekhuyse RM, Kuhlmann ED, Winkens HJ. 1992a. Experimental autoimmune anterior uveitis (EAAU), II Dose dependent induction and adoptive transfer using a melanin-bound antigen of the retinal pigment epithelium. Exp Eye Res 55:401–411.

Broekhuyse RM, Kuhlmann ED, Winkens HJ. 1992b. Experimental autoimmune uveitis accompanied by epithelioid cell accumulation (EAPU): a new type of experimental ocular disease induced by immunisation with PEP-65, a pigment epithelial polypeptide preparation. Exp Eye Res 55:818–829.

Broekhuyse RM, Kuhlmann ED, Winkens HJ. 1993. Experimental autoimmune anterior uveitis (EAAU): induction by melanin antigen and suppression by various treatments. Pigment Cell Res 6:1–6.

Caffe AR, Szel A, Juliusson B, van Veen T. 1993. Hyperplastic neuroretinopathy and disorder of pigment epithelial cells precede accelerated retinal degeneration in the SJL/N mouse. Cell and Tissue Res 271:297–307.

Campochiario PA, Jerdan JA, Glaser BM. 1986. The extracellular matrix of human retinal pigment epithelial cells in vivo and its synthesis in vitro. Invest Ophthalmol Vis Sci 27:1615–1621.

Caspi RR, Roberge RG, Nussenblatt RB. 1987. Organ resident nonlymphoid cells suppress proliferation of autoimmune T helper lymphocytes. Science 237:1029–1032.

Chan C-C, Detrick B, Nussenblatt RB, Palestine A, Fujikawa LS, Hooks JJ. 1986a. HLA-DR antigens on retinal pigment epithelial cells from patients with uveitis. Arch Ophthalmol 104:725–729.

Chan C-C, Hooks JJ, Nussenblatt RB, Detrick B. 1986b. Expression of Ia antigen on retinal pigment epithelium in experimental autoimmune uveoretinitis. Curr Eye Res 5:325–330.

Connor TB, Roberts AB, Sporn MB, Danielpour D, Dart LL, Michels RG, de Bustros S, Enger C, Kato H, Lansing H, Glaser BM. 1989. Correlation of fibrosis and transforming growth factor-b type 2 levels in the eye. J Clin Invest 83:1661–1666.

Cousins SW, McCabe MM, Danielpour D, Steilein W. 1991. Identification of TGF-β as an immunosuppressive factor in aqueous humor. Invest Ophthalmol Vis Sci 32:2201–2211.

Crane IJ, Kuppner MC, McKillop-Smith S, Forrester JV. 1998. Cytokine regulation of RANTES production by human retinal pigment epithelial cells. Cell Immunol. in press.

De Kozak Y, Naud MC, Bellot J, Faure JP, Hicks D. 1994. Differential tumor necrosis factor expression by resident retinal cells from experimental uveitis-susceptible and resistant rats. J Neuroimmunol 55:1–9.

De Vos AF, Hoekzema R, Kijlstra A. 1992. Cytokines and uveitis, a review. Curr Eye Res 6:581–597.

De Vos AF, Van Haren MAC, Verhagen C, Hoekzema R, Kijlstra A. 1994a. Kinetics of intraocular TNF and IL-6 in endotoxin induced uveitis in the rat. Invest Ophthalmol Vis Sci 35:1100–1106.

De Vos AF, Klaren VNA, Kijlstra A. 1994b. Expression of multiple cytokines and interleukin-1 receptor antagonist in the uvea and retina during endotoxin-induced uveitis in the rat. Invest Ophthalmol Vis Sci 35:3873–3883.

De Vos AF, Van Haren MAC, Verhagen C, Hoekzema R, Kijlstra A. 1995. Systemic anti-tumor necrosis factor antibody treatment exacerbates endotoxin-induced uveitis in the rat. Exp Eye Res 61:667–675.

Devine L, Lightman SL, Greenwood J. 1996. Role of LFA-1, ICAM-1, VLA-4 and VCAM-1 in lymphocyte migration across retinal pigment epithelial monolayers in vitro. Immunology 88:456–462.

Dicou E, Nerriere V, Naud NC, de Kozak Y. 1994. NGF involvement in ocular inflammation: secretion by rat resident retinal cells. Neuroreport 6:26–28.

Dick, AD. 1995. Retinal antigen-specific T cells mediate experimental autoimmune uveoretinitis (EAU) in PVG rats. Ocular Immunol & Inflammation 3:261–270.

Dua HS, McKinnon A, McMenamin PG, Forrester JV. 1991. Ultrastructural pathology of the barrier sites in experimental autoimmune uveitis and experimental autoimmune pinealitis. Br J Ophthalmol 75:391–397.

Dua HS, Lee RH, Lolley RN, Barrett JA, Abrahams M, Forrester JV, Donoso LA. 1992. Induction of experimental autoimmune uveitis by the retinal photoreceptor cell protein, phosducin. Curr Eye Res 11(suppl):107–111.

Duguid IGM, Boyd AW, Mandel TE. 1991. The expression of adhesion molecules in the human retina and choroid. Aust and New Zealand J Ophthalmol 19:309–316.

Dutt K, Waldrep JC, Kaplan HJ, Del Monte M, Semple E, Verly G. 1989. In vitro phenotypic and functional characterisation of human pigment epithelial cell lines. Curr Eye Res 8:435–440.

Eckert CG, Hafeman DB. 1986. Search for Fc and C3b receptors on black-eyed RCS rat RPE cells. Curr Eye Res 5:911–917.

Elner SG, Elner VM, Nielsen JC, Torczynski E, Riley Y, Franklin WA. 1992a. CD68 antigen expression by human retinal pigment epithelial cells. Exp Eye Res 55:21–28.

Elner SG, Elner VM, Pavilack MA, Todd RF, Mayobond L, Franklin WA, Streiter RM, Kunkel SL, Huber AR. 1992b. Modulation and function of intercellular adhesion molecule-1 (CD54) on human retinal pigment epithelial cells. Lab Invest 66:200–211.

Elner VM, Schaffer T, Taylor K, Glagov S. 1981. Immunophagocytic properties of retinal pigment epithelial cells. Science 211:74–76.

Elner VM, Streitter, RM, Elner SG, Lindley L, Kunkel SL. 1990. Neutrophil chemotactic factor (IL-8) gene expression by cytokine activated retinal epithelial cells. Am J Pathol 136:745–750.

Elner VM, Elner SG, Standiford TJ, Lukacs NW, Steiter RM, Kunkel SL. 1996. Interleukin 7 (IL-7) induces retinal pigment epithelial cell MCP-1 and IL-8. Exp Eye Res 63:297–303.

Faure J-P. 1980. Autoimmunity and the retina. Curr Top Eye Res 2:215–302.

Ferguson TA, Herndon JM. 1994. The immune response and the eye: the ACAID inducing signal is dependent on the nature of the antigen. Invest Ophthalmol Vis Sci 35:3085–3093.

Ferguson TA, Waldrep JC, Kaplan HJ. 1987. The immune response and the eye II. The nature of T suppressor cell induction in anterior chamber associated immune deviation (ACAID). J Immunol 139:352–357.

Fergusson TA, Herndon JM, Dube P. 1994. The immune response and the eye: a role for TNF-α in ACAID. Invest Ophthalmol Vis Sci 35:2643–2651.

Ferrick MR, Thurau SR, Oppenheim MH. 1991. Ocular inflammation stimulated by intravitreal interleukin-8 and interleukin-1. Invest Ophthalmol Vis Sci 32:1534–1539.

Forrester JV, Borthwick GM, McMenamin PG. 1985. Ultrastructural pathology of S-antigen uveoretinitis. Invest Ophthalmol Vis Sci 26:1281–1292.

Forrester JV, Liversidge J, Dua HS, Dick AD, Harper F, McMenamin PG. 1992. Experimental Autoimmune Uveoretinitis: a model system for immunointervention. Curr Eye Res 11(suppl):33–40.

Forrester JV, McMenamin PG, Holthouse I, Lumsden L, Liversidge J. 1994. Localisation and characterisation of major histocompatibility complex Class II positive cells in the posterior segment of the eye: implications for the induction of autoimmune uveoretinitis. Invest Ophthalmol Vis Sci 35:64–77.

Forrester JV, Lumsden L, Liversidge J, Kuppner M, Mesri M. 1995. Immunoregulation of uveoretinal inflammation. Prog Ret Res 14:393–412.

Foulds WS. 1976. Clinical significance of trans-scleral fluid transfer. Trans Ophthalmol Vis Sci 96:290–308.

Fu Y, Blankenhorn EP. 1992. Nitric oxide-induced anti-mitogenic effects in high and low responder rat strains. J Immunol 148:2217–2222.

Gery I. 1986. Retinal antigens and the immunopathologic process they provoke. Prog Ret Res 5:75–109.

Gery I, Chanaud NP, Anglade E. 1994. Recoverin is highly uveitogenic in Lewis rats. Invest Ophthalmol Vis Sci 35:3342–3345.

Gordon S. 1986. The biology of the macrophage. J Cell Sci 4 (suppl):267–286.

Goureau O, Le Poivre M, Courtois Y. 1992. Lipopolysaccharide and cytokines induce a macrophage-type of nitric oxide synthase in bovine retinal pigmented epithelial cells. Biochem Biophys Res Comm 186:854–859.

Goureau O, Lepoivre M, Becquet F, Courtois Y. 1993. Differential regulation of inducible nitric oxide synthase by fibroblast growth factors and transforming growth factor b in bovine retinal pigmented epithelial cell: inverse correlation with cellular proliferation. Proc Nat Acad Sci USA 90:4276–4280.

Goureau O, Hicks D, Courtois Y. 1994. Human retinal pigment epithelial cells produce nitric oxide in response to cytokines. Biochem Biophys Res Comm 198:120–126.

Goureau O, Bellot J, Thillaye B, Courtois Y, De Kozac Y. 1995a. Increased nitric oxide production in endotoxin-induced uveitis: reduction of uveitis by an inhibitor of nitric oxide synthase. J Immunol. 154:6518–6523.

Goureau O, Faure V, Courtois Y. 1995b. Fibroblast growth factors decrease inducible nitric oxide synthase mRNA accumulation in bovine retinal pigment epithelial cells. Eur J Biochem 2230: 1046–1052.

Greenwood J, Howes R, Lightman S. 1994. The blood-retinal barrier in experimental autoimmune uveoretinitis. Lab Invest 70:39–52.

Hara Y, Caspi RR, Wiggert B, Chan C-C, Wilbanks GA, Steilein JW. 1992. Suppression of experimental autoimmune uveitis in mice by induction of anterior chamber-associated immune deviation with interphotoreceptor retinoid-binding protein. J Immunol 148:1685–1692.

Hayes KC, Lindsey S, Stephan ZF, Brecker D. 1989. Retinal pigment epithelium possesses both LDL and scavenger receptor activity. Invest Ophthalmol Vis Sci 30:225–232.

Helbig H, Gurley RC, Palestine AG, Nussenblatt RB, Caspi RR. 1990. Dual effect of ciliary body cells on T lymphocyte proliferation. Eur J Immunol 20:2457–2463.

Hoekzema R, Murray PI, Kijlstra A. 1990. Cytokines and intraocular inflammation. Curr Eye Res 9(suppl):207–211.

Hoey S, Grabowski PS, Ralston S, Forrester JV, Liversidge J. 1997. Nitric Oxide accelerates the onset and increases the severity of experimental autoimmune uveoretinitis through an interferon-γ dependent mechanism. J Immunol. 159:5132–5142.

Hooks JJ, Percopo C, Wang Y, Detrick B. 1993. Retina and retinal pigment epithelial cell autoantibodies are produced during murine coronavirus retinopathy. J Immunol 156:3381–3389.

Jaffe GF, Roberts WL, Wong HL, Yurochko AD, Cianciolo GJ. 1995. Monocyte-induced cytokine expression in cultured human retinal pigment epithelial cells. Exp Eye Res 60:533–543.

Jaffe GJ, Van Le L, Valea F, Haskill S, Roberts W, Arend WP, Stuart A, Peters WP. 1992. Expression of Interleukin-1a, interleukin-1b and an interleukin-1 receptor antagonist in human retinal pigment epithelial cells. Exp Eye Res 55:325–335.

Jiang LQ, Jorquera M, Streilein JW. 1993. Subretinal space and vitreous cavity as immunologically privileged sites for retinal allografts. Invest Ophthalmol Vis Sci 34:3347–3354.

Keizer GD, Velde AA, Schwarting R, Figdor CG, De Vreis JE. 1987. Role of p150,95 in adhesion, migration, chemotaxix and phagocytosis of human monocytes. Eur J Immunol 17:1317–1322.

Konda BR, Pararajasegaram G, Wu GS, Stanforth D, Rao NA. 1994. Role of retinal pigment epithelium in the development of experimental autoimmune uveoretinitis. Invest Ophthalmol Vis Sci 35:40–47.

Kumaki N, Anderson DM, Cosman D, Kumaki S. 1996. Expression of interleukin-15 and its receptor by human fetal retinal pigment epithelial cells. Curr Eye Res 15:876–882.

Kuppner MC, Liversidge J, McKillop-Smith S, Lumsden L, Forrester JV. 1993. Adhesion molecule expression in acute and fibrotic sympathetic ophthalmia. Curr Eye Res 10:923–934.

Kuppner MC, McKillop-Smith S, Forrester JV. 1995. TGF-β and IL-1β act in synergy to enhance IL-6 and IL-8 mRNA levels and IL-6 production by human retinal pigment epithelial cells. Immunology 84:265–271.

Kutty RK, Kutty G, Hooks JJ, Wiggert B, Nagineni CN. 1995. Transforming growth factor β inhibits the cytokine-mediated expression of the inducible nitric oxide synthase mRNA in human retinal pigment epithelial cells. Biochem Biophys Res Comm 215:386–393.

Limb GA, Brown KA, Wolstencroft RA, Ellis BA, Dumonde DC. 1988. Modulation of Fc and C3b receptor expression on guinea-pig macrophages by lymphokines. Clin Exp Immunol 74:171–176.

Lipton SA, Chol Y-B, Pan ZH, Lel SZ, Chen HS, Sucher NJ, Loscalzo J, Singel DJ, Stamler JS. 1993. A redox based mechanism for the neuroprotective and neurodestructive effects of nitric oxide and related compounds. Nature 364:626–632.

Liversidge J, Forrester JV. 1990. Are accessory cells implicated in activation of T cells at the blood-retinal barrier? Curr Eye Res 9 (suppl):131–134.

Liversidge J, Forrester JV. 1991. Changes in RPE cell morphology, behaviour and function is a result of modulated gene expression in response to altered environmental influences. Invest Ophthalmol Vis Sci 32:1376.

Liversidge J, Forrester JV. 1992. Antigen processing and presentation in the eye, a review. Curr Eye Res 11(suppl):49–58.

Liversidge J, Sewell HF, Forrester JV. 1988a. Human retinal pigment epithelial cells differentially express MHC class II (HLA DP, DR, DQ) antigens in response to in vitro stimulation with lymphokine or purified IFN-γ. Clin Exp Immunol 73:489–494.

Liversidge J, Sewell H, Thomson AW, Forrester JV. Lymphokine-induced MHC Class II antigen expression on cultured retinal pigment epithelial cells and the influence of cyclosporin-A. Immunology 63: 313–317.

Liversidge J, Sewell HF, Forrester JV. 1990. Interactions between lymphocytes and cells of the blood-retina barrier: mechanisms of T lymphocyte adhesion to human retinal capillary endothelial and retinal pigment epithelial cells in vitro. Immunology 71:390–396.

Liversidge J, McKay D, Mullen G, Forrester JV. 1993a. Retinal pigment epithelial cells modulate lymphocyte function at the blood-retina barrier by autocrine PGE2 and membrane bound mechanisms. Cell Immunol 149:315–330.

Liversidge J, Dick AD, Cheng Y-F, Scott GB, Forrester JV. 1993b. Retinal antigen specific lymphocytes, TCR-γδ T cells and CD5+ve B cells cultured from the vitreous in acute sympathetic ophthalmitis. Autoimmunity 15:257–266.

Liversidge J, Grabowski P, Ralston S, Benjamin N, Forrester JV. 1994a. Rat retinal pignment epithelial cells express an inducible form of nitric oxide synthase and produce nitric oxide in response to inflammatory cytokines and activated T cells. Immunology 83: 404–409.

Liversidge J, Grabowski P, Ralston S, Benjamin N, Forrester JV. 1994b. Human retinal pigment epithelial cells produce nitric oxide in the presence of activated T lymphocytes. In: The Biology of Nitric Oxide Immunology and Inflammation. 378–383.

Liversidge J, Dawson R, McKay D, Hoey S, Forrester JV. 1996. CD59 and CD48 expressed by rat retinal pigment epithelial cells are major ligands for the CD2-mediated alternative pathway of T cell activation. J Immunol 156:3696–3703.

Marrs JA, Andersson Fisone C, Jeong MC, Cohen Gould L, Zurzolo C, Nabi IR, Rodriguez Boulan E, Nelson WJ. 1995. Plasticity in epithelial cell phenotype: modulation by expression of different cadherin cell adhesion molecules. J Cell Biol 129:507–519.

Martini B, Wang HM, Lee MB, Ogden TE, Ryan SJ, Sorgente N. 1991. Synthesis of extracellular matrix by macrophage modulated retinal pigment epithelium. Arch Ophthalmol 109:576–580.

McLaughlin BJ, Tarnowski BI, Shepherd VL. 1987. Idenification of mannose 6-phosphate and mannose receptors in dystrophic and normal retinal pigment epithelium. Prog Clin Biol Res 247–257.

McMenamin PG, Holthouse I. 1992. Immunohistochemical characterisation of dendritic cells and macrophages in the aqueous outflow pathways of the rat eye. Exp Eye Res 55:315–324.

McMenamin PG, Broekhuyse RM, Forrester JV. 1992. Ultrastructural pathology of experimental autoimmune uveitis: a review. Micron 24:521–546.

McMenamin PG, Crewe J, Morrison S, Holt PG. 1994. Immunomorphological studies of macrophages and MHC Class II positive dendritic cells in the iris and ciliary body of the rat, mouse and human eye. Invest Ophthalmol Vis Sci 35:3234–3250.

Mesri M, Liversidge J, Forrester JV. 1994a. ICAM-1/LFA-1 interactions in T lymphocyte activation and adhesion to cells of the blood-retina barrier in the rat. Immunology 83:52–57.

Mesri M, Liversidge J, Grabowski P, Benjamin N, Forrester JV. 1994b. Nitric oxide production by blood-retinal barrier cells and its modulation by cytokines. Reg Immunol 6:169–172.

Mesri M, Liversidge J, Forrester JV. 1996. Prostaglandin E2 and monoclonal antibody differentially inhibit migration of T lymphocytes across microvascular retinal endothelial cells in rat. Immunology 88:471–477.

Mills CD. 1990. Molecular basis of suppressor macrophages: arginine metabolism via the nitric oxide synthase pathway. J Immunol 146:2719–2723.

Moncada S, Palmer RMJ, Higgs EA. 1991. Nitric oxide: physiology, pathophysiology and pharmacology. Pharmacol Rev 43:109–142.

Murphy PM. 1994. The molecular biology of leukocyte chemoattractant receptors. Ann Rev Immunol 12:593–633.

Nathan C. 1992. Nitric oxide as a secretory product of mammalial cells. Fed Am Soc Exp Biol J 6:3051–3064.

Neidercorn JY. 1990. Immune privilege and immune regulation in the eye. Adv Immunol 48:191–226.

Opdenakker G, van Damme J. 1994. Cytokine regulated proteases in autoimmune diseases. Immunol Today 15:103–107.

Oppenheimer-Marks N, Davis LS, Bogue DT, Ramberg J, Lipsky PE. 1991. Differential utilisation of ICAM-1 and VCAM-1 during the adhesion and transendothelial migration of human T lymphocytes. J Immunol 147:2913–2921.

Osusky R, Soriano D, Ye J, Ryan SJ. 1994. Cytokine effect on fibronectin release by retinal pigment epithelial cells. Curr Eye Res 13:569–574.

Pasquale LM, Dorman-Pease ME, Lutty GA, Quigley HA, Jampel HD. 1993. Immunolocalisation of TGF-β1, TGF-β2 and TGF-β3 in the anterior segment of the eye. Invest Ophthalmol Vis Sci 34:23–30.

Percopo CM, Hooks JJ, Shinohara T, Caspi RR, Detrick B. 1990. Cytokine activation of a neuronal resident cell mediates antigen presentation. J Immunol 145:4101–4107.

Planck SR, Dang TT, Graves D, Tara D, Ansel JC, Rosenbaum JT. 1992. Retinal pigment epithelial cells secrete interleukin-6 in response to interleukin 1. Invest Ophthalmol Vis Sci 33:78–82.

Planck SR, Huang XN, Robertson JE, Rosenbaum JT. 1993. Retinal pigment epithelial cells produce interleukin-1β and granulocyte-macrophage colony-stimulating factor in response to interleukin-1α. Curr Eye Res 12:205–212.

Platts KF, Benson MT, Rennie IG, Sharrard RM, Rees RC. 1995. Cytokine modulation of adhesion molecule expression on human retinal pigment epithelial cells. Invest Ophthalmol Vis Sci 36:2262–2269.

Polans AS, Burton MD, Haley TL, Crabb JW, Palcewski K. 1993. Recoverin, but not visinin, is an autoantigen in the human retina identified with a cancer associated retinopathy. Invest Ophthalmol Vis Sci 34:81–82.

Powrie F, Menon S, Coffman RL. 1993. Interleukin 4 and interleukin 10 synergise to inhibit cell mediated immunity in vivo. Eur J Immunol 23:2223–2229.

Rao NA, Wu GS, Zhang J. 1996. Up-regulation of a novel RPE protective protein in experimental uveitis. Invest Ophthalmol Vis Sci 37:S919.

Reid DM, Loeffler KU, Campbell AM, Forrester JV. 1987. Electron immunocytochemical localisation of retinal S-antigen with a rat monoclonal antibody. Exp Eye Res 45:731–745.

Robbins SG, Brem RB, Wilson DJ, O'Rourke LM, Robertson JE, Westra I, Planck SR, Rosenbaum JT. 1994. Immunolocalisation of integrins in proliferative retinal membranes. Invest Ophthalmol Vis Sci 35:3475–3485.

Roberge FC, Caspi RR, Nussenblatt RB. 1988. Glial retinal muller cells produce IL-1 activity and have a dual effect on autoimmune T helper lymphocytes. J Immunol 140:2193–2196.

Schleiffenbaum B, Moser R, Patarroyo M, Fehr J. 1989. The cell surface glycoprotein Mac-! (Cd11b/CD18) mediates neutrophil degranulation independently of its quantitative cell surface expression. J Immunol 142:3537–3545.

Shinohara T, Donoso LA, Tsuda M, Yamaki K, Singh VK. 1988. S-antigen : structure, function and experimental autoimmune uveoretinitis. Prog Ret Res 8:51–56.

Sippy BD, Hofman FM, He S, Osusky R, Sheu SJ, Walker SM, Ryan SJ, Hinton DR. 1995. SV-40 immortalised and primary cultured human retinal pigment epithelial cells share similar patterns of cytokine-receptor expression and cytokine responsiveness. Curr Eye Res 14:495–503.

Shattuck RL, Wood LD, Jaffe GJ, Richmond A. 1994. MGSA/GRO transcription is differentially regulated in normal retinal pigment epithelial and melanoma cells. Mol Cell Biol 14:791–802.

Springer T. 1990. Adhesion receptors of the immune system. Nature 346:425–434.

Streilien JW, Willbanks GA, Cousins S. 1992a. Immunoregulatory mechanisms of the eye. J Neuroimmunol 39:185–200.

Streilien JW, Willbanks GA, Taylor A, Cousins S. 1992b. Eye derived cytokines and the immunosuppressive microenvironment: a review. Curr Eye Res 11(suppl):41–47.

Tanihara H, Yoshida M, Matsumoto M, Yoshimura N. 1993. Identification of transforming growth factor β expressed in cultured human retinal pigment epithelial cells. Invest Ophthalmol Vis Sci 34:413–419.

Taylor AW, Streilein JW, Cousins SW. 1992. Identification of alpha melanocyte stimulating hormone as a potential immunosuppressive factor in aqueous humour. Curr Eye Res 11:1199–1206.

Taylor AW, Steilein JW, Cousins SW. 1994. Immunoreactive vasoactive intestinal peptide contributes to the immunosuppressive activity of the normal aqueous humour. J Immunol 144:1080–1086.

Tompsett E, Al-hanna D, Wakefield D. 1990. Immunological privilege in the eye. Curr Eye Res 12:1141–1145.

Vodovotz Y, Bogdan C, Paik J, Xie Q-W, Nathan C. 1993. Mechanisms of suppression of macrophage nitric oxide release by transforming growth factor β. J Exp Med 178:605–613.

Wacker WB. 1991. Experimental allergic uveitis: investigations of retinal autoimmunity and the immunopathologic responses evoked. Invest Ophthalmol Vis Sci 32:3119–3128.

Wahl SM, McCartney-Francis N, Mergenhagen SE. 1989. Inflammatory and immunomodulatory roles of TGF-β. Immunol Today 10:258–261.

Whitcup SM, Chan CC, Li Q, Nussenblatt RB. 1992. Expression of cell adhesion molecules in posterior uveitis. Arch Ophthalmol 110:662–666.

Whitcup SM, DeBarge LR, Casoi RR, Harning R, Nussenblatt RB, Chan C-C. 1993. Monoclonal antibodies against ICAM-1(CD54) and LFA-1 (CD 11a/CD18) inhibit autoimmune uveitis. Clin Immunol Immunopathol 67:143–150.

Willbanks GA, Streilein JW. 1991. Studies on the induction of anterior chamber-associated immune deviation: Evidence that an antigen specific, ACAID inducing, cell associated signal exists in peripheral blood. J Immunol 146:2610–2617.

Young E, Lutty GA. 1987. Modulation of human lymphocyte proliferation by normal bovine vitreous. Invest Ophthalmol Vis Sci 28P:753–756.

Young RW. 1974. Biogenesis and renewal of visual cell outer segment membranes. Exp Eye Res 18:215–223.

Zhou Y, Dziak E, Unnasch TR, Opas M. 1994. Major retinal components recognised by onchocerciasis sera are associated with the cell surface and nucleoli. Invest Ophthalmol Vis Sci 35:1089–1099.

27. Inflammations and infections of the retinal pigment epithelium

NARSING A. RAO

The retinal pigment epithelium (RPE), via the generation of either proinflammatory or antiinflammatory agents, plays an active role in the modulation of intraocular inflammations and infections. The RPE may proliferate, undergo atrophic changes or become necrotic in response to inflammation. The proinflammatory agents produced by the RPE, which include among others interleukins, adhesion molecules, and oxygen metabolites, may play a role in the elimination of pathogens present in the RPE or adjacent tissue, by enhancing the inflammatory process. The antiinflammatory agents generated, including transforming growth factor beta and antioxidant enzymes, may act in the down-regulation of the inflammation to limit the damaging effects of the process. These responses may be followed by a reactive proliferation of the RPE, leading to the formation of chorioretinal scars, or the RPE may atrophy. This type of involvement of the RPE is evident in various intraocular conditions such as sympathetic ophthalmia, Vogt-Koyanagi-Harada syndrome, and other uveitis entities, as well as in infections of the RPE and adjacent tissues.

UVEITIS

The intraocular inflammation commonly known as uveitis is a complex, local inflammation, primarily involving the uvea. There is also extension of the process to the RPE and the retina, as well as to other sites. Clinical features typically include loss of vision and altered blood–ocular barrier in the retinal vasculature and the anterior uvea at the level of the RPE. In association with these changes there is the presence of cellular exudate in the intraocular cavities. From a histopathologic perspective, in the vast majority of patients, the cellular infiltration is observed predominantly in the uvea, although other intraocular structures, including the RPE and retina, can be invaded by acute or chronic inflammatory cells. Less commonly, the inflammatory cell infiltration may extend to the sclera or the cornea in addition to the uveal tract.

Classification of Uveitis

In general, based on clinical and histological features, uveitis is classified as either a granulomatous or a nongranulomatous process. From a clinical standpoint, granulomatous uveitis is characterized by the presence of large keratic precipitates on the posterior surface of the cornea or by the presence of tiny nodules made up of aggregated inflammatory cells in the iris stroma or other sites. If these signs are absent, the uveitis is classified as nongranulomatous. A finding of epithelioid cells in the inflammatory infiltrate on histopathologic examination is considered pathognomonic of granulomatous uveitis, whereas the absence of such cells in the inflammation is considered a sign of nongranulomatus uveitis.

The epithelioid cells are known to be derived from macrophages, some of which display major histocompatibility complex class II molecules (MHC-II) while others do not. The primary function of the MHC-II molecule is to act as a co-recognition element during antigen-specific interaction of helper–inducer T-lymphocytes with dendritic antigen-presenting cells, activated macrophages, or B-lymphocytes. The MHC-II-positive dendritic cells or macrophages ingest and process the antigen and present it to lymphocytes, thus initiating and maintaining the immune (or allergic) process. Like the MHC-II-positive macrophages, the MHC-II-negative macrophages can ingest and degrade the antigenic material; but the MHC-II-negative macrophages do not present that antigen to lymphocytes, thus eliminating noxious antigenic material at the site of its release and breaking the cycle of hypersensitivity reaction. It is possible that the initiation, persistence, and termination of a granulomatous process is determined in part by the balance of the class-II-positive and -negative macro-phages.

Granulomatous and nongranulomatous uveitis or related intraocular inflammations result from diverse causes. Broadly, the causes can be classified as traumatic, autoimmune, or infectious in nature. Infectious agents such as viruses, bacteria, fungi, and parasites are well recognized as etiologic agents of uveitis (Henderly et al., 1987).

Uveitis Entities

Sympathetic ophthalmia. Although either blunt or surgical trauma can induce uveitis, such cases are usually self-limited. In very rare instances a penetrating ocular injury can lead to a chronic, recalcitrant, and visually disabling bilateral granulomatous intraocular inflammation known as sympathetic ophthalmia (Goto and Rao, 1990). This bilateral intraocular inflammation appears to be a result of autoimmunity against intraocular antigen(s) (Marak, 1979).

Clinicopathologic evaluation of human eyes enucleated during the early and late stages of uveitis have revealed the importance of RPE in modulation of uveitis and its response to acute and chronic intraocular inflammation. During early stages of posterior uveitis or panuveitis, RPE may show focal areas of damage. Such damaged sites can be detected by fluorescein angiography or by other clinical investigations (Fig. 27-1). In

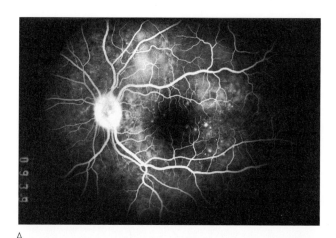

A

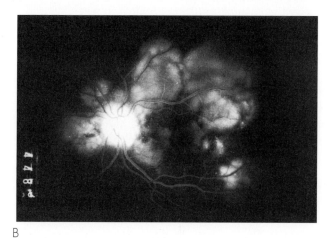

B

FIGURE 27-1. Fluorescein angiography in the arteriovenous phase of Vogt-Koyanagi-Harada syndrome shows hyperfluorescent dots at the level of RPE during early phase (A); subsequent collection of the fluid in the subretinal space during late phase (B).

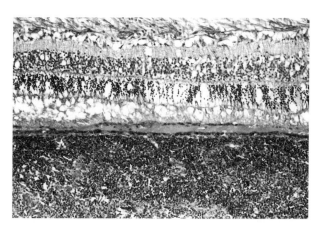

FIGURE 27-2. Sympathetic ophthalmia. Note granulomatous choroiditis with preservation of choriocapillaris, RPE, and retina from inflammatory cell infiltration. H&E; magnification ×200.

chronic stages of uveitis RPE may undergo atrophy or focal areas of hyperplasia. Such RPE changes can be readily detected by either clinical examination or by histologic examination when the eye is enucleated late for various complications related to uveitis. However, in patients with sympathetic ophthalmia the traumatized eye is usually submitted for histopathologic examination during the early stages of uveitis.

Histologically, sympathetic ophthalmia is characterized by a diffuse granulomatous inflammation that involves the entire uveal tract. The inflammatory infiltrate is primarily made up of T-lymphocytes admixed with histiocytes and epithelioid cells. Even though the uveal tract is heavily infiltrated by these cells, the choriocapillaris, RPE, and retina are usually spared from extension of the inflammatory process (Fig. 27-2). However, focal collections of macrophage/epithelioid cells may be noted along Bruch's membrane underneath a dome-shaped elevation of the RPE (Dalen-Fuchs nodule). The retinal photoreceptors and the remainder of the retina are not invaded by macrophages even at these sites. These histologic changes suggest that RPE may play a protective function in preventing migration of the inflammatory cells into the retina.

Vogt-Koyanagi-Harada syndrome. Another bilateral granulomatous uveitis, Vogt-Koyangi-Harada (VKH) syndrome, shows histologic features identical to sympathetic ophthalmia; however, the former condition develops in the absence of any penetrating injury and is believed to be an autoimmune disorder. In VKH various morphologic changes are observed in the RPE, particularly during the chronic stage of this disorder (Moorthy et al., 1995). The RPE may show foci of atrophy or hyperplasia. The hyperplastic areas appear as pigment

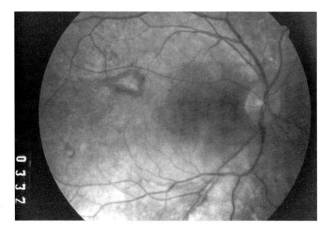

FIGURE 27-3. Chronic Vogt-Koyanagi-Harada syndrome. The RPE shows foci of atrophy and foci of hyperplasia.

clumps in some patients (Fig. 27-3). In others, the hyperplastic epithelium undergoes a fibrous metaplasia (Fig. 27-4), extending into the subretinal space in a condition which is clinically recognized as "subretinal fibrosis."

Infectious uveitis. In infectious uveitis, RPE may be damaged directly by the infectious agent or by extension of the inflammatory process from the adjacent choroid or retina. There are several viral infections that involve RPE, resulting in necrosis of these epithelial cells. In other infections, focal areas of choroid, RPE, and overlying retina are damaged, resulting in chorioretinal scars, with surrounding areas of RPE hyperplasia. Such changes are typically seen in *Toxoplasma gondii* infections.

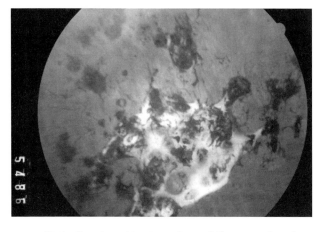

FIGURE 27-4. Chronic uveitis. Note subretinal fibrosis resulting from changes in RPE.

MODULATION OF UVEITIS BY RPE

The RPE cells are believed to play a pivotal role in the induction and perpetuation of uveitis. This belief is based on several in vitro studies (Detrick et al., 1985; Percopo et al., 1990). In the presence of interferon-γ and tumor necrosis factor α (TNFα), cultured RPE cells express MHC class II molecules and these cells may present retinal antigens to CD4+T cells (Detrick et al., 1985; Percopo et al., 1990). Additionally, the RPE cells produce a potent leukocyte chemotactic factor, interleukin-8 (IL-8), and in response to interleukin-1 (IL-1), they secrete interleukin-6 (IL-6) (Elner et al., 1990; Planck et al., 1992).

Production of IL-8 by the RPE may enhance the inflammation due to the potent chemotactic function of the cytokine (Elner et al., 1990). Similarly, IL-6 generated by the RPE may potentiate the inflammation (Planck et al., 1992). In addition to the generation of cytokines such as IL-1, IL-6, and IL-8, RPE cells can produce platelet-derived growth factor (PDGF)—like protein and granulocyte macrophage-colony stimulating factor (GM-CSF). These factors may enhance ongoing intraocular inflammation and uveitis. Moreover, cultured RPE cells express the adhesion molecule CD54 and intercellular adhesion molecule-1 (ICAM-1), both of which play a role in leukocyte trafficking and in amplification of the inflammatory process (Elner et al., 1992).

RPE cells can release superoxide during phagocytosis (Dorey et al., 1989). This oxygen metabolite can amplify inflammation and cause retinal damage by peroxidation of retinal cell membrane lipids (Rao, 1990). Such peroxidation may take place from the hydroxyl radicals, derived from superoxide and hydrogen peroxide in the presence of free iron or other metals. Hydroperoxides thus generated from lipid peroxidation can function as chemotactic agents and may amplify intraocular inflammation and uveitis (Goto et al., 1991). Generation of these oxygen metabolites, various cytokines and adhesion molecules by the RPE supports the hypothesis that the RPE may contribute to the pathogenesis of immune-mediated uveitis and to the perpetuation and amplification of intraocular inflammation.

Paradoxically, the enucleated eyes of patients with uveitis (sympathetic ophthalmia and Vogt-Koyanagi-Harada syndrome) show preservation of the retina and choriocapillaris at the site of intact RPE, even though the choroid is heavily infiltrated by macrophages, lymphocytes and other inflammatory cells (Green, 1985). These morphologic observations do not support the above-mentioned in vitro findings suggesting the proinflammatory function of RPE. It appears that, in a manner similar to macrophages, RPE cells may modulate uveal inflammation, i.e., enhance it by releasing various cytokines or suppress the process by releasing antiinflammatory factors.

Those antiinflammatory factors that the RPE is known to generate include transforming growth factor-beta (TGF-β), and antioxidant enzymes such as superoxide dismutase, catalase, 75 kDa protein known as RPE protective protein (RPP) and others (Rao, 1990; Wu and Rao, 1996; Wu et al., 1996). In vitro the RPP inhibits neutrophil and macrophage generation of superoxide (Wu and Rao, 1996). It is believed that this protein may prevent retinal damage in uveitis and related intraocular inflammation by inhibiting the phagocyte generation of oxygen metabolites (Wu and Rao, 1996; Wu et al., 1996). TGF-β, RPP, and antioxidants may play a role in down-regulating the inflammation and protecting the photoreceptors and choriocapillaris in cases of severe uveitis, such as sympathetic ophthalmia and Vogt-Koyanagi-Harada syndrome. It appears that a balance between the production and catabolism of proinflammatory and antiinflammatory factors by RPE may play a role in modulation of uveitis and in protection or degeneration of retinal tissue and adjacent choriocapillaris.

ANIMAL MODELS OF UVEITIS

Attempts at induction of uveitis in various laboratory animals have resulted in the discovery of various intraocular proteins that act as potent uveitogenic antigens (Gery et al., 1986). Several animal models of uveitis have been developed utilizing sensitization with these antigens to produce an organ-specific autoimmune intraocular inflammation (Rao et al., 1979; Gery et al., 1986; Schalken et al., 1988; Dua et al., 1992; Brockhuyse et al., 1992; Gery et al., 1994). These uveitis models are induced by retinal soluble protein known as S-antigen, rhodopsin, interphotoreceptor retinoid-binding protein, melanin-associated protein obtained from RPE or uvea, lens protein, and others. A second group of models is produced by intraocular injection of nonocular proteins such as heterologous albumin or gamma globulins. A third group of experimental models is produced by intravitreal injection of cytokines or complement products. A fourth group includes intravitreal injection of endotoxin (Rosenbaum et al., 1980), and a fifth group utilizes injection of xanthine and xanthine oxidase to generate reactive oxygen metabolites (Sery and Petrillo, 1984). One major disadvantage of all of these intravitreal injection models is that the primary inflammatory response consists of an acute vitritis rather than uveitis; thus, these intravitreal injection models do not provide a clinically relevant model for uveitis studies.

Of all the above experimental models, uveitis induced by retinal soluble protein, interphotoreceptor retinoid-binding protein, and melanin-associated protein have been studied most extensively and have been well characterized clinically, morphologically, and immunologically. Moreover, these models offer several similarities in clinical and pathologic features to those observed in various uveitis entities noted in humans (Gery et al., 1986). These retinal, RPE, and choroidal antigen-induced intraocular inflammations have increased our understanding of the role of autoimmunity in the development of uveitis and have allowed us to study the effects of various new therapeutic agents in the treatment of autoimmune uveitis.

Retinal antigen-induced uveitis. Multiple retinal proteins can induce uveitis/intraocular inflammation in laboratory animals when sensitized by these proteins. These antigenic proteins include retinal soluble protein, interphotoreceptor retinoid-binding protein, rhodopsin, and phosducin, a 33 K retinal phosphoprotein involved in phototransduction (Rao et al., 1979; Gery et al., 1986; Schalken et al., 1988; Brockhuyse et al., 1992; Dua et al., 1992; Gery et al., 1994).

Retinal soluble antigen (S-antigen) is considered to be a photoreceptor arrestin. It is a 48 kDa protein that is relatively specific for binding retinol used in the visual cycle. This protein is associated with the plasma membrane of the photoreceptor cells. This antigen can induce intraocular inflammation in guinea pigs, Lewis rats, and other animals within two weeks, when the animals are immunized with the protein along with complete Freund's adjuvant. Induction of uveitis in these animals is highly reproducible. In guinea pigs, smaller quantities of S-antigen (one microgram) lead to a nongranulomatous focal uveitis. At an intermediate dose range of 5 to 10 micrograms, the animals develop granulomatous panuveitis and other histologic features of sympathetic ophthalmia (Rao et al., 1979). Unlike guinea pigs, Lewis rats immunized with this antigen develop retinitis along with panuveitis (Fig. 27-5A). Such rats have been extensively utilized in various immunologic investigations which have revealed that the uveitis is a T-cell-mediated disease, where CD4+ T-cells recognize the antigen in the form of peptides associated with MHC-II molecules. Several uveitogenic peptides of S-antigen that can induce uveitis in submicrogram doses have been identified in these rats.

Interphotoreceptor retinoid-binding protein (IRBP) is the major soluble protein of the interphotoreceptor ma-

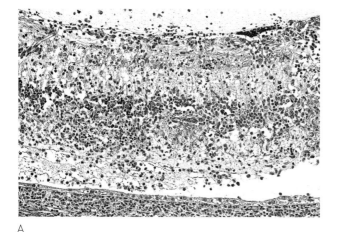

A

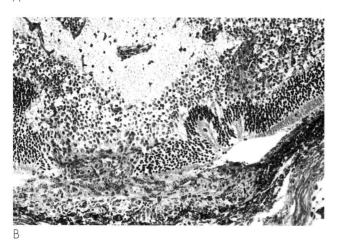

B

FIGURE 27-5. (A) Lewis rat immunized with S-antigen shows retinitis and choroiditis. H&E; magnification ×250. (B) B10A mouse with IRBP induced uveitis shows granulomatous choroiditis, which involves RPE and the retina. H&E; magnification ×250.

trix of vertebrate retinas. This 140 kDa glycoprotein is believed to function in the transport of retinoids between the neural retina and RPE. It is highly uveitogenic in various laboratory animals, and in particular, in Lewis rats (Gery et al., 1986).

Rats with IRBP-induced uveitis show retinitis, iridocyclitis, and choroiditis. There is cellular exudate in the anterior chamber and the vitreous cavity. The target of the inflammation, however, is the photoreceptors, which are destroyed in this uveitis (Gery et al., 1986). Usually RPE is also damaged at these sites. Mice immunized with IRBP readily develop granulomatous choroiditis (Fig. 27-5B), retinitis, and retinal vasculitis. Primates and rabbits also develop uveitis on immunization with this protein. Like the uveitis induced by S-antigen, IRBP-induced uveitis is a T-cell-mediated process. Similar to S-antigen and IRBP, several retinal proteins, including rhodopsin, phosducin, and others mentioned

above can induce uveitis. In all cases, the uveitis appears to develop from delayed hypersensitivity to the respective retinal proteins.

Uveitis induced by melanin-associated protein. A melanin-associated protein obtained from either RPE or uveal melanocytes can readily induce a primarily anterior uveitis in Lewis rats, when these animals are injected with this protein in an emulsion of complete Freund's adjuvant (Brockhuyse et al., 1992). This uveitogenic antigen is present in the RPE of various species, and in iris, choroid, and skin. The induced uveitis is characterized by infiltrations of polymorphonuclear leukocytes and mononuclear inflammatory cells in the iris and ciliary body with exudation into the anterior and posterior chambers. The choroid may be minimally involved with the mononuclear cell infiltration. Retina and RPE are usually spared from inflammatory cell infiltration. Similar to retinal antigen-induced uveitis, the melanin-associated protein-induced uveitis is found to be a T-cell process that can be adoptively transferred by sensitized CD4+ lymphocytes (Brockhuyse et al., 1992).

The above animal models show some similarities to those observed in humans with uveitis. Animals with melanin-associated protein-induced uveitis develop anterior uveitis (Brockhuyse et al., 1992); IRBP-induced uveitis in mice shows features of Dalen-Fuchs-like nodules (Rao et al., 1993); and guinea pigs with S-antigen-induced uveitis demonstrate several features of sympathetic ophthalmia, including granulomatous panuveitis, pigment phagocytosis by epithelioid cells, and presence of Dalen-Fuchs nodules (Rao et al., 1979). Patients with uveitis similar to that seen in the animal studies reveal in vitro lymphocyte activation/proliferation in the presence of various retinal antigens. Such activation is observed with S-antigen and with IRBP, in patients with posterior uveitis including sympathetic ophthalmia, Vogt-Koyanagi-Harada syndrome, and others. It appears that one or more of the intraocular antigens may play a role in the induction or perpetuation of some forms of uveitis observed in humans.

INFECTIONS OF RPE

Various infectious agents affect choroid, retina, or RPE, altering the functions of the RPE or causing morphologic damage to these pigmented cells. Those infectious agents which affect RPE include viruses, bacteria, protozoa, and fungi. Many of these agents primarily infect the retina or choroid with subsequent involvement of RPE. Unlike bacterial or fungal infections, the intraocular infections caused by viruses or protozoa *(Toxo-*

plasma gondii) are known to cause in utero infection leading to congenital abnormalities and/or sight-threatening complications. These agents are also the leading causes of life-threatening and sight-threatening infections in the epidemic of the acquired immunodeficiency syndrome (AIDS), as well as in individuals on immunosuppressive therapy for organ transplantation or in patients undergoing high-dose chemotherapy for various malignancies.

Viral infections. The DNA and RNA viral agents which affect RPE include the herpes family, rubella, rubeola, and influenza A among others (Yoser et al., 1993). The herpes viral infections of the retina and RPE are commonly seen in the ophthalmic clinics. Rubella ocular infections, on the other hand, are rarely seen, but this virus affects RPE without inducing any changes in the sensory retina. Recently, involvement of RPE in retroviral infections such as HIV and HTLV-1 has also been reported (Kumar et al., 1994). All of these viral agents involve RPE either by directly invading the RPE cells or by secondarily causing damage to RPE through the release of inflammatory mediators during the retinal viral infections. Among the members of herpes virus family, cytomegalovirus (CMV) and herpes simplex virus (HSV) cause both congenital and acquired infections of the retina and RPE.

Cytomegalovirus infection. Cytomegaolvirus infects almost the entire population at some time in their life: it has been estimated that at least 80% to 85% of adults are infected by age 40 (Yoser et al., 1993). The virus is usually transmitted by close or intimate individuals who are shedding the virus in urine, stool, saliva, and or excretions. Other modes of transmission are venereal spread; in utero, natal, or perinatal exposure; and via transfusion of blood products, transplanted organs, or breast milk.

Usually, CMV infection in an immunocompetent individual is a benign asymptomatic infection, rarely leading to ocular involvement. But CMV is a potent opportunistic infection in immunocompromised individuals, particularly during the late stages of AIDS (Rao, 1994).

Most newborns who are infected with CMV in utero remain asymptomatic, although 5% to 20% of those who shed virus will develop symptoms. Symptomatic infants present with low birth weight, hepatosplenomegaly, jaundice, microcephaly, and intracranial calcification, along with retinitis or other ocular findings (Birdsong et al., 1956). The retinitis is usually accompanied by choroiditis and involvement of RPE. During resolution of the infection, at the site of retinitis, chorioretinal scarring is noted and the RPE exhibits prolifera-

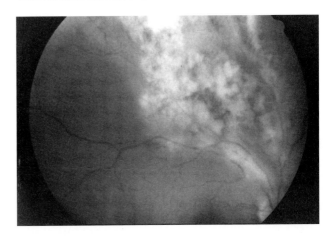

FIGURE 27-6. CMV retinitis. Necrotizing retinitis with foci of hemorrhages is present.

tion at the margin of the lesion. At the center of the lesion, the RPE cells are either necrotic or are replaced by chorioretinal scarring (Yoser et al., 1993).

In adults, CMV infection usually occurs in an individual with an immune system compromised by, for example, human immunodeficiency viral (HIV) infection, lymphoma/leukemia, or chemotherapy used to treat malignancies or to suppress organ graft rejection. Between 15% and 40% of individuals with HIV infection develop intraocular CMV infection, particularly during the severe immunodeficiency state, AIDS (Rao, 1994). Such ocular involvement is seen in only about 1% to 2% of renal transplant cases (Yoser et al., 1993).

Although the intraocular CMV infection clinically presents with features of retinitis (Fig. 27-6), the virus usually affects the RPE also. On histologic examination, a full-thickness retinal and RPE necrosis is noted at the site of the retinitis. Typically, the necrosis shows large cells with intranuclear inclusion bodies (Cowdry type A) and basophilic intracytoplasmic inclusion bodies (Fig. 27-7). Such megalic cells are observed in all layers of the involved retina, including the RPE (Rajeev and Rao, 1995). Cytomegalovirus can be detected in these cells by electron microscopy, immunohistochemistry, and in situ DNA hybridization (Henderly et al., 1988). Viral cultures and polymerase chain reaction (PCR) also reveal the presence of CMV at the site of retinitis (Biswas et al., 1993).

Electron microscopy may reveal necrotic RPE, with some of the cells containing virus particles in their nuclei or cytoplasm. Unlike the congenital CMV infection of the retina and retinal pigment epithelium, RPE in adults rarely shows proliferation at the site of resolution. Usually these sites show markedly atrophic retina and retinal pigment epithelium with glial scarring (Rao, 1994).

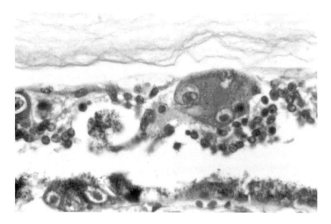

FIGURE 27-7. Histologic appearance of CMV retinitis. Large cells containing intranuclear and intracytoplasmic inclusion are present. Note RPE with intranuclear viral inclusions. H&E; magnification ×240.

In the United States, there are three currently approved medications for treatment of CMV retinitis: ganciclovir, foscarnet, and cidofovir. In the vast majority of the patients, all these agents are administered intravenously. However, these agents are also found therapeutically useful when injected intravitreally (Diaz-Llopis et al., 1992). There is an oral form of ganciclovir that is useful in the maintenance therapy of CMV infection; and there are reports indicating promising results in controlling CMV retinitis with long-term intraocular delivery using ganciclovir implants (Anand et al., 1993).

The intravenous ganciclovir treatment consists of an initial two-week high-dose induction therapy of 5 mg/kg twice daily followed by long-term maintenance therapy of 5 mg/kg once daily seven days a week or 6 mg/kg once daily five days a week. The primary side effect of ganciclovir therapy is myelosuppression. Concomitant use of granulocyte colony stimulating factor can reduce neutropenia, the most serious component of myelosuppression, and may allow continuation of ganciclovir. Foscarnet is also administered intravenously, in a two-week high-dose induction of 60 mg/kg every eight hours followed by long-term maintenance therapy of 90–120 mg/kg daily five or seven days a week. This agent is toxic to the kidneys (Yoser et al., 1993; Rao, 1994). Other anti-CMV therapies currently under investigation include intravenous agents such as cytosine dihydrate and oral agents such as valaciclovir.

Herpes simplex virus (HSV). Herpes simplex virus is a double-stranded DNA packaged within an icosahedral capsid with an outer covering of lipid membrane. Originally, neutralization antibody tests revealed the presence of two antigenic types of the herpes simplex virus: HSV-1 and HSV-2. Both of these subtypes can cause mucocutaneous and visceral infections which are clinically indistinguishable from each other. Infection of certain cells with HSV, neurons in particular, does not always result in virus replication and cell death. Rather, the virus may be maintained in a latent state, with repression of the viral genome compatible with survival and normal cell activity. Subsequent reactivation of the viral genome can occur, resulting in virus relocation and, in some cases, redevelopment of herpetic lesions (Yoser et al., 1993).

Type 1 HSV is the main agent responsible for the majority of cases of herpetic eye disease in all age groups. However, rarely type 2 HSV has been recovered, from eyes of both adults and neonates with ocular disease (Yoser et al., 1993). Neonatal HSV 1 infections are usually acquired either postnatally through contact with immediate family members who have oral-labial HSV-1 infection or by nosocomial transmission. In neonates, ocular manifestations of HSV infection include conjunctivitis, keratitis, necrotizing retinitis associated with damage to RPE and choroidal inflammation, optic neuritis, cataracts, and microphthalmos. The retinal and RPE findings may include whitish-yellow, punctate lesions in both the macula and posterior pole, perivascular sheathing, and scarring with variable pigmentation from hyperplastic RPE at the border of the lesions. In a study of 32 children with virologically verified HSV infection, the presence of chorioretinal scars was noted more frequently than other ocular findings (el Azazi et al., 1990).

In children and adults, HSV ocular infection manifests similar to those seen in neonates. The most common manifestation is keratitis, heralded by acute onset of pain, blurry vision, chemosis, conjunctivitis, and characteristic dendritic lesions of the cornea. Herpes simplex retinitis primarily occurs in healthy individuals. Funduscopic examination in the early stages shows patches of necrotic retina, perivenous sheathing, flame-shaped hemorrhages, and vitreous opacities (Yoser et al., 1993). Progression of the disease can lead to papilledema and retinal vascular occlusion, along with retinal pigment epithelial and choroidal atrophy. Some patients with retinal necrosis may present with all the features typical of acute retinal necrosis (ARN) syndrome (Duker and Blumenkranz, 1991). With appropriate antiviral treatment the retinal necrosis may regress, leaving glial scars with focal areas of hyperpigmentation from RPE hyperplasia.

Histopathologic examination of HSV retinitis generally reveals full-thickness retinal necrosis with the necrotic process involving the adjacent retinal pigment

INFLAMMATIONS AND INFECTIONS OF THE RPE

epithelium. Fibrinoid necrosis and occlusion of retinal arteries and veins with acute and chronic inflammatory cell infiltration in the retina and choroid may be observed (Yoser et al., 1993). Intranuclear inclusions are occasionally seen within retinal cells; these are basophilic Feulgen-positive inclusions (Cowdry type A), containing viral DNA. Electron microscopy readily reveals the presence of virus particles measuring about 100 nm in the nuclear debris of retinal cells and in many RPE cells. Immunofluorescent studies (using monoclonal antibodies) can readily detect herpes simplex antigens in all layers of the retina, including the RPE (Yoser et al., 1993).

Herpes simplex retinitis is mainly treated by acyclovir; the dose for this agent is 30 mg/kg per day (Corey, 1987). Early diagnosis of HSV infection and administration of this agent may decrease the likelihood of ocular morbidity.

Varicella/herpes zoster virus (VZV).

VZV is a member of the herpes virus family which causes varicella or herpes zoster. Varicella is generally a benign illness, primarily of childhood. This illness is characterized by an exanthematous, vesicular rash. Herpes zoster develops from reactivation of latent VZV in sensory ganglionic neurons, most commonly in adults. This disease presents as a dermatomal, vesicular rash and is usually associated with severe pain.

Congenital varicella is a rare infection associated with a high mortality rate. Ocular manifestations include microphthalmos, cataract, Horner's syndrome, and chorioretinitis (Lambert et al., 1989). On resolution, the chorioretinitis leads to chorioretinal scars consisting of white elevated, gliotic centers, each surrounded by an irregular ring of black pigment caused by hyperplasia of RPE.

Acquired varicella/herpes zoster infection can present with retinitis, usually in association with the maculopapular and vesicular skin lesions of chickenpox or herpes zoster ophthalmicus. Recent studies suggest that in AIDS patients this retinitis presents with distinct clinical features and it is known as progressive outer retinal necrosis (PORN) (Forster et al., 1990). Varicella-zoster virus is also a major cause of the acute retinal necrosis (ARN) syndrome (Duker and Blumenkranz, 1991). This necrotizing retinitis is found in otherwise healthy individuals without the accompanying skin changes of the above-noted infections.

In immunocompetent individuals, the retinal manifestations of VZV include blurry vision, decreased visual acuity, eye pain and signs of intraocular inflammation. Initially, retinitis is seen mainly in the periphery where the entire thickness of the retina may be necrot-

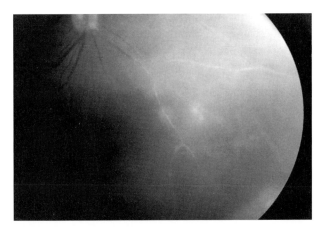

FIGURE 27-8. Acute retinal necrosis from VZV infection shows sheathing of retinal vessels and retinitis.

ic. The retinal vessels are either sheathed or occluded (Fig. 27-8). Retinal tears and detachment may develop during resolution of the retinitis. These findings may be either unilateral or bilateral, and the retinitis may spontaneously regress in occasional cases. Similar clinical findings are observed in ARN syndrome.

In HIV-infected individuals, the VZV retinitis (PORN) characteristically is rapidly progressive, with clinical features indicative of outer retinal necrosis (Forster et al., 1990). The process may begin in the posterior or peripheral retina while the retinal vessels and paravascular retina appear to be free from inflammatory damage (Fig. 27-9). Vitritis and papillitis are rare in this condition; however, like ARN patients, HIV-infected individuals with PORN usually develop a rhegmatogenous retinal detachment.

The most frequently used investigations for assessing host infectivity are immunofluorescent detection of antibodies to VZV membrane antigens. Unequivocal con-

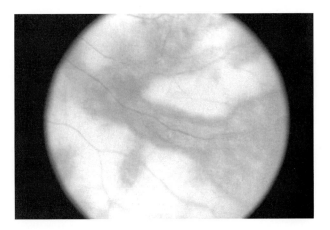

FIGURE 27-9. Note necrotizing retinitis with apparent sparing of the retinal vessels in progressive outer retinal necrosis.

firmation of the diagnosis is possible through the isolation of VZV, or by the demonstration of either seroconversion or a fourfold or greater rise in antibody titer. Immunofluorescence, in situ nucleic acid hybridization, or polymerase chain reaction (PCR) may also confirm the diagnosis (Yoser et al., 1993).

Histopathologic specimens obtained from immunocompetent individuals with acquired zoster retinitis reveal full-thickness necrotizing retinitis, retinal vasculitis, and mononuclear inflammatory cell infiltration, primarily in the choroid. Areas of necrosis are sharply demarcated, and intranuclear inclusions may be found in the inner retinal layers. Retinal pigment epithelial cells occasionally contain eosinophilic intranuclear inclusion bodies. Electron microscopy may reveal the presence of herpes virus particles and immunohistochemical methods can detect VZV antigens in retinal tissue. Staining with an antibody that detects the major gp 98/gp 62 VZV glycoprotein complex has been found useful (Yoser et al., 1993).

Varicella zoster virus retinitis and acute retinal necrosis syndrome are treated primarily with intravenous acyclovir. The recommended intravenous dose of acyclovir is 30 mg/kg in three divided doses per day for 7 days followed by 7–14 days of oral acyclovir, 400–600 mg five times a day (Blumenkranz et al., 1986). There is no satisfactory treatment for progressive outer retinal necrosis. Various combinations of antivirals, ganciclovir, foscarnet, acyclovir, and others have been tried with limited success.

Epstein-Barr virus.

Epstein-Barr Viral (EBV) infections account for a wide range of clinical conditions, such as infectious mononucleosis, Burkitt's lymphoma, anaplastic nasopharyngeal carcinoma, and possibly, some of the B-cell malignancies encountered in immunosuppressed individuals (Schooley, 1987). This virus is made up of a double-stranded DNA core surrounded by a nucleocapsid and complex envelope.

Ocular manifestations of EBV are diverse. Follicular conjunctivitis is the most common; others include keratitis, uveitis, episcleritis, dacryoadenitis, cranial nerve palsies, and oculoglandular syndrome. There are a few case reports associating chorioretinitis with EBV infection. A case of punctate outer retinitis was reported in a patient with acute EBV infection and infectious mononucleosis (Raymond et al., 1987). The patient had retinal pigment epithelial clumping and depigmentation near the macula. There were gray-white deep retinal lesions with indistinct borders in the peripheral retina and inflammatory cells in the vitreous.

Antibodies to several EBV-specific antigens appear during primary EBV infection. These include IgM anti-

bodies to the viral capsid antigen (VCA), IgG antibodies to VCA, and antibodies to diffuse early antigens (EA-D), restricted early antigens (EA-R), and Epstein-Barr nuclear antigens (EBNA). The presence of IgM anti-VCA antibodies and seroconversion to EBNA is diagnostic of a primary EBV infection. Patients with defects in cellular immunity may fail to make antibodies to EBNA (Yoser et al., 1993).

Therapeutic considerations for slowly resolving EBV choroiditis or retinitis would include use of acyclovir or alpha interferon. Both these agents are active inhibitors of EBV replication in vitro. However, most intraocular infections from EBV appear to be self-limiting. Corticosteroids are likely to be of limited benefit.

Measles virus.

Measles virus is an RNA virus with a helically arranged protein coat surrounded by a lipid envelope. The virus is classified as a paramyxovirus and measures about 120–200 nm in diameter. The virus, which causes an acute febrile eruption called *measles* or *rubeola,* is transmitted by nasopharyngeal secretions. The disease typically occurs during childhood.

Measles virus can be transmitted from a pregnant woman to her fetus. Malformations attributed to maternal measles include cardiopathy, cataract, pyloric stenosis, dacryostenosis, deafness, mongolism, cleft lip and cleft palate, rudimentary ear and pigmentary retinopathy. The retinopathy, which is present bilaterally with equal involvement of the posterior pole and periphery, shows a fine, scattered pigmentary pattern (Yoser et al., 1993).

Acquired measles is usually a benign self-limiting disease but may be associated with complicated illnesses like subacute sclerosing panencephalitis (SSPE). This late complication of measles is a rare entity with an incidence of about one per million and a male-to-female ratio of approximately 4:1. The disease is more common in rural areas. Children with SSPE may present with visual problems, behavior disorders, memory impairment, spastic quadriparesis, and dementia. Decerebrate rigidity and coma usually develop, leading to fatality within 5 to 12 months (Yoser et al., 1993).

The retinopathy is more common with acquired than with congenital measles. It may be associated with encephalitis and SSPE, but is often seen in otherwise uncomplicated cases. During the acute stage of retinopathy, the fundus shows attenuated vessels, especially arterioles, and diffuse retinal edema. Retinal hemorrhages, exudative stellate macular lesion and swollen optic disc may be present. As the symptoms of measles resolve, a secondary pigmentary retinopathy with a "salt and pepper" or a "bone corpuscle" pigment pattern appears in association with RPE changes, and the stellate exudate in the macula usually resolves. As a late sequela of retinitis, paravenous atrophy of RPE and bone spicule pigment deposition may be observed along the course of retinal veins (Foxman et al., 1985).

Since SSPE and measles encephalomyelitis are frequently fatal, postmortem retinal tissue has been available for histologic examination. Histologically, the retinal tissue usually shows focal necrosis with invasion of pigment-laden macrophages. The RPE may show a patchy loss of pigment. In SSPE, the inflammation involves the retina, RPE, and adjacent choriocapillaris. The rod and cone layer shows focal areas of degeneration. The RPE a lso exhibits degeneration, and large clumps of pigment granules are seen attached to the degenerated photoreceptor segments (Font et al., 1973). Intranuclear inclusions can be seen in ganglion cells and the inner nuclear layers of the retina. Occasionally, multinucleated syncytial giant cells containing numerous intranuclear eosinophilic inclusions surrounded by marginated nuclear chromatin are observed in areas of retinal atrophy. Electron microscopic studies have revealed the presence of filamentous microtubular structures of the paramyxovirus in the inclusion bodies. With immunofluorescent techniques, these sites are found to be positive for measles antigen (Font et al., 1973).

Serologic confirmation of measles can be carried out with complement fixation, enzyme immunoassay, and immunofluorescent and hemagglutination inhibition tests. In acute cases of retinopathy, electroretinography (ERG) is extinguished. As the retinitis resolves and vision improves, the ERG may show a return of activity. Although corticosteroids have been tried, there is no specific antiviral therapy for the retinopathy (Yoser et al., 1993).

Rubella virus. Rubella virus is an RNA virus and a member of the togavirus family, which measures 60 to 70 nm in diameter. It usually causes a benign febrile exanthem known as *rubella*. Acquired infections are common in children and young adults. In an infected individual, the virus is present in blood and throat secretions, and occasionally in feces. The virus most likely induces infection by instillation in the nasopharynx.

Congenital infection results from transplacental transmission of virus to the fetus from the infected mother during the first trimester of pregnancy. Such infection leads to chronic fetal infection and malformations, commonly known as congenital rubella syndrome. This syndrome consists of deafness, microcephaly, heart malformations, mental retardation, and eye lesions, including microphthalmia and pigmentary retinopathy.

Pigmentary retinopathy is the most common ocular complication of congenital rubella. The pigmentary changes may be observed throughout the fundus, but these changes are most marked in the macular region and may involve both eyes. The pigment disturbance consists of small, black, irregular masses, varying in size, commonly referred to as *salt and pepper retinitis* or *moth-eaten changes*. Rarely, subretinal neovascularization and hemorrhage may develop, particularly in the macula, later developing into a disciform scar (Menne, 1986). The individuals with the pigmentary retinopathy may have normal ERG and EOG (Krill, 1972). Histopathologic examination of pigmentary retinopathy reveals changes confined to the RPE. Some areas show increased pigmentation in the RPE and others reveal decrease in pigmentation or atrophy. These RPE changes are more prominent posterior to the equator (Zimmerman, 1968). Cataract is the second most common ocular problem seen with congenital rubella. Other common ocular abnormalities are microphthalmia and glaucoma.

Acquired rubella infection may also cause retinitis or chorioretinitis, leading to retinal and RPE detachments. Depigmentation and atrophy of RPE may be present at the sites of resolved bullous detachments of the retina.

A definitive diagnosis of rubella can be made only by virus isolation or by changes in antibody titers. The titers are usually determined by rubella hemagglutination-inhibiting antibodies, complement fixation, enzyme-linked immunosorbent assay, fluorescence immunoassay, radioimmunoassay and a variety of IgM- specific antibody tests. The presence of IgM-specific antibodies suggests recent rubella infection.

There is no specific antiviral therapy for either the congenital or the acquired form of rubella retinitis. Corticosteroids may be of some benefit in the management of retinitis, particularly in patients with bullous retinal detachment.

Human immunodeficiency virus (HIV). The illness that results from HIV infection varies from one individual to another. However, there are several predictable stages that lead invariably to death. Initially, infected individuals experience an acute primary infection, followed by a relatively asymptomatic infection that can include generalized lymphadenopathy. Subsequently, the disease progresses with a decline in T-helper lymphocytes and eventually reaches the advanced stage with the development of opportunistic infections, malignancies, or both. It is this advanced stage that is recognized as the acquired immunodeficiency syndrome (AIDS).

HIV is a member of the Lentivirinae subfamily. Two lentiviruses are currently known to infect humans: HIV-1 is more prevalent and is seen worldwide; HIV-2 is isolated primarily in West Africa. There is roughly 40%

homology in nucleotide sequences between HIV-1 and HIV-2. Both HIV-1 and HIV-2 measure 100 nm in diameter. The virion of HIV has a cylindrical nucleocapside that contains a single-stranded RNA along with viral enzymes, proteinase, integrase, and reverse transcriptase. Surrounding the capsid is a lipid envelope, derived from the infected host cell, containing virus-encoded glycoproteins. These glycoproteins are encoded by three structural genes: *gag, pol,* and *env.* In addition to these structural genes, HIV contains six additional regulatory genes, *tat, rev, nef, vif, vpr,* and *vpu.* The *tat* and *rev* genes are essential for virus replication (Kessler et al., 1992).

The pathogenesis of HIV infection includes attachment of the virus to T-cells and monocytes/macrophages that display CD4 surface molecules. After attachment, the viral core enters the cell cytoplasm; uncoating and transcription then take place, resulting in a complementary strand of DNA. This DNA becomes double-stranded and circular and enters into the cell nucleus. In the nucleus, the viral DNA integrates into the host cellular genome by means of viral endonuclease. This host cell can be either latently or actively infected. The infected cells gradually decrease in number from the cytopathic effects of virus replication. The decrease in T-cells eventually leads to a variety of opportunistic infections and the development of neoplasias such as Kaposi's sarcoma and lymphomas (Kessler et al., 1992).

Human immunodeficiency viral retinopathy is the most common ocular finding in patients with AIDS, occurring in about 50% to 70% of cases. The retinopathy is characterized by evanescent cotton-wool spots (Fig. 27-10), retinal hemorrhages, and microaneurysms. The cotton-wool spots appear as discrete, fluffy opacities in the superficial retina, usually localized in the posterior pole adjacent to the major vascular arcades. These retinal hemorrhages, which are seen in 15% to 40% of patients with AIDS, appear as flame-shaped or as blot hemorrhages. Retinal microaneurysms occur in about 20% of patients. These vascular changes are usually associated with capillary telangiectasia, focal areas of nonperfusion, and capillary loss (Rajeev and Rao, 1995).

Histopathologic examination of postmortem eyes with HIV retinopathy shows the presence of cytoid bodies at the site of cotton-wool spots. These cytoid bodies primarily involve the nerve fiber layer, which is focally thickened by a sharply circumscribed disciform lesion containing globular eosinophilic bodies that measure 10 to 20 μm in diameter (Rajeev and Rao, 1995). Particles and/or antigens of HIV-1 have been demonstrated in the retina, including the retinal vascular endothelium and the RPE at the sites of retinal changes.

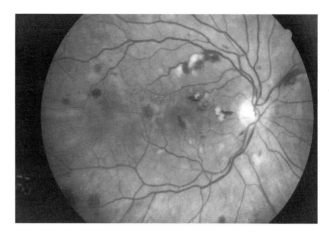

FIGURE 27-10. Cotton-wool spots and focal hemorrhages are noted in HIV retinopathy.

There is no specific therapy for HIV retinopathy. Usually, the cotton-wool spots resolve in about 6 to 12 weeks. Similarly, other retinal alterations either become less prominent or progress to further capillary closure during progression of the HIV infection. Although several antiretrovirals, such as zidovudine (AZT), dideoxyinosine (DDI), and dideoxycytidine, have been used in the treatment of HIV infection, many patients fail to respond to such therapy. In part, such treatment failures could be due to the emergence of drug-resistant viruses. Such resistance appears to be more common in the later stages of the disease (Kessler, 1992).

Human T-cell lymphotropic virus-type 1 (HTLV-1). HTLV-1 is a retrovirus associated with a wide range of ocular conditions, including inflammatory, infectious, and neoplastic lesions. This viral infection, which is endemic in southwest Japan, the Caribbean islands, and part of central Africa, is a known cause of adult T-cell leukemia-lymphoma and myelopathy.

Various ocular manifestations have been described in individuals infected with HTLV-1. Such ocular manifestations include retinal vasculitis, cotton-wool spots, uveitis, ocular adnexal lymphomas, orbital T-cell lymphoma, and intraocular T-cell lymphoma (Kumar et al., 1994; Mochizuki et al., 1992). The latter is characterized by the collections of neoplastic T cells primarily below the RPE, detaching thee epithelial cells from Bruch's membrane.

Treatment of HTLV-1-related T-cell lymphoma remains a challenge, with several modes of therapy under investigation. These experimental treatments include multiagent chemotherapy, monoclonal antibodies to the interleukin-2 receptor, zidovudine, interferon, and radiation therapy (Kumar et al., 1994).

Bacterial infections. RPE may be involved in a variety of gram-positive or gram-negative bacterial infections; however, the involvement is usually secondary to infections affecting the retina and/or choroid. Most intraocular bacterial infections lead to inflammation predominantly involving the vitreous and the anterior chamber. Such inflammations are classified as infectious endophthalmitis. These infections are caused either by introduction of organisms intraocularly during accidental or surgical trauma or by endogenous spread of the organism through circulation. The inflammatory process in endophthalmitis is usually diffuse, resulting in extensive damage to the retina and RPE. On resolution of the inflammation, the damaged retina and RPE are replaced by fibroglial tissue.

In contrast to the fulminating and purulent intraocular infections, certain bacteria, particularly acid-fast organisms, may cause localized chorioretinitis. At these sites, the choroid shows a necrotizing granulomatous inflammation, and the adjacent RPE and retina may be involved in the inflammation. When such lesions heal, the RPE at these sites shows foci of atrophy or proliferation resulting in pigmented chorioretinal scars.

Fungal infections. Fungal intraocular infections also result either from exogeneous causes, such as penetrating ocular injury, or from endogenous dissemination of the organism through the blood stream. In endogenous mycotic intraocular infections, the enucleated globes may show the organisms in the vitreous, retina, choroid and other sites; however, large numbers of these organisms are seen along the RPE in the subretinal space (L. E. Zimmerman, personal communication). At the subretinal site, the organisms appear to thrive, unlike in the retina, choroid, or other intraocular sites. Such findings suggest that the RPE may play a role either in preventing antimycotic functions of phagocytic inflammatory cells or in enhancing the growth of the fungi. Cytokines, such as TGF-β, generated by RPE have an antiinflammatory function. Similarly, RPE is a rich source of antioxidant enzymes and other antioxidants that may down-regulate oxygen metabolites. These metabolites are known antimicrobial agents, which are released locally by activated neutrophils and macrophages.

Parasitic diseases. Like the above-noted bacterial and fungal infections, parasitic infections can cause RPE changes, usually as an extension of the inflammatory process from either the retina or choroid. Such a process is typically seen in *Toxoplasma gondii* infection primarily involving the retina. During the active stage of inflammation, there is retinitis and choroiditis, with dam-

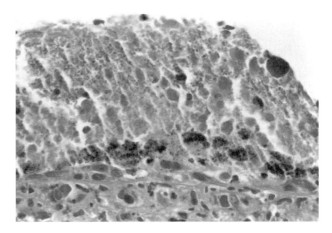

FIGURE 27-11. Necrotizing retinitis from *Toxoplasma gondii* infection. Note damage to the retinal pigment epithelium. H&E; magnification ×360.

age to the RPE (Fig. 27-11) at the site of the retinitis. When the inflammation subsides, the retinitis is replaced by a glial scar, and the RPE is either absent or markedly atrophic. At the edges of this retinal scar, however, the RPE shows hyperplastic changes that are clinically recognized as a ring of dark pigment surrounding the whitish glial scar (Fig. 27-12).

Secondary degenerative changes in the RPE are also noted in other parasitic diseases. For example, in ocular onchocerciasis, the choriocapillaris and choroid are found to be atrophic. In association with these changes, there is atrophy of the overlying RPE. The choroidal changes are believed to occur from local infection caused by microfilariae of *Onchocerca volvulus* (Paul and Zimmerman, 1970).

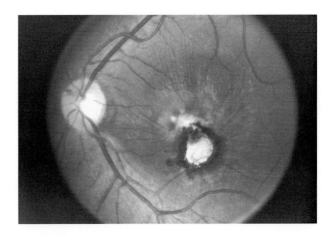

FIGURE 27-12. Toxoplasma retinochoroiditis. Scar tissue resulting from necrotizing retinal inflammation and subsequent resolution of the inflammation. RPE proliferation is present around the chorioretinal scar.

SUMMARY

The RPE actively participates in modulation of uveitis and other intraocular inflammations, including various intraocular infections. The pigmented cells enhance uveitis, either by expressing various surface proinflammatory molecules such as MHC-class II and adhesion molecules or by producing cytokines, such as IL-1, IL-6, IL-8, PDGF, and others. These cells can also downregulate the uveitis by the release of TGF-β and the actions of various antioxidant enzymes.

The RPE is a source of uveitogenic proteins; one specific protein associated with the melanin of these cells is a potent uveitogenic agent in laboratory animals and can readily induce severe anterior uveitis with mild choroiditis. RPE may also play a role in exposing other uveitogenic retinal proteins to the immune system by phagocytosis of photoreceptor outer segments.

Various DNA and RNA viruses infect RPE. Such infected cells may either undergo necrotic change or may harbor the virus without undergoing cytopathic changes. In parasitic intraocular infections, the RPE exhibits foci of either necrosis, atrophy, or hyperplasia. Typically in *Toxoplasma* retinochoroiditis, the pigmented cells undergo necrotic change in the center of the retinochoroiditis, while at the edges of these lesions, the RPE shows hyperplasia. During the resolution of infection and inflammation these pigmented cells participate in the formation of chorioretinal scars and in the development of subretinal fibrosis.

REFERENCES

Anand R, Nightingale SD, Fish RH, et al. 1993. Control of cytomegalovirus retinitis using sustained release of intraocular ganciclovir. Arch Ophthalmol 3:223–227.

Birdsong M, Smith DE, Mitchell FN, Coreh JR Jr. 1956. Generalized cytomegalic inclusion disease in newborn infants. JAMA 162:1305–1308.

Biswas J, Mayr AJ, Martin WJ, Rao NA. 1993. Detection of human cytomegalovirus in ocular tissue by polymerase chain reaction and in-situ DNA hybridization: a comparative study. Graefe's Arch Clin Exp Ophthalmol 231:66–70.

Blumenkranz MS, Culbertson WW, Clarkson JG, Dix R. 1986. Treatment of the acute retinal necrosis syundrome with intravenous acyclovir. Ophthalmology 93:296–300.

Broeckhuyse RM, Kuhlmann ED, Winkens HJ. 1992. Experimental autoimmune anterior uveitis (EAAU): II. Dose-dependent induction and adoptive transfer using a melanin-bound antigen of the retinal pigment epithelium. Exp Eye Res 55:401–411.

Corey L. 1987. Herpes simplex viruses. In: Braunwald E, Isselbacher KJ, Petersdorf RG, et al, eds, Harrison's Principles of Internal Medicine, 11th ed. New York: McGraw-Hill, 692–697.

Detrick B, Newsome DA, Percopo CM, Hooks JJ. 1985. Class II antigen expression and gamma interferon modulation of monocytes and retinal pigment epithelial cells from patients with retinitis pigmentosa. Clin Immunol Immunopathol 36:201–211.

Diaz-Llopis M, Chipont E, Sanchez S, et al. 1992. Intravitreal foscarnet for cytomegalovirus retinitis in a patient with acquired immunodeficiency syndrome. Am J Ophthalmol 114:742–747.

Dorey CK, Khouri GG, Syniuta LA, Curran SA, Weiter JJ. 1989. Superoxide production by porcine retinal pigment epithelium in vitro. Invest Ophthalmol Vis Sci 30:1047–1054.

Dua HS, Lee RH, Lolley RN, Barrett JA, Abrams M, Forrester JV, Donoso LA. 1992. Induction of experimental autoimmune uveitis by the retinal photoreceptor cell protein, phosducin. Curr Eye Res 11(suppl):107–111.

Duker JS, Blumenkranz MS. 1991. Diagnosis and management of the acute retinal necrosis (ARN) syndrome. Surv Ophthalmol 35:327–343.

el Azazi M, Malm G, Forsgren M. 1990. Late ophthalmic manifestations of neonatal herpes simplex virus infection. Am J Ophthalmol 109:1–7.

Elner SG, Elner VM, Pavilack MA, Todd RF III, Mayo-Bond L, Franklin WA, Strieter RM, Kunkel SL, Huber AR. 1992. Modulation and function of intercelular adhesion molecule 1 (CD54) on human retinal pigment epithelial cells. Lab Invest 66:200–211.

Elner VM, Strieter RM, Elner SG, Baggiolini M, Lindley I, Kunkel SL. 1990. Neutrophil chemotactic factor (IL-8) gene expression by cytokine-treated retinal pigment epithelial cells. Am J Pathol 136:745–750.

Font RL, Jenis EH, Tuck KD. 1973. Measles maculopathy associated with subacute sclerosing panencephalitis: immunofluorescent and immuno-ultrastructural studies. Arch Pathol 96:168–174.

Forster DJ, Dugel PU, Frangieh GT, Liggett PE, Rao NA. 1990. Rapidly progressive outer retinal necrosis in the acquired immunodeficiency syndrome. Am J Ophthalmol 110:342–348.

Foxman SG, Heckenlively JR, Sinclair SH. 1985. Rubeola retinopathy and pigmented paravenous retinochoroidal atrophy. Am J Ophthalmol 99:605–606.

Gery I, Mochizuki M, Nussenblatt RB. 1986. Retinal specific antigens and immunopathogenic process they provoke. Prog Ret Res 5:75–109.

Gery I, Chanaud NP III, Anglade E. 1994. Recoverin is highly uveitogenic in Lewis rats. Invest Ophthalmol Vis Sci 35:3342–3345.

Goto H, Rao NA. 1990. Sympathetic ophthalmia and Vogt-Koyanagi-Harada Syndrome. Int Ophthalmol Clin 30:279–285.

Goto H, Wu GS, Gritz DC, Atalla LR, Rao NA. 1991. Chemotactic activity of the peroxidized retinal lipid membrane in experimental autoimmune uveitis. Curr Eye Res 10:1009–1014.

Green WR. 1985. Uveal tract. In: Spencer WH, ed, Ophthalmic Pathology: An Atlas and Textbook. Philadelphia: Saunders, 1923–1932.

Henderly DE, Genstler AJ, Smith RE, Rao NA. 1987. Changing patterns of uveitis. Am J Ophthalmol 103:131–136.

Kessler HA, Bick JA, Pottage JC Jr, et al. 1992. AIDS: part II. Dis Mon 38:691–764.

Krill AE. 1972. Retinopathy secondary to rubella. Int Ophthalmol Clin 12:89–103.

Kumar SR, Gill PS, Wagner DG, Dugel PU, Moudgil T, Rao NA. 1994. Human T-cell lymphotropic virus type 1-associated retinal lymphoma. A clinicopathologic report. Arch Ophthalmol 112:954–959.

Lambert SR, Taylor D, Kriss A, Holzel H, Heard S. 1989. Ocular manifestations of the congenital varicella syndrome. Arch Ophthalmol 107:52–56.

Marak GE Jr. 1979. Recent advances in sympathetic ophthalmia. Surv Ophthalmol 24:141–156.

Menne K. 1986. Congenital rubella retinopathy—a progressive disease. Klinische Monatsablatt fur Augenheilkunde 189(4):436–439.

Mochizuki M, Watanabe T, Yamaguchi K, Yoshimura K, Nakashima S, Shirao M, Araki S, Takatsuki K, Mori S, Miyata N. 1992. Uveitis associated with human T-cell lymphotropic virus type 1. Am J Ophthalmol 114:123–129.

Moorthy RS, Inomata H, Rao NA. 1995. Vogt-Koyanagi-Harada syndrome. Surv Ophthalmol 39:265–292.

Paul EV, Zimmerman LE. 1970. Some observations on the ocular pathology of onchocerciasis. Human Pathol 1:581–589.

Percopo CM, Hooks JJ, Shinohara T, Caspi R, Detrick B. 1990. Cytokine-mediated activation of a neuronal retinal resident cell provokes antigen presentation. J Immunol 145:4101–4107.

Planck SR, Dang TT, Graves D, Tara D, Ansel JC, Rosenbaum JT. 1992. Retinal pigment epithelial cells secrete interleukin-6 in response to interleukin-1. Invest Ophthalmol Vis Sci 33:78–82.

Rajeev B, Rao NA. 1995. Advances in ocular pathology in AIDS. In: Advances in Ophthalmic Pathology. Ophthalmol Clinics of North America. Philadelphia: Saunders, 129–132.

Rao NA. 1990. Role of oxygen free radicals in retinal damage associated with experimental uveitis. Tr Am Ophthalmol Soc 88:797–850.

Rao NA. 1994. Acquired immunodeficiency syndrome and its ocular complications. Ind J Ophthalmol 42:51–63.

Rao NA, Wacker WB, Marak GE Jr. 1979. Experimental allergic uveitis. Clinicopathologic features associated with varying doses of S antigen. Arch Ophthalmol 97:1954–1958.

Rao NA, Naidu YM, Bell R, Lindsey JW, Pararajasegaram G, Sun Y, Steinman L. 1993. Usage of T cell receptor β-chain variable gene is highly restricted at the site of inflammation in murine autoimmune uveitis. J Immunol 150:5716–5721.

Raymond LA, Wilson CA, Linnemann CC Jr, Ward MA, Bernstein DI, Lovd DC. 1987. Punctate outer retinitis in acute Epstein-Barr virus infection. Am J Ophthalmol 104:424–426.

Rosenbaum JT, McDevitt HO, Gus RB, Egbert PR. 1980. Endotoxin-induced uveitis in rats as a model for human disease. Nature 268:611–613.

Schalken JJ, Winkens HJ, Van Vugt AHM, Bovée-Geurts PHM, de Grip WJ, Broekhuyse RM. 1988. Rhodopsin-induced experimental autoimmune uveoretinitis: dose-dependent clinicopathological features. Exp Eye Res 47:135–145.

Schooley RT. 1987. Epstein-Barr virus infections, including infectious mononucleosis, In: Braunwald E, Isselbacher KJ, Petersdorf RG, et al., eds, Harrison's Principles of Internal Medicine, 11th ed. New York: McGraw-Hill, 699–703.

Sery TW, Petrillo R. 1984. Superoxide anion radical as an indirect mediator in ocular inflammatory disease. Curr Eye Res 3:243–252.

Wu GS, Rao NA. 1996. A novel retinal pigment epithelial protein suppresses neutrophil superoxide generation. I. Characterization of the suppression factor. Exp Eye Res 63:713–725, 1996.

Wu GS, Swiderek KM, Rao NA. 1996. A novel retinal pigment epithelial protein suppresses neutrophil superoxide generation. II: Purification and microsequencing analysis. Exp Eye Res 63:727–737, 1996.

Yoser SL, Forster DJ, Rao NA. 1993. Systemic viral infections and heir retinal and choroidal manifestations. Surv Ophthalmol 37:313–346.

Zimmerman LE. 1968. Histopathologic basis for ocular manifestations of congenital rubella syndrome. Am J Ophthalmol 65:837–862.

28. Multifocal chorioretinopathy syndromes

SAM E. MANSOUR

The rare disorders grouped as multifocal chorioretinopathy syndromes involve a primary pathological process occurring at or near the level of the retinal pigment epithelium (RPE) with or without choriocapillaris involvement. Ultimately, the etiology is presumed to be either a vasculitic obstruction of the choriocapillaris with secondary infarction of the overlying RPE or possibly an immunological response directed at the RPE itself. Many of the clinical features of these individual entities overlap, causing much confusion. As such, it is still unknown whether these conditions represent distinct entities or whether some may be parts of a spectrum of the same basic disease. There are other conditions of choroiditis with overlying RPE involvement that will not be described in this section, yet they are important to consider in the differential diagnosis of these more atypical choroiditides such as tuberculosis, histoplasmosis, syphilis, posterior scleritis, reticulum cell sarcoma, lymphoid neoplasia, and Lyme disease, or the idiopathic syndromes such as central serous retinochoroidopathy, sarcoidosis, Vogt-Koyanagi-Harada syndrome, and sympathetic ophthalmia.

CLASSIFICATION: THE PROBLEM OF THE "ONE AND MANY"

In an attempt to find common characteristics among these myriad disorders, Gass (Gass, 1993) has grouped multiple evanescent white dot syndrome (MEWDS), acute idiopathic blind spot enlargement syndrome (AIBSES), acute macular neuroretinopathy (AMN) and multifocal choroiditis (MFC) or pseudo-presumed ocular histoplasmosis (pseudo-POHS) under the term *acute zonal occult outer retinopathy* (AZOOR). This inclusion group arose primarily from the observation of a few case reports where two or three of these entities had coincident manifestation in the same patient (Gass, 1993). AZOOR is characterized by the following common clinical features: minimal initial ophthalmoscopic changes followed later by signs of retinochoroidal degeneration, rapid reduction in one or more parameters of the visual field, photopsia, and abnormalities on electrophysiolog-

ical testing (Gass, 1993). AIBSES appears to be not so much a distinct and separate entity but rather a manifestation of some of the other conditions listed. AMN, a bilateral condition affecting otherwise healthy young adults, appears to involve a pathological process occurring more in the middle and outer retinal layers than in the RPE and choriocapillaris. As such, both AIBSES and AMN will not be discussed in the present section.

This grouping of AZOOR disorders is not universally accepted, however, as there are other authors who believe that the aforementioned entities are sufficiently distinct as to preclude any effective single inclusion group. (Jampol and Wiredu, 1995). The main problem for these disorders at present is the absence of any significant histopathologic material and serological findings. Thus these conditions not only present a classification problem, but also remain poorly understood with regards to etiology or pathogenesis. The present discussion of multifocal choroidopathy syndromes in this chapter will consider each entity separately and defer the problematic issue of classification.

MULTIFOCAL CHOROIDITIS AND PANUVEITIS (MCP)

Since the initial description of the disease by Nozik and Dorsch in 1973, there have been approximately 120 patients reported in the literature with multifocal choroiditis and panuveitis. As mentioned earlier, many investigators have lately suspected the MCP is one and the same with several other disorders, all representing various stages of the same basic clinical entity, the recently termed acute zonal occult outer retinopathy (AZOOR). With further follow-up of some of these patients, it is hoped that this spectrum of clinical manifestations of multifocal choroiditis will become better defined.

The disease affects young, otherwise healthy patients in their third decade (average age 34 years; range 6–74 years) with an incidence of bilateral involvement of 80%. There is a moderate racial and gender predisposition; approximately 66% of patients are Caucasian patients and 80% are female. As well, myopia is present in over 85% of these individuals.

Signs and Symptoms

The principal presenting symptom is usually that of blurry vision with or without photophobia. There may be mild ocular pain and complaints of metamorphopsia, floaters, scotomas, and photopsia.

Presenting visual acuity may vary from 20/20 to light perception with an average of somewhere around 20/100. Clinical examination reveals a mild-to-moderate aqueous inflammation with cell and flare in approximately 50%–60% of patients. Small-to-medium-sized keratic precipitates may be present as well as posterior synechiae and iris atrophy with nodule formation. There are vitreous cellular infiltrates in over 90% of patients.

Fundus examination reveals multiple, small, discrete yellow to gray-white spots which are typically round and may be polygon or oval in shape (Fig. 28-1). These lesions are approximately 200 μm in diameter, but can vary from 50 to 1000 μm in size. The lesions tend to scatter predominantly in the periphery rather than in the macula and are located at the level of the RPE and choriocapillaris. There may be multiple active lesions at any one time. During the late stage of the disease, the spots may become atrophic with a rim of hyperpigmentation. These can assume the classic "punched-out" appearance with bands of subretinal fibrosis at their margins (Fig. 28-2A). During the acute phase there may be optic disc edema, which later develops to peripapillary scarring, assuming a characteristic "napkin ring" subretinal fibrosis. Periphlebitis is often present, with resultant retinal vasculature narrowing (Schenck and Boke, 1990). Cystoid macular edema is present in approximately 10%–20% of patients, and the incidence of choroidal neovascular membrane formation varies somewhere from 25%–40% (Krill and Archer, 1970).

Fluorescein Angiography

During the early stage the active lesions exhibit blockage of the early fluorescence, followed by late staining (Fig. 28-1B). There may or may not be a rim of hyperfluorescence around the lesions. With the late stage of the disease, the most predominant feature is that of RPE window defects corresponding to the areas of the lesions (Fig. 28-2B). Similar findings are noted on Indocyanine Green angiography, where early lesions of MCP are hypofluorescent, in contrast with those of POHS which tend to be hyperfluorescent (Jampol and Wiredu, 1995).

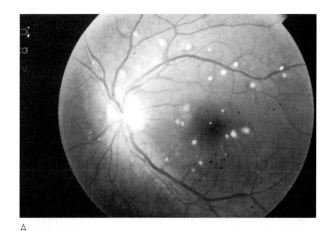

A

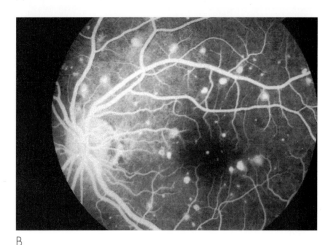

B

FIGURE 28-1. Multifocal choroiditis and panuveitis (MCP). (A) Multiple discrete lesions appearing in the early stage of the disease. (B) Fluorescein angiogram of same eye demonstrating punctate hyperfluorescence due to staining of the lesions.

Electrophysiological and Psychophysical Studies

The electroretinogram (ERG) is normal in approximately 50% of patients with MCP. However, a recent report by Jacobson and colleagues (1995) that looked at ERG testing in patients with AZOOR which included patients with MCP, revealed interocular asymmetry in all patients tested with full-field ERGs. In addition, moderate abnormalities in the a-wave suggest that there is dysfunction at the level of the photoreceptor outer segment. Similar findings have been noted in MEWDS and AMN, involving both the a-wave and early-receptor-potential recordings (Sieving et al., 1984; 1984b). The electrooculogram (EOG) is abnormal in approximately 60% of patients studied. Visual field testing sometimes demonstrates increased blind spot size (Khorram et al., 1991). Scotomata are associated with

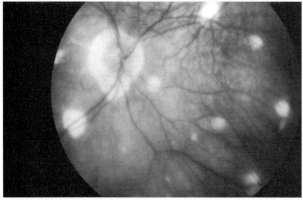

A

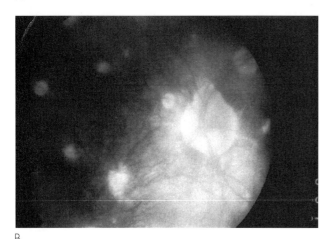

B

FIGURE 28-2. Multifocal choroiditis and panuveitis (MCP). (A) Late stage of disease manifesting atrophic, "punched-out" lesions. (B) Fluorescein angiogram demonstrating late-phase transmission hyperfluorescence of lesions.

clinical retinal lesions. Visual-field pattern abnormalities correlate well with ERG a-wave amplitude (Jacobson et al., 1995). In addition, large temporal field defects that do not correspond to clinical lesions have also been noted.

Etiology

The etiology of MPC remains unknown. Extensive systemic medical evaluations have not yet identified a single common cause for MPC. Unlike POHS, where there is a 90% positive histoplasmin skin test, only 25% of patients with MPC exhibit positive reactions to the histoplasmin skin test (Dreyer, Gass, 1984). Positive treponemal serology is evident in up to 27% of patients with MPC, yet no modification of the disease with penicillin treatments have been achieved to date.

Radiological investigations of patients with MPC have demonstrated hilar adenopathy in a small minority of patients (approximately 4%) along with pulmonary calcification (approximately 10%). In conjunction with this, approximately 20% of patients with MPC have a positive Mantoux test. Half of those patients, when treated with antituberculous medications, have a decrease in the ocular inflammation. Sarcoidosis has also been diagnosed in over one-third of patients with MPC.

Other infections that have been associated with MPC include herpes simplex, herpes zoster, Epstein-Barr virus, Lyme disease, and *Toxocara canis* (Bloom and Snady-McCoy, 1989; Bodine et al., 1992; Frau et al., 1990; Spaide et al., 1991; Tiedeman, 1987). Despite this, it is still felt by the majority of investigators that MPC is the result of an underlying autoimmune mechanism possibly triggered by an infectious agent. Histopathological studies of ocular specimens from patients with MPC have revealed a predominant B-lymphocyte and plasma cell infiltrate of the choroid and choriocapillaris (Palestine et al., 1985). In addition, a deposition of complement and immunoglobulins at or above Bruch's membrane has also been noted. There is a proliferation of the pigment epithelium with hyperplastic changes and migration into the neurosensory retina (Palestine et al., 1985).

Disease Course and Prognosis

Unfortunately, recurrence is very high in MPC and the visual prognosis remains poor (Joondeph and Tessler, 1991) (Morgan and Schatz, 1986). Peripapillary atrophy with progressive subretinal fibrosis results in enlargement of a blind spot in approximately 43% of patients. Unlike the aforementioned conditions, the major cause of central visual loss is due to subretinal neovascular membrane formation (~45%) and not due to cystoid macular edema (~13%) (Watzke and Claussen, 1981). Rarely may MPC lead to serous retinal detachments. Approximately one-third of patients are able to maintain their initial visual acuity at onset, while another third will lose on average at least two Snellen lines with MPC.

Treatment of MPC remains problematic. In a few cases there is often a prompt response in the acute phase to high systemic corticosteroids with subsequent improvement in visual acuity. In some instances, amelioration of the subretinal neovascular membrane has also been noted with corticosteroid therapy (Morgan and Schatz, 1986). However, with each recurrence there is a progressive diminution in the effect of corticosteroid treatment.

DIFFUSE SUBRETINAL FIBROSIS SYNDROME (DSFS)

DSFS, a very rare and incompletely characterized entity was first described in 1982 (Doran and Hamilton, 1982). Many investigators have lately suspected that DSFS represents a variation of multifocal choroiditis and panuveitis. As well, this condition shares many features of punctate inner choroidopathy and other similar diseases in the AZOOR grouping.

Diffuse subretinal fibrosis syndrome typically affects otherwise healthy individuals in their second decade (average age is approximately 20 years; range 14–34 years). The condition is often bilateral. There is some questionable association with axial myopia.

Signs and Symptoms

Patients typically present with central visual loss and complaints of metamorphopsia. Clinical examination during the acute phase reveals multiple small, yellow stellate lesions scattered throughout the posterior pole (Fig. 28-3A). There may be a mild vitritis at the time with isolated pockets of subretinal fluid. In the chronic phase, the lesions become discrete with sharply angulated subretinal scar formation. In the macula, the lesions tend to coalesce, forming broad zones of subretinal fibrosis. Later complications can include serous and hemorrhagic macular detachment.

Fluorescein Angiography

As mentioned earlier, this condition shares many clinical features with that of multifocal choroiditis and panuveitis. This is also reflected in the fluorescein angiogram. The distinct features of DSFS on angiography is an early-phase hypofluorescence in the areas of subretinal fluid loculation. During the late phase of the angiogram, there is extensive leakage at these sites that may, in some cases, suggest subretinal neovascularization (Doran and Hamilton, 1982) (Fig. 28-2B and 28-2C).

Electrophysiological and Psychophysical Studies

The findings on the ERG and the EOG are notoriously variable in this condition, with surprisingly intact studies in individuals with both acute and chronic involvement. Visual-field testing reveals constriction peripherally with central scotomata that often correlate with the clinical lesions.

Etiology

As with multifocal choroiditis, there have been no systemic associations with DSFS. Earlier suggestions that

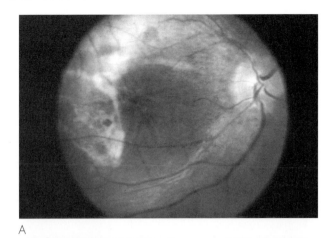

A

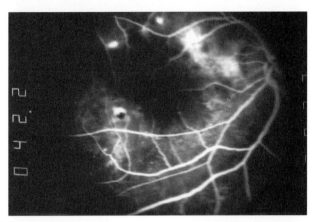

B

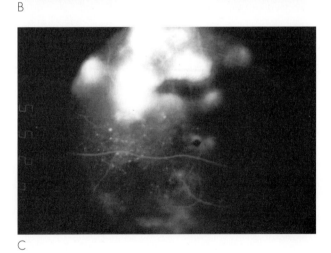

C

FIGURE 28-3. Diffuse subretinal fibrosis syndrome (DSFS). (A) This patient's right eye shows the typical subretinal angulated scar formation. (B) and (C) Mid and late phases of the fluorescein angiogram demonstrating progressive leakage hyperfluorescence.

this condition may be due to as yet unknown hormonal irregularities in young women (Salvador et al., 1994) have not developed into any trend of significance. In view of the clinical and angiographic findings, it is likely this condition's clinical appearance is secondary to a primary RPE hyperplastic process (Cantrill and Folk, 1986).

Disease Course and Prognosis

This condition is characterized by recurrent episodes with the fellow eye becoming involved within a six-month period. Management of DSFS involves the use of corticosteroids early in the disease. This is useful in sparing visual loss largely in the contralateral eye. Cyclosporin may be useful in those cases where steroid has failed to control the disease.

PUNCTATE INNER CHOROIDOPATHY (PIC)

First described by Watzke and colleagues in 1984, PIC is a syndrome that typically affects young, moderately myopic women who present with typical signs of ocular histoplasmosis, but have negative serology or skin test for histoplasmosis (Morgan and Schatz, 1986). This rare condition is also one of the entities in the AZOOR group. Other terms used to describe this condition include *multifocal inner choroiditis* and *pseudohistoplasmosis*. The average age of patients with PIC is 27 years, with a range of 16 to 40 years. Females represent 90% of the patients with PIC, and usually have bilateral ocular involvement (Gass, 1987).

Signs and Symptoms

Patients present with the usual blurred vision, photopsia, and central and peripheral scotomata. However, there is no history of any viral prodrome. It is important to note that PIC differs from POHS in that patients afflicted with the latter tend to be more assymptomatic with regards to scotomata. As well, chronic chorioretinal scars tend to be more stable in POHS than in PIC. The initial visual acuity at presentation varies from 20/50 to 20/400. There are no anterior segment or external ocular signs of inflammation. The characteristic lesion of PIC is essentially identical to that seen in ocular histoplasmosis with multiple (approximately 2–6) yellow-white spots (100–300 μm) of the inner choroid and retina largely confined to the posterior pole (Fig. 28-4). These lesions tend to assume a linear branching pattern. During the late stage of the disease, the spots become atrophic and pigmented. The classic triad of punched-out peripheral lesions in association with peripapillary atrophic scar formation and disciform macular scar seen in POHS is often present in patients with PIC. Small serous retinal detachments may form, but

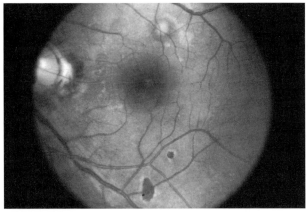

A

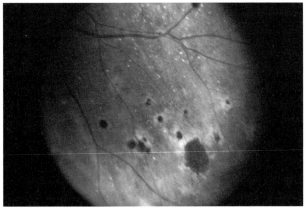

B

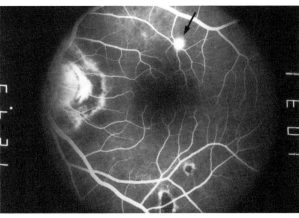

C

FIGURE 28-4. Punctate inner choroidopathy (PIC). (A) Pigmented central lesions in association with peripapillary scarring are also seen in conjunction with similarly pigmented peripheral lesions (B). (C) Late-phase fluorescein angiogram of same patient demonstrating "halo" hyperfluorescence of both the peripapillary and inferior macular scars, which are more chronic relative to the more active superior macular lesion *(arrow)* demonstrating leakage hyperfluorescence.

they resolve spontaneously and usually require no treatment. Both optic-disc edema and the presence of vitreous cells appear to be a variable finding in patients with PIC. There is a 25–40% occurrence of subretinal neovascular membranes in this condition.

Fluorescein Angiography

Again, paralleling the findings in ocular histoplasmosis, the early phase of the angiogram demonstrates hyperfluorescence of the lesions and the late phase is marked by leakage at the lesions (Fig. 28-4C).

Electrophysiological and Psychophysical Studies

The ERG is infrequently subnormal in patients with PIC. The EOG demonstrates very mild abnormalities of the Arden ratio. Visual-field testing demonstrates central and paracentral scotomas. There may or may not be an enlarged blind spot.

Etiology

It is likely that PIC represents a variant of multifocal choroiditis. It may represent either an inflammatory or infectious thrombosis of the choriocapillary layer by an as yet unidentified organism that behaves very similarly to histoplasmosis.

Disease Course and Prognosis

Recurrences are common in PIC, usually occurring within the first three months (Morgan and Schatz, 1986). Despite this, visual outcome is good, with approximately 50%–75% of eyes having vision better than 20/25, especially if uncomplicated with choroidal neovascular membrane formation.

There is a variable response to systemic corticosteroids depending on the stage of the disease. Laser photocoagulation has been used for the management of subretinal neovascular membranes.

MULTIPLE EVANESCENT WHITE DOT SYNDROME (MEWDS)

Described in 1984, MEWDS is a self-limited condition that afflicts young, otherwise healthy patients, usually in their second decade (average age 28 years; range 14–57 years) (Jampol et al., 1984). MEWDS shares many clinical and electrophysiological features with AIBSES and for that matter with other entities in the AZOOR grouping. Despite that commonality, however, MEWDS

is still felt to be uniquely distinguishable, warranting its own separate identification (Jampol and Wiredu, 1995). The condition usually presents unilaterally with few instances of later contralateral ocular involvement (Aaberg et al., 1985). The majority of patients appear to be women (approximately 75%). There is no racial predilection.

Signs and Symptoms

In addition to presenting with blurred vision and multiple paracentral scotomata, patients also, when questioned, report symptoms of flulike illness (approximately 25%–50%). Initial visual acuities on presentation vary from 20/25 to 20/300 (average 20/100). Vitreous cells are noted in approximately 50% of patients, this despite the absence of any anterior segment or external ocular signs of inflammation. The characteristic lesions in MEWDS consist of multiple small (approximately 100–200 μm in diameter), gray-white patches, each patch comprising smaller white to light orange dots (Figs. 28-5, 28-6; plate 28-I). These appear to be at the level of the RPE and outer retina and are typically distributed in the perifoveal and peripapillary regions with rare involvement of the fovea itself. In the periphery, the dots become sparse and assume a somewhat radial pattern, in some instances paralleling the retinal vasculature.

Later, the macula often exhibits a fine, granular, white, or orange-speckled appearance. These specks are much smaller than the white dots and are often associated with an irregular light reflex of the internal limiting membrane. Other posterior pole findings include splinter hemorrhages, venous sheathing, hyperemia or edema of the optic nerve head, and, very rarely, subreti-

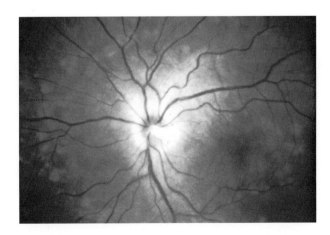

FIGURE 28-5. Multiple evanescent white dot syndrome (MEWDS). Acute manifestation of deep, white spots scattered throughout the posterior pole.

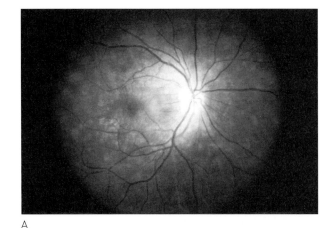

A

B

FIGURE 28-6. Multiple evanescent white dot syndrome (MEWDS). (A) Another patient with similar spots as in Figure 28-5. (B) Fluorescein angiogram of same patient demonstrating the characteristic late-phase mottled hyperfluorescence and staining of the optic disc.

nal neovascular membrane formation (Callanan and Gass, 1992; McCollum and Kimble, 1992).

Fluorescein Angiography

In the early phase of the angiogram, there is a punctate hyperfluorescence of the gray-white patches, which often display a "wreath-shaped" pattern. Leakage of dye at the optic disc is present in approximately 60% of patients (Fig. 28-6B). During the late phase of the angiogram, there is a patchy, mottled pattern of hyperfluorescence throughout the posterior pole with staining of the optic nerve head (Fig. 28-6B).

With resolution of the acute episode, the angiographic findings become much less prominent, but usually subtle RPE window defects persist.

Recent ICG angiography studies demonstrate multi-ple deep, small, round, hypofluorescent lesions that appear early and persist into the late phases (Ie et al., 1994). It is interesting to note that there were many more lesions seen on ICG angiography than were visible by clinical examination or fluorescein angiography.

Electrophysiological and Psychophysical Studies

Electrophysiological abnormalities are prominent during the active phase of MEWDS. Electroretinography demonstrates a marked reduction in the a- and b-waves, which gradually recover as the white dots disappear (Fig. 28-7). The early receptor potential (ERP) is also abnormal, suggesting not only photoreceptor malfunction but also abnormal visual pigment regeneration kinetics (Horiguchi et al., 1993; Sieving et al., 1984b). EOG testing demonstrates a moderate reduction of the Arden ration. Visual-field testing can demonstrate central and peripheral scotomas, and the blind spot is often enlarged (Dodwell et al., 1990; Hamed et al., 1989).

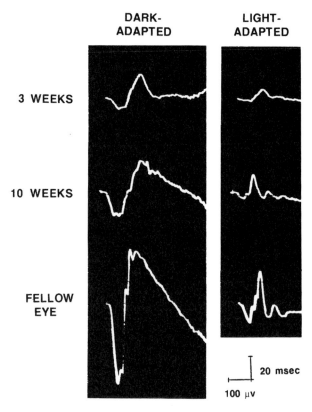

FIGURE 28-7. Multiple evanescent white dot syndrome (MEWDS). Electroretinogram of a patient with unilateral disease demonstrating marked reduction of both the a- and b-waves of the affected eye in comparison to the unaffected fellow eye. At 10 weeks partial recovery is evident. (Courtesy of Michael F. Marmor M.D.)

Etiology

The etiology of MEWDS remains unknown. The possibility of a viral cause has been entertained in view of the elicitation of a history of flulike viral illness in a significant proportion of patients. The high prevalence of MEWDS in female patients also suggests that hormonal factors may play a role in this condition. Despite a report of increased serum immunoglobulins, IgM and IgG, in MEWDS (Chung et al., 1987), workup for systemic disease in MEWDS is usually negative.

Disease Course and Prognosis

The disease usually has a very self-limited course with good visual recovery, typically occurring within a 2-month period from the onset of symptoms (varies from 2 to 16 weeks). Approximately 90% of patients will have better than 20/30 final visual acuity. Although late recurrences may occasionally occur (Tsai et al., 1994), MEWDS is characterized by recovery of visual function and normalization of ERG findings. There is a return of normal peripheral funduscopic appearance, although macular changes may persist. Because of its self-limited course, no treatment for MEWDS is currently indicated.

ACUTE POSTERIOR MULTIFOCAL PLACOID PIGMENT EPITHELIOPATHY (APMPPE)

APMPPE was first described by Gass in 1968 (Gass 1968). This typically afflicts young or middle-aged, otherwise healthy adults (average age approximately 25 years; range 8–57 years) who experience an acute loss of visual acuity in one or both eyes. There appears to be neither a racial nor a gender predilection for this condition. There is a slight preponderance of bilateral involvement. The condition tends to resolve itself after approximately 7 to 11 weeks with near normal return of visual function. Although the RPE changes remain visible, there are no other ocular or systemic disturbances. The typical course of the disease suggests an underlying viral inflammatory disorder (Holt et al., 1976).

Signs and Symptoms

Typically, there is a rapid reduction in visual acuity with or without a history of a preceding flulike illness or respiratory infection, often treated with systemic antibiotics. Clinically, APMPPE presents as multiple well-circumscribed, flat subretinal lesions at the level of the RPE and choriocapillaris (Fig. 28-8; Plate 28-II). These le-

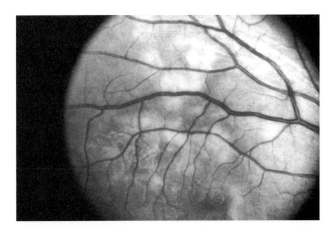

FIGURE 28-8. Acute posterior multifocal placoid pigment epitheliopathy (APMPPE). Lesions are typically creamy white and are scattered throughout the posterior pole. (Courtesy of Everett Ai, M.D.)

sions range from approximately $\frac{1}{8}$ to 1 disc diameter in size and may be confluent. They typically scatter in the midperiphery and the posterior pole. Initially, they appear cream colored or grayish-white in color. There is minimal evidence of anterior segment inflammation, although vitreous cells are present in up to 50% of the patients. This is likely the result of a mild periphlebitis with exudation. In addition to vascular inflammation, there is also mild optic disc edema noted. Very rarely, the condition can result in retinal edema, retinal hemorrhage, and subretinal neovascular membrane formation with hemorrhage.

Fluorescein Angiography

The initial phase of the angiogram sometimes demonstrates prolonged filling of the choroidal vasculature. There is often an early hypofluorescence that is attributed to a combination of both incomplete and irregular filling of the choriocapillaris in conjunction with a masking effect produced by the edematous, swollen RPE cells. This is followed in a late phase with evidence of leakage and staining at the lesion sites (Fig. 28-9).

Electrophysiological and Psychophysical Studies

The majority of patients with APMPPE have normal EOG findings. However, some patients have diminished, subnormal EOGs during the acute phase of the disease and occasionally exhibit subnormal cone and rod ERGs. Permanent scotomata on visual field testing are often present that may or may not be coincident with the observable clinical lesions.

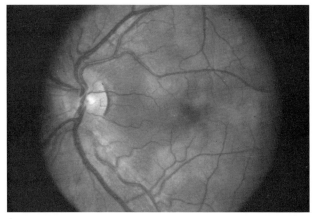

A

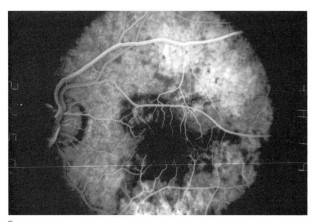

B

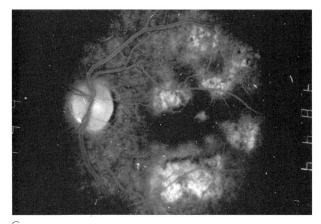

C

FIGURE 28-9. Acute posterior multifocal placoid pigment epitheliopathy (APMPPE). (A) Another patient with more central and confluent lesions. Early (B) and late (C) phases of the fluorescein angiogram of the same patient demonstrating the typical early masking but late leakage and staining of the lesions. (Courtesy of Lee Jampol M.D.)

Etiology

Gass originally felt that APMPPE was a primary disease of the RPE (Gass, 1968). However, others (Deutman et al., 1972; Van Buskirk, 1971) have argued that APMPPE represents a primary obstruction of the choroidal circulation with secondary RPE degeneration. This view is supported by more recent Indocyanine Green (ICG) angiographic evidence (Howe et al., 1995; Park et al., 1995). In view of this condition's association with a viral flulike illness, it is possible that an immune reaction to shared viral and RPE antigens, with or without modification by the usage of antibiotics, might be underlying the choroidal or RPE involvement. Interestingly enough, of all the conditions to be described in this section, APMPPE has the greatest variety of associations with other systemic conditions (see Table 28-1).

Disease Course and Prognosis

Fortunately the prognosis for visual recovery is good, with the vast majority of patients (>80%) having better than 20/30 vision (Wolf et al., 1991). Over a two to six week period, the lesions begin to fade, leaving atrophic, geographic-shaped lesions at the level of the RPE. Improvement in visual acuity often lags the resolution of the RPE lesions, which can take from weeks to months. Recurrences, unlike other conditions in these syndromes, are rare and usually occur within the first six months (Saraux and Pelosse, 1987). If there is initial unilateral presentation, the second eye often lags from the first eye within a few days or weeks. Treatment with corticosteroids has not been demonstrated to influence the outcome of this condition.

TABLE 28-1. *Systemic associations with APMPPE*

Reaction to swine flu vaccine
Platelet aggregation abnormalities
Systemic mycobacterial infections
Erythema nodosum
Cerebrovasculitis
Microvascular nephropathy
Adenovirus type V
Thyroiditis
Lymphadenopathy
Hepatomegaly
Regional enteritis
Sarcoidosis
Dysacusis
Spinal fluid pleocytosis and elevated CSF protein

ACUTE RETINAL PIGMENT EPITHELIITIS (ARPE), (KRILL'S DISEASE)

ARPE or Krill's disease, an extremely rare RPE disease which occurs in young adults (median age of onset approximately 45 years; range 16 to 75 years), was first described by Krill and Deutman in 1972. There is a preponderance of involvement in males (approximately two-thirds). There is no racial predilection, and the condition is bilateral in approximately 40% of patients.

Signs and Symptoms

Half of the patients are asymptomatic at the time of presentation, with others describing a sudden decrease in vision with or without central scotomata and metamorphopsia. Unlike APMPPE, the majority of patients have visual acuities around 20/30. The lesions are small, discrete clusters of spots in the macula that appear dark gray to black in color with a yellow-white halo and are typically between 50 and 100 μm in size (Fig. 28-10A). With resolution, the spots may either darken or lighten, but the halos remain. Extramacular lesions are rare, and with time a pattern of RPE migration may develop at the sites of the spots. Very rarely can this condition result in macular edema or be a precursor of central serous chorioretinopathy (Jamison, 1979).

Fluorescein Angiography

During the active phase of the disease there is hyperfluorescence in the center of spots with normal halos. With time, the center of the spots may either remain hyperfluorescent or become hypofluorescent while the halos might demonstrate hyperfluorescence, which is largely due to window defect pattern rather than due to any leakage (Fig. 28-10B).

Electrophysiological and Psychophysical Studies

On Amsler grid testing, these patients sometimes describe central scotomas and, as well, mild color vision abnormalities have also been described with this condition. EOG testing has yielded a variety of results from essentially normal to subnormal depending on the extent of RPE involvement in the macula. With resolution of the disease, there is a high rate of conversion back to normal in all tests.

Etiology

To date, systemic investigations of patients with this rare condition have failed to yield any conclusive viral

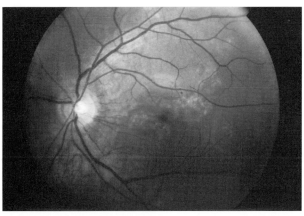

A

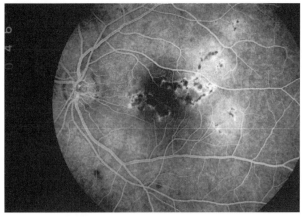

B

FIGURE 28-10. Acute retinal pigment epitheliitis (ARPE). (A) Fundus photograph. (B) Late-phase fluorescein angiogram in ARPE displaying transmission hyperfluorescence.

etiology, although that is clearly what is suspected. Associations with rubella, *Borrelia burgdorferi* (Lyme disease), and hepatitis C have been made (Bialasiewicz and Schonherr, 1990; Quillen et al., 1994). As well, this condition in some instances is thought to be a harbinger of central serous retinal choroidopathy (CSR) (Piermarocchi et al., 1983).

Disease Course and Prognosis

ARPE has a very self-limited course, usually with complete resolution over a 6 to 12 week period (Prost, M 1989). Recurrences are very rare (Chittum, ME and Kalina, RE 1987). There are currently no therapeutic modalities recommended.

SERPIGINOUS (GEOGRAPHIC) CHOROIDITIS

Serpiginous or geographic helicoid peripapillary choroidopathy is a rare, progressive choroiditis that manifests a characteristic snakelike or propeller-like pattern of RPE and choriocapillaris atrophy. This condition was first described in 1932 by Junius, but it was not until 1974 that Shatz, Maumenee, and Patz characterized the condition (Schatz et al., 1974). Hamilton and Bird also described this condition in the same year (Hamilton and Bird, 1974). The disease typically affects patients in their fourth to sixth decades who are otherwise healthy. It is more prevalent in Caucasians and has no gender predilection. The condition may present initially as unilateral, but with time, eventually all cases become bilateral. The interval between the primary and contralateral eye involvement may be several years.

Signs and Symptoms

Patients typically complain of blurred vision in association with metamorphopsia and scotomas, mostly central or paracentral. The initial visual acuity varies according to the extent of foveal involvement (average approximately 20/40; range from 20/20 to counting fingers). There may occasionally be an associated papillitis or a nongranulomatous uveitis, but the anterior segment and external ocular examinations are usually unremarkable (Masi et al., 1978). Vitritis may be present in 25%–30% of patients.

The characteristic early lesion in serpiginous choroiditis is that of a yellow to gray geographic pattern, usually with well-defined borders (Fig. 28-11). The lesion typically arises from the peripapillary region and spreads centrifugally in pseudopod or a geographic-like fashion. Regions of quiescent atrophy are present in the wake of the advancing active border of the lesion. There may also be some noncontiguous areas of activity. With time, there is pigment clumping and hypopigmentation of the RPE with clear visibility of the underlying large choroidal vessels within these atrophic patches (Chisholm et al., 1976). Despite bilateral involvement, there is often a high degree of asymmetry between both eyes. Unfortunately, this condition has a predilection for the temporal rather than the nasal fundus. Although the overlying retina is usually edematous and may progress to serous detachment, the retinal vessels and the optic nerve head usually appear normal throughout the disease. Choroidal neovascularization develops in approximately 25% of patients (Jampol et al., 1979; Blumenkranz et al., 1982). Other rare associations with serpiginous choroiditis include retinal periphlebitis, retinal and disc neovascularization, branch retinal vein occlu-

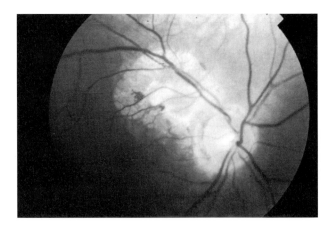

FIGURE 28-11. Serpiginous (geographic) choroiditis. This patient shows an old, inactive serpiginous scar extending in a pseudopod-like fashion from the optic disc. (Courtesy of Patrick Monahan, M.D.)

sion, and RPE detachment (Laatikainen and Erkkila, 1982) (Friberg, 1988).

Fluorescein Angiography

The lesions of serpiginous choroiditis in the acute phase of the disease demonstrate blockage of fluorescence during the early transit phase of the angiogram. Eventually there is staining during the late phases. The hypofluorescence during the acute phase is attributed to a combination of RPE cell edema and choriocapillaris nonperfusion. Staining of the vein walls may be demonstrated when focal areas of retinal phlebitis are present.

The inactive phase is characterized by a patchy diminution of the early choroidal flush due to the destruction of the choriocapillaris. There is unmasking of the underlying choroidal vessel fluorescence, this occurring in areas of healed lesions which become atrophic scars (Fig. 28-12). The staining at the margins of inactive lesions results from leakage of adjacent preserved choriocapillaris. In the very late phases of the angiogram, there is a diffuse hyperfluorescence of the lesions due to staining of the sclera and fibrous tissues. The staining typically progresses from the peripheral margins toward the center, similar to that seen in APMPPE.

Electrophysiological and Psychophysical Studies

The ERG amplitude and implicit time responses are abnormal in approximately 11% of patients with serpiginous. The EOG is likewise abnormal in 25% of patients (Hamilton and Bird, 1974; Chisholm et al., 1976). The degree of ERG and EOG abnormality is closely correlated with the extent of clinically involved retina. Visu-

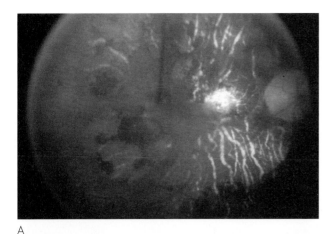

A

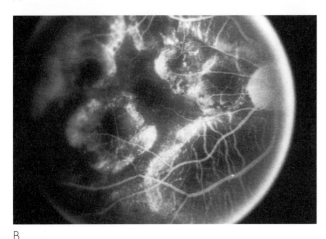

B

FIGURE 28-12. Serpiginous (geographic) choroiditis. (A) Chronic atrophic lesions displaying widespread geographic chorioretinal atrophy with moderate foveal sparing. (B) The transit-phase fluorescein angiogram demonstrates leakage and staining hyperfluorescence at the margins of the atrophic lesions. The underlying large choroidal vessels are easily seen within the atrophic lesions.

al-field testing reveals absolute or relative scotomata also corresponding with clinical retinal lesions. Central, cecocentral, and paracentral scotomata are the predominant feature on visual-field testing.

Etiology

The etiology of serpiginous choroiditis remains elusive. It is known that the lesions appear to be at the level of the RPE and choriocapillaris. Histopathological studies reveal that the disease is primarily a nongranulomatous choroiditis (Wu et al., 1989). The suggestion that serpiginous may be due to immunologic mechanisms is strengthened by its association with the HLA-A2 and HLA-B7 histocompatibility antigen (Laatikainen and Erkkila, 1982) and also by the occurrence of other in-

flammatory lesions in the involved eye. Other associations with serpiginous choroiditis include sarcoidosis (Edelsten et al., 1994), extrapyramidal dystonia (Richardson et al., 1981) and elevated Factor VIII–Von Willebrand factor (King et al., 1990).

Disease Course and Prognosis

The disease is characterized by an episodic and indolent course, with recurrences often going undetected unless there is macular involvement. There can be reactivation of quiescent borders of single lesions and, as well, new activity may arise from independent foci in the peripheral fundus. Fibrous metaplasia of the RPE develops within the area of chorioretinal atrophy in approximately 50% of patients. This is particularly prominent nasally and in the peripapillary region. The prognosis for retaining good visual acuity is poor, with only 45% of patients maintaining normal visual acuity. The contralateral eye may be involved within months or several years following the initial process in the involved eye.

Most investigators currently agree that the efficacy of any therapeutic agent has not yet been established in serpiginous choroiditis. Laser photocoagulation treatment does not appear to slow the progression of this disease. Treatments employing systemic corticosteroids, Chlorambucil, and Cyclosporine-A have variable responses (Secchi et al., 1990). Combination therapy with Azathioprine, Cyclosporine-A, and Prednisone may hold promise (Hooper and Kaplan, 1991).

BIRDSHOT (VITILIGINOUS) RETINOCHOROIDOPATHY:

Birdshot, or vitiliginous, retinochoroidopathy was first named by Ryan and Maumenee to describe a rare, acquired, bilateral intraocular inflammatory disease (Ryan and Maumenee, 1980). It typically involves middle- to late-age patients (average age approximately 52 years; range 23–70 years). The disease primarily affects Caucasians and, in the older age groups, especially beyond the fourth decade, female cases outnumber males.

Signs and Symptoms

Patients typically present with not only decreased visual acuity, but also complain of symptoms of nyctalopia and dyschromatopsia. Rarely, patients may complain also of photophobia and a reduction in visual field. The condition is painless. On clinical examination, there is minimal to no anterior segment inflammation. Visual acuities may vary at onset from 20/20 to 20/800, with most patients having a visual acuity of around 20/50.

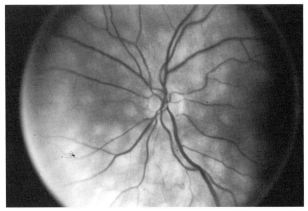

A

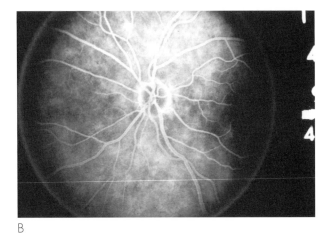

B

FIGURE 28-13. Birdshot (vitiliginous) retinochoroidopathy. (A) Multiple, uniformly hypopigmented lesions with mild disc swelling. (B) Late-phase fluorescein angiogram demonstrating patchy hyperfluorescence.

The characteristic appearance of lesions in birdshot consist of multifocal patches of RPE and choroidal depigmentation (Fig. 28-13A; Plate 28-III). Unlike other conditions in these syndromes, there is an absence of a halo of hyperpigmentation within or at their margins. Individual lesions are typically one-quarter disc diameter in size and have a certain uniformity in appearance. They can be cream colored or depigmented and round to oval, and they typically do not have a well-defined border. Hyperpigmentation may occur in some lesions in the late stages of the disease. The lesions are typically scattered throughout the postequatorial fundus in a pattern analogous to a shotgun blast of birdshot. There is initial foveal sparing. Birdshot can be associated with other retinal and ocular abnormalities (Barondes et al., 1989; Soubrane et al., 1983) (see Table 28-2).

TABLE 28-2. *Ocular abnormalities associated with birdshot retinochoroidopathy*

Cystoid macular edema
Retinovascular sheathing
Epiretinal membrane formation
Optical atrophy
Retinovascular attenuation
Retinal and vitreous hemorrhages
Glaucoma
Optic disc edema
Retinal neovascularization
*Subretinal neovascularization
*Rhegmatogenous retinal detachment
*Serous macular detachment

*Very rare.

Fluorescein Angiography

The key fluorescein angiographic finding in birdshot retinochoroidopathy is due to vascular leakage. This is quite pronounced in the perifoveal region with resultant cystoid macular edema. Acutely, the patches in birdshot are surprisingly silent, showing no abnormality. With time and enlargement of the patches, the individual lesions behave as window defects, transmitting underlying fluorescence from the choroid. In the early phase of the angiogram, there is a delay in retinal arteriole filling and circulation time, although retinal capillary nonperfusion is not typically seen with this disease. During this phase, the lesions are either not evident or are hypofluorescent. Choroidal vessels are often visible through the hypofluorescent lesions. With the late phase, the patches become hyperfluorescent (Fig. 28-13B) with staining of the larger retinal veins and pooling, particularly in the setting of cystoid macular edema.

Electrophysiological and Psychophysical Studies

The ERG in birdshot typically displays moderate to severe abnormalities of both rod and cone function (up to 80% of patients). At certain stages there can be a disproportionate decrease in the amplitude of the b-wave compared with the a-wave and some have felt this to be the distinguishing feature of the disease (Hirose et al., 1991). Later ERG abnormalities tend to be nonspecific. The EOG may be either normal or slightly subnormal (70% of patients), and, similarly, dark-adaptation studies may show subnormal rod function. Patients may also exhibit nonspecific color vision defects.

The visual field demonstrates a generalized constriction of peripheral fields with central scotomas or enlarged blind spots. Interestingly enough, these scotomas do not correspond to the birdshot lesion distribution, clinically.

Etiology

Birdshot is felt to be the result of a pathological process occurring not only in the photoreceptor-RPE-choroid complex, but also more diffusely throughout the neural layers of the retina. A genetic predisposition has been suggested since the incidence of the HLA-A29 marker is present in approximately 85% of patients with birdshot retinochoroidopathy. This is to be contrasted with 7% prevalence in the normal population (Nussenblatt et al., 1982). An autoimmune mechanism as the cause of birdshot is supported by in vitro studies demonstrating immune responses to retinal-S antigen (>90% of patients tested) (Priem and Oosterhuis, 1988). In addition, histological examination reveals focal depigmentation of the choroidal melanocytes. As well, birdshot has been associated with cutaneous vitiligo and elevated C_4 complement. Therefore, it is likely that some sort of altered immune mechanism is responsible for the clinical findings of this disease.

Disease Course and Prognosis

Birdshot, unlike the aforementioned conditions, is a fairly chronic disease with slow progression. It can be active for three to four years before finally going into remission (Priem and Oosterhuis, 1988). It is characterized by exacerbations and remissions. Although 73% of eyes have a visual acuity better than 20/60, ultimately 33% of patients will have a final visual acuity of less than 20/200. Not surprisingly, the most significant cause of central visual loss in patients with birdshot is the presence of cystoid macular edema (60% of patients). There is no therapy that has proven effective for the treatment of this condition. A variety of steroidal and nonsteroidal antiinflammatory drugs, as well as immunosuppressives and antibiotics, have been tried with none having any significant long term efficacy. There is a partial transient response to corticosteroid treatment, and Cyclosporine is currently being investigated as a treatment for this condition.

DIFFUSE UNILATERAL SUBACUTE NEURORETINTIS (DUSN)

DUSN, which is caused by the chronic subretinal migration of one of at least two species of nematodes, char-

acteristically involves children or young adults with a slight male preponderance among patients. The patients are otherwise healthy and are often asymptomatic at time of presentation.

Signs and Symptoms

The patients often present quite late in the disease with typically poor visual acuities, usually less than 20/200. Those few cases which have presented during the acute period have demonstrated a moderate degree of vitritis with optic disc swelling and a variable anterior chamber reaction, with or without hypopyon. The characteristic posterior pole findings are those of focal, gray-white or yellow-white spots developing in the deep layers of the retina and also at the level of the RPE. These normally develop within several days to weeks from the onset of symptoms. The lesions tend to cluster in the macula or juxtamacular region and typically last several days before fading. Occasionally, a subretinal worm (500–2000 μm length and 25 μm in width) can be seen (Fig. 28-14).

In the inactive phase, the posterior pole exhibits extensive mottling of the RPE assuming a "pseudo–retinitis pigmentosa" appearance (Fig. 28-15). There is also extensive retinovascular narrowing and sheathing with optic atrophy. Subretinal neovascularization may develop at this stage. A mild to moderate anterior chamber and vitreous cell reaction may be present even in the inactive stage. The patient often has an afferent pupillary defect.

Fluorescein Angiography

In the very early stage of the disease, the angiogram may be entirely normal. If lesions are present, they hypofluoresce during the early phase of the angiogram and typically stain during the late phase. In addition, there is leakage from the capillaries overlying the optic nerve and more-diffuse perivenous leakage occurring in the retina.

In a more typical late stage of the disease, there is an increase in the background choroidal fluorescence due to extensive RPE dropout and loss of pigmentation (Fig. 28-15B). Hypofluorescence, indicative of RPE atrophy, occurs in the periphery as well as the peripapillary regions, exhibiting fine, mottled hyperfluorescence, particularly in the macular region. If a worm is present, it can be seen as a hypofluorescent lesion.

Electrophysiological and Psychophysical Studies

Moderate to severe reductions in the ERG can be seen, depending on the extent of involvement. A dispropor-

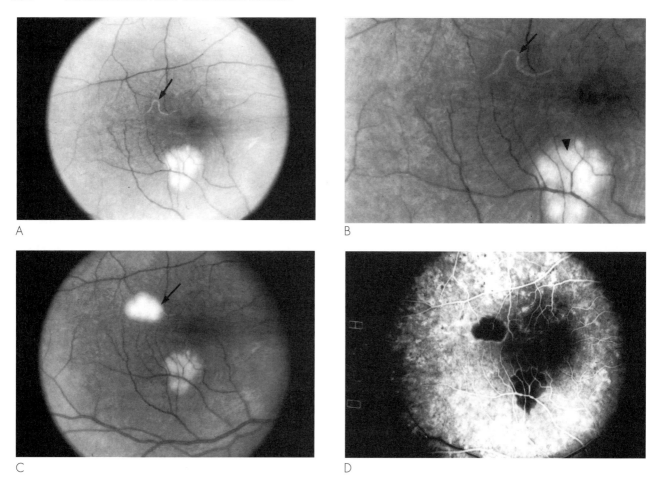

FIGURE 28-14. Diffuse unilateral subacute neuroretinitis (DUSN). (A) Attempted focal laser photocoagulation of a subretinal nematode suspected of being *Baylisascaris procyonis (arrow)*. (B) The worm *(arrow)* was only later discovered to have migrated from the original site, which was initially targeted for laser treatment *(arrowhead)*. (C) A second laser treatment was successful at destroying the worm *(arrow)*. (D) Fluorescein angiogram performed on the same eye immediately after second laser treatment showing not only the hypofluorescent laser-treated areas but also the characteristic mottled hyperfluorescence of diffuse RPE and choriocapillaris destruction. (Courtesy of Everett Ai, M.D.)

tionate decrease of the b-wave relative to the decrease in the a-wave amplitudes can sometimes be present. In rare instances, the ERG may be extinguished.

Etiology

Leading the list of suspected causative agents in this disease are the three nematodes *Toxocara canis* (dog roundworm), *Ancylostoma caninum* (dog hookworm) (Gass, 1987), and *Baylisascaris procyonis* (raccoon intestinal nematode) (Goldberg, 1993). Clinically, there appear to be two types of worms that have been described with this condition. They are differentiated by length. Smaller worms (400–1000 μm) and longer worms (1500–2000 μm) may wander in the subretinal space for many years and cause progressive ocular damage. It is important to note that the nematode may be found during any stage of the disease. The worm is often located in the deep, white retinal exudative lesions. Recent surgical removal of a subretinal nematode in a patient with DUSN identified the causative organism as a third-stage *Toxocara canis* larva (De Sousa and Nakashima, 1995). It should be noted, however, that serological testing for Toxocara is typically negative in patients with DUSN. The damage caused by the organisms appears to involve a local toxic tissue reaction in the outer retina caused by the worm's by-products in addition to a more diffuse toxic reaction affecting both the inner and outer retinal tissues that is felt to be due to the host's immunologic defenses. Eosinophilia is infre-

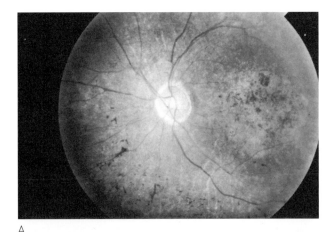

A

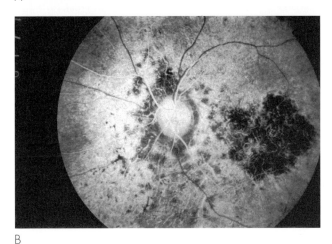

B

FIGURE 28-15. Diffuse unilateral subacute neuroretinitis (DUSN). (A) Late stage of the disease presenting the characteristic "pseudo–retinitis pigmentosa" features. (B) Fluorescein angiogram of same eye demonstrating peripapillary and macular mottled hyperfluorescence due to atrophy of the RPE and the choriocapillaris.

quently detected, and the patients do not manifest evidence of systemic disease.

Histopathological examination of the few eyes that have been examined with DUSN reveals a largely nongranulomatous vitritis, retinitis, and retinal and optic nerve perivasculitis. As well, there is a low-grade patchy nongranulomatous choroiditis. There is extensive degeneration of the peripheral retina, particularly of the posterior region within the arcades. Mild to moderate degenerative changes in the RPE have also been described. Not surprisingly, optic atrophy is a common feature of these eyes.

Disease Course and Prognosis

Following the acute phase of the disease, focal and more diffuse depigmentation of the RPE develops over weeks

or months. There is pigment migration into the overlying retina with a gradual narrowing of the retinal vasculature. Retinal hemorrhages may be the result of choroidal neovascularization and can also result in occasional serous retinal detachments.

Management of patients with DUSN has not yet been optimized to date. There are three modalities of treatment, of which a combination is usually applied. Argon laser photocoagulation is effective in destroying the worm and causing minimal inflammatory reaction. Surgical (transvitreal) removal of a subretinal nematode elicits less inflammatory response, but is accompanied by the risks inherent to this treatment. Medicinals such as antihelmintics (Thiabendazole, Diethylcarbamazine) or antifilarial agents such as Ivermectin may be used as adjunctive treatment.

CONCLUSION

With the exception of diffuse unilateral subacute neuroretinitis (DUSN), the idiopathic multifocal chorioretinopathy syndromes discussed remain problematic not only from an etiological point of view, but also from a classification point of view. Although there is a practical benefit to lumping these entities into groups, such as AZOOR or multifocal choroidopathy, there are still unique characteristics to each of these conditions that make them distinct from each other. At the same time, there are also instances where patient symptomatology and clinical findings overlap between these entities. Although the majority of findings point toward an infectious and/or immunological mechanism as the cause of these conditions, no conclusive evidence for either has been demonstrated.

REFERENCES

Aaberg TM, Campo RV, Joffe L. 1985. Recurrences and bilaterality in the multiple evanescent white-dot syndrome. Am J Ophthalmol 100(1):29–37.

Barondes MJ, Fastenberg DM, Schwartz PL, Rosen DA. 1989. Peripheral retinal neovascularization in birdshot retinochoroidopathy. Ann Ophthalmol 21(8):306–308.

Bialasiewicz, AA, Schonherr U. 1990. Choriocapillaritis (so-called pigment epitheliitis) in Borrelia burgdorferi seroconversion. Klin Monatsbl Augenheilkd 1996(6):481–483.

Blinder KJ, Peyman GA, Paris CL. 1994. Diffuse posterior punctate pigment epitheliopathy. Retina 14(1):31–35.

Bloom SM, Snady-McCoy L. 1989. Multifocal choroiditis uveitis occurring after herpes zoster ophthalmicus. Am J Ophthalmol 108(6):733–735.

Blumenkranz MS, Gass JD, Clarkson JG. 1982. Atypical serpiginous choroiditis. Arch Ophthalmol 100(11):1773–1775.

Bodine SR, Marino J, Camisa TJ, Salvate AJ. 1992. Multifocal choroiditis with evidence of Lyme disease. Ann Ophthalmol 24(5): 169–173.

Callanan D, Gass JD. 1992. Multifocal choroiditis and choroidal neovascularization associated with the multiple evanescent white dot and acute idiopathic blind spot enlargement syndrome. Ophthalmology 99(11):1678–1685.

Cantrill HL, Folk JC. 1986. Multifocal choroiditis associated with progressive subretinal fibrosis. Am J Ophthalmol 101(2):170–180.

Chisholm IH, Gass JD, Hutton WL. 1976. The late stage of serpiginous (geographic) choroiditis. Am J Ophthalmol 82(3):343–351.

Chittum ME, Kalina RE. 1987. Acute retinal pigment epitheliitis. Ophthalmology 94(9):1114–1119.

Chung YM, Yeh TS, Liu JH. 1987. Increased serum IgM and IgG in the multiple evanescent white-dot syndrome. Am J Ophthalmol 104(2):187–188.

Cunha de Souza E, Nakashima Y. 1995. Diffuse unilateral subacute neuroretinitis: report of transvitreal surgical removal of a subretinal nematode. Ophthalmology 102(8):1183–1186.

Deutman AF, Oosterhuis JA, Boen-Tan TN, Aan de Kerk AL. 1972. Acute posterior multifocal placoid pigment epitheliopathy. Pigment epitheliopathy of choriocapillaritis? Br J Ophthalmol 65(12):863–874.

Dodwell DG, Jampol LM, Rosenberg M, Berman A, Zaret CR. 1990. Optic nerve involvement associated with the multiple evanescent white-dot syndrome. Ophthalmology 97(7):862–868.

Doran RML, Hamilton AM. 1982. Disciform macular degeneration in young adults. Trans Ophthalmol Soc UK 102:471–480.

Dreyer RF, Gass DJ. 1984. Multifocal choroiditis and panuveitis: a syndrome that mimics ocular histoplasmosis. Arch Ophthalmol 102(12):1776–1784.

Edelsten C, Stanford MR, Graham EM. 1994. Serpiginous choroiditis: an unusual presentation of ocular sarcoidosis. Br J Ophthalmol 78(1):70–71.

Frau E, Dussaix E, Offret H, Bloch-Michel E. 1990. The possible role of herpes viruses in multifocal choroiditis and panuveitis. Int Ophthalmol 14(5–6):365–369.

Friberg TR. 1988. Serpiginous choroiditis with branch vein occlusion and bilateral periphlebitis: case report. Arch Ophthalmol 106(5):585–586.

Gass JD. 1968. Acute posterior multifocal placoid pigment epitheliopathy. Arch Ophthalmol 80:177.

Gass JDM. 1987. Stereoscopic Atlas of Macular Diseases: Diagnosis and Treatment, 3rd ed. St Louis: Mosby - Year Book.

Gass, J. D. 1993. Acute zonal occult outer retinopathy. J Clin Neuroophthalmol 13:79–97.

Goldberg MA, Kazacos KR, Boyce WM, Ai E, Katz B. 1993. Diffuse unilateral subacute neuroretinitis: morphometric, serologic and epidemiologic support for Baylisascaris as a causative agent. Ophthalmology 100(11):1695–1701.

Hamed LM, Glaser JS, Gass JD, Schatz NJ. 1989. Protracted enlargement of the blind spot in multiple evanescent white dot syndrome. Arch Ophthalmol 107(2):194–198.

Hamilton AM, Bird AC. 1974. Geographical choroidopathy Br J Ophthalmol 58:784–797.

Hirose T, Katsumi O, Pruett RC, Sakaue H, Mehta M. 1991. Retinal function in birdshot retinochoroidopathy. Acta Ophthalmol (Copenh) 69(3):327–337.

Holt WS, Regan CD, Trempe C. 1976. Acute posterior multifocal placoid pigment epitheliopathy. Am J Ophthalmol 81(4):403–412.

Hooper PL, Kaplan HJ. 1991. Triple agent immunosuppression in serpiginous choroiditis. Ophthalmology 98(6):944–951; discussion 951–952.

Horiguchi M, Miyake Y, Nakamura M, Fujii Y. 1993. Focal electroretinogram and visual field defect in multiple evanescent white dot syndrome. Br J Ophthalmol 77(7):452–455.

Howe LJ, Woon H, Graham EM, Fitzke F, Bhandari A, Marshall J. 1995. Choroidal hypoperfusion in acute posterior multifocal placoid pigment epitheliopathy. Ophthalmology 102:790–798.

Ie D, Glaser BM, Murphy RP, Gordon LW, Sjaarda RN, Thompson JT. 1994. Indocyanine green angiography in multiple evanescent white-dot syndrome. Am J Ophthalmol 117(1):7–12.

Jacobson SG, Morales DS, Sun XK, Feuer WJ, Cideciyan AV, Gass DM, Milam AH. 1995. Pattern of retinal dysfunction in acute zonal occult outer retinopathy. Ophthalmology 102(8):1187–1197.

Jamison RR. 1979. Acute retinal pigment epitheliitis with macular edema. Ann Ophthalmol 11(3):359–361.

Jampol LM, Wiredu A. 1995. MEWDS, MFC, PIC, AMN, AIBSE, and AZOOR: One disease or many? [editorial]. Retina 15(5):373–378.

Jampol LM, Orth D, Daily MJ, Rabb MF. 1979. Subretinal neovascularization with geographic (serpiginous) choroiditis. Am J Ophthalmol 88(4):683–689.

Jampol LM, Sieving PA, Pugh D, Fishman GA, Gilbert H. 1984. Multiple evanescent white dot syndrome. I. Clinical findings. Arch Ophthalmol 102(5):671–674.

Joondeph BC, Tessler HH. 1991. Clinical course of multifocal choroiditis: photographic and angiographic evidence of disease recurrence. Ann Ophthalmol 23(11):424–429.

Khorram KD, Jampol LM, Rosenberg MA. 1991. Blind spot enlargement as a manifestation of multifocal choroiditis. Arch Ophthalmol 109(10):1403–1407.

King DG, Grizzard WS, Sever RJ, Espinoza L. 1990. Serpiginous choroidopathy associated with elevated factor VIII-von Willebrand factor antigen. Retina 10(2):97–101.

Krill AE, Archer D. 1970. Choroidal neovascularization in multifocal (presumed histoplasmin) choroiditis. Arch Ophthalmol 84(5):595–604.

Krill AE, Deutman AF. 1972. Acute retinal pigment epitheliitis. Am J Ophthalmol 74:193.

Laatikainen L, Erkkila H. 1982. Subretinal and disc neovascularisation in serpiginous choroiditis. Br J Ophthalmol 66(5):326–331.

Masi RJ, O'Connor GR, Kimura SJ. 1978. Anterior uveitis in geographic or serpiginous choroiditis. Am J Ophthalmol 86(2):228–232.

McCollum CJ, Kimble JA. 1992. Peripapillary subretinal neovascularization associated with multiple evanescent white-dot syndrome [letter, comment]. Arch Ophthalmol 110(1):13–14.

Morgan CM, Schatz H. 1986. Recurrent multifocal choroiditis. Ophthalmology 93(9):1138–1147.

Nozik RA, Dorsch WA. 1973. A new chorioretinopathy associated with anterior uveitis. Am J Ophthalmol 76:758–762.

Nussenblatt RB, Mittal KK, Ryan S, Green WR, Maumenee AE. 1982. Birdshot retinochoroidopathy associated with HLA-A29 antigen and immune responsiveness to retinal S-antigen. Am J Ophthalmol 94(2):147–158.

Palestine AG, Nussenblatt RB, Chan CC, Hooks JJ, Friedman L, Kuwabara T. 1985. Histopathology of the subretinal fibrosis and uveitis syndrome. Ophthalmol 92:838–844.

Park D, Schatz H, McDonald R, Johnson RN. 1995. Indocyanine green angiography of acute multifocal posterior placoid pigment epitheliopathy. Ophthalmol 102:1877–1883.

Piermarocchi S, Corradini R, Midena E, Segato T. 1983. Correlation between retinal pigment epitheliitis and central serous chorioretinopathy. Ann Ophthalmol 15(5):425–428.

Priem HA, Oosterhuis JA. 1988. Birdshot chorioretinopathy: clinical characteristics and evolution. Br J Ophthalmol 72(9):646–659.

Prost, M. 1989. Long-term observations of patients with acute retinal pigment epitheliitis. Ophthalmologica 199(2–3):84–89.

Quillen DA, Zurlo JJ, Cunningham D, Blankenship GW. 1994. 118(1):120–121.

Richardson RR, Cooper IS, Smith JL. 1981. Serpiginous choroiditis and unilateral extrapyramidal dystonia. Ann Ophthalmol 13(1): 15–19.

Ryan SJ, Maumenee AE. 1980. Birdshot retinochoroidopathy. Am J Ophthalmol 89:31–45.

Salvador F, Garcia-Arumi J, Mateo C, Rouras A, Corcostegui B. 1994. Multifocal choroiditis with progressive subretinal fibrosis: report of two cases. Ophthalmologica 208(3):163–167.

Saraux H, Pelosse B. 1987. Acute posterior multifocal placoid pigment epitheliopathy: a longterm follow-up. Ophthalmologica 194 (4):161–163.

Schatz H, Maumenee AE, Patz A. 1974. Geographical helicoid peripapillary choroidopathy: clinical presentation and fluorescein angiographic findings. Trans Am Acad Ophthalmol Otolaryngol 78:747–761.

Schenck F, Boke W. 1990. Retinal vasculitis with multifocal retinochoroiditis. Int Ophthalmol 14(5–6):401–404.

Secchi AG, Tognon MS, Maselli C. 1990. Cyclosporine-A in the treatment of serpiginous choroiditis. Int Ophthalmol 14(5–6):395–399.

Sieving PA, Fishman GA, Jampol LM, Pugh D. 1984a. Multiple evanescent white dot syndrome. II. Electrophysiology of the photoreceptors during retinal pigment epithelial disease. Arch Ophthalmol 102(5):675–679.

Sieving PA, Fishman GA, Saizano T, Rabb MF. 1984b. Acute macular

neuroretinopathy: Early receptor potential change suggests photoreceptor pathology. Br J Ophthalmol 68:229–234.

Soubrane G, Coscas G, Binaghi M, Amalric P, Bernard JA. 1983. Birdshot retinochoroidopathy and subretinal new vessels. Br J Ophthalmol 67(7):461–467.

Spaide RF, Sugin S, Yannuzzi LA, DeRosa JT. 1991. Epstein-Barr virus antibodies in multifocal choroiditis and panuveitis. Am J Ophthalmol 112(4):410–413.

Tiedeman JS. 1987. Epstein-Barr viral antibodies in multifocal choroiditis and panuveitis. Am J Ophthalmol 103(5):659–663.

Tsai L, Jampol LM, Pollock SC, Olk J. 1994. Chronic recurrent multiple evanescent white dot syndrome. Retina 14(2):160–163.

Van Buskirk EM, Lessel S, Friedman E. 1971. Pigment epitheliopathy and erythema nodosum Arch Ophthalmol 85:369.

Watzke RC, Claussen RW. 1981. The long-term course of multifocal choroiditis (presumed ocular histoplasmosis). Am J Ophthalmol 91(6):750–760.

Watzke RC, Packer AJ, Folk JC, et al. 1984. Punctate inner choroidopathy. Am J Ophthalmol 98:572–84.

Wolf MD, Alward WL, Folk JC. 1991. Long-term visual function in acute posterior multifocal placoid pigment epitheliopathy. Arch Ophthalmol 109(6):800.

Wu JS, Lewis H, Fine SL, Grover DA, Green WR. 1989. Clinicopathologic findings in a patient with serpiginous choroiditis and treated choroidal neovascularization. Retina 9(4):292–301.

VIII | EXOGENOUS INFLUENCES

29. Light damage to retina and retinal pigment epithelium

CHARLOTTE E. REMÉ, FARHAD HAFEZI, ANDREAS MARTI,
KURT MUNZ, AND JÖRG J. REINBOTH

LIGHT AS A MODULATOR AND DAMAGING AGENT IN RETINA AND RETINAL PIGMENT EPITHELIUM

The universal effect of light in the retina is to create the visual signal. Apart from this primary function, however, light can distinctly modify structure and physiology by altering molecular and cellular mechanisms (Remé et al., 1991). Laboratory studies reveal that different ambient illuminances alter the length of rod outer segments, the content of the visual pigment rhodopsin, photoreceptor phospholipid fatty acid composition, antioxidant state (Penn and Anderson, 1991; Penn et al., 1987; 1992; Penn and Williams, 1986) and the levels of key molecules involved in the visual transduction cascade (Farber et al., 1991; Organisciak et al., 1991). Photostasis of the retina is a basic regulative process which ensures that a "set" number of photons per day is absorbed in a given eye. This is achieved by light-dependent and gene-regulated processes (Penn et al., 1986; Schremser and Williams, 1995a; 1995b). Among the physiological systems subject to such regulatory gates are circadian and circannual rhythms, major features in chronobiology (Cahill and Besharse, 1995; Remé et al., 1991).

Apart from such adaptive interactions of light with physiology, ultraviolet (UV) and visible radiation can damage and destroy the retina and pigment epithelium (PE). This apparent paradox has been observed already in ancient history in humans, but systematic research has been incited by Noell's work on light damage in laboratory animals (Noell et al., 1966). Because retina and PE represent a structural unit with functional cross-talk, both will be considered in this article, with the main focus on the PE. There is a variety of extensive reviews on light damage, which will be briefly summarized with their specific emphases outlined.

OVERVIEWS ON RETINAL LIGHT DAMAGE

Comprehensive reviews covering basic mechanisms and clinical aspects including major historical perspectives are given by Lanum, 1978; Organisciak and Winkler, 1994; Sperling, 1980. Discussions on photochemical, photophysical, and general damage mechanisms are found in Andley, 1987; Dillon, 1991; Ham and colleagues, 1984; Handelman and Dratz, 1986; Lawwill, 1982; Williams and Baker, 1980. Action spectra and damage types are analyzed in Kremers and Van Norren, 1988; Zigman, 1993. Prevention of light-induced lesions and possible therapeutic strategies are shown in Gerster, 1991; Tso, 1989. Extensive discussions on instrument hazards are provided in *Ophthalmology*, 1983. Finally, clinical, epidemiological, and age-related aspects are reviewed in Marshall, 1983; 1985; Miller, 1987; Remé and colleagues, 1995a; Terman and colleagues, 1990; Waxler and Hitchins, 1986; Weale, 1989; Young, 1988; 1994.

Studies on human light damage include prospective and retrospective analyses, epidemiological surveys and case reports. The spectral composition of the damaging light source, including sunlight and retinal irradiance levels, varies considerably depending on exposure conditions, the involved individuals, and the methods of analysis. Epidemiological studies are concerned with a potential causal relation of UV and visible radiation to eye diseases such as corneal and conjunctival degenerations, cataracts, retinal and PE degenerative diseases, and retinal aging. There are major discrepancies between epidemiological evidence for such relations and the results obtained in laboratory studies, giving rise to critical views by epidemiologists (Dolin, 1994; Remé and colleagues, 1995a). Irrespective of those discussions, much can be learned from light damage observations in humans, most notably that UV and visible radiation does indeed injure the retina and PE acutely and chronically. Further, human observations may lead the way to the design of controlled laboratory experiments that can avoid the above-mentioned uncertainties and approach basic underlying mechanisms.

Laboratory studies in animals or in vitro systems can control at least some of the confounding factors that complicate human studies. Earlier light damage work in animals displays a broad spectrum of experimental conditions which renders comparisons a difficult task. Nevertheless, fundamental regimens can be distinguished. These include exposure to diffuse, white light, or green light for varying time periods; exposure to constant diffuse, white light, again for varying time periods; exposure to focussed white light or specific wavelengths for short time periods in the hours range; exposure to laser light and to UV light. Whereas the exposure to diffuse, white light may represent the most naturalistic condition, elucidation of action spectra obviously is precluded. An advantage of such regimen is the fact that relatively low light doses can be applied, permitting the analysis of subtle threshold changes on a morphological and biochemical level that may not be readily apparent in funduscopy or electrophysiological testing. Thus, any of these light exposure regimens permits, in its own way, the approach to basic underlying mechanisms, by the analysis of action spectra and potential chromophores, by a dose–response function, by molecular and tissue changes, or by lesion-enhancing or lesion-reducing factors. By far the most frequently applied analytical tool is the evaluation of damage in light and electron microscopic preparations.

Human as well as laboratory studies thus describe light damage as a phenomenon in its own right or as a model system to study retinal and PE diseases including degenerations and dystrophies. As mentioned above, an important aspect perhaps not fully recognized among vision scientists and clinicians is the modulation by light of retinal physiology. This is of particular relevance for circadian rhythm research, because light processed by the visual system represents a crucial zeitgeber signal for the "master clock" in the hypothalamic suprachiasmatic nuclei. Therefore, light that alters the retinal input stage may change the photic signal to the rhythm-generating master clock (Remé et al., 1991). Within a clinical setting one should be aware that diagnostics and therapies involving the exposure to bright light sources may transiently or permanently alter retinal functions. Clinicians investigating retinal physiology and function would be prudent to remember that several basic features can distinctly vary over a 24-hour period as well as within annual seasons (Remé et a., 1991).

LIGHT DAMAGE IN HUMANS

Acute and Chronic Exposure to Sunlight

Several studies report the effects of chronic exposure to sunlight that lead to reduced visual acuity, an elevated threshold of dark adaptation, and reduced night vision (Clark et al., 1946; Hecht et al., 1948; Marlor et al.,

1973). A selective loss of blue-cone sensitivity (Werner et al., 1989) and increased incidence of cystic macular edema (Kraff et al., 1985) were found in eyes bearing intraocular lenses without UV filters. An extensive epidemiological survey of watermen in the Chesapeake Bay area concluded that chronic exposure to blue light or visible light, respectively, may be related to the development of age-related macular degeneration, despite the relatively small number of individuals with severe geographic atrophy or disciform scar (Taylor et al., 1992). Acute solar retinopathy is a well-known phenomenon and has been observed in patients after sunbathing, sun gazing, or other outdoor activities (Gladstone and Tasman, 1978; Sadun et al., 1984; Yannuzzi et al., 1987). Of particular interest is the description of histological changes in retina and PE after voluntary sun gazing, because they closely resemble alterations amply documented in animal light damage studies (Hope-Ross et al., 1993).

Acute and Chronic Exposure during Therapeutic Regimens

Chronic cumulative exposure to argon laser blue light reduced the color contrast sensitivity of the treating ophthalmologists (Berninger et al., 1989). Numerous studies describe damage inflicted by ophthalmological instruments, particularly the operating microscope in apparently normal or predisposed eyes (Davidson and Sternberg, 1993; Michels and Sternberg, 1990). Safety recommendations include the use of filters in operating microscopes and the avoidance of coaxial illumination when possible. Endoillumination during vitrectomy may also present a potential hazard (Kuhn et al., 1991). Support for observations in humans comes from studies in monkeys, which were exposed to the light of an operating microscope with lesions in photoreceptors and PE resembling those seen in blue-light injuries (Irvine et al., 1984). Photic maculopathy affecting photoreceptors and PE was induced by an indirect ophthalmoscope (Tso, 1973); repeated exposures to an indirect ophthalmoscope produced more severe lesions than a single exposure of the same retinal irradiance (Borges et al., 1990).

A recently developed therapeutic strategy prompts attention to retinal and PE safety. Exposure of patients to bright artificial light with illuminance ranges of 2500 to 10,000 lux for up to eight hours is used to treat winter depression (seasonal affective disorder, SAD), circadian sleep-phase disorders, shift-work and jet-lag maladaptation (Terman et al., 1990; Remé et al., 1996). Light regimens may be used for half of the year for periods of decades and more. At present, no ocular lesions have been observed in patients, but long-term observations are lacking and the question of cumulative subthreshold lesions thus remains (Gallin et al., 1995).

Relevant aspects for all light-induced retinal lesions in humans include predisposing factors such as genetic ones on the one hand and drug-induced photosensitization, eye color, pupil size, or environmental conditions and exposure geometry on the other hand. The latter two conditions are of particular importance and unfortunately often underestimated in epidemiological studies evaluating radiation effects on ocular pathology such as cataracts (Sliney, 1992; 1994).

LIGHT DAMAGE TO RETINA AND PIGMENT EPITHELIUM IN LABORATORY STUDIES

Considering the close anatomical association and functional interdependence of retina and PE it appears problematic to clearly separate light damage in the PE from that in the neural retina in vivo. Only in vitro studies examining the PE in cell culture or the isolated incubated retina may shed light on separate damage mechanisms. A presumed primary lesion in one tissue will lead to responses in the other. For example, a light-induced release of signalling molecules in the retina may alter PE functions such as disk shedding and phagocytosis. (For detailed review, especially on PE lesions, see Waxler et al., 1986.)

Elusive Chromophores and Action Spectra

Retinal and PE light damage is modulated by the absorption and transmission properties of the cornea and mainly, the lens. Therefore, action spectra for retinal and PE light damage will be dependent on those characteristics. For example, human lens absorption significantly changes with age and thus the action spectra in young eyes may be distinctly different from those in older eyes. Similarly, lens transmission varies greatly in animal species: whereas the rodent lens transmits blue and UVA to a high degree (Gorgels and van Norren, 1992), the yellow squirrel lens can act as an efficient UV and blue filter (Collier et al., 1989). This latter observation led to the design of UV- and blue-filtering protective and vision-enhancing spectacle lenses (Zigman, 1990). The UV transmission of rodent lenses is mirrored in photoreceptors that are maxiamlly sensitive to UV (Jacobs et al., 1991).

An *action spectrum* is defined as the light dose that is required to obtain the same biological effect at different wavelengths. There are stringent criteria for elucidating a true action spectrum, which is then called an *analyti-*

cal action spectrum. The conditions for an action spectrum to be considered analytical include: the same mechanism and the same quantum yield is present at all wavelengths tested; the absorption spectrum of the chromophore in question is the same in vivo and in vitro; the absorption of inactive chromophores and light scattering is negligible. Finally, not more than half of the incident quanta should be absorbed by the sample in the wavelength range of interest and the effect must be the same regardless of the rate at which the light is provided, that is, the effect should not change whether a given light dose is applied in a short time or over a longer time period. By contrast, a higher level of complexity is encountered in multicellular systems which restrain the elucidation of individual chromophores and yield polychromatic action spectra (Coohill, 1992; Grossweiner, 1989). In practice, most light damage studies have been done in a way that precludes an analytical action spectrum. For the retina, the visual pigments are primary candidates for triggering light damage. However, numerous studies reveal that some types of light damage may be potentiated and perhaps in some cases initiated by several other chromophores (see below).

Visual pigments. Visual pigments as chromophores for retinal light damage may present a confusing enigma for physiologists and clincians. Why would the visual cells that are exquisitely designed for photon absorption be damaged by light? In humans, there may be a variety of damage-promoting conditions either endogenously present or induced by therapeutic or other manipulations (see below). Animal models or in vitro preparations, as many other model systems, may exaggerate their variables (such as the light dose) in order to obtain unequivocal effects. Changes observed in such "exaggerated" models may be qualitatively similar in the human eye; they may occur, however, over extended time periods at low levels and gradually develop into manifest lesions corresponding to those observed in animal models. Thus, such model systems are indispensable tools to unravel pathogenetic mechanisms in humans.

Using diffuse green light of varying intensities, W. Noell distinguished type I and type II damage. Type I lesions were found in retina and PE after short exposures to high light levels, whereas type II lesions occured after extended exposures to low illuminances. Both were rhodopsin mediated (Noell et al., 1966). The work of van Norren and colleagues distinguishes class I and class II lesions. Class I is created by diffuse visible light applied in low doses and is probably rhodopsin mediated, class II injuries peak in the UVA and blue wavelengths range (Gorgels and van Norren, 1995; Kremers et al.,

1988; Kremers and van Norren, 1989—for extensive review and discussion the reader is referred to Organisciak et al., 1994).

Diffuse green or white light at relatively low doses used for extended time periods in various rodent models is one of the most frequently applied paradigms and is characterized in detail by Organisciak and colleagues (1994). The studies of T. P. Williams and his colleagues contributed classical concepts for this model system and developed the principle of photostasis (Penn et al., 1986) that may not be limited to the albino rat model but may gain a broad significance for several biological systems such as invertebrates and plants (T. P. Williams, personal communication). In the rodent retina, cones appear to be less susceptible to damage than the predominant rods (LaVail, 1976) and genetic regulation determines the extent of damage (LaVail and Gorrin, 1987). Diffuse green light is used in the analysis of damage mechanisms and damage prevention (Fu et al., 1992; Li et al., 1993; Organisciak et al., 1994).

Light-induced lesions to cones were investigated in primates, with blue cones being selectively damaged by intermittent, focused, narrow-band blue light. By contrast, damage to PE prevailed when the light was applied continuously (Kalloniatis and Harwerth, 1993; Sperling, 1980; Sperling et al., 1980). Pigeon cones but not rods were damaged by diffuse light of 3000 nits applied for 6–48 hours (Marshall et al., 1972). Similarly, cone thresholds were lower in monkeys for exposure to diffuse white light, as evaluated by light and electron microscopy (Sykes et al., 1981). In the rabbit retina, rods, cones, and the pigment epithelium were injured by focussed blue-green light as assessed by light and electron microscopy (Hoppeler et al., 1988).

The blue-light mystery. Whereas earlier studies had appeared to limit blue-light-induced lesions exclusively to the primate retina, more recent developments clearly showed similar mechanisms in rodents and other species (van Norren and Schellekens, 1990). Apart from blue-cone lesions, the hazard presented by laser light in earlier studies was thought to affect mainly the PE photochemically—and, at longer wavelengths, thermally (Ham and Mueller, 1976; Ham et al., 1978; 1979). Mediators of blue-light lesions other than the visual pigments may include chromophores which may reside in the PE, in photoreceptors and perhaps in other retinal layers. To date, no key chromophores directly linked to blue-light lesions have been identified, however. On the other hand, there are numerous studies providing indirect evidence for the existence of molecules that could mediate blue- and UV-induced lesions, respectively. Such chromophores may also act as "adjuvants", potentiating rather than initiating the lesions.

In their study using cultured bovine PE exposed to 435 nm light, Crockett and Lawwill (1984) suggested several chromophores in the PE that could mediate oxygen-dependent photodynamic reactions, such as amino acids, flavins and hemoproteins. In the isolated bovine pigment epithelium, exposure to blue light reduced the transepithelial potential and the short circuit current and induced morphological changes in mitochondria. The action spectrum of changes closely matched that of the respiratory mitochondrial enzyme cytochrome oxidase c and possibly other hemoproteins (Pautler et al., 1990). Exposure of rats to focused narrow-band blue light in vivo inhibited cytochrome oxidase in retina and PE and led to retinal damage as quantified by morphometry, histochemistry, and microradiography (Chen, 1993). A photosensitivity with a peak at 520 nm of the isolated bovine PE was found, resulting in the release of arachidonic acid and increasing the ethanol-induced transepithelial response (Pautler, 1994). Similarly, irradiation of pigment epithelial cells in culture with near UV caused severe damage that was reduced by the addition of catalase (Liu et al., 1995). Light damage was also observed in temperature-controlled pigment epithelium cultures upon irradiation with different wavelengths (Olsen et al., 1995). Narrow-band blue light of 439 nm was most effective in the induction of blood–retina-barrier-dysfunction as assessed morphologically and with fluorometry with no differences in pigmented versus albino rabbits (Putting et al., 1994). Focused UVA and blue-light-inflicted lesions in the rat retina similar to those noted in earlier work as assessed by funduscopy (van Norren et al., 1990). When the effects of collimated UVA light and green light were compared by light and electron microscopy, a remarkable similarity of lesions emerged, indicating the possibility of common underlying mechanisms (Rapp and Smith, 1992b). However, UVA light was more effective in causing photoreceptor cell death. Furthermore, the synthesis of new rod outer segment disks was slowed after UV exposure (Rapp et al., 1994). Both the retina and PE were heavily injured after exposure to collimated monochromatic UV light of 366 nm in aphakic gray squirrels, whereas phakic animals remained uninjured due to the UV-absorbing property of the squirrel lens (Collier et al., 1989). The chromophore for lesions induced exclusively by UV without visible light remains to be elucidated, however.

Recent studies in our laboratory indicate that monochromatic blue light (403 nm, 10nm bandwidth) can induce the so called photoreversal of rhodopsin bleaching in vivo. After bleaching of rhodopsin by intense green light (550 nm, 10 nm bandwidth, 47mW/cm^2) followed by blue light (403nm, 10 nm bandwidth, 33mW/cm^2) about 30% of rhodopsin was regenerated in the living animal. The evaluation of retinal morphology in animals exposed under the same conditions revealed no damage after green light exposure, whereas massive apoptotic cell death was seen in retinas exposed to blue. The photoreversal has long been known to occur in vitro, whereas photoreversal in vivo has not been shown previously. Our data thus suggest that a long-lived blue absorbing photoproduct is generated from rhodopsin, and this absorber photoregulates rhodopsin when it absorbs blue light (Remé et al., 1998; Williams et al., 1998). We conclude that either rhodopsin itself or a blue-absorbing photoproduct induces the massive apoptotic cell death observed after exposure to blue. Green light, which did not cause apoptosis, was unable to photoregenerate rhodopsin and did not appear to react with any photoproduct.

Pigment epithelial chromophores as candidates involved in light damage.

In recent studies, attention has been focused on components in PE lipofuscin as potential chromophores that may participate in initiating or promoting light damage. Lipofuscin has long been suspected to contribute significantly to retinal aging and to age-related macular degeneration. It was assumed that the granule burden in PE cells would partially or totally hamper important PE functions. It remained unclear, however, how PE and photoreceptor cell death was brought about and how the well-known alterations of Bruch's membrane occurred. Photophysical studies on purified intact human lipofuscin granules from different age groups revealed a distinct increase in fluorescence with age and demonstrated three different fluorophores emitting in the blue, yellow, and orange ranges (Docchio et al., 1991). Furthermore, a wavelength-dependent oxygen uptake of PE cells with the generation of singlet oxygen, superoxide anion, hydrogen peroxide, and enhanced lipid peroxidation was shown (Rozanowska et al., 1995). Time-resolved experiments monitored fluorescence decay, UV-visible absorption of longer-lived excited states, and the formation and decay of singlet oxygen in extracts from human lipofuscin, synthetic lipofuscin, and a synthetic orange-emitting fluorophore. The experiments demonstrated that all three compounds absorb in the UV and visible range and can act as sensitizers for creating reactive oxygen species (a triplet state, a radical, singlet oxygen). They may thus be involved in age-related cell loss and degeneration including apoptotic cell death and their relation to light

exposure in that they can potentiate light-induced lesions (Gaillard et al., 1995). Those studies shed new light on mechanisms of retinal and PE aging and degenerative changes. Because lipofuscin occurs in vast amounts and accumulates already in young eyes, its sensitizing action might represent a property fundamental to human disease. In vivo fluorescence measurements in human eyes confirm the spectral characteristics of lipofuscin and may thus represent a valuable diagnostic and prognostic tool for evaluation of age-related and other degenerative changes (Delori et al., 1995). Lipids in human lipofuscin fractions, compared with those from rod outer segments, show a different composition that is more pronounced with age, supporting the concept that lipofuscin does not merely reflect rod outer segments but is the result of complex chemical reactions (Bazan et al., 1990). Recent studies demonstrated a blue- and UV-absorbing opsin in the PE. This opsin is distinct from rhodopsin and cone visual pigments, contains the all-trans-retinal Schiff base and has absorption maxima at 469 and 370 nm (Hao and Fong, 1996). Those molecules may thus represent further candidates for promoting blue-light lesions. An important autofluorescent component of PE lipofuscin was recently isolated, purified, and characterized. It is a pyridinium bis-retinoid (N-retinylidene-N-retinyletha-nolamine, A2-E) that exhibits detergent properties and inhibits lysosomal functions (Eldred and Lasky, 1993; Kopitz et al., 1996). Due to its properties, it may contribute to changes leading to PE diseases such as age related macular degeneration. In addition, it may act as a chromophore, absorbing light in the UV and visible part of the spectrum. Our laboratory developed a specific and sensitive quantitative assay to monitor this compound, which was found to increase significantly with age in the rat (Reinboth et al., 1997).

PE melanin has long been claimed as a chromophore for blue-light damage because it absorbs exponentially more in the blue and UV spectral range (Ham et al., 1986). By the same mechanism it was suggested that PE melanin protects against damage (Sanyal and Zeilmaker, 1988). However, other studies could not confirm this protective role but rather found no difference in the amount of light damage in pigmented versus albino eyes (Hoppeler et al., 1988; LaVail et al., 1987; Putting et al., 1994; Rapp and Smith, 1992a) or in heavily pigmented fundus areas as compared to lightly pigmented ones (Howell et al., 1982; Lawwill, 1973). When exposure to light in albino and pigmented rats was equated in terms of its effectiveness to bleach rhodopsin, damage was equal in the two strains of rats (Rapp and Williams, 1980). Notably, the pigmentation of the iris may well protect against incident light and thus act in a protec-

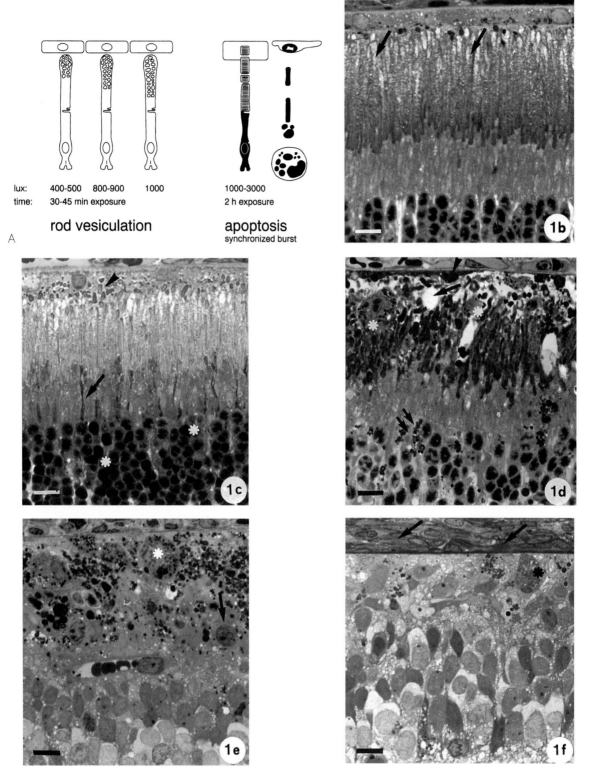

FIGURE 29-1. (a)Schematic drawing indicating photoreceptor changes as a function of illuminance duration and intensity, illustrated for the albino rat retina. Lesions are confined to rod outer segments (ROS) after exposures of 500–1000 lux for 30–45 minutes. Exposure to 1000 lux for 2 hours represents a turning point, with apoptotic cell death occuring in the lower central retina, followed by massive cellular decay, apoptotic bodies and macrophage invasion at later time points after exposure (>24 hours). Exposure to 3000 lux for 2 hours results in qualitatively identical changes as observed after 1000 lux for 2 hours, however the lesions are now spread over the entire ocular fundus except the far periphery.

Light microscopic pictures illustrating ROS lesions as well as the turning point with apoptotic lesions and scar formation in the albino rat retina. (b) ROS alterations (↑) seen immediately after exposure to

tive manner. In light of those studies, melanin might be considered an ambivalent compound with potentially protective, damage enhancing, or neutral qualities. Similar observations were made in the skin and expressed in the following way: "Is melanin photoprotective? Sometimes yes, sometimes no." (Giacomoni, 1995).

Exogenous photosensitizing chromophores. There is a vast amount of drugs which potentially could act as photosensitizer for retina and PE, provided that they pass the blood–retina interface, absorb in the near UV and visible range, and either have a cationic-amphiphilic nature, show a porphyrin-like structure, or show a tricyclic-heterocyclic ring system. A number of them have been shown relevant for the eye (Roberts et al., 1992). Clinical observations diagnosed a pigment retinopathy in patients treated with the antiarrhythmic amiodarone. Subsequent laboratory studies revealed a photosensitization of PE cells with increased cell death after irradiation with visible blue and UV light (Dinda et al., 1992; Minelli et al., 1991). The well-known sensitizer phenothiazine can also affect the pigment epithelium (Fox et al., 1993), as can the diuretic hydrochlorothiazide (Hartzer et al., 1993). Rose bengal, a strong sensitizer and closely related to fluorescein, which is known to every ophthalmologist for fluorescence angiography, was found to sensitize the PE by forming reactive oxygen species (Menon et al., 1992). Therapeutic strategies using various porphyrins span a wide area of clinical and laboratory investigations (Gomer, 1991) and porphyrins are suggested to contribute to hematogenous photosensitization of the outer retina (Gottsch et al., 1990). The addition of protoporphyrin IX to pigment epithelium in culture that was irradiated with blue light caused an increase in light damage, supporting the idea that hematogenous photosensitization may occur under certain circumstances (Bynoe et al., 1995). Investigators using the rodent model for light damage studies should remember the Harderian gland, located at the posterior pole of the eye in the orbit, which is a source of a number of different porphyrins (Shirama and Hokano, 1991) and may thus sensitize retina and PE. The importance of photosensitizing drugs should be borne in

mind by various clinical disciplines such as ophthalmology and dermatology, but also psychiatry, internal medicine, and others.

Different Light Exposures Answer Different Questions

White light or broad spectral ranges can be applied as collimated beam or as diffuse radiation. Light focussed on the retina will mostly cover a small area and is applied in a high dose within relatively short time periods to anesthetized animals with dilated pupils. Those regimens often mimick instrument hazards such as the operating microscope or the indirect ophthalmoscope. Diffuse white or green light is used for extended time periods or constantly over days to weeks; light doses vary per experiment and, obviously, with the time period of application. The animals are not anesthetized. Quantitative analyses frequently measure the end stage of injury, namely, the reduction or loss of the outer nuclear layer of the retina. This type of paradigm crudely mimicks outdoor exposure (without exactly paralleling a given solar spectrum).

Our laboratory developed a rat model where low light doses are applied for short time periods (Fig. 29-1a). Initial changes are confined to rod outer segments and are reversible within one week. At higher doses, apoptotic death of single cells is observed in photoreceptors and PE, whereas at still higher illuminances, massive apoptosis leading to large areas of decay prevails in the acute stage, followed by a marked macrophage response, proliferative changes and scar formation replacing photoreceptors and PE (Hafezi et al., 1997a; Szczesny et al., 1995). This model does not allow the definition of action spectra, but it permits a detailed analysis of the threshold for individual changes and the determination of their time course in the range of minutes, hours, and days (Fig. 29-1b–f).

Extended exposure durations in any of the above regimens will allow a host of secondary changes to occur and may thus obscure primary events for analysis. For example, it may be impossible to determine whether the PE or the retina is initially and mainly affected by a given light exposure.

500–1000 lux for 30–45 minutes. Lesions are reversible within one week. (c) Changes observed immediately after exposure to 3000 lux for 2 hours. Nuclear (*) and cytoplasmic (↑) condensations indicating apoptosis are seen in photoreceptors. Note the abundance of newly shed phagosomes in the PE (∇), indicating that a shedding burst can be elicited by bright light irrespective of the circadian disk-shedding rhythm. (d) 36–48 hours after exposure to 3000 lux for 2 hours, edema (↑) and macrophages (*) are seen in the area of ROS, PE cells show apoptotic condensation of nuclei (∇) and cytoplasm, and numerous

apoptotic bodies (↑↑) appear in the outer nuclear layer. (e) 72 hours after exposure to 3000 lux for 2 hours, most of the photoreceptor nuclei and the PE have vanished. Large macrophages (*), mitotic figures (↑), and abundant cellular debris are seen. (f) 6 days after exposure to 3000 lux for 2 hours, most of the debris has been removed; the choroid shows a dense network of cells and fibers (↑). Some macrophages and glia cells appear in the region of the outer retina (*). Bar represents 10 μm.

Notably, not even diffuse white light creates uniform changes in the retina or PE despite a uniform rhodopsin bleaching (Williams and Webbers, 1995). The work of T. P. Williams and colleagues analyzed in detail the classical sensitive area in the upper temporal region of the rat retina that differs in biochemical and structural parameters from the remaining fundus and is most affected after diffuse white-light exposure (Rapp et al., 1980). In our rat light-damage model, where the light source is mounted above the exposure chambers and shielded by a diffusing screen, the lower central retina shows stronger responses than the other parts at threshold illuminances and short exposure durations (30 minutes–2 hours). In light-damage studies in rats with a transsection of the optic nerve, it is suggested that dopaminergic neurons in the sensitive area may exert protective effects (Bush and Williams, 1991).

Methods of Damage Evaluation

Qualitative and quantitative estimates of lesions span a wide range including psychophysical and electrophysiological methods, fundus reflectometry and spectrophotometry, funduscopy, light and electron microscopy, and biochemistry. The choice of method will depend on the given clinical or experimental situation. It is likely, though, that certain experimental paradigms such as the damage threshold and magnitude, the time course of lesion, and the qualitiy of a change may depend on the method of evaluation. Among other reasons this renders comparisons of data between laboratories rather complex. When large fields of monkey retinas were illuminated by broad-spectrum fluorescent light for 12 hours, the threshold for cones was 6000 to 11,000 lux and for rods 11,000–19,000 lux with histological evaluation 15 hours after exposure (Sykes et al., 1981). The exposure of small patches of monkey retinas under Maxwellian view with a xenon arc light source resulted in a threshold irradiant dose of 230 J/cm^2 for exposures from 10 minutes to 12 hours. The evaluation was by funduscopy and densitometry. Distinct funduscopically visible lesions occured two days after exposure (Kremers et al., 1989). Kremers and van Norren calculated the threshold irradiant dose in Sykes's experiments to be 16 J/cm^2. The distinctly lower threshold in Sykes's experiments may be due, at least in part, to the method of evaluation: light and electron microscopy is likely to reveal subtle changes that will remain unnoticed with funduscopy. Furthermore, a distinction between rod and cone lesions is possible. In addition, the timing of evaluation may be crucial. Whereas funduscopic lesions are clearest 2 days after exposure, the morphological changes are seen already 15 hours following the retinal illumination.

In our rat model, apoptotic cell death occurs in photoreceptors immediately after light exposure, whereas the pigment epithelium consistently shows a time lag of at least 5 hours (Hafezi et al., 1997a). An analysis of only early postexposure time points would find the pigment epithelium uninjured. By contrast, evaluation time points later than 24 hours after exposure reveal lesions of both photoreceptors and pigment epithelium with massive cell death and macrophage responses. Thus, the quality of a change may vary as distinctly as the threshold, depending on the method and the timing of an analysis.

MOLECULAR, CELLULAR, AND TISSUE RESPONSES IN LIGHT DAMAGE

In the human eye, damage mechanisms obviously cannot be evaluated as extensively and systematically as in laboratory studies. Clinically, functional and funduscopic changes of the acute solar retinopathy are reported, whereas photochemical and biochemical data are lacking. There are reports, however, on histological changes after sunlight exposure (Hope-Ross et al., 1993).

Molecular Mechanisms in Light Damage

Initial light damage mechanisms on a molecular level still remain unclear, even though there is a large number of studies devoted to different aspects of light-induced lesions (reviewed in detail in Organisciak et al., 1994). Photochemical events may include the formation of singlet oxygen, hydroxyl radical, hydrogen peroxide, and other toxic photoproducts as shown by the experimental application of various antioxidants that reduce light damage (Dillon, 1991; Organisciak et al., 1994). In those studies, the protective agents served as experimental tools that suggested underlying processes. Of special interest is the role of ascorbate that may predominantly protect the pigment epithelium (Organisciak et al., 1994).

Hemoxygenase is the rate-limiting enzyme in heme degradation and is induced in many cell types by oxidative stress (Stocker, 1990). Hemoxygenase I was induced by exposure to intense green light in the rat retina, and this effect was suppressed by the antioxidant dimethylurea (Kutty et al., 1995). When human pigment epithelial cells in culture were transfected with adenovirus-hemoxygenase 1-construct, the cells overexpressed human hemoxygenase 1 and were protected against the toxicity of heme/hemoglobin that was added to the culture (Dunn et al., 1995). Notably, the cytokine transforming growth factor-β induced hemoxygenase 1 in human pigment epithelial cells (Kutty et al., 1994). The mechanisms involved in the protective effects of growth factors on chronic light-induced lesions are unknown (Collins et al., 1994; Faktorovich et al., 1992; LaVail et al., 1992). Conceivably, the suppression of apoptotic cell death may be involved (Collins et al., 1994). An elevated level of the protein clusterin was observed in light-induced lesions in the rat retina and this increase was reduced by the anitoxidant dimethylurea (Wong et al., 1995a). Increased clusterin levels are also associated with apoptotic cell death in the *rd* mouse model of human retinitis pigmentosa (Wong, 1994).

Particular attention has been paid to the role of lipids and lipid peroxydation in retinal and pigment epithelial light damage (Organisciak et al., 1994; Penn et al., 1991; Wiegand et al., 1983). The retina normally contains more than 60 mol% of polyunsaturated fatty acids, the most abundant ones are arachidonic acid (AA; 20:4 n-6) and docosahexaenoic acid (DHA; 22:6 n-3) (Fliesler and Anderson, 1983). Dietary manipulation of fatty acids, particularly DHA, altered the susceptibility to light-induced lesions. When retinal DHA was lowered (Organisciak et al., 1987) or practically absent (Bush et al., 1991), light damage was significantly reduced or absent, respectively. Paradoxically, in animals with significantly reduced retinal DHA levels showing no acute light damage, the rhodopsin content was distinctly increased. In those animals, however, the rhodopsin regeneration rate was slowed and the photon catch during light exposure reduced to half of controls, implicating a reduced retinal light sensitivity and possibly a role of DHA in normal pigment epithelial physiologic phenomena, such as the visual cycle, shedding, and phagocytosis or fatty acid esterification (Bush et al., 1994). No increase in acute retinal and PE light damage and virtually no peroxidized lipids in vivo were observed in rats fed a diet enriched in DHA and its precursor eicosapentaenoic acid (EPA; 20:5 n-3). However, the ratio of EPA to AA was increased in fish-oil-fed rats, indicating that AA, the precursor of potent and harmful inflammatory mediators, was reduced. Furthermore, a moderately protective effect in fish-oil-fed rats was observed in quantitative analysis (Remé et al., 1994). This apparently contradictory observation supports the idea that mechanisms other than lipid peroxidation may be the primary events in light damage. In a series of chronic experiments, rats fed a diet rich in n-3 fatty acids were more susceptible to a light exposure of 24 hours followed by 10 days of dim cyclic light (Koutz et al., 1995; Wiegand et al., 1995). These observations may indicate that lipid peroxidation occurs within longer experimental periods, perhaps secondary to other, initial events.

Fatty Acid Metabolites as Inflammatory Mediators and Cellular Signaling Molecules

Histological evaluation in numerous light damage studies reveals subacute and chronic changes that show some characteristics of an inflammatory response, such as edema, cell death, cell proliferation, and presence of mononuclear cells (Hoppeler et al., 1988; O'Steen and Karcioglu, 1974; Tso, 1973). The mediators of such changes are not known in detail. AA is the precursor molecule of a variety of inflammatory mediators (Samuelsson, 1991) and is also directly involved in cellular signaling (Axelrod et al., 1988). Furthermore, lipoxygenase products of AA play a role in neuronal transmembrane signaling (Piomelli and Greengard, 1990). The retinal phospholipids are rich in AA and thus furnish ample substrate molecules for cyclooxygenase and lipoxygenase, the major metabolizing enzymes that produce the eicosanoids. A light-induced release of AA was shown in the isolated rat retina (Jung and Remé, 1994) and isolated rod outer segments (Birkle and Bazan, 1989). Recent studies also demonstrate a light-induced release of the lipoxygenase product leukotriene B_4 (LTB_4) in vitro (Reinboth et al., 1995). The releases of both AA and LTB_4 were intensity and time dependent and were inhibited in part by the phospholipase A_2 inhibitor quinacrine and the lipoxygenase inhibitor zileuton, respectively, suggesting finely tuned light-regulated release mechanisms (Jung et al., 1994; Reinboth et al., 1995). In addition, DHA is released by light exposure with kinetics similar to that of AA, implying a further source of inflammatory mediators, albeit less potent, the docosanoids (Reinboth et al., 1996). It is tempting to speculate that there is a functional interaction between AA and DHA release mechanisms. Indeed, preliminary data show an inhibition of AA release by free DHA or free AA in the retina vitro, suggesting the existence of an interaction of free PUFAs with phospholipases as observed in other systems (Reinboth et al., in preparation).

The observations on light-evoked release of lipid mediators led us to propose a concept for retinal light damage mechanisms and possibly other ocular disease processes (Fig. 29-2). The light-released fatty acids and their enzymatically peroxidized metabolites subserve messenger functions and mediate inflammatory and immune responses. Once triggered by light, the mediators may stimulate the PE (Jaffe et al., 1995) or retinal Müller cells (Drescher and Whittum-Hudson, 1996) to release cytokines. Furthermore, the invasion of mononuclear cells is initiated, as documented in histological sections of different light damage models. The mononuclear cells themselves may also release cy-

Effect of light exposure on retina and pigment epithelium

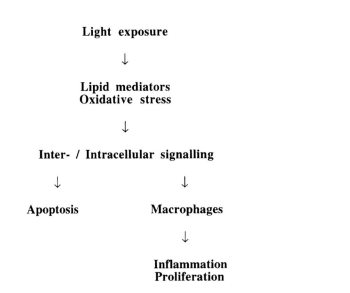

Light exposure

↓

**Lipid mediators
Oxidative stress**

↓

Inter- / Intracellular signalling

↓   ↓

Apoptosis   **Macrophages**

↓

**Inflammation
Proliferation**

FIGURE 29-2. Cascade of events that could lead to different cellular responses after light exposure. Lipid mediators and molecules of oxidative stress arising after light exposure can initiate different intracellular signaling pathways (such as the release of certain cytokines) that may activate effectors of apoptosis. Lipid mediators are also messengers for the induction of macrophage responses and/or the release of cytokines, which may then lead to inflammatory and proliferative tissue reactions. The conditions that could lead to one or the other of the above described cascades remain to be elucidated.

tokines, which could sustain a cascade of different cellular reactions (Planck et al., 1993; Rappolee and Werb, 1992; Rosenbaum, 1993; Rosenbaum et al., 1987; Wiedemann, 1992). For example, the cytokine interleukin-1β is released by monocytes/macrophages. It can induce the hydrolysis of phospholipids with production of diacylglycerol (Rosoff et al., 1988), protein phosphorylation and cellular signaling via G-protein coupling or transcription factor phosphorylation in various tissues (Dinarello, 1994), and an inflammatory response in ocular tissues (Claudio et al., 1994; Kulkarni and Mancino, 1993; Martiney et al., 1992) as well as cytokine production (Yarosh, 1994) in the skin, indicating the potential for similar responses to radiation in both the eye and the skin.

Vascular endothelial growth factor (VEGF) gene expression is induced in the retinal pigment epithelium (Shima et al., 1995) and other retinal cells (Pe'er et al., 1995; Pierce et al., 1995) by hypoxia in vivo and in vitro. Pigment epithelial cells in vitro stimulate vessel formation from choroidal endothelial cells, an effect that is inhibited by antibodies against various cytokines including VEGF (Sakamoto et al., 1995). In the developing retina, VEGF is expressed by glia cells at certain stages, possibly induced by tissue hypoxia preceding vessel formation (Hata et al., 1995; Stone et al., 1995). Because molecular and cellular responses in hypoxia/ischemia and light damage show striking similarities—such as the hydrolysis and the metabolization of phospholipids, altered levels of intracellular calcium, and proliferative changes—it is tempting to assume that in chronic light damage, too, VEGF gene expression is induced, perhaps mediated by cytokines. IL-1 gene expression was indeed observed in retinal ischemia (Hangai et al., 1995). Furthermore, growth factors provide protection in retinal ischemia (Unoki and LaVail, 1994; Zhang et al., 1994) similar to light damage (Faktorovich et al., 1992; LaVail et al., 1992). The cellular mechanisms by which growth factors can rescue the retina and photoreceptors are unclear to date. It is well known, however, that individual as well as groups of cytokines can have a variety of different effects (Dinarello, 1994) consistent with their potential involvement in light damage as promoters as well as protectors.

In view of dietary modification of retinal light damage susceptibility, it is important to note that supplementation with n-3 long-chain fatty acids like DHA, EPA, or their precursors, suppress the formation of some cytokines such as IL-1 and tumor necrosis factor (Endres et al., 1989; Meydani et al., 1993). It remains to be seen in animal models of light damage or in human ocular pathology whether n-3 fatty acid supplementation can influence disease processes. The importance of n-3 fatty acids for retinal and brain development and function has been repeatedly demonstrated (Hoffmann et al., 1993; Neuringer et al., 1986). The dietary supplementation with n-3 long-chain fatty acids for inflammatory and immune responses in eye diseases may represent an important therapeutic strategy in the future. Recent data from our laboratory showing that DHA can inhibit the release of AA in the light-exposed retina in vitro supports this notion (Reinboth et al., in preparation). With the suppression of AA release the precursor molecule for potent inflammatory and immune mediators would be eliminated or reduced, respectively, and replaced by the precursor of less potent messengers.

Apart from the induction of cytokine responses by lipid mediators, apoptotic cell death also could be incurred. Lipid mediators and some of their intermediates as well as molecules of oxidative stress (such as NO) were observed to induce apoptosis in nonocular tissues (Buttke and Sandstrom, 1994) (see "Potential Gene Expression . . ." below). The intracellular pathways leading to the execution of apoptosis may include signaling by cytokines via membrane receptors (Barinaga, 1996; Martin and Green, 1995).

In the context of retinal light damage, both of the hypothetical cascades may occur after the light-induced release of lipid mediators. It remains to be seen which conditions would lead toward the apoptosis cascade and which toward the chronic proliferative changes.

Modes of Cell Death: Apoptosis and Necrosis

Cell death by means of apoptosis is of outstanding interest for scientists in a large variety of research fields including cancer research, immunology, virology, degenerative diseases, and radiobiology. The unique mode of this cell death appears to stimulate the imagination as illustrated in phrases such as "death by informed consent" (Gregory and Bird, 1995), "death at an early age" (Papermaster and Windle, 1995), "no self-respecting cell would be seen dead other than by apoptosis these days" (Allen and Goldberg, 1995), "cellular suicide," "altruistic cell death," and others.

The term "programmed cell death" (PCD) was originally used in development to describe a tightly regulated process in organ and tissue remodeling in response to physiological stimuli, requiring de novo gene expression. PCD is not identical to apoptosis, nevertheless the terms are often used interchangeably. Most apoptotic phenomena require de novo gene expression (Schwartz and Osborne, 1993). In many mammalian cells the effectors for apoptosis are continuously present and are activated by several mechanisms (Weil et al., 1996).

Apoptosis can clearly be distinguished from necrosis, the latter involving lysis of cells and organelles and collateral tissue responses. By contrast, characteristic features of apoptosis are the death of individual cells with condensation of chromatin and cytoplasm with relatively well-preserved organelles, followed by fragmentation of the cell and phagocytosis of the apoptotic bodies by macrophages or neighboring cells (Steller, 1995; Wyllie et al., 1980) (Fig. 29-3). Besides light- and electron microscopy, there is the histochemical demonstration of apoptosis by in situ labeling of DNA nick ends by the TUNEL method (terminal transferase-dUTP nick-end labeling) (Gavrieli et al., 1992) or modifications thereof. During apoptosis, the nuclear DNA is fragmented into regular subunits of about 200 base pairs (bp) or their multiples and these fragments can be visualized by gel electrophoresis forming the so-called ladder. For unequivocal confirmation of apoptosis, at least two of those methods should demonstrate the described changes.

The expression of several genes coincides with apoptosis, for example, stromelysin, ubiquitin, clusterin, and others. The expression of other genes appears to be involved in the regulation of cell death, either preventing or promoting the death program, for example, c-myc, glucocorticoid receptor, p53, bcl-2, and others (Gavrieli et al., 1992; Reed, 1994; Schwartz et al., 1993; Steller, 1995). There is a wide variety of tissues in which apoptosis occurs and an equally large number of endogenous and exogenous stimuli and mediators (Schwartzman and Cidlowski, 1993; Thompson, 1995). Intracellular signaling pathways may include increased calcium levels, protein kinase C (PKC), phosphatidylinositol-3-kinase (PI-3 kinase), oxidative stress and lipid hydroperoxides, and activation of endogenous endonucleases. Recent evidence indicates that the small family of transcription factor proteins Fos and Jun (AP-1) may regulate apoptosis in several systems (Colotta et al., 1992; Hafezi et al., 1997b; Marti et al., 1994; Preston et al., 1996). An important regulative role for apoptosis is also ascribed to the transcription factor proteins Myc and Max (Amati et al., 1993). To date, numerous effector molecules have been identified that are essential for the basic death program. Intracellular proteases and nucleases are thought to be crucial components. For example, family members of the protease IL-1β-converting enzyme (ICE) appear to be key enzymes to execute apoptosis (Martin et al., 1995).

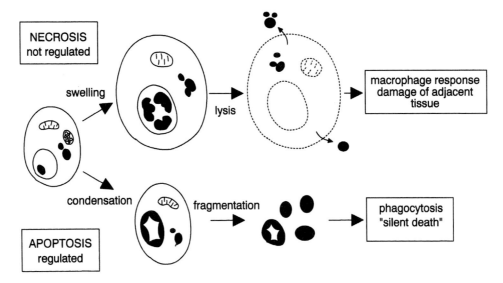

FIGURE 29-3. Schematic drawing illustrating the different modes of cell death in necrosis versus apoptosis. Necrosis includes swelling and disruption of cells and organelles, causing collateral reactions in the adjacent tissue. Apoptosis, by contrast, implies condensation and shrinkage of nucleus and cytoplasm followed by fragmentation and phagocytosis of fragments by adjacent cells or macrophages.

Retinal Dystrophies

In the eye, apoptosis is observed in the developing mouse retina (Young, 1984) and in rat retinas that have been exposed to lead during development (Poblenz et al., 1995), in retinoblastoma (Howes et al., 1994), and in some animal models of retinitis pigmentosa (Chang et al., 1993; Gregory et al., 1995; Lolley, 1994; Papermaster et al., 1995; Portera-Cailliau et al., 1994; Tso et al., 1994; Wong et al., 1995b). Furthermore, apoptosis is found in donor eyes from patients that had suffered from retinitis pigmentosa (Li and Milam, 1995). The discovery of apoptosis in those animal models with diverse genotypic and phenotypic characteristics may indicate a final common pathway during the course of the retinal dystrophy. Which gene mutations and their molecular consequences acutally may induce the apoptotic death pathway is unknown. Several genes have been investigated for a potential involvement in retinal apoptosis, such as clusterin, *c-fos,* and p53 (Wong et al., 1995a; review: Remé et al., 1998).

Several factors induce apoptosis in the pigment epithelium in vitro, such as tumor necrosis factor-α (TNF-α, staurosporine, anti-Fas antibody). Apoptosis was prevented by bFGF and PDGF (He et al., 1995). The well-know photosensitizer and antidepressant hypericin, contained in St. John's wort, or *Hypericum perforatum* (Duran and Song, 1986), induces apoptosis in the PE at higher concentration, possibly via an inhibition of PKC.

Light-Induced Apoptosis in Retina and Pigment Epithelium

It is noteworthy but perhaps not surprising that apoptotic cell death in the retina can be evoked by light. Exposure to intense green light for prolonged periods (Abler et al., 1996) and exposure to diffuse white light of relatively low intensity for short time periods (Remé et al., 1995b) elicits an apoptotic response. The amount of apoptosis in the retina is strain dependent (Lai et al., 1995), can be ameliorated by different agents (Chang et al., 1994), and occurs sooner after exposure to intermittent light than continuous light of the same final irradiant dose (Li et al., 1994).

In our model of acute threshold light damage in the albino rat, apoptosis in photoreceptors and pigment epithelium is seen in the lower central retina after exposure of dark-adapted animals to diffuse white fluorescent light of 1000 lux for two hours, whereas even more apoptosis occurs after exposure to 3000 lux for two hours. In the retina of pigmented mice, distinct apoptosis is seen after exposure to 5000–6000 lux for two hours (Fig. 29-4a, b). Addressing the question of apoptosis in cones, we observed ample apoptotic cells in the retina of the thirteen-lined ground squirrel, which has an all-cone retina, in animals living in a normal light/ dark cycle shortly before entering hibernation (Fig. 29-3c).

Detailed time course studies show that in the rat retina a massive and immediate apoptotic response at the end of light exposure is followed by an almost complete

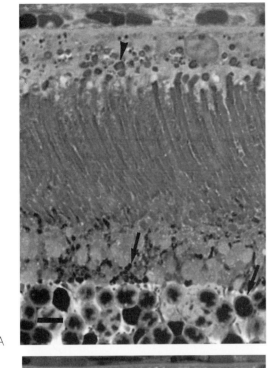

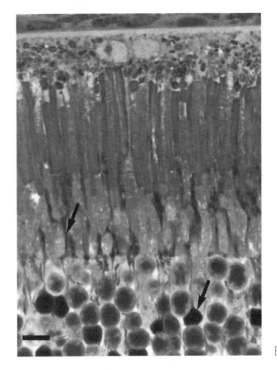

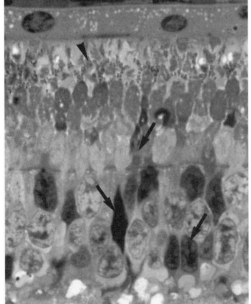

FIGURE 29-4. Light micrographs showing apoptosis in photoreceptors immediately after light exposure and under a regular light/dark cycle, respectively. (a) Albino rat, killed immediately after exposure to 3000 lux for 2 hours. Distinct condensations of photoreceptor nuclei (↑) and inner segments (↑) appear, indicating apoptotic cell death. Note the abundance of newly shed phagosomes (▽). (b) Pigmented mouse, killed immediately after exposure to 5000 lux for 2 hours. Numerous condensed nuclei (↑) and inner segments (↑) are seen indicating apoptotic cell death. (c) Thirteen-lined ground squirrel, killed shortly before hibernation during the regular 12:12 light/dark cycle (L: 100 lux at cage level). Numerous cones in the outer nuclear display apoptotic changes with condensed nuclei (↑) and inner segments (↑). The outer segments appear short with diminished disk membranes (▼). Bar represents 10 μm.

decay of photoreceptors about 24–36 hours after light exposure. This is confirmed by gel electrophoresis. TUNEL labeling reveals distinct staining within the entire outer nuclear layer, in contrast to the staining of fewer cells at earlier time points (Fig. 29-5a–c). At early time points during and after light exposure, such as 30, 60, 90 minutes *during* exposure and 0, 60, 120 min-

utes *following* exposure, electron micrographs show clear signs of chromatin condensation and inner segment densifications in photoreceptors, but gel electrophoresis is negative for apoptotic signs (Fig. 29-6a–i). TUNEL staining reveals few positive nuclei in the outer nuclear layer at zero hours after exposure, distinctly fewer positive cells than morphology reveals. This dis-

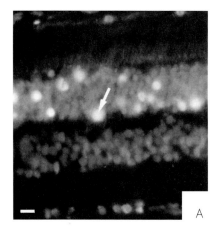 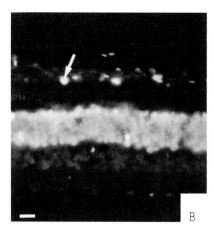 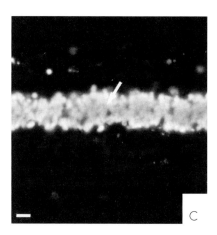

FIGURE 29-5. TUNEL staining demonstrating apoptosis at different times after exposure to 3000 lux for 2 hours in the albino rat retina. (A) Positive TUNEL staining of some nuclei (↑) in the ONL 5 hours after exposure. Bar represents 10 μm. (B) Positive TUNEL staining of nuclei (↑) in the PE 10 hours after exposure. Bar represents 20 μm. (C) Massive TUNEL staining of the ONL 24 hours after exposure. Bar represents 20 μm.

crepancy may indicate that DNA fragmentation occurs in several steps with a cleavage into large fragments in the kilobase range preceding the internucleosomal fragmentation that produces the positive nick-end labeling and the ladder in gel electrophoresis. This has been observed by other laboratories in nonocular tissues (Cohen et al., 1992; Oberhammer et al., 1993) and in the lead-exposed developing retina (Poblenz et al., 1995). The endonucleases performing DNA fragmentation have not yet been characterized in detail, DNase-I may be involved (Peitsch et al., 1993).

The morphological picture of massive and rather simultaneous decay of photoreceptors following at 24 hours after bright light exposure may be interpreted as a tissue necrosis, because macrophages are beginning to invade the area of lesion and only a few viable cells can be distinguished. However, recent studies in our laboratory using mice lacking the gene *c-fos* clearly demonstrate a complete prevention of acute and delayed apoptosis in the retina after exposure to 5000-lux for 2 hours. Therefore, the massive cellular decay seen in the rat model and in control wild-type mice is interpreted as apoptotic (Hafezi et al., 1997b).

In notable contrast to photoreceptors, the pigment epithelium shows a different time course of apoptosis. In electron micrographs, peripheral chromatin clumping followed by cytoplasmic condensation is seen at 5–24 hours after light exposure. TUNEL staining shows distinctly positive PE nuclei about 10 hours after exposure. These different timing patterns in the retina and the PE may indicate that trigger mechanisms, messengers, and gene expression are not identical (Fig. 29-7). Possibly, the rapid death of photoreceptor cells repre-

sents a major mechanism to trigger apoptosis and cell death in the PE. Furthermore, following light exposure, cytokines may be induced in the retina and/or the PE, which could trigger a delayed apoptotic response (see "Fatty Acid Metabolites . . ." above) (Hafezi et al., 1997a). In nonocular systems, cytokines act as proapoptotic factors (Han et al., 1996).

Potential Gene Expression, Messengers, and Inducers in Light-Evoked Apoptosis

As mentioned earlier, there is a multitude of agents that can induce apoptosis in nonocular tissues, whereas for the eye, these processes are just beginning to be investigated. Similarly, potential messengers and potential genes involved in apoptosis are barely unraveled. Light damage studies in the zebrafish by means of microscopy, western blotting, and differential display polymerase chain reaction (DDPCR) disclosed novel genes potentially involved in light damage. Furthermore, the transcription factors c-Fos and c-Jun were elevated (Robinson et al., 1995). In the rat retina, the expression of clusterin correlated with light damage and the levels of expression reflected the severity of lesions (Wong et al., 1995a). In the normal mouse retina, *c-fos* is expressed in a diurnal manner with high levels in the dark but not in the light (Nir and Agarwal, 1993; Yoshida et al., 1993), whereas in the *rds* mouse, the levels of c-Fos were high throughout the light/dark cycle, indicating that it may be a signal for the apoptotic pathway (Agarwal et al., 1995). A detailed study of the expression of c-Fos was performed in the *rd* mouse. An aberrant expression of the c-Fos protein was found in photoreceptors im-

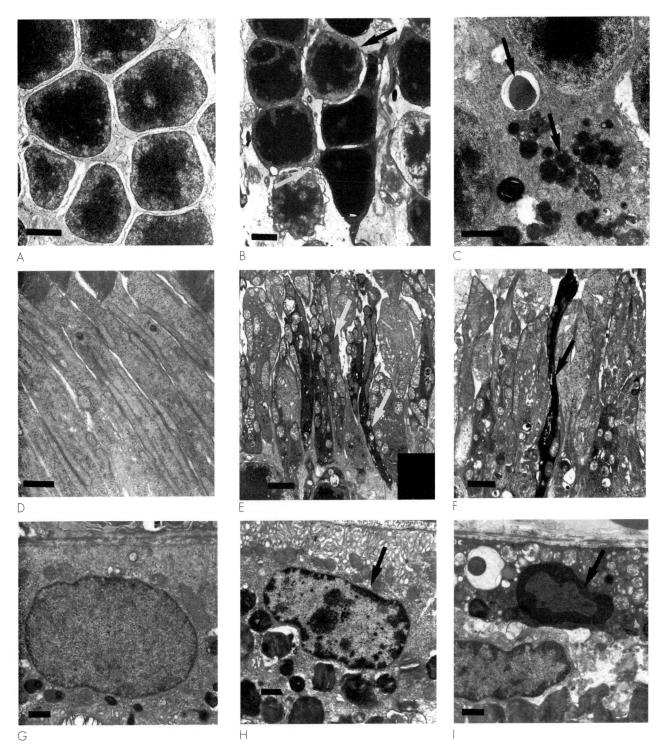

FIGURE 29-6. Electron micrographs depicting apoptotic changes in photoreceptor and PE nuclei and cytoplasm at different time points after exposure to 3000 lux for 2 hours in the albino rat retina. (a) Unexposed control nuclei of photoreceptors showing the regular pattern of chromatin. Bar represents 2 μm. (b) Early (↑) and intermediate (↑) stages of chromatin condensation in the ONL. Bar represents 2 μm. (c) Apoptotic bodies (↑) among normal photoreceptor nuclei. Bar represents 2 μm. (d) Unexposed control photoreceptor inner segments. Bar represents 1 μm. (e) Early stages of cytoplasmic condensation of photoreceptor inner segments (↑). Bar represents 2 μm. (f) Late stage of cytoplasmic condensation of a photoreceptor inner segment (↑). Bar represents 2 μm. (g) Unexposed control nucleus of the PE. Bar represents 3 μm. (h) Early stage of peripheral chromatin condensation (↑) in a PE nucleus. Bar represents 1 μm. (i) Late stage of peripheral nuclear chromatin condensation (↑) and cytoplasmic condensation in a PE cell. Bar represents 2 μm.

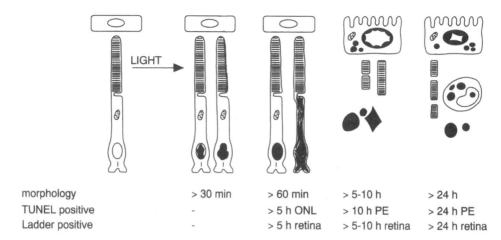

morphology	> 30 min	> 60 min	> 5-10 h	> 24 h
TUNEL positive	-	> 5 h ONL	> 10 h PE	> 24 h PE
Ladder positive	-	> 5 h retina	> 5-10 h retina	> 24 h retina

FIGURE 29-7. Schematic drawing summarizing an approximate time course of apoptotic changes in photoreceptors and PE after exposure to 3000 lux for 2 hours in the albino rat retina. Morphological signs of ONL chromatin condensation occur as early as 30 minutes after the onset of light exposure followed by cytoplasmic condensation at 60 minutes during light exposure. 5 hours after exposure apoptotic bodies appear in the ONL and progressive chromatin condensation occurs in the PE. 24 hours and later, the PE shows distinct apoptotic signs; the ONL reveals massive cellular decay, apoptotic bodies, and macrophages. TUNEL staining appears in the ONL from 5 hours after exposure and from 10 hours after exposure in the PE. Ladder formation in gel electrophoresis is seen from 5 hours after exposure.

mediately prior to their death by apoptosis, suggesting the possibility that c-Fos may be involved in triggering apoptosis (Rich et al., 1997). In several tissues, the gene *bcl-2* was found to protect against apoptotic cell death (Reed, 1994), possibly among other mechanisms via antioxidant pathways (Hockenbery et al., 1993). In mice with inherited retinal degenerations, *bcl-2* overexpression slightly retarded the apoptotic death of photoreceptor cells. Similarly, *bcl-2* overexpression diminished but did not prevent photoreceptor death in mice exposed to constant light (Chen et al., 1996).

Studies in our laboratory using mice lacking a functional protooncogene *c-fos* (c-fos knockout mice) revealed a striking scarcity of apoptosis in knockout mice after 2 hours of exposure to 5000 lux white fluorescent light and the complete absence of severe lesions in retina and PE at 12 and 24 hours after light exposure. By contrast, control littermates showed distinct and irreversible lesions (Hafezi et al., 1997b). Those studies imply a functional role of *c-fos* in retinal apoptosis and show a complete protection against light-induced cell loss in the absence of *c-fos*. In view of those studies, apoptosis may be considered as a major underlying mechanism of retinal light damage. To date, the exact role of *c-fos* in the apoptosis pathway is not known. It is conceivable that *c-fos* or the lack of *c-fos* modify retinal physiology and thus alter the susceptibility to light-induced apoptosis. Alternatively, *c-fos* may be a specific gene for some apoptosis pathways.

The cysteine protease IL-1β-converting enzyme (ICE) is thought to play a key role in apoptosis in nonocular tissues and corresponds to the cell death gene *ced-3* of the nematode, *Caenorhabditis elegans*. ICE may activate other proteases and/or endonucleases but may also have further unidentified functions in the pathway of apoptosis (Allen et al., 1995; Vaux et al., 1994). Thus, it will be important to investigate whether the ICE family of proteases is involved in retinal apoptosis.

In nonocular tissues, oxidative stress was found to mediate apoptotic cell death (Buttke et al., 1994; Ratan et al., 1994; McGowan et al., 1996). Furthermore, enzymatically peroxidized metabolites of arachidonic acid were found to induce apoptosis in various experimental models (Agarwal et al., 1993; Haliday et al., 1991; Horiguchi et al., 1989; Sandstrom et al., 1994). Because oxidative stress is thought to be one of the hallmarks in the course of retinal and PE light damage, this process is a likely candidate for the induction of apoptosis in light-induced lesions. Notably, light can release arachidonic acid and docosahexaenoic acid and its metabolites in the retina (Jung et al., 1994; Reinboth et al., 1996; Reinboth et al., 1995). Indeed, preliminary studies in our laboratory revealed an induction of apoptosis by AA metabolites in the retina in vitro (Hafezi et al., 1998). Thus, reactive oxygen species as well as PUFAs and their metabolites may well subserve important messenger functions in the apoptosis pathway in retinal light damage (Fig. 29-2). The suppression of light-induced apoptosis by antioxidants, by oxidative enzyme inhibitors, or by phospholipase inhibitors will strengthen this notion. The light-evoked retinal messengers may also act as messengers for the PE. This can be tested in experimental models using PE cells in culture.

LIGHT DAMAGE IN THE CONTEXT OF HUMAN RETINAL PATHOPHYSIOLOGY

Are there relevant relations between light damage and human retinal pathophysiology? One must distinguish acute and chronic light-induced lesions in order to answer this question. The solar retinopathy is a typical example of an acute lesion that may or may not leave a small central scar and functional disturbances. The pathogenesis of cystic macular edema and proliferative vitreoretinopathy (PVR) is a subject for intense discussion. In view of our observations that light can release cellular mediators in the retina and light exposure creates an apoptotic response with macrophage invasion in the retina and PE potentially followed by the release of cytokines, a causal relation seems plausible but needs further experimental and clinical support.

An intriguing but unanswered question is whether exposure to light during a lifetime can accelerate or even partially cause aging changes in the retina and PE. Detailed studies in autopsy eyes demonstrate a selective loss of rods in the central fundus while the number of cones remains remarkably stable. It is tempting to speculate that light exposure is a causative or contributory factor for this phenomenon. The question then arises, however, why rods but not cones are diminished with age even though they are likely to receive the same amount of light and are in a similar metabolic situation (Curcio et al., 1993). An analogy may be found in the rat retina, where cones survived significantly longer from the exposure to constant bright light (LaVail, 1976). Rods may die through an apoptotic mechanism triggered among other potential causes by light and the threshold for apoptosis may be lower in rods than in cones. In aging Fisher rats, cell loss includes apoptosis (Fan et al., 1995). However, a relation of age-related rod loss with light exposure remains to be elucidated.

The accumulation of PE lipofuscin, the retinal "age pigment," has been tentatively related to light exposure (Weale, 1989). The steep increase in PE lipofuscin content during the first two decades of life may be due to a high lens transmission, with increased exposure of the retina to short wavelength visible light and UVA. The second rise in lipofuscin content from the fifth decade onward that follows a plateau may be the result of augmented light exposure due to an increase in lens transmission by means of a dislocation of the mainly absorbing nucleus (Weale, 1989).

Bruch's membrane shows distinct alterations with age and some of them include inflammatory signs such as macrophages (Bird, 1992). Again it is open for speculation whether light-evoked inflammatory mediators and cytokines contribute to such changes.

What is the role of light exposure in retinal degenerations and dystrophies? There is much discussion about the potential role of light in the pathogenesis of age-related macular degeneration (AMD) (Young, 1987; 1988). It is well known that AMD is a multifactorial disease that may be associated with environmental and endogenous risk factors. However, genetic disposition may also contribute. Indeed, mutations of the Stargardt disease gene have now been observed in 16% of a population of unrelated AMD patients (Allikmets et al., 1997). Despite of a lack of direct epidemiological or clinical evidence, laboratory studies suggest the possibility that light may be a contributory environmental factor.

Geographic Atrophy

The "silent death" by apoptosis may diminish photoreceptors and PE, leaving the well-recognized central geographic atrophy in AMD. In the macula, apoptosis would have to include rods and primarily cones. Pilot studies in our laboratory in the thirteen-lined ground squirrel clearly show apoptotic cell death of cones, indicating that cones can indeed die by apoptotic mechanisms (Fig. 29-3c). The signalling for apoptosis remains to be investigated, but light exposure initiating a messenger cascade cannot be excluded (Fig. 29-2).

Deposits and Drusen

Deposit and drusen formation in the area of Bruch's membrane may be considered from a novel vantage point in the context of apoptosis and AMD. In nonocular epithelial and endothelial cells, apoptosis is induced by deprivation of extracellular matrix anchorage and extracellular signaling molecules (Frisch and Francis, 1994; Meredith et al., 1993; Ruoslahti and Reed, 1994). With drusen and deposits in Bruch's membrane, a similar deprivation mechanism could act on PE cells, causing them to undergo apoptotic death with subsequent loss of overlying photoreceptors. This notion is supported by observations that demonstrate apoptotic cell death in photoreceptors of mice deficient for the adhesion molecule on glia (AMOG) (Molthagen et al., 1996). Detailed mechanisms of formation of drusen and deposit are unknown but PE-cell-derived cytoplasmic debris may represent a pathogenetic factor: The accumulation of lipofuscin granules and other phagocytic material in the PE has long been suspected to contribute to the formation of drusen. In view of lipofuscin as a candidate photosensitizer in light damage which initiates free-radical reactions upon light exposure, such a cause for cellular dysfunction or death seems plausible. This cell death may include apoptosis. The described mechanisms would imply a self-sustaining vicious circle between drusen and deposit formation on the one hand and apoptosis on the other hand.

Subretinal Neovascularization

Chronic inflammatory and proliferative changes may be induced and maintained via the release of inflammatory lipid mediators, mononuclear cells, and cytokines, and the cascade may be initiated by light exposure. Subretinal neovascularization may be stimulated when inflammatory cytokines and VEGF predominate. Several conditions are known to evoke VEGF (see "Fatty Acid Metabolies . . ." above). Retinal neovascularization was inhibited when the adhesion receptor system for newly forming vessels such as various integrins was inhibited (Hammes et al., 1996).

The route and end stage of AMD—atrophic or proliferative—may depend on genetic factors, ocular defense systems, and exogenous factors such as light exposure and others.

Animal Models of Human Retinitis Pigmentosa

Apoptosis was recently discovered and assumed to represent a final common death pathway in diverse genetic mutations in animal models for human retinitis pigmentosa. Because light can induce apoptosis in the human retina and PE and light exposure was shown to induce apoptosis genes in animals (Hafezi et al., 1997b), light exposure of humans or animal models suffering from retinitis pigmentosa may thus lead to an acceleration of apoptotic cell death. This assumption can be tested in the laboratory and may have distinct clinical significance for retinitis pigmentosa patients.

CONCLUSION

An important and perhaps underestimated insight thus emerges from recent research on retinal light damage and light-induced apoptosis: the retina and the PE possess the inherent property to respond to light exposure with the release of cellular mediators, signaling molecules, and cell death by apoptosis. When several of those factors act in concert, such as light exposure and surgical trauma, light exposure and an insufficient defense system, light exposure and photosensitization, or bright light exposure to a completely dark-adapted eye, pathological cascades may be initiated and may lead to retinal dysfunction. On these bases, new therapeutic strategies can be developed from the knowledge of cellular mediators and regulative mechanisms of apoptotic cell death.

ACKNOWLEDGMENTS

We would like to thank Prof. W. R. Lee, Pathology Department, Western Infirmary, Glasgow, GB; Prof. T. P. Williams, Biological Sciences, Florida State University, Tallahassee; and Richard W. Young, Los Angeles, for many stimulating discussions. Our work was supported by the Swiss National Science Foundation, grant Nr. 3100-040791.94/1; Bruppacher Stiftung, Zürich; Sandoz-Stiftung, Basel; Wilhelm-Sander-Stiftung, Munich.

REFERENCES

Abler AS, Chang CJ, Ful J, Tso MOM, Lam TT. 1996. Photic injury triggers apoptosis of photoreceptor cells. Res Comm Molecular Pathol Pharmacol 92:177–189.

Agarwal ML, Larkin HE, Zaidi SIA, Mukhtar H, Oleinick NL. 1993. Phospholipase activation triggers apoptosis in photosensitized mouse lymphoma cells. Cancer Res 53:5897–5902.

Agarwal N, Patel H, Brun A-M, Nir I. 1995. Alteration of c-fos by light/dark in rds mouse retina: possible involvement in apoptosis of photoreceptors. Invest Ophthalmol Vis Sci 36:2921.

Allen TD, Goldberg MW. 1995. Four functions and a funeral: mitosis, replication, transcription, transport and apoptosis in the nucleus. Trends Cell Biol 5:176–178.

Allikmets R, Shroyer NF, Singh N, Seddon JM, Lewis RA, Bernstein PS, Pfeiffer A, Zabriskie NA, Li Y, Hutchinson A, Dean M, Lupski JR, Leppert M. 1997. Mutation of the Stargardt Disease Gene (ABCR) in age-related macular degeneration. Science 277:1805–1807.

Amati B, Littlewood TD, Evan GI, Land H. 1993. The c-Myc protein induces cell cycle progression and apoptosis through dimerization with Max. EMBO J 12:5083–5087.

Andley UP. 1987. Photodamage to the eye. Photochem Photobiol 46:1057–1066.

Axelrod J, Burch RM, Jelsema CL. 1988. Receptor-mediated activation of phospholipase A2 via GTP-binding proteins: arachidonic acid and its metabolites as second messenger. Trends Neurol Sci. 11:117–123.

Barinaga M. 1996. Forging a path to cell death. Science 273:735–737.

Bazan HE, Bazan NG, Feeney-Burns L, Berman ER. 1990. Lipids in human lipofuscin-enriched subcellular fractions of two age populations: comparison with rod outer segments and neural retina. Invest Ophthalmol Vis Sci 31:1433–1443.

Berninger TA, Canning CR, Gündüz K, Strong N, Arden GB. 1989. Using argon laser blue light reduces ophthalmologists' color contrast sensitivity. Arch Ophthalmol 107:1453–1458.

Bird AC. 1992. Bruch's membrane change with age. Br J Ophthalmol 76:166–168.

Birkle DL, Bazan NG. 1989. Light exposure stimulates arachidonic acid metabolism in intact rat retina and isolated rod outer segments. Neurochem Res 14:185–190.

Borges J, Li ZY, Tso MO. 1990. Effects of repeated photic exposures on the monkey macula. Arch Ophthalmol 108:727–733.

Bush RA, Williams TP. 1991. The effect of unilateral optic nerve section on retinal light damage in rats. Exp Eye Res 52:139–153.

Bush RA, Malnoe A, Remé CE. 1991. Light damage in the rat retina: the effect of dietary deprivation of N-3 fatty acids on acute structural alterations. Exp Eye Res 53:741–752.

Bush RA, Malnoe A, Remé CE, Williams TP. 1994. Dietary deficiency of N-3 fatty acids alters rhodopsin content and function in the rat retina. Invest Ophthalmol Vis Sci 35:91–100.

Buttke TM, Sandstrom PA. 1994. Oxidative stress as a mediator of apoptosis. Immunology Today 15:7–10.

Bynoe LA, Del Priore LV, Hornbeck R. 1995. Blue light-dependent destruction of the retinal pigment epithelium (RPE) by Protoporphyrin IX. Invest Ophthalmol Vis Sci 36:861.

Cahill GM, Besharse JC. 1995. Circadian rhythmicity in vertebrate retinas: regulation by a photoreceptor oscillator. In: Osborne NN, Chader GJ, eds, Progress in Retinal and Eye Research. Oxford: Pergamon Press, 268–291.

Chang CJ, Li SH, Abler AS, Zhang SR, Tso MOM. 1994. Inhibitory effects of aurintricarboxylic acid and phorbol ester on light-induced apoptosis of photoreceptor cells. Invest Ophthalmol Vis Sci 35 (suppl):1518.

Chang GQ, Hao Y, Wong F. 1993. Apoptosis: final common pathway of photoreceptor death in rd, rds, and rhodopsin mutant mice. Neuron 11:595–605.

Chen E. 1993. Inhibition of cytochrome oxidase and blue-light damage in rat retina. Graefes Arch Clin Exp Ophthalmol 231:416–423.

Chen J, Flannery J, LaVail MM, Steinberg R, Xu J, Simon MI. 1996. bcl-2 overexpression reduces apoptotic photoreceptor death in three different retinal degenerations. Proc Natl Acad Sci USA 93:7042–7047.

Clark BC, Johnson ML, Dreher RE. 1946. The effect of sunlight on dark adaptation. Am J Ophthalmol 29:828–836.

Claudio L, Martiney JA, Brosnan CF. 1994. Ultrastructural studies of the blood-retina barrier after exposure to interleukin-1 beta or tumor necrosis factor-alpha. Lab Invest 70:850–861.

Cohen GM, Sun XM, Snowden RT, Dinsdale D, Skilleter DN. 1992. Key morphological features of apoptosis may occur in the absence of internucleosomal DNA fragmentation. Biochem J 286:331–334.

Collier RJ, Waldron WR, Zigman S. 1989. Temporal sequence of changes to the gray squirrel retina after near-UV exposure. Invest Ophthalmol Vis Sci 30:631–637.

Collins MK, Perkins GR, Rodriguez Tarduchy G, Nieto MA, Lopez Rivas A. 1994. Growth factors as survival factors: regulation of apoptosis. Bioessays 16:133–138.

Colotta F, Polentarutti N, Sironi M, Mantovani A. 1992. Expression and involvement of c-fos and c-jun protooncogenes in programmed cell death induced by growth factor deprivation in lymphoid cell lines. J Biol Chem 167:18278–18283.

Coohill TP. 1992. Action spectra revisited. J Photochem Photobiol B 13:95–98.

Crockett RS, Lawwill T. 1984. Oxygen dependence of damage by 435 nm light in cultured retinal epithelium. Curr Eye Res 3:209–215.

Curcio CA, Millican CL, Allen KA, Kalina RE. 1993. Aging of the human photoreceptor mosaic: evidence for selective vulnerability of rods in central retina. Invest Ophthalmol Vis Sci 34:3278–3296.

Davidson PC, Sternberg P Jr. 1993. Potential retinal phototoxicity. Am J Ophthalmol 116:497–501.

Delori FC, Dorey CK, Staurenghi G, Arend O, Goger DG, Weiter JJ. 1995. In vivo fluorescence of the ocular fundus exhibits retinal pigment epithelium lipofuscin characteristics. Invest Ophthalmol Vis Sci 36:718–729.

Dillon J. 1991. The photophysics and photobiology of the eye. J Photochem Photobiol B 10:23–40.

Dinarello CA. 1994. Interleukin-1. In: Dinarello CA, ed, The Cytokine Handbook, 2nd ed. New York: Academic Press, 31–56.

Dinda S, Minelli E, Bolon M, Hartzer M, Blumenkranz M. 1992. Photosensitization thresholds for retinal pigment epithelial cells are decreased by amiodaronew. Invest Ophthalmol Vis Sci 33:918.

Docchio F, Boulton M, Cubeddu R, Ramponi R, Barker PD. 1991. Age-related changes in the fluorescence of melanin and lipofuscin granules of the retinal pigment epithelium: a time-resolved fluorescence spectroscopy study. Photochem Photobiol 54:247–253.

Dolin PJ. 1994. Ultraviolet radiation and cataract: a review of the epidemiological evidence. Br J Ophthalmol 78:478–482.

Drescher KM, Whittum-Hudson JA. 1996. Herpes simplex virus type 1 alters transcript levels of tumor necrosis factor-alpha and interleukin-6 in retinal glial cells. Invest Ophthalmol Vis Sci 37:2302–2312.

Dunn MW, Lavrovsky Y, Stoltz RA, Abraham NG. 1995. Protection of human retinal epithelial (RPE) cells from hemoglobin toxicity by adenovirus-mediated transfer of human heme oxygenase cDNA. Invest Ophthalmol Vis Sci 36:519.

Duran N, Song PS. 1986. Hypericin and its photodynamic action. Photochem Photobiol 43:677–680.

Eldred GE, Lasky MR. 1993. Retinal age pigments generated by self-assembling lysosomotropic detergents. Nature 361:724–726.

Endres S, Ghorbani R, Kelley VE, Georgilis K, Lonnemann G, van der Meer JW, Cannon JG, Rogers TS, Klempner MS, Weber PC, et al. 1989. The effect of dietary supplementation with n-3 polyunsaturated fatty acids on the synthesis of interleukin-1 and tumor necrosis factor by mononuclear cells. N Eng J Med 320:265–271.

Faktorovich EG, Steinberg RH, Yasumura D, Matthes MT, LaVail MM. 1992. Basic fibroblast growth factor and local injury protect photoreceptors from light damage in the rat. J Neurosci 12:3554–3567.

Fan W, Wordinger RJ, Agarwal N, Turner JE. 1995. Age-related changes in retina of Fischer 344 rats: degeneration may involve apoptosis. Invest Ophthalmol Vis Sci 36:304.

Farber DB, Danciger JS, Organisciak DT. 1991. Levels of mRNA encoding proteins of the cGMP cascade as a function of light environment. Exp Eye Res 52:781–786.

Fliesler SJ, Anderson RE. 1983. Chemistry and metabolism of lipids in the vertebrate retina. Prog Lipid Res 22:79–131.

Fox GM, Magat CB, Cheng N, Werner J, Blumenkranz M, Hartzer M. 1993. High oxygen tension enhances the cytotoxic damage to retinal pigment epithelial cells by Phenothiazines and UV light. Invest Opthalmol Vis Sci 34:1434.

Frisch SM, Francis H. 1994. Disruption of epithelial cell-matrix interactions induces apoptosis. J Cell Biol 124:619–626.

Fu J, Lam TT, Tso MO. 1992. Dexamethasone ameliorates retinal photic injury in albino rats. Exp Eye Res 54:583–594.

Gaillard ER, Atherton SJ, Eldred G, Dillon J. 1995. Photophysical studies on human retinal lipofuscin. Photochem Photobiol 61:448–453.

Gallin PF, Terman M, Remé CE, Rafferty AB, Terman JS, Burde RM. 1995. Ophthalmological examination of patients with seasonal affective disorder, before and after bright light therapy. Am J Ophthalmol 119:202–210.

Gavrieli Y, Sherman Y, Ben-Sasson SA. 1992. Identification of programmed cell death in situ via specific labeling of nuclear DNA fragmentation. J Cell Biol 119:493–501.

Gerster H. 1991. Review: antioxidant protection of the ageing macula. Age Ageing, 20:60–69.

Giacomoni PU. 1995. Open questions in photobiology. III. Melanin and photoprotection. J Photochem Photobiol B-Biology 29:87–89.

Gladstone GJ, Tasman W. 1978. Solar retinitis after minimal exposure. Arch Ophthalmol 96:1368–1369.

Gomer CJ. 1991. Preclinical examination of first and second generation photosensitizers used in photodynamic therapy. Photochem Photobiol 54:1093–1107.

Gorgels TGMF, van Norren D. 1992. Spectral transmittance of the rat lens. Vision Res 32:1509–1512.

Gorgels TGMF, Van Norren D. 1995. Ultraviolet and green light cause different types of damage in rat retina. Invest Ophthalmol Vis Sci 36:851–863.

Gottsch JD, Pou S, Bynoe LA, Rosen GM. 1990. Hematogenous photosensitization. A mechanism for the development of age-related macular degeneration. Invest Ophthalmol Vis Sci 31:1674–1682.

Gregory CY, Bird AC. 1995. Cell loss in retinal dystrophies by apoptosis-death by informed consent. Br J Ophthalmol 79:186–190.

Grossweiner LI. 1989. Photophysics. In: Smith KC, ed., The Science of Photobiology. New York: Plenum Press, 1–45.

Hafezi F, Marti A, Munz K, Remé CE. 1997a. Light-induced apoptosis: differential timing in the retina and pigment epithelium. Exp Eye Res 64:963–970.

Hafezi F, Steinbach JP, Marti A, Munz K, Wang Z-Q, Wagner EF, Aguzzi A, Remé CE. 1997b. Retinal degeneration: lack of c-fos prevents delayed light-induced apoptotic cell death of photoreceptors in vivo. Nature Medicine 3:346–349.

Hafezi F, Reinboth JJ, Wenzel A, Munz K, Remé CE. 1998. HPETE, ein Arachidonsäure-Metabolit, induziert Apoptose in der Rattennetzhaut in vitro. Klin Monatsbl Augenheilk 212, in press.

Haliday EM, Chakkodabylu SR, Ringold G. 1991. TNF induces c-fos via a novel pathway requiring conversion of arachidonic acid to a lipoxygenase metabolite. EMBO J 10:109–115.

Ham WT, Mueller HA. 1976. Retinal sensitivity to damage from short wavelength light. Nature 260:153–155.

Ham WT, Ruffolo JJ, Mueller HA, Clarke AM, Moon ME. 1978. Histologic analysis of photochemical lesions produced in rhesus retina by short-wavelength light. Invest Ophthalmol Vis Sci 17:1029–1035.

Ham WT, Mueller HA, Ruffolo JJ, Clarke AM. 1979. Sensitivity of the retina to radiation damage as a function of wavelength. Photochem Photobiol 29:735–743.

Ham WT, Jr, Mueller HA, Ruffolo JJ Jr, Millen JE, Cleary SF, Guerry RK, Guerry DD. 1984. Basic mechanisms underlying the production of photochemical lesions in the mammalian retina. Curr Eye Res 3:165–174.

Ham WT, Allen RG, Feeney-Burns L, Marmor MF, Parver LM, Proctor PH, Sliney DH, Wolbarsht ML. 1986. The involvement of the retinal pigment epithelium. In: Waxler M, Hitchins VM, eds, Optical Radiation and Visual Health. Boca Raton, FL: CRC Press, 44–67.

Hammes H-P, Brownlee M, Jonczyk A, Sutter A, Preissner K. 1996. Subcutaneous injection of a cyclic peptide antagonist of vitronectin receptor-type integrins inhibits retinal neovascularization. Nature Medicine 2:529–533.

Han X, Becker K, Degen HJ, Jablonowski H, Strohmeyer G. 1996. Synergistic stimulatory effects of tumor necrosis factor alpha and interferon gamma on replication of human immunodeficiency virus type 1 and on apoptosis of HIV-1-infected host cells. Eur J Clin Invest 26:286–292.

Handelman GJ, Dratz EA. 1986. The role of antioxidants in the retina and retinal pigment epithelium and the nature of prooxidant-induced damage. Adv Free Radical Biology & Medicine 2:1–89.

Hangai M, Yoshimura N, Yoshida M, Yabuuchi K, Honda Y. 1995. Interleukin-1 gene expression in transient retinal ischemia in the rat. Invest Ophthalmol Vis Sci 36:571–578.

Hao W, Fong HKW. 1996. Blue and ultraviolet light-absorbing opsin from the retinal pigment epithelium. Biochemistry 35:6251–6256.

Hartzer M, Desai S, Bolon M, Cheng M. 1993. Hydrochlorothiazide-increased human retinal epithelial cell toxicity following low-level UV A irradiation. Invest Opthalmol Vis Sci 34:1436.

Hata Y, Nakagawa K, Ishibashi T, Inomata H, Ueno H, Sueishi K. 1995. Hypoxia-induced expression of vascular endothelial growth factor by retinal glial cells promotes in vitro angiogenesis. Virchows Arch 426:479–486.

He S, Law R, Couldwell WT, Ryan SJ, Hinton DR. 1995. Induction and inhibition of RPE cell apoptosis in vitro. Invest Ophthalmol Vis Sci 36:583.

Hecht S, Hendley CD, Sherman R, and Richmond PN. 1948. The effect of exposure to sunlight on night vision. Am J Ophthalmol 31:1573–1580.

Hockenbery DM, Oltvai ZN, Yin XM, Milliman CL, Korsmeyer SJ. 1993. bcl-2 functions in an antioxidant pathway to prevent apoptosis. Cell 75:241–251.

Hoffmann DR, Birch EB, Birch DG, Uauy RD. 1993. Effects of supplementation with ω3 long-chain polyunsaturated fatty acids on retinal and cortical development in premature infants. Am J Clin Nutr 57:807–812.

Hope-Ross MW, Mahon GJ, Gardiner TA, Archer DB. 1993. Ultrastructural findings in solar retinopathy. Eye 7:29–33.

Hoppeler T, Hendrickson P, Dietrich C, Remé CE. 1988. Morphology and time course of defined photochemical lesions in the rabbit retina. Curr Eye Res 7:849–859.

Horiguchi J, Spriggs D, Imamura K, Stone R, Luebbers R, Kufe D. 1989. Role of arachidonic acid metabolism in transcriptional induction of tumor necrosis factor gene expression by phorbol ester. Mol Cell Biol. 9:252–258.

Howell WL, Rapp LM, Williams TP. 1982. Distribution of melanosomes across the retinal pigment epithelium of a hooded rat: implications for light damage. Invest Ophthalmol Vis Sci 22:139–144.

Howes KA, Ransom N, Papermaster DS, Lasudry GH, Albert DM, Windle JJ. 1994. Apoptosis or retinoblastoma: alternative fates of photoreceptors expressing the HPV-16 E7 gene in the presence or absence of p53. Genes & Develop 8:1300–1310.

Irvine AR, Wood I, Morris BW. 1984. Retinal damage from the illumination of the operating microscope: an experimental study in pseudophakic monkeys. Trans Am Ophthalmol Soc 82:239–263.

Jacobs GH, Neitz J, Deegan JFD. 1991. Retinal receptors in rodents maximally sensitive to ultraviolet light. Nature 353:655–666.

Jaffe GL, Roberts WL, Wong HL, Yurochko AD, Cianciolo GJ. 1995. Monocyte-induced cytokine expression in cultured human retinal pigment epithelial cells. Exp Eye Res 60:533–543.

Jung H, Remé CE. 1994. Light-evoked arachidonic acid release in the retina: illuminance/duration dependence and the effects of quinacrine, mellitin and lithium. Graefes Arch Clin Exp Ophthalmol 232:167–175.

Kalloniatis M, Harwerth RS. 1993. Modelling sensitivity losses in ocular disorders: colour vision anomalies following intense blue-light exposure in monkeys. Ophthalmic Physiol Opt 13:155–167.

Kochevar IE, Granstein R, Moran M. 1994. UVR-induced mediators in photoaging. Photochem Photobiol 56:65.

Kopitz J, Monahan D, Stogsdill PL, Cantz M, Eldred GE. 1996. Evidence that an unprecedented vitamin A derivative may underlie the leading cause of age-related blindness. Am J Pathol 148:1–7.

Koutz CA, Wiegand RD, Rapp LM, Anderson RE. 1995. Effect of dietary fat on the response of the rat retina to chronic and acute light stress. Exp Eye Res 60:307–316.

Kraff MC, Sanders DR, Jampol LM, Lieberman HL. 1985. Effect of an ultraviolet-filtering intraocular lens on cystoid macular edema. Ophthalmology 92:366–369.

Kremers JJ, van Norren D. 1988. Two classes of photochemical damage of the retina. Lasers Light in Ophthalmol 2:41–52.

Kremers JJ, van Norren D. 1989. Retinal damage in macaque after white light exposures lasting ten minutes to twelve hours. Invest Ophthalmol Vis Sci 30:1032–1040.

Kuhn F, Morris R, Massey M. 1991. Photic retinal injury from endoillumination during vitrectomy. Am J Ophthalmol 111:42–46.

Kulkarni PS, Mancino M. 1993. Studies on intraocular inflammation produced by intravitreal human interleukins in rabbits. Exp Eye Res 56:275–279.

Kutty RK, Nagineni CN, Kutty G, Hooks JJ, Chader GJ, Wiggert B. 1994. Increased expression of heme oxygenase-1 in human retinal pigment epithelial cells by transforming growth factor-beta. J Cell Physiol 159:371–378.

Kutty RK, Kutty G, Wiggert B, Chader GJ, Darrow RM, Organisciak DT. 1995. Induction of heme oxygenase 1 in the retina by intense visible light: suppression by the antioxidant dimethylthiourea. Proc Natl Acad Sci USA 92:1177–1181.

Lai WW, Chang CJ, Abler AS, Tso MOM. 1995. A comparative study of apoptosis of photoreceptor cells following light injury to four strains of inbred albino rats. Invest Ophthalmol Vis Sci 36:306.

Lanum J. 1978. The damaging effects of light on the retina: empirical findings, theoretical and practical implications. Surv Ophthalmol 22:221–249.

LaVail MM. 1976. Survival of some photoreceptor cells in albino rats following long-term exposure to continuous light. Invest Ophthalmol 15:64–70.

LaVail MM, Gorrin GM. 1987. Protection from light damage by ocular pigmentation: analysis using experimental chimeras and translocation mice. Exp Eye Res 44:877–889.

LaVail MM, Unoki K, Yasumura D, Matthes MT, Yancopoulos GD, Steinberg RH. 1992. Multiple growth factors, cytokines, and neurotrophins rescue photoreceptors from the damaging effects of constant light. Proc Natl Acad Sci USA 89:11249–11253.

Lawwill T. 1973. Effects of prolonged exposure of rabbit retina to low-intensity light. Invest Ophthalmol 12:45–51.

Lawwill T. 1982. Three major pathologic processes caused by light in the primate retina a search for mechanisms. Tr Am Ophthalm Soc 80:517–579.

Li J, Edward DP, Lam TT, Tso MO. 1993. Amelioration of retinal photic injury by a combination of flunarizine and dimethylthiourea. Exp Eye Res 56:71–78.

Li S, Chang CJ, Abler AS, Fu J, Tso MOM. 1994. A comparison of continuous versus intermittent light exposure on induction of apoptosis in photoreceptor cells of rat retina. Invest Ophthalmol Vis Sci 35(suppl):1516.

Li Z-Y, Milam A. 1995. Apoptosis in retinitis pigmentosa In: Anderson RE, LaVail MM, Hollyfield JG, eds, (Degenerative Diseases of the Retina.), 1–8. New York: Plenum Press, 1995.

Liu X, Yanoff M, Li W. 1995. Characterization of lethal action of near ultraviolet (NUV) on retinal pigment epithelial (RPE) cells in vitro. Invest Ophthalmol Vis Sci 36:519.

Lolley RN. 1994. The rd gene defect triggers programmed rod cell death. Invest Ophthalmol Vis Sci 35:4182–4191.

Marlor RL, Blais BR, Preston FR, Boyden DG. 1973. Foveomacular retinitis, an important problem in military medicine: epidemiology. Invest Ophthalmol 12:5–16.

Marshall J. 1983. Light damage and the practice of ophthalmology. In: Rosen ES, Maining WM, Arnott EJ, eds, Intraocular Lens Implantation. St Louis: Moseby, 182–207.

Marshall J. 1985. Radiation and the ageing eye. Ophthalmic Physiol Opt 5:241–263.

Marshall J, Mellerio J, Palmer DA. 1972. Damage to pigeon retinae by moderate illumination from fluorescent lamps. Exp Eye Res 14:164–169.

Marti A, Jehn B, Costello E, Keon N, Ke G, Martin F, Jaggi R. 1994. Protein kinase A and AP-1 (c-Fos/Jun D) are induced during apoptosis of mouse mammary epithelial cells. Oncogene 9:1213–1223.

Martin SJ, Green DR. 1995. Protease activation during apoptosis: death by a thousand cuts? Cell 82:349–352.

Martiney JA, Berman JW, Brosnan CF. 1992. Chronic inflammatory effects of interleukin-1 on the blood-retina barrier. J Neuroimmunol 41:167–176.

McGowan AJ, Ruiz-Ruiz MC, Gorman AM, Lopez-Rivas A, Cotter TG. 1996. Reactive oxygen intermediate (s) (ROI): common mediators of poly(ADP-ribose)polymerase (PARP) cleavage and apoptosis. FEBS lett 392:299–303.

Menon IA, Basu PK, Persad SD, Das A, Wiltshire JD. 1992. Reactive oxygen species in the photosensitization of retinal pigment epithelial cells by rose bengal. J Toxicol Cut Ocular Toxicol. 11: 269–283.

Meredith JE, Jr, Fazeli B, Schwartz MA. 1993. The extracellular matrix as a cell survival factor. Mol Biol Cell 4:953–961.

Meydani SN, Lichtenstein AH, Cornwall S, Meydani M, Goldin BR, Rasmussen, H, Dinarello CA, Schaefer EJ. 1993. Immunologic effects of national cholesterol education panel step-2 diets with and without fish-derived N-3 fatty acid enrichment. J Clin Invest 92: 105–113.

Michels M, Sternberg P, Jr. 1990. Operating microscope-induced retinal phototoxicity: pathophysiology, clinical manifestations and prevention. Surv Ophthalmol 34:237–252.

Miller D, ed. 1987. Clinical Light Damage to the Eye. New York: Springer Verlag, 3–225.

Minelli E, Hartzer M, Blumenkranz M. 1991. Amiodarone: increased retinal epithelial cell toxicity following low-level near UV irradiation. Invest Ophthalmol Vis Sci 32:1097.

Molthagen M, Schachner M, Barsch U. 1996. Apoptotic cell death of photoreceptor cells in mice deficient for the adhesion molecule on glia (AMOG, the beta-2 subunit of the Na,K-ATPase). J Neurocytology 25:243–255.

Neuringer M, Connor WE, Lin DS, Barstad L, Luck S. 1986. Biochemical and functional effects of prenatal and postnatal omega 3 fatty acid deficiency on retina and brain in rhesus monkeys. Proc Natl Acad Sci USA 83:4021–4025.

Nir I, Agarwal N. 1993. Diurnal expression of c-fos in the mouse retina. Mol Brain Res 19:47–54.

Noell WK, Walker, VS, Kang BS, Berman S. 1996. Retinal damage by light in rats. Invest Ophthalmol 5:450–473.

O'Steen WK, Karcioglu ZA. 1974. Phagocytosis in the light-damaged albino rat eye: light and electron microscopic study. Am J Anat 139:503–517.

Oberhammer F, Wilson JW, Dive C, Morris ID, Hickman JA, Wakeling AE, Walker PR, Sikorska M. 1993. Apoptotic death in epithelial cells: cleavage of DNA to 300 and/or 50 kb fragments prior to or in the absence of internucleosomal fragmentation. Embo J 12:3679–3684.

Olsen TW, Jones DP, Reed RL, Sternberg P Jr. 1995. The effects of light on cultured human retinal pigment epithelium in vitro. Invest Ophthalmol Vis Sci 36:519.

Ophthalmology. 1983. Potential retinal hazards. Ophthalmology 90: 927–972.

Organisciak DT, Winkler BS. 1994. Retinal light damage: practical and theoretical considerations. In (Osborne NN, Chader GJ), eds, Progress in Retinal and Eye Research. Oxford: Pergamon Press, 1–29.

Organisciak DT, Wang WM, Noell WK. 1987. Aspects of the ascor-

bate protective mechanism in retinal light damage of rats with reduced ROS docosahexaenoic acid. In: Hollyfield JG, Anderson RE,
and LaVail MM, eds, Degenerative Retinal Disorders: Clinical and
Laboratory Investigations. New York: Liss.

Organisciak DT, Xie A, Wang H-M, Jiang Y-L, Darrow RM, Donoso
LA. 1991. Adaptive changes in visual cell transduction protein levels: effect of light Exp Eye Res 53:773–779.

Papermaster DS, Windle J. 1995. Death at an early age: apoptosis in
inherited retinal degenerations. Invest Ophthalmol Vis Sci 36:977–
983.

Pautler EL. 1994. Photosensitivity of the isolated pigment epithelium
and arachidonic acid metabolism: preliminary results. Curr Eye Res
13:687–695.

Pautler EL, Morita M, Beezley D. 1990. Hemoprotein(s) mediate blue
light damage in the retinal pigment epithelium. Photochem Photobiol 51:599–605.

Pe'er J, Shweiki D, Itin A, Hemo I, Gnessin H, Keshet E. 1995. Hypoxia-induced expression of vascular endothelial growth factor by
retinal cells is a common factor in neovascularizing ocular diseases.
Lab Invest 72:638–645.

Peitsch MC, Polzar B, Stephan H, Crompton T, MacDonald HR,
Mannherz HG, Tschopp J. 1993. Characterization of the endogenous deoxyribonuclease involved in nuclear DNA degradation during apoptosis (programmed cell death). Embo J 12:371–377.

Penn JS, Anderson RE. 1991. Effects of Light History on the Rat Retina. In: Osborne NN, Chader GJ, eds, Progress in Retinal Research.
Oxford: Pergamon Press, 76–97.

Penn JS, Williams TP. 1986. Photostasis: regulation of daily photon
catch by rat retinas in response to various cyclic illuminances. Exp
Eye Res 44:915–928.

Penn JS, Naash MI, Anderson RE. 1987. Effect of light history on retinal antioxidants and light damage susceptibility in the rat. Exp Eye
Res 44:779–788.

Penn JS, Tolman BL, Thum LA, Koutz CA. 1992. Effect of light history on the rat retina: timecourse of morphological adaptation and
readaptation. Neurochem Res 17:91–99.

Pierce EA, Avery RL, Foley ED, Aiello LP, Smith LE. 1995. Vascular
endothelial growth factor/vascular permeability factor expression
in a mouse model of retinal neovascularization. Proc Nat Acad Sci
USA 92:905–990.

Piomelli D, Greengard P. 1990. Lipoxygenase metabolites of arachidonic acid in neuronal transmembrane signalling. Trends Pharmacol Sci 11:367–373.

Planck SR, Huang XN, Robertson JE, Rosenbaum JT. 1993. Retinal
pigment epithelial cells produce interleukin-1 beta and granulocyte-
macrophage colony-stimulating factor in response to interleukin-1
alpha. Curr Eye Res 12:205–212.

Poblenz AT, Singh S, Campbell AS, Fox DA. 1995. Apoptosis in retinas of developmentally lead-exposed rats produces 50-700 kbp, but
not internucleosomal, DNA fragments. Invest Ophthalmol Vis Sci
36:2917.

Portera-Cailliau C, Sung CH, Nathans J, Adler R. 1994. Apoptotic
photoreceptor cell death in mouse models of retinitis pigmentosa.
Proc Nat Acad Sci USA 91:974–978.

Preston GA, Lyon TT, Yin Y, Lang JE, Solomon G, Annab L, Srini-
vasan DG, Alcorta DA, Barrett JC. 1996. Induction of apoptosis by
c-Fos protein. Mol Cell Biol 16:211–218.

Putting BJ, Van Best JA, Vrensen GF, Oosterhuis JA. 1994. Blue-light-
induced dysfunction of the blood-retinal barrier at the pigment epithelium in albino versus pigmented rabbits. Exp Eye Res 58:31–40.

Rapp LM, Fisher PL, Dhindsa HS. 1994. Reduced rate of rod outer
segment disk synthesis in photoreceptor cells recovering from UVA
light damage. Invest Ophthalmol Vis Sci 35:3540–3548.

Rapp LM, Smith SC. 1992a. Evidence against melanin as the mediator of retinal phototoxicity by short-wavelength light. Exp Eye Res
54:55–62.

Rapp LM, Smith SC. 1992b. Morphologic comparisons between
rhodopsin-mediated and short-wavelength classes of retinal light
damage. Invest Ophthalmol Vis Sci 33:3367–3377.

Rapp LM, Williams TP. 1980. A parametric study of retinal light dam-
age in albino and pigmented rats. In: Williams TP, Baker BN, eds,
The Effects of Constant Light on Visual Processes. New York:
Plenum Press, 135–139.

Rappolee DA, Werb Z. 1992. Macrophage-derived growth factors.
Curr Topics Microbiol Immunol 181:87–140.

Ratan RR, Murphy TH, Baraban JM. 1994. Macromolecular synthesis inhibitors prevent oxidative stress-induced apoptosis in embryonic cortical neurons by shunting cysteine from protein synthesis to
glutathione. J Neurosci 14:4385–4392.

Reed JC. 1994. Bcl-2 and the regulation of programmed cell death. J
Cell Biol 124:1–6.

Reinboth JJ, Gautschi K, Clausen M, Remé CE. 1995. Lipid mediators in the rat retina: light exposure and trauma elicit leukotriene B
4 release in vitro. Curr Eye Res 14:1001–1008.

Reinboth JJ, Clausen M, Remé CE. 1996. Light elicits the release of
docosahexaenoic acid from membrane phospholipids in the rat retina in vitro. Exp Eye Res 63:277–284.

Reinboth JJ, Gautschi K, Munz K, Eldred GE, Remé, ChE. 1997.
Lipofuscin in the retina: Quantitative assay for an unprecedented
autofluorescent compound (pyridinium bis-retinoid, A2-E) of ocular age pigment. Exp Eye Res. 65:639–643.

Remé CE, Wirz-Justice A, Terman M. 1991. The visual input stage of
the mammalian circadian pacemaking system: I. Is there a clock in
the mammalian eye? J Biol Rhythms 6:5–29.

Remé CE, Malnoë A, Jung HH, Wei Q, Munz K. 1994. Effect of dietary fish oil on acute light-induced photoreceptor damage in the
rat retina. Invest Ophthalmol Vis Sci 35:78–90.

Remé ChE, Grimm Ch, Hafezi F, Marti A, Wenzel A. 1998. Apoptotic cell death in retinal degenerations. In: Chader GJ, Osborne NN,
eds, Progress in Retinal and Eye Res, in press.

Remé CE, Reinboth JJ, Clausen M, Hafezi F. 1995a. Light damage revisited: Converging evidence, diverging views? Graefes Arch Clin
Exp Ophthal 234:2–11.

Remé CE, Weller M, Szczesny P, Munz K, Hafezi F, Reinboth JJ,
Clausen M. 1995b. Light-induced apoptosis in the rat retina in vivo:
morphological features, threshold and time course. In: Anderson
RE, LaVail MM, Hollyfield JG, eds, Degenerative Diseases of the
Retina. New York: Plenum Press, 19–25.

Remé CE, Rol P, Grothmann K, Kaase H, Terman M. 1996. Bright
light therapy in focus: lamp emission spectra and ocular safety.
Technology and Health Care 9:1–11.

Remé CE, Williams TP, Rol P, Grimm C. 1998. Blue-light damage re-
visitied: abundant retinal apoptosis after blue-light exposure, little
after green. Invest Ophthalmal Vis Sci 39:S128.

Rich KS, Zhan Y, Blanks JC. 1997. Aberrant expression of c-Fos accompanies photoreceptor cell death in the *rd* mouse. J Neurobiol
32:593–611.

Roberts JE, Remé CE, Dillon J, Terman M. 1992. Exposure to bright
light and the concurrent use of photosensitizing drugs [letter]. N
Eng J Med 326:1500–1501.

Robinson J, Janssen-Bienhold U, Dowling JE. 1995. Light-damage alters gene expression in the zebrafish (Danio rerio) retina. Invest
Ophthalmol Vis Sci 36:3939.

Rosenbaum JT. 1993. Cytokines: the good, the bad, and the unknown. Invest Ophthalmol Vis Sci 34:2389–2391.

Rosenbaum JT, O'Rourke L, Davies G, Wenger C, David L, Robertson JE. 1987. Retinal pigment epithelial cells secrete substances that are chemotactic for monocytes. Curr Eye Res 6:793–800.

Rosoff PM, Savage N, Dinarello CA. 1988. Interleukin-1 stimulates diacylglycerol production in T lymphocytes by a novel mechanism. Cell 54:73–81.

Rozanowska M, Jarvis-Evans J, Korytowski W, Boulton ME, Burke JM, Sarna T. 1995. Blue light-induced reactivity of retinal age pigment. J Biol Chem 270:18825–18830.

Ruoslahti E, Reed JC. 1994. Anchorage dependence, integrins, and apoptosis. Cell 77:477–478.

Sadun AC, Sadun AA, Sudan LA. 1984. Solar retinopathy: a biophysical analysis. Arch Ophthalmol 102:1510–1512.

Sakamoto T, Sakamoto H, Murphy TL, Spee C, Soriano D, Ishibashi T, Hinton DR, Ryan SJ. 1995. Vessel formation by choroidal endothelial cells in vitro is modulated by retinal pigment epithelial cells. Arch Ophthalmol 113:512–520.

Samuelsson B. 1991. Arachidonic acid metabolism: role in inflammation. Z Rheumatol 50:3–6.

Sandstrom PA, Tebbey PW, Van Cleave S, Buttke TM. 1994. Lipid hydroperoxides induce apoptosis in T cells displaying a HIV-associated glutathione peroxidase deficiency. J Biol Chem 269:798–801.

Sanyal S, Zeilmaker GH. 1988. Retinal damage by constant light in chimaeric mice: implications for the protective role of melanin. Exp Eye Res 46:731–743.

Schremser JL, Williams TP. 1995a. Rod outer segment (ROS) renewal as a mechanism for adaptation to a new intensity environment. I. Rhodopsin levels and ROS length. Exp Eye Res 61:17–24.

Schremser JL, Williams TP. 1995b. Rod outer segment (ROS) renewal as a mechanism for adaptation to a new intensity environment. II. Rhodopsin synthesis and packing density. Exp Eye Res 61:25–32.

Schwartz LM, Osborne BA. 1993. Programmed cell death, apoptosis and killer genes. Immunol Today 14:582–590.

Schwartzman RA, Cidlowski JA. 1993. Apoptosis: the biochemistry and molecular biology of programmed cell death. Endocr Rev 14:133–151.

Shima DT, Adamis AP, Ferrara N, Yeo K-T, Yeo T-K, Allende I. 1995. Hypoxic induction of vascular endothelial cell growth factors in the retina: identification and characterization of vascular endothelial growth factor (VGEF) as the sole mitogen. Mol Med 2:64–71.

Shirama K, Hokano M. 1991. Electron-microscopic studies on the maturation of secretory cells in the mouse Harderian gland. Acta Anat Basel 140:304–312.

Sliney DH. 1992. The potential ocular hazards of viewing bright light sources. In: Holick MF, Kligman AM, eds, Biologic Effects of Light. Berlin: Walter de Gruyter, 230–244.

Sliney DH. 1994. Epidemiological studies of sunlight and cataract: the critical factor of ultraviolet exposure geometry. Ophthalmic Epidemiology 1:107–119.

Sperling HG, ed. 1980. Intense Light Hazards in Ophthalmic Diagnosis and Treatment. Vol. 20. Oxford: Pergamon Press, 1033–1203.

Sperling HG, Johnson C, Harwerth RS. 1980. Differential spectral photic damage to primate cones. Vision Res 20:1117–1125.

Steller H. 1995. Mechanisms and genes of cellular suicide. Science 267:1445–1449.

Stocker R. 1990. Induction of heme oxygenase as a defense against oxidative stress. Free Rad Res Commun 9:101–112.

Stone J, Itin A, Alon T, Pe'er J, Gnessin H, Chang-Ling T, Keshet E. 1995. Development of retinal vasculature is mediated by hypoxia-induced vascular endothelial growth factor (VEGF) expression by neuroglia. J Neurosci 15:4738–4747.

Sykes SM, Robison W Jr, Waxler M, Kuwabara T. 1981. Damage to the monkey retina by broad-spectrum fluorescent light. Invest Ophthalmol Vis Sci 20:425–434.

Szczesny PJ, Munz K, Remé CE. 1995. Light damage in the rat retina: patterns of acute lesions and recovery. In: Pleyer U, Schmidt K, Thiel HJ, eds, Cell and Tissue Protection in Ophthalmology. Stuttgart: Hippokrates Verlag, 163–175.

Taylor HR, West S, Munoz B, Rosenthal FS, Bressler SB, Bressler NM. 1992. The long-term effect of visible light on the eye. Arch Ophthalmol 110:99–104.

Terman M, Remé CE, Rafferty B, Gallin PF, Terman JS. 1990. Bright light therapy for winter depression: potential ocular effects and theoretical implications. Photochem Photobiol 51:781–792.

Thompson CB. 1995. Apoptosis in the pathogenesis and treatment of disease. Science 267:1456–1462.

Tso MO. 1989. Experiments on visual cells by nature and man: in search of treatment for photoreceptor degeneration. Friedenwald lecture. Invest Ophthalmol Vis Sci 30:2430–2454.

Tso MOM. 1973. Photic maculopathy in rhesus monkey: a light and electron microscopic study. Invest Ophthalmol 12:17–34.

Tso MOM, Zhang C, Abler AS, Chang, CJ, Wong F, Chang GQ, Lam TT, 1994. Apoptosis leads to photoreceptor degeneration in inherited retina dystrophy of RCS rats. Invest Ophthalmol Vis Sci 35:2693–2699.

Unoki K, LaVail MM. 1994. Protection of the rat retina from ischemic injury by brain-derived neurotrophic factor, ciliary neurotrophic factor, and basic fibroblast growth factor. Invest Ophthalmol Vis Sci 35:907–915.

van Norren D, Schellekens P. 1990. Blue light hazard in rat. Vision Res 30:1517–1520.

Vaux DL, Haecker G, Strasser A. 1994. An evolutionary perspective on apoptosis. Cell 76:777–779.

Waxler M, Hitchins VM, 1986. Optical Radiation and Visual Health, Boca Raton, FL: CRC Press.

Weale RA. 1989. Do years or quanta age the retina? Photochem Photobiol 50:429–438.

Weil M, Jacobson MD, Coles HSR, Davies TJ, Gardener RL, Raff KD, Raff MC. 1996. Constitutive expression of the machinery for programmed cell death. J Cell Biol 133:1053–1059.

Werner JS, Steele VG, Pfoff DS. 1989. Loss of human photoreceptor sensitivity associated with chronic exposure to ultraviolet radiation. Ophthalmology 96:1552–1558.

Wiedemann P. 1992. Growth factors in retinal diseases: proliferative vitreoretinopathy, proliferative diabetic retinopathy, and retinal degeneration. Surv Ophthalmol 36:373–384.

Wiegand RD, Giusto NM, Rapp LM, Anderson RE. 1983. Evidence for rod outer segment lipid peroxidation following constant illumination of the rat retina. Invest Ophthalmol Vis Sci 24:1433–1435.

Wiegand RD, Koutz CA, Chen H, Anderson RE. 1995. Effect of dietary fat and environmental lighting on the phospholipid molecular species of rat photoreceptor membranes. Exp Eye Res 60:291–306.

Williams TP, Baker BN, eds. 1980. The Effects of Constant Light on Visual Processes. New York: Plenum Press, 3–453.

Williams TP, Webbers JP. 1995. Photometer for measuring intensity and rhodopsin distributions in intact eyes. Applied Optics 34:5720–5724.

Williams TP, Remé CE, Rol P. 1998. Blue-light damage revisited: rhodopsin might be the chromophore. Invest Ophthalmol Vis Sci 39:S128.

Wong P. 1994. Apoptosis, retinitis pigmentosa, and degeneration. Biochem Cell Biol 72:489–498.

Wong P, Kutty RK, Darrow RM, Shivaram S, Kutty G, Fletcher RT, Wiggert B, Chader G, Organisciak DT. 1995a. Changes in clusterin expression associated with light-induced retinal damage in rats. Biochem Cell Biol 72:499–503.

Wong P, Ulyanova T, Darrow R, Shivaram S, van Veen T, Chader G, Organisciak DT. 1995b. Correlation of light-induced retinal damage in rats with changes in TRPM-2/clusterin (TRPM-2) expression. Invest Ophthalmol Vis Sci 36:3941.

Wyllie AH, Kerr JFR, Currie AR. 1980. Cell death: the significance of apoptosis. Int Rev Cytol 68:251–306.

Yannuzzi LA, Fisher YL, Krueger A, Slakter J. 1987. Solar retinopathy: a photobiological and geophysical analysis. Trans Am Ophthalmol Soc 85:120–158.

Yarosh DB. 1994. Induction of cytokines by UV. Photochem Photobiol 59:2S.

Yoshida K, Kawamura K, Imaki J. 1993. Differential expression of c-fos mRNA in rat retinal cells: regulation by light/dark cycle. Neuron 10:1049–1054.

Young RW. 1984. Cell death during differentiation of the retina in the mouse. J Comp Neurol 229:362–373.

Young RW. 1987. Pathophysiology of age-related macular degeneration. Surv Ophthalmol 31:291–306.

Young RW. 1988. Solar radiation and age-related macular degeneration. Surv Ophthalmol 32:252–269.

Young RW. 1994. The family of sunlight-related eye diseases. Optom Vis Sci 71:125–144.

Zhang C, Takahashi K, Lam TT, Tso MO. 1994. Effects of basic fibroblast growth factor in retinal ischemia. Invest Ophthalmol Vis Sci 35:3163–3168.

Zigman S. 1990. Vision enhancement using a short wavelength light-absorbing filter. Optom Vis Sci 67:100–104.

Zigman S. 1993. Ocular light damage. Photochem Photobiol 57:1060–1068.

30. Laser interactions with the retina and retinal pigment epithelium

CAROLINE R. BAUMAL AND CARMEN A. PULIAFITO

The ocular effects of radiant energy were noted by Socrates as the occurrence of solar retinopathy after direct viewing of an eclipse. In 1945, Meyer-Schwickerath noted a similarity between macular lesions occurring after observation of a solar eclipse and lesions produced by diathermy (Meyer-Schwickerath, 1959). He investigated many sources including the sun, mercury lamps and carbon arcs in an effort to deliver radiant energy to the retina for therapeutic purposes. In 1956, the xenon arc was utilized to produce retinal photocoagulation. The ruby laser was introduced in 1963 as the first commercial laser available for ophthalmologic use (Campbell et al., 1963; Kapany et al., 1963). Improvements in technology quickly replaced the xenon and ruby sources with argon, krypton, dye and diode lasers, which are presently used for retinal photocoagulation. Lasers permit efficient and precise delivery of energy to the target tissue, thus minimizing damage to adjacent areas. The optical properties of the eye, the accessibility of the retina to laser therapy and the unique properties of retinal chromophores make laser therapy particularly suitable for ophthalmologic use.

LASER THEORY

The electromagnetic spectrum is composed of a broad range of radiation extending from short cosmic waves to long radio waves (Fig. 30-1). Currently available laser outputs include ultraviolet, visible, and infrared radiation. Electromagnetic radiation has both wave-like and particle-like properties. Wave theory is useful to describe refraction and interference phenomena while particle properties are responsible for light absorption and emission by atoms and molecules. Radiation of a given wavelength is associated with photons of a corresponding energy, defined by $E = h\nu = hc/\lambda$ where h = Planck's constant (6.626×10^{-34} J/sec), ν = frequency, c = speed of light (3×10^8 m/sec), and λ = wavelength. As the wavelength increases, the frequency and energy of the photons decrease.

The processes of spontaneous emission, absorption, and stimulated emission were described by Albert Einstein in 1917. Spontaneous emission occurs when an atom falls from a higher energy state to a lower level, and the resultant energy is spontaneously emitted as a photon of electromagnetic radiation. The frequency of this radiation is proportional to the difference between the two energy levels. Absorption occurs when the incident energy causes the atom to ascend to its excited state. When an excited atom is struck by an incoming photon possessing energy equal to the difference between the atom's higher and lower energy levels, the atom returns to its ground state by releasing a photon. This newly emitted photon has the same energy, direction, and phase as the incoming photon that triggered its release. This is the process of stimulated emission, where the incoming photon stimulates emission of another photon and results in the production of two photons that are identical with respect to wavelength, direction, and phase.

LASER CONSTRUCTION

Laser is the acronym for *light amplification by stimulated emission of radiation*. A laser selectively amplifies energy transitions produced by stimulated emission, creating a chain reaction or cascade of photons with identical properties. The three components required to produce laser activity are (1) an active medium that undergoes stimulated emission, (2) a mechanism for energy input, known as *pumping* and (3) a resonant cavity to allow oscillation, amplification, and selective release of photons produced by stimulated emission (Steinert and Puliafito, 1985).

Most atoms (or molecules) of a gas or crystal exist in their unexcited ground state. In order to produce laser activity with a particular medium, its atoms must have an excited energy state with a comparatively long lifetime, known as the *metastable state*. The active medium of the laser supports the process of stimulated emission by allowing a large number of atoms to exist in their metastable state. The wavelength emitted is a function

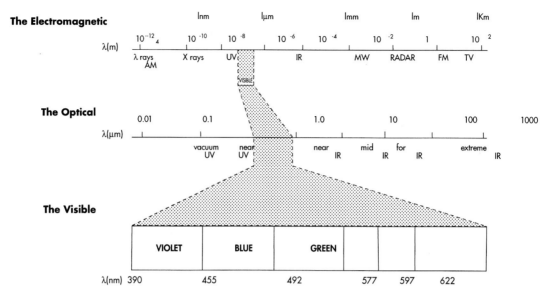

FIGURE 30-1. The electromagnetic spectrum.

of the laser cavity's active medium, which may be gas (argon, krypton, carbon dioxide, helium with neon), liquid (organic dye), solid (an active element supported by a crystal such as neodymium with yttrium-aluminum-garnet [Nd:YAG]), or a semiconductor (diode) (Table 30-1). Population inversion occurs when more atoms in the active medium have electrons in their excited energy level than in a lower energy configuration. Pumping, the energy input required to create population inversion, can be produced with an electric current as in gas lasers, or with a flash lamp as in solid crystal lasers. Dye lasers are often pumped by other lasers, such as an argon source.

When population inversion has been accomplished, the atoms (or molecules) of the active medium are primed for stimulated emission, whereby photons from atoms relaxing from the excited state stimulate neighboring excited atoms to emit their energy as photons. Optical feedback is produced by a resonant cavity that selectively amplifies the photons produced by stimulated emission along a single axis. Mirrors at each end of a resonant cavity allow these photons to oscillate back and forth through the active medium, which the pumping mechanism maintains in a state of population inversion. One of the mirrors is only partially reflecting, known as the output coupler, allowing some of the photons traveling along the axis to escape and form the laser beam. A prism or filter in the cavity is used to deviate photons with any wavelength other than that desired.

In the laser cavity, resonant waves travel between the mirrors in slightly different directions. The interference between these waves produces well-defined patterns of intensity classified by transverse modes (Peyman et al.,

1984). The transverse electromagnetic (TEM) mode describes the energy configuration across the beam, and determines the spatial distribution of laser light and the characteristics of the laser focus. The fundamental mode (noted by TEM_{00}) is a transverse mode characterized by an intensity concentrated only along its axis with a Gaussian (normal) distribution of energy in the beam profile, producing low beam divergence. In contrast, the multimode configuration produces an irregular beam profile. The fundamental mode is often used due to its precise focusing capability; however, it represents only a small portion of the laser output and may not be desirable when very high energy levels are required.

LASER OUTPUT

Laser output may be delivered at a continuous power level (continuous wave, CW), in a single pulse, or as a series of pulses. Gas lasers such as argon or krypton run only in the continuous mode, while solid and liquid lasers may be pulsed. The continuous laser beam has a uniform power and the duration of exposure is controlled by a external shutter. The pulse mode allows energy to be concentrated and delivered over a short time period, resulting in average and peak powers. The rate of energy delivery is the radiant power, which is equal to energy measured in joules divided by the pulse duration in seconds. An increase in power can be achieved by either shortening pulses or increasing the energy. Various methods are available to achieve compression of laser pulses, including Q switching and mode locking. Q switching utilizes an intracavitary shutter called a Q

TABLE 30-1. *Ophthalmologic lasers in clinical use and their wavelengths*

Laser	Wavelength
Argon blue-green	488.0 nm blue and 514.5 nm green
Argon green	514.5 nm
Carbon dioxide	10.6 μm
Diode	Variable range: 780–850 nm
Dye (tunable)	Variable range: 570–630 nm
Double frequency Nd:YAG	532.0 nm
Erbium: YAG	2.94 μm
Erbium: YSSG	2.78 μm
Excimer	
Argon fluoride	193 nm
Krypton fluoride	248 nm
Xenon chloride	308 nm
Holmium	2.1 μm
Krypton red	647.1 nm
Krypton yellow	568.2 nm
Nd:YAG	1064.0 nm
Ruby	694.3 nm

switch to permit rapid release of the energy produced by population inversion. The Q in the term Q *switch* stands for "quality factor" of the laser cavity, which is the ratio of the energy stored in the cavity to the energy lost per cycle. The typical Q switch pulse duration is in the range of 2 to 30 nanoseconds (1 ns = 10^{-9} second) (Mainster et al., 1983). Mode locking produces ultrashort pulses in the picosecond (1 ps = 10^{-12} seconds) to femtosecond (1 fs = 10^{-15} seconds) range by synchronizing the phase relationships within the laser cavity (Lin, 1993). A typical mode-locked pulse train consist of seven to ten pulses spaced over a total of 35 to 50 nanoseconds, where the typical pulse width is 30 picoseconds (Mainster et al., 1983). Mode locking potentially produces pulses of higher power than Q switching, due to its shorter pulse duration.

PROPERTIES OF LASER LIGHT

Laser properties include monochromaticity, directionality, spatial and temporal coherence, polarization, and intensity (Steinert and Puliafito, 1985; Lin, 1993). These unique properties allow precise and efficient delivery of laser light, making it suitable for ophthalmologic use.

Monochromaticity refers to the discrete wavelength(s) of light emitted by the laser. This occurs due to the limited number of efficient electron transitions from the excited to lower-lying electron energy levels. Monochromaticity allows selection of a particular wavelength to

enhance absorption by the target tissue. *Directionality* means that there is little divergence of the laser beam output, allowing the laser light to travel for considerable distances without widening. A high degree of collimation is produced, as the resonant chamber only amplifies photons traveling along a very narrow path between the mirrors. This property permits effective focusing of the laser beam to a small spot size with high irradiance. *Coherence* describes the spatial and temporal synchronicity of the photons produced and amplified within the resonant cavity of the laser. *Polarization* of light emitted by the laser is often incorporated into the system to allow maximum energy transmission through the laser medium without loss due to reflection.

A variety of radiometric terms are used to describe the electromagnetic radiation produced by medical lasers. Radiant energy is measured in *joules* (J, 1 joule = 1 watt × 1 second) and radiant power is measured in *watts* (W, 1 watt = 1 joule/1 second). *Intensity* is the power in a beam of a given angular size, and *brightness* is the intensity per unit area. Laser irradiance is the power incident per unit area (W/cm^2), while radiant energy density is the energy per unit area (J/cm^2).

MECHANISM OF LASER ACTION

The tissue effects of laser may be divided into the following three categories: photochemical, ionizing and thermal. These effects are differentiated by the laser irradiance, wavelength, and duration of exposure.

Photochemical reactions occur at a low to moderate irradiance below coagulation thresholds and are often associated with a short wavelength and an exposure duration longer than one microsecond (Mainster, 1983). Absorption of a photon by the outer electrons creates an excited molecular state to drive a chemical reaction. An example of this effect is photoablation produced by the excimer laser for phototherapeutic keratectomy. During photoablation, short pulses of ultraviolet radiation are applied to precisely shape the cornea without adjacent thermal damage (Puliafito et al., 1985). Similarly, photodynamic therapy utilizes a photochemical reaction for its effect and will be described in a subsequent section.

Ionization requires high laser irradiances produced by a short exposure time in the nanosecond or picosecond range (Mainster et al., 1983). Energy strips the electrons from atoms and molecules, resulting in ionization and disintegration of target tissue into ions and electrons called plasma. This process produces mechanical effects in the target tissues. The commonest example of ionization is photodisruption produced by the Nd:YAG laser (Puliafito and Steinert, 1984). This laser delivers a near infrared wavelength of 1024 nm to target tissues, with a small spot size and brief exposure. Therapeutic applications include posterior capsulotomy and peripheral iridectomy.

Thermal effects include both photocoagulation and photovaporization, which occur with a moderate irradiance, an exposure duration greater than one microsecond and a laser wavelength longer than that required for photochemical effects (Mainster, 1985). Photovaporization occurs as excessive absorption of laser energy raises the tissue temperature to the boiling point of water, producing tissue disruption (Peyman et al., 1984). The carbon dioxide laser utilizes this mechanism for tissue incision.

Photocoagulation is the commonest therapeutic application for retinal lasers and its effect results from focal heating of the retina and choroid. Photocoagulation occurs when photon absorption or molecular vibrations produce a critical temperature rise sufficient to denature biomolecules, resulting in thermally induced structural changes in the target tissue. A 10–20°C rise in retinal temperature produces enzyme inactivation and protein denaturation, resulting in cellular necrosis, hemostasis and coagulation (Priebe et al., 1975; White et al., 1971; Birngruber et al., 1985). In practice, the peak temperature achieved at the center of a retinal lesion after photocoagulation may be in excess of 100°C (Vander Zypen 1985; Jacques and Prahl, 1987). Photocoagulative lesions are immediately visible due to cellular necrosis and mechanical disruption of the adjacent neurosensory retina that decreases its regular transparency. Delayed effects result from inflammation and repair processes such as cellular proliferation, migration, and scar formation. For example, the mechanism for occlusion of choroidal neovascularization (CNV) involves thrombus formation and collagen shrinkage in vascular walls and surrounding connective tissue induced by laser-generated heat (Boergen et al., 1981; Gorish and Boergen, 1982).

Factors that influence the photocoagulative results for a given power are the amount of energy conducted by a specific wavelength, the duration of exposure, light scattering during transmission through the eye, and the optical and thermal properties of absorbing tissue (Mainster, 1986; Mainster et al., 1970). Most lasers employed for photocoagulation use radiation in the visible portion of the electromagnetic spectrum, with the exception of the diode and long-pulsed Nd:YAG lasers. The thermal damage to the retina is proportional to the magnitude and duration of tissue temperature increase (Mainster, 1986). For a burn of given intensity, decreasing the temperature rise in the target tissue increases the duration of exposure required. The tissue temperature

rise is also proportional to the laser irradiance (which is equal to the power incident per unit area). In ophthalmologic lasers, the spot size is the diameter of the focused beam and its area is calculated by πr^2. Cooling of the center of a large spot is less effective, because its immediately adjoining areas are also hot, while small spots are more affected by heat dissipation to surrounding tissues. For this reason, small spots require higher irradiance to achieve the same central effect as larger spots. For an increase in the laser spot size by two (which increases the area by four), less than four times as much power is required to reach the same temperature (March, 1990). A higher temperature rise produces the appearance of an immediate photocoagulation lesion while a lower temperature rise may result in delayed appearance of the burn by hours. The temperature rise in the periphery of the burn may be lower than in the center for a variety of reasons, including laser light scattering and eye movements (Mainster, 1986). In addition, heat may be transferred beyond the immediate target size by passive thermal diffusion or convection due to blood flow (Boergen et al., 1981). These factors may account for delayed burn expansion based on a subthreshold temperature increase at the margin of a laser spot (Dastgheib et al., 1993).

LASER ABSORPTION BY THE RETINA AND RPE

In addition to the mechanism of laser action, the effect of laser light also depends on the properties of the target tissue. Laser light encountering biological tissue may be absorbed, transmitted, scattered, or reflected. For retinal therapy, the laser must be able to adequately penetrate the ocular media to interact with the target tissue. The ocular media effectively transmits wavelengths from 380 nm to 1400 nm, allowing therapy by a transpupillary route. Wavelengths shorter than 380 nm are limited by ultraviolet-absorbing properties of the lens and cornea, while wavelengths longer than 1400 nm are restricted by water absorption. There is approximately 75% to 90% transmission of electromagnetic radiation with a wavelength of 400 nm to 1064 nm through the ocular media (Boettner and Wolter, 1962). Scattering by the ocular media is dependent on the wavelength of incident light, the size and refractive index of the scattering particles, and the age of the patient (Pomerantzeff et al., 1976). In general for small particles, shorter wavelengths are scattered more than longer wavelengths. When laser light reaches the target tissue, its effect is dependent primarily upon its absorption. For photocoagulation, the tissue temperature rise is proportional to the light absorption in the target tissues, which is determined by how effectively its molecules absorb photons of a given wavelength (Mainster, 1985).

The ability of a target to absorb radiation is measured by the attenuation of incident radiation after a certain length of the material has been traversed (Krauss and Puliafito, 1995). The absorbance (A) of a material is defined as $A(d) = \log[I_o/I(d)] = \epsilon cd$, where I_o = initial intensity, $I(d)$ = intensity at distance d, ϵ = absorptivity of the material, and c = molarity of the material. Transmission is the portion of incident energy that is not absorbed after traversing a particular target thickness. It is described by T(d), where $T(d) = 10^{-A(d)} = e^{-\alpha d}$, where $\alpha d = 2.3A$ defines the absorption coefficient α. α describes the fraction of incident energy that is absorbed per unit length of target material in units of cm^{-1}. The thermal susceptibility of the irradiated tissue is denoted by the thermal relaxation time (τ), which represents the time required for the irradiated target tissue to carry away heat energy by conduction. It is proportional to $1/4\alpha^2\kappa$ where κ represents tissue diffusivity in cm^2/s and is wavelength dependent.

The absorption maximum of a compound is the wavelength in the electromagnetic spectrum that has the highest probability of absorption. A plot of absorption versus wavelength produces an absorption spectrum that is characteristic of the chemical composition of the material (Fig. 30-2). Quantum yield measures the efficiency with which absorbed radiation produces chemical changes. The action spectrum is a plot of the relative efficiency of the photoreaction versus the wavelength. The differences in spectral absorption of different molecules allow selective damage to specific components of the target tissue. A chromophore is a molecule or a portion of it that absorbs photons of particular energy. In principle, selection of a laser whose wavelength matches the absorption characteristics of the target ocular tissue maximizes the therapeutic effect and minimizes potential side effects.

In the macular region, laser light may potentially be absorbed by five different pigments: hemoglobin in retinal and choroidal blood vessels, melanin in the retinal pigment epithelium (RPE) and choroidal melanocytes, lipofuscin in the RPE, xanthophyll in the inner and outer plexiform layers, and rhodopsin and cone photopigments in the photoreceptors (Mainster, 1985). The three primary absorbers involved in the process of photocoagulation are melanin, xanthophyll, and hemoglobin. In elderly eyes, lipofuscin may be a potential chromophore for photocoagulation (Dillon, 1991; Gaillard et al., 1995).

Melanin is the main site of energy absorption for laser photocoagulation. Melanin absorption is maximal between 400 nm and 700 nm, absorbing blue, green, yellow, and red wavelengths in decreasing order (Peyman

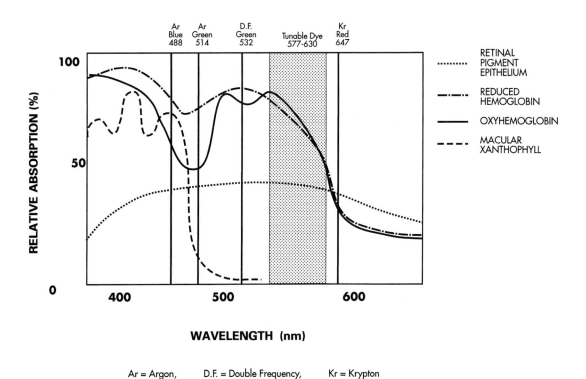

FIGURE 30-2. Relative absorption versus wavelength for various intraocular chromophores.

et al., 1984). Approximately 50% of incident 514 nm laser light is absorbed by the RPE. At longer wavelengths, melanin absorption decreases, resulting in deeper chorioretinal burns. Only 15% of the infrared wavelength is absorbed by RPE melanin. Argon green is absorbed at the level of the RPE, krypton red produces a deeper burn, and Nd:YAG causes primarily choroidal and even scleral effects (Coscas and Soubrane, 1983). In general, a deeper burn is more painful and less prominent on clinical examination.

Hemoglobin in the inner retinal circulation and the choroidal vessels is often targeted to destroy or occlude leaky vessels. Hemoglobin has strong absorption for all colors with wavelengths shorter than red. Thus, it absorbs blue, green, and yellow wavelengths well, with poor absorption of red and infrared wavelengths. The absorption spectrum of hemoglobin varies with its amount of oxygen saturation. Oxyhemoglobin has poorer absorption of red than reduced hemoglobin, which accounts for the increased prominence of retinal veins on clinical examination. The two absorption maxima for oxyhemoglobin are at 542 nm (green) and 577 nm (yellow), while reduced hemoglobin absorbs maximally at 555 nm (yellow) (Mainster, 1986). Blue, green, and yellow wavelengths produce maximal effects on hemoglobin-containing structures, which are visible clinically as vasospasm (Peyman et al., 1984). However, vasospasm can be produced by longer wavelengths in attached retina by absorption of laser light in the underlying RPE with subsequent heat production and transfer to adjacent retinal vessels.

Yellow xanthophyll pigment in the perifoveal region absorbs strongly below, but not above 500 nm. Therefore, it absorbs blue strongly, green minimally, and yellow and red light negligibly. Due to this property, the blue wavelength emitted by the argon blue-green laser is absorbed by the inner retina as well as the RPE, while longer wavelengths such as argon green or krypton red avoid this effect (Trempe et al., 1982; Marshall et al., 1974).

LASER SELECTION FOR RETINAL THERAPY

Lasers are often classified by their active medium, but it is the wavelength that is critical in determining absorption by ocular pigments. A variety of lasers are available for ocular photocoagulation with wavelengths ranging from 488 nm to 1064 nm (Table 30-1). Factors to be considered when selecting a laser wavelength for optimal retinal photocoagulation are effective transmission through the ocular media, low absorption by macular xanthophyll during macular photocoagulation, and ef-

fective penetration through hemorrhage or fluid anterior to the target tissue (Mainster, 1986).

Although no longer widely used in North America, the xenon arc photocoagulator provides a source of monochromatic white light, emitting wavelengths from 400 nm to 1600 nm (Blankenship, 1991). The clinical result is a full-thickness retinal burn. Other disadvantages of xenon include lack of collimation and a long exposure duration of several seconds. Moreover, the procedure is painful, requiring retrobulbar anesthesia. The ruby crystal laser is no longer widely used in North America. There is an increased risk of subretinal hemorrhage with the ruby laser, due to its short pulse duration and its longer red wavelength emission. It is not useful for direct treatment of blood vessels.

The argon laser was introduced by L'Esperance in 1968 (L'Esperance, 1968). The argon laser emits either blue-green (488 nm and 514.5 nm) or green (514.5 nm) wavelengths. The standard argon blue-green produces 60% to 70% blue light. Due to its short wavelength, blue light is scattered more by media opacities and may be absorbed by yellow lenticular changes. Blue light in the perifoveal region is absorbed by xanthophyll in the inner retina, producing undesirable neurosensory retinal damage (Marshall et al., 1975). In addition, damage to the internal limiting membrane may precipitate epiretinal membrane formation. The white inner retinal burn that is produced may induce light scattering, preventing deeper laser penetration to the RPE with repeated laser applications and obscuring post-treatment fluorescein angiographic visualization of persistent CNV (Marshall and Bird, 1979). There is a concern that the prolonged use of blue light may decrease color discrimination in a tritan color-confusion axis in ophthalmologists (Arden et al., 1991; Berninger et al., 1989). Argon blue-green photocoagulation performed after fluorescein angiography in patients with increased vitreous fluorescence (for example, diabetics with defective vascular tight junctions) may increase the surgeon's exposure to laser light due to the similar wavelengths of fluorescein excitation and argon blue-green (Friberg et al., 1995). At present, there is no role for the blue wavelength in treatment of macular disorders.

Argon green is well absorbed by hemoglobin and melanin, with minimal xanthophyll absorption. This is useful for direct coagulation of retinal vessels, but does not permit this wavelength to penetrate through retinal hemorrhage to the underlying RPE or choroid. A moderate argon green laser burn in the absence of a large retinal vessel produces a cone-shaped lesion with relative sparing of the inner retina (Apple et al., 1973; Swartz, 1986).

The krypton laser was introduced in 1972 and emits

either red (647.1 nm) or yellow (568.2 nm) wavelengths. Krypton red has no hemoglobin absorption, negligible xanthophyll absorption, and has deeper penetration than argon green. Thus, krypton red is useful primarily for treatment of the RPE and choroid. Closure of CNV by krypton red is most likely due to light absorption by melanin in the choroid and RPE with thermal transfer to adjacent vessels (Mainster, 1986; Weider et al., 1981). Advantages of krypton red include better penetration than shorter wavelengths through lenticular nuclear sclerosis, mild vitreous hemorrhages, and shallow subretinal hemorrhages. Disadvantages include increased risk of choroidal hemorrhage and disruption of Bruch's membrane due to deeper laser penetration and patient discomfort. In the event of an inadvertent hemorrhage, the red wavelength is unable to directly coagulate vessels. Krypton yellow causes less RPE damage than krypton red but may produce inner retinal damage: specifically, nerve fiber layer and ganglion cell edema and coagulation at the border between the outer plexiform and nuclear layers (Peyman et al., 1984; Pomerantzeff et al., 1983).

The tunable dye laser provides a range of monochromatic wavelengths throughout much of the visible spectrum (Romanelli and Puliafito, 1990). Dye lasers utilize the molecular transitions of an organic liquid dye (the active medium) and are designed so a given frequency can be isolated from the many different wavelengths it can produce. Dye lasers can produce yellow (575 nm), orange (590–600 nm), and red, (630 nm) wavelengths, in addition to the blue (488 nm) and green (514 nm) that are produced by the argon laser used to pump the dye. In principle, this allows selection of the most suitable wavelength for the clinical treatment based on the transparency and absorption characteristics of the target tissue. Dye yellow (577 nm) absorption is negligible for xanthophyll, moderate for melanin (41% absorption), and maximal for oxyhemoglobin (70% absorption) and deoxyhemoglobin (82% absorption) (L'Esperance, 1985a). This is useful for direct therapy of abnormal retinal or choroidal vasculature. Controversy regarding the safety of dye orange (600 nm) has limited its current clinical use, as high-intensity juxtafoveal dye orange burns were noted to produce inner retinal damage in the primate retina (Smiddy et al., 1988; Brooks et al., 1989). This may be due to an unknown retinal chromophore with maximal absorption at this wavelength or due to an additive effect of chromophore absorption at this wavelength. Low-power tunable dye laser lesions (100 mW, 0.1 seconds, 100 μm spot size), produced by yellow, orange, and red wavelengths in the primate retina, produce similar histopathologic damage to the RPE, the inner choroid, and the photoreceptor nuclei and

outer segments, while the inner nuclear, gangion cell, and plexiform layers remain intact (Figure 30-3).

Nd:YAG radiation at 1064 nm is poorly absorbed by melanin, resulting in deep choroidal penetration. A crystal of potassium-titanium-phosphate may be used to double the frequency of the Nd:YAG laser, thus decreasing the wavelength in half to 532 nm in the green range. This double-frequency Nd:YAG output is more highly absorbed by the RPE and hemoglobin than argon green and is close to absorption peaks of oxyhemoglobin and deoxyhemoglobin (L'Esperance, 1985b). Vasoocclusive effects are achieved efficiently with the double frequency Nd:YAG with lower power requirements than other lasers.

The semiconductor diode laser is capable of emitting longer wavelengths in the infrared region, producing damage in the outer retina and choroid while sparing the inner retina and nerve fiber layer (McHugh et al., 1988). Most commercial versions have only a single emission at 810 nm and are not tunable. Advantages of the diode laser include its high electrical efficiency, compact size, portability, and ability to be powered from an ordinary electrical wall current. Clinical benefits include minimal absorption by intraocular media opacities and excellent penetration through serous fluid or retinal edema (Balles and Puliafito, 1990). However, the diode laser requires greater power and a longer exposure duration to create clinical photocoagulation than argon green (Balles et al., 1990a). Pain is a common complaint when the diode is used for panretinal photocoagulation.

Clinical trials have shown that retinal photocoagulation is beneficial therapy for diabetic macular edema, retinal neovascularization, and CNV (ETDRSRG, 1981; 1985; BVOSG, 1986; MPSG, 1986). Photocoagulation is also useful to form a chorioretinal adhesion around retinal breaks and areas of retinal detachment. The therapeutic effect of retinal photocoagulation is often not caused by the immediate photocoagulation burn but by the secondary tissue response induced by thermal damage. In proliferative diabetic retinopathy, the therapeutic effect is due to either the removal of oxygen-consuming photoreceptors and their replacement by a glial scar or the regeneration of the RPE (Wolbarsht and Landers, 1980; Tso et al., 1980). RPE cells may release inhibitors of intraocular neovascularization (Glaser et al., 1987). Stimulation and restoration of the RPE barrier after laser photocoagulation is postulated to produce the therapeutic effect in central serous chorioretinopathy and diabetic macular edema (Wallow, 1984).

Selection of the most suitable laser wavelength for retinal therapy should consider the location and characteristics of the target tissue and the presence of associated ocular pathology such as lens opacity, vitreous hemorrhage,

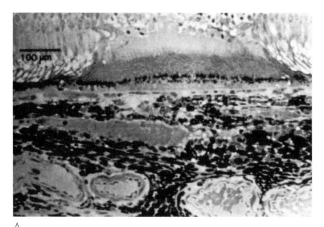

A

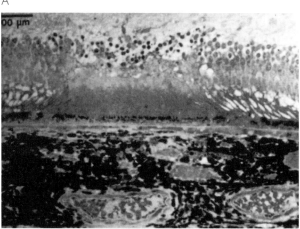

B

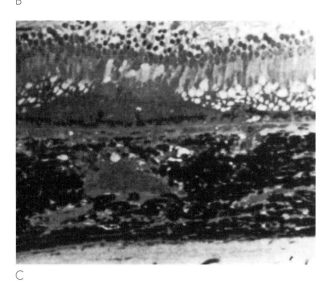

C

FIGURE 30-3. Low-power laser lesions (100 mW) produced by the different wavelengths of a tunable dye laser in the primate eye. A lightly visible white lesion was produced with a power of 100 mW, a duration of 0.1 second and a 100 μm spot size with each wavelength. Each lesion shows damage to the RPE, the inner choroid, and the photoreceptor nuclei and outer segments. The inner retinal layers are intact. (A) 577 nm yellow; (b) 590 nm orange; (c) 630 nm red. (Reprinted from Romanelli and Puliafito, 1990.)

intraretinal fluid or hemorrhage, and serous retinal detachment. In principle, selection from a wide variety of available laser wavelengths and parameters allows maximal damage to the target tissue with minimal effect on adjacent normal tissue. A wavelength should be chosen to limit inner retinal and nerve fiber layer damage; thus, argon blue-green should be avoided for macular photocoagulation. However, excessively heavy photocoagulation with any wavelength can produce varying degrees of full-thickness retinal damage due to heat conduction to the inner retina (Smiddy et al., 1988).

When retinal or choroidal vascular closure is desired, direct hemoglobin absorption by the shorter wavelengths may be advantageous. For therapy of CNV, the yellow wavelength may be beneficial due to minimal xanthophyll and cataract uptake with moderate melanin and maximal hemoglobin absorption. Argon green may be more effective than longer wavelengths for therapy of CNV overlying poorly pigmented areas of RPE and choroid, and for treating CNV with large-caliber vessels. If hemorrhage is associated with CNV, a wavelength should be selected to minimize hemoglobin absorption and heating, which may result in inner retinal damage. Thus, longer wavelengths such as krypton red and diode are favored over argon green. Folk and colleagues (1985) demonstrated that the krypton red wavelength penetrated a thin layer of hemorrhage better than argon wavelengths in the primate retina, although neither argon (blue-green or green) nor krypton red had effective energy penetration if the specimen of hemorrhage was four cell layers thick (Folk et al., 1985).

Longer wavelengths such as krypton red and diode are useful in the presence of lens opacity and vitreous or retinal hemorrhage, as they are scattered less than shorter wavelengths and are absorbed poorly by hemoglobin. In the presence of poor fundus pigmentation, longer wavelengths such as krypton red require higher energy levels to produce a photocoagulative lesion. The use of excessive photocoagulation energy may cause retraction of a fibrovascular CNV or a tear in the RPE before producing significant whitening in the overlying retina, as well as increase the risk of choroidal hemorrhage and rupture of Bruch's membrane.

HISTOPATHOLOGIC STUDIES OF LASER PHOTOCOAGULATION

Many histopathologic studies have been performed in animals and humans to study the effect of the various laser wavelengths used for photocoagulation (Coscas and Soubrane, 1983; Marshall and Bird, 1979; Apple et al., 1973; 1976; Romanelli and Puliafito, 1990; Brooks et al., 1989; Folk et al., 1985; Campbell et al., 1969;

L'Esperance, 1969; Bresnick et al., 1970; Powell et al., 1971; Wallow and Tso, 1973; Weingeist, 1974; Peyman et al., 1981; 1983; Juarez et al. 1982; Thomas et al., 1984; Smiddy et al., 1984a; 1984b; 1985; 1988; Borges et al., 1987; Puliafito et al., 1987; Vogel et al., 1989; Brancato et al., 1989; Benner et al., 1992; Roider et al., 1993; McHugh et al., 1995). The laser wavelength and results are summarized in Table 30-2. However, the clinical significance of these studies is uncertain. Laser therapy is often performed in eyes with concurrent ocular pathology (such as retinal edema, hemorrhage, and pigmentary disturbances) that may interfere with laser absorption and effect. At the pulse duration used for conventional retinal photocoagulation, heat dissipates out of the RPE to damage the adjacent choroid and neural retina. While few clinical trials have compared the therapeutic effect of different wavelengths, a significant difference has not been found. Olk (1990) found no difference between krypton red or argon green treatment of diabetic macular edema with regards to visual outcome or scotoma. Coscas (1983) showed that both krypton red and argon green can effectively close juxtafoveal CNV. The Macular Photocoagulation Study (MPSG, 1991) found no difference in clinical outcome between argon green or krypton red treatment of subfoveal CNV. Both argon blue-green and krypton red have proven equally effective in producing regression of diabetic retinal neovascularization (KARNSRG, 1993). Further evaluation is required to assess the therapeutic effect of different wavelengths for various retinal diseases.

REPAIR OF THE RPE AFTER LASER PHOTOCOAGULATION

Laser-photocoagulation burns acutely damage the outer blood–retinal barrier at the level of the RPE (Ohkuma et al., 1983). Subsequent healing of laser lesions is accompanied by regeneration of the RPE cells and the appearance of scattered foci of subretinal neovascularization (Pollack and Korte, 1990). Factors affecting RPE healing are the intensity and the size of the laser burn.

Reestablishment of the RPE barrier has been observed after moderately intense laser burns in the primate retina, but was not noted after high-intensity laser burns (Wallow, 1984; Peyman and Bok, 1972). After krypton laser photocoagulation in the rat, RPE regeneration occurs from surviving RPE cells at the periphery of the burn. A continuous epithelial sheet is re-formed by a morphologically heterogeneous population of RPE cells along Bruch's membrane. This sheet relines most small laser burns by 14 to 21 days after laser and zonulae occludens between regenerated RPE cells restore the outer blood–retinal barrier (Pollack and Korte, 1990). This

has been demonstrated experimentally by the lack of diffusion of horseradish peroxidase through this barrier into the retina (Pollack and Korte, 1993). Thus, the continuity of the regenerated RPE cells appears to play a role in repair of the outer blood–retinal barrier. In large burns, regenerated RPE cells are seen only at the margin of the burn and a glial scar is present centrally where the outer blood–retinal barrier is not repaired.

While the regenerated RPE cells appear normal by light microscopy, these cells are distinguished from normal RPE cells by irregular arrangement of their apical villi and melanosomes. Three morphological types of regenerated RPE cells have been identified during RPE healing in the rat: RPE-like macrophages, electron dense cells, and electron lucent cells (Pollack and Korte, 1990). Variations in the appearance of the regenerated RPE may reflect the multiple functions of a single RPE cells. Evaluation of growth factors and cytokines in cultured human RPE cells after laser photocoagulation demonstrated an increased production of transforming growth factor (TGF)-β2 (Matsumoto et al., 1994). TGF-β2 inhibits proliferation of vascular endothelial cells and may play a role in regression of neovascularization after laser photocoagulation.

COMPLICATIONS OF RETINAL LASER THERAPY

Laser-induced complications may be secondary to improper technique or inappropriate use of the laser parameters. Argon blue-green in the macular region may damage the neurosensory retina and nerve fiber layer. Excessive or extensive use of laser energy may cause exudative retinal detachment, epiretinal membrane formation, or tears in the RPE (Han et al., 1988). The laser energy may rupture through Bruch's membrane, producing choroidal hemorrhage or possibly late choroidal neovascularization (Grabowski et al., 1984). This most often occurs with a small spot size of 100 μm or less, a short duration time, or longer wavelengths in the red or near infrared range. To avoid this complication, it is preferable to prolong the exposure time rather than increasing the power when an increase in the intensity of photocoagulation is desired. Excessive therapy to retinal vessels can produce vascular occlusions and retinal or vitreous hemorrhage.

NEW DEVELOPMENTS IN RETINAL LASER THERAPY

Targeting of retinal and choroidal components is ideally based on laser wavelength and the distribution and absorption by tissue chromophores. During photocoagulation, laser energy is transformed into heat within the

TABLE 30-2. *Histopathological studies of laser photocoagulation*

Study	Laser	Species	Results
Campbell et al., 1969	Argon blue vs. argon green	Chinchilla rabbits	No wavelength difference detected clinically or histologically.
L'Esperance, 1969	Krypton 647 nm, 568 nm, 530 nm Argon 488 nm, 457 nm	Chinchilla rabbits	A greater response in the RPE and choroid and acute nerve fiber layer edema occurred with longer wavelengths compared to shorter wavelengths.
Bresnick et al., 1970	Argon green	Rhesus monkeys	No difference between macular and paramacular exposures. RPE damage occured prior to sensory retinal damage.
Powell et al., 1971	Argon blue vs. argon green	Rhesus monkeys	No histological difference noted between argon blue or green. Site of lesion not specified. RPE seemed to be the principal site of damage.
Apple et al., 1973	Argon blue-green	Humans	Lesions to papillomacular bundle show damage to nerve fibers.
Wallow and Tso, 1973	Xenon Arc	Rhesus monkeys	Moderate lesions destroyed the outer retina up to the middle limiting membrane. Severe lesions destroyed full-thickness retina, but some of Bruch's membrane, internal limiting membrane, and retinal vessels remained intact.
Weingeist, 1974	Argon blue-green	Humans	Damage centered on RPE and choroid. Low power spared inner retina. Increased nerve fiber layer damage with high power.
Apple et al., 1976	Argon blue-green	Rhesus monkeys	Direct photocoagulation of temporal arcade vessels led to permanent perivascular axonal destruction. Variable inner retinal damage within the macula.
Marshall and Bird, 1979	Argon blue-green vs. krypton red	Humans	Low- and high-energy krypton lesions were similar when greater than 2 μm from the fovea. Within 2 μm of fovea, argon affected inner nuclear, plexiform, and ganglion cell layers. Krypton spared inner retina with deeper choroidal penetration.
Peyman et al., 1981	Argon blue-green vs. krypton red	Cynomolgus monkeys	In the fovea, argon had more inner retinal damage than krypton. In parafoveal lesions, both spared inner retina. Krypton showed increased choroidal penetration.
Juarez et al., 1982	Argon blue-green vs. krypton red	Cynomolgus monkeys	Retina experimentally detached prior to photocoagulation. Argon blue-green damaged inner and outer retina in foveal area. Krypton spared sensory retina.
Coscas and Soubrane, 1983	Argon green vs. krypton red	Baboons	Both laser wavelengths spared inner retina. Maximal damage at RPE with argon green and at internal choroid with krypton red.
Peyman et al., 1983	Continuous Wave (CW) Nd:YAG (1060 nm) vs. argon green vs. krypton red	Cynomolgus monkeys, pigmented rabbits	5 to 10 times more energy required for transpupillary CW YAG coagulation than argon green or krypton red. Nerve fiber damage only observed when coagulating vessels with argon green.
Thomas et al., 1984	Argon blue-green vs. krypton red	Humans	Krypton red penetrated deeper into choroid than argon.

(*continued*)

TABLE 30-2. (*Continued*)

Study	Laser	Species	Results
Smiddy et al., 1984a	Argon blue-green vs. argon green vs. krypton red	Cynomolgus monkeys	Full-thickness retinal damage with argon blue-green. Argon green produced less severe ganglion cell loss. Krypton red spared ganglion layer with some inner nuclear layer damage.
Smiddy et al., 1984b	Argon green vs. krypton red	Humans	Krypton red spared inner nuclear and ganglion layer compared to argon.
Smiddy et al., 1985	Argon blue-green vs. argon green vs. krypton red	Cynomolgus monkeys	Krypton spared ganglion cell layer while argon green and blue-green caused ganglion cell loss. All lasers damaged inner nuclear layers.
Folk et al., 1985	Argon blue-green vs. argon green vs. krypton red	Cynomolgus monkeys, rabbits	Neither argon nor krypton could penetrate a moderately thick preretinal hemorrhage to produce an underlying retinal burn. Krypton penetrated intraretinal hemorrhage to produce a burn in the RPE/choroid, while argon did not.
Borges et al., 1987	Dye green vs. dye yellow vs. dye red vs. dye orange	Cynomolgus monkeys	Greater damage to inner retina and deep choroid with red than green, yellow, or orange at 24 hours, but not detectable at 31 days after treatment. Green, yellow, and orange lesions similar.
Puliafito et al., 1987	Semiconductor diode endophoto-coagulation, 808 nm, 818 nm	Pigmented rabbits	Localized injury to outer retina, with alteration and disorganization of photoreceptors.
Smiddy et al., 1988	Dye orange vs. dye red vs. krypton red (Range from 560 to 630 nm)	Cynomolgus monkeys	Comparable histopathological effects of krypton red and dye red. Inner retinal damage with high-energy 600 nm orange burns. At lower energy, 600 nm effects were similar to other wavelengths.
Brooks et al., 1989	Dye yellow vs. dye red vs. dye orange	Humans	At high levels, orange wavelength produces more severe inner retinal damage.
Vogel et al., 1989	570 to 630 nm	Rabbits	No difference in effect of various wavelengths noted immediately or after 3 weeks.
Brancato et al., 1989	Diode vs. argon blue-green	Chinchilla rabbits	Argon damaged inner and outer retinal layers. Diode damaged outer retina and choroid.
Romanelli and Puliafito, 1990	Dye red vs. dye orange vs. dye yellow	Cynomolgus monekys	No wavelength difference detected clinically or histologically. Lesions affected choroid, RPE, and outer retina. Low-energy lesions spared inner retina, High-energy lesions caused minimal inner retinal edema.
Benner et al., 1992	Laser indirect ophthalmo-scope:Argon green vs. krypton red vs. diode	Pigmented rabbits	Argon spared inner choroid and sclera while krypton and diode caused choroidal and inner scleral effects. More energy required to make equivalent diode burns when compared to argon and krypton.
Roider et al., 1993	Argon green—, short vs. long pulses	Chinchilla rabbits	Selective RPE damage with sparing of the neural retina occurred only with repetitive short laser pulses
McHugh et al., 1995	Diode vs. Nd:YAG (continuous wave)	Pigmented and albino rabbits	Pigmented rabbits: damage to RPE, middle choroid, and outer retina produced by both lasers, higher power required for Nd:YAG. Albino rabbits: Nd:YAG at 10W produced damage, while diode at maximum power of 1.2 W did not produce discernible lesions.

absorbing structures, and the thermal effects are temperature and time dependent. As the length of exposure increases, the thermal effects are often not confined to the absorbing area but dissipate into surrounding tissues. At the duration of exposure presently used for retinal photocoagulation, the nonabsorbing neural retina is often thermally damaged due to its position adjacent to the RPE, which may adversely affect the final visual outcome. Selective damage to a specific retinal component, such as the RPE or choroidal vasculature, may be desirable. Spatial confinement of thermal effects may be produced by selecting the appropriate pulse duration or by controlling the temperature rise in the target house. Several investigational techniques have been developed to enhance target specificity of ophthalmic lasers, such as selective photothermolysis, short-pulse lasers, dye enhancement, and photodynamic therapy.

SELECTIVE PHOTOTHERMOLYSIS

Anderson and Parrish coined the term *selective photothermolysis* to describe thermally confined injury of pigmented target tissue caused by selective absorption of brief pulses of radiation (Parrish and Deutsch, 1984). Selective thermal injury is produced by the unique properties of the target tissue, rather than precise aiming of the laser beam. After laser exposure, the target begins to dissipate heat by conduction to adjacent tissues. Selective target heating may be achieved when the energy is deposited at a rate faster than the rate of cooling. In order to achieve this effect, the pulse duration must be equal to or less than the target's thermal relaxation time. The length of exposure is determined by the target size. Other requirements include a wavelength that reaches and is preferentially absorbed by the target structure and a fluence sufficient to cause thermal damage. This method has produced selective damage to blood vessels (3.0×10^{-7} s, 577 nm) and melanocytes (2.0×10^{-8} s, 351 nm) and in principle, is applicable at the subcellular level (Anderson and Parrish).

SHORT-PULSE LASERS

At a pulse duration of 100 milliseconds or greater, heat dissipates out of the RPE during and after irradiation to damage the adjacent neurosensory retina. The heat flux is negligible if very short pulse durations are used. With short pulses, high temperatures are required to produce similar thermal effects as with long pulses. To avoid the thermomechanical damage induced by high temperatures, subthreshold pulses are applied repeatedly to compensate for the lower pulse energy. Multiple short

laser pulses can confine injury to absorbing structures with pulse energies below the threshold energy for single-pulse damage. Selective RPE destruction with minimal damage to adjacent neural retina and choroid has been produced in the rabbit retina with multiple subthreshold short laser exposures (514 nm, 5 μs, 1–500 pulses at 500 Hz, 2–10 μJ pulse energy (Roider et al., 1993). Lesions were often not visible clinically due to decreased damage to the adjacent neurosensory retina. In contrast, it was not possible to selectively affect the RPE using continuous wave laser exposures ranging from 50 milliseconds to 1 second, without damage to adjacent structures.

The healing response of the RPE to selective photocoagulation was evaluated in rabbits (Roider et al., 1992). The RPE was re-formed by a single sheet of hypertrophic RPE cells within two weeks with minimal associated inflammatory cells. RPE cells showed signs of viability, such as phagocytosis of photoreceptor outer segments. The RPE barrier was restored within four weeks with resolution of local photoreceptor and subretinal edema. As short-pulse laser photocoagulation spares the photoreceptors, this may prevent the scotomas that occur after laser photocoagulation. No damage was produced in Bruch's membrane by short-pulse lasers. This may prevent the CNV that is occasionally induced after conventional laser therapy. The reformation of the RPE may restore the function of the outer blood–retinal barrier and play a role in recovery of diabetic macular edema.

Ultrashort pulses in the picosecond to femtosecond range produce extremely high peak laser intensity with minimal pulse energy. Retinal damage mechanisms and thresholds produced by a femtosecond pulse laser (single 80 fs pulse, 625 nm) have been reported in rabbits (Birngruber et al., 1987). ED_{50} injury thresholds of 0.75 μJ and 4.5 μJ were measured for fluorescein angiographic and ophthalmoscopic visibility criteria, respectively. However, exposures greater than 100 times the energy threshold in the 50 to 100 μJ range did not produce significantly more damage or hemorrhage, suggesting that energy deposition and damage is nonlinear in the femtosecond range. Ultrastructural studies have revealed that melanin is the primary absorber of the femtosecond pulse. Therefore, for equal pulse or peak intensities, the ultrashort pulse has lower energy and produced fewer nonspecific thermal effects due to nonlinear damage mechanisms.

DYE ENHANCEMENT

Dye enhancement is based on similar wavelengths of absorption of a dye that concentrates in the target tissue and emission from the laser. Exogenous dyes such as sodium fluorescein and indocyanine green (ICG) have been utilized to enhance retinal laser therapy. Fluorescein dye has been used to enhance argon laser therapy of retinal angiomas outside the macular region (Gorin, 1992). Fluorescein effectively absorbs the blue wavelength emitted from argon blue-green laser, decreasing the amount of laser energy required for vascular closure. However, fluorescein laser enhancement is rarely used, due to the potential ocular toxicity associated with the blue laser wavelength.

ICG is a water soluble tricarbocyanine intravenous dye used as an angiographic agent in ophthalmology. ICG enhances visualization of the choroidal circulation and has been used to characterize occult CNV and other choroidal disorders. (Guyer et al., 1992a; 1992b; Destro and Puliafito, 1989; Lim et al., 1991). ICG is approximately 98% protein bound. Due to this property, ICG is essentially a nondiffusible dye in the normal retinal vasculature. In the choroidal circulation, ICG dye leaks less from the fenestrated choriocapillaris than fluorescein and has a predilection to concentrate in CNV (Destro and Puliafito, 1989). ICG has peak absorption (805 nm) and emission (835 nm) in the near infrared range: these longer wavelengths may allow improved florescence of the choroidal vasculature through hemorrhage, fluid, and pigment. As the wavelength of ICG absorption is similar to that of diode laser emission (810 nm), intravenous ICG administration (5 mg/kg) immediately prior to diode laser treatment may permit selective photocoagulation of ICG-filled CNV with lower energy requirements, thus limiting laser damage to the adjacent normal retina (Guyer et al., 1992a). The endpoint of ICG-enhanced diode photocoagulation of CNV is a deep, light gray burn. This is a lighter color than the heavy white burns achieved in the Macular Photocoagulation Studies and is presumably due to minimal damage to the neurosensory retina and RPE. This technique may be useful when ICG shows better demarcation of CNV than fluorescein angiography, and when CNV is associated with an overlying serious fluid or hemorrhage.

In the primate model, ICG-enhanced diode laser photocoagulation has successfully closed CNV with lower energy requirements than for diode laser treatment alone (Balles et al., 1996). Histopathologic studies in animals treated with ICG-enhanced diode photocoagulation revealed full-thickness choroidal damage with minimal neurosensory retinal damage (Matsumoto et al., 1993). Reichel and colleagues (1994) reported stabilization of visual acuity within two lines of presenting vision in nine of ten patients with poorly defined subfoveal CNV after ICG-enhanced diode laser therapy. While ICG dye-enhancement appears to be promising

for therapy of CNV, larger prospective clinical trials are required to assess the efficacy of this technique.

PHOTODYNAMIC THERAPY

Photodynamic therapy (PDT) is a therapeutic modality that utilizes low-intensity light of an appropriate wavelength to activate an exogenous photosensitizing agent. A photochemical interaction between the photosensitizer and the light leads to in situ production of singlet oxygen and superoxide anions, which interact with cellular components such as lipid membranes, proteins, and nucleic acids (Weishoupt et al., 1976). This results in intracellular damage and cellular death, and is evident as vascular thrombosis and occlusion in the target tissue (Nelson et al., 1988). It has been demonstrated that vascular injury plays a major role in tumor destruction following PDT and endothelial cells are particularly sensitive to the effects of photosensitization. The wavelength of light utilized depends on the absorption spectrum of the photosensitizer. PDT potentially allows selective tissue targeting, as the photosensitizer preferentially concentrates and is retained longer in hyperproliferating and neoplastic tissues than in surrounding normal (Henderson and Dougherty, 1992). Thermal damage to adjacent normal retina is minimized by the direct application of low-intensity light. Various photoactive agents have been utilized for ablation of systemic and cutaneous malignancies. In ophthalmology, PDT has been used to treat patients with intraocular melanomas and retinoblastoma, as well as experimental CNV (choroidal neovascularization) in animal models (Murphee et al., 1987; Gonzalez et al., 1995; Kliman et al., 1994; Miller et al., 1995).

Most medical experience with PDT has been with the photosensitizer hematoporphyrin derivative (HPD) and its derivatives. HPD preferentially localizes in tumors and absorbs at wavelengths of 402 nm and 624 nm. HPD has been utilized with variable success in small series of patients with choroidal, ciliary body, and iris melanomas (Davidorf and Davidorf, 1992; Tse et al., 1994; Favilla et al., 1992). Clinical regression was achieved in some eyes with lightly pigmented small and medium-sized melanomas. Retinoblastomas without vitreous seeds initially responded to PDT, although the therapeutic effect did not persist. Vitreous seeds of retinoblastoma did not respond to PDT, possibly due to an inadequate HPD concentration or insufficient oxygen availability (Murphee et al., 1987).

Newer second-generation photosensitizers have been synthesized that are activated by longer wavelengths and potentially have more selective target tissue uptake with diminished cutaneous photosensitivity. The longer wavelength absorption may improve penetration through tissues, pigment, and blood and be activated by low-energy diode sources. These agents include chloroaluminum sulfonated phthalocyanine (CASPc), benzoporphyrin derivative monoacid ring A (BPD-MA) and tin etiopurpurin (SnET2) which are activated by light of 675 nm, 692 nm, and 664 nm, respectively (Fisher et al., 1995). Both CASPc and BPD have produced regression of experimental choroidal melanomas in rabbits (Panagopoulos et al., 1989). As vascular occlusion is produced by PDT, it is presently being investigated for therapy for ocular neovascularization. In animal models, PDT with SnET2, CASPc and BPD has successfully induced closure of experimental choroidal neovascularization in primates (Kliman et al., 1994; Miller et al., 1995; Baumal et al., 1996). While further investigation regarding the clinical applications of PDT is necessary, its use in ophthalmology is promising due to the optical properties of the eye and the accessibility of the eye to light irradiation by the transpupillary route.

Further studies are required to evaluate the effect of different laser wavelengths for therapy of retinal diseases. New developments in laser technology may increase the specificity of tissue damage, and may be applicable to the cellular or subcellular level. While the desired histopathological result is selective treatment of retinal pathology without damage to adjacent tissues, the significance of this result with respect to visual outcome remains to be determined.

REFERENCES

Anderson RR, Parrish JA. 1983. Selective photothermolysis: precise microsurgery by selective absorption of pulsed radiation. Science 220:524–527.

Apple DJ, Goldberg MF, Wyhinny G. 1973. Histopathology and ultrastructure of the argon laser lesion in human retinal and choroidal vasculatures. Am J Ophthalmol 75:595–609.

Apple DJ, Wyhinny G, Goldberg MF, Polley EH, Bizzell JW. 1976. Experimental argon laser photocoagulation. I. Effects on retinal nerve fiber layer. Arch Ophthalmol 94:137–144.

Arden GB, Berninger T, Hogg CR, Perry S. 1991. A survey of color discrimination in German ophthalmologists: changes associated with the use of lasers and operating microscopes. Ophthalmology 98:567–575.

Balles MW, Puliafito CA. 1990. Semiconductor diode lasers: a new laser light source in ophthalmology. Int Ophthalmol Clin 30:77–83.

Balles MW, Puliafito CA, D'Amico DJ, Jacobson JJ, Birngruber R. 1990a. Semiconductor diode laser photocoagulation in retinal vascular disease. Ophthalmology 97:1553–1561.

Balles MW, Puliafito CA, Kliman GH, El-Koumy HA, Reidy WT. 1990b. Indocyanine green dye enhanced diode laser photocoagulation of subretinal neovascular membranes. Invest Ophthalmol Vis Sci (ARVO Abstract) 31(suppl):282.

Baumal CR, Puliafito CA, Pieroth L, Schuman JS, Lahav M, Pedut-Kloizman T, Kiernan C, Coker JG, Wilkins JR, Fujimoto JG, Crean DH. 1996. Photodynamic therapy (PDT) of experimental choroidal neovascularization with tin ethyl etiopurpurin. Invest Ophthalmol Vis Sci (ARVO Abstract) 37(suppl):S122.

Benner JD, Huang M, Morse LS, Hjelmeland LM, Landers MB III. 1992. Comparison of photocoagulation with the argon, krypton and diode laser indirect ophthalmoscopes in rabbit eyes. Ophthalmology 99:1554–1563.

Berninger TA, Canning CR, Gunduz K, Strong N, Arden GB. 1989. Using argon laser blue light reduces ophthalmologists' color contrast sensitivity: argon blue and surgeons' vision. Arch Ophthalmol 107:1453–1458.

Birngruber R, Hillenkamp, F, Gabel VP. 1985. Theoretical investigations of laser thermal retinal injury. Health Phys 48:781–796.

Birngruber R, Puliafito CA, Gawande A, Lin WZ, Schoenlein RW, Fujimoto JG. 1987. Femtosecond laser-tissue interactions: retinal injury studies. IEEE J Quantum Electronics QE-23:1836–1844.

Blankenship GW. 1991. Fifteen-year argon laser and xenon photocoagulation results of Bascom Palmer Eye Institute's patients participating in the diabetic retinopathy study. Ophthalmology 98:125–128.

Boergen KP, Birngruber R, Hillenkamp F. 1981. Laser-induced endovascular thrombosis as a possibility of selective vessel closure. Ophthalmic Res 13:139–150.

Boettner EA, Wolter JR. 1962. Transmission of the ocular media. Invest Ophthalmol 1:776–783.

Borges JM, Charles HC, Lee CM, Smith RT, Cunha-Vaz JG, Goldberg MF, Tso MO. 1987. A clinicopathological study of dye laser photocoagulation on primate retina. Retina 7:46–57.

Brancato R, Pratesi R, Leoni G, Trabucchi G, Vanni U. 1989. Histopathology of diode and argon laser lesions in rabbit retina: a comparative study. Invest Ophthalmol Vis Sci 30:1504–1510.

Bresnick GH, Frisch GD, Powell JO, Landers MB, Holst GC, Dallas AG. 1970. Ocular effects of argon laser radiation. I. Retinal damage threshold studies. Invest Ophthalmol 9:901–910.

Brooks HL Jr, Eagle RC Jr, Schroeder RP, Annesley WH, Shields JA, Augsburger JJ. 1989. Clinicopathologic study of organic dye laser in the human fundus. Ophthalmology 96:822–834.

[BVOSG] Branch Vein Occlusion Study Group. 1986. Argon laser scatter photocoagulation for prevention of neovascularization and vitreous hemorrhage in branch vein occlusion: a randomized clinical trial. Arch Ophthalmol 104:34–41.

Campbell CJ, Rittler MC, Koester CJ. 1963. The optical maser as a retinal coagulator: an evaluation. Trans Am Acad Ophthalmol Otolaryngol 67:58–67.

Campbell CJ, Rittler MC, Swope CH, Wallace RA. 1969. The ocular effects produced by experimental lasers. IV. The argon laser. Am J Ophthalmol 67:671–681.

Coscas G, Soubrane G. 1983. The effects of red krypton and green argon laser on the foveal region: a clinical and experimental study. Ophthalmology 990:1013–1022.

Dastgheib K, Bressler SB, Green WR. 1993. Clinicopathologic correlation of laser lesion expansion after treatment of choroidal neovascularization. Retina. 13:345–352.

Davidorf J, Davidorf F. 1992. Treatment of iris melanoma with photodynamic therapy. Ophthalmic Surg 23:522–527.

Destro M, Puliafito CA. 1989. Indocyanine-green videoangiography of choroidal neovascularization. Ophthalmology 96:846–853.

Dillon J. 1991. The photophysics and photobiology of the eye. J Photochem Photobiol B Biol 10:23–40.

[DRSRG] Diabetic Retinopathy Study Research Group. 1981. Photocoagulation treatment of proliferative diabetic retinopathy: clinical application of Diabetic Retinopathy Study (DRS) findings. DRS report number 8. Ophthalmology 88:583–600.

[ETDRSRG] Early Treatment Diabetic Retinopathy Study Research

Group. 1985. Photocoagulation for diabetic macular edema. Early treatment of diabetic retinopathy study report number 1. Arch Ophthalmol 103:1796–1806.

Favilla I, Barry WR, Gosbell A, Ellims P, Burgess F. 1991. Phototherapy of posterior uveal melanomas. Br J Ophthalmol 75:718–721.

Fisher AMR, Murphree AL, Gomer CJ. 1995. Clinical and preclinical photodynamic therapy. Lasers Surg Med 17:2–31.

Folk JC, Shortt SG, Kleiber PD. 1985. Experiments on the absorption of argon and krypton laser by blood. Ophthalmology 92:100–108.

Friberg TR, Novak KD, Rehkopf PG, Bower KS. 1995. Recent fluorescein angiography increases the risk of harmful light exposure during retinal laser photocoagulation. Lasers Light Ophthalmol 7:31–36.

Gaillard ER, Atherton SJ, Eldred G, Dillon J. 1995. Photophysical studies on human retinal lipofuscin. Photochem Photobiol 61:448–453.

Glaser BM, Campochiaro PA, Davis JL, Jerdan JA. 1987. Retinal pigment epithelial cells release inhibitors of neovascularization. Ophthalmology 94:780–784.

Gonzalez VH, Hu LK, Theodossiadis PG, Flotte TJ, Gragoudas ES, Young LHY. 1995. Photodynamic therapy of pigmented choroidal melanomas. Invest Ophthalmol Vis Sci 36:871–878.

Gorin MB. 1992. Von-Hippel Lindau disease: clinical considerations and the use of fluorescein-potentiated argon laser therapy for treatment of retinal angiomas. Sem Ophthalmol 7:182–191.

Gorish W, Boergen KP. 1982. Heat induced contraction of blood vessels. Lasers Surg Med 2:1–13.

Grabowski WM, Decker WL, Annesley WH Jr. 1984. Complications of krypton red laser photocoagulation to subretinal neovascular membranes. Ophthalmology 91:1587–1591.

Guyer DR, Duker JS, Puliafito CA. 1992a. Indocyanine green angiography and dye-enhanced diode laser photocoagulation. Sem Ophthalmol 7:172–176.

Guyer DR, Puliafito CA, Mones JM, Friedman E, Chang W, Verdooner SR. 1992b. Digital indocyanine-green angiography in chorioretinal disorders. Ophthalmology 99:287–291.

Guyer DR, Yannuzzi LA, Slatker JS, Sorenson JA, Hope-Ross M, Orlock DR. 1994. Digital indocyanine-green videoangiography of occult choroidal neovascularization. Ophthalmology 101:1727–1737.

Han DP, Folk JC, Bratton AR. 1988. Visual loss after successful photocoagulation of choroidal neovascularization. Ophthalmology 95:1380–1384.

Henderson BW, Dougherty TJ. 1992. How does photodynamic therapy work? Photochem Photobiol 55:145–157.

Jacques SL, Prahl SA. 1987. Modelling optical and thermal distributions in tissue during laser irradiation. Laser Surg Med 6:494–503.

Juarez CP, Peyman GA, Raichand M. 1982. Effects of argon and krypton laser on experimentally detached retinas. Ophthalmic Surg 113:928–933.

Kapany NS, Peppers NA, Zweng HC, Flocks M. 1963. Retinal photocoagulation by lasers. Nature 199:146–149.

[KARNSRG] Krypton Argon Regression Neovascularization Study Research Group. 1993. Randomized comparison of krypton versus argon scatter photocoagulation for diabetic disc neovascularization. The krypton argon regression neovascularization study report number 1. Ophthalmology 100:1655–1664.

Kliman GH, Puliafito CA, Stern D, Borirakchanyavat S, Gregory WA. 1994. Phthalocyanine photodynamic therapy: New strategy for closure of choroidal neovacularization. Lasers Surg Med 15:2–10.

Krauss JM, Puliafito CA. 1995. Lasers in ophthalmology. Lasers Surg Med 17:102–159.

L'Esperance FA Jr. 1968. An ophthalmic argon laser photocoagulation system: design, construction and laboratory investigations. Trans Am Ophthalmol Soc 66:827–904.

L'Esperance FA Jr. 1969. The ocular histopathologic effect of krypton and argon laser radiation. Am J Ophthalmol 68:263–273.

L'Esperance FA Jr. 1985a. Clinical photocoagulation with the organic dye laser. A preliminary communication. Arch Ophthalmol 103:1312–1316.

L'Esperance FA Jr. 1985b. New laser systems and their potential clinical usefulness. In: Transactions of the New Orleans Academy of Ophthalmology: Symposium on the Laser in Ophthalmology and Glaucoma Update. St Louis: Mosby, 182–209.

Lim JI, Sternberg P Jr, Capone Aaberg TM, Gilman JP. 1995. Selective neovascularization. Am J Ophthalmol 120:75–82.

Lin CP. 1993. Laser-tissue interactions: basic principles. Ophthalmol Clin North Am 6:381–391.

Mainster MA. 1985. Ophthalmic laser surgery: principles, technology and technique. In: Transactions of the New Orleans Academy of Ophthalmology. Symposium on the Laser in Ophthalmology and Glaucoma Update. St. Louis: Mosby, 81–101.

Mainster MA. 1986. Wavelength selection in macular photocoagulation. Tissue optics, thermal effects and laser systems. Ophthalmology 93:952–958.

Mainster MA, White TJ, Allen RG. 1970. Spectral dependence of retinal damage produced by intense light sources. J Opt Soc Am 60:848–855.

Mainster MA, Sliney DA, Belcher CD, Buzney SM. 1983. Laser photodisruptors: damage mechanisms, instrument design and safety. Ophthalmology 90:973–991.

March WF. 1990. Fundamental concepts. In: March WF, ed, Ophthalmic Lasers: A Second Generation. Thorofare, NJ: Slack Inc, 7–12.

Marshall J, Bird AC. 1979. A comparative histopathological study of argon and krypton laser irradiation of the human retina. Br J Ophthalmol 63:657–668.

Marshall J, Hamilton AM, Bird AC. 1974. Intra-retinal absorption of argon laser irradiation in human and monkey retinae. Experientia 30:1335–1337.

Marshall J, Hamilton AM, Bird AC. 1975. Histopathology of ruby and argon laser lesions in monkey and human retina: a comparative study. Br J Ophthalmol 59:610–630.

Matsumoto M, Miki T, Obana A, Shiraki K, Sakamoto T. 1993. Choroidal damage in dye-enhanced photocoagulation. Lasers Light Ophthalmol 5:157–165.

Matsumoto M, Yoshimura N, Honda Y. 1994. Increased production of transforming growth factor-b2 from cultures human retinal pigment epithelial cells by photocoagulation. Invest Ophthalmol Vis Sci 35:4245–4252.

McHugh JDA, Marshall J, Capon M, Rothery S, Raven A, Naylor RP. 1988. Transpupillary retinal photocoagulation in the eyes of rabbit and humans using a diode laser. Lasers Light Ophthalmol 2:125–143.

McHugh D, England C, Van der Zypen E, Marshall J, Fankhauser F, Fankhauser-Kwansnieska S. 1995. Irradiation of rabbit retina with diode and Nd:YAG lasers. Br J Ophthalmol 9:672–677.

Meyer-Schwickerath G. 1959. Indications and limitations of light coagulation of the retina. Trans Am Acad Ophthalmol Otolaryngol 63:725–738.

Miller JW, Walsh AW, Kramer M, Hasan T, Michaud N, Flotte TJ, Haimovici R, Gragoudas ES. 1995. Photodynamic therapy of experimental choroidal neovascularization using lipoprotein-delivered benzoporphyrin. Arch Ophthalmol 113:810–818.

[MPSG] Macular Photocoagulation Study Group. 1986. Argon laser photocoagulation for neovascular maculopathy: three-year results from randomized clinical trials. Arch Ophthalmol 104:694–701.

[MPSG] Macular Photocoagulation Study Group. 1991. Laser photocoagulation for subfoveal neovascular lesions of age related macular degeneration: results of a randomized clinical trial. Arch Ophthalmol 109:1219–1231.

Murphee AL, Cote M, Gomer CJ. 1987. The evolution of photodynamic therapy in the treatment of intraocular tumors. Photochem Photobiol 46:919–923.

Nelson JS, Liaw LH, Orenstein A. 1988. Mechanism of tumor destruction following photodynamic therapy with hematoporphyrin derivative, chlorin and phthalocyanine. J Nat Cancer Inst 80:1599–1605.

Ohkuma H, et al. 1983. Experimental subretinal neovascularization in the monkey: permeability of new vessels. Arch Ophthalmol 101:1102–1110.

Olk RJ. 1990. Argon green (514 nm) vs krypton red (647 nm) modified grid laser photocoagulation for diffuse diabetic macular edema. Ophthalmology 97:1101–1112.

Panagopoulos JA, Svitra PP, Puliafito CA, Gragoudas ES. 1989. Photodynamic therapy for experimental intraocular melanoma using chloroaluminum sulfonated phthalocyanine. Arch Ophthalmol 107:886–890.

Parrish JA, Deutsch TF. 1984. Laser photomedicine. IEEE J Quantum Electronics QE-20:1386–1396.

Peyman GA, Bok D. 1972. Perioxidase diffusion in the normal and laser-coagulated primate retina. Invest Ophthalmol Vis Sci 11:35–45.

Peyman GA, Li M, Yoneya S. 1981. Fundus photocoagulation with the argon and krypton lasers: a comparative study. Ophthalmic Surg 12:481–490.

Peyman GP, Conway MD, House B. 1983. Transpupillary CW YAG laser coagulation. A comparison with argon green and krypton red lasers. Ophthalmology 90:992–1002.

Peyman GA, Raichand M, Zeimer RC. 1984. Ocular effects of various laser wavelengths. Surv Ophthalmol 28:391–404.

Pollack A, Korte GE. 1990. Repair of the retinal pigment epithelium and its relationship with capillary endothelium after krypton laser photocoagulation. Invest Ophthalmol Vis Sci 31:890–898.

Pollack A, Korte GE. 1993. Restoration of the outer blood-retinal barrier after krypton laser photocoagulation. Ophthalmic Res 25:201–209.

Pomerantzeff O, Kaneko H, Donovan RH, Schepens CL, McMeel JW. 1976. Effect of the ocular media on the main wavelengths of argon laser emission. Invest Ophthalmol Vis Sci 15:70–77.

Pomerantzeff O, Wang GJ, Pankratov M, Schneider J. 1983. A method to determine correct photocoagulation dose. Arch Ophthalmol 101:949–953.

Powell JO, Bresnick GH, Yanoff M, Frisch GD, Chester JE. 1971. Ocular effects of argon laser radiation. II. Histopathology of chorioretinal lesions. Am J Ophthalmol 71:1267–1276.

Priebe LA, Cain CP, Welch AJ. 1975. Temperature rise required for the production of minimal lesions in the Macaca mulatta retina. Am J Ophthalmol 79:405–413.

Puliafito CA, Steinert RF. 1984. Short-pulsed Nd:YAG laser microsurgery of the eye: biophysical considerations. IEEE J Quantum Electronics QE-20:1442–1448.

Puliafito CA, Steinert RF, Deutsch TF, Hillenkamp F, Dehm EJ, Adler CM. 1985. Excimer laser ablation of the cornea and lens: experimental studies. Ophthalmology 92:741–748.

Puliafito CA, Deutsch TF, Boll J, To K. 1987. Semiconductor laser endophotocoagulation of the retina. Arch Ophthalmol 105:424–427.

Reichel E, Puliafito CA, Duker JS, Guyer DR. 1994. Indocyanine green dye-enhanced diode laser photocoagulation of poorly defined subfoveal choroidal neovascularization. Ophthalmic Surg 25:195–201.

Roider J, Michaud NA, Flotte TJ, Birngruber R. 1992. Response of the retinal pigment epithelium to selective photocoagulation. Arch Ophthalmol 110:1786–1792.

Roider J, Hillenkamp F, Flotte T, Birngruber R. 1993. Microphotocoagulation: selective effects of repetitive short laser pulses. Proc Natl Acad Sci USA 90:8643–8647.

Romanelli JF, Puliafito CA. 1990. Metabolic studies of dye laser retinal photocoagulation. Int Ophthalmol Clin 30:95–101.

Smiddy WE, Fine SL, Quigley HA, Hohman RM, Addicks EA. 1984a. Comparison of krypton and argon laser photocoagulation. Results of stimulated clinical treatment of primate retina. Am J Ophthalmol 102:1086–1092.

Smiddy WE, Fine SL, Green WR, Glaser BM. 1984b. Clinicopathologic correlation of krypton red, argon blue-green, and argon green laser photocoagulation in the human fundus. Retina 4:15–21.

Smiddy WE, Fine SL, Quigley HA, Hohman RM, Dunkelberger G. 1985. Simulated treatment of recurrent choroidal neovascularization in primate retina. Comparative histopathologic studies. Arch Ophthalmol 103:428–433.

Smiddy WE, Patz A, Quigley HA, Dunkelberger GR. 1988. Histopathology of the effects of tunable dye laser on the monkey retina. Ophthalmology 95:956–963.

Steinert RF, Puliafito CA. 1985. The Nd-YAG Laser in Ophthalmology: Principles and Clinical Applications of Photodisruption. Philadelphia: Saunders.

Swartz M. 1986. Histology of macular photocoagulation. Ophthalmology 93:959–963.

Thomas EL, Apple DJ, Swartz M, Kavka-Van Norman D. 1984. Histology and ultrastructure of krypton and argon laser lesions in human retina-choroid. Retina. 4:22–39.

Trempe CL, Mainster MA, Pomerantzeff O, Avila MO, Jalkh AE, Weiter JJ, McMeel JW, Schepens CL. 1982. Macular photocoagulation: optimal wavelength selection. Ophthalmology 89:721–729.

Tse DT, Dutton JJ, Weingeist TA, Hermsen VM, Kersten RC. 1984. Hematoporphyrin photoradiation therapy for intraocular and orbital malignant melanoma. Arch Ophthalmol 102:833–838.

Tso MO, Cunha-Vaz JG, Shih C, Jones CW. 1980. Clinicopathologic study of blood retinal barrier in experimental diabetes mellitus. Arch Ophthalmol 98:2032–2040.

Van der Zypen E. 1985. The use of laser in eye surgery: morphological principles. Int Ophthalmol Clin 26:21–52.

Vogel M, Schafer FP, Stuke M, Muller K, Theuring S, Morawietz A. 1989. Animal experiments for the determination of an optimal wavelength for retinal coagulations. Graefes Arch Clin Exp Ophthalmol 227:277–280.

Wallow IH. 1984. Repair of the pigment epithelial barrier following photocoagulation. Arch Ophthalmol 102:126–135.

Wallow IHL, Tso MOM. 1973. Repair after xenon arc photocoagulation: a clinical and light microscopic study of the evolution of retinal lesions in the rhesus monkey. Am J Ophthalmol 75:610–626.

Wieder M, Pomerantzeff O, Schneider J. 1981. Retinal vessel photocoagulation. A quantitative comparison of argon and krypton laser effects. Invest Ophthalmol Vis Sci 20:418–424.

Weingeist TA. 1974. Argon laser photocoagulation of the human retina. I. Histopathologic correlation of chorioretinal lesions in the region of the maculopapillar bundle. Invest Ophthalmol 13:1024–1032.

Weishaupt KR, Gomer CJ, Dougherty TJ. 1976. Identification of singlet oxygen as the cytotoxic agent in photo-inactivation of murine tumor. Cancer Res 36:2326–2329.

White TJ, Mainster MA, Wilson PW, Tips JH. 1971. Chorioretinal temperature increases from solar observation. Bull Math Biophys. 33:1–17.

Wolbarsht MT, Landers MB. 1980. The rationale of photocoagulation therapy for proliferative diabetic retinopathy a review and model. Ophthalmic Surg 11:235–245.

31. Pharmacology of the retinal pigment epithelium

THOMAS J. WOLFENSBERGER

In view of the manifold physiological roles of the retinal pigment epithelium (RPE), there are many different mechanisms by which RPE function can be modulated pharmacologically. Many compounds have been evaluated and used in studies on RPE physiology, and a few may be important clinically. The experimental modulation of ion and fluid transport across the RPE, for example (see Chapter 6), has led to new concepts about the treatment of intraretinal and subretinal fluid. Another expanding field of RPE pharmacology is concerned with the pharmacological inhibition of RPE proliferation in the treatment of proliferative vitreoretinopathy (see Chapter 23). This chapter will review the major drug classes that affect RPE function, and will consider clinical effects of these pharmacological agents where possible.

DRUG TARGETING TO THE RPE

The drug delivery to the posterior segment for the treatment of retinal pathologies has been the subject of several studies (Lee et al., 1989). It is even more problematic for a drug to be targeted specifically at the RPE. There exist two basic routes that may be taken to achieve this: either the drug can be applied directly to the cells (such as in cell cultures, or during surgery with subretinal injection), or it can be given systemically and carried to the RPE by the blood stream with the aim that it attaches itself preferentially to the RPE. Whether the active components of locally applied eyedrops reach the RPE by direct diffusion is still an area of debate. Recent studies on rabbit eyes showed that drug concentration in the retina was due to systemic absorption and redelivery, rather than direct diffusion of the drug (Conroy et al., 1994).

Of course, clinical systemic application of a drug to treat only the RPE is not highly efficient, and systemic side effects of the drug may have to be tolerated in the course of such a treatment. In view of these obstacles, special drug targeting directly to the RPE has been sought. One approach is the delivery of drugs encapsulated in biodegradable polylactide microspheres (Moritera et al., 1994) with intracellular drug release after phagocytosis by RPE cells (Kimura et al., 1994). It appears possible to control the release rate of drugs from these microspheres by changing the molecular weight of the polymer, which would make it possible to time the duration of a treatment. It has been reported, for example, that the microspheres may remain intracellularly for up to four weeks, although exocytosis of microspheres was observed thereafter (Ogura and Kimura, 1995).

Some drugs attach themselves preferentially to the RPE. A possible mechanism for this is affinity to melanin (Lindquist, 1973; Mason, 1977; Persad et al., 1986; Larsson, 1993). Especially polycyclic cationic compounds with a coplanar ring structure (phenothiazines, thioxanthenes, 4-aminoquinolines, and amitriptyline) (Larsson and Tjalve, 1979), monocyclic sympathomimetic amines, and other basic and hydrophobic drugs such as chlorpromazine, diethylstilbestrol, 19-nortestosterone, salbutamol, salicylic acid, and trenbolone (Howells et al., 1994), as well as beta adrenergic agonists (clenbuterol and salmeterol) and antagonists (propranolol and carazolol) (Sauer and Anderson, 1994) can bind firmly to melanin in the uvea and RPE. These binding properties of the drugs mentioned above have not been exploited pharmacologically to date (except as a concern over toxic effects), and melanin binding has proved to be a nonspecific effect without clear correlation with either enhanced pharmacological or toxicological action. An extended discussion of the different binding strategies of different drugs and metals can be found in the chapters on RPE toxicology (Chapter 32) and on the role of melanin in the RPE (Chapter 4).

ADRENERGIC AGENTS

The autonomous sympathomimetic nervous system contains two major receptor systems, alpha and beta, through which neural transmission is effected; both receptor types also express subtypes 1 and 2. The pharmacological modulation of these receptors in ophthalmology has been exploited mostly for effects on aqueous humor production and pupillary movements. Experimental studies have, however, suggested a direct effect

TABLE 31-1. *Adrenergic drugs modulating RPE function*

Alpha agonists
  Phenylephrine
  Epinephrine
Alpha antagonists
  Prazosin
Beta blockers
  Timolol
  Bisoprolol
  Propranolol
Adenylate cyclase activators
  Forskolin
  Isoproterenol

of adrenergic agents on the RPE (Table 31-1) given the presence of alpha-2 adrenergic receptors in the RPE of human eyes (Matsuo and Cynader, 1992; Horie et al., 1993; and Quinn and Miller, 1992), a receptor which has recently been identified as the alpha-2D subtype (Berlie et al., 1995). Retinal pigment epithelium in culture also expresses a distinct beta-2-adrenergic receptor which is coupled to adenylate cyclase (Koh and Chader, 1984; Tran, 1992), whose activators will also be discussed below. Similar receptors have also been found on cultured fetal human retinal pigment epithelium (Frambach et al., 1990). Pharmacologic modulation of the adrenergic system in the RPE has been implicated in the stimulation of fluid absorption across the RPE, and a more detailed account of these actions may be found in Chapter 6.

Alpha Receptor Agents

Alpha receptor agents such as *epinephrine* have been implicated in the modulation of K^+ and Cl^- transport across bovine RPE (Joseph and Miller, 1992), but the most interesting observation clinically has been the demonstration of epinephrine-stimulated fluid absorption across bovine RPE (Edelman and Miller, 1991). This increase in fluid absorption was completely abolished by addition of 1 μM of the alpha-1-adrenergic antagonist *prazosin*. These results must be reconciled with the evidence that increased serum levels of catecholamines seem to be related to the development of central serous chorioretinopathy and the accumulation of subretinal fluid (Yoshioka et al., 1982). The blood–retinal barrier (BRB) breakdown caused by catecholamines may not be mediated by direct adrenergic action but by stimulation of adenylate cyclase, given that epinephrine as well as *isoproterenol* and *norepi-*

nephrine have been shown to stimulate adenylate cyclase *and* cause transient intravitreous fluorescein leakage, whereas *phenylephrine,* an adrenergic agent that is a poor stimulator of adenylate cyclase, caused only minimal leakage (Sen and Campochiaro, 1991).

Beta Receptor Agents

In the context of the evaluation of cAMP as a potent inhibitor of RPE cell migration, timolol has been shown to block the isoproterenol-induced stimulation of RPE adenylate cyclase, and the drug attenuated the ability of isoproterenol to inhibit RPE migration (Hackett et al., 1986). Despite the accumulation of beta-adrenergic agents at the level of the outer blood–retinal barrier, an accumulation that may be linked to melanin affinity, other effects of these drugs on the RPE are not known. High concentrations of bisoprolol, for example, were detected in pigmented ocular structures of the beagle after 4 weeks of conjunctival and oral administration of the drug (Steiner et al., 1990) with a half-time of about 7 days. Other beta blockers such as timolol and befunolol show similar half lives of melanin binding, although the clinical implications of this effect are not known.

Adenylate Cyclase Activators

Forskolin has been known for several years as a potent stimulator of adenylate cyclase activity in the RPE (Miller and Farber, 1984), and given the central role of this enzyme in cell metabolism, its effect on RPE physiology are manifold. The drug has been shown to inhibit phagocytosis of latex particles by chick (Ogino et al., 1984) and rat RPE (Hall et al., 1993), as well as the uptake of retinal outer segments by cultured human RPE cells (Miceli and Newsome, 1994). This forskolin-induced cAMP increase was more markedly reduced in RPE cells from Royal College of Surgeons (RCS) rat than in controls, suggesting a defect in the adenylyl cyclase signaling pathway in dystrophic RPE cells (Gregory et al., 1992). A similar drop in forskolin-induced increase of cAMP has been demonstrated in the presence of melatonin (Nash and Osborne, 1995). Forskolin has also been implicated in the blockage of thrombin-induced intercellular gap formation in confluent cultured bovine retinal pigment, which suggests that this effect is mediated at least in part through a cAMP-dependent pathway (Sakamoto et al., 1994). Other observed effects after application of forskolin include the induction of pigment aggregation in the teleost RPE, which could not be suppressed by inhibitors of organic anion transport like probenecid and sulfinpyrazone

(Burnside et al., 1982; Burnside and Basinger, 1983; Garcia and Burnside, 1994), and the increase of insulin-like growth-factor-binding protein secretion (Feldman and Randolph, 1994). Forskolin also induces several electropysiological RPE-specific responses (Hughes and Segawa, 1993; Kuntz et al., 1994), which are discussed in detail in Chapters 9 and 10.

ANTIINFLAMMATORY DRUGS

Corticosteroids

Corticosteroids modulate cellular metabolism by acting on a nuclear receptor in the RPE (He, 1994), and their role in the modulation of RPE function seems to be twofold. On one hand, these agents may be beneficial in the prevention of light-induced retinal and RPE damage, and on the other, they may suppress RPE proliferation, an effect that has gained importance in the treatment of proliferative vitreoretinopathy.

Methylprednisolone, for example, was shown to be beneficial in argon-laser-induced retinal injury (Lam et al., 1993) if the treatment of 5.4 mg/kg/hour was started just before the treatment and continued for at least 4 days. Methylprednisolone has therefore also been investigated in the use for the treatment of solar retinopathy. A dose of 160 mg/kg/day was more effective in preserving the photoreceptor and RPE layer than in controls (Rosner et al., 1992). *Dexamethasone* has also shown a potential role in the amelioration of photic injury in albino rats, an effect that may be mediated through inhibition of lipid peroxidation (Fu et al., 1992). After daily doses of 1 mg/kg/day starting 1 day before the light damage and lasting for 3 days, structural damage to the retina and light-induced vacuolization of the RPE was markedly reduced.

The corticosteroid's more important role, however, is found in the modulation of RPE proliferation. The repairing processes of RPE after photocoagulation with krypton red laser, for example, was markedly inhibited in monkeys with intramuscular *betamethasone* (0.5 mg/kg) administered every day for 1–14 days, and no metaplasia of RPE cells into fibroblast-like cells was observed (Kishimoto et al., 1993). This effect of steroids is being studied in the treatment of proliferative vitreoretinopathy, and treatment with *methylprednisolone* has been shown for example to suppress RPE platelet-derived growth factor (PDGF) gene expression during experimental PVR (Cousins et al., 1996). Steroid treatment also slows the accumulation of PDGF mRNA under detached retina and prevents PDGF gene activation from spreading to the RPE under attached retina. Simi-

lar suppressive effects on RPE cell proliferation have recently been shown for *dexamethasone* (Koutsandra et al., 1991) and *hydrocortisone* (Chiba et al., 1993). These antiproliferative effects stand, however, in contrast to other in vitro observations, which showed no effect on cell growth in cultures of rabbit RPE (Fiscella et al., 1985; Campochiaro and Glaser, 1986; He, 1994) and in chick RPE (La Rocca and Rafferty, 1982), and it is not known whether this is a species-dependent phenomenon.

There is also an isolated report on a suppressive effect of dexamethasone on urokinase and plasminogen activator inhibitor-1 messenger RNA levels in RPE cells, which may have implications for the role of the RPE in the regulation of choroidal neovascularization (Hackett and Campochiaro, 1993).

Nonsteroidal Antiinflammatory Drugs

The major roles of nonsteroidal antiinflammatory drugs on the RPE seem to be the suppression of phagocytosis and the modulation of prostaglandin-mediated immune responses at the level of the RPE (see Chapter 26). *Aspirin* as well as *indomethacin* have been shown to reduce the ability of the bovine RPE to phagocytose latex particles labeled with iodinie-125, as measured by the gamma emissions from the RPE cup (Goldhar et al., 1984). Furthermore, daily administration of acetyl salicylic acid and *ibuprofen* have been demonstrated to lead to an appreciable retardation in the process of retinal degeneration in the RCS rat, an effect which is dose dependent. Phagolysosomal structures which are not otherwise apparent in this strain of rats are detected only in the RPE cells of animals treated with high doses (el-Hifnawi et al., 1992).

Further studies have demonstrated that nonsteroidal antiinflammatory agents profoundly, but reversibly, suppress lymphocyte proliferation to antigen, mitogen, and interleukin (IL-2) stimulation in an in vitro system of RPE cells. Indomethacin restored proliferative responses of cocultured lymphocytes to specific antigens and mitogens, and it was suggested that the soluble component of suppression was mediated in part by prostaglandin (PGE_2) production by the RPE (Liversidge et al., 1993). Further studies on the effect of cytokines and prostaglandins revealed that PGE_1, PGE_2, and PGF_2 alpha suppressed RPE cell growth, whereas indomethacin did not affect the spontaneous RPE cell growth at 10^{-7}–10^{-9} M. However, 10^{-7} M indomethacin enhanced RPE cell growth stimulated by cytokines synergistically, an enhancement which could be blocked by addition of PGF_2 alpha. RPE cells stimulated by cytokines produced PGF_2. These results suggest that RPE cells produce prostaglandins, which have a negative regulatory role in RPE cell growth (Kishi et al., 1994). Disruption of the outer blood–retinal barrier, causing the liberation of prostaglandins which induce an inflammatory reaction, has been demonstrated in cystoid macular edema after cataract extraction and in traumatic retinal edema. Cyclooxygenase inhibitors such as indomethacin may reduce the production of the prostaglandins and maintain the patency of the blood–retinal barrier. Topical administration of these drugs has been widely used clinically in these disorders.

Immunosuppressive Drugs

Cyclosporine has been used for the treatment of different general autoimmune disorders as well as in the therapy of uveitis. Apart from delaying histopathological changes at the level of the RPE in spontaneous posterior uveitis (Fite et al., 1986), the drug has also been shown to influence MHC II antigen expression of cultured RPE cells (Liversidge et al., 1988). Recently, cyclosporine has been introduced successfully as an adjunct in the prevention of RPE transplant rejection (Gouras et al., 1992; Sheng et al., 1995). A recent report also investigated the effects of long-term treatment with cyclosporine. Biodegradable nanoparticles as a controlled release device for cyclosporine have also been investigated to prevent RPE xenograft rejection after transplantation, which allows the achievement of therapeutic levels without toxic high initial peaks of the drug (Rodriguez-Ares et al., 1995).

ALDOSEREDUCTASE INHIBITORS

Glucose-induced sugar alcohol (sorbitol) accumulation is mediated by aldose reductase and its intracellular accumulation has been invoked in the pathogenesis of retinal diabetic complications. Aldose reductase inhibitors, such as *sorbinil*, have therefore been evaluated for the prevention of such pathologies. The drug can inhibit polyol synthesis in human RPE cells (Reddy et al., 1992; Nakamura et al., 1994) and block glucose induced time- and dose-dependent increases in sorbitol content and decreases in myoinositol (Del Monte et al., 1991). Treatment with sorbinil has also been shown to partly prevent thickening of the basal laminae and vacuolization of the RPE, as well as preventing outer blood–retinal barrier breakdown in diabetic and galactosemic rats (Vinores and Campochiaro, 1989; Vinores et al., 1990). Furthermore, treatment with sorbinil arrested the deterioration of the RPE-generated c-wave in the electroretinogram (ERG) of diabetic rats (MacGregor and Matschinsky, 1985). Whether aldose reductase inhibitors will be useful in man is not yet determined.

ANTIOXIDANTS AND VITAMINS

In the past few years, public interest in antioxidants and vitamins has grown immensely, and their use in the prevention of disease has been investigated extensively. Furthermore, different vitamins have been evaluated as prophylactic treatment for several dystrophic disorders of the retina and the RPE (Table 31-2), although there is no conclusive evidence that they are of clinical benefit.

Vitamins

The role of the lipid-soluble *vitamin A* in the modulation of RPE function is complex. Of prime importance is its metabolism in the RPE for the regeneration of rhodopsin, which is well documented (Bok, 1993). An in-depth study of this action is provided in Chapter 7 of this volume. Another function of vitamin A also seems to be to influence the amount of lipofuscin granules accumulating in the RPE (Robison et al., 1982). In this context evidence was put forward that dietary vitamin A (in the metabolizable form of retinyl palmitate, but not in the form of retinoid acid, which does not support visual function) is directly involved in RPE lipofuscin fluorophore formation (Katz and Norberg, 1992). Dietary supplementation to combat retinal dystrophies seems not to be significantly beneficial, since vitamin A treatment (50,000 IU/d for 14 days) could not shorten the dark adaptation in Stargardt's dystrophy (Glenn et al., 1994) and excessive vitamin A ingestion had little, if any, effect on RPE retinyl ester content or composition (Katz et al., 1987). A large masked trial on the treatment of retinitis pigmentosa (Berson et al., 1993) showed only a very small effect that has been questioned

TABLE 31-2. *Vitamins and antioxidants modulating RPE function*

Vitamins
    Vitamin A
    Ascorbate
    Vitamin E
Antioxidants
    Selenium
    Superoxide dismutase
    Catalase
    Mannitol
    Beta-carotene
    Centrophenoxine

by others (Norton et al., 1993). Vitamin A also seems to have antiproliferative effects. In an in vitro wound-healing experiment, 5–20 μ/ml vitamin A significantly inhibited wound closure by reducing cell migration and proliferation (Verstraeten et al., 1992). Similar doses of vitamin A also inhibited cell contractility, and indirect immunofluorescence patterns of fibronectin, actin, tubulin, and vimentin were altered after exposure to vitamin A. All these effects were reversible after removal of the drug. *Ascorbate* (vitamin C) acts as an antioxidant in the retina, where it scavenges superoxide radicals and hydroxyl radicals, quenches singlet oxygen and reduces hydrogen peroxide, all of which are formed in retinal photic injury. Vitamin C–deficient animals have been shown to exhibit much more severe retinal photic damage than normal animals, and it was suggested that the basic mechanism by which ascorbate mitigates retinal photic injury depends on its redox properties (Tso, 1987; Li et al., 1985). Furthermore, it has been shown in a rat model that ascorbate treatment prevents accumulation of phagosomes in RPE in light damage (Blanks et al., 1992). The antioxidant *vitamin E* is found in considerable concentration in the outer segments to minimize autooxidative damage. Vitamin E deficiency can thus lead to a retinopathy which has been described in different species (Riis et al., 1981; Robison et al., 1979) and in man (Berger et al., 1991). The deficiency induces disintegration of rod outer segment membranes and accelerates the accumulation of aging pigments in the RPE. Addition of vitamin E to the culture medium of bovine RPE cells also prevented the loss of phagocytic activity induced by free radicals (Becquet et al., 1994). Despite the fact that vitamin E has been shown to accumulate in RPE over time (Organisciak et al., 1987), dietary vitamin E supplements do not appear to provide significant protection of the retina from light damage (Robison et al., 1982). Vitamin E has also been shown to inhibit RPE cell proliferation in vitro (Mojon et al., 1994), with a maximal inhibition at 100 μM. Given that supplemental oral administration of vitamin E can raise the RPE concentration of alpha-tocopherol well above this level, and in view of the fact that supplementation is not associated with any clinically relevant adverse effect, it was suggested that vitamin E could be beneficial in the treatment of PVR. Vitamin E has also been shown to delay the onset of melanin-antigen-induced experimental autoimmune anterior uveitis (EAAU) (Broekhuyse et al., 1993) although the mechanism involved is not clear.

Other Antioxidants

The RPE has been reported to be particularly sensitive to in vivo lipid peroxidation linked to experimental an-

tioxidant deficiencies, and pharmacological supplementation has been beneficial. *Selenium* deficiency, for example, led to a large decrease in polyunsaturated fatty acids in the RPE, a small decrease in the retinal rod outer segments but no change in the liver when compared to tissues from animals fed the selenium-supplemented control diet. These results suggest that changes in fatty acid composition are not generalized to all tissues in severely antioxidant-deficient animals (Farnsworth et al., 1979). The large decrease of fatty acids in the RPE has also been shown to appear parallel to the accumulation of a yellow autofluorescent pigment generally thought to be indicative of membrane autooxidation (Katz et al., 1978). The autofluorescence produced in the RPE by antioxidant deficiency was again more concentrated than autofluorescence produced in other organs of the body, suggesting that the RPE is particularly sensitive to physiological antioxidant deficiencies. Further ultrastructural studies of selenium-deficient rats showed a decreased number of inner nuclear layer nuclei, although photoreceptor nuclei were kept normal in number. After 1.5 years there was prominent decrease in photoreceptor cells but no increase of lipofuscin granules in the RPE (Amemiya, 1985). *Superoxide dismutase* (SOD) occurs in all cells exposed to an oxygen-containing environment, including the RPE. The enzyme is present in two distinct species located in the cytosol and the mitochondria (Newsome et al., 1990), and its role lies in the control of reactive oxygen radicals that can harm cells. The beneficial effect of SOD on the RPE is twofold. On one hand, it has been shown, along with *catalase,* to prevent blue-light-induced (425–500 nm at 42 J/cm^2) inhibition of growth of RPE cells in vitro, providing evidence of a photooxidative mechanism (Dorey et al., 1990). Addition of SOD, as well as catalase, also caused significant improvement in growth of porcine RPE cells but had no significant effects on bovine RPE cells (Akeo et al., 1992). On the other hand, intravenous injection of SOD (10,000 IU/kg) induces total recovery of the c-wave after 30 minutes of ischemia in the cat (Yamamoto et al., 1994), compared with 50% recovery in the untreated eyes. High levels of SOD may also protect mitochondria from oxidative damage (Oliver and Newsome, 1992). *Mannitol* is both an osmotic agent and a free-radical scavenger, and intravenous injection of this drug has been shown to minimize ischemic damage to the RPE and the retina in a rabbit model (Gupta and Marmor, 1993). A similar antiischemic effect could be obtained with the injection of catalase in rabbit (Gupta and Marmor, 1993) and in cat (Yamamoto et al., 1994). Mannitol has also been shown to increase retinal adhesiveness in vitro (Yao et al., 1991) (see Chapter 19), and the compound is also used to elicit nonphotic responses in the EOG for the diagnosis of RPE pathologies (see

Chapter 10). Alteration of macular pigment optical density (MPOD) is a potential therapeutic approach to preventing retinal degenerative disease. Recently, it has been shown that by adding *beta-carotene*-rich foods to the diet xanthophylls responded and MPOD increased significantly from baseline (Edwards et al., 1996). Confirmation of such a possible effect has also come from a study in rats which demonstrated a sharp increase in beta-carotene levels in the RPE (35 times higher than in the retina) after supplementation (Rapp et al., 1996). *Centrophenoxine* had held much promise as an antioxidant agent that could potentially slow the formation of lipofuscin formation in vivo, especially in neurons of lower mammals. However, the accumulation of lipofuscin could not be prevented in a monkey model by addition of 80 mg/kg of centrophenoxine (Andrews and Brizzee, 1986), and even the ultrastructure of lipofuscin granules stayed the same (Katz and Robison, 1983). The development of the lipofuscin-like inclusions in an in vitro model could also not be halted by the addition of this drug (Boulton et al., 1989).

ANTIPROLIFERATIVE DRUGS

The RPE has been shown–among other cells such as glia and macrophages—to play an important role in membrane formation associated with proliferative vitreoretinopathy (PVR) (see Chapter 24). These RPE cells undergo a transformation into fibroblast-like cells which can proliferate and contract, leading ultimately to retinal traction and detachment (see chapter 24). Apart from surgical excision and peeling of these membranes, several agents have been evaluated experimentally to curb proliferative activity of these cells (Table 31-3). Most pharmacologic compounds thus investigated in the treatment of experimental PVR are water-soluble drugs. Given that surgical excision of these membranes is often combined with silicon oil tamponade of the reti-

TABLE 31-3. *Antiproliferative drugs modulating RPE function*

BCNU
Crovidisin
Interferon beta
Proteinkinase C inhibitors
Aclacinomycin
Mitomycin
Thiotepa
5-FU
Hypericin
Retinoic acid
Colchicine

na, the use of these hydrophilic drugs may be limited in these cases, although recently a lipophilic agent, carmustine (*BCNU*), has been developed (Chung et al., 1988).

Generally speaking, the effect of antiproliferative agents of RPE physiology may be mediated by several different mechanisms. On one hand, the agent may inhibit RPE-mediated collagen adhesion and vitreous contraction, as was shown for a collagen-binding snake venom protein, crovidisin, which in an in vitro assay could inhibit bovine RPE-cell-mediated collagen adhesion and vitreous contraction (Yang et al., 1996). On the other hand, the antiproliferative effect may also be mediated by affecting the proliferative cell cycle as well as the synthesis of growth factors and their receptors. Most antiproliferative agents fall into this category, and the biggest group is represented by the classic antineoplastic drugs that have been used widely in oncology. There are several other less well known antiproliferative agents with inhibitory effects on RPE, which have been summarized in Table 31-4.

Daunomycin has been described as having cytotoxic effects on the RPE in vitro (Weller et al., 1987) and may be useful in the pharmacological treatment of human proliferative retinopathy (Wiedemann et al., 1989; Mietz et al., 1994). However, since it has a very narrow therapeutic safety range, its delivery to the posterior pole is difficult (Rahimy et al., 1994). In view of associated important side effects, such as a sharp increase of histone-associated DNA fragments in the RPE as an indicator of apoptosis (Lebek et al., 1996), focus has recently shifted to better-tolerated drugs.

Aclacinomycin A is an anthracycline that, by contrast to daunomycin, lacks carcinogenicity, and it is less toxic to the retina than daunomycin. It has been used for the treatment of acute myeloblastic leukemia but may hold some promise in treating PVR. A recent in vitro study of RPE cell culture showed that a single exposure of the cells to aclacinomycin A for five minutes at a concentration of 5 μg/ml appears sufficient to achieve long-term inhibition of in vitro cell proliferation without destroying the cell population completely (Schmidt and Löffler, 1995). *Doxorubicin* (Adriamycin) has also been reported to be a very efficient chemotherapeutic agent to inhibit cellular proliferation of rabbit RPE cells (Fiscella, 1985) without inducing toxic changes in the retina (Vernot et al., 1985; Barrada et al., 1984). Doxorubicin encapsulated in biodegradable microspheres, which may reduce the toxicity of the drug even further, has also been investigated for the treatment of PVR (Moritera et al., 1992). A derivative of doxorubicin, called *N,N-dimethyladriamycin,* exhibits even less mutagenicity and carcinogenicity than the parent compound. Its suitability for treatment of PVR has been

TABLE 31-4. *Other drugs with antiproliferative effects on the RPE*

Agent	Effect	Species	Reference
Interferon beta	In vitro inhibition of RPE proliferation	Human	Yamada et al., 1995
	In vivo tightening of blood retinal barrier	Human	Gillies, 1996
Staurosporine	RPE Proteinkinase C	Human	Hirakata et al., 1996
Hypericine	Inhibition in vitro with antiproliferative effect	Human	Harris et al., 1995
Ciprofloxacin	In vitro inhibition of RPE proliferation	Human	Koutsandrea et al., (1991)
Retionoic acid	In vitro inhibition of RPE proliferation	Human	Kothary and Del Monte (1995)
Cytochalasin B	In vitro inhibition of RPE proliferation	Chick Bovine	Crawford, 1979 Verstraeten et al., 1990 Campochiaro and Glaser, 1986

evaluated in experimental studies where antiproliferative effects were observed with no ultrastructural retinal and RPE damage (Steinhorst et al., 1993).

5-Fluorouracil has also been shown to inhibit migration and proliferation of RPE cells in vitro completely (10 µg/ml) (Verstraeten et al., 1990). Similar data was obtained from fluorouridine, an intracellular metabolite of fluorouracil, which is nearly 100 times more potent than fluorouracil and its deoxymetabolite (Blumen-kranz et al., 1987). Recent investigations have demonstrated that 5-FU in a concentration of 10 mg/ml for 5 days caused marked inhibition of cultured human RPE for at least 14 days after stopping the treatment (DeLuca et al., 1995). RPE monolayers were also exposed to single 30-minute treatments of either 5-FU or thiotepa, both of which significantly inhibited the proliferation of RPE cells and the contraction of collagen lattices containing RPE cells at concentrations above 0.25 mg/ml and 0.06 mg/ml, respectively (Kon et al., 1996). Intravitreal injection of 0.375 and 1.0 mg of 5-FU has been shown to be well tolerated by the normal retina in a rabbit model (Vernot et al., 1985), whereas a combination of 250 µg 5-FU with 0.15 or 0.1 µg vincristine caused toxic effects (Barrada et al., 1984). Long-term application of *mitomycin* on cultured human RPE at a concentration of 34.0 ng/ml for 5 days caused marked inhibition of cultured human RPE for at least 14 days after stopping the treatment (Lin et al., 1996; Cardillo et al., 1996). *Colchicine,* which blocks cytoskeleton assembly, is also a potent inhibitor of RPE cell migration (Campochiaro and Glaser, 1986; Lemor et al., 1986a). The ensuing in vivo studies of experimental PVR in rabbits could also demonstrate a decreased incidence and severity of traction retinal detachment in animals receiving oral colchicine (Lemor et al., 1986b). However, there was no therapeutic effect of colchicine on

proliferative vitreoretinopathy in a clinical study (Berman and Gambos, 1989).

CALCIUM CHANNEL BLOCKERS

The calcium channel blockers have been widely employed in cardiology, and *verapamil, nifedipin,* and *diltiazem* have also been used to characterize calcium conductances in normal rat RPE and in the RCS rat (Strauss et al., 1993; Strauss et al., 1994; Ramachandran et al., 1993). An L-type calcium channel in the rat RPE was postulated with an increased membrane conductance for calcium in the RCS rat, and calcium antagonists were able to block these channels in micromolar concentrations. A detailed discussion of these calcium channels can be found in Chapter 6.

Calcium antagonists and drugs such as *minoxidil,* a hypertensive agent, may in the future also be useful in the treatment of proliferative diseases such as PVR and bleb scarring after trabeculectomy. *Verapamil* significantly inhibits human fetal RPE cell growth in a dose-dependent manner with concentrations equivalent to a clinically therapeutic dose of the drug (Hoffmann et al., 1996), whereas verapamil and *diltiazem* have also been shown to significantly inhibit gel contraction by rabbit RPE, and tritiated thymidine uptake showed significant dose-related inhibition of cell proliferation (Hahn et al., 1996). Minoxidil has also been shown to suppress proliferation of cultured human RPE cells (Handa et al., 1993; 1994). The antiproliferative effect of two slightly altered compounds, which do not exhibit antihypertensive effects, called 3'-hydroxyminoxidil (0.25 mM) and 4'-hydroxyminoxidil (0.5 mM) persisted even after the drug was removed from the culture medium.

DIURETICS

Carbonic Anhydrase Inhibitors

The effect of carbonic anhydrase (CA) inhibitors on transepithelial fluid transport has been known for several decades. The discovery of the CA enzyme in the ciliary body by Wistrand in 1955 led to one of the major discoveries in ophthalmology, the suppression of aqueous humor production with CA inhibition (Becker, 1954). Given the known role of the RPE in fluid transport, several authors have since then investigated the effects of CA inhibitors on the outer blood–retinal barrier. Electrophysiologic data on CA activity in the RPE was recorded as early as twenty years ago with the detection of the transepithelial potential (TEP) changes in the frog after application of the lipophilic carbonic anhydrase (CA) inhibitor *acetazolamide* (Miller and Steinberg, 1977) (further details see Chapter 9). More recently the drug has been shown to enhance subretinal fluid absorption and retinal adhesiveness (Marmor and Maack, 1982; Marmor et al., 1980; Tsuboi and Pederson, 1987), as well as improve cystoid macular edema (CME) from various etiologies (Cox et al., 1988; Fishman et al., 1989; Chen et al., 1990; Marmor, 1990). However, its clinical use is limited by frequent and bothersome side effects (Lichter, 1981). The underlying mechanisms for the action of CA inhibitors is still not entirely clear, but given that acetazolamide decreases the pH in the subretinal space of the cat (Yamamoto and Steinberg, 1992) and the chick (Wolfensberger et al., 1996), volume changes may be preceded by local changes in acid–base balance that influence transport capacity (Edelman et al., 1994).

As mentioned above, acetazolamide is lipophilic, and thus readily diffusing through cell membranes into the cytosol of cells (Travis et al., 1964). The well-known systemic side effects are thought to be a result of inhibiting intracellular CA isoenzymes (Travis, 1969), which represents the bulk of CA enzyme in the body (Dodgson, 1991). However, intracellular CA seems not to play a major role in RPE function, since the membrane-bound form of CA (CA IV) is the predominant isozyme in the human RPE (Wolfensberger et al., 1994). Since fluid transport from the subretinal space to the choroid (which is driven to a large extent by active ion transport through the RPE [Negi and Marmor; 1986; Frambach and Marmor, 1982]) can be enhanced experimentally by acetazolamide, membrane-bound CA may be instrumental in this process. This suggests that treatment with a membrane-limited CA inhibitor may be sufficient to elicit effects on subretinal fluid transport similar to the ones induced by acetazolamide, and may

avoid systemic side effects from intracellular CA inhibition. *Benzolamide* (CL 11,366) is a hydrophilic CA inhibitor which does *not* readily penetrate the cell membrane due to its very high degree of ionization (Travis et al., 1964), thus it is believed to act predominantly upon membrane-bound CA. The drug is almost completely ionized at physiologic pH (pK = 3.2) and is poorly lipid soluble with a very low ether partition coefficient. Acetazolamide, in contrast, is readily lipid soluble with a much higher ether partition coefficient, which allows it to enter the lipid bilayer of the cell membrane easily (Travis et al., 1964). This property of benzolamide severely restricts its diffusibility across biologic membranes, and in particular across a polarized epithelial cell layer (Wistrand et al., 1960). On this basis the drug has been used to differentiate intracellular from extracellular CA inhibition in vivo (Travis et al., 1964) and in vitro (Saarikoski and Kaila, 1992). Benzolamide has been shown to have a qualitatively similar effect as the lipophilic acetazolamide on the enhancement of subretinal fluid absorption, retinal adhesiveness, and acidification of the subretinal space (Wolfensberger et al., 1995; 1996), which suggests that inhibition of membrane-bound CA inhibitor may be sufficient for these RPE-mediated effects. This confirms previous findings that intracellular CA may not play a role in this RPE function (Wolfensberger et al., 1994), and it might be, therefore, advantageous clinically if one could use a membrane-acting CA inhibitor like benzolamide, that had the desired effects on RPE function and on intraocular pressure without incurring side effects from intracellular CA inhibition.

Acetazolamide has also been shown to enhance the strength of retinal adhesion (measured as the percentage of peeled retina covered by RPE pigment) which usually drops from 100% immediately after enucleation to half within a few minutes (Endo et al., 1988). However, eyes from animals given intravenous acetazolamide (20 mg/kg) or benzolamide (20 mg/kg) 30 minutes before enucleation showed a slower rate of adhesive failure. This protective effect was most accentuated after a very high dose of benzolamide (50 mg/kg), which preserved nearly 85% pigment adherence 2.5 minutes after enucleation (Wolfensberger et al., 1995). Metabolic factors contribute to retinal adhesion, presumably through the enhancement of active fluid transport of subretinal fluid (Marmor et al., 1980; Kita and Marmor 1992a). It is likely that CA inhibitors act upon this mechanism through inhibition of CA at the basolateral cell membrane, since acetazolamide administered to the apical side of the RPE has no apparent effect on retinal adhesion both in vivo (Kita and Marmor, 1992a) and in vitro (Marmor et al., 1980; Endo et al., 1988), whereas intravenous injection of the drug enhances adhesiveness (Marmor and Maack, 1982; Endo et al., 1988; Kita and Marmor 1992b).

Loop Diuretics

Furosemide is a diuretic that inhibits the active resorption of sodium and chloride in the ascending limb of Henle's loop. The compound has been used extensively to study RPE physiology, and furosemide-sensitive Na^+-dependent Cl^- flux across the apical membrane of the RPE in the chick and frog was described several years ago (Frambach and Misfeldt, 1983; DiMattio et al., 1983; Wiederholt and Zadunaisky, 1984). While this flux could not be observed in rabbit RPE (Frambach et al., 1988), further studies on bovine RPE showed a reduction of transepithelial potential without affecting the resistance when applied to the apical side of the RPE, but no effect when applied to the basal side of the preparation (Frambach et al., 1989a). Despite the promising effect of the other diuretics, such as carbonic anhydrase inhibitors, furosemide seems to have an inhibitory effect on trans-RPE flow of fluid and Cl^- in the isolated dog RPE (Tsuboi et al., 1986; Tsuboi, 1987), in a model of experimental retinal detachment in cynomolgous monkeys (Tsuboi and Pederson, 1986), and in frog RPE (La Cour, 1992). Recent in vivo studies have also shown a decrease in retinal adhesive force after subretinal injection of furosemide in rabbits (Kita and Marmor, 1992b).

Amiloride, an inhibitor of the Na^+/H^+ exchanger, has a similar action as the loop diuretics; it not only inhibits the *resorption* of sodium, chloride, and water, but also the potassium *secretion* in the distal tubule. This drug has been shown to diminish the TEP of the rabbit RPE without affecting the electrical resistance (Frambach et al., 1988), although the drug had no effect when applied to either surface of the chick RPE (Frambach and Misfeldt, 1983). Furthermore, amiloride has been used to characterize trans-RPE ion flow (Khatami, 1990), cell volume regulation (Civan, 1994), and intracellular pH regulation (Lin and Miller, 1991; Lin et al., 1992) (see Chapter 6). Similarly to furosemide, in vivo subretinal injection of amiloride has been shown in the rabbit to decrease retinal adhesiveness (Kita and Marmor, 1992b).

DOPAMINERGIC SYSTEM

Dopamine and its antagonists have been used mainly in the modulation of RPE function in respect to electrophysiological recordings (Gallemore and Steinberg,

1990) as well as in the modulation of circadian rhythms of illumination-associated changes in the morphology of RPE cells of lower vertebrates (Dearry and Burnside, 1986). The retinae of these animals undergo a number of structural changes during light adaptation, including the dispersion of melanin granules into processes of the pigment epithelium that extend between photoreceptors, a process called pigment screening. Under photopic conditions the pigment migrates vitreally, in the dark-adapted state it aggregates sclerally. The application of dopamine, as well as of serotonin (which is thought to increase endogenous dopamine release), to dark-adapted retinae has been reported to produce the same morphological changes that are characteristic of light adaptation (Dearry and Burnside, 1986; 1988; 1989). These effects can be blocked by the dopamine receptor antagonists *haloperidol* and *sulpiride* in goldfish RPE (Ball et al., 1993), suggesting that dopamine acting on D2 receptors is sufficient to induce pigment migration. Similar results have been obtained in isolated teleost (Garcia and Burnside, 1994) and in frog RPE (Dearry et al., 1990). For further details of the action of dopamine on RPE function the reader is referred to Chapters 3, and 6.

METABOLIC INHIBITORS

This group of agents encompasses several different drugs which have been used to evaluate RPE physiology (Table 31-5), although a few of them may also be important clinically in the future.

Ion Transport Blocker

Ion transport blockers have been used extensively to characterize the physiology of the RPE cells, and an extensive discussion of these agents can be found in Chapter 6. From a clinical standpoint the most interesting effects of these compounds concern changes in transepithelial fluid absorption. Although these drugs have been very useful in determining certain mechanisms of RPE-modulated fluid transport, they have not yet found a pharmacological application in clinical terms.

Bumetanide is a blocker of $Na^+K^+2Cl^-$ channels that has been widely used in the characterization of ion flux in the RPE of different species (Joseph and Miller, 1991; Quinn and Miller 1992; Kennedy, 1992). Epinephrine-induced stimulation of fluid absorption across bovine RPE, for example, can be inhibited by apical bumetanide (0.1 mM), suggesting that the mechanisms underlying fluid absorption include an apical bumetanide-inhibitable membrane Na^+-K^--$2Cl^-$ cotransporter (Edelman and Miller, 1991). The observation

TABLE 31-5. *Metabolic inhibitors modulating RPE function*

Ion transport blocker
  Bumetanide
  Ouabain
  Barium
  Tetrodotoxin
IPM modulators
  β-D-xylopyranoside
Metabolic inhibitors
  Cyanide
  Dinitrophenol
  Strychnine
Organic acid transport inhibitors
  Probenecid
  Hippurate
  Iodipamide
Phosphodiesterase inhibitors
  Aminophylline
  Methylxanthine
Protease inhibitors
  Leupeptin
  Pepstatin
Oligosacharide synthesis
  Tunicamycin
  Swainsonine

that increased trans-RPE Cl^- absorption after HCO_3^- removal from the bathing media was also inhibited by apical bumetanide has undergirded this hypothesis (Edelman et al., 1994). Bumetanide has also been shown to inhibit the increase in active K^+ absorption in the RPE induced by barium and epidermal growth factor (Miller and Edelman, 1990; Arrindell et al., 1992).

Ouabain has been known for many years as a potent inhibitor of Na^+-K^+-ATPase. In contrast to most other polarized epithelial cells in the body, the RPE expresses the $Na^+/K^+/ATPase$ on the apical membrane, and ouabain labeling has thus been used as an indicator of pump site, number, and distribution of the apical membranes of RPE cells (Burke, 1991a). Given the importance of the Na^+-K^+-ATPase for cell survival, the effects of ouabain on RPE physiology and biochemistry are crucial. The drug may decrease the outward permeability of fluorescein (Koyano et al., 1993) and ascorbic acid (DiMattio and Streitman, 1991), suggesting an active mechanism for outward transport dependent on Na^+-K^+-ATPase. Ouabain has also been shown to increase retinal adhesiveness (Kita and Marmor, 1992), but this may be a result of cellular swelling from sodium pump

dysfunction (Marmor and Yao, 1989). Ouabain can also inhibit myoinositol accumulation in the RPE (Khatami, 1990). Electrophysiological investigations have demonstrated an irreversible ouabain-induced depolarization of the apical membrane (Griff, 1990a), as well as a decrease in the TEP (Hu et al., 1994).

Barium has also been used to block K^+ conductance in the RPE of different species (Griff, 1990b; Miller and Edelman, 1990; Quinn and Miller, 1992; Fox and Steinberg, 1992; Strauss et al., 1994; Hernandez et al., 1995; Hughes et al., 1995). Similar findings have been reported in cultured RPE from RCS rats (Strauss and Weinrich, 1993). Barium has also been employed to characterize volume regulatory mechanisms in response to hypertonic and hypotonic challenge. Both the regulatory volume decrease and the hypotonically activated Rb^+ efflux were inhibited by the K^+ channel blocker barium. On the other hand, hypotonically activated Rb^+ influx was increased by barium treatment, suggesting the presence of a barium-inhibitable, hypotonically activated K^+ efflux pathway as part of the volume regulation in cultured human RPE cells (Kennedy et al., 1994).

Tetrodotoxin (TTX) has been investigated as a Ca^{2+} channel blocker in the RPE (Strauss and Weinrich, 1994; Strauss et al., 1994), as well as an inhibitor of voltage-activated Na^+ channels in RPE cultures of neonatal rats (Botchkin and Matthews, 1994). This TTX channel was not found in any freshly isolated fetal or adult RPE cells using the whole-cell version of the patch-clamp technique (Wen et al., 1994). It was hypothesized that expression of this Na^+ current in culture is regulated by an intrinsic program related to cell differentiation that may represent a tendency of proliferating RPE cells to dedifferntiate toward a more embryonic and neuroepithelial phenotype.

Metabolic Inhibitors

Metabolic inhibitors display a high toxicity for the general metabolism of all cells, and the pharmacologic specificity of these drugs for the RPE is minimal. However, these compounds have been useful in the investigation of physiological principles concerning RPE transport. *Cyanide* has been shown to reversibly inhibit a basal membrane response that was evoked by changing the apical potassium concentration (Griff, 1990a), whereas only a very little suppressive effect on $Na^+K^+2Cl^-$ cotransport activity in cultured monkey RPE was demonstrated (Kennedy, 1992). It also diminishes adhesion of the RPE to the retina, and the rate of fluid absorption across the RPE (Marmor et al., 1980). *Dinitrophenol,* a nonspecific metabolic toxin, significantly decreased the outward permeability of fluorescein across the RPE-choroid by about 50%, though the inward permeability was not affected (Koyano et al., 1991a,b; 1993). This suggests that the fluorescein movement in the retina–choroidal direction depends on an active metabolic transport system, whereas inward movement depends on a passive transport mechanism. Active transport of ascorbic acid across the RPE of the bullfrog has also been demonstrated to be markedly reduced by dinitrophenol (DiMattio and Streitman, 1991), and the drug has also been shown to decrease retinal adhesiveness to unmeasurable levels if injected into the subretinal space, supporting the concept that metabolic factors contribute to retinal adhesion in vivo (Kita and Marmor, 1992). Although *strychnine* binding sites have been described in membranes prepared from RPE of several species (Bondy et al., 1982; Lopez-Colome et al., 1991), the physiological significance of these receptors is not yet clear (Lopez-Colome et al., 1994).

Modulators of the Interphotoreceptor Matrix (IPM)

β-D-*xylopyranoside* is a specific inhibitor of chondroitin sulfate proteoglycan synthesis. After intravitreal injection this agent may selectively affect the IPM in micropigs by disrupting the cone-matrix-sheath-associated proteoglycan synthesis and thus inducing retinal detachment. These findings support the hypothesis that RPE–outer segment attachment is dependent upon continuous synthesis of cone-matrix-sheat-associated proteoglycans (Lazarus and Hageman, 1992). Intravitreal or subretinal injection of such different enzymes as *chondroitinase ABC, neuraminidase,* and testicular *hyaluronidase,* which degrade oligosaccharides, has also been shown to cause diffuse loss of adhesion, albeit without affecting photoreceptor function (Yao et al., 1992; Hageman et al., 1995). Whether some of these agents may be useful in the iatrogenic induction of posterior vitreous detachment is not yet clear.

Inhibitor of Organic Acid Transport

Probenecid is an inhibitor of organic anion transport, and has been used to characterize proton-lactate cotransport in the apical membrane of the RPE of different species (Lin et al., 1994; La Cour et al., 1994). Probenecid has also been shown to inhibit the cAMP-induced pigment granule aggregation in the RPE of the green sunfish (Garcia and Burnside, 1994), which suggests that cAMP can gain access to the cytoplasm of isolated RPE cells via organic anion transporters. Probenecid also significantly decreases the outward permeability of fluorescein and carboxyfluorescein across the

RPE-choroid preparation of different species including primates, whereas the inward permeability was not affected (Tsuboi and Pederson, 1986b; 1987; Koyano, 1993; 1991). A similar decrease of fluorescein permeability has also been shown with *hippurate* and *iodipamide* (Koyano et al., 1993; 1991a,b). These findings suggest that the fluorescein movement in the retina–choroidal direction depends on an active metabolic transport system, whereas inward movement depends on a passive transport mechanism. Similarly, in vivo intravitreal injection of 10^{-4} M probenecid has been shown to inhibit active outward transport of fluorescein (Tsuboi and Pederson, 1986).

Phosphodiesterase Inhibitors

Aminophyllin is a phosphodiesterase inhibitor that is widely used in the treatment of asthma. In vitro it induces a suppressive effect on retinal outer segment uptake by the RPE cells (Miceli and Newsome, 1994), although there is no clinical significance known for this effect. The effects of *3-Isobutyl-1-methylxanthine* (IBMX) on the RPE range from altering membrane potentials (Nao-i et al., 1990) (see Chapter 6) to affecting net fluid absorption by the RPE (Miller et al., 1982). Furthermore, IBMX has been demonstrated to induce dark-adaptive dopamine-inhibited cone and RPE retinomotor movements in isolated light-adapted green sunfish retinas cultured in constant light (Dearry and Burnside, 1985). In addition, IBMX also acts on adenylatecyclase by increasing its activity significantly in the frog (Miller and Farber, 1984) and rabbit RPE (Blazynski and Cohen, 1984).

Inhibitors of Lysosomal Enzymes

Given the high concentration of lysosomal enzymes in the RPE, several agents that suppress their activity have been investigated in order to elucidate the pathophysiology of lipofuscin accumulation at the level of the RPE. Generally speaking, these inhibitors lead in the end to an increased accumulation of lipofuscin-like material. *Pepstatin,* an aspartic protease inhibitor, has been shown, for example, to inhibit cathepsin D, a major lysosomal enzyme in the bovine RPE (Hayasaka et al., 1975a), and thus the cathepsin-associated degradation of photoreceptor outer segments (Hayasaka et al., 1975b). Along with *leupeptin* (a cystein protease inhibitor), pepstatin has also been shown to reduce rod outer segment digestion by the human RPE in vitro (Kennedy et al., 1994). Intravitreal injection of leupeptin has been demonstrated to induce widespread accumulation throughout the RPE cytoplasm of inclusions that resembled lipofuscin associated with an increase in cell height and a displacement of melanin from the apical cell border, however, without changes in RPE physiology (Rapp et al., 1994). Lipofuscin-like autofluorescence, correlating with leupeptin-induced inclusions in the RPE, has also been causally linked to a diet rich in retinyl palmitate (which can be converted metabolically into the retinoids involved in vision) suggesting that retinoids involved in the visual process are probably directly involved in the RPE lipofuscin fluorophore formation (Katz and Norberg, 1992).

Inhibitors of Oligosaccharide Synthesis

Given that many receptors that mediate rod outer segment (ROS) phagocytosis by the RPE are glycoproteins the effect of inhibitors of glycoprotein synthesis and processing on this process has been investigated. *Tunicamycin* (an inhibitor of N-linked oligosaccharide synthesis), for example, has clearly been shown to inhibit the phagocytosis of ROS by initially reducing ROS binding and consequently their subsequent ingestion. By contrast, *castanospermine* and *swainsonine* (inhibitors of oligosaccharide processing) had no effect on the ability of RPE to phagocytose ROS. These results support the hypothesis that ROS phagocytosis is mediated by a specific glycoprotein receptor. N-glycosylation of these receptors is probably required for their function, or for their insertion into the plasma membrane, whereas processing of the N-linked oligosaccharide chains seems not to be crucial for ROS phagocytosis by RPE cells (Hall et al., 1990). However, this concept has been questioned in other reports in which *swainsonine* has been shown to reduce ROS ingestion by the rat (Boyle and McLaughlin, 1990) and human RPE in vitro (Kennedy et al., 1994).

REFERENCES

Akeo K, et al. 1992. Comparison of effects of oxygen and antioxidative enzymes on cell growth between retinal pigment epithelial cells and vascular endothelial cells in vitro. Ophthalmic Res 24:357–364.

Amemiya T. 1985. Retinal changes in the selenium deficient rat. Intern J Vit Nutr Res 55:233–237.

Andress LD, Brizzee KR. 1986. Lipofuscin in retinal pigment epithelium of rhesus monkey: lack of diminution with centrophenoxine treatment. Neurobiol Aging 7:107–113.

Arrindell EL, et al. 1992. Modulation of potassium transport in cultured retinal pigment epithelium and retinal glial cells by serum and epidermal growth factor. Exp Cell Res 203:192–197.

Ball AK, Baldridge WH, Fernback TC. 1993. Neuromodulation of pigment movement in the RPE of normal and 6-OHDA-lesioned goldfish retinas. Vis Neurosci 10:529–540.

Barrada A, et al. 1984. Evaluation of intravitreal 5-fluorouracil, vin-

cristine, VP-16, doxorubicin and thiotepa in primate eyes. Ophthalmic Surg 15:767–769.

Becker B. 1954. Decrease in intraocular pressure in man by a carbonic anhydrase inhibitor. Am J Ophthalmol 37:13–15.

Becquet F, et al. 1994. Superoxide inhibits proliferation and phagocytic internalization of photoreceptor outer segments by bovine retinal pigment epithelium in vitro. Exp Cell Res 212:374–382.

Berger AS, Tychsen L, Rosenblum JL. 1991. Retinopathy in human vitamin E deficiency. Am J Ophthalmol 111:774–775.

Berlie JR, et al. 1995. Alpha-2 adrenergic receptors in the bovine retina. Invest Ophthalmol Vis Sci 36:1885–1892.

Berman DH, Gombos GM. Proliferative vitreoretinopathy: does oral low-dose colchicine have an inhibitory effect? A controlled study in humans. Ophthalmic Surg 20:268–272.

Berson EL, et al. 1993. A randomized trial of vitamin A and vitamin E supplementation for retinitis pigmentosa. Arch Ophthalmol 111:761–772.

Blanks JC, Pickford MS, Organisciak DT. 1992. Ascorbate treatment prevents accumulation of phagosomes in RPE and light damage. Invest Ophthalmol Vis Sci 33:2814–2821.

Blazynski C, Cohen AI. 19984. Cyclic nucleotide distribution in identified layers of suprafused rabbit retinas. Exp Eye Res 38:279–290.

Blumenkranz MS, Hartzer MK, Hajek AS. 1987. Selection of therapeutic agents for intraocular proliferative disease. Arch Ophthalmol 105:396–399.

Bok D. 1993. The retinal pigment epithelium: a versatile partner in vision. J Cell Sci 17(suppl):189–195.

Bondy SC, et al. 1982. Retinal pigment epithelium contains a distinctive strychnine-binding site. Neurochem Res 7:1445–1452.

Botchkin LM, Matthews G. 1994. Voltage-dependent sodium channels develop in rat retinal pigment epithelium cells in culture. Proc Nat Acad Sci 91:4564–4568.

Boulton M, et al. 1989. The formation of autofluorescent granules in cultured human RPE. Invest Ophthalmol Vis Sci 30:28–89.

Boyle L, McLaughlin BJ. 1990. The effect of swainsonine on the phagocytosis of rod outer segments by rat ROE. Curr Eye Res 9:407–414.

Broekhuyse RM, Kuhlmann ED, Winkens HJ. 1993. Experimental autoimmune anterior uveitis (EAAU): induction by melanin antigen and suppression by various treatments. Pigm Cell Res 6:1–6.

Burke JM, Jaffe GJ, Brzeski CM. 1991a. The effect of culture density and proliferation rate on the expression of ouabain-sensitive Na/K ATPase pumps in cultured human retinal pigment epithelium. Exp Cell Res 194:190–194.

Burke JM, McKay BS, Jaffe GJ. 1991b. Retinal pigment epithelial cells of the posterior pole have fewer Na/K ATPase pumps than peripheral cells. Invest Ophthalmol Vis Sci 32:2042–2046.

Burnside B, et al. 1982. Induction of dark-adaptive retinomotor movement (cell elongation) in teleost retinal cones by cyclic adenosine 3′, 5′-monophosphate. J Gen Physiol 79:759–774.

Burnside B, Basinger S. 1983. Retinomotor pigment migration in the teleost retinal pigment epithelium. II. Cyclic-3′,5′-adenosine monophosphate induction of dark-adaptive movement in vitro. Invest Ophthalmol Vis Sci 24:16–23.

Campochiaro PA, Glaser BM. 1986. Mechanisms involved in retinal pigment epithelial cell chemotaxis. Arch Ophthalmol 104:277–280.

Cardillo JA, et al. 1996. The potential of mitomycin C in the treatment of experimental proliferative vitreoretinopathy. Invest Ophthalmol Vis Sci 37(suppl):S392.

Chen JC, Fitzke FW, Bird AC. 1990. Long term effect of acetazolamide in a patient with retinitis pigmentosa. Invest Ophthalmol Vis Sci 31:1914–1918.

Chiba K, Inada K, Sakamoto S. 1993. Human cultured retinal pigment epithelial cells produce interleukin-6. Nippon Ganka Gakkai Zasshi 97:29–35.

Chung H, et al. 1988. BCNU silicone oil in proliferative vitreoretinopathy: I. Solubility, stability and antiproliferative studies. Curr Eye Res 7:1199–1206.

Civan MM, et al. 1994. Prolonged incubation with elevated glucose inhibits the regulatory response to shrinkage of cultured human retinal pigment epithelial cells. J Membr Biol 139:1–13.

Conroy CW, Wynns GC, Maren TH. 1994. Carbonic anhydrase inhibitors do not reach the retina by the topical route. Invest Ophthalmol Vis Sci 35(suppl):2220.

Cousins SW, et al. 1996. RPE platelet-derived growth factor (PDGF) gene expression is suppressed by corticosteroid therapy during experimental PVR. Invest Ophthalmol Vis Sci 37(suppl):S392.

Cox SN, Hay E, Bird AC. 1988. Treatment of chronic macular edema with acetazolamide. Arch Ophthalmol 106:1190–1195.

Crawford B. 1979. Cloned pigmented retinal epithelium: the role of microfilaments in the differentiation of cell shape. J Cell Biol 81: 301–315.

Dearry A, Burnside B. 1985. Dopamine inhibits forskolin- and 3-isobutyl-1-methylxanthine-induced dark-adaptive retinomotor movements in isolated teleost retinas. J Neurochem 44:1753–1763.

Dearry A, Burnside B. 1986. Dopaminergic regulation of cone retinomotor movement in isolated teleost retinas: I. Induction of cone contraction is mediated by D2 receptors. J Neurochem 46:1006–1021.

Dearry A, Burnside B. 1988. Stimulation of distinct D2 dopaminergic and alpha 2-adrenergic receptors induces light adaptive pigment dispersion in teleost retinal pigment epithelium. J Neurochem 51: 1516–1523.

Dearry A, Burnside B. 1989. Light-induced dopamine release from teleost retinas acts as a light-adaptive signal to the retinal pigment epithelium. J Neurochem 53:870–878.

Dearry A, et al. 1990. Dopamine induces light-adaptive retinomotor movements in bullfrog cones via D2 receptors and in retinal pigment epithelium via D1 receptors. J Neurochem 54:1367–1378.

Del Monte MA, et al. 1991. Sorbitol, myo-inositol, and rod outer segment phagocytosis in cultured human RPE cells exposed to glucose. In vitro model of myo-inositol depletion hypothesis of diabetic complications. Diabetes 1335–1345.

DeLuca RL, Hu DN, McCormick SA. 1995. Long-term effect of 5-FU on cultured human retinal pigment epithelium. Invest Ophthalmol Vis Sci 36(suppl):S751.

DiMattio J, Streitman J. 1991. Active transport of ascorbic acid across the retinal pigment epithelium of the bullfrog. Curr Eye Res 10:959–965.

DiMattio J, Degnan KJ, Zadunaisky JA. 1983. A model for transepithelial ion transport across the isolated retinal pigment epithelium of the frog. Exp Eye Res 37:409–414.

Dodgson SJ. 1991. The carbonic anhydrases: overview of their importance in cellular physiology and in molecular genetics. In Dodgson SJ, et al., eds, The Carbonic Anhydrases: Cellular Physiology and Molecular Genetics. New York: Plenum, 3–13.

Dorey CK, Delori FC, Akeo K. 1990. Growth of cultured RPE and endothelial cells is inhibited by blue light but not green or red light. Curr Eye Res 9:549–559.

Edelman JL, Miller SS. 1991. Epinephrine stimulates fluid absorption across bovine retinal pigment epithelium. Invest Ophthalmol Vis Sci 32:3033–3040.

Edelman JL, Lin H, Miller SS. 1994. Acidification stimulates chloride and fluid absorption across frog retinal pigment epithelium. Am J Physiol 266:C946–956.

Edwards RB, et al. 1996. Dietary modification of macular pigment density. Invest Ophthalmol Vis Sci 37(suppl):S914.

el-Hifnawi ES, et al. 1992. The effect of cyclooxygenase inhibitors on the course of hereditary retinal dystrophy in RCS rats. Anatom Anz 174:251–258.

Endo EG, Yao X-Y, Marmor MF. 1988. Pigment adherence as a measure of retinal adhesion: dependence on temperature. Invest Ophthalmol Vis Sci 29:1390–1396.

Farnsworth CC, Stone WL, Dratz EA. 1979. Effects of vitamin E and selenium deficiency on the fatty acid composition of rat retinal tissues. Biochim Biophys Acta 552:281–293.

Feldman EL, Randolph AE. 1994. Regulation of insulin-like growth factor binding protein synthesis and secretion in human retinal pigment epithelial cells. J Cell Physiol 158:198–204.

Fiscella R, et al. 1985. In vitro evaluation of cellular inhibitory potential of various antineoplastic drugs and dexamethasone. Ophthalmic Surg 16:247–249.

Fishman GA, et al. 1989. Acetazolamide for treatment of chronic macular edema in retinitis pigmentosa. Arch Ophthalmol 107: 1445–1452.

Fite KV et al. 1986. Effects of cyclosporine in spontaneous posterior uveitis. Current Eye Res 5:787–796.

Fox JA, Steinberg RH. 1992. Voltage-dependent currents in isolated cells of the turtle retinal pigment epithelium. Pflugers Arch 420: 451–460.

Frambach DA, Marmor MF. 1982. The rate and route of fluid resorption from the subretinal space of the rabbit. Invest Ophthalmol Vis Sci 22:292–302.

Frambach DA, Misfeldt DS. 1983. Furosemide-sensitive Cl transport in embryonic chick retinal pigment epithelium. Am J Physiol 244: F679–685.

Frambach DA, Valentine JL, Weiter JJ. 1988. Initial observations of rabbit retinal pigment epithelium-choroid-sclera preparations. Invest Ophthalmol Vis Sci 29:814–817.

Frambach DA, Valentine JL, Weiter JJ. 1989a. Furosemide-sensitive Cl- transport in bovine retinal pigment epithelium. Invest Ophthalmol Vis Sci 30:2271–2274.

Frambach DA, et al. 1989b. Precocious retinal adhesion is affected by furosemide and ouabain. Curr Eye Res 8:553–556.

Frambach DA, et al. 1990. Beta adrenergic receptors on cultured human retinal pigment epithelium. Invest Ophthalmol Vis Sci 31: 1767–1772.

Fu J, Lam TT, Tso MO. 1992. Dexamethasone ameliorates retinal photic injury in albino rats. Exp Eye Res 54:583–594.

Gallemore RP, Steinberg RH. 1990. Effects of dopamine on the chick retinal pigment epithelium. Invest Ophthalmol Vis Sci 31:67–80.

Garcia DM, Burnside B. 1994. Suppression of cAMP-induced pigment granule aggregation in RPE by organic anion transport inhibitors. Invest Ophthalmol Vis Sci 35:178–188.

Gillies MC. 1996. Orbital interferon alpha 2b for cystoid macular edema recalcitrant to conventional treatment. Invest Ophthalmol Vis Sci 37(suppl):S590.

Glenn AM, et al. 1994. Effect of vitamin A treatment on the prolongation of dark adaptation in Stargardt's dystrophy. Retina 14:27–30.

Goldhar SW, Basu PK, Ranadive NS. 1984. Phagocytosis by retinal pigment epithelium: evaluation of modulating agents with an organ culture model. Can J Ophthalmol 19:33–35.

Gouras P, et al. 1992. The ultrastructure of transplanted rabbit retinal epithelium. Graefes Arch Clip Exp Ophthalmol 230:468–475.

Gregory CY, Abrams TA, Hall MO. 1992. cAMP production via the adenylyl cyclase pathway is reduced in RCS rat RPE. Invest Ophthalmol Vis Sci 33:3121–3124.

Griff ER. 1990a. Metabolic inhibitors reversibly alter the basal membrane potential of the gecko retinal pigment epithelium. Exp Eye Res 50:99–107.

Griff ER. 1990b. Response properties of the toad retinal pigment epithelium. Invest Ophthalmol Vis Sci 31:2353–2360.

Gupta LY, Marmor MF. 1993. Mannitol, dextromethorphan, and catalase minimize ischaemic damage to retinal pigment epithelium and retina. Arch Ophthalmol 111:384–388.

Hackett SF, Campochiaro PA. 1993. Modulation of plasminogen activator inhibitor-1 and urokinase in retinal pigmented epithelial cells. Invest Ophthalmol Vis Sci 34:2055–2061.

Hackett S, Friedman Z, Campochiaro PA. 1986. Cyclic 3′5′-adenosine monophosphate modulates retinal pigment epithelial cell migration in vitro. Arch Ophthalmol 104:1688–1692.

Hageman GS, et al. 1995. The interphotoreceptor matrix mediates primate retinal adhesion. Arch Ophthalmol 113:655–660.

Hahn JM, et al. 1996. Calcium channel blocker mediated inhibition of retinal pigment epithelial cell contraction of collagen gels. Invest Ophthalmol Vis Sci 37(suppl):S393.

Hall MO, et al. 1990. The effect of inhibitors of glycoprotein synthesis and processing on the phagocytosis of rod outer segments by cultured retinal pigment epithelial cells. Glycobiology 1:51–61.

Hall MO, Abrams TA, Mittag TW. 1993. The phagocytosis of rod outer segments is inhibited by drugs linked to cyclic adenosine monophosphate production. Invest. Ophthalmol Vis Sci 34:2329–2401.

Handa JT, Murad S, Jaffe GJ. 1993. Minoxidil inhibits ocular cell proliferation and lysyl hydroxylase. Invest Ophthalmol Vis Sci 34:567–575.

Handa JT, Murad S, Jaffe GJ. 1994. Inhibition of cultured human RPE cell proliferation and lysyl hydroxylase. Invest Ophthalmol Vis Sci 35:463–469.

Harris M, et al. 1995. Hypericin inhibits retinal pigment epithelium cell proliferation through a protein kinase C pathway and induces apoptosis. Invest Ophthalmol Vis Sci 36(suppl):S753.

Hayasaka S, Hara S, Mizuno K. 1975a. Partial purification and properties of cathepsin D in the retinal pigment epithelium. Invest Ophthalmol Vis Sci 14:617–620.

Hayasaka S, Hara S, Mizuno K. 1975b. Degradation of rod outer segment proteins by cathepsin D. J Biochem 78:1365–1375.

He S, et al. 1994. Dexamethasone induced proliferation of cultured retinal pigment epithelial cells. Curr Eye Res 13:257–261.

Hernandez EV, et al. 1995. Potassium conductances in cultured bovine and human retinal pigment epithelium. Invest Ophthalmol Vis Sci 36:113–122.

Hirakata A, et al. 1996. Effects of protein kinase inhibitors on wound closure in cultured human retinal pigment epithelial cells. Invest Ophthalmol Vis Sci 37(suppl):S381.

Hoffmann S, et al. 1996. Effect of the calcium-antagonist verapamil on the serum induced proliferation of RPE cells in vitro. Invest Ophthalmol Vis Sci, 37(suppl):S389.

Horie K, et al. 1993. Identification of alpha 1C-adrenergic receptor mRNA in bovine retinal pigment epithelium. Invest Ophthalmol Vis Sci 34:2769–2775.

Howells L, Godfrey M, Sauer MJ. 1994. Melanin as an absorbent for drug residues. Analyst 119:2691–2693.

Hu JG, et al. 1994. Localization of Na-K-ATPase on cultured human retinal pigment epithelium. Invest Ophthalmol Vis Sci 35:3582–3588.

Hughes BA, Segawa Y. 1993. cAMP-activated chloride currents in amphibian retinal pigment epithelial cells. J Physiol 466:749–766.

Hughes BA, Shaikh A, Ahmad A. 1995. Effects of Ba^{2+} and Cs^+ on apical membrane K^+ conductance in toad retinal pigment epithelium. Am J Physiol 268:C1164–1172.

Joseph DP, Miller SS. 1991. Apical and basal membrane ion transport mechanisms in bovine retinal pigment epithelium. J Physiol 435:439–463.

Joseph DP, Miller SS. 1992. Alpha-1-adrenergic modulation of K^+ and Cl^- transport in bovine retinal pigment epithelium. J Gen Physiol 99:263–290.

Katz ML, Norberg M. 1992. Influence of dietary vitamin A on autofluorescence of leupeptin-induced inclusions in the retinal pigment epithelium. Exp Eye Res 54:239–246.

Katz ML, Robison WG, Jr. 1983. Lipofuscin response to the "aging-reversal" drug centrophenoxine in rat retinal pigment epithelium and frontal cortex. J Gerontol 38:525–531.

Katz ML, Stone WL, Dratz EA. 1978. Fluorescent pigment accumulation in retinal pigment epithelium of antioxidant-deficient rats. Invest Ophthalmol Vis Sci 17:1049–1058.

Katz ML, Drea CM, Robison WG. 1987. Dietary vitamins A and E influence retinyl ester composition and content of the retinal pigment epithelium. Biochim Biophys Acta 924:432–441.

Kennedy BG. 1992. Rubidium transport in cultured monkey retinal pigment epithelium. Exp Eye Res 55:289–296.

Kennedy BG. 1994. Volume regulation in cultured cells derived from human retinal pigment epithelium. Am J Physiol 266:C676–683.

Kennedy CJ, et al. 1994. Kinetic studies on phagocytosis and lysosomal digestion of rod outer segments by human retinal pigment epithelial cells in vitro. Exp Cell Res, 210:209–214.

Khatami M. 1990. Regulation of myo-inositol transport in retinal pigment epithelium by sugars, amiloride, and pH gradients: potential impairment of pump-leak balance in diabetic maculopathy. Membr Biochem 9:279–292.

Kimura H, et al. 1994. In vitro phagocytosis of polylactide microspheres by retinal pigment epithelial cells and intracellular drug release. Curr Eye Res 13:353–360.

Kishi H, Mishima HK, Yamashita U. 1994. Effect of cytokines and prostaglandins on the growth of chick retinal pigment epithelial cells. Curr Eye Res 13:833–837.

Kishimoto N, et al. 1993. The effect of corticosteroid on the repair of the retinal pigment epithelium. Nippon Ganka Gakkai Zasshi 97:360–369.

Kita M, Marmor MF. 1992a. Retinal adhesive force in living rabbit, cat, and monkey eyes. Invest Ophthalmol Vis Sci 33:1879–1882.

Kita M, Marmor MF. 1992b. Effects on retinal adhesive force in vivo of metabolically active agents in the subretinal space. Invest Ophthalmol Vis Sci 33:1883–1887.

Koh SW, Chader GJ. 1984. Retinal pigment epithelium in culture demonstrates a distinct beta-adrenergic receptor. Exp Eye Res 38:7–13.

Kon CH, et al. 1996. Thiotepa: possible use in the treatment and prevention of proliferative vitreoretinopathy (PVR). Invest Ophthalmol Vis Sci 37(suppl):S390.

Kothary PC, Del Monte MA. 1995. Mechanism of growth inhibition of cultured human retinal pigment epithelial cells by retinoic acid. Invest Ophthalmol Vis Sci 36(suppl):S99.

Koutsandrea CN, et al. 1991. Ciprofloxacin and dexamethasone inhibit the proliferation of human retinal pigment epithelial cells in culture. Curr Eye Res 10:249–258.

Koyano S Eguchi S, Araie M. 1991a. Analysis of transport of fluorescein across the isolated retinal pigment epithelium-choroid using an Ussing type chamber. Nippon Ganka Gakkai Zasshi 95:434–440.

Koyano S, Eguchi S, Araie M. 1991b. Kinetic study of movement of fluorescein across the isolated rabbit retinal pigment epithelium-choroid. Nippon Ganka Gakkai Zasshi 95:428–433.

Koyano S, Araie M, Eguchi S. 1993. Movement of fluorescein and its glucuronide across retinal pigment epithelium-choroid. Invest Ophthalmol Vis Sci 34:531–538.

Kuntz CA, et al. 1994. Modification by cyclic adenosine monophosphate of basolateral membrane chloride conductance in chick retinal pigment epithelium. Invest Ophthalmol Vis Sci 35:422–433.

La Cour M. 1992. Cl- transport in frog retinal pigment epithelium. Exp Eye Res 54:921–931.

La Cour M. et al. 1994. Lactate transport in freshly isolated human fetal retinal pigment epithelium. Invest Ophthalmol Vis Sci 35:434–442.

Lam TT, et al. 1993. Methylprednisolone therapy in laser injury of the retina. Graefes Arch Clin Exp Ophthalmol 231:729–736.

La Rocca PJ, Rafferty KA. 1982. Kinetics of chick embryo cell types in culture. J Cell Physiol 113:203–210.

Larsson BS. 1993. Interaction between chemicals and melanin. Pigment Cell Res 6:127–133.

Larsson B, Tjalve H. 1979. Studies on the mechanism of drug binding to melanin. Biochem Pharmacol 28:1181–1187.

Lazarus HS, Hageman GS. 1992. Xyloside-induced disruption of interphotoreceptor matrix proteoglycans results in retinal detachment. Invest Ophthalmol Vis Sci 33:364–376.

Lebek J, et al. 1996. Daunomycin induces apoptosis in retinal pigment epithelial cells. Invest Ophthalmol Vis Sci 37(suppl):S390.

Lee VHI, et al. 1989. Drug delivery to the posterior segment. In Ryan SJ, ed, Retina. St Louis: Mosby 483–498.

Lemor M, de Bustros S, Glaser BM. 1986a. Low-dose colchicine inhibits astrocyte, fibroblast, and retinal pigment epithelial cell migration and proliferation. Arch Ophthalmol 104:1223–1225.

Lemor M, Yeo JH, Glaser BM. 1986b. Oral colchicine for the treatment of experimental traction retinal detachment. Arch Ophthalmol 104:1226–1229.

Li ZY, et al. 1985. Amelioration of photic injury in rat retina by ascorbic acid: a histopathologic study. Invest Ophthalmol Vis Sci 26:1589–1598.

Lichter PR. 1981. Reducing side effects of carbonic anhydrase inhibitors. Ophthalmology 88:266–269.

Lin H, Miller SS. 1991. pHi regulation in frog retinal pigment epithelium: two apical membrane mechanisms. Am J Physiol 261:C132–142.

Lin H, Kenyon E, Miller SS. 1992. Na-dependent pHi regulatory mechanisms in native human retinal pigment epithelium. Invest Ophthalmol Vis Sci 33:3528–3538.

Lin H, et al. 1994. Proton-lactate cotransport in the apical membrane of frog retinal pigment epithelium. Exp Eye Res 59:679–688.

Lin JY, Hu DN, McCormick SA. 1996. Long-term effect of mitomycin on cultured human retinal pigment epithelium. Invest Ophthalmol Vis Sci 37(suppl):S390.

Lindquist NG. 1973. Accumulation of drugs in melanin. Acta Radiol (Stockholm) 325:1–92.

Liversidge J, et al. 1988. Cyclosporine A, experimental autoimmune uveitis, and major histocompatibility class II antigen expression of cultured retinal pigment epithelial cells. Transplantation Proceedings 20:163–169.

Liversidge J, et al. 1993. Retinal pigment epithelial cells modulate lymphocyte function at the blood-retina barrier by autocrine PGE_2 and membrane-bound mechanisms. Cell Immunol 149:315–330.

Lopez-Colome AM, Fragoso G, Salceda R. 1991. Taurine receptors in membranes from retinal pigment epithelium cells in culture. Neurosci 41:791–796.

Lopez-Colome AM, Salceda R, Fragoso G. 1994. Specific interaction of glutamate with membranes from cultured retinal pigment epithelium. J Neurosci Res 34:454–461.

MacGregor LC, Matschinsky FM. 1985. Treatment with aldose reductase inhibitor or with myo-inositol arrests deterioration of the electroretinogram of diabetic rats. J Clin Invest 76:887–889.

Marmor MF. 1990. Hypothesis concerning carbonic anhydrase treatment of cystoid macular edema: example with epiretinal membrane. Arch Ophthalmol 108:1524–1525.

Marmor MF, Maack T. 1982. Enhancement of retinal adhesion and subretinal fluid resorption by acetazolamide. Invest Ophthalmol Vis Sci 23:121–124.

Marmor MF, Yao XY. 1989. The enhancement of retinal adhesiveness by ouabain appears to involve cellular edema. Invest Ophthalmol Vis Sci 30:1511–1514.

Marmor MF, Abdul-Rahim AS, Cohen DS. 1980. The effect of metabolic inhibitors on retinal adhesion and subretinal fluid resorption. Invest Ophthalmol Vis Sci 19:893–903.

Mason CG. 1977. Ocular accumulation and toxicity of certain systemically administered drugs. J Toxicol Env Health 2:977–995.

Matsuo T, Cynader MS. 1992. Localization of alpha-2 adrenergic receptors in the human eye. Ophthalmic Res 24:213–219.

Miceli MV, Newsome DA. 1994. Insulin stimulation of retinal outer segment uptake by cultured human retinal pigment epithelial cells redetermined by a flow cytometric method. Exp Eye Res 59:271–280.

Mietz H, et al. 1994. Histopathologic study of epiretinal proliferations after vitrectomy with daunomycin and silicone oil. Retina 14:425–429.

Miller SS, Edelman JL. 1990. Active ion transport pathways in the bovine retinal pigment epithelium. J Physiol 424:283–300.

Miller SS, Farber D. 1984. Cyclic AMP modulation of ion transport across frog retinal pigment epithelium: measurements in the short-circuit state. J Gen Physiol 83:853–874.

Miller SS, Steinberg RH. 1977. Active transport of ions across frog retinal pigment epithelium. Exp Eye Res 25:235–248.

Miller SS, Hughes BA, Machen TE. 1982. Fluid transport across retinal pigment epithelium is inhibited by cyclic AMP. Proc Nat Acad Sci 79:2111–2115.

Mojon D, et al. 1994. Vitamin E inhibits retinal pigment epithelium cell proliferation in vitro. Ophthalmic Res 26:304–309.

Moritera T, et al. 1992. Biodegradable microspheres containing adriamycin in the treatment of proliferative vitreoretinopathy. Invest Ophthalmol Vis Sci 33:3125–3130.

Moritera T, et al. 1994. Feasibility of drug targeting to the retinal pigment epithelium with biodegradable microspheres. Curr Eye Res 13:171–176.

Nakamura J, Lattimer SA, Greene DA. 1994. Transphosphatidylation of sugar alcohols and its implications for the pathogenesis of diabetic complications. Diabetologia 37:1147–1153.

Nao-i N, Gallemore RP, Steinberg RH. 1990. Effects of cAMP and IBMX on the chick retinal pigment epithelium. Membrane potentials and light-evoked responses. Invest Ophthalmol Vis Sci 31:54–66.

Nash MS, Osborne NN. 1995. Pertussis toxin sensitive melatonin receptors negatively coupled to adenylate cyclase associated with cultured human and rat retinal pigment epithelial cells. Invest Ophthalmol Vis Sci 36:95–102.

Negi A, Marmor MF. 1986. Quantitative estimation of metabolic transport of subretinal fluid. Invest Ophthalmol Vis Sci 27:1564–1568.

Newsome DA, et al. 1990. Human retinal pigment epithelium contains two distinct species of superoxide dismutase. Invest Ophthalmol Vis Sci 31:2508–2513.

Norton EWD, et al. 1993. A randomized trial of vitamin A and vitamin E supplementation for retinitis pigmentosa [letters]. Arch Ophthalmol 111:1460–1463.

Ogino N, et al. 1984. Forskolin inhibits phagocytosis of latex particles by cultured chick retinal pigment epithelial cells. Nippon Ganka Gakkai Zasshi 88:974–976.

Ogura Y, Kimura H. 1995. Biodegradable polymer microspheres for targeted drug delivery to the retinal pigment epithelium. Surv Ophthalmol 39(suppl 1):S17–S24.

Oliver PD, Newsome DA. 1992. Mitochondrial superoxide dismutase in mature and developing human retinal pigment epithelium. Invest Ophthalmol Vis Sci 33:1909–1918.

Onoe S, et al. 1988. The effect of beta-blocker on ERG c-wave of the rabbit. Doc Ophthalmol 68:337–348.

Organisciak DT, et al. 1987. Vitamin E in human neural retina and retinal pigment epithelium: effect of age. Curr Eye Res 6:1051–1055.

Persad S, et al. 1986. Binding of imipramine, 8-methoxypsoralen, and epinephrine to human blue and brown eye melanins. J Toxicol Cutaneous Toxicol 5:125–132.

Quinn RH, Miller SS. 1992. Ion transport mechanisms in native human retinal pigment epithelium. Invest Ophthalmol Vis Sci 33:3513–3527.

Rahimy MH, et al. 19994. Effects of an intravitreal daunomycin implant on experimental proliferative vitreoretinopathy: simultaneous pharmacokinetic and pharmacodynamic evaluations. J Ocular Pharmacol 10:561–570.

Ramachandran E, Frank RN, Kennedy A. 1993. Effects of endothelin on cultured bovine microvascular pericytes. Invest Ophthalmol Vis Sci 34:586–595.

Rapp LM, Fisher PL, Sheinberg CH. 1994. Impact of lipofuscin on the retinal pigment epithelium: electroretinographic evaluation of a protease inhibition model. Graefes Arch Clin Exp Ophthalmol 232:232–237.

Rapp LM, Choi JH, Singh SH. 1996. Retinal pigment epithelium has relatively high levels of beta-carotene in supplemented animals. Invest Ophthalmol Vis Sci 37(suppl):S1144.

Reddy VN, et al. 1992. The efficacy of aldose reductase inhibitors on polyol accumulation in human lens and retinal pigment epithelium in tissue culture. J Ocular Pharmacol 8:43–52.

Riis RC, et al. 1981. Vitamin E deficiency retinopathy in dogs. Am J Vet Res 42:74–86.

Robison WG, Kuwabara T, Bieri JG. 1979. Vitamin E deficiency and the retina: photoreceptor and pigment epithelial changes. Invest Ophthalmol Vis Sci 18:683–690.

Robison WG, Kuwabara T, Bieri JG. 1982. The roles of vitamin E and unsaturated fatty acids in the visual process. Retina 2:263–281.

Rodriguez-Ares MT, et al. 1995. Retinal toxicity of intravitreal nanoencapsulated cyclosporin A. Invest Ophthalmol Vis Sci 36:S157.

Rosner M, Lam TT, Tso MO. 1992. Therapeutic parameters of methylprednisolone treatment for retinal photic injury in a rat model. Res Com Chem Pathol Pharmacol 77:299–311.

Saarikoski J, Kaila K. 1992. Simultaneous measurement of intracellular and extracellular carbonic anhydrase activity in intact muscle fibres. Pflügers Arch 421:357–363.

Sakamoto T, et al. 1994. Intercellular gap formation induced by thrombin in confluent cultured bovine retinal pigment epithelial cells. Invest Ophthalmol Vis Sci 35:720–729.

Sauer MJ, Anderson SP. 1994. In vitro and in vivo studies of drug residue accumulation in pigmented tissues. Analyst 119:2553–2556.

Schmidt J, Löffler KU. 1995. Toxicity and antiproliferative effect of aclacinomycin A on RPE cells in vitro. Invest Ophthalmol Vis Sci 36(suppl):S747.

Sen HA, Campochiaro PA. 1991. Stimulation of cyclic adenosine monophosphate accumulation causes breakdown of the blood-retinal barrier. Invest Ophthalmol Vis Sci 32:2006–2010.

Sheng Y, et al. 1995. Intravitreal cyclosporine prevents RPE xenograft rejection in rabbit retina. Invest Ophthalmol Vis Sci 36(suppl):S250.

Steiner K, Buhring KU, Merck E. 1990. The melanin binding of bisoprolol and its toxicological relevance. Lens Eye Tox Res 7:319–333.

Steinhorst UH, et al. 1993. N,N-dimethyladriamycin for treatment of experimental proliferative vitreoretinopathy: efficacy and toxicity on the rabbit retina. Exp Eye Res 56:489–495.

Strauss O, Weinrich M. 1993. Cultured retinal pigment epithelial cells from RCS rats express an increased calcium conductance compared with cells from non-dystrophic rats. Pflügers Arch 425:68–76.

Strauss O, Weinrich M. 1994. Ca^{2+}-conductances in cultured rat retinal pigment epithelial cells. J Cell Physiol 160:89–96.

Strauss O, Richard G, Wienrich M. 1993. Voltage-dependent potassium currents in cultured human retinal pigment epithelial cells. Biochem Biophys Res Com 191:775–781.

Strauss O, Weiser T, Weinrich M. 1994. Potassium currents in cultured cells of the rat retinal pigment epithelium. Comp Biochem Physiol 109:975–983.

Tran VT. 1992. Human retinal pigment epithelial cells possess beta 2-adrenergic receptors. Exp Eye Res 55:413–417.

Travis DM. 1969. Renal Carbonic Anhydrase Inhibition by Benzolamide (CL 11,366) in Man. J Pharmacol Exp Ther 167:253–264.

Travis DM, et al. 1964. Selective Renal Carbonic Anhydrase Inhibition without Respiratory Effect: Pharmacology of 2-benzenesulfonamido-1,3,4-thiadiazole 5-sulfonamide (CL 11,366). J Pharmacol Exp Ther 143:383–394.

Tso MO. 1987. Retinal photic injury in normal and scorbutic monkeys. Trans Am Ophthalmol Soc 85:498–556.

Tsuboi S. 1987. Measurement of the volume flow and hydraulic conductivity across the isolated dog retinal pigment epithelium. Invest Ophthalmol Vis Sci 28:1776–1782.

Tsuboi S, Pederson JE. 1986. Experimental retinal detachment. XI. Furosemide-inhibitable fluid absorption across retinal pigment epithelium in vivo. Arch Ophthalmol 104:602–603.

Tsuboi S, Pederson JE. 1987. Acetazolamide effect on the inward permeability of the blood-retinal barrier to carboxyfluorescein. Invest Ophthalmol Vis Sci 28:92–95.

Tsuboi S, Manabe R, Iizuka S. 1986. Aspects of electrolyte transport across isolated dog retinal pigment epithelium. Am J Physiol 250:F781–784.

Vernot J, et al. 1985. Effects of selected repeated intravitreal chemotherapeutic agents. Intern Ophthalmol 8:193–198.

Verstraeten TC, et al. 1990. Retinal pigment epithelium wound closure in vitro: pharmacologic inhibition. Invest Ophthalmol Vis Sci 31:481–488.

Verstraeten T, et al. 1992. Effects of vitamin A on retinal pigment epithelial cells in vitro. Invest Ophthalmol Vis Sci 33:2830–2838.

Vinores SA, Campochiaro PA. 1989. Prevention or moderation of some ultrastructural changes in the RPE and retina of galactosemic rats by aldose reductase inhibition. Exp Eye Res 49:495–510.

Vinores SA, et al. 1990. Ultrastructural localization of blood-retinal barrier breakdown in diabetic and galactosemic rats. J Histochem Cytochem 38:1341–1352.

Weller M, Heimann K, Wiedemann P. 1987. Cytotoxic effects of daunomycin on retinal pigment epithelium in vitro. Graefes Arch Clin Exp Ophthalmol 225:235–238.

Wen R, Lui GM, Steinberg RH. 1994. Expression of a tetrodotoxin-sensitive Na^+ current in cultured human retinal pigment epithelial cells. J Physiol 476:187–196.

Wiedemann P, et al. 1989. A fluorescein angiographic study on patients with proliferative vitreoretinopathy treated by vitrectomy and intraocular daunomycin. Int Ophthalmol 13:211–216.

Wiederholt M, Zadunaisky JA. 1984. Decrease of intracellular chloride activity by furosemide in frog retinal pigment epithelium. Curr Eye Res 3:673–675.

Wistrand PJ, Rawls JA, Maren TH. 1960. Sulphonamide carbonic anhydrase inhibitors and intra-ocular pressure in rabbits. Acta Pharmacol Toxicol 17:337–355.

Wolfensberger TJ, et al. 1994. Membrane-bound carbonic anhydrase in human retinal pigment epithelium. Invest Ophthalmol Vis Sci 35:3401–3407.

Wolfensberger TJ, et al. 1995. Inhibition of membrane-bound carbonic anhydrase enhances subretinal fluid absorption and retinal adhesiveness. Invest Ophthalmol Vis Sci 36(suppl):S921.

Wolfensberger TJ, et al. 1996. Inhibition of membrane-bound carbonic anhydrase decreases subretinal volume and pH. Invest Ophthalmol Vis Sci 37(suppl):S1109.

Yamada H, et al. 1995. Inhibition of proliferation of human retinal pigment epithelium by beta-interferon in vitro. Invest Ophthalmol Vis Sci 36(suppl):S99.

Yamamoto F, Steinberg RH. 1992. Effects of intravenous acetazolamide on retinal pH in the cat. Exp Eye Res 54:711–718.

Yamamoto F, Hiroi K, Honda Y. 1994. Effects of intravenous superoxide dismutase and catalase on the ERG in the cat post-ischaemic retina. Ophthalmic Res 26:163–168.

Yang CH, et al. 1996. Inhibition of retinal pigment epithelial cell mediated matrix adhesion and vitreous contraction by crovidisin, a collagen-binding snake venom protein. Invest Ophthalmol Vis Sci 1996. 37(suppl):S387.

Yao XY, Moore KT, Marmor MF. 1991. Systemic mannitol increases retinal adhesiveness measured in vitro. Arch Ophthalmol 109:275–277.

Yao XY, Hageman GS, Marmor MF. 1992. Recovery of retinal adhesion after enzymatic perturbation of the interphotoreceptor matrix. Invest Ophthalmol Vis Sci 33:498–503.

Yoshioka H, Katsume Y, Akune H. 1982. Experimental central serous chorioretinopathy in monkey eyes: fluorescein angiographic findings. Ophthalmologica 185:168–178.

32. Toxicology of the retinal pigment epithelium

THOMAS J. WOLFENSBERGER

The retinal pigment epithelium (RPE) is responsible for many different functions, such as rhodopsin and photoreceptor renewal, ion and fluid transport, production of interphotoreceptor matrix, and maintenance of retinal adhesion, photochemical activities, and the blood–retinal barrier. Toxic effects on this cell layer may be as manifold as its functions. Furthermore, as the retina and the RPE act as a physiological unity these changes in RPE functions may in turn also give rise to altered retinal function or morphology so much so that what started as an isolated RPE-related phenomenon may end in generalized retinal dysfunction. On the other hand, primary retinal toxicity may in the end also affect the RPE both physiologically and morphologically. Despite these closely linked interactions it has nevertheless been possible in some cases to isolate the pathogenesis of RPE-specific toxicity. The earliest observations of a toxic effect on the RPE date back to the early years of this century, when retinal and RPE degenerations were described in siderosis (Wagenmann, 1913). Chemical iodate intoxication with subsequent RPE and retinal degeneration, a side effect from a then prevalent treatment of septicemia, was recognized a few years later (Schimmel, 1926). The first toxic effects on the RPE induced by newer pharmaceutical products sold on a large scale were reported in the 1950s, when compounds such as chloroquine and phenothiazines became widely used. Since then several other pathological changes at the level of the RPE have been recorded and more data has become available on the toxicity of different substances at a cellular and subclinical level. This chapter will review experimental data from more recent in vivo and in vitro studies which have investigated the toxic effects of different substances on the RPE. Where possible this information will be reconciled with clinical observations.

ANESTHETICS

Several anesthetic agents have been found to influence the RPE in an experimental setting, although very few clinically relevant complications have been documented to date. The changes have mostly been demonstrated by electrophysiology and histology using different in vivo models. Electrophysiological data differed quite substantially, depending on the species used and the effects on the c-wave of the electroretinogram (ERG), which depends to a significant degree upon the RPE (see Chapter 9) are summarized in Table 32-1. The only experimentally and clinically important toxic effects on the RPE are induced by urethane and methoxyflurane.

Urethane is an anesthetic widely used for in vivo animal studies but not in humans. Several toxic effects on the retina and the RPE have been reported which are important for the interpretation of ocular observations obtained in animals under urethane anesthesia. The major effect seems to lie in the induction of new vessel formation at the level of the RPE. 1 mg/kg subcutaneous urethane once a week for eight weeks postpartum induces a severe retinopathy in newborn rats (Korte et al., 1984) which is characterized by late-stage ingrowth of retinal blood vessels through the RPE where they proliferate (Burns and Tyler, 1990). Some of these vessels within the RPE change their phenotype from continuous to fenestrated endothelial cells and may influence the polarity of the RPE (Korte et al., 1986; Burns and Hartz, 1992). The RPE may undergo focal hyperplasia and loss of blood–retinal barrier function at the site of the capillary invasion (Korte et al., 1986; Kritzinger and Bellhorn, 1982), although it retains the properties of the blood–retinal barrier in the nonaffected areas.

In contrast to urethane, *methoxyflurane* is an anesthetic used in humans. It is not directly toxic to the RPE but may lead to renal failure and hyperoxaluria with a resultant secondary toxic deposition of oxalate crystals in the RPE and retina. Two metabolites of methoxyflurane, fluoride and oxalic acid, are known nephrotoxins, and renal failure has been reported as a rate complication of this kind of general anesthesia. In a patient who had undergone prolonged abdominal surgery under methoxyflurane anesthesia, following which he developed acute irreversible renal failure, autopsy showed widespread oxalosis including crystals in the RPE and some in the neural retina (Bullock and Albert, 1975; Al-

TABLE 32-1. *Effect of anesthetics on the c-wave of the ERG*

Drug	ERG change	Species	Reference
Barbiturates	Transient c-wave decrease	Sheep	Knave et al., 1974
		Chick	Wioland et al., 1984
		Dog	Dawson et al., 1983
	No c-wave decrease	Rabbit	Lurie and Marmor, 1979
Halothane	C-wave decrease	Dog	Dawson et al., 1983
Ketamin	C-wave decrease	Chick	Wioland et al., 1984
	No c-wave decrease	Rabbit	Lurie and Marmor, 1979
Urethane	C-wave decrease	Chick	Wioland et al., 1984
	No c-wave decrease	Rabbit	Lurie and Marmor, 1979

bert et al., 1975). Illicit inhalational methoxyflurane abuse can also lead to secondary hyperoxaluria in which there is widespread retinal distribution of birefringent crystalline deposits, especially along the retinal arteries and arterioles but also at the level of the RPE (Novak et al., 1988). This distribution is almost identical to the fundus changes seen in primary hyperoxaluria and the crystalline deposits may induce hypertrophy or hyperplasia of the RPE with a resultant black macular lesion (Meredith et al., 1984).

ANTIINFECTIOUS DRUGS

Several categories of antiinfectious agents have been demonstrated to be toxic to the RPE, as shown in Table 32-2. After first reports were published on the toxicity of antimalarial therapy with quinoline derivates, many other and newer antibiotics have been investigated for the treatment of endophthalmitis. Most of these compounds lead to cellular dysfunction of the RPE and the retina with important clinical complications if a critical dose is reached.

Antibiotics

Intravenous and intravitreal injection of antibiotics have become indispensable in the treatment of endophthalmitis in recent years. Given their potency and use in close proximity to the retina and the RPE, such therapies carry considerable toxic risks which have been investigated among other techniques with electrophysiology. Table 32-3 shows effects on one ERG component, the c-wave, which reflects activity of the RPE. Safe doses have been investigated and demonstrated both in vivo and in vitro. Some overdoses may affect retina primarily, for example by an ischemic retinopathy, with secondary involvement of the RPE. However, specific alterations in RPE morphology and biochemistry have also been documented with some compounds.

Aminoglycosides. Most aminoglycosides may induce lysosomal inclusions in the RPE as their earliest sign of toxicity and, although they display marked differences (Table 32-4), their deleterious effects on the retinal vasculature after administration of higher doses are well known: gentamicin is considered the most toxic compound, followed—as toxicity decreases—by tobramy-

TABLE 32-2. *Antiinfectious drugs with toxic effects on the RPE*

Antibiotics
    Aminoglycosides
        Gentamicin
        Tobramycin
        Netilmicin
        Amikacin
    Glycopolypeptides
        Vancomycin
    Cephalosporins
        Cephaloridine
    Betalactam
        Penicillin
    Quinolones
        Norfloxacin
        Oxfloxacin
        Flumequine
        Levofloxacin
Antimicobacterial drugs
    Rifampicin
    Clofazimine
Antiviral drugs
    Didanosine
    Ganciclovir
Quinolines
    Chloroquine
    Hydroxychloroquine
    Quinine

TABLE 32-3. *Effects of antibiotics on the c-wave of the ERG*

Drug	ERG change	Species	Reference
Gentamicin	C-wave abolished Doses > 0.2 mg intravitreal	Rabbit	Kawasaki et al., 1990
Tobramycin	C-wave normal Doses < 0.08 mg intravitreal	Rabbit	Kawasaki et al., 1990
Netilmicin	C-wave decrease reversible Doses > 0.2 mg intravitreal	Rabbit	Kawasaki et al., 1990
Disodium Sulbenicillin	C-wave normal Doses < 2 mg intravitreal	Rabbit	Kawasaki et al., 1990
Cephaloridine	ERG abolished Doses > 0.5 mg intravitreal	Rabbit	Graham et al., 1975
Procain Penicillin G	C-wave decrease 0.85 mM intravitreal	Human (in vitro)	Kawasaki and Ohnogi, 1988
Norfloxaxin	C-wave decrease Doses > 500 µg intravitreal	Rabbit	Yamashita et al., 1995
Oxfloxacin	No ERG change	Rabbit	Kawasaki et al., 1990

cin, netilmicin, and amikacin (D'Amico et al., 1985). "Safe doses" for intravitreal injections have been advocated; however, there are several reports that have illustrated that even much smaller doses of different drugs may trigger widespread toxic changes in susceptible patients (Campochiaro and Lim, 1994; Piguet et al., 1996). These potent agents have thus to be used with great care.

Gentamicin is considered the most toxic compound, and it has been suggested that the clinically most important toxic effect of high-dose intravitreal gentamicin is a complete shutdown of retinal blood flow, probably by granulocytic plugging in the capillary bed as shown in primates (Conway et al., 1989; Hines et al., 1993) which is thought to be responsible for the ischemic retinopathy feared by clinicians (Campochiaro and Lim, 1994). On the other hand, at lower doses the drug may also induce intracellular lysosomal inclusions in the RPE associated with a few focal areas of RPE necrosis and hyperplasia—comparable to inclusions reported in kid-

TABLE 32-4. *Minimal intravitreal dosages of antibiotics to induce retinal and RPE changes*

Drug	Lysosomal overloading of the RPE	Photoreceptor death	Full-thickness retinal necrosis
Gentamicin	0.2 mg	0.4 mg	0.8 mg
Netilmicin	0.1 mg	0.8 mg	1.0 mg
Tobramycin	0.5 mg	0.8 mg	1.6 mg
Amikacin	0.75 mg	1.5 mg	3.0 mg
Kanamycin	0.75 mg	1.5 mg	3.0 mg

Source: D'Amico et al., 1985.

ney and other tissues as manifestations of gentamicin toxicity (D'Amico et al., 1984)—as early as three days after intravitreal injection in rabbit eyes (100–500 µg). This possible RPE-specific effect may come about by the binding of gentamicin to the RPE, an effect which seems to be strong, as the drug could be localized primarily in the RPE and choriocapillaris with only occasional staining in the neurosensory retina 12–24 hours following a single intravitreal injection of 400 µg (Tabatabay et al., 1990). However, other authors have conversely suggested that ocular pigmentation may paradoxically protect from gentamicin-induced toxicity (Zemel et al., 1995) by binding the drug to melanin, which thereby reduces the concentration of free gentamicin (Barza et al., 1976; Kane et al., 1981). From a clinical point of view the combination of gentamicin with other antibiotics such as clindamycin (McDonald et al., 1986) or 1 mg vancomycin with 100 µg gentamicin in aphakic and vitrectomized eyes (Oum et al., 1992) and their repeated intravitreal injection may be very problematic with deleterious effects on retinal perfusion, retinal outer segments, and the RPE. A few reports have also been published on poorly understood effects of gentamicin on the RPE, such as enhanced RPE phagocytosis (Markowitz et al., 1981) and an induction of a pigmentary change in the ocular fundus after an intravitreal injection of 0.2 mg (Kawasaki et al., 1990). Interestingly, gentamicin has also been shown to neutralize the RPE-selective toxic effects of an orally administered rat poison, N-3-pyridylmethyl-N'-p-nitrophenylurea (PNU) (Mindel et al., 1988), although the mechanism involved is elusive.

Tobramycin is the second most toxic aminoglycoside (D'Amico et al., 1985). Retinal and RPE toxicity (such as intracellular membranous inclusions) has been shown from intravitreal doses as small as 0.5 mg (Moschos et al., 1990). Contrary to the findings with gentamicin, tobramycin does not seem to have an inhibitory effect on the lysosomal enzymes in the RPE at low concentrations (Hayasaka et al., 1988), and intravitreal injections of a small dose (0.08 mg) did not alter the c-wave of the ERG (Kawasaki et al., 1990). Only larger doses of 0.5 mg and more have been associated experimentally with lysosomal inclusions in the RPE (D'Amico et al., 1985), and a clinical report has documented the deleterious effects of a high dose of intravitreal injection (20 mg) of tobramycin with ensuing retinal degeneration and optic atrophy (Balian, 1983).

Netilmicin has about the same toxicity as tobramycin and displays its adverse effects far less in the retinal vasculature but more specifically in the RPE by producing an accumulation of membrane-limited osmiophilic lamellated inclusions in this cell layer. The inclusions measure from 1–3 microns in diameter, exhibit acid hydrolase activity, and seem to represent residual bodies, suggesting that these accumulations are responsible for the observed cellular lipidosis (Tabatabay et al., 1987). Only as much as 0.2 mg netilmicin did suppress the c-wave in the rabbit ERG reversibly (Kawasaki et al., 1990), and a dose of more than 0.5 mg led to damage of outer segments and RPE (Takeichi et al., 1991). This damage to the RPE could be prevented by addition of calcium (CaCl$_2$) to the intravitreal injection, although the mechanism for this rescue is not quite clear (Takeichi et al., 1994).

Amikacine exhibits even lower toxicity and toxic effects only appear after intravitreal doses of more than 1.5 mg (Talamo et al., 1985), whereas a single combined injection of 0.4 mg amikacin with 1 mg of vancomycin is considered safe (Oum et al., 1989). However, repeated intravitreal injection of 0.4 mg amikacin with 1 mg of vancomycin also triggered a severe ischemic retinopathy with reduced ERG and grossly abnormal electrooculogram (EOG), hinting at secondary RPE dysfunction. (Oum et al., 1989; Habib et al., 1994). A similarly deleterious effect of amikacin was documented in a series of susceptible patients who developed macular infarction after receiving intravitreal injections of a dose, previously thought safe, of 0.2 or 0.4 mg (Campochiaro and Lim, 1994).

Glycopolypeptide. *Vancomycin,* in contrast to the aminoglycosides, is generally regarded as an agent with low toxicity for the retina–RPE interface (Pflugfelder et al., 1987). However, intravitreal injection of vancomycin in combination with aminoglycosides can enhance the toxicity of the latter, as discussed above. Intravitreal injection of 1 mg vancomycin alone caused no ERG changes for 8 weeks after the injection. Increasing the dose to 10 mg, however, abolished all ERG responses 1–4 weeks after the injection, whereafter only the c-wave recovered (Kawasaki et al., 1990). The pathophysiology of this selective recovery of the c-wave is not well understood.

Cephalosporins. Cephalosporins have been advocated as less toxic alternatives to aminoglycosides for intravitreal injection, for example in combination with vancomycin (Campochiaro and Lim, 1994). However, an older generation of this drug class, such as *cephaloridine,* may in higher intravitreal doses (0.5–10 mg) in the rabbit induce clumping of the outer segments and destruction of the RPE with first ERG changes ten minutes after the intravitreal injection followed by an extinguished ERG after 24 hours (Graham et al., 1975). A more recent experimental study in rabbits has also demonstrated that by the second day numerous specks of pigment were scattered about over the whole fundus with larger clumps of pigment in the periphery against a background of extensive atrophy of the RPE (Turut and Malthieu, 1980). Despite this well-defined and severe toxic reaction from *intravitreal* injection, no retinotoxic effect was detected after intravenous, subconjunctival, or intracameral injection of the drug (Graham et al., 1975). This stands in contrast to a clinical report that documented a pigmentary retinopathy and loss of vision in four patients who had received a subconjunctival or intracameral injection of the drug (Turut et al., 1979).

Beta-lactam antibiotics. Previous experiments have established that *penicillin* is actively transported across the RPE and competes with fluorescein transport (Cunha-Vaz et al., 1967). Furthermore, penicillin has been shown to significantly inhibit phagocytosis by the RPE in bovine organ culture, although the exact mechanism is unclear (Markowitz et al., 1981). Further evidence of an effect on the RPE has been demonstrated in an in vitro eyecup preparation of a human eye, where procaine penicillin-G suppressed the ERG c-wave as well as the oscillatory potentials (Kawasaki and Ohnogi, 1988), whereas other penicillin derivatives such as cloxacillin did not have this effect. There is no clinical significance known to date for these toxic effects.

Quinolones. Quinolone antibiotics are bactericidal agents that interfere with the activity of DNA gyrase, a bacterial enzyme, and thus inhibit DNA synthesis. *Norfloxacin,* for example, has been shown to induce retinal edema and diminish the b- and c-waves of the ERG in the rabbit after intravitreal injection at a concentration of 500 µg weekly for four weeks. Electron microscopy demonstrated swelling of the RPE cells with enlarged smooth endoplasmic reticulum containing osmiophilic material as well as focal retinal destruction (Yamashita et al., 1995). *Flumequine* is another quinolone that has been implicated in RPE dysfunction. Several patients have developed bilateral serous detachment of the RPE and retina after administration of 1.2 g/day flumequine during three days for urinary tract infection. All the patients had prior chronic renal failure. When the treatment was discontinued, the bullae in the macula disappeared within five days (Sirbat et al., 1983). Whether these effects are due to direct drug toxicity to RPE transport function or linked to vascular changes in the choriocapillaris is not known. Fluoroquinolones have a strong affinity for melanin and drugs such as *levofloxacin* may thus be deposited in the uvea and the RPE. However, no toxic effects have been shown to date (Ohkubo et al., 1995).

Antimycobacterial Agents

Clofazimine is an iminophenazine dye with antimycobacterial activity which has been used to treat leprosy and psoriasis for several decades. Recently its use has also been advocated for the treatment of mycobacterium avium complex infection in patients with AIDS. Reddish-brown pigmentary skin changes have been well known for several decades but ocular side effects of clofazimine were only recently reported for the first time by Ohman and Wahlberg (1975); and later a classic bull's-eye retinopathy was characterized (Craythorn et al., 1986; Cunningham et al., 1990; Forster et al., 1992) (Fig. 32-1a and b). In one case retinotoxicity appeared after an eight-month treatment with clofazimine at the dose of 200 mg/day (total dose of 48 g) (Cunningham et al., 1990); in another 300 mg/day given for five months was sufficient (Craythorn et al., 1986). Electrophysiological examination showed generalized reduction in retinal function although the EOG was normal. The treatment was discontinued soon after the fundus changes appeared, but there was no long-term follow-up due to the death of the patients. Autopsy was not granted in either of the cases.

Rifampicin, another tuberculostatic drug, has been shown to selectively alter the c-wave in the ERG without concomitant changes in the a- or b-waves (Knave et al., 1973; Calissendorff, 1976a). There have been no data on the clinical significance of these findings, although there is evidence that rifampicin exhibits an increased affinity for melanin in the uvea and the RPE of the human fetal eye (Boman, 1973).

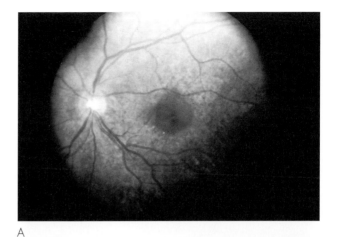

A

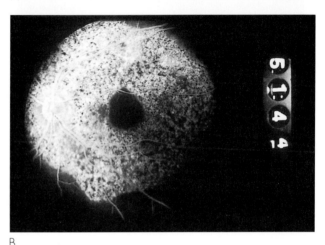

B

FIGURE 32-1. Clofazimine retinopathy. (A) Fundus photograph: note bull's-eye-like appearance of the macula with normal or slightly increased pigment centrally surrounded by a broad zone of hypopigmentation and pigment mottling. (B) Fluorescein angiogram: note the broad annular window defect due to retinal pigment epithelial depigmentation. Centrally there is increased hypofluorescence as a result of mild hyperpigmentation in that area. (Courtesy of Ronald E. Carr, M.D.)

Antiviral Agents

Didanoside is a purine analog with antiretroviral activity which is used as a second-line drug in the treatment of diseases associated with the human immunodeficiency virus. Several side effects, such as peripheral neuropathy and retinopathy, have been reported in children (Whitcup et al., 1992). The retinal complications were characterized by multiple well-circumscribed depigmented lesions in the midperipheral retina (Fig. 32-2). Histopathological investigation showed these areas to represent RPE atrophy, sometimes surrounded by areas of hypertrophy or hypopigmentation of the RPE. Partial loss of the choriocapillaris and neurosensory retina were

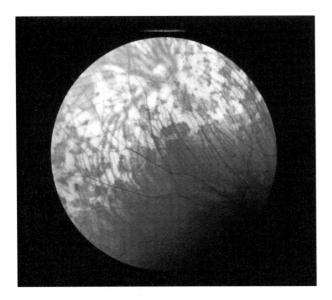

FIGURE 32-2. Retinal changes associated with didanosine therapy. Well-circumscribed depigmented retinal lesions are evident in the mid-periphery of the retina. (Courtesy of Scott M. Whitcup, M.D.)

also observed in the region of diseased RPE. Electron microscopy demonstrated membranous lamellar inclusions in the RPE. It was concluded that the primary tissue that is affected in didanoside retinopathy is the RPE, with the choriocapillaris and retina consequently affected in areas of diseased RPE (Whitcup et al., 1994).

Parenteral and intravitreal *ganciclovir* are currently used in the treatment of cytomegalo virus (CMV) retinitis. The pattern of accumulation of ganciclovir in the retina of human eyes treated for CMV retinitis (Park et al., 1995) seems to be confined to the RPE and photoreceptor outer segments, whereas there was no accumulation in eyes treated with foscarnet or in patients who received the drug without the presence of CMV retinitis. This difference in drug accumulation is not yet fully understood. Recently new data has become available on 2'-nor cyclic GMP, a nucleotide anolog and a cyclic phosphate derivative of ganciclovir which has been encapsulated into a multivesicular liposome system (Shakiba et al., 1993). Toxicity of this compound could be shown in a rabbit model after intravitreal injection of concentrations above 50 mg with loss of ERG amplitude and increased vacuolization of the RPE as well as shortening of the outer photoreceptor segments.

Quinolines

Quinoline derivatives represent a group of drugs with a related structure: the quinoline ring. However, depending on the substitutes around the ring, different agents exhibit a wide range of effects. The toxic changes mediated by chloroquine, for example, are not limited to the retina but can also become manifest in the cornea and the lens. With a slight alteration in the quinoline ring of hydroxychloroquine these extraretinal manifestations are, however, much less frequent.

Chloroquine was introduced earlier this century for the treatment and prophylaxis of malaria, but it was not until after the Second World War that the first description of a retinopathy associated with the use of this drug was published (Goldman and Preston, 1957). Later, chloroquine diphosphate (Resochin) and chloroquine sulfate (Nivaquine) were introduced as potent agents in the treatment of lupus erythematosis and rheumatoid arthritis. Chloroquine has been gradually replaced by hydroxychloroquine for these latter clinical uses due to the fewer side effects (Shearer and Dubois, 1967), although the mode of action and the toxicity of these two compounds are eventually very similar.

Mechanisms of toxicity. The physiologic effects and pharmacokinetics of chloroquine and hydroxychloroquine are similar, whereby the half-life of the drug is increasing parallel with the increase of the dose given (Frisk-Holmberg et al., 1979). The general mechanism of chloroquine toxicity has been ascribed to acute inhibition of lysosomal enzyme activity (Homewood et al., 1972) or protein synthesis (Roskoski and Jaskunas, 1972). The drug-induced lysosomal abnormalities include diminished vesicle fusion, and diminished exocytosis. In the eye the RPE seems to be the most susceptible organ, followed by astroglia or neuronal cells from the retina (Bruinink et al., 1991), with RPE lysosomal enzyme activity such as N-acetyl-beta-glucosaminidase being reduced (Toimela et al., 1995). The RPE seems to be compromised not only biochemically but also physiologically, as a breakdown of the outer blood–retinal barrier (BRB) could be demonstrated fluorophotometrically in symptomatic patients whereas the BRB remained intact in asymptomatic patients who were receiving the drug (Raines et al., 1989). Other authors have demonstrated that the primary insult in albino rats and cats may be in the ganglion cells, with secondary degeneration of the photoreceptors (Rosenthal et al., 1978; Ivanina et al., 1983), and similar studies in the mouse have demonstrated morphological and biochemical signs of phospholipidosis in the neuroretina with relative sparing of the RPE after more than 6 months of treatment with chloroquine (Hallberg et al., 1990).

RPE-specific toxicity of chloroquine has been linked to melanin binding of the drug (Rosenthal et al., 1978), and the major reason for accumulation of these drugs seems to be uptake involving a charge transfer (Mason, 1977), although binding may be via multiple sites (Larsson and Tjalve, 1979). However, melanin binding does not necessarily make drugs available for toxic damage, and could in fact be a protective mechanism for the eye (Zemel et al., 1995). Affinity to melanin-containing cells per se is therefore not sufficient to class a substance as potentially harmful to vision. Furthermore, the binding of the enantiomers of hydroxychloroquine and its metabolites to ocular structures showed that the drug accumulated both in pigmented *and* nonpigmented tissues (Wainer et al., 1994). Further detailed information on binding of chloroquine can be found in the chapter on RPE and Melanin. Apart from histological investigations, RPE-specific chloroquine toxicity has also been evaluated by electrophysiological studies, and there is experimental evidence that intravenous injection of chloroquine in small doses induces a delayed selective drop in c-wave amplitude in sheep. Larger doses (such as 3 mg/kg) also had an immediate effect on the b- and c-wave (Calissendorff, 1976b). Recently, the protective effect of a platelet-activating factor (PAF) antagonist against these chloroquine-induced ERG changes has been reported, although the mechanisms involved are not known (Doly et al., 1993).

Clinical manifestations of chloroquine. Reports on the incidence of chloroquine retinopathy range from 3%–10% of treated patients (Bernstein, 1983). Despite the heterogeneity of the statistics, it is evident that the retinopathy gets worse with increased dose and duration of treatment (Bernstein, 1983). Daily oral doses associated with a very low incidence of retinopathy are 250 mg for chloroquine diphosphate and 200 mg for chloroquine sulfate (3.5–4 mg/kg). A cumulative dose of less than 100 g and a duration of treatment less than one year have also been associated with a very low incidence of toxic changes (Bernstein, 1983). In the prophylaxis of malaria much lower doses of the drug are employed than in the treatment of the collagen disorders (such as 300 mg per week), but with even these very low doses toxic effects have been observed sporadically, especially in children (Cordier et al., 1981). Early visual complaints may start after ingestion of as little as 500–700 mg per day (2–3 times the daily dose) and include blurring and sometimes diplopia. These early complaints are usually the result of accidental overdosage and have been reversible upon cessation of treatment. Symptoms of the chronic exposure retinopathy range from central or paracentral scotoma to photophobia, nyctalopia, and photopsias to an asymptomatic state with visible retinopathy, pigment mottling, and loss of foveal reflex. Pigment irregularity tends to be more prominent in the inferior macula with the final picture of a horizontally oval bull's-eye lesion (Hart et al., 1984). At about the

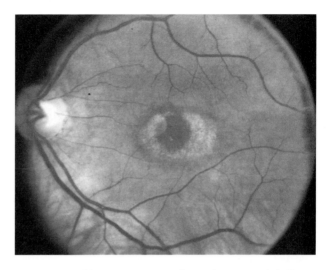

FIGURE 32-3. Chloroquine retinopathy with a typical bull's-eye pattern. (Courtesy of Michael F. Marmor, M.D.)

same time parafoveal retinal function changes subtly while central visual acuity remains normal. The typical bull's-eye pattern becomes more obvious as time goes on, which is usually associated with an annular scotoma of 2–3 degrees from fixation (Fig. 32-3). If the process develops further, peripheral pigmentary irregularity and bone spicule formation may ensue with vascular attenuation and disc pallor. Functional deficits have been reported to regress somewhat after cessation of the therapy, this being mostly the case in mild and early damage. However, even if the treatment is stopped early in the disease residual loss of vision may be permanent. Furthermore, there are also cases of progression of retinopathy despite discontinuation of medication, an observation made mostly in very advanced stages of the disease (Brinkley et al., 1979). There have also been some cases reported where the disease started months to years after the treatment had been stopped (Ogawa et al., 1979; Sassani et al., 1983).

Given these important toxic effects of chloroquine, regular follow-up of these patients is mandatory. Evidence for early stages of retinopathy, when patients are still asymptomatic and the fundus appearance is nonspecific, can be found by central threshold fields (Hart et al., 1984) or Amsler grid testing (Easterbrook, 1984). Electrodiagnostic testing with the EOG has also been advocated for detection of early chloroquine-induced changes; however, its usefulness or specificity as a screening test is questioned by many (Arden and Kolb, 1966; Pinkers and Broekhuyse, 1983). For practical clinical purposes, the measuring of visual fields and color vision and detailed ophthalmoscopy should be done about once a year, and for patients on high doses or after many years of usage a baseline ERG and EOG should be obtained.

Hydroxychloroquine retinopathy was shown in one study to develop after a total dose of more than 800 g (Mills et al., 1981), whereas a total cumulative dose of 200 g was not associated with an elevated risk of retinopathy. Another larger study found a total drug accumulation of up to 700 g safe with minimal changes of visual fields in 4% patients, changes which regressed upon discontinuation of the drug (Tobin et al., 1982). Daily oral doses associated with a very low incidence of retinopathy are 400 mg (6.0–6.5 mg/kg) (Mackenzie, 1983). The risk of retinopathy associated with the chronic use of hydroxychloroquine at these doses has been reported to be almost nonexistent (Spalton et al., 1993). However, even with adherence to the clinically recommended therapeutic guidelines, elderly patients have been reported with typical maculopathy (Falcone et al., 1993).

Clinical manifestations of hydroxychloroquine. The clinical picture of hydroxychloroquine retinopathy resembles very closely the changes induced by chloroquine. The typical bull's-eye appearance may also present, or sometimes a more diffuse form.

The current guidelines suggested for the follow-up of patients treated with hydroxychloroquine are similar to those for chloroquine. However, the economy of regular screening of patients has been questioned as a whole on the basis of an almost nonexistent risk for retinopathy (Morsman et al., 1990), at least in the first two years on standard doses.

Quinine has been used in the treatment of malaria for well over a century, and first reports of retinotoxic effects date back to the beginning of this century. Since quinine binds to uveal tissue in vitro, the RPE may be affected selectively after intoxication. In sheep, for example, intravenous injection of quinine in small doses induces a delayed selective drop in c-wave amplitude (Calissendorff, 1976b), and experimental EOG examination has shown a rapid selective inversion of the c-wave in the rabbit (Junemann and Schulze, 1968). Similar EOG changes have been recorded in patients during the initial acute phase of visual loss, but they subsequently returned to normal (Behrman and Mushin, 1968). However, clinical observations and examination with fluorescein angiography have also demonstrated marked constriction of retinal vessels associated with retinal ischaemia and reversible reduction in ERG a- and b-waves (Yospaiboon et al., 1984; Bacon et al., 1988), and damage to retinal tissue seems thus more generalized (Nusinowitz et al., 1996). The therapeutic dose for quinine is less than 1 g/day and even this has

proved toxic to some patients, but toxicity has more often been seen with overdoses of 2–5 grams. A clinically detectable pigmentary retinopathy has also been described after ingestion of excessive amounts (more than 300 mg/day) of quinine in the form of tablets (Dekking, 1949) or in the form of excessive drinking of Indian tonic water, which contains 80 mg/l quinine (Horgan and Williams, 1995).

ANTIINFLAMMATORY DRUGS

Corticosteroids

Intensive systemic steroid therapy has been linked to the occasional development or aggravation of central serous chorioretinopathy (Gass, 1987; Polak et al., 1995; Chaine et al., 1995). The mechanisms of these effects are still not entirely clear, but may relate to the potentiating effect that steroids exhibit on catecholamines, which in turn have been implicated in the pathogenesis of central serous chorioretinopathy (Yoshioka et al., 1982; Yannuzzi, 1986).

Nonsteroidal Antiinflammatory Drugs (NSAIDs)

NSAIDs are widely used for their antiinflammatory, antipyretic, and analgesic effect, often for prolonged periods. Despite the ubiquitous consumption of this agent, retinal toxicity is very rare. Some experimental studies have investigated the effect of NSAID on RPE function.

Several clinical observations have suggested a retinotoxic effect from indomethacin. The lesions usually comprise diffuse pigment scattering of the RPE perifoveally as well as fine areas of depigmentation around the macula (Graham and Blach, 1988), although the changes may be more marked in the periphery of the retina (Henkes et al., 1972). Color vision deficiency of the blue-yellow type has been found (Palimeris et al., 1972). After discontinuation of treatment, visual acuity, the reduced EOG and ERG, and pigment alterations may improve over several months (Henkes et al., 1972; Palimeris et al., 1972). A patient with a total cumulative dose of 100 g of indomethacin over four years has also been reported to show RPE stippling as well as an abnormal EOG (Buchanan and Archer, 1978). The pathogenesis of this toxic effect is not entirely clear but a direct effect on the RPE has been postulated (Henkes et al., 1972; Palimeris et al., 1972). Indeed, indomethacin has been shown to depress the ability of RPE to phagocytose latex particles labelled with iodine 125 (Goldhar et al., 1984), but whether this explains the clinical retinopathy is not known.

Aspirin has been shown to depress the ability of RPE to phagocytose latex particles labelled with iodine 125 (Goldhar et al., 1984) although there are no reports of clinical RPE toxicity and the functional significance of these results remains unclear.

CRYSTAL-INDUCING DRUGS

Canthaxanthin (b,b-carotene-4,4'-dione) is an internationally used food color that has also been incorporated into compounds used for tanning. In early 1980 an association between the ingestion of tanning tablets—for cosmetic reasons or for the treatment of various light sensitive dermatoses—and fine glistening yellow or gold-colored particles in the macula was described for the first time (Cortin et al., 1982). The clinical entity has since been recognized by several authors. The treatment has been combined with beta-carotene (standard human dose 2 mg/kg), which itself does not cause any crystalline deposits. Intake of high doses of canthaxanthin has also been associated with the ingestion of food additives where the compound is used to produce a more desirable color of fish (Oosterhuis et al., 1989) in which cauthaxanthine is already a minor component of the flesh pigmentation of, for example, wild salmon and trout (Sharkey, 1993). The occurrence of deposits is strongly correlated with the total dose of ingested drug. Thirty-seven grams of canthaxanthine induced retinal deposits in 50% of patients (Boudreault et al., 1983) and a dose of 60 g in 100% of patients (Metge et al., 1984).

The investigation of autopsy specimens has demonstrated the deposits as red, birefringent, lipid-soluble crystals in the inner layer of the entire retina with a predilection of the macula. Clinically these deposits are only seen when they are packed most densely (Daicker et al., 1987). The deposits may develop until they are about 10–14 μm in size and are located principally in a ring-shaped area between 5 and 10 degrees around the fovea, although irregular dissemination in the posterior fundus has also been observed (Fig. 32-4 and Plate 32-I). Usually, patients are asymptomatic and visual loss has not been associated with the deposits. However, there have been some reports of subnormal ERGs and higher thresholds in static perimetry. A- and b-waves which were depressed during therapy returned to normal levels shortly after withdrawal of the drugs (Weber et al., 1992). The EOG is usually normal or subnormal (Metge et al., 1984). Changes in retinal function disappear after withdrawal of the drug, but the crystals dissolve rather slowly (Harnois et al., 1989), sometimes needing several years and at times leaving minor defects

at the level of the RPE. Ultrastructural studies of the RPE have shown an increase in cell height and a regional vacuolization due to an enlargement and disruption of some phagolysosomes (Scallon et al., 1988) as well as enlarged lipid droplets (Weber et al., 1987). Canthaxanthine retinopathy has also been described with an asymmetric appearance in an eye with a branch retinal vein occlusion (Chang et al., 1995), although the reason for this association is not clear.

Tamoxifen is a nonsteroidal antiestrogen which binds to estrogen receptor proteins in the cytoplasm. It is primarily used in the treatment of metastatic breast cancer in postmenopausal patients, and is usually given as a daily dose of 10–20 mg/day. Chemically, it has cationic amphiphillic properties like those of other compounds, including chloroquine, thioridazine, chlorpromazine, and amiodarone (Burke et al., 1987). These agents are characterized by a hydrophobic moiety and a positively charged hydrophilic side chain on the same molecule (Bockhardt and Lullmann-Rauch, 1978), which allow them to reversibly form polar lipid complexes which are then accumulated in lysosomes (Lullmann-Rauch, 1981) or incorporated into biological membranes (Custodio et al., 1993). The toxicity of tamoxifen may be due to decreasing the activity of lysosomal enzymes such as N-acetyl-beta-glucosaminidase and cathepsin D as shown in an in vitro RPE cell culture model (Toimela et al., 1995). A profound decrease of enzyme activities started only after therapeutic doses were exceeded (concentration of tamoxifen >10 μM).

Since its first description (Kaiser-Kupfer and Lippman, 1978) tamoxifen retinopathy has become a recognized clinical entity (McKeown et al., 1981). The clinical picture is characterized by crystalline refractile deposits found in the retina and at the level of the RPE after ingestion of a cumulative dose of 90–230 g of tamoxifen or a daily dose of 60–90 mg (Fig. 32-5). However, retinopathy is extremely rare in large series of patients taking the currently recommended dose of 30 mg per day (Winding and Nielsen, 1983). Screening for ocular toxicity in asymptomatic patients has demonstrated a prevalence of 1%–2% (Heier et al., 1994; Kalina and Wells, 1995). The cumulative doses in these patients were between 10 and 22 g, whereas in the other asymptomatic patients the cumulative dose was a mean of 17 g with a standard deviation of 13. Given these uncommon findings and the large variations in the doses needed to induce pathology, special screening of patients does not seem to be warranted if they receive the recommended dose of 10–20 mg/day (Heier et al., 1994).

Cystoid macular edema and visual-field loss may develop both peripherally and centrally. Visual acuity is reduced and retinal vessels may appear mildly narrowed.

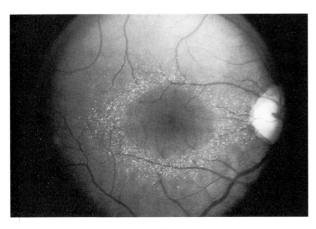

FIGURE 32-4. Extensive deposits of refractile canthaxanthin crystals in the perifoveal region. (See also Plate 32-I.) (Courtesy of Michael F. Marmor, M.D.)

Fluorescein angiography demonstrates hypofluorescent granular areas with border hyperfluorescence and no evidence of late leakage. ERG investigations in patients treated with tamoxifen have shown that rod amplitudes and rod b-wave implicit time may be compromised without the presence of visible fundus changes (Berezovsky et al., 1996), and a reduction in oscillatory potential has also been reported (Burke et al., 1987).

CYTOSTATIC DRUGS

Several effects of cytostatic drugs on the RPE have been investigated recently to evaluate inhibition of pathological RPE proliferation, which could be exploited in the treatment of proliferative disorders at the level of the

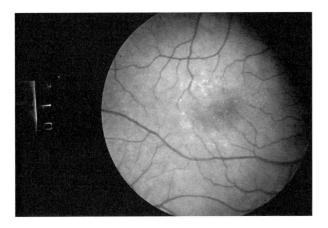

FIGURE 32-5. Tamoxifen retinopathy. Fundus of right eye with multiple tiny refractile, intraretinal lesions and larger granular areas at the level of the retinal pigment epithelium. (Courtesy of Michael F. Marmor, M.D.)

TABLE 32-5. *Cytostatic drugs with toxic effects on the RPE*

Tamoxifen
Mitomycin C
Methotrexate
Vincristine
Carmustine
Tilorone

retina and RPE (see Chapter 32). Once a critical concentration is surpassed, however, toxic effects on healthy RPE and retinal cells become evident with the use of some compounds, as shown in Table 32-5. For some widely used local and systemic cytostatic drugs these effects can be deleterious.

Mitomycin C is a widely used antiproliferative drug to suppress scarring and to enhance the success rate of filtering surgery in glaucoma, and several studies have addressed its toxicity on the retina. Intravitreal injection of mitomycin C (40 mg/ml) in rats, for example induced a decrease of the b-wave in the ERG after 2 days, and after day 7 the a-wave was diminished too. No recovery was seen after 1 month. Electron microscope findings showed mild degeneration of the RPE and disarrangement of the disc structure of photoreceptor outer segments at day 2. On day 28 the outer layer was completely destroyed, although some of the cellular components in the inner layer were relatively intact (Adachi-Usami et al., 1995). Other investigators have found that subretinal injection of 0.004 mg/ml had no effect, 0.4 mg/ml triggered moderate disruption of the outer segments and a concentration of 40 mg/ml mitomycin C induced panretinal atrophy and RPE hypertrophy (Casey et al., 1995).

In patients who received *methotrexate* treatment for intracranial malignant neoplasms via the internal carotid or vertebral artery, ipsilateral retinal pigment epitheliopathy has been described (Millay et al., 1986). This was, however, associated with minimal functional loss which was therefore not a limiting factor with this therapeutic modality.

Vincristine sulfate is the salt of an alkaloid from the periwinkle plant and has been shown to stop mitosis at the stage of the metaphase. This compound has been reported to induce night blindness in man, and experimental evaluation has demonstrated reduced ERG b-waves as well as a rapid fall in the c-wave. Ultrastructural damage is, however, mostly confined to the photoreceptors and other retinal neurons. Experimental studies in rabbits have demonstrated that intravitreal injection of 0.1–0.2 mg/ml vincristine sulfate produced histologic changes in the rabbit retina and RPE within 24 hours (Vrabec et al., 1968). Doses of 1–4 mg/ml did not change the ERG nor did they induce morphologic changes (Barrada et al., 1983). The drug seems to interfere with microtubules and impair axonal transport as well as the functional integrity of the transport system by which synaptic activity is maintained (Green, 1975; Ripps et al., 1989). A case report has been described with RPE degeneration, retinal atrophy, and a macular hole in an acute lymphocytic leukemia which was treated with methotrexate, vincristine, cyclophosphamide, and prednisone, however the causal relationship to this combination of drugs is not entirely clear (Inkeles and Friedman, 1975). The described effects of vincristine on the photoreceptor outer segments were recently inhibited by a platelet aggregating factor (PAF) antagonist in the rat, suggesting that the toxic effect is an inflammatory process involving PAF (Doly et al., 1992).

Carmustine has been used for several years as a therapeutic agent for malignant gliomas of the central nervous system, metastatic breast cancer, and leukemia. To increase its bioavailability this drug has also been infused into the internal carotid artery for the treatment of brain tumors fed by this vessel. This has been associated with ocular toxicity in some patients (Grimson et al., 1981). Retinal complications range from changes at the level of the RPE to retinal infarction and macular edema. These side effects can, however, be avoided by passing the infusion catheter beyond the origin of the ophthalmic artery (Chrousos et al., 1986). More recently, carmustine (BCNU) has also been described as a new antiproliferative drug that is lipid soluble and thus very suitable for use in combination with silicone oil (Chung et al., 1988).

Tilorone is an antitumor drug which boosts natural killer cell activity. Two patients have been reported who developed corneal infiltrates and a toxic retinopathy characterized by fine pigment mottling of the peripheral fundus and macula with mild arteriolar narrowing after a total oral dose of 152 g. Although visual acuity remained stable at 6/6 throughout treatment, Goldmann visual fields showed marked peripheral constriction of the visual fields and ERG and EOG amplitudes were abnormal. It has been suggested that tilorone may act as an antioxidant that affects the free-radical-scavenging mechanism of the RPE (Weiss et al., 1980).

DRUGS ACTING ON THE CENTRAL NERVOUS SYSTEM

Antipsychotic and Hypnotic Drugs

Most toxic effects of antipsychotic agents have been documented in experimental studies (see Table 32-6)

TABLE 32-6. *Drugs acting on the central nervous system with toxic effects on the RPE*

Antipsychotic and hypnotic drugs	Hallucinogenic drugs
Benzodiazepines	LSD
Diazepam	
Flunitrazepam	
Phenothiazines	
Chlorpromazine	
Thioridazine	
Fluphenazine	
Tricyclic antidepressants	
Imipramine	
Amitryptiline	
Piperidindiones	
Thalidomid	
Amphiphilic cationic drugs	
Citalopram	
Chlorphentermine	
Zimelidine	

and the only drug that gives rise to a clinically significant disorder is thioridazine.

Benzodiazepines. The majority of specific benzodiazepine binding sites in the rat, monkey, and human retina are found in the inner plexiform layer, although relatively high levels were also found in the RPE (Zarbin and Anholt, 1991). The physiological role of these receptors is still debated. They do not seem to influence visually induced preganglionic retinal activity, as it has been shown both in rats and cats that neither acute nor chronic administration of benzodiazepines or their antagonists altered the retinal functions as determined by the ERG (Robbins and Tkeda, 1989). Other authors have, however, found changes in the EOG after a single injection of 20 mg *diazepam* (Müller and Haase, 1975), and also in the ERG and visual fields (Jaffe et al., 1989; Elder, 1992).

The clinical significance of these findings is undetermined. Manners reported on one case where a treatment over years with high doses of diazepam (30 mg/day) was associated with a maculopathy characterized by RPE mottling and atrophy (Manners and Clarke, 1995), although in view of the widespread use of diazepam this association may be entirely fortuitous.

Although *flunitrazepam* has similar melanin-binding characteristics as chloroquine, it does not induce the structural alterations in retinal and RPE cells observed in chloroquine retinopathy, as shown in a mouse and cat model which were both fed clinical doses of chloroquine and flunitrazepam for a period of 6–12 months (Kuhn et al., 1981). Augmentation of lysosomal structures in the eye could only be seen in the melanin-free region of the pigment epithelium.

Phenothiazines. The phenothiazine derivatives, first synthesized in 1883, have been used for several decades in the treatment of schizophrenia and other psychoses with the first report of an associated retinopathy appearing in the 1950s (Kinross-Wright et al., 1956; Verrey, 1956). Serious toxic effects and pigmentary retinopathy have been reported only with thioridazine. All phenothiazines have a three-ringed structure in which two benzene rings are linked. The derivatives can be divided into different classes according to the substitution of the N atom in position 10. This is of great importance since the substitution of a piperidyl side chain enhances the toxicity of these compounds considerably more than substitution with an aliphatic side chain.

Chlorpromazine was the first widely used phenothiazine derivative for the treatment of schizophrenia. There are manifold studies on the long-term effect of the drug on the retina but even in large series clear-cut retinotoxicity has not been found (McClanahan et al., 1966). Nevertheless, a small number of single cases have been recorded in which pigmentary changes might be attributed to chlorpromazine therapy. It is very difficult, however, to ascertain whether these changes were really due to the drug, since many of these patients had concomitantly taken other phenothiazine derivatives, such as thioridazine, which unequivocally give rise to a pigmentary retinopathy (Zelickson and Zeller, 1964).

Mechanisms of toxicity. Toxic effects of chlorpromazine may involve the accelerated release of lysosomal enzymes cathepsin D and arylsulfatase from bovine RPE lysosomes in a dose-dependent fashion (Shiono et al., 1984), although the agent showed only minimal inhibitory effects on the activities of lysosomal enzymes such as acid phosphatase, beta-D-glucuronidase and alpha-L-fucosidase (Hayasaka, 1988). Furthermore, phototoxic properties of the compound (at concentrations above 25 mg/ml in the growth media) may be responsible for cell lysis upon exposure to light, which was prevented by addition of vitamin E (Persad et al., 1988). Chlorpromazine and fluphenazine also show a dose-dependent inhibition of phagocytosis of latex particles by cultured chick RPE cells (Matsumura et al., 1986).

Clinical manifestations of chlorpromazine. Intravenous injection of chlorpromazine in sheep induces a decrease in ERG b-wave and c-wave amplitude followed by cyclic amplitude changes (Calissendorff, 1976a); previous experimental work has demonstrated a marked reduction of the Arden ratio of the EOG.

Thioridazine, mainly used as an antipsychotic in the treatment of schizophrenia, is used because of its lower level of general systemic side effects than other phenothiazines such as chlorpromazine. It is the only phenothiazine in current use that unquestionably causes a pigmentary retinopathy. This complication has been known for several decades and involves progressive chorioretinopathy and atrophy of the RPE, abnormal dark adaption, and a decreased ERG and EOG in the late stages (Meredith et al., 1978). Toxicity is closely related to the dose, and patients may develop visual symptoms within just a few weeks of taking excess levels. In most cases a total daily dose of 800 mg had been exceeded when a retinopathy developed, although there have been cases reported of pigment changes with lower doses of about 700 mg (Reboton et al., 1962; Kozy et al., 1984) and one associated with very low dose thioridazine (100–400 mg/day and total dose of 45 g) (Sousa Neves et al., 1990).

Mechanisms of toxicity. The exact mechanisms of thioridazine toxicity are still elusive, although there is evidence that the chemical composition of the piperidyl side chain attached to a dimethyl group at the 10 position is responsible for the toxic effect. The same side chain was also a characteristic feature in NP-207, a highly retinotoxic phenothiazine (Kinross-Wright, 1956; Verrey, 1956), which was as a consequence abandoned before it became commercially available. As the drug may also accumulate over long time in the uveal tissues and the RPE (Kimbrough and Campbell, 1981), these toxic effects mostly take place at the level of the outer blood–retinal barrier. The binding of the drug to melanin per se does not, however, induce toxic effects, since such binding has been observed with many phenothiazines and with other drugs which do not trigger a clinically discernible retinopathy.

Clinical manifestations. The pigmentary changes begin as a coarse brownish stippling in the macula, sometimes extending into the periphery (Fig. 32-6a and b and Color Plate 32-II). Over several months pigmentation evolves into large hypopigmented plaques with areas of hyperpigmentation extending into the midperiphery (Davidorf, 1973; Kozy et al., 1984), sometimes called a *nummular retinopathy*. In the late stages the fundus may exhibit a diffusely atrophic appearance with vascular narrowing (Fig. 32-6c and d and Color Plate 32-III). Onset of toxicity usually coincides with blurred vision, and discontinuation of the drug is imperative. Visual acuity may improve after the drug is stopped despite the accumulation of pigment, but peripheral scotomas may remain. Fluorescein angiography may show more widespread clinically evident changes of the RPE, as well as loss of choriocapillaris (Kozy et al., 1984). The ERG is subnormal acutely but can improve or become normal

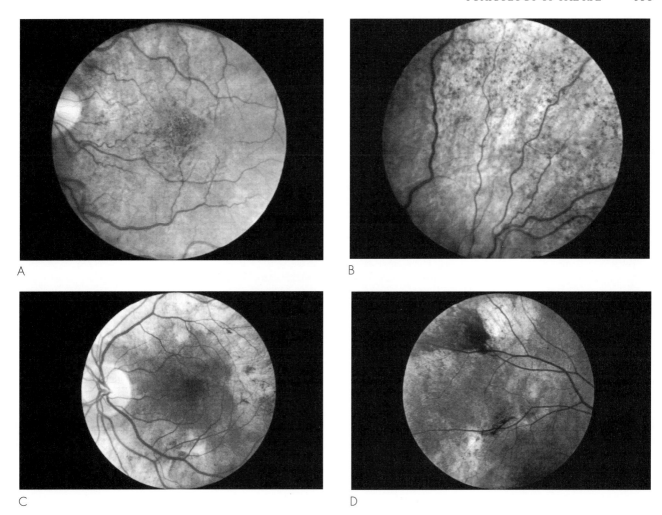

A

B

C

D

FIGURE 32-6. Thioridazine retinopathy. (A and B) Patient with early pigmentary changes. These begin as a coarse brownish stippling that may be prominent in the macula. Patient with late retinopathy (C and D). The pigmentation evolves into large hypopigmented plaques with areas of hyperpigmentation extending into the midperiphery. In the end stage the fundus may be diffusely atrophic with vascular narrowing. (See also Plates 32-II and 32-III.) (Courtesy of Michael F. Marmor, M.D.)

over several months after the treatment is stopped. However, the chorioretinal atrophy and pigmentary degeneration will sometimes progress again, very slowly, many years later (Davidorf, 1973). There is little evidence for continuing drug-related progression (Marmor, 1990), and the late atrophy may represent decompensation of RPE cells that were injured years previously. Pathology of advanced retinopathy is characterized by multiple confluent areas of hypopigmentation and choroidal atrophy posterior to the equator as well as atrophy of the photoreceptor outer segments, the RPE, and the choriocapillaris (Miller et al., 1982). Electrophysiological evaluation of patients have ranged from normal ERG and EOG in early and mild cases (Davidorf, 1973) to impaired dark adaptation and a severely reduced ERG and EOG (Meredith et al., 1978; Marmor, 1990).

A maculopathy after unprotected exposure to a welding arc has been described in a patient who had received chronic *fluphenazine* for several years, and the hypothesis was put forward that the drug, having accumulated in the RPE, may have rendered the patient particularly susceptible to retinal photic damage (Power et al., 1991). Fluphenazine has also been shown to inhibit the phagocytosis of latex particles by cultured chick RPE cells in a dose-dependent fashion (Matsumura et al., 1986), although the clinical significance of this finding is not yet understood.

Tricyclic antidepressants. Treatment of albino rats with high oral doses of *iprindole, 1-chloroamitriptyline, imipramine,* or *clomipramine* for several weeks induced an increased size of RPE cells due to deposition of excessive amounts of abnormal cytoplasmic inclusions of a crystalloid substructure. These inclusions were suggested to contain nondigestible phospholipids which originate mainly from phagocytosed outer segment discs in the RPE. The alterations disappeared after discontinuation of the treatment (Lullmann-Rauch, 1976). No clinical correlate to these ultrastructural changes have been described to date.

Piperidindiones. *Thalidomide* is a sedative and hypnotic which was widely used in the 1950s causing severe congenital abnormalities in babies of women who took this medication early in pregnancy. It is being considered currently as an antiproliferative agent to suppress subretinal neovascularization. Congenital ocular abnormalities include retinal dysplasia, peripheral pigmentary retinopathy, and atrophic retinopathy, as reported by several authors (Cullen, 1964; Schutte et al., 1977).

Amphiphilic cationic drugs. *Citalopram* is a potential antidepressant and an amphiphilic cationic compound which can induce generalized lipidosis in animals. Mild lysosomal alterations were found in RPE in female rats which had been treated with a single oral dose (Lullmann-Rauch and Nussberger, 1983). These changes were reversible within 2–4 weeks after cessation of the drug. No clinical correlate to these ultrastructural changes have been described to date.

Chronic administration of the cationic amphiphilic anorexogenic drug *chlorphentermine* (30–45 mg/kg) for 4–16 weeks can induce ocular lipidosis in rats. This is associated with a large number of lysosomal cytoplasmic inclusions of polar lipids in the RPE which show a crystalline-like internal structure. Freeze-fracture images indicate that they consist of phospholipids organized in a hexagonal phase (Lullmann-Rauch, 1981). Deposits have also been demonstrated in the neurosensory retina leading to an isolated depression of the b-wave in the ERG (Duncker and Bredehorn, 1994). As soon as the treatment is discontinued, the alterations recede completely (Daxecker and Bilcher, 1993). The clinical significance of this lipidosis remains to be clarified.

Zimelidine has also been shown to induce lipidosis-like cellular alteration of the RPE in rats though of much milder degree than the other amphiphilic cationic drugs (Bockhardt and Lullmann-Rauch, 1980).

Hallucinogenic Drugs

Pigment screening occurs in the retina of lower vertebrates and consists of the bidirectional migration of melanin granules into the processes of the pigment epithelium that extend between the photoreceptors in response to changes in the illumination conditions (for de-

tails see Chapter 3). It has been shown in frog retina that intravenous injection of *lysergic acid diethlyamide* (LSD), *d-amphetamine, lisuride,* and the LSD derivative *2-bromolysergic acid* modified this migration both vitreally and sclerally (Kemalie et al., 1983). Maternal LSD ingestion during the first trimester of pregnancy has been reported to induce severe ocular anomalies with a persistent hyperplastic primary vitreous and retinal dysplasia (Chan et al., 1978). However, in vivo evaluation of the toxicity of amphetamines after 10 mg/kg given daily to dogs for three months showed only slight blanching of the fundus as seen by ophthalmoscopy but no histologic change in the retina or at the level of the RPE (Delahunt et al., 1963).

INDUSTRIAL TOXINS

Several industrial chemicals, metals, and chelators may exhibit potent toxicity toward the RPE (see Table 32-7).

Industrial Dye

Naphthalene is a compound that has been used industrially as a dye-intermediate as well as a component of moth balls. Systemic poisoning from ingestion, inhalation, or absorption through the skin causes nausea, acute hemolysis, and eventually coma. Ocular toxic effects have mostly been seen in the lens as cataracts, but abnormalities have also been described at the level of the RPE in a rabbit model. Circular patches of pigment epithelial changes were visible both opthalmoscopically and in the flat preparation, and damage to the RPE preceded damage to the retina (Pirie, 1968). Napthalene diol, a metabolite of naphthalene, has also been reported to produce retinal lesions when injected systemically in rabbits (van Heyningen, 1979).

Pesticides

Retina and RPE changes in workers occupationally exposed to pesticides such as *fenthion*, a DDT analog,

TABLE 32-7. *Industrial chemicals, metals, and chelators with toxic effects on the RPE*

Industrial toxins	Metals and chelators
Industrial dye	Metals
Naphthalene	Iron
Pesticides	Copper
Fenthion	Lead
Rodenticide	Zinc
Pyridylmethyl-nitrophenylurea	Chelators
	Penicillamine
	Desferrioxamine
	Zinc chelator

have been reported in a few studies from Japan (Misra et al., 1985). These macular lesions were characterized by perifoveal irregularity of pigmentation and areas of hypopigmentation after a mean exposure time of about eight years. Symptoms included loss of visual acuity, photophobia, flashes, and floaters. The pathogenetic mechanisms of this disease are not yet fully understood. There is experimental evidence that fenthion (100 mg/kg subcutaneously) decreases the muscarinic receptor function over several days in the adult rat retina (Tandon et al., 1994). At the same time, increased immunoreactivity for glial fibrillary acidic protein within the retina was noted, which persisted for more than 50 days. Other reports from Japan have hinted at the association of exposure to organophosphate pesticides in agriculture with myopia and advanced visual problems (Saku disease) (Dementi, 1994). Funduscopically, a degeneration of the retina was observed, and histology demonstrated marked abnormalities in the retina and RPE. Levels of butylcholinesterase in plasma and liver were extremely reduced after three months of fenthion treatment and preceded structural damage in the retina.

Rodenticide

Ingestion of the rat poison *N-3-Pyridylmethyl-N'-p-nitrophenylurea* (PNU) produces ocular toxicity in humans and in an animal model of the Dutch belted rabbit (Mindel et al., 1988). The ERG b-wave was attenuated by the effects of the poison and histological investigations showed that the RPE appeared to be the target tissue. The poison had to be administered orally and not parenterally to have an effect. Gentamicin or L-tryptophan administered together with PNU prevented ocular toxicity. While L-tryptophan is a known antidote for the lethal effects of PNU, the action of gentamicin seems to lie in the eradication of those gastrointestinal bacteria responsible for PNU's metabolism into an ocular toxin.

METALS AND CHELATORS

Metals may accumulate in melanin granules over a lifetime (Ulshafer et al., 1990; Larsson, 1993), and the mechanisms of metal ion binding seem to be pH dependent. An extended discussion of metal binding properties and mechanisms is presented in Chapter 4. The following section focuses on the clinical effects of metal toxicity.

Metals

Copper has been identified as a normal component of the retinal outer nuclear layer, photoreceptor inner and outer segments, the RPE, and the choroid, suggesting a role for copper as a component of some metalloenzymes (Hirayama, 1990). Retinal toxicity of excess intraocular copper has been known for almost over a century. Clinical experience and experiments in animals have demonstrated that the toxicity of an intraocular foreign body is less pronounced the more it is distanced from the retina (Brunette et al., 1980). Pure copper seems to be tolerated surprisingly well, with good ERG responses despite the presence of deposits in the macula. These lesions range from RPE clumping to a copper-colored sheen and early granular deposits of copper in the internal limiting membrane (Rosenthal et al., 1974). The reasons for some toxic results are unclear. Excess amounts of copper have also been implicated in retinal damage (Reim et al., 1989) including liquefaction of the vitreous accompanied by retinal necrosis and a marked increase in lysosomal and cellular enzymes such as LDH, GAPDH, G-6-PDH, although these effects may have been triggered by the associated inflammation. There have been some reports on a maculopathy that may be produced by copper and reversed by removal of the metallic foreign body, but there is still little information available on this subject (Delaney, 1975; Rosenthal et al., 1979). ERG experiments showed that changes in amplitude appear within a week or less (Brunette et al., 1980). There is also experimental evidence that systemic injection of copper sulfate may induce photoreceptor and pigment epithelial degeneration (Gahlot et al., 1976). Interestingly, copper deficiency has also been associated with RPE changes such as irregular melanin granules associated with the presence of electron-dense inclusion bodies and an abnormal elastic layer in Bruch's membrane (Dingle and Havener, 1978; Wray et al., 1976). A few years ago there was a controversy whether or not systemic copper metabolism is affected in retinitis pigmentosa patients (Gahlot et al., 1976), but evidence was put forward that this was not the case (Marmor et al., 1978; Rao et al., 1981).

Although *iron* constitutes an integral part of the RPE, being present in considerable amounts in melanosomes (Ulshafer et al., 1990), excess of this metal has been implicated in toxic changes at the level of the RPE. Clinically, it has been recognized for many years that in ocular siderosis with foreign bodies there may be a retinal degeneration with fine irregular pigmentation and loss of the macular reflex in late stages (Wagenmann, 1913). A proliferation of peripheral pigment epithelium has also been observed similar to that seen in retinitis pigmentosa (Karpe, 1948; Cibis et al., 1957). The pathogenesis of ion toxicity appears to involve ferrous ions that promote reduction of molecular oxygen. The hydrogen peroxide and hydroxyl radicals that are formed this way depolymerize the hyaluronate and attack the collagen of the vitreous humor (Hofmann and Schmut, 1980). Ferric ions may thus be less toxic than iron, since they are already fully oxidized and cannot promote the reduction of molecular oxygen to form toxic intermediates. Intravitreal injection of iron (ferrous sulfate, a catalyst that promotes nonenzymatic oxidation of photoreceptor outer segments in RPE lipofuscin formation) has been shown to induce fluorophore formation in the photoreceptor outer segments followed by an accumulation of inclusions with lipofuscin-like fluorescence in the RPE. This effect is vitamin A–dependent (Katz et al., 1993; 1994). It has also been shown that RPE cells remove iron from diferric transferrin in a low pH compartment and subsequently release it in a low-molecular-weight form that can be chelated by apotransferrin (Davis and Hunt, 1993). Another underlying mechanism of iron toxicity may be lying in a proliferative response. The effect of ferrous iron injected intravitreally for example in an in vivo model of penetrating injury showed iron to be an important stimulus for inflammation and membrane formation (Vergara et al., 1989). Retinal proliferation in response to intravitreous iron (FeSO4) has also been described in a rabbit model (Burke and Smith, 1981). Damage caused by iron on the outer blood–retinal barrier also includes the destruction of anionic sites at the basement membrane of the RPE with an end stage of a disorganized retina with a proliferating RPE (Kishimoto et al., 1991).

Clinically, the retinopathy is associated with hemeralopia and visual-field constrictions but may also entail loss of central visual acuity which may progress to total blindness. Ophthalmoscopically generalized atrophy of the retina can be observed mixed with patchy areas of RPE proliferation and an irregular fine pigmentation of the fovea. Clinical evaluation may be helped with electroretinographic follow-up (ERG changes preceding visual defects) and analysis of early receptor potentials (Sieving et al., 1983).

A clinical case has been described of pigment epitheliopathy with serous detachment of the retina in a young man following a total dose infusion of iron dextran for erythropoetin-induced iron deficiency in chronic renal failure (Hodgkins et al., 1992). There was visual loss to 6/60, a reduced EOG with almost normal ERG, and serum iron levels were increased to over 300 μmol/l (norm 13–40 μmol/l). Fluorescein angiography showed slow choroidal filling and leakage through multiple RPE defects, with pooling in the subretinal space. Vision returned to normal over a period of two weeks, with the remaining fundal abnormality being patchy depigmentation at the posterior poles. Fluorescein angiography three months later showed recovery of choroidal perfusion with complete resolution of the pigment epitheliopathy. EOG abnormalities completely recovered as well. EOG abnormalities have been observed with iron overload in siderosis (Good and Gross, 1988) and desferrioxamine therapy (Pall et al., 1989), which may be due to iron-promoted oxidative damage to RPE cell membranes and photoreceptor outer segments, both of which have long-chain polyunsaturated fatty acids (Good and Gross, 1988). Another case of pigmentary retinal degeneration has been noted (Fraunfelder, 1996). Ocular siderosis from systemic iron is extremely rare but has been described after over one hundred blood transfusions (Cibis et al., 1957). One unusual patient had bilateral pigmentary retinopathy but normal ERG after weekly intramuscular injection of iron-dextran and cyanocobalamine for twenty years for pernicious anemia (Syversen, 1979).

Ocular symptoms of systemic poisoning from *lead* have been reported for several centuries (Uhthoff, 1911). In addition to the well-known toxic effect on the brain and optic nerve, retinal and RPE damage have been recognized recently. In rabbits the RPE has been demonstrated to become greatly swollen by accumulation of granules of lipofuscin without changes in the ERG, EOG, or ophthalmoscopic appearance (Brown, 1974). Later degeneration of photoreceptor cells may occur (Hughes and Coogan, 1974). This phenomenon may be specific for rabbits, as it could not be induced in rats and monkeys. The rods seems to be affected preferentially by lead and dysfunction could be detected in mesopic conditions (Fox and Sillman, 1979; Cavalleri et al., 1982). Chronic lead administration in neonatal rats has also demonstrated necrosis of photoreceptor cells and cells of the inner nuclear layer associated with increased permeability of the retinal vessels and pigment epithelium to horseradish peroxidase (Santos-Anderson et al., 1984). Clinically important visual loss in humans after lead poisoning is usually related to encephalopathy and optic neuropathy, with no known case of pigmentary retinopathy.

Zinc constitutes an integral part of the RPE being present in considerable amounts in melanosomes (Ulshafer et al., 1990). Both deficiency and excess of this metal have been implicated in toxic changes at the level of the RPE. The effect of severe zinc deficiency on the morphology of RPE has been investigated in rats showing an accumulation of osmiophilic inclusion bodies in the RPE. At seven weeks there were marked ultrastructural alterations of the RPE with vesiculation and degeneration of the photoreceptor outer segments (Leure-duPree and McClain, 1982). The mechanisms of zinc binding in the RPE include a low-molecular-weight protein with a high capacity for zinc binding that is dependent on available sulfhydryl groups (Oliver and Newsome, 1992). Zinc has also been shown to be taken up by in vitro human RPE by a facilitated transport independent of NaKATPase (Newsome and Rothman, 1987). A proposed treatment of macular degeneration by oral zinc (Newsome et al., 1988) has been questioned by many and epidemiological evidence is marginal (see Chapter 37).

Chelators

Several metal chelators, such as *diethyldithiocarbamate, dithizone, edetate, ethambutol, ethylenediamine derivatives, imidazo quinazoline, oxypertine,* and *pyrithione,* have been implicated in experimental degeneration of the tapetum in certain animals (Grant, 1986). A few other clinically important chelators that have been shown to induce a pigmentary retinopathy in man will be discussed below.

D-Penicillamine is a chelating agent for copper and heavy metals and has been extensively used in the treatment of Wilson's disease (hepatolenticular degeneration), rheumatoid arthritis, and cystinuria. There have been rare cases of a retinopathy associated with this drug. Defects in the RPE were seen to develop after seven years of medication, giving the impression of drusen-like lesions in dense white clusters throughout the posterior poles, associated with normal visual acuity (Dingle and Havener, 1978). Another case has also been described with bilateral serous macular detachments and rapid decrease of visual acuity but fast recovery after discontinuation of penicillamine (Klepach and Wray, 1981).

The iron chelator *desferrioxamine* (Desferal, deferoxamine) has been used clinically in systemic iron overload but also locally in the eye for ocular siderosis and iron foreign bodies. Retinal toxicity has only been described with parenteral administration. Excessive intravenous treatment with desferrioxamine can induce xanthopsia and diffuse macular pigment mottling (Charton et al., 1990). Another study has found, in up to 35% of patients who are treated with desferrioxamine, changes in the RPE and tortuosity of retinal vessels, deficiency in color vision, and changes in EOG and reduction of ERG responses (Dennerlein et al., 1995). These changes appear similar to those seen in hemochromatosis (Arden et al., 1984). Discussed mechanisms of toxicity are induction of oxidation, damage of the blood–retinal barrier, and reduction in other metal ions such as copper or zinc (Pall et al., 1989). Oculotoxicity seems to be dose related; side effects are partly reversible after discontinuation of the drug. Pigmentary changes at the level of the RPE (Fig. 32-7a and b, and Color Plate 32-IV) have

been described in a series of patients after total dose of 12–96 g (Lakhanpal et al., 1984). In a postmortem specimen obtained after several years of desferrioxamine therapy, light and electron microscopy showed loss of microvilli from the apical surface of the RPE, patchy depigmentation, vacuolation of the cytoplasm, swelling and calcification of mitochondria, and disorganization of the plasma membrane (Rahi et al., 1986). In addition, Bruch's membrane overlying degenerate RPE cells appeared abnormally thickened. Electrooculographic monitoring of desferrioxamine therapy has been tried (Potamitis et al., 1996); it showed a return from abnormal EOG to normal values after cessation of desferrioxamine therapy. Retinal toxicity of another novel orally absorbed iron chelator, *1,2-demethyl-3-hydroxypyrid-4-one,* or L1, has been investigated in an albino rat model (Purple et al., 1995), which showed less short-

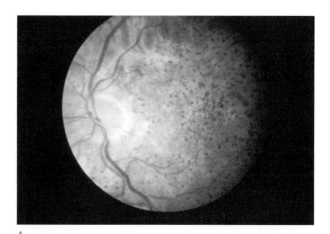

A

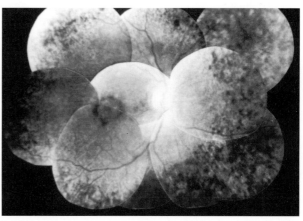

B

FIGURE 32-7. Desferrioxamine-induced retinal pigment epitheliopathy. (A) Pigment mottling in the posterior pole. (B) Composite photograph to show peripheral pigmentation. (See also Plate 32-IV.) (From Lakhanpal et al., 1984.)

term retinal dysfunction than desferrioxamine, although systemic toxicity unfortunately precludes the use of this agent.

The zinc chelator *dithizone* has been known for several decades to induce a retinopathy in rabbits and rats by causing destruction of the tapetum, which is rich in zinc (Sorsby and Harding, 1962). Intravenous administration of 50–100 mg/kg causes disappearance of the ERG within a few hours. Histopathological changes at the level of the retina and RPE are seen within 40 hours as a degeneration of Müller cells, migration of RPE cells, and proliferation of glia. In the rat, treatment with chelators of zinc such as dithizone and *1,10-phenanthroline* have been shown to induce dose-dependent electron-opaque inclusions in the RPE (Leure-duPree, 1981). Ethylenediamine derivatives have also been implicated as zinc chelators that can induce tapetal depigmentation in dogs (Kaiser, 1963). The eyes of monkeys and humans have no zinc-containing tapetum and seem therefore not to be affected by dithizone. There are to date no data on a clinically apparent retinopathy related to this compound.

PHOTOSENSITIZERS

Early studies on the phototoxic effects of *Rose Bengal*, a fluorescein derivative used as a vital stain in the diagnosis of certain external ocular disease, on RPE cells in vitro have shown cell lysis in up to 43% of cells (Menon et al., 1989). The lysis progressively increased when the exposure time was varied from 10 to 40 minutes. A relatively short period of irradiation in the presence of Rose Bengal was sufficient to produce sublytic cellular injury, which could subsequently lead to complete cell lysis even in the absence of the photochemical treatment. This reaction in the dark was time dependent and reached a maximum for a given irradiation period (Menon et al., 1989). Rose Bengal has been used more often to injure capillary endothelium and produce rapid occlusion of choroidal and retinal circulation. Of course the RPE invariably shows ischemic damage over occluded areas of choriocapillaris. Focal ischemic injury to the choriocapillaris causes the formation of overlying serous detachments (Wilson et al., 1991; Marmor and Yao, 1994).

Recently the use of *benzophorphyrines* in the treatment of subretinal new vessels has been advocated. Although photodynamic therapy is promising for a localized occlusion of choroidal vessels some unwanted damage to the adjacent RPE is hard to avoid (Lin et al., 1994) (Schmidt-Erfuhrt et al., 1994). Further studies have shown that other photosensitizers such as *proto-*porphyrin and *8-methoxypsoralen* can bind to melanin and may thus bind more preferentially to the RPE predisposing to collateral RPE damage, even though the laser energy is aimed at the underlying choroidal vessels (Persad et al., 1986).

RPE TOXINS

Knowledge on the ocular toxic effect of *sodium iodate* dates back to the early 1920s when vision loss was described as a result of intravenous injection of an antiinfective solution known as Septojod (Roggenkämper, 1927). In some visual acuity improved but the majority had a residual central scotoma with persistent disseminated pigmentation of the retina. It was later widely agreed that the prime injury is to the RPE, with rod and cone degeneration ensuing later (Noell, 1953).

Investigation into sodium iodate toxicity in the last decades has been largely due to the selective use of this compound in modeling outer blood–retinal barrier (BRB) damage. Intravenous injection of sodium iodate selectively destroys the RPE and this destruction leads to secondary choriocapillaris atrophy (Korte et al., 1984). Intravitreous and intravenous injection of iodate seem to induce similar RPE lesions (Orzalesi et al., 1967), which are characterized histologically by marked destruction of the RPE, which may be replaced with a new layer of different cells that form a more or less tight epithelium (Ringvold et al., 1981). For unknown reasons the juxtapapillary portion of the RPE seems to have a greater resistance to iodate than the rest of the pigment epithelium (Flage, 1983). The predilection of iodate for the RPE entails a destruction of anionic sites in the outer BRB (Kishimoto et al., 1990b), suggesting a decreased barrier function which facilitates subretinal fluid flow to the choroid according to oncotic pressure (Negi and Marmor, 1983). This loosened barrier function also induces a marked decrease in retinal adhesion within one hour after administration of the drug (Ashburn et al., 1980; Yoon and Marmor, 1993). As a consequence, transport properties of sodium-iodate-damaged RPE may also be compromised. Intravitreal injection of sodium iodate was used to determine outward permeability; intravenous injection was used to investigate inward permeability. Both showed a clearly decreased active transport after iodate application (Kitano et al., 1988; Grimes, 1988). Sucrose permeability of the BRB was also compromised after iodate, whereas the blood–brain barrier was entirely intact (Ennis and Betz, 1986). A similar observation for *D-glucose* has been made recently (Taarnhoj and Alm, 1992). This iodate induced decrease in active transport across the RPE is also associated with an acidification of the subretinal space (Yamamoto et al., 1993), suggesting that the RPE may actively transport acids from the subretinal space to the choroid.

The biochemical activity of sodium iodate on the RPE comprises the inhibition of lysosomal enzyme activity in the crude extract of bovine RPE in concentrations of 10^{-4}–10^{-6} M (Hayasaka et al., 1988). The polarized distribution of other enzymes such as Na^+-K^+-ATPase are lost with RPE degeneration but the ensuing regeneration of an epithelial sheet starts to exhibit this polarized distribution (Korte and Wanderman, 1993). In vitro evaluation of iodate effects on melanin have shown a ten times greater ability of melanin to convert glycine to glyoxylate, suggesting that this mechanism may be at least partly responsible for the specific iodate toxicity to the RPE (Baich and Ziegler, 1992). It has been suggested that preinjection of L-cystein can protect the RPE from acute iodate toxicity as well as from late development of pigmentary degeneration (Sorsby and Harding, 1960; Heike and Marmor, 1990).

Noell showed many years ago that iodate given intravenously rapidly and selectively eliminated the c-wave of the ERG, leaving a large, negative slow PIII response (Noell, 1953). More recent work has shown that there may be a paradoxical enhancement of the ERG c-wave by a small dose (20 mg/kg) of sodium iodate, whereas administration of 30 mg/kg decreased the c-wave clearly and replaced it by a potential of opposite polarity (Nao-i et al., 1986). The same group has also provided evidence that intravitreal administration of iodate (0.5–3.5 mM) produced complete suppression of intraretinal b-wave without remarkable changes of slow PIII and light-evoked K^+ decrease in the subretinal space, whereas intravenous iodate (30 mg/kg) also showed the suppression of b-waves, suggesting that iodate not only acts as a poison to the RPE but also might block the postsynaptic response (Yamamoto et al., 1993). The loss of the c-wave and the exposure of the slow PIII (which represents a retinal Müller cell response (Faber, 1969) may occur because of a large decrease in the transepithelial resistance (Kiryu et al., 1992).

Iodate-induced destruction of the RPE has also been linked to proliferation of RPE cells in the posterior pole. Vitreous removed from eyes after intravenous injection of 30 mg/kg of sodium iodate caused significant stimulation of RPE migration by about 500% while control vitreous and saline-injected vitreous caused only 90% stimulation, implying that RPE damage or BRB destruction may be imperative for the development of PVR (Campochiaro et al., 1986).

Recently, a clinical entity of *potassium iodate* toxicity by ingestion was described (Singalavanija et al., 1994) with visual acuity reduced to perception of hand motion, retinal edema, and subsequent pigmentary change at the macula and the level of the RPE resembling retinitis pigmentosa. Fluorescein angiography and electrophysiologic studies showed degenerative changes of the RPE and photoreceptor cells.

Hemicholinium-3 is a choline analog that can interfere with the retina's synthesis of new phosphatidylcholine from extracellular choline (Pu and Masland, 1984). This disrupts the process by which a new membrane is added to the rod photoreceptor outer segments and eventually causes outer segment degeneration. There is also evidence of an early effect of hemicholinium on the RPE. Injected intravitreally, the drug induced a decreased c-wave amplitude and a clinically apparent pigmentary retinopathy in the fundus of pigmented rabbits (White et al., 1990). Later experiments revealed that intravitreal injection of the drug causes loss of photoreceptor outer segments as well as RPE damage with ensuing pigmentary changes in the fundus and weakened retinal adhesiveness (Negi et al., 1993). Furthermore, it was demonstrated that the drug can weaken the adhesion of RPE to Bruch's membrane in a rabbit model (Yoon and Marmor, 1993).

Cytoskeleton Disrupting Agents

Colchicine is the water-soluble alkaloid of the plant *Colchicum autumnale* which inhibits the spindle formation during mitosis, leading to disassembly of the microtubules. The drug has been a useful tool to study microtubules; for example, in vitro evaluation of the effects of colchicine on the microtubule network of cultured pig RPE cells has shown a dose-dependent (1–100 nM) inhibition of microtubule network formation by depolymerization (Devin et al., 1995). Furthermore, colchicine may also inhibit phagocytic activity of RPE, as shown by a reversibly inhibitable phagosome–lysosome interaction when added at 5×10^{-5} M to the growth medium (Keller and Leuenberger, 1977; Ogino et al., 1980). In vivo colchicine hastens the RPE cell rounding that occurs after retinal separation in the rabbit (Immel et al., 1986). Studies with mouse RPE have also shown that 10 mg/kg colchicine given intraperitoneally prior to peak phagocytosis (4 hours before light onset) resulted in a marked increase in the number of phagosomes and a decrease in the number of microtubules. On the other hand, when colchicine was given during the period in which phagocytosis is inactive (8 hours after light onset), it induced only a slight increase in the number of phagosomes which recovered to the normal level earlier than the above, suggesting that the effect of colchicin on rod outer segment phagocytosis by RPE might depend on the functional state of RPE during the light cycle (Suzuki et al., 1987). Colchicine has also been used to characterize the retinomotor pigment migration in response to changes in light conditions in the teleost RPE (Burnside and O'Connor, 1983). Light-induced pigment dispersion as well as maintenance of the fully dispersed light-adapted position appear to require actin-dependent processes. Recently, this drug has also been evaluated as an antiproliferative agent for the treatment of PVR (see Chapter 31).

Cytochalasins are metabolites from fungi which are able to cross cell membranes. These agents have been used extensively to characterize intracellular actin-mediated processes (Ohmori et al., 1992). These processes serve mainly the maintenance of epithelial integrity as well as phagocytosis, disk shedding, and light-induced migration of pigment granules in fish RPE. High concentrations of cytochalasin induce gaps in well-differentiated RPE cells (Sakamoto et al., 1994), as well as disrupt both zonulae occludentes and adherentes in cultured RPE (Owaribe et al., 1979), suggesting that the breakdown of actin filaments impaired the maintenance of epithelial integrity. In addition, the drug may also disrupt circumferential microfilament bundles (Owaribe et al., 1979) by inducing contraction of these bundles to masses which accumulate at the subapical region of the RPE cells (Owaribe, 1988). After acute detachment of rabbit retina in vivo, cytochalasin D caused bulging and prominence of tufts of apical RPE microvilli (Immel et al., 1986). Furthermore, the drug reversibly weakens the adhesive force between retina and RPE (Chiang et al., 1995).

The drug has also been shown to inhibit migration of pigment granules in fish RPE (Burnside et al., 1983) and engulfment of rod outer segment packets or foreign particles during phagocytosis by RPE cells (Besharse and Dunis, 1982). Other studies on pigment dispersion have demonstrated that dopamine-induced dispersion was also inhibited by cytochalasin D in isolated RPE sheets of green sunfish, suggesting that dopamine mimics the effect of light on cone and RPE retinomotor movement and that different cytoskeletal mechanisms may be used to affect pigment transport (Dearry et al., 1990).

In cultured RPE cells cytochalasin B has also been shown to induce morphologic alteration in the microvilli with thinning, elongation, and honeycomb-like changes (Matsumura et al., 1986), as well as to reversibly inhibit phagocytosis of cultured RPE (Ogino et al., 1980).

Recently, several newer compounds have been described which can also sever actin filaments such as latrunculin (Spector et al., 1989), tolytoxin (Patterson et

al., 1993), and swinholide A (Bubb et al., 1995), although no data is yet available on the action of these drugs on the RPE. Cytochalasin has also been reported to inhibit RPE cell migration in vitro (Campochiaro et al., 1986) and wound closure in epithelial monolayers of cultured RPE (Verstraeten et al., 1990), and it has therefore been investigated as an antiproliferative agent in the treatment of PVR (see Chapter 31).

Nacodazole is also a microtubule-disrupting agent in the RPE. It acts as inhibitor of RPE pigment granule aggregation but not dispersion (Troutt and Burnside, 1989). However, overexpression of microtubule-associated protein renders the cells' microtubules nocodazole insensitive, indicating increased stability. Nacodazole binds to a similar site on the tubulin dimer as colchicine and has similar effects on microtubules but may have fewer side effects.

Taxol blocks many microtubule-dependent processes by binding to and stabilizing the microtubule polymer, thus preventing microtubule disassembly. Taxol may also block mitosis, indicating that not only assembly but also disassembly are critical to many microtubule functions (Mitchison, 1992). In vitro evaluation of the effects of taxol on the microtubule network of cultured pig RPE cells has shown a dose-dependent (1–100 nM) inhibition of microtubule network formation by stabilization.

INTRAOCULAR AGENTS FOR VITREORETINAL SURGERY

Oil

Since its introduction into vitreoretinal surgery, *silicone oil* has been used for the treatment of complicated retinal detachments. Although treatment with silicone oil is very beneficial in counteracting tractional forces, long-term toleration of this compound by the retina is not without problems (Gonvers et al., 1986; Eckhardt et al., 1993; Doi et al., 1995). Complications seem to be directed mostly to the inner retinal layers. However, after subretinal injection of silicone oil massive subretinal and epiretinal membrane proliferation was seen, which suggests a proliferogenic action of the oil on the RPE (Shikishima et al., 1992). More basic in vitro studies addressing this effect of silicone oil on the RPE have shown that emulsified oil seemed to have less of a proliferation-inducing effect than unemulsified oil for a short time, a difference which disappeared after a few weeks. Neither fluorination nor viscosity had a significant effect, and there was no difference between medical-grade and severe purified oils. However, contaminated oil was associated with a significantly higher proliferation index (Friberg et al., 1991). Another group has also shown in an in vitro model that exposure of RPE cell cultures to silicone oil or hyaluronic acid induced multilayer sheets of cells and a decrease of cell polarity (Verstraeten et al., 1990). Silicone-filled vitreous has also been shown to increase mitogenic activity for RPE cells compared with gas-filled or fluid-filled vitreous (Lambrou et al., 1987). The mechanisms for this action may include stimulation of the release of different mitogenic factors and concentrating active factors into a smaller volume near the retina.

Gas

Intravitreal gas is commonly used in the treatment of retinal detachment, but, due to its toxicity, injection always has to be diluted in air. Several different kinds of gases have been proposed for clinical use.

Perfluoropropane (C_6F_8) has been evaluated in a rabbit model. After intravitreal injection of 0.4 ml of 50% or 100% C_6F_8, RPE destruction could be observed histologically after four days (Iwasaki et al., 1996). Eyes injected with 100% C_6F_8 had a significant reduction in ERG a- and b-waves.

Injection of *sulfur hexafluoride* (SF_6) induced a decrease of BRB function as assessed by the cationic probe polyethyleneimine until 7 days after SF-6 injection. BRB function returned to normal at 14 days. Injection of the same amount of air reduced BRB function only briefly; it returned to normal levels within 7 days (Kishimoto et al., 1990a).

REFERENCES

Adachi-Usami E, et al. 1995. Effects of mitomycin on the retina of rat. Invest Ophthalmol Vis Sci 36(suppl):S918.

Albert DM, et al. 1975. Flecked retina secondary to oxalate crystals from methoxyflurane anesthesia: clinical and experimental studies. Trans Am Acad Ophthalmol Otolaryngol 79:OP817.

Arden GB, Kolb H. 1966. Antimalarial therapy and early retinal changes in patients with rheumatoid arthritis. Br Med J 29:270.

Arden GB, et al. 1984. Ocular changes in patients undergoing long-term desferrioxamine treatment. Br J Ophthalmol 68:873–877.

Ashburn FS, et al. 1980. The effects of iodate and iodoacetate on the retinal adhesion. Invest Ophthalmol Vis Sci 19:1427–1432.

Bacon P, Spalton DJ, Smith SE. 1988. Blindness from quinine toxicity. Br J Ophthalmol 72:219–224.

Baich A, Ziegler M. 1992. The effect of sodium iodate and melanin on the formation of glyoxylate. Pigm Cell Res 5:394–395.

Balian JV. 1983. Accidental intraocular tobramycin injection: a case report. Ophthalmic Surg 14:353.

Barrada A, et al. 1983. Toxicity of antineoplastic drugs in vitrectomy infusion fluids. Ophthalmic Surg 14:845–847.

Barza M, Baum J, Kane A. 1976. Inhibition of antibiotic activity in vitro by synthetic melanin. Antimicrob Agents Chemother 10:569–570.

Behrman J, Mushin A. 1968. Electrodiagnostic findings in quinine amblyopia. Br J Ophthalmol 52:925–928.

Berezovsky A, Middendorf RC, Birch DG. 1996. Electroretinographic findings in patients treated with tamoxifen. Invest Ophthalmol Vis Sci 37(suppl):S345.

Bernstein HN. 1983. Ophthalmic considerations and testing in patients receiving long-term antimalarial therapy. Am J Med 75:25.

Besharse JC, Dunis DA. 1982. Rod photoreceptor shedding in vitro: inhibition by cytochalasin and activation by colchicine. In Hollyfield JG, ed, The Structure of the Eye. New York: Elsevier, 85–96.

Bockhardt H, Lullmann-Rauch R. 1980. Zimelidine-induced lipidosis in rats. Acta Pharmacol Toxicol 47:45–48.

Bockhardt H, Drenckhahn D, Lullmann-Rauch R. 1978. Amiodarone-induced lipidosis-like alterations in ocular tissues of rats. Graefes Arch Clin Exp Ophthalmol 207:91–96.

Boman G. 1973. Melanin affinity of a new antituberculous drug, rifampicin, investigated by whole body autoradiography. Acta Ophthalmol 51:367–370.

Boudreault G, et al. 1983. La rétinopathie à la canthazanthine: étude clinique de 51 consommateurs. Can J Ophthalmol 18:325–328.

Brinkley JR, Dubois EL, Ryan SJ. 1979. Long-term course of chloroquine retinopathy after cessation of medication. Am J Ophthalmol 88:1.

Brown DvL. 1974. Reaction of the rabbit retinal pigment epithelium to systemic lead poisoning. Trans Am Ophthalmol Soc 72:404–447.

Bruinink A, Zimmermann G, Riesen F. 1991. Neurotoxic effects of chloroquine in vitro. Arch Toxicol 65:480–484.

Brunette JR, Wagdi S, Lafond G. 1980. Electroretinographic alterations in retinal metallosis. Can J Ophthalmol 15:176–178.

Bubb MR, et al. 1995. Swinholide A is a microfilament disrupting marine toxin that stabilizes actin dimers and severs actin filaments. J Biol Chem 270:3463–3466.

Buchanan T, Archer D. 1978. Indomethacin retinopathy. Irish J Med Sci 147:255–256.

Bullock JD, Albert DM. 1975. Flecked retina: appearance secondary to oxalate crystals from methoxyflurane anesthesia. Arch Ophthalmol 93:26–31.

Burke E, et al. 1987. The retinotoxic effects of oncological agents. Bull Soc Bel Ophthalmol 224:77–79.

Burke JM, Smith JM. 1981. Retinal proliferation in response to vitreous hemoglobin or iron. Invest Ophthalmol Vis Sci 20:582–592.

Burns MS, Hartz MJ. 1992. The retinal pigment epithelium induces fenestration of endothelial cells in vivo. Curr Eye Res 11:863–873.

Burns MS, Tyler NK. 1990. Selective neovascularization of the retinal pigment epithelium in rat photoreceptor degeneration in vivo. Current Eye Res 9:1061–1075.

Burnside B, Adler R, O'Connor P. 1983. Retinomotor pigment migration in the teleost retinal pigment epithelium. I. Roles for actin and microtubules in pigment granule transport and cone movement. Invest Ophthalmol Vis Sci 24:1–15.

Calissendorff B. 1976a. Melanotropic drugs and retinal functions. II. Effects of phenothiazine and rifampicin on the sheep ERG. Acta Ophthalmologica 54:118–128.

Calissendorff B. 1976b. Melanotropic drugs and retinal functions I. Effects of quinine and chloroquine on the sheep ERG. Acta Ophthalmologica 54:109–117.

Campochiaro PA, Lim JI. 1994. Aminoglycoside toxicity in the treatment of endophthalmitis. Arch Ophthalmol 112:48–53.

Campochiaro PA, et al. 1986. Intravitreal chemotactic and mitogenic activity: implications of blood-retinal barrier breakdown. Arch Ophthalmol 104:1685–1687.

Casey RC, et al. 1995. Toxicity of subretinal mitomycin C. Invest Ophthalmol Vis Sci 36(suppl):S161.

Cavalleri A, Trimarchi F, et al. 1982. Effects of lead on the visual system of occupationally exposed subjects. Scand J Work Environ Health 8(suppl 1):148–151.

Chaine GJ, Badelon I, Favard CM. 1995. Systemic steroid therapy and central serous detachment. Ophthalmology 102(9A suppl):118.

Chan CC, Fishman M, Egbert PR. 1978. Multiple ocular anomalies associated with maternal LSD ingestion. Arch Ophthalmol 96:282–284.

Chang TS, et al. 1995. Asymmetric canthaxanthin retinopathy. Am J Ophthalmol 119:801–802.

Charton N, Sahel JA, Flament J. 1990. Poisoning of retinal pigment epithelium by deferoxamine. Bull Soc Ophthalmol France 90:599–602.

Chiang RK, et al. 1995. Cytochalasin D reversibly weakens retinal adhesiveness. Curr Eye Res 14:1109–1113.

Chrousos GA, et al. 1986. Prevention of ocular toxicity of carmustine (BCNU) with supraophthalmic intracarotid infusion. Ophthalmology 93:1471–1475.

Chung H, et al. 1988. BCNU in silicone oil in proliferative vitreoretinopathy: I. Solubility, stability and antiproliferative studies. Curr Eye Res 7:1199–1206.

Cibis PA, Brown EB, Hong SM. 1957. Ocular effects of systemic siderosis. Am J Ophthalmol 44:158–172.

Conway BP, et al. 1989. Gentamicin toxicity in the primate retina. Arch Ophthalmol 107:107–112.

Cordier C, Raspiller A, Lepori JC. 1981. Childhood form of chloroquine retinopathy. Bull Soc Ophthalmol Fr 81:647–650.

Cortin P, et al. 1982. Maculopathie en paillettes d'or. Can J Ophthalmol 17:103–106.

Craythorn JM, Swartz M, Creel DJ. 1986. Clofazimine-induced bull's-eye retinopathy. Retina 6:50–52.

Cullen JF. 1964. Ocular defects in thalidomide babies. Br J Ophthalmol 48:151–153.

Cunha-Vaz JG, Maurice DM. 1967. The active transport of fluorescein by the retinal vessels and the retina. J Physiol 191:467.

Cunningham CA, Friedberg DN, Carr RE. 1990. Clofazimine-induced generalized retinal degeneration. Retina 10:131–134.

Custodio JBA, Almeida LM, Madeira VMC. 1993. The active metabolite of the anticancer drug tamoxifen induces structural changes in membranes. Biochim Biophys Acta 1153:308–314.

Daicker B, et al. 1987. Canthaxanthin retinopathy. Graefes Arch Clin Exp Ophthalmol 225:189–197.

D'Amico DJ, et al. 1984. Retinal toxicity of intravitreal gentamicin: an electron microscopic study. Invest Ophthalmol Vis Sci 25:564–572.

D'Amico DJ, et al. 1985. Comparative toxicity of intravitreal aminoglycoside antibiotics. Am J Ophthalmol 100:264–275.

Davidorf FH. 1973. Thioridazine pigmentary retinopathy. Arch Ophthalmol 90:251–255.

Davis AA, Hunt, RC. 1993. Transferrin is made and bound by photoreceptor cells. J Cell Physiol 156:280–285.

Dawson WW, et al. 1983. The canine c-wave: breed and anesthetic dependent variations. Doc Ophthalmol Proc Series 37:57–64.

Daxecker F, Bichler E. 1993. Experimental chlorphentermine lipidosis of the retina in albino rats. Ophthalmologica 206:102–106.

Dearry A, et al. 1990. Dopamine induces light-adaptive retinomotor movements in bullfrog cones via D2 receptors and in retinal pigment epithelium via D1 receptors. J Neurochem 54:1367–1378.

Dekking HM. 1949. Pigmentary degeneration of the retina after quinine intoxication. Ophthalmologica 118:743.

Delahunt CS, et al. 1963. Toxic retinopathy following prolonged treatment with dl(p-trifluoromethyl (phenyl) isopropylamine hydrochloride (P-1727) in experimental animals. Toxicol Appl Pharmacol 5:298–305.

Delaney WV. 1975. Presumed ocular chalcosis and reversible maculopathy. Ann Ophthalmol 7:378–380.

Dementi B. 1994. Ocular side effects of organophosphates: a historical perspective of Saku disease. J Appl Toxicol 14:119–129.

Dennerlein JA, et al. 1995. Ocular findings in desferrioxamine therapy. Ophthalmologe 92:38–42.

Devin FC, et al. 1995. In vitro evaluation of the effects of colchicine and taxol on the microtubule network of cultured pig RPE cells by immunofluorescence microscopoy. Invest Ophthalmol Vis Sci 36(suppl):S753.

Dingle J, Havener WH. 1978. Ophthalmoscopic changes in a patient with Wilson's disease during long-term penicillamine therapy. Ann Ophthalmol 10:1227–1230.

Doi M, Refojo MF, Uji Y. 1995. Histopathology of silicone/fluorosilicone copolymer oil as six month internal retinal tamponade in rabbits. Invest Ophthalmol Vis Sci 36(suppl):S745.

Doly M, et al. 1992. Inhibition of vincristine-induced retinal impairments by a specific PAF antagonist. Lens Eye Tox Res 9:529–535.

Doly M, et al. 1993. Prevention of chloroquine-induced ERG damage by a new platelet-activating factor antagonist, BN 50730. Ophthalmic Res 25:314–318.

Duncker G, Bredehorn T. 1994. Chlorphentermine-induced lipidosis in the rat retina: a functional and morphological study. Graefes Arch Clin Exp Ophthalmol 232:368–372.

Easterbrook M. 1984. The use of Amsler grids in early chloroquine retinopathy. Ophthalmology 91:1368.

Eckhardt C, et al. 1993. Ocular tissue after intravitreous silicone oil injection: histologic and electron microscopy studies. Ophthalmologe 90:250–257.

Elder MJ. 1992. Diazepam and its effects on visual fields. Aust NZ J Ophthalmol 20:267–270.

Ennis SR, Betz AL. 1986. Sucrose permeability of the blood-retinal and blood-brain barriers: effects of diabetes, hypertonicity, and iodate. Invest Ophthalmol Vis Sci 27:1095–1102.

[ESG] Endophthalmitis Vitrectomy Study Group. 1995. Results of the Endophthalmitis Vitrectomy Study Group. Arch Ophthalmol 113:1479–1496.

Faber DS. 1969. Analysis of the slow transretinal potentials in response to light. PhD dissertation. State University of New York at Buffalo.

Falcone PM, Paolini L, Lou PL. 1993. Hydroxychloroquine toxicity despite normal dose therapy. Ann Ophthalmol 25:385–388.

Flage T. 1983. Changes in the juxtapapillary retinal pigment epithelium following intravenous injection of sodium iodate: a light and electron microscopic study using horseradish peroxidase as a tracer. Acta Ophthalmol 61:20–28.

Forster DJ, Causey DM, Rao NA. 1992. Bull's eye retinopathy and clofazimine. Ann Int Med 116:876–877.

Fox DA, Sillman AJ. 1979. Heavy metals affect rod, but not cone photoreceptors. Science 206:78–80.

Fraunfelder FT. 1996. Drug-Induced Ocular Side Effects and Drug Interactions. Philadelphia: Lea & Febiger, 193–194.

Friberg TR, Verstraeten TC, Wilcox DK. 1991. Effects of emulsification, purity and fluorination of silicone oil on human retinal pigment epithelial cells. Invest Ophthalmol Vis Sci 32:2030–2034.

Frisk-Holmberg M, et al. 1979. Chloroquine serum concentration and side-effects: evidence for dose-dependent kinetics. Clin Pharmacol Ther 25:347.

Gahlot DK, et al. 1976. Effect of copper on rabbit retina. Exp Ophthalmol 2:76–78.

Gass JDM. 1987. Stereoscopic Atlas of Macular Diseases: Diagnosis and Treatment. St Louis: Mosby Year Book, 46–59.

Goldhar SW, Basu PK, Ranadive NS. 1984. Phagocytosis by retinal pigment epithelium: evaluation of modulating agents with an organ culture model. Can J Ophthalmol 19:33–35.

Goldman L, Preston RH. 1957. Reactions to chloroquine observed during the treatment of various dermatologic disorders. Am J Trop Med Hyg 6:654.

Gonvers M, Hornung JP, de Courten C. 1986. The effect of liquid silicone on the rabbit retina: histologic and ultrastructural study. Arch Ophthalmol 104:1057–1062.

Good P, Gross K. 1988. Electrophysiology and metallosis: support for an oxidative (free radical) mechanism in the human eye. Ophthalmologica 196:204–209.

Graham CM, Blach RK. 1988. Indomethacin retinopathy: case report and review. Br J Ophthalmol 72:434–438.

Graham RO, Peyman GA, Fishman G. 1975. Intravitreal injection of cephaloridine in the treatment of endophthalmitis. Arch Ophthalmol 93:56–61.

Grant WM. 1986. Toxicology of the Eye. 3rd ed. Springfield, IL: Thomas.

Green WR. 1975. Retinal and optic nerve atrophy induced by intravitreous vincristine in the primate. Trans Am Ophthalmol Soc 73:389–416.

Grimes PA. 1988. Carboxyfluorescein transfer across the blood-retinal barrier evaluated by quantitative fluorescence microscopy: comparison with fluorescein. Exp Eye Res 46:769–783.

Grimson BS, et al. 1981. Ophthalmic and central nervous system complications following intracarotid BCNU (carmustine). J Clin Neuro-Ophthalmol 1:261–264.

Habib NE, et al. 1994. Toxic retinopathy secondary to repeat intravitreal amikacin and vancomycin. Eye 8:700–702.

Hallberg A, Naeser P, Andersson A. 1990. Effects of long-term chloroquine exposure on the phospholipid metabolism in retina and pigment epithelium of the mouse. Acta Ophthalmol 68:125–130.

Harnois C, et al. 1989. Canthaxanthine retinopathy anatomic and functional reversibility. Arch Ophthalmol 106:58–60.

Hart WM, et al. 1984. Static perimetry in chloroquine retinopathy: perifoveal patterns of visual field depression. Arch Ophthalmol 102:377–380.

Hayasaka S, Noda S, Setogawa T. 1988. Effect of drugs in vitro on lysosomal enzyme activities in bovine retinal pigment epithelial cells. Jpn J Ophthalmol 32:316–321.

Heier JS, et al. 1994. Screening for ocular toxicity in asymptomatic patients treated with tamoxifen. Am J Ophthalmol 117:772–775.

Heike M, Marmor MF. 1990. L-cystein protects the pigment epithelium from acute sodium iodate toxicity. Doc Ophthalmol 75:15–22.

Henkes HE, van Lith GHM, Canta LR. 1972. Indomethacin retinopathy. Am J Ophthalmol 73:846–856.

Hines J, Vinores SA, Campochiaro PA. 1993. Evolution of morphologic changes after intravitreous injection of gentamicin. Current Eye Res 12:521–529.

Hirayama Y. 1990. Histochemical localization of zinc and copper in rat ocular tissues. Acta Histochem 89:107–111.

Hodgkins PR, et al. 1992. Pigment epitheliopathy with serous detachment of the retina following intravenous iron dextran. Eye 6:414–415.

Hofmann H, Schmut O. 1980. The inability of superoxide dismutase to inhibit the depolymerization of hyaluronic acid by ferrous ions and ascorbate. Graefes Arch Clin Exp Ophthalmol 214:181–185.

Homewood CA, et al. 1972. Lysosomes, pH and the antimalarial action of chloroquine. Nature 235:50–52.

Horgan SE, Williams RW. 1995. Chronic retinal toxicity due to quinine in Indian tonic water. Eye 9:637–638.

Hughes WF, Coogan P. 1974. Pathology of the retinal pigment epithelium and retina in rabbits poisoned with lead. Am J Path 77:237–254.

Immel J, Negi A, Marmor MF. 1986. Acute changes in RPE apical morphology after retinal detachment in rabbit. Invest Ophthalmol Vis Sci 27:1770–1776.

Inkeles DM, Friedman AH. 1975. Retinal pigment epithelial degeneration, partial retinal atrophy and macular hole in acute lymphocytic leukemia. Graefes Arch Clin Exp Ophthalmol 194:253–261.

Ivanina TA, et al. 1983. Ultrastructural alterations in cat and rat retina and pigment epithelium induced by chloroquine. Graefes Arch Clin Exp Ophthalmol 220:32.

Iwasaki T, et al. 1996. The retinal changes following intravitreal gas injection in rabbits. Invest Ophthalmol Vis Sci 37(suppl):S196.

Jaffe MJ, et al. 1989. Attenuating effects of diazepam on the electroretinogram of normal humans. Retina 9:216–225.

Junemann G, Schulze J. 1968. Electroretinographic studies of the development of quinine and chloroquine retinopathy. Klin Mbl Augenheilk 152:562–566.

Kaiser JA. 1963. Tapetal depigmentation in dogs produced by ethylenediamines. Fed Proc 22:369.

Kaiser-Kupfer MI, Lippman ME. 1978. Tamoxifen retinopathy. Cancer Treat Rep 62:315–320.

Kalina RE, Wells CG. 1995. Screening for ocular toxicity in asymptomatic patients treated with tamoxifen. Am J Ophthalmol 119:112–113.

Kane A, Barza M, Baum J. 1981. Intravitreal injection of gentamicin in rabbits: effects of inflammation and pigmentation on half-life and ocular distribution. Invest Ophthalmol Vis Sci 20:593.

Karpe G. 1948. Early diagnosis of siderosis retinae by the use of electroretinography. Doc Ophthalmol 2:277–296.

Katz ML, et al. 1993. Iron-induced accumulation of lipofuscin-like fluorescent pigment in the retinal pigment epithelium. Invest Ophthalmol Vis Sci 34:3161–3171.

Katz ML, et al. 1994. Iron-induced fluorescence in the retina: dependence on vitamin A. Invest Ophthalmol Vis Sci 35:3613–3624.

Kawasaki K, Ohnogi J. 1988. Nontoxic concentration of antibiotics for intravitreal use evaluated by human in-vitro ERG. Documenta Ophthalmologica 70:301–308.

Kawasaki K, et al. 1990. Electroretinographical changes due to antimicrobials. Lens Eye Toxicity Res 7:693–704.

Keller G, Leuenberger PM. 1977. Effects of colchicine on phagosome-lysosome interaction in retinal pigment epithelium. II. In vitro observations on histio-organotypical retinal pigment epithelial cells of the pig. Graefes Arch Clin Exp Ophthalmol 203:253–259.

Kemali M, Milici N, Kemali D. 1983. Modification of the pigment screening of the frog retina following administration of neuroactive drugs. Exp Eye Res 37:493–498.

Kimbrough BO, Campbell RJ. 1981. Thioridazine levels in the human eye. Arch Ophthalmol 99:2188–2189.

Kinross-Wright V. 1956. Clinical trial of a new phenothiazine compound: NP-207. Psychiatr Res 4:89–94.

Kiryu J, Yamamoto F, Honda Y. 1992. Effects of sodium iodate on the electroretinogram c-wave in the cat. Vision Res 32:2221–2227.

Kishimoto N, Ohkuma H, Uyama M. 1990a. Effect of intravitreal gas on the destruction of anionic sites in the outer blood-retinal barrier. Nippon Ganka Gakkai Zasshi 94:654–662.

Kishimoto N, et al. 1990b. Early effects of sodium iodate shown by detection of the destruction of anionic sites in outer blood-retinal barrier. Nippon Ganka Gakkai Zasshi 94:25–32.

Kishimoto N, Ohkuma H, Uyama M. 1991. Detection of destruction of anionic sites in the outer blood-retinal barrier and damage caused by iron. Nippon Ganka Gakkai Zasshi 95:130–139.

Kitano S, Hori S, Nagataki S. 1988. Transport of fluorescein in the rabbit eye after treatment with sodium iodate. Exp Eye Res 46:863–870.

Klepach GL, Wray SH. 1981. Bilateral serous retinal detachment with thrombocytopenia during penicillamine therapy. Ann Ophthalmol 13:201–203.

Knave B, et al. 1973. Selective effect of a new antituberculous drug, rifampicin, on the c-wave of the sheep electroretinogram. Acta Ophthalmol 51:371–374.

Knave B, Persson HE, Nilsson SEG. 1974. The effect of barbiturate on retinal functions. II. Effects on the c-wave of the electroretinogram and the standing potential of the sheep eye. Acta Physiol Scand 91:181–186.

Korte GE, Hirsch D. 1986. Intercellular junctions of hyperplastic retinal pigment epithelium. Experientia 42:812–815.

Korte GE, Wanderman MC. 1993. Distribution of Na-K-ATPase in regenerating retinal pigment epithelium in the rabbit. Exp Eye Res 56:219–229.

Korte GE, Bellhorn RW, Burns MS. 1984. Urethane-induced rat retinopathy. Plasticity of the blood-retinal barrier in disease. Invest Ophthalmol Vis Sci 25:1027–1034.

Korte GE, Bellhorn RW, Burns MS. 1986. Remodeling of the retinal pigment epithelium in response to intraepithelial capillaries: evidence that capillaries influence the polarity of epithelium. Cell Tissue Res 245:135–142.

Kozy D, Doft BH, Lipkowitz J. 1984. Nummular thioridazine retinopathy. Retina 4:253–256.

Kritzinger EE, Bellhorn RW. 1982. Permeability of blood-retinal barriers in urethane-induced rat retinopathy. Br J Ophthalmol 66:630–635.

Kuhn H, et al. 1981. Lack of correlation between melanin affinity and retinopathy in mice and cats treated with chloroquine or flunitrazepam. Graefes Arch Clin Exp Ophthalmol 216:177–190.

Lakhanpal V, Schocket SS, Jiji R. 1984. Deferoxamine (Desferal) - induced toxic retinal pigmentary degeneration and presumed optic neuropathy. Ophthalmology 91:443–451.

Lambrou FH, Burke JM, Aaberg TM. 1987. Effect of silicone oil on experimental traction retinal detachment. Arch Ophthalmol 105:1269–1272.

Larsson BS. 1993. Interaction between chemicals and melanin. Pigment Cell Res 6:127–133.

Larsson B, Tjalve H. 1979. Studies on the mechanism of drug binding to melanin. Biochem Pharmacol 28:1181–1187.

Leure-duPree, AE. 1981. Electron-opaque inclusions in the rat retinal pigment epithelium after treatment with chelators of zinc. Invest Ophthalmol Vis Sci 21:1–9.

Leure-duPree AE, McClain CJ. 1982. The effect of severe zinc deficiency on the morphology of the rat retinal pigment epithelium. Invest Ophthalmol Vis Sci 23:425–434.

Lin SC, et al. 1994. The photodynamic occlusion of choroidal vessels using benzoporphyrin derivatives. Curr Eye Res 13:513–522.

Lullmann-Rauch R. 1976. Retinal lipidosis in albino rats treated with chlorphentermine and with tricyclic antidepressants. Acta Neuropathol 35:55–67.

Lullmann-Rauch R. 1981. Experimentally induced lipidosis in rat retinal pigment epithelium. Graefes Arch Clin Exp Ophthalmol 215:297–303.

Lullmann-Rauch R, Nussberger L. 1983. Citalopram-induced generalized lipidosis in rats. Acta Pharmacol Toxicol 52:161–167.

Lurie M, Marmor MF. 1979. Light integrating capacity of the ERG c-wave under different anesthesia. Proc 16th ISCEV Symp Mirioka, Jpn J Ophthalmol 16:129–133.

Mackenzie AH. 1983. Pharmacologic actions of 4-aminoquinoline compounds. Am J Med 75:5–10.

Manners TD, Clarke MP. 1995. Maculopathy associated with Diazepam. Eye 9:660–662.

Markowitz S, et al. 1981. Enhancement and inhibition of phagocytic activity in the retinal pigment epithelium. Can J Ophthalmol 16:187–191.

Marmor MF. 1990. Is thioridazine retinopathy progressive? Relationship of pigmentary changes to visual function. Br J Ophthalmol 74:739–742.

Marmor MF, Yao XY. 1994. Conditions necessary for the formation of serous detachment: experimental evidence from the cat. Arch Ophthalmol 112:830–838.

Marmor MF, Nelson JW, Levin AS. 1978. Copper metabolism in American retinitis pigmentosa patients. Br J Ophthalmol 62:168– 171.

Mason CG. 1977. Ocular accumulation and toxicity of certain systemically administered drugs. J Toxicol Env Health 2:977–995.

Matsumura M, et al. 1986. Effects of phenothiazines on cultured retinal pigment epithelial cells. Ophthalmic Res 18:47–54.

McClanahan WS, et al. 1966. Ocular manifestations of chronic phenothiazine derivative administration. Arch Ophthalmol 75:319–325.

McDonald HR, et al. 1986. Retinal toxicity secondary to intraocular gentamicin injection. Ophthalmology 93:871.

McKeown CA, et al. 1981. Tamoxifen retinopathy. Br J Ophthalmol 65:177–179.

Menon IA, et al. 1989. A study on the sequence of phototoxic effects of rose bengal using retinal pigment epithelial cells in vitro. Exp Eye Res 49:67–73.

Meredith TA, Aaberg TM, Willerson WD. 1978. Progressive chorioretinopathy after receiving thioridazine. Arch Ophthalmol 96:1172–1176.

Meredith TA, et al. 1984. Ocular involvement in primary hyperoxaluria. Arch Ophthalmol 102:584–587.

Metge P, Mandirac-Bonnefoy C, Bellaube P. 1984. Thésaurismose rétinienne à la canthaxanthine. Bull Mem Soc Fr Ophthalmol 95:547–549.

Millay RH, et al. 1986. Maculopathy associated with combination chemotherapy and osmotic opening of the blood-brain barrier. Am J Ophthalmol 102:626–632.

Miller FS, Bunt-Milam AH, Kalina RE. 1982. Clinical-ultrastructural study of thioridazine retinopathy. Ophthalmology 89:1478–1488.

Mills PV, Beck M, Power BJ. 1981. Assessment of the retinal toxicity of hydroxychloroquine. Trans Ophthalmol Soc UK 101:109–113.

Mindel JS, et al. 1988. N-3-pyridylmethyl-N'-p-nitrophenylurea ocular toxicity in man and rabbits. Br J Ophthalmol 1988. 72:584–590.

Misra UK, et al. 1985. Some observations on the macula of pesticide workers. Human Toxicol 4:135–145.

Mitchison TJ. 1992. Compare and contrast actin filaments and microtubules. Mol Biol Cell 3:1309–1315.

Morsman CD, et al. 1990. Screening for hydroxychloroquine retinal toxicity: is it necessary? Eye 4:572–576.

Moschos M, et al. 1990. ERG and electron microscopic findings after intravitreal use of aminoglycosides. Ann Ophthalmol 22:255–258.

Müller W, Haase E. 1975. Fragen zur Beeinflussung des Elektrooculogramms durch Diazepam. Graefes Arch Clin Exp Ophthalmol 197:159–164.

Nao-i N, Kim SY, Honda Y. 1986. Paradoxical enhancement of the ERG c-wave by a small dose of sodium iodate. Acta Ophthalmol 64:206–211.

Negi A, Marmor MF. 1983. The resorption of subretinal fluid after diffuse damage to the retinal pigment epithelium. Invest Ophthalmol Vis Sci 24:1475–1479.

Negi A, White MP, Marmor MF. 1993. Effects of hemicholinium-3, a photoreceptor and pigment epithelial toxin on retinal adhesiveness and subretinal fluid absorption. Doc Ophthalmol 83:331–336.

Newsome DA, Rothman RJ. 1987. Zinc uptake in vitro by human retinal pigment epithelium. Invest Ophthalmol Vis Sci 28:1795–1799.

Newsome DA, et al. 1988. Oral zinc in macular degeneration. Arch Ophthalmol 106:192–198.

Nijman NN, et al. 1989. Canthaxanthin Retinopathie. Klin Mbl Augenheilk 194:48–51.

Noell WK. 1953. Studies on the Electrophysiology and the Metabolism of the Retina. US Air Force SAM Project No. 21-1201-004.

Novak MA, Roth AS, Levine MR. 1988. Calcium oxalate retinopathy associated with methoxyflurane abuse. Retina 8:230–236.

Nusinowitz S, et al. 1996. Characteristic electroretinographic findings in quinine retinal toxicity. Invest Ophthalmol Vis Sci 37(suppl):S344.

Ogawa S, et al. 1979. Progression of retinopathy long after cessation of chloroquine therapy. Lancet 1:1408.

Ogino N, et al. 1980. Reversible inhibition of phagocytosis of cultured retinal pigment epithelial cells by cytochalasin B and colchicine. Nippon Ganka Gakkai Zasshi 84:2108–2112.

Ohkubo S, et al. 1995. Effects of intravitreal levofloxacin on the rabbit retina. Invest Ophthalmol Vis Sci 36:S742.

Ohman L, Wahlberg I. 1975. Ocular side-effects of clofazimine. Lancet 7941:933–934.

Ohmori H, Toyama S, Toyama S. 1992. Direct proof that the primary site of action of cytochalasin on cell motility processes is actin. J Cell Biol 116:933–941.

Oliver PD, Newsome DA. 1992. Mitochondrial superoxide dismutase in mature and developing human retinal pigment epithelium. Invest Ophthalmol Vis Sci 33:1909–1918.

Oosterhuis JA, et al. 1989. Canthaxanthin retinopathy without intake of canthaxanthin. Klin Mbl Augenheil 194:110–116.

Orzalesi N, Grignolo A, Calabria A. 1967. Experimental degeneration of the rabbit retina induced by sodium fluoride. Exp Eye Res 6:165–170.

Oum BS, D'Amico DJ, Wong KW. 1989. Intravitreal antibiotic therapy with vancomycin and aminoglycoside. An experimental study of combination and repetitive injections. Arch Ophthalmol 107:1055–1060.

Oum BS, et al. 1992. Intravitreal antibiotic therapy with vancomycin and aminoglycoside: examination of the retinal toxicity of repetitive injections after vitreous and lens surgery. Graefes Arch Clin Exp Ophthalmol 230:56–61.

Owaribe K, Araki M, Eguchi G. Cell shape and actin filaments. in Hatano S, Ishikawa H, and Sato H. eds, 1979. Cell Motility: Molecules and Organization. Tokyo: University of Tokyo Press, 491–500.

Owaribe K. 1988. The cytoskeleton of retinal pigment epithelial cells. In Osborne N, Chader J, eds, Progress in Retinal Research. New York: Pergamon Press, 23–49.

Palimeris G, Koliopoulos J, Velissaropoulos P. 1972. Ocular side effects of indomethacin. Ophthalmologica 164:339–353.

Pall H, et al. 1989. Ocular toxicity of desferrioxamine—an example of copper promoted auto-oxidative damage? Br J Ophthalmol 73:42–47.

Park SS, et al. 1995. Immunohistological localization of ganciclovir in human eyes treated with intravenous or intravitreal ganciclovir. Ophthalmology 102(9A suppl):162–163.

Patterson GM, et al. 1993. Action of tolytoxin on cell morphology, cytoskeletal organization, and actin polymerization. Cell Motil Cytoskeleton 24:39–48.

Persad S, et al. 1986. Binding of imipramine, 8-methoxypsoralen, and epinephrine to human blue and brown eye melanins. J Toxicol-Cutaneous Toxicol 5:125–132.

Persad S, et al. 1988. Phototoxicity of chlorpromazine on retinal pigment epithelial cells. Current Eye Res 7:1–9.

Pflugfelder SC, et al. 1987. Intravitreal vancomycin. Retinal toxicity, clearance, and interaction with gentamicin. Arch Ophthalmol 105:831–837.

Piguet B, Chobaz C, Grounauer PA. 1996. Rétinopathie toxique sur injection intravitrénne d'Amikacine et Vancomycine. Klin Mbl Augenheil 208:358–359.

Pinkers A, Broekhuyse RM. 1983. The EOG in rheumatoid arthritis. Acta Ophthalmol 61:831.

Pirie A. 1968. Pathology in the eye of the naphthalene-fed rabbit. Exp Eye Res 7:354–357.

Polak BCP, Baarsma GS, Snyers B. 1995. Diffuse retinal pigment epitheliopathy complicating systemic corticosteroid treatment. Br J Ophthalmol 79:922–925.

Potamitis T, et al. 1996. EOG monitoring of desferrioxamine treatment. Invest Ophthalmol Vis Sci 37(suppl):S344.

Power WJ, Travers SP, Mooney DJ. 1991. Welding arc maculopathy and fluphenazine. Br J Ophthalmol 75:433–435.

Pu GA, Masland RH. 1984. Biochemical interruption of membrane phospholipid renewal in retinal photoreceptor cells. J Neurosci 4:1559–1576.

Purple RL, Schauer BA, Gehlbach PL. 1995. Retinal toxicity of the iron chelator 1,2-dimethyl-3-hydroxyprid-4-one, (L1) in an albino rat model. Invest Ophthalmol Vis Sci 36(suppl):S163.

Rahi AH, Hungerford JL, Ahmed AI. 1986. Ocular toxicity of desferrioxamine: light microscopic histochemical and ultrastructural findings. Br J Ophthalmol 70:373–381.

Raines MF, Bhargava SK, Rosen ES. 1989. The blood-retinal barrier in chloroquine retinopathy. Invest Ophthalmol Vis Sci 30:1726–1731.

Rao SS, Satapathy M, Sitaramayya A. 1981. Copper metabolism in retinitis pigmentosa patients. Br J Ophthalmol 65:127–130.

Reboton J, et al. 1962. Pigmentary retinopathy and iridocycloplegia in psychiatric patients. J Neuropsych 3:311–316.

Reim M, Lukow K, Weber H. 1989. Enzyme activities of the retina and vitreous body following experimental implantation of a brass splinter. Klin Mbl Augenheilk 195:363–367.

Ringvold A, Olsen EG, Flage T. 1981. Transient breakdown of retinal pigment epithelium diffusion barrier after sodium iodate. Exp Eye Res 33:361–369.

Ripps H, et al. 1989. Vincristine-induced changes in the retina of the isolated arterially-perfused cat eye. Exp Eye Res 48:771–790.

Robbins J, Ikeda H. 1989. Benzodiazepines and the mammalian retina. I. Autoradiographic localisation of receptor sites and the lack of effect on the electroretinogram. Brain Res 479:313–322.

Roggenkämper W. 1927. Akuter Pigmentzerfall in der Netzhaut infolge Septojod intoxikation. Klin Mbl Augenheilk 79:827–828.

Rosenthal AR, Hopkins JL, Appleton B. 1974. Studies on intraocular copper foreign bodies. Arch Ophthalmol 92:431–436.

Rosenthal AR, et al. 1978. Chloroquine retinopathy in the rhesus monkey. Invest Ophthalmol Vis Sci 17:1158–1175.

Rosenthal AR, et al. 1979. Chalcosis—a study of natural history. Ophthalmology 86:1956–1972.

Roskoski R, Jaskunas SR. 1972. Chloroquine and primaquine inhibition of rat liver cell-free polynucleotide-dependent polypeptide synthesis. Biochem Pharmacol 21:391–399.

Sakamoto T, et al. 1994. Intercellular gap formation induced by thrombin in confluent cultured bovine retinal pigment epithelial cells. Invest Ophthalmol Vis Sci 35:720–729.

Santos-Anderson RM, et al. 1984. Chronic lead administration in neonatal rats: electron microscopy of the retina. J Neuropathol Exp Neurol 43:175–187.

Sassani JW, et al. 1983. Progressive chloroquine retinopathy. Ann Ophthalmol 15:19–22.

Scallon LJ, et al. 1988. Canthaxanthine-induced retinal pigment epithelial changes in the cat. Current Eye Res 7:687–693.

Schimmel R. 1926. Augenschädigungen nach Septojodinjektionen. Münch Med Wochenschr 73:590.

Schmidt-Erfuhrt U, et al. 1994. Vascular targeting in photodynamic occlusion of subretinal vessels. Ophthalmology 101:1953–1961.

Schutte E, Klaas D, Lizin F. 1977. Serial studies in thalidomide damaged children. Ber Dtsch Ophthalmol Ges 74:578–580.

Shakiba S, et al. 1993. Evaluation of retinal toxicity and liposome encapsulation of the anti-CMV drug 2'-nor-cyclic GMP. Invest Ophthalmol Vis Sci 34:2903–2910.

Sharkey JA. 1993. Idiopathic canthaxanthine retinopathy. Eur J Ophthalmol 3:226–228.

Shearer RV, Dubois EL. 1967. Ocular changes induced by long-term hydroxychloroquine (Plaquenil) therapy. Am J Ophthalmol 64:245–252.

Shikishima K, et al. 1992. Effects and distribution of intravitreally or subretinally injected silicone oil identified in rabbit retina using osmium tetroxide method. Jpn J Ophthalmol 36:469–478.

Shiono T, Hayasaka S, Mizuno K. 1984. Effect of chlorpromazine in vitro on release of enzymes from lysosomes of the bovine retinal pigment epithelium. Invest Ophthalmol Vis Sci 25:115–117.

Sieving PA, et al. 1983. Early receptor potential measurements in human ocular siderosis. Arch Ophthalmol 101:1716–1720.

Singalavanija A, Dongosintr N, Dulayajinda D. 1994. Potassium iodate retinopathy. Acta Ophthalmol 72:513–519.

Sirbat D, et al. 1983. Serous detachment of macular neuro-epithelium and flumequine. J Fr Ophthalmol 6:829–836.

Sorsby A, Harding R. 1960. Experimental degeneration of the retina. Br J Ophthalmol 43:559–565.

Sorbsy A, Harding R. 1962. Experimental degeneration of the retina-VIII Dithizone retinopathy: its independence of the diabetogenic effect. Vision Res 2:149–155.

Sousa Neves M, Jordan K, Dragt H. 1990. Extensive chorioretinopathy associated with very low dose thioridazine. Eye 4:767–770.

Spalton DJ, Verdon-Roe GM, Hughes GR. 1993. Hydroxychloroquine, dosage parameters and retinopathy. Lupus 2:355–358.

Spector I, et al. 1989. Latrunculins-novel marine macrolides that disrupt microfilament organization and affect cell growth. Cell Motil Cytoskeleton 13:127–144.

Suzuki J, et al. 1987. The effect of colchicine on the diurnal variation of phagocytosis in mouse retinal pigment epithelium. Exp Eye Res 44:755–765.

Syversen, K. 1979. Intramuscular iron therapy and tapetoretinal degeneration. Acta Ophthalmol 57:358–361.

Taarnhoj J, Alm A. 1992. The effect of sodium iodate on the blood-retinal and blood-brain barriers. Graefes Arch Clin Exp Ophthalmol 230:589–591.

Tabatabay CA, et al. 1987. Experimental drusen formation induced by intravitreal aminoglycoside injection. Arch Ophthalmol 105:826–830.

Tabatabay CA, et al. 1990. Immunocytochemical localization of gentamicin in the rabbit retina following intravitreal injection. Arch Ophthalmol 108:723–726.

Takeichi Y, Miki K, Uyama M. 1991. Morphological changes in the retina following one-shot injection of netilmicin sulfate into the vitreous. Nippon Ganka Gakkai Zasshi 95:669–677.

Takeichi Y, Miki K, Uyama M. 1994. Morphological change in the retina after injection of calcium and netilmicin sulfate in the rabbit vitreous body. Nippon Ganka Gakkai Zasshi 98:150–156.

Talamo JH, et al. 1985. The influence of aphakia and vitrectomy on experimental retinal toxicity of aminoglycoside antibiotics. Am J Ophthalmol 100:840–847.

Tandon P, et al. 1994. Fenthion produces a persistent decrease in muscarinic receptor function in the adult rat retina. Toxicol Appl Pharmacol 125:271–280.

Tobin DR, Krohel GB, Rines RI. 1982. Hydroxychloroquine: seven-year experience. Arch Ophthalmol 100:81.

Toimela T, Tähti H, Salminen L. 1995. Retinal pigment epithelium cell culture as a model for evaluation of the toxicity of tamoxifen and chloroquine. Ophthalmic Res 27:150–153.

Troutt LL, Burnside B. 1989. Role of microtubules in pigment granule migration in teleost retinal pigment epithelial cells. Exp Eye Res 48:433–443.

Turut P, Florin P, Malthieu D. 1979. Pigmentary pseudo-retinitis from Ceporine; 4 observations. Bull Soc Fr Ophtalmol 79:1095–1098.

Turut P, Malthieu D. 1980. Ocular toxicity of cephaloridine: clinical and experimental study. J Fr Ophtalmol 3:401–408.

Uhthoff W. 1911. Augenstörungen bei Vergiftungen In: Graefe A, Sämisch T, eds, Graefe-Sämisch Handbuch der Augenheilkunde. Vol. XI. Berlin, 62–75.

Ulshafer RJ, Allen CB, Rubin ML. 1990. Distribution of elements in the human retinal pigment epithelium. Arch Ophthalmol 108:113–117.

van Heyningen R. 1979. Naphthalene cataract in rats and rabbits: a resume. Exp Eye Res 28:435–439.

Vergara O, Ogden T, Ryan S. 1989. Posterior penetrating injury in the rabbit eye: effect of blood and ferrous ions. Exp Eye Res 49:1115–1126.

Verrey F. 1956. Dégénérescence pigmentaire de la rétine d'origine médicamenteuse. Ophthalmologica 131:296–303.

Verstraeten TC, et al. 1990. Retinal pigment epithelium wound closure in vitro: pharmacologic inhibition. Invest Ophthalmol Vis Sci 31:481–488.

Vrabec F, Obenberger J, Bolkova A. 1968. Effect of intravitreous vincristine sulfate on the rabbit retina. Am J Ophthalmol 66:199–204.

Wagenmann A. 1913. Die Verletzungen des Auges durch chemische Einwirkung. In: Graefe A, Sämisch T, eds, Handbuch der Augenheilkunde. Vol. IX. Leipzig: Wilhelm Engelmann, 1531–1636.

Wainer IW, et al. 1994. Distribution of the enantiomers of hydroxychloroquine and its metabolites in ocular tissues of the rabbit after oral administration of racemic-hydroxychloroquine. Chirality 6:347–354.

Weber U, et al. 1987. Experimental carotenoid retinopathy. Graefes Arch Clin Exp Ophthalmol 225:198–205.

Weber U, et al. 1992. Canthaxanthine retinopathy. Follow-up of over 6 years. Klin Mbl Augenheilk 201:174–177.

Weiss JN, et al. 1980. Retinopathy after tilorone hydrochloride. Am J Ophthalmol 90:846–853.

Whitcup SM, et al. 1992. Retinal toxicity in human immunodeficiency virus infected children treated with 2',3'-dideoxyinosine. Am J Ophthalmol 113:1–7.

Whitcup SM, et al. 1994. A clinicopathologic report of the retinal lesions associated with didanosine. Arch Ophthalmol 112:1594–1598.

White MP, Negi A, Hock PA. 1990. Effects of hemicholinium-3 on the pigmented rabbit retina and pigment epithelium. Curr Eye Res 9:669–676.

Wilson CA, et al. 1991. Exudative retinal detachment after photodynamic injury. Arch Ophthalmol 109:125–134.

Winding T, Nielsen NV. 1983. Retinopathy caused by treatment with tamoxifen in low dosage. Acta Ophthalmol 61:45–50.

Wioland N, et al. 1984. Pharmacologic sensitivity of the photopic c-wave in the ERG of the chicken. II. Effects of sodium iodate and general anesthesia. Comptes Rendus de l'Academie des Sciences 299:799–804.

Wray SH, Kuwabara T, Sanderson P. 1976. Menkes' kinky hair disease: a light and electron microscopic study of the eye. Invest Ophthalmol Vis Sci 15:128–138.

Yamada H, et al. 1995. Inhibition of proliferation of human retinal pigment epithelium by beta-interferon in vitro. Invest Ophthalmol Vis Sci 36(suppl):S99.

Yamamoto F, Kiryu J, Kiroi K. 1993. Effects of iodate on intraretinal b- and c-waves of the cat electroretinogram. Ophthalmologica 206:152–157.

Yamashita Y, et al. 1995. Effects of intravitreal injection of norfloxacin on rabbit retina. Invest Ophthalmol Vis Sci 36(suppl): S918.

Yannuzzi LA. 1986. Type A behavior and central serous chorioretinopathy. Trans Am Ophthalmol Soc 84:799–845.

Yoon YH, Marmor MF. 1993. Retinal pigment epithelium adhesion to Bruch's membrane is weakened by hemicholinium-3 and sodium iodate. Ophthalmic Res 25:386–392.

Yoshioka H, Katsume Y, Akune H. 1982. Experimental central serous chorioretinopathy in monkey eyes: fluorescein angiographic findings. Ophthalmologica 185:168–178.

Yospaiboon Y, Lawatiantong T, Chotibutr S. 1984. Clinical observations of ocular quinine intoxication. Jpn J Ophthalmol 28:409–415.

Zarbin MA, Anholt RR. 1991. Benzodiazepine receptors in the eye. Invest Ophthalmol Vis Sci 32:2579–2587.

Zelickson AS, Zeller HC. 1964. A new and unusual reaction to chlorpromazine. JAMA 188:394–396.

Zemel E, et al. 1995. Ocular pigmentation protects the rabbit retina from gentamicin-induced toxicity. Invest Ophthalmol Vis Sci 36:1875–1884.

IX | AGING AND DEGENERATION

33. Lipofuscin and other lysosomal storage deposits in the retinal pigment epithelium

GRAIG E. ELDRED

Residual lysosomal storage granules, varying in form and composition, accumulate within the retinal pigment epithelium (RPE) under the influence of a number of factors. These include normal aging, modified diets, specific classes of pharmaceuticals, and certain genetically inherited disease processes.

The impact of the lysosomal storage granules on the physiology of the RPE is largely unknown. It has long been suspected that lipofuscin granules (age pigments) are involved in the early biochemical processes that ultimately lead to age-related macular degeneration (AMD). However, good models for lipofuscinogenesis are lacking, and this has impeded progress in our understanding of how this pigment is formed and how it influences retinal pathophysiology. Many of the experimentally induced lysosomal storage granules that had been considered to be good models for RPE lipofuscin are now known to be quite different from the true RPE age pigments. Some disease-related storage granules once thought to be lipofuscin granules are proving not to be, while others have not yet been characterized fully enough to draw firm conclusions as to their relatedness to RPE lipofuscin. Therefore, a great deal of caution needs to be applied in calling any RPE lysosomal storage deposit "lipofuscin-like."

As AMD becomes ever more prevalent, it is becoming increasingly important to clarify the mechanisms of formation of lipofuscin in the RPE and to identify valid models for studies into the role that it may play in this and other disease processes. It is the purpose of this review to cover what is currently known of lipofuscin and the other lysosomal storage granules that are seen in the RPE.

RPE LIPOFUSCIN

The term *lipofuscin* is derived from both Greek and Latin roots: *lipos* meaning "fatty," and *fuscus* meaning "dark." True RPE lipofuscin granules are very specific subcellular structures with unique characteristics. Lipofuscin granules from other tissues differ from RPE lipofuscin in extractability, buoyant density, and composition (Siakotos and Kopang, 1973; Elleder, 1981; Brizzee and Ordy, 1981; Eldred, 1987).

Histochemical Description and Ultrastructural Appearance

The earliest descriptions of RPE lipophilic granules were reviewed by Streeten in 1961 in her seminal work on the histochemistry of human RPE lipofuscin. Prior to her work, the prevalence and nature of the material was unclear. She was the first to distinguish these particles as unique sudanophilic granules, clearly distinguishable from RPE melanin in unstained tissue sections. She showed that they accumulate with age (Fig. 33-1 and Plate 33-I) starting in the basal and peripheral portions of normal, nondiseased RPE as early as 16 months of age. The granules gradually increase in size and number until the bottoms of the cells became filled. Then they begin to extend up among the more apically located melanin granules by the fifth decade. Staining characteristics indicated that the material is lipidic with a high degree of unsaturation. The granules tested negative for sulfhydryl compounds, cholesterol, and glycolipids, and were quite resistant to extraction with fat solvents. Streeten pointed out that these pigment granules were very likely to be the same as ones described in 1912 by Kreibich, who called them *myeloid granules related to the lipofuscins* or "wear and tear" pigments. By 1961, further histochemical characterizations of other tissue lipofuscins had occurred, and Streeten, too, concluded that these sudanophilic RPE granules most closely resembled the lipofuscins in their resistance to chemicals and staining characteristics.

Ultrastructurally, the mature lipofuscin granules (Fig. 33-2) appear quite homogenous (Feeney et al., 1965; Feeney, 1978), showing little substructure as compared to the lipofuscin of other tissues (Brizzee and Ordy,

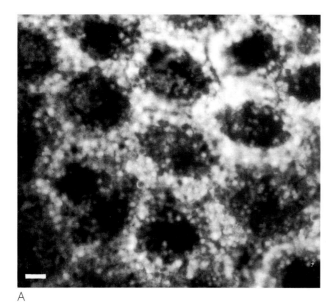

A

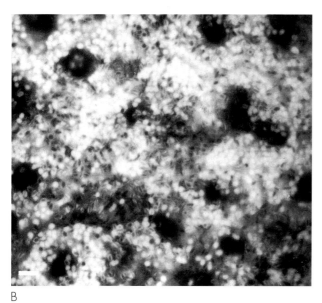

B

FIGURE 33-1. Fluorescence light micrographs of flat mounts of human pigment epithelium. (a) From a 45-year-old individual, showing the margin of cells filled with fluorescent granules. (b) From a 82-year-old individual, showing the entire cells filled with fluorescent granules. Bar represents 5 μm.

1981). With increasing age an increasing number of granules appear containing incorporated melanin granules (Feeney, 1978; Feeney-Burns, 1980).

Rate and Distribution of Accumulation

Although in 1961 Streeten noted the age-related accumulation of lipofuscin granules, it was not until 1984 that the first quantitative morphometric study was per-

formed to trace the rate of lipofuscin buildup in the RPE (Feeney-Burns et al., 1984). Surprisingly, it was found that the increase in lipofuscin granules followed a sigmoidal time course. During the first decade of life lipofuscin accumulates quite slowly, then a large increase occurs from ages 10 to 20 years, followed by a slower increase throughout most of the remainder of life. As the number of lipofuscin granules increases, the number of RPE melanin granules decreases, with a corresponding increase in the number of complexed melanolipofuscin granules (Feeney-Burns et al., 1984; Feeney-Burns and Katz, 1992).

Geographically, the greatest accumulation of lipofuscin and melanolipofuscin granules occurs in the posterior pole of the eye, especially in the macula (Wing et al., 1978; Feeney-Burns et al., 1984; Weiter et al., 1986), and in a pattern that correlates remarkably well with the distribution of degenerative changes associated with AMD (Weiter et al., 1988; Dorey et al., 1989).

Autophagic and Heterophagic Origins

Streeten (1961) pointed out that the staining characteristics of RPE lipofuscin granules were similar to some of those of the photoreceptor outer segments (POS), giving the first clue of common compositions. In 1965, Feeney and colleagues described the ultrastructure of the lipofuscin granules and other granules in the apical portion of the RPE that appeared to be broken or detached por-

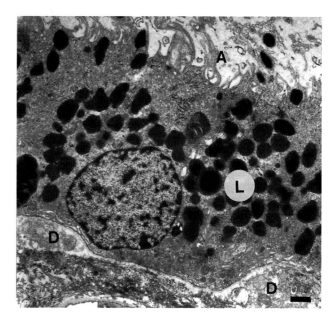

FIGURE 33-2. Electron micrograph showing lipofuscin granules (L) in the human pigment epithelium. (D) drusen and deposits in Bruch's membrane; (A) apical PE processes. Bar represents 1 μm.

tions of rod and cone outer segments engulfed by the RPE. She postulated that over time, fragments of outer segment are phagocytosed and only partially broken down by enzymatic digestion, leaving residues to accumulate as lipofuscin granules. Shortly thereafter Young (1967) and Young and Bok (1969) demonstrated the renewal and shedding of POS and confirmed the phagocytosis of shed tips by the RPE (Bosch et al., 1993). Auto-phagic contributions to RPE lipofuscin were evidenced by the presence of complex granules containing both lipofuscin and melanin (Feeney et al., 1965; Remé, 1977).

Subsequent observations have confirmed that most of the materials accumulating in RPE lipofuscin granules originate from the phagocytosis of the shed photoreceptor materials. The RPE of Royal College of Surgeons (RCS) rats, that are unable to phagocytose POS except at very low levels, do not accumulate the same amount of lipofuscin as seen in congenic age-matched control animals (Katz et al., 1986a). When photoreceptors are eliminated by photic damage, the RPE does not accumulate the same amount of lipofuscin as seen in dim-light-reared animals (Katz and Eldred, 1989). Boulton and Marshall (1986) demonstrated that cultured human RPE cells fed daily doses of isolated rod outer segments for 0.5 to 3 months developed intracellular granules whose characteristics are similar to lipofuscin. These results have been confirmed by others (Boulton et al., 1989; Rakoczy et al., 1992; Kennedy et al., 1994; Wrigstad et al., 1995).

Enzyme Cytochemistry

Essner and Novikoff (1960; 1961) were the first to definitively demonstrate that lipofuscin granules of the human liver and brain arise as residual bodies of the lysosomal system. Ishikawa and Yamada (1970) demonstrated by enzyme cytochemistry acid phosphatase activity in both the phagolysosomes and lipofuscin granules of human RPE. Feeney (1978) demonstrated both acid phosphatase and arylsulfatase activity in RPE lipofuscin granules and showed that lysosomes continue to add digestive enzymes to not only the nascent phagosomes, but also mature lipofuscin granules, melanin granules, and melanolipofuscin granules (Feeney-Burns, 1980; Feeney-Burns and Eldred, 1983).

RPE Lysosomal Enzymes

With continual lysosomal attack, why do materials accumulate? Is something lacking in the RPE lysosomal enzyme system that is required for the complete degradation of the phagocytosed outer segments?

There are more than sixty lysosomal enzymes known to cell biology (Dean and Barrett, 1976; Bohley and Seglen, 1992). Many of these enzymes have been identified in RPE lysosomes by both histochemical and enzymological techniques (Abraham et al., 1969; Berman, 1971; Hayasaka, 1974). Those identified include acid phosphatase (Lessell and Kuwabara, 1964; Shantha-veerappa and Bourne, 1964; Marshall, 1970; Feeney, 1973), acid lipase (Rothman et al., 1976; Hayasaka et al., 1977); phospholipase (Swartz and Mitchell, 1973; Berman, 1979; Zimmerman et al., 1983), arylsulfatases (Hara et al., 1979; Noji, 1980), glycosidases (Berman, 1971; Lentrichia et al., 1978; Hayasaka and Shiono, 1982), and proteases (Hayasaka et al., 1975b; Hayasaka and Hayasaka, 1978; Rakoczy et al., 1994).

The mix of lysosomal enzymes in the RPE seems to be ideally suited to the task of outer segment degradation. The acid hydrolases in the lysosomal fraction of RPE are seven times more active than those in liver lysosomal fractions in degrading isolated POS (Zimmerman et al., 1983).

Opsin, the main glycoprotein present in the photoreceptor outer segment, is degraded completely by cathepsin D and other RPE lysosomal enzymes (Hayasaka et al., 1975a; Regan et al., 1980; Kean et al., 1983). Cathepsins D and S appear to be the most important proteinases in the process of outer segment digestion by RPE cells (Rakoczy et al., 1994). When these enzymes and/or other cysteine proteases are inhibited, by genetic manipulation or administration of leupeptin, nondegraded residues accumulate within the RPE lysosomes (Ivy et al., 1990; Katz and Shanker, 1989; Rakoczy et al., 1994), but they do not appear to be similar to the products that accumulate within lipofuscin granules (Ikegami et al., 1995).

The POS lipids are degraded by phospholipases and acid lipases (Swartz and Mitchell, 1973; Hayasaka et al., 1977). As the engulfed membrane phospholipids are degraded, fatty acids, especially docosahexaenoic acid, leave the lysosomal compartment and are recycled from the phagosome for reuse in the construction of nascent photoreceptor outer segment disks (Gordon et al., 1992; Gordon and Bazan, 1993). Cytochemical studies showed active acid lipases even in the oldest samples (Feeney, 1978). No defect in normal lipid catabolism or turnover has been reported with increased age.

There is an uneven distribution of lysosomal enzymes across the back of the eye (Boulton et al., 1994), but the specific activities of acid phosphatase, cathepsin D, and arylsulfatase are actually highest in the macula, where lipofuscin granules accumulate to the greatest extent (Hayasaka et al., 1981; Burke and Twining, 1988). The total cellular activity of cathepsin D and n-acetyl-β-glucosaminidase in cultured RPE cells does not vary with the donor age (Wilcox, 1988). Therefore, the accumulation of lipofuscin granules does not seem to be correlated with the distribution or age-related changes of any known lysosomal enzyme.

Lipid, Protein, and Carbohydrate Analysis

Not every known lysosomal enzyme has been analyzed in the RPE with respect to presence, distribution, and age-related changes. The possibility remains that one or more not yet studied may be defective and responsible for lipofuscin accumulation. If this were the case, one might expect the accumulation of a predominant specific substrate in the lysosomal residual bodies. The RPE is particularly susceptible to genetically inherited lysosomal storage diseases (Aguirre and Stramm, 1991). In any genetic lysosomal storage disease, specific substrates accumulate.

Analysis of RPE lipofuscin contents reveals no such predominant substrate accumulation, however. Antigenic sites on opsin are cleaved rapidly upon digestion in the phagolysosome, and none remains in the lipofuscin granule (Feeney-Burns et al., 1988). This does not rule out the possibility that hydrophobic components remain undigested. Data of Bazan and colleagues (1990) suggest that peptides accumulate over time in the lipofuscin granule to a greater extent than do lipidic components (Fig. 33-3). SDS-PAGE of the peptides of lipofuscin granules reveal thirty or more discrete bands that remain in the granule at all ages tested (Feeney-Burns et

al., 1988). No single component predominates. Lipids of the lipofuscin granule are complex and differ in relative proportion to the lipids of the POS (Bazan et al., 1990). Again, no specific lipid species accumulates in preference to others.

Carbohydrate analyses have not been performed on the RPE lipofuscin granules. While Streeten (1961) showed negative periodic acid-Schiff (PAS) reactions for glycosylated compounds (not to be confused with positive fuchsin reactions for specific unsaturated phospholipids), all others demonstrate positive PAS reactivity. The source of the positivity is unknown. The antigenic glycopeptide components of opsin are known to be rapidly cleaved by lysosomal digestion both in vivo and in vitro, and none remains in the lipofuscin granules (Regan et al., 1980; Hara et al., 1983; Kean et al., 1983; Feeney-Burns et al., 1988).

In short, no specific substrate appears to accumulate in RPE lipofuscin, as would be expected for a defect in a specific lysosomal enzyme.

Autofluorescence and the Putative Role of Lipid Autoxidation

The only other feature of RPE lipofuscin granules that could not readily be accounted for was their autofluorescence (Fig. 33-1). The lipofuscin granules from the RPE emit a characteristic golden yellow fluorescence when stimulated by 366 nm light (Feeney, 1978). The chemical nature of the fluorophores involved and their role in the accumulation of lipofuscin granules have been the source of much speculation, and the source of a great deal of confusion in the field for many years.

As early as 1952, all tissue lipofuscin pigments were widely considered to arise as a result of the oxidation of unsaturated fatty acids (Gomori, 1952). Published in 1969 was a key paper that served as the cornerstone for the lipid oxidation theory of lipofuscin formation (Chio et al., 1969). In this study lipid peroxidation reactions were induced in suspensions of isolated subcellular organelles. Uncorrected fluorescence excitation and emission spectra of aqueous supernatants from these suspensions were then reported to be very similar to previously reported uncorrected fluorescence spectra of chloroform extracts of age pigments. It was suggested that the fluorescent materials accumulating in age pigments were likely to be products of membrane lipid peroxidation. That paper was followed by another influential paper that likened the fluorescent reaction products of malonaldehyde and several amino acids to the fluorophores reported by others in age pigment extracts (Chio and Tappel, 1969).

In 1980 it was shown that chloroform extracts of hu-

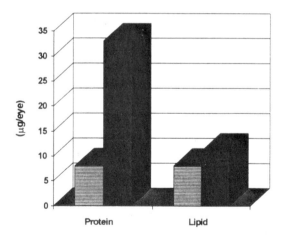

FIGURE 33-3. Human retinal pigment epithelium lipofuscin protein and lipid analyses. The peptide components of RPE lipofuscin accumulate over time to a greater extent than do the lipid components. Determinations were performed on RPE lipofuscin from individuals under 40 *(light bars)* or over 50 *(dark bars)* years of age. (Data from Bazan et al., 1990.)

man RPE lipofuscin granules also exhibited uncorrected fluorescence spectra that appeared similar to those reported for the in vitro lipid oxidation products (Feeney-Burns et al., 1980). In addition, dietary antioxidant deficiency studies had recently shown that deposits of pigment granules in the RPE fluoresced in situ with the same golden yellow emissions as those of RPE lipofuscin (Hayes, 1974; Katz et al., 1978; Robison et al., 1979). The high abundance of polyunsaturated fatty acids in the POS and the photic and oxygen-rich environments in which they function (Fliesler and Anderson, 1983; Handelman and Dratz, 1986), also strongly suggested that lipid oxidation was a very likely explanation for RPE lipofuscinogenesis. This lipid oxidation theory for RPE lipofuscin formation was formalized by Feeney-Burns and colleagues (1980), and has been widely held ever since.

However, no lipid oxidation product or aldehyde/amine reaction product had ever been isolated and identified from any source of lipofuscin. Furthermore, there was a discrepancy between the emission properties reported for the extracts and those reported for the in situ granules. While every description of autofluorescent emissions from the in situ granules reported a golden yellow fluorescence (corresponding to a wavelength centered around 575 nm), the instrumental determinations always reported peak emissions in the vicinity of 430–470 nm (corresponding to blue emitted light) (see Appendix, "Lipofuscin in UV Vision?"). This discrepancy was resolved when it was demonstrated that instruments used at that time were usually about one hundred times more sensitive to blue emissions than yellow or red emissions (Eldred et al., 1982; Stark et al., 1984). Correction of the instrumental bias demonstrated that the extracts of human RPE lipofuscin actually do emit yellow to orange light. Later, it was shown that oxidation of retinal homogenates using either iron ascorbate or oxygen caused the formation of only the blue-emitting fluorophores that are known to be lipid oxidation products (Eldred and Katz, 1989; 1991). Similar results were obtained when iron ascorbate was injected intravitreally in rat eyes (Katz et al., 1994).

The lipid oxidation theory of lipofuscinogenesis as widely held predicts that the contents of the granule will be a cross-linked, polymerized mixture of components of no definite structure (Eldred, 1987). However, when separated by thin-layer chromatography, distinct well-defined autofluorescent components are seen in RPE lipofuscin granules (Eldred and Katz, 1988a).

Similarly, the vitamin E deficiency pigments that accumulate in the RPE proved not to be extractable, and could therefore not be considered a good model for natural RPE lipofuscin granules (Eldred and Katz, 1988b).

Nor could vitamin E deficiency be considered a good model for other tissue lipofuscin deposits. The tissue distribution of age pigments is entirely different from that of the vitamin E deficiency pigments (Katz et al., 1984). In fact, many investigators now believe that those pigments arising either as a result of antioxidant deficiency or under prooxidant conditions should be considered ceroid pigments rather than lipofuscin pigments (Jolly et al., 1993).

In view of these findings, serious doubts exist as to the validity of the lipid oxidation mechanism of lipofuscinogenesis as originally proposed for the RPE (Eldred, 1987; 1991a). There still remains, however, the possibility that lipid oxidation plays a role in the promotion of lipofuscin formation in some yet to be determined way (Katz et al., 1994).

Autofluorescence and Vitamin A

The importance of adequate vitamin A nutrition to the functional and structural integrity of the retina had been known for quite some time (Dowling and Wald, 1958; 1960; Dowling and Gibbons, 1961; Carter-Dawson et al., 1979). But a role for vitamin A in RPE lipofuscin formation was not revealed until the studies by Robison and colleagues (1979; 1980) into the influence of vitamin A nutrition on the deposition of vitamin E deficiency pigments in the rat RPE. In these studies, the presence of adequate vitamin A in the diet dramatically increased the intensity of in situ fluorescence from both normal lipofuscin and vitamin E deficiency pigments.

It was also found that the photoreceptor outer segment debris that accumulates above the RPE in RCS rats evolves an in situ fluorescence similar to that of lipofuscin (Katz et al., 1986a). This fluorescence, too, was dramatically reduced in vitamin A deficiency (Katz et al., 1987). These results suggested again that the precursors for RPE lipofuscin are present in the POS but it could not be concluded whether these fluorophores were vitamin A compounds themselves, or whether vitamin A played some vital role in the metabolic formation of unrelated chemical compounds. The yellow fluorescence of RPE lipofuscin granules and RCS rat outer segment debris is very different from the rapidly fading green fluorescence of retinol and retinyl esters.

A technique was developed for the thin-layer chromatographic separation of the autofluorescent components of RPE lipofuscin (Eldred et al., 1982; Eldred and Katz, 1988a). It provided a fingerprint of lipofuscin fluorophore composition that has proven useful for comparing the compositions of experimentally induced and disease-related pigments, and for monitoring the course of development of specific fluorophoric components.

Among the prominent fluorophores of lipofuscin granules are green-emitting retinol and retinyl esters (Eldred, 1991; Eldred and Lasky, 1993). It appears that normal vitamin A derivatives may preferentially partition into the lipophilic environment of the lipofuscin granule. This could also account for much of the influence of dietary vitamin A on the fluorescence seen in hydrophobic residues that accumulate as the result of vitamin E deficiency pigments (Robison et al., 1979; 1980) and leupeptin-induced pigments (Katz and Norberg, 1992). A potentially interesting question is whether natural RPE lipofuscin granules serve as an exchangeable storage pool for retinol and retinyl esters, or as an irretrievable sink that could interfere with the normal turnover of vitamin A in the visual process.

The remainder of the fluorophores are strictly age related and range in emissions from yellow-green to orange. Although relative proportions of the fluorophores may vary slightly with age (Docchio et al., 1991), there is almost no qualitative variation in the fluorophoric composition between individuals or age groups. (However, in human RPE extracts, occasional autofluorescent drugs appear in extract chromatograms that had probably been bound to melanin.) The age-related bands are also present in aging rat RPE lipofuscin, and have been seen in every other aged species that we have had a chance to analyze (dog, hamster, guinea pig). The nature of the remaining fluorophores is only now being revealed, and evidence is beginning to point toward a more direct role for unusual vitamin A derivatives in the formation of lipofuscin and in the possible link between lipofuscin accumulation and the early stages of AMD.

After retinol and retinyl esters, the next most prominent fluorophores in the thin-layer chromatograms of lipofuscin are two orange-emitting fluorophores: one prominent low-migrating orange-emitting compound, and one of much lesser quantity that migrates higher on the chromatograms (Eldred and Katz, 1988a). These age-related fluorophores are virtually eliminated in rats raised on a vitamin A–deficient diet (Katz et al., 1986b).

Similar orange-emitting fluorophores are seen in the POS debris that accumulates above the RPE in RCS rats (Katz et al., 1986a), but in this case, the high-migrating fluorophore predominates over the low-migrating one. When RCS rats are raised on vitamin A–deficient diets, the orange-emitting fluorophore in the photoreceptor outer segment debris is greatly reduced (Katz et al., 1987). In age series studies, this outer segment debris orange-emitting fluorophore disappears as the debris zone is resorbed and as it disappears, the low-migrating orange-emitting fluorophore more prominent in RPE age pigments appears, suggesting that the outer segment flu-

orophore is converted into the age pigment fluorophore (Eldred, 1991b).

These experiments again suggested an involvement of vitamin A in the formation of the orange-emitting fluorophores, but they did not clarify whether vitamin A is a direct precursor or a controlling factor at one step in some other unidentified chemical or metabolic pathway.

The major orange-emitting fluorophores of both the RCS POS debris and the RPE age pigments have now been identified (Eldred and Lasky, 1993; Eldred, 1993b). Using fast atom bombardment tandem mass spectrometry, the dominant orange-emitting fluorophore of human RPE was identified as a quaternary nitrogen compound apparently derived from sequential Schiff base reactions between two molecules of retinaldehyde (A) and one molecule of ethanolamine (E): A2-E. Based on the deduced structure, the compound could be synthesized and shown to be identical to the lipofuscin-derived fluorophore. In that the likely source of the ethanolamine moiety of the molecule was the POS disk membrane phosphatidylethanolamine (PE), retinaldehyde was similarly reacted with PE, and the product proved to be very similar in fluorescence properties and chromatographic mobility to the orange-emitting compound in the RCS rat outer segment debris. By removing the phosphoglycerolipid component, A2-E would remain (Eldred and Lasky, 1993).

Questions were raised with regard to the structures originally proposed for this compound (Eldred, 1993a). Subsequent nuclear magnetic resonance work has identified it as a highly unusual *bis*-retinoid pyridinium salt, never before reported (Fig. 33-4) (Sakai et al., 1996). An acid-catalyzed reaction mechanism has been proposed that would be consistent with its formation within the acidic environment of the lysosome. Similar disruption of the membrane structure and acidic conditions in the decaying RCS outer segment debris would promote the formation of A2-PE there.

It should also be noted that other products yet to be identified arise in this reaction mixture, which appear to be related to some of the other fluorophores of RPE lipofuscin. These other RPE fluorophores never appear in the absence of A2-E, so it is likely that they are structurally related.

Theory of A2-E Formation in the RPE.

A chemical reaction mechanism has been proposed for the in vitro synthesis of A2-E (Eldred, 1995). Briefly, it involves a five-step mechanism where *trans*-retinaldehyde reacts with ethanolamine in an acid-catalyzed reaction to form a protonated Schiff base that undergoes

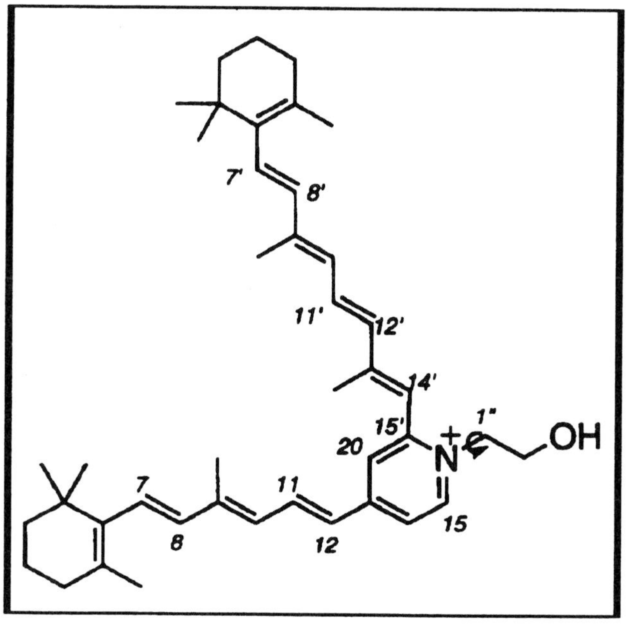

FIGURE 33-4. A2-E: A *bis*-retinoid pyridinium salt with amphiphilic properties.

a rearrangement to yield an enamine intermediate. This then reacts with a second molecule of *trans*-retinaldehyde to form an imminium base that subsequently cyclizes and aromatizes to yield the final pyridinium structure.

The formation of this compound in the retina under rare but physiological conditions has been proposed (Eldred, 1993b). There are several requirements for the reaction to proceed: (1) vitamin A must be present in the aldehyde form, (2) the aldehyde end must be able to physically approach the reactive amine group, (3) acidic conditions are required, and (4) excess water will reverse the initial Schiff base reaction and should, therefore, be absent (Layer, 1963; Dayagi and Degani, 1970).

The rare survival of *trans*-retinaldehyde is probably a key factor in the slow in vivo formation of A2-E and lipofuscin accumulation. Normally, when *trans*-retinaldehyde is released from the visual pigment upon photoisomerization, it is immediately converted to retinol through the action of *trans*-specific, POS retinol dehydrogenase (oxidoreductase). The proton is provided by NADPH (Zimmerman et al., 1975).

Transient elevated ambient light may play a role in A2-E formation. Normally, the retina has adaptive mechanisms to compensate for a variety of lighting conditions, including adjusting the length of the POS and adjusting the visual pigment densities in the outer segment disks (Penn and Anderson, 1991; Schremser and

Williams, 1995a; 1995b). These adaptive mechanisms require a relatively long period of time, however. On an acute basis, it has been shown that elevated ambient light levels can be expected to overwhelm the dehydrogenase pathway (Palczewski et al., 1994). There may also be lighting conditions in which NADPH supplies are inadequate. There is some evidence that short-term exposure to elevated light levels will accelerate lipofuscin granule deposition in quail RPE (Fite et al., 1993).

Surviving retinaldehyde can be expected to either remain buried within the hydrophobic domain of the disk membrane (Robert et al., 1983), or relink to opsin to form a nonfunctional visual pigment (Hofmann et al., 1992). Only when the membrane is disrupted (as in the RCS retinal debris, or in the RPE lysosome, or possibly in threshold light damage (Bush et al., 1991) can the aldehyde group approach the ethanolamine moiety of phosphatidylethanolamine or free ethanolamine. The acidic and hydrophobic conditions provided by the RPE lysosome would be well suited for the promotion of the A2-E synthetic reaction. Self-assembly of other aldehyde/amine Schiff base reaction products within the lysosomal compartment has been utilized pharmaceutically for the selective formation of certain toxic chemotherapeutic agents (Rideout et al., 1988).

Effects of A2-E on Lysosomal Function

A2-E is a permanently charged, amphiphilic cation that will remain within the lysosome, much as charged protonated ammonium compounds become trapped within lysosomes (deDuve et al., 1974; Seglen, 1983). These latter compounds are weak bases that, by virtue of their ability to titrate hydrogen ions, have been demonstrated to be capable of elevating lysosomal pH beyond the optimum required for full lysosomal enzyme activity (Ohkuma and Poole, 1978). As a result, substrates accumulate, and residual storage granules form. Chloroquine is an example of this type of compound, and it is known to cause lysosomal disruption both in the retina and RPE (Ramsey and Fine, 1972; Rosenthal et al., 1978; Raines et al., 1989). Other cationic drugs are known to have similar effects on the RPE (Lüllmann-Rauch, 1981).

Unlike these lysosomotrophic amines, however, A2-E is a quaternary nitrogen compound with a fixed positive charge and no exchangeable hydrogen. If hydroxyl ion were its counterion, it could be expected to exhibit even stronger base properties. But hydroxyl ion does not exist under physiological conditions. The likely counterion is more likely the chloride ion that is known to be cotransported with protons by the actions of the lysosomal membrane proton pumps (Mulberg et al., 1991; Van Dyke and Rost, 1993; Tapper and Sundler, 1995). Thus, in the RPE lipofuscin granule, A2-E would be a neutral salt.

Nonetheless, quaternary nitrogen compounds are also known to inhibit lysosomal function, but by mechanisms that have yet to be determined (Matsumoto et al., 1989). Cationic amphiphiles are known to bind strongly to anionic compounds to form complexes (Okuzaki and Osada, 1995; Mel'nikov et al., 1995). Certain cationic compounds have been proposed to bind sulfated glycosaminoglycans in the RPE lysosomal compartment and cause the inhibition of their degradation (Lüllmann-Rauch, 1994). Special fixation procedures are required to demonstrate these effects, and such procedures have not yet been applied to RPE lipofuscin granules.

A2-E has been tested for its ability to inhibit lysosomal proteolysis (Eldred, 1995). A2-E has a low water solubility, and its delivery directly to the lysosomal compartment requires a carrier. By loading A2-E onto low-density lipoproteins, it was possible to utilize receptor-mediated endocytic transport to deliver A2-E to human fibroblast lysosomes. It was demonstrated that lysosomal degradation of endogenous proteins is inhibited at least 60% by A2-E. Extralysosomal proteolysis remained unaffected. The presence of A2-E in RPE lysosomes can be expected to have a similar effect and could help account for the enhanced accumulation of peptides over lipids in RPE lipofuscin (Fig. 33-3). The effect of A2-E on the degradation of other classes of compounds is not currently known.

Possible Eventual Leakage of A2-E from Lysosomes

The amphiphilic structure of A2-E classifies it as a detergent. Other compounds called *lysosomotrophic detergents* display very characteristic patterns of effect within lysosomes. They exhibit sigmoidal dose–response curves (Firestone et al., 1979; Pisano and Firestone, 1981; Miller et al., 1983). The compounds accumulate with little effect until a critical concentration is reached related to the compound's critical micelle concentration. At this stage, the detergents begin to interact with the lysosomal membrane, causing leakage and eventual cell death. It is interesting to note that the accumulation of RPE lipofuscin exhibits a sigmoidal time course (Fig. 33-5). It is possible that A2-E may also accumulate benignly until it reaches a critical concentration, at which point it might start to leak from the lysosomal compartment. This means that the number of lipofuscin granules may be less important than the actual concentration of A2-E within each granule.

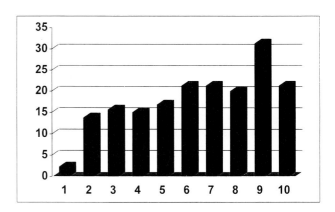

FIGURE 33-5. Plot of number macular lipofuscin granules in the human RPE vs. decade of life. Accumulation of macular lipofuscin granules in human RPE follows a sigmoidal pattern. During the first decade of life, very little accumulates, then there is a rapid accumulation during the second decade, followed by a much slower accumulation thereafter. It is during the slow accumulation that A2-E may begin to gradually leak from the lipofuscin granule and trigger basal deposit formation. (Data plotted from Feeney-Burns et al., 1984.)

Another mechanism that might cause A2-E leakage from the lysosome involves a photodynamic effect. The lysosomally targeted drugs used in photodynamic therapy of tumor tissues are known to have two effects that may be significant to the RPE story. First, illumination of these compounds generates free radicals that have a rapid inhibitory effect on lysosomal enzymes (Berg and Moan, 1994). Second, upon illumination, these compounds leak from the lysosome and redistribute throughout the cell (Berg et al., 1993). Wrigstad and colleagues (1995) have demonstrated that illumination of cultured RPE cells loaded with autofluorescent pigments causes leakage and redistribution of granule markers. Others (Boulton et al., 1993; Rózanowska et al., 1995; Gaillard et al., 1995) have established that illumination of human lipofuscin granules and/or their extracts can induce free-radical formation. A2-E and other reaction products may be responsible for these reactions. Light of the proper wavelength does reach the RPE (van Norren and Vos, 1974), so these reactions are possible in vivo.

If A2-E did leak from the granules by either detergent or photodynamic mechanisms, then some extralysosomal effects that could prove to be very important to the mechanism of AMD may be initiated.

A2-E in AMD: A Potential Link between Lipofuscin and Basal Deposit Formation

Slowly progressing age-related changes in the RPE and Bruch's membrane are believed to lead to AMD. One of the earliest changes seen in the retina is the accumulation of lipofuscin granules within the RPE cells (Feeney-Burns et al., 1984). Later, a variety of ultrastructural and histochemical changes are detectable underneath the RPE cells, especially in the macular region. Materials start to accumulate between the basal plasma membrane of the RPE and its basement membrane (basal laminar deposits), and within the inner collagenous zone of Bruch's membrane (basal linear deposits) (Sarks, 1976; Green and Key, 1977; Sarks et al., 1980; Green et al., 1985; Loeffler and Lee, 1986; Bressler et al., 1992). Eventually, the deposits become sites for localized areas of detachment, seen clinically as soft drusen, which are positively correlated with the occurrence of choroidal neovascularization, disciform scarring, and visual loss (Green and Enger, 1993).

The debris-like materials that make up the basal laminar and basal linear deposits appear to comprise both extracellular matrix materials (collagen, laminin, fibronectin) and organelle-like vesiculoid elements and membrane-bound structures (Loeffler and Lee, 1986; Green and Enger, 1993; Kliffen et al., 1994). Most of these membranous materials are thought to arise when the overlying RPE cells evaginate their basal membranes and pinch off portions of their cytoplasm (Burns and Feeney-Burns, 1980; Feeney-Burns and Ellersieck, 1985; Ishibashi et al., 1986; Killingsworth, 1987). The stimulus for this cellular shedding has long been thought to be an excessive burden of lipofuscin granules within the RPE (Hogan, 1972; Dorey et al., 1993). But the biochemical connection between lipofuscin granule accumulation and this shedding activity has remained obscure.

There is evidence now that if A2-E leaked from the lipofuscin granule, then it could be responsible for this shedding activity (Eldred, 1993b; Eldred, 1995). Similar amphiphilic compounds are known to be capable of selective insertion into one or the other of the hemileaflets of cellular plasma membrane bilayers (Sheetz and Singer, 1974). When they do, they induce a change in the curvature of the membrane and, thereby, a change in the shape of the cell. Depending upon several factors, such as the charge and shape of the inserting compound, either an evagination or an invagination of the membrane may result. Ultimately, small, membranous vesicles may break away either externally or internally (Hagerstrand and Isomaa, 1992).

A2-E has been tested for its ability to induce shape changes and vesiculation in the best-characterized membrane system used to demonstrate this phenomenon, the red cell model (Eldred, 1995). A2-E was seen to insert into the plasma membrane of red blood cells (RBCs). As a consequence, the cells initially undergo a concentra-

tion-dependent, stomatocytic (cup-shaped) transformation. Eventually, portions of the membrane internalize as small vesicles.

A2-E can be classified as an inverted conical molecule; the cross-section of its shape is larger at the hydrophobic end than at the hydrophilic end (Israelachvili et al., 1980). That A2-E does assume this shape has been tested by molecular modeling. When bond relaxation rules are applied and energies are minimized, the molecule takes on such an inverted conical configuration.

Typically, when cylindrical or normal conical molecules are preferentially inserted into the outer hemileaflet of the RBC membranes, there is an expansion of that leaflet while the inner leaflet remains unchanged. As a consequence, the membrane bends outward and, in red cell model membranes, spiculated echinocytes form. Similarly, if such molecules are introduced preferentially into the inner leaflet, a reversed bending occurs and stomatocytes form. The theoretical basis for this phenomenon was first posited by Sheetz and Singer (1974) as the bilayer couple hypothesis (Fig. 33-6). Its predictive value for the effects of membrane insertion by many cylindrical or conical molecules has been tested extensively and proven repeatedly through the intervening years (Isomaa and Paatero, 1981; Fujii et al., 1979; Ferrell et al., 1988; Palek and Jarolim, 1993).

In contrast, when an inverted conical molecule is inserted into one side of a membrane bilayer, there is an expansion of the hydrophobic domain of that single hemileaflet in relation to the hydrophilic domain, and the single-layer bending forces dominate over the bilay-

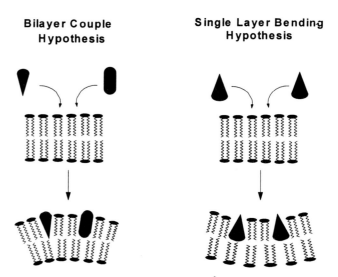

FIGURE 33-6. Membrane bending by insertion of amphiphilic compounds. Two mechanisms have been proposed that depend on the geometry and charge of the inserting amphiphile (see text).

er couple bending forces. This results in bending in the opposite direction of that predicted by the bilayer couple hypothesis (Fig. 33-6). This has been demonstrated in RBCs experimentally (Kuypers et al., 1984) and mathematically (Fischer, 1993). Thus, when the inverted cone of A2-E inserts into the external leaflet of the red cell plasma membrane, the shape change predicted by the single-layer bending effect (i.e., stomatocytosis) is seen experimentally.

Eventually, portions of the membrane are seen to break off to form small vesicles. Typically these vesicles differ in their composition from the normal plasma membrane in that they lack their cytoskeletal elements (Snyder et al., 1978; Weitz et al., 1982; Maher and Singer, 1983). The final vesiculation process requires membrane fusion and is probably facilitated by lateral redistribution of the lipids (Takahashi et al., 1983; Müller et al., 1981; Sackmann et al., 1986) and/or aggregation of proteins (Wilbers et al., 1979). This vesiculation occurs without hemolysis in the case of the red cell (Frenkel et al., 1986) and is seen in many cell types (Kobayashi et al., 1986).

A2-E has now been demonstrated to be capable of causing such membrane vesiculation. In the red cell experiments, A2-E was applied to the outside hemileaflet and induced primarily endovesicle formation. In the case of the RPE, the source of A2-E in vivo would be the intracellular lipofuscin granule. Therefore, insertion of A2-E into the inner, cytoplasmic hemileaflet of the basal plasma membrane will be expected to cause an evagination and eventual shedding like that reported during drusen formation (Burns and Feeney-Burns, 1980; Ishibashi et al., 1986). Additionally, disturbing the basal attachments of the RPE cell could stimulate the cells to overproduce the extracellular matrix materials that are seen in the basal deposits as well.

If this mechanism is at play in the RPE, then many questions remain to be addressed. First, one would expect any A2-E that leaked from the lipofuscin granule to distribute throughout the membrane system of the RPE cell. If this is true, then why is the effect seen only basally? The answer likely resides with the fact that other factors also come into play in the determination of cell shape. Unlike the case of the RBC, the RPE cell is a highly polarized epithelial cell. The apical surface of the RPE cell has different integral membrane components and more cytoskeletal involvement than does the basolateral membrane (Okami et al., 1990; Rizzolo and Heiges, 1991; Sugasawa et al., 1994; Burnside and Laties, 1979). Both cytoskeletal attachments and integral membrane proteins can profoundly influence membrane rigidity and mechanical stability (Mohandas and Chasis, 1993). These elements may reduce the deformability and, hence, the effect of A2-E membrane in-

sertion at the apical membrane of the RPE cell. Also, the turnover rate of the apical membrane is likely to be much higher because of the phagocytic activity of the cell, and A2-E is probably removed at a rapid rate by this mechanism. This could help explain why exovesicle formation is favored in the basal area of the RPE plasma membrane.

If A2-E is inserting into the basal membrane and is the main driving force for shedding, why are significant amounts of A2-E not detectable by fluorescence in drusen deposits? There are several possible explanations for this as well. First, very few molecules of inserting compound are required to induce dramatic shape changes in membranes. It has been estimated that less than 1.5% of the total composition of the membrane need be represented by the inserting molecule to induce the shape change (Ferrell et al., 1988; Lange and Slayton, 1982; Ferrell et al., 1985). Thus, unlike the case for lipofuscin granule fluorescence where A2-E accumulates and is concentrated, very little A2-E may enter the drusen deposits, and that which is present would likely be widely dispersed. Second, as the drusen deposits "mature" the membranous components are seen to fragment and disappear by mechanisms that have yet to be identified. It is not inconceivable that A2-E might be carried away by serum retinol binding proteins. In structure-binding specificity studies with serum RBPs, it has been firmly established that modifications in the cyclohexene ring can readily inhibit retinoid binding, but addition of side groups to the terminal carbon (as is the case with A2-E) barely affect binding by RBP (Berni et al., 1993; Zanotti et al., 1994). It is known that RBPs coupled with transthyretin diffuse readily from the choriocapillaris capillaries through Bruch's membrane to the basal membrane of the RPE cell to deliver retinol (Bok and Heller, 1976). Thus, any A2-E deposited in Bruch's membrane could conceivably be removed by this carrier as well.

Prior to the pathologic changes clinically identified with AMD (especially neovascularization), the number of RPE cells overlying drusen declines (Dorey et al., 1989; Feeney-Burns et al., 1990). The mode of elimination of these cells is not yet clear. A2-E in the lipofuscin granules might contribute to RPE cell death in two ways. First, a rupture of the lysosomal membrane would lead to death by autolytic necrosis. Necrotic cell death, however, might be expected to be proliferative and inflammatory and extend to surrounding cells. While this type of process can be seen in advanced stages of AMD, this is not what is typically seen chronically in the RPE overlying drusen. Here single cells apparently selectively die out. This form of selective cell death is referred to as *apoptosis*. It proceeds by an entirely different mechanism from cellular necrosis (Buja et al., 1993), and the morphological manifestations are often difficult to detect because so few cells are undergoing the process at any given time. The trigger for this type of cell death has yet to be determined. Epithelial and endothelial cells denied anchorage can undergo apoptosis (Frisch and Francis, 1994). The controlling factor has been implied to be an integrin-mediated signal (Meredith et al., 1993; Rouslahti and Reed, 1994). The integrins comprise a diverse family of cell adhesion proteins that mediate cell–cell and cell–basement membrane interactions (Albeda and Buck, 1990). The reason for the diversity is in their different signaling functions (Hynes, 1992). One characteristic of mature RPE is the basal distribution of integrin (Philp and Nachmias, 1987; Rizzolo et al., 1994). If the loss of basal plasma membrane through the shedding phenomenon that is seen during drusen formation causes a loss of integrin or a disruption in its association with its basement membrane components, then this could be a triggering mechanism for apoptotic loss of the involved RPE cell. Such an RPE cell loss is seen over drusen in AMD (Delori et al., 1994).

These findings lend additional credence to the notion that RPE lipofuscin accumulation is directly related to soft drusen formation and AMD. It is hypothesized that A2-E is formed slowly in a reaction between retinaldehyde and membrane-phospholipid-derived ethanolamine in the acidic environment of the lysosome, as has been previously described (Eldred 1993b; Eldred and Lasky, 1993; Eldred 1995). This compound is not likely to be benign. It has been demonstrated to inhibit lysosomal proteolysis, thereby probably playing a key role in the initial formation of lipofuscin within the RPE. Through either photochemical or detergent effects, it can also be expected to eventually leak from the lipofuscin granule. If any of the A2-E escapes and reaches the basal plasma membrane, it can be expected to insert into the cytoplasmic hemileaflet. By a single-layer bending effect, it can cause an evagination and eventual shedding of membrane vesicles. Basal laminar and linear deposits will start to form. Disruption of basement membrane attachments may trigger an overproduction of extracellular matrix material by the RPE and/or an integrin-mediated induction of apoptotic cell death. The stage is then set for the subsequent progressive clinical changes seen in AMD.

DISEASE-RELATED PIGMENTS WITH LIPOFUSCIN-LIKE APPEARANCE

As more is understood about the biochemical mechanisms of normal RPE lipofuscin accumulation and its implications for AMD, it becomes more pressing to identify those genetically inherited diseases that may involve similar biochemical mechanisms. Accelerated accumulation of autofluorescent granules has been reported in Batten's disease, Best's vitelliform dystrophy, and Stargardt's disease (fundus flavimaculatus). In one case, it is now known that the autofluorescent pigment granules are nothing like lipofuscin pigments; in another, evidence exists that would indicate a greater similarity to lipofuscin; while in the others, there is simply not enough evidence to yet draw any conclusions as to the nature of the deposits.

Batten's Disease (Neuronal Ceroid Lipofuscinosis; NCL)

The various forms of Batten's disease are characterized by the intralysosomal accumulation of residues in a variety of tissues including nerves of the brain and eye (Traboulsi et al., 1987).

The Batten's disease granules exhibit yellow emissions in situ when observed by fluorescence microscopy at 366 nm illumination. The nature of the fluorophores in this disease has not yet been determined, but it is now clear that the source of the fluorescence is much different from that of normal RPE lipofuscin. It has been argued that optical interference phenomena may be responsible for an illusory fluorescent emission that does not exist upon further examination (Palmer et al., 1993). However, in the canine form, genuine autofluorescent molecules are present, but only a very small proportion is extractable (Katz et al., 1988). Therefore, the fluorophoric component of these granules behaves more akin to vitamin E deficiency pigments (i.e., ceroid) than lipofuscin pigments. However, much is now known of the nature of Batten's pigments, and it has been concluded that all foregoing terminology is misleading, in that the pigments are neither ceroid- nor lipofuscin-like.

A tremendous breakthrough in our understanding of this disease came with the discovery of a specific predominant storage product in the lysosomes: subunit c of mitochondrial ATP synthase (Palmer et al., 1986; 1989). A variety of animal models for Batten's disease have now been shown to accumulate this peptide (Jolly and Palmer, 1995). Other components that have been demonstrated to accumulate to a lesser extent are the peptides that activate the lysosomal hydrolases required for sphingolipid degradation (SAPs: sphingolipid activator proteins) (Tyynelä et al., 1993; 1995).

The cause for this accumulation has not yet been determined. It could indicate a defect in the intracellular processing of hydrophobic proteins. Katz has suggested that an unspecified lysosomal enzyme responsible for its degradation is methylated at a lysine residue, rendering it ineffective (Katz, 1993). However, others have found that the lysine methylation reported is variable and also occurs in nondiseased tissues (Palmer et al., 1993). Still others argue that a defect in a lysosomal protease is not likely to account for subunit c accumulation (Ezaki et al., 1993).

Progress is being made in the genetic analysis of these diseases. At least four gene loci are known to be associated with different forms of human NCL. The gene involved in the juvenile form has been mapped to chromosome 16 (Mitchison et al., 1993), and a microdeletion has been identified (Taschner et al., 1995). The peptide coded by the gene remains to be determined.

In sum, these pigments arise largely as a very specific lysosomal storage product in a genetically inherited disease, and are quite unique from either ceroid or lipofuscin granules. It has been suggested that they would more appropriately be referred to as *proteolipid proteinosis pigments* (Jolly and Dalefield, 1990; Jolly et al., 1993).

Best's Vitelliform Macular Dystrophy

Histopathologic studies of eyes with Best's vitelliform macular dystrophy have demonstrated large accumulations of lipofuscin and melanolipofuscin in the RPE (Weingeist et al., 1982; Frangieh et al., 1982; O'Gorman et al., 1988). Identity as lipofuscin is based on location within the RPE, in situ autofluorescence, positivity for Sudan Black and periodic acid-Schiff stains, and ultrastructural morphology. The RPE lipofuscin, however, should be distinguished from the large deposits of extracellular material seen clinically as vitelliform or "egg yolk" lesions and the yellow material that pools in pseudohypopyon in certain stages of this disease (Mohler and Fine, 1981). As with AMD, the large macular accumulations of autofluorescent pigments in the RPE are thought to stimulate the deposition of large mounds of extracellular matrix material in the sub-RPE space. As with AMD, these deposits do not contain lipofuscin or melanolipofuscin.

In that the pigments that are stimulated by vitamin E deficiency appear identical to lipofuscin pigments in the RPE, it will be important to test the extractability and fluorophoric compositions of the RPE pigments in Best's disease to clarify this question. The results could have important implications for the pathogenetic mechanisms of the disease (i.e., lipid autoxidation vs. A2-E formation).

If the RPE pigments in Best's disease are true lipofuscin granules, one would expect elevated levels of A2-E at the early stages. Clinical instruments (see Chapter 11) are being developed that could allow longitudinal monitoring of the buildup of A2-E in the living patient (Delori et al., 1995a; von Rückmann et al., 1995). Candidate genes could include those potentially involved in

the initial formation of A2-E such as that for *trans*-specific retinol dehydrogenase, or ones involved in the supply of NADPH. Progress is being made along these lines, in that the gene for Best's disease has now been linked to chromosome 11q13 (Stone et al., 1992).

Stargardt's Macular Dystrophy (Fundus Flavimaculatus; Juvenile Macular Degeneration)

As with Best's vitelliform dystrophy, massive accumulations of pigment granules accumulate within the macular RPE in Stargardt's disease. Similarity to lipofuscin is based on fluorescence and staining properties. However, these pigment granules may differ slightly from normal age-related pigments in their ultrastructural morphology, being slightly more heterogeneous and less electron dense (Eagle et al., 1980). Unlike in Best's disease and AMD, however, the pigment accumulation does not seem to lead to large sub-RPE deposits of extracellular matrix or other material.

Again, it would be advantageous to be able to compare extractability and fluorophoric composition with normal age pigments and vitamin E deficiency pigments to gain a better understanding of the nature of the pigments present. One study has now been able to demonstrate that the granules that accumulate do exhibit A2-E fluorescence in vivo (Staurenghi et al., 1993; Delori et al., 1995b).

The gene in this disease has been mapped to chromosome 1p13 (Kaplan et al., 1994). Thus far, geneticists have ruled out the involvement of certain retinoid binding proteins (Yuan et al., 1994) and the cone-specific α-subunit of transducin (Rozet et al., 1995). No studies have investigated the potential candidate genes that would lead to early and accelerated A2-E formation.

CONCLUSION

The chemistry of lipofuscin formation is only now becoming clear. A highly unusual and potentially toxic retinoid has now been discovered that may play a key role in certain of the macular degenerative processes. This retinoid can now be synthesized and used to develop good models of RPE lipofuscin accumulation, and perhaps models for the onset of the changes seen in AMD. At the same time, powerful new clinical instruments are becoming available that allow the monitoring of lipofuscin and specific fluorophoric components in the RPE of patients with both age-related and disease-related accumulations of these compounds (Delori et al., 1995a; von Rückmann et al., 1995). With these new insights and developments, for the first time, hope for a new understanding into possible preventions and/or cures for some of the age-related degenerative processes in the human retina may be on the horizon.

APPENDIX: LIPOFUSCIN IN UV VISION?

The discrepancy between what had been reported in the literature for emissions from extracts and the emissions from in situ granules first came to my attention as a question relating to ultraviolet vision in humans.

Dr. Feeney-Burns had recently moved to the University of Missouri-Columbia, Department of Ophthalmology, and was presenting a seminar at the Department of Biology showing her microscopic and spectral work on human RPE lipofuscin. At the end of her talk, Dr. William S. Stark rose and asked about the discrepancy between the blue peak in the emission spectra of lipofuscin extracts as opposed to the vivid golden yellow emissions displayed by the in situ granules as seen by fluorescence microscopy.

Dr. Stark's interest in this problem was personal. As a child, he had been building a "soap box" car and a nail had flown up into his eye resulting in the loss of his lens. This was before intraocular lenses were widely used, therefore he grew up experiencing the ability to see near ultraviolet light in his aphakic eye. Curiosity drove him to study UV vision in *Drosophila*.

His question to Dr. Feeney-Burns was, "When I see ultraviolet light, I perceive an unsaturated blue color. Is this a primary photoreceptor response, or am I seeing the re-emission of light from lipofuscin granules in the RPE? If they really emit light at 340 nm, then this may be what I see. If they emit yellow light, then the fluorescence of lipofuscin granules cannot account for my UV light perception."

They suggested that I study the reason for this discrepancy, and our collaborations resulted in the discovery that color bias of the spectrophotometric equipment was responsible. Drs. Stark and Tan (1982) went on to demonstrate that UV perception in aphakic humans is, in fact, a primary photoreceptor response.

REFERENCES

Abraham R, Hume M, Smith J. 1969. A histochemical study of lysosomal enzymes in the retina of the rat. Histochemie 18:195–201.

Aguirre GC, Stramm LE. 1991. The RPE: a model system for disease expression and disease correction: the use of inherited mutations of the lysosomal system to probe RPE-matrix interactions. Prog Retinal Res 11:153–191.

Albeda SM, Buck CA. 1990. Integrins and other cell adhesion molecules. FASEB J 4:2868–2880.

Bazan HEP, Bazan NG, Feeney-Burns L, Berman ER. 1990. Lipids in human lipofuscin-enriched subcellular fractions of two age populations: comparison with rod outer segments and neural retina. Invest Ophthalmol Vis Sci 31:1433–1443.

Berg K, Moan J. 1994. Lysosomes as photochemical targets. Int J Cancer 59:814–822.

Berg K, Prydz K, Moan J. 1993. Photochemical treatment with the lysosomally localized dye tetra(4-sulfonatophenyl)porphine results in lysosomal release of the dye but not of β-N-acetyl-D-glucosaminidase activity. Biochim Biophys Acta 1158:300–306.

Berman ER. 1971. Acid hydrolases of the retinal pigment epithelium. Invest Ophthalmol Vis Sci 10:64–68.

Berman ER. 1979. Biochemistry of the retinal pigment epithelium. In: Zinn KM, Marmor MF, eds., The Retinal Pigment Epithelium. Cambridge (MA): Harvard University Press, 83–102.

Berni R, Zanotti G, Sartori G, Monaco HL. 1993. Plasma retinol-binding protein and its interaction with transthyretin. In: Livrea MA, Packer L, eds., Progress in Research and Clinical Applications. Marcel Dekker, New York, 91–102.

Bohley P, Seglen PO. 1992. Proteases and proteolysis in the lysosome. Experientia 48:151–157.

Bok D, Heller J. 1976. Transport of retinol from the blood to the retina: an autoradiographic study of the pigment epithelial cell surface receptor for plasma retinol-binding protein. Exp Eye Res 22:395–402.

Bosch E, Horwitz J, Bok D. 1993. Phagocytosis of outer segments by retinal pigment epithelium: phagosome-lysosome interaction. J Histochem Cytochem 41:253–263.

Boulton M, Marshall J. 1986. Effects of increasing phagocytic inclusions on human retinal pigment epithelial cells in culture: a model for ageing. Br J Ophthalmol 70:801–815.

Boulton M, McKechnie NM, Breda J, Bayly M, Marshall J. 1989. The formation of autofluorescent granules in cultured human RPE. Invest Ophthalmol Vis Sci 30:82–89.

Boulton M, Dontsov A, Jarvis-Evans, J, Ostrovsky M, Svistunenko D. 1993. Lipofuscin is a photoinducible free radical generator. J Photochem Photobiol B Biol 19:201-204.

Boulton M, Moriarity P, Jarvis-Evans J, Marcyniuk B. 1994. Regional variation and age-related changes of lysosomal enzymes in the human retinal pigment epithelium. Br J Ophthalmol 78:125–129.

Bressler SB, Silva JC, Bressler NM, Alexander J, Green WR. 1992. Clinicopathologic correlation of occult choroidal neovascularization in age-related macular degeneration. Arch Ophthalmol 110:827–832.

Brizzee KR, Ordy JM. 1981. Cellular features, regional accumulation, and prospects of modification of age pigments in mammals. In: Sohal RS, ed, Age Pigments. Amsterdam: Elsevier/North Holland Biomedical Press, 101–154.

Buja LM, Eigenbrodt ML, Eigenbrodt EH. 1993. Apoptosis and necrosis: basic types and mechanisms of cell death. Arch Pathol Lab Med 117:1208–1214.

Burke JM, Twining SS. 1988. Regional comparisons of cathepsin D activity in bovine retinal pigment epithelium. Invest Ophthalmol Visual Sci 29:1789–1793.

Burns RP, Feeney-Burns L. 1980. Clinico-morphologic correlations of drusen of Bruch's membrane. Trans Am Ophthalmol Soc 78:206–225.

Burnside B, Laties AM. 1979. Pigment movement and cellular contractility in the retinal pigment epithelium. In: Zinn K, Marmor MF, eds., The Retinal Pigment Epithelium. Cambridge, MA: Harvard University Press, 175–191.

Bush A, Remé CE, Malnöe A. 1991. Light damage in the rat retina: the effect of dietary deprivation of n-3 fatty acids on acute structural alterations. Exp Eye Res 53:741–752.

Carter-Dawson L, Kuwabara T, O'Brien PJ, Bieri JG. 1979. Structural and biochemical changes in vitamin A deficient rat retinas. Invest Ophthalmol Vis Sci 18:437–446.

Chio KS, Tappel AL. 1969. Synthesis and characterization of fluorescent products derived from malonaldehyde and amino acids. Biochemistry 8:2821–2827.

Chio KS, Reiss U, Fletcher B, Tappel AL. 1969. Peroxidation of subcellular organelles: formation of lipofuscinlike fluorescent pigments. Science 166:1535–1536.

Dayagi S, Dengani Y. 1970. Methods of formation of the carbon-nitrogen double bond. In: Patai S, ed., Chemistry of the Carbon-Nitrogen Double Bond. New York: Interscience, 61–147.

Dean RT, Barrett AJ. 1976. Lysosomes. Essays Biochem 12:1–40.

deDuve C, deBarsy T, Poole B, Trouet A, Tulkens P, Van Hoof F. 1974. Lysosomotropic agents. Biochem Pharmacol 23:2495–2531.

Delori FC, Arend O, Staurenghi G, Goger D, Dorey CK, Weiter JJ. 1994. Lipofuscin and drusen fluorescence in aging and age-related macular degeneration. Invest Ophthalmol Vis Sci 35(4):2145.

Delori FC, Dorey CK, Staurenghi G, Arend O, Goger DG, Weiter JJ. 1995a. In vivo fluorescence of the ocular fundus exhibits retinal pigment epithelium lipofuscin characteristics. Invest Ophthalmol Vis Sci 36:718–729.

Delori FC, Staurenghi G, Arend O, Dorey CK, Goger DG, Weiter JJ. 1995b. In vivo measurement of lipofuscin in Stargardt's disease—fundus flavimaculatus. Invest Ophthalmol Vis Sci 36:2327–2331.

Docchio F, Boulton M, Cubeddu R, Ramponi R, Barker PD. 1991. Age-related changes in the fluorescence of melanin and lipofuscin granules of the retinal pigment epithelium: a time-resolved fluorescence spectroscopy study. Photochem Photobiol 54:247–253.

Dorey CK, Wu G, Ebenstein D, Garsd A, Weiter JJ. 1989. Cell loss in the aging retina: relationship to lipofuscin accumulation and macular degeneration. Invest Ophthalmol Vis Sci 30:1691–1699.

Dorey CK, Staurenghi G, Delori FC. 1993. Lipofuscin in aged and AMD eyes. In: Hollyfield JG, LaVail MM, Anderson RE, eds., Retinal Degeneration: Clinical and Laboratory Applications. New York: Plenum, 3–14.

Dowling JE, Gibbons IR. 1961. The effect of vitamin A deficiency on the fine structure of the retina. In: Smelser GK, ed, The Structure of the Eye. New York: Academic Press, 85–99.

Dowling JE, Wald G. 1958. Vitamin A deficiency and night blindness. Proc Nat Acad Sci USA 44:648–661.

Dowling JE, Wald G. 1960. The biological function of vitamin A acid. Proc Nat Acad Sci USA 46:587–608.

Eagle RC, Lucier AC, Bernadino VB, Janoff M. 1980. Retinal pigment epithelial abnormalities in fundus flavimaculatus: a light and electron microscopic study. Ophthalmology 87:1189–1200.

Eldred GE. 1987. Questioning the nature of the fluorophores in age pigments. In: Totaro EA, Glees P, Pisanti FA, eds., Advances in Age Pigments Research. Oxford: Pergamon Press, 23–36.

Eldred GE. 1991a. Questioning the nature of age pigment (lipofuscin) in the human retinal pigment epithelium and its relationship to age-related macular degeneration. In: Armstrong D, Marmor MF, Ordy J, Harman D, Benedetto MD, eds., Environmental Design for Optimal Vision in the Elderly, New York: Plenum Press, 133–142.

Eldred GE. 1991b. The fluorophores of the RCS rat retina and implications for retinal degeneration. In: Anderson RE, Hollyfield JG, LaVail MM, eds., Retinal Degenerations. Boca Raton, FL: CRC Press, 173–181.

Eldred GE. 1993a. Age pigment structure. Nature 364:396.

Eldred GE. 1993b. Retinoid reaction products in age related retinal degeneration. In: Hollyfield JG, LaVail MM, Anderson RE, eds., Retinal Degeneration: Clinical and Laboratory Applications. New York: Plenum, 15–24.

Eldred GE. 1995. Lipofuscin fluorophore inhibits lysosomal protein degradation and may cause early stages of macular degeneration. Gerontology 41(suppl. 2):15–28.

Eldred GE, Katz ML. 1988a. Fluorophores of the human retinal pigment epithelium: separation and spectral characterization. Exp Eye Res 47:71–86.

Eldred GE, Katz ML. 1988b. Vitamin E-deficiency pigment and lipofuscin (age) pigment from the retinal pigment epithelium differ in fluorophoric composition. Invest Ophthalmol Vis Sci 29(suppl):92.

Eldred GE, Katz ML. 1989. The autofluorescent products of lipid peroxidation may not be lipofuscin-like. Free Radical Biol Med 7:157–163.

Eldred GE, Katz ML. 1991. The lipid peroxidation theory of lipofuscinogenesis cannot yet be confirmed. Free Radical Biol Med 10:445–447.

Eldred GE, Lasky MR. 1993. Retinal age pigments generated by self-assembling lysosomotropic detergents. Nature 361:724–726.

Eldred GE, Miller GV, Stark WS, Feeney-Burns L. 1982. Lipofuscin: resolution of discrepant fluorescence data. Science 216:757–759.

Elleder M. 1981. Chemical characterization of age pigments. In: Sohal RS, ed., Age Pigments. Amsterdam: Elsevier/North Holland Biomedical Press, 203–241.

Essner E, Novikoff AB. 1960. Human hepatocellular pigments and lysosomes. J Ultrastruc Res 3:374–391.

Essner E, Novikoff AB. 1961. Localization of acid phosphatase activity in hepatic lysosomes by means of electron microscopy. J Biophys Biochem Cytol 9:773–784.

Ezaki J, Wolfe LS, Kominami E. 1993. Molecular basis of lysosomal accumulation of subunit c of mitochondrial ATP synthase in neuronal ceroid lipofuscinosis. J Inherited Metab Dis 16:296–298.

Feeney L. 1973. The phagolysosomal system of the pigment epithelium: a key to retinal disease. Invest Ophthalmol 12:635–638.

Feeney L. 1978. Lipofuscin and melanin of human retinal pigment epithelium: fluorescence, enzyme cytochemical, and ultrastructural studies. Invest Ophthalmol Vis Sci 17:583–600.

Feeney L, Grieshaber JA, Hogan MJ. 1965. Studies on human ocular pigment. In: Rohen JW, ed., The Structure of the Eye. Stuttgart: Schattauer-Verlag, 535–548.

Feeney-Burns L. 1980. The pigments of the retinal pigment epithelium. Curr Topics Eye Res 2:119–178.

Feeney-Burns L, Eldred GE. 1983. The fate of the phagosome: conversion to "age pigment" and impact in human RPE. Trans Ophthalmol Soc UK 103:416–421.

Feeney-Burns L, Ellersieck MR. 1985. Age-related changes in the ultrastructure of Bruch's membrane. Am J Ophthalmol 100:686–697.

Feeney-Burns L, Katz ML. 1992. Retinal pigment epithelium. In: Tasman W, Jaeger E, eds, Duane's Foundations of Clinical Ophthalmology. Lippincott: Philadelphia, 1–20.

Feeney-Burns L, Berman ER, Rothman H. 1980. Lipofuscin of human retinal pigment epithelium. Am J Ophthalmol 90:783–791.

Feeney-Burns L, Hildebrand ES, Eldridge S. 1984. Aging human RPE: morphometric analysis of macular, equatorial, and peripheral cells. Invest Ophthalmol Vis Sci 25:195–200.

Feeney-Burns L, Gao C-L, Berman ER. 1988. The fate of immunoreactive opsin following phagocytosis by pigment epithelium in human and monkey retinas. Invest Ophthalmol Visual Sci 29:708–719.

Feeney-Burns L, Burns RP, Gao C-L. 1990. Age-related macular changes in humans over 90 years old. Am J Ophthalmol 109:265–278.

Ferrell JE Jr, Lee K-J, Huestis WH. 1985. Membrane bilayer balance and erythrocyte shape: a quantitative assessment. Biochemistry 24:2849–2857.

Ferrell JE Jr, Mitchell KT, Huestis WH. 1988. Membrane bilayer balance and platelet shape: morphological and biochemical responses to amphipathic compounds. Biochim Biophys Acta 939:223–237.

Firestone RA, Pisano JM, Bonney RJ. 1979. Lysosomotropic agents. 1. Synthesis and cytotoxic action of lysosomotropic detergents. J Med Chem 22:1130–1133.

Fischer TM. 1993. Bending stiffness of lipid bilayers: IV. Interpretation of red cell shape change. Biophys J 65:687–692.

Fite KV, Bengston L, Donaghey B. 1993. Experimental light damage increases lipofuscin in the retinal pigment epithelium of Japanese quail *(Coturnix coturnix Japonica)*. Exp Eye Res 57:449–460.

Fliesler SJ, Anderson RE. 1983. Chemistry and metabolism of lipids in the vertebrate retina. Prog Lipid Res 22:79–131.

Frangieh GT, Green WR, Fine SL. 1982. A histopathologic study of Best's macular dystrophy. Arch Ophthalmol 100:1115–1121.

Frenkel EJ, Kuypers FA, Op den Kamp JAF, Roelofsen B, Ott P. 1986. Effect of membrane cholesterol on dimyristoylphosphatidylcholine-induced vesiculation of human red blood cells. Biochim Biophys Acta 855:293–301.

Frisch SM, Francis H. 1994. Disruption of epithelial cell-matrix interactions induces apoptosis. J Cell Biol 124:619–626.

Fujii T, Sato T, Tamura A, Wakatsuki M, Kanaho Y. 1979. Shape changes of human erythrocytes induced by various amphipathic drugs acting on the membrane of the intact cells. Biochem Pharmacol 28:613–620.

Gaillard ER, Atherton SJ, Eldred GE, Dillon J. 1995. Photophysical studies on human retinal lipofuscin. Photochem Photobiol 61:448–453.

Gomori G. 1952. Microscopic Histochemistry: Principles and Practice. Chicago: University of Chicago Press, 91–94.

Gordon WC, Bazan NG. 1993. Visualization of [^{3}H]docosahexaenoic acid trafficking through photoreceptors and retinal pigment epithelium by electron microscopic autoradiography. Invest Ophthalmol Vis Sci 34:2402–2411.

Gordon WC, Rodriguez de Turco EB, Bazan NG. 1992. Retinal pigment epithelial cells play a central role in the conservation of docosahexaenoic acid by photoreceptor cells after shedding and phagocytosis. Curr Eye Res 11:73–83.

Green WR, Enger C. 1993. Age-related macular degeneration, histopathologic studies. Ophthalmology 100:1519–1535.

Green WR, Key SN III. 1977. Senile macular degeneration: histopathologic study. Trans Am Ophthalmol Soc 75:180–254.

Green WR, McDonnell PJ, Yeo JH. 1985. Pathologic features of senile macular degeneration. Ophthalmology 92:615–627.

Hagerstrand H, Isomaa B. 1992. Morphological characterization of exovesicles and endovesicles released from human erythrocytes following treatment with amphiphiles. Biochim Biophys Acta 1109:117–126.

Handelman GJ, Dratz EA. 1986. The role of antioxidants in the retina and retinal pigment epithelium and the nature of pro-oxidant induced damage. Adv Free Radical Biol Med 2:1–89.

Hara S, Hayasaka S, Mizuno K. 1979. Distribution and some properties of lysosomal arylsulfatases in the bovine eye. Exp Eye Res 28:641–650.

Hara S, Plantner JJ, Kean EL. 1983. The enzymatic cleavage of rhodopsin by the retinal pigment epithelium. I. Enzyme preparation, properties and kinetics: characterization of the glycopeptide product. Exp Eye Res 36:799–816.

Hayasaka S. 1974. Distribution of lysosomal enzymes in the bovine eye. Jpn J Ophthalmol 18:233–239.

Hayasaka S, Hayasaka I. 1978. The distribution and properties of collagenolytic cathepsin in the bovine eye. Albrecht von Graefes Arch Klin Exp Ophthalmol 206:163–168.

Hayasaka S, Shiono T. 1982. α-Fucosidase, α-mannosidase and β-N-acetylglucosaminidase of the bovine retinal pigment epithelium. Exp Eye Res 34:565–569.

Hayasaka S, Hara S, Mizuno K. 1975a. Degradation of rod outer segment proteins by cathepsin D. J Biochem 78:1365–1367.

Hayasaka S, Hara S, Mizuno K. 1975b. Distribution and some properties of cathepsin D in the retinal pigment epithelium. Exp Eye Res 21:307–313.

Hayasaka S, Hara S, Mizuno K, Aizu S. 1977. In vitro degradation of rod outer segment lipid by acid lipase. Jpn J Ophthalmol 21:342–347.

Hayasaka S, Shiono T, Hara S, Mizuno K. 1981. Regional distribution of lysosomal enzymes in the retina and choroid of human eyes. Graefes Arch Klin Exp Ophthalmol 216:269–273.

Hayes KC. 1974. Retinal degeneration in monkeys induced by deficiencies of vitamin E or A. Invest Ophthalmol 13:499–510.

Hofmann KP, Pulvermuller A, Buczylko J, Van Hooser P, Palczewski K. 1992. The role of arrestin and retinoids in the regeneration pathway of rhodopsin. J Biol Chem 267:15701–15706.

Hogan MJ. 1972. Role of the retinal pigment epithelium in macular disease. Trans Am Acad Ophthalmol Otolaryngol 76:64–80.

Hynes RO. 1992. Integrins: versatility, modulation, and signaling in cell adhesion. Cell 69:11–25.

Ikegami Y, Dorey CK, Obin M, Delori FC, Taylor A. 1995. Leupeptin induced changes in the composition of photoreceptor derived lipofuscin in cultured rat RPE cells. Invest Ophthalmol Vis Sci 36:S769.

Ishibashi T, Patterson R, Ohnishi Y, Inomata H, Ryan SJ. 1986. Formation of drusen in the human eye. Am J Ophthalmol 101:342–353.

Ishikawa T, Yamada E. 1970. Degradation of the photoreceptor outer segment within the pigment epithelial cell of rat retina. J Electronmicrosc 19:85–99.

Isomaa B, Paatero G. 1981. Shape and volume changes in rat erythrocytes induced by surface-active alkyltrimethylammonium salts and sodium dodecyl sulphate. Biochim Biophys Acta 647:211–222.

Israelachvili JN, Marcelja S, Horn RG. 1980. Physical principles of membrane organization. Q Rev Biophys 13:121–200.

Ivy GO, Kanai S, Ohta M, Smith G, Sato Y, Kobayashi M, Kitani K. 1990. Lipofuscin-like substances accumulate rapidly in brain, retina and internal organs with cysteine protease inhibition. In: Porta EA, ed, Lipofuscin and Ceroid Pigments. New York: Plenum Press, 31–47.

Jolly RD, Dalefield RR. 1990. Lipopigments in veterinary pathology. In: Porta EA, ed, Lipofuscin and Ceroid Pigments. New York: Plenum Press, 157–167.

Jolly RD, Palmer DN. 1995. The neuronal ceroid-lipofuscinoses (Batten disease): comparative aspects. Neuropathol Appl Neurobiol 21:50–60.

Jolly RD, Dalefield RR, Palmer DN. 1993. Ceroid, lipofuscin and the ceroid-lipofuscinoses (Batten disease). J Inher Metab Dis 16:280–283.

Kaplan J, Gerber S, Rozet JM, Larget Piet D, Dollfus H, Munnich A. 1994. A gene for Stargardt's disease maps on the short arm of chromosome 1. Invest Ophthalmol Vis Sci 35(4):1715.

Katz ML. 1993. Hereditary ceroid lipofuscinosis. Methylated amino acids in storage body proteins. J Inherited Metab Dis 16:305–307.

Katz ML, Eldred GE. 1989. Retinal light damage reduces autofluorescent pigment deposition in the retinal pigment epithelium. Invest Ophthalmol Vis Sci 30:37–43.

Katz ML, Norberg M. 1992. Influence of dietary vitamin A on autofluorescence of leupeptin-induced inclusions in the retinal pigment epithelium. Exp Eye Res 54:239–246.

Katz ML, Shanker MJ. 1989. Development of lipofuscin-like fluorescence in the retinal pigment epithelium in response to protease inhibitor treatment. Mech Ageing Dev 49:23–40.

Katz ML, Stone WL, Dratz EA. 1978. Fluorescent pigment accumulation in retinal pigment epithelium of antioxidant-deficient rats. Invest Ophthalmol Vis Sci 17:1049–1058.

Katz ML, Robison WG Jr, Herrmann RK, Groome AB, Bieri JG. 1984. Lipofuscin accumulation resulting from senescence and vitamin E deficiency: spectral properties and tissue distribution. Mech Ageing Devel 25:149–159.

Katz ML, Drea CM, Eldred GE, Hess HH, Robison WG Jr. 1986a. Influence of early photoreceptor degeneration on lipofuscin in the retinal pigment epithelium. Exp Eye Res 43:561–573.

Katz ML, Drea CM, Robison WG Jr. 1986b. Relationship between dietary retinol and lipofuscin in the retinal pigment epithelium. Mech Ageing Devel 35:291–305.

Katz ML, Eldred GE, Robison WG Jr. 1987. Lipofuscin autofluorescence: evidence for vitamin A involvement in the retina. Mech Ageing Devel 39:81–90.

Katz ML, Eldred GE, Siakotos AN, Koppang N. 1988. Characterization of disease-specific brain fluorophores in ceroid-lipofuscinosis. Am J Med Genetics 5(suppl):253–264.

Katz ML, Christianson JS, Gao C-L, Handelman GJ. 1994. Iron-induced fluorescence in the retina: dependence on vitamin A. Invest Ophthalmol Vis Sci 35:3613–3624.

Kean EL, Hara S, Mizoguchi A, Matsumoto A, Kobata A. 1983. The enzymatic cleavage of rhodopsin by the retinal pigment epithelium. II. The carbohydrate composition of the glycopeptide cleavage product. Exp Eye Res 36:817–825.

Kennedy CJ, Rakoczy PE, Robertson TA, Papadimitriou JM, Constable IJ. 1994. Kinetic studies on phagocytosis and lysosomal digestion of rod outer segments by human retinal pigment epithelial cells in vitro. Exp Cell Res 210:209–214.

Killingsworth MC. 1987. Age-related components of Bruch's membrane in the human eye. Graefes Arch Clin Exp Ophthalmol 255:406–412.

Kliffen M, Mooy CM, Luider TM, de Jong PTVM. 1994. Analysis of carbohydrate structures in basal laminar deposit in aging human maculae. Invest Ophthalmol Vis Sci 35:2901–2905.

Kobayashi T, Yamada J-I, Setaka M, Kwan T. 1986. Effects of chlorpromazine and other calmodulin antagonists on phosphatidylcholine-induced vesiculation of platelet plasma membranes. Biochim Biophys Acta 855:58–62.

Kuypers FA, Roelofsen B, Berendsen W, Op den Kamp JAF, van Deenen LLM. 1984. Shape changes in human erythrocytes induced by replacement of the native phosphatidylcholine with species containing various fatty acids. J Cell Biol 99:2260–2267.

Lange Y, Slayton JM. 1982. Interaction of cholesterol and lysophosphatidylcholine in determining red cell shape. J Lipid Res 23:1121–1127.

Layer RW. 1963. The chemistry of imines. Chem Rev 63:489–510.

Lentrichia BB, Bruner WE, Kean EL. 1978. Glycosidases of the retinal pigment epithelium. Invest Ophthalmol Visual Sci 17:884–895.

Lessell S, Kuwabara T. 1964. Phosphatase histochemistry of the eye. Arch Ophthalmol 71:851–860.

Loeffler KU, Lee WR. 1986. Basal linear deposit in the human macula. Graefes Arch Clin Exp Ophthalmol 224:493–501.

Lüllmann-Rauch R. 1981. Experimentally induced lipidosis in rat retinal pigment epithelium: a brief review. Albrecht von Graefes Arch Klin Ophthalmol 215:297–303.

Lüllmann-Rauch R. 1994. Drug-induced intralysosomal storage of sulfated glycosaminoglycans (GAGs): a methodical pitfall occurring with acridine derivatives. Exp Toxic Pathol 46:315–322.

Maher P, Singer SJ. 1984. Structural changes in membranes produced

by the binding of small amphipathic molecules. Biochemistry 23:232–240.

Marshall J. 1970. Acid phosphatase activity in the retinal pigment epithelium. Vision Res 10:821–824.

Matsumoto Y, Watanabe T, Suga T, Fujitani H. 1989. Inhibitory effects of quaternary ammonium compounds on lysosomal degradation of endogenous proteins. Chem Pharm Bull 37:516–518.

Mel'nikov SM, Sergeyev VG, Yoshikawa K. 1995. Discrete coil-globule transition of large DNA induced by cationic surfactant. J Am Chem Soc 117:2401–2408.

Meredith JE, Fayeli B, Schwartz MA. 1993. The extracellular matrix as a cell survival factor. Mol Biol Cell 4:953–961.

Miller DK, Griffiths E, Lenard J, Firestone RA. 1983. Cell killing by lysosomotropic detergents. J Cell Biol 97:1841–1851.

Mitchison HM, Thompson AD, Mulley JC, Kozman HM, Richards RI, Callen DF, Stallings RL, Doggett NA, Attwood J, McKay TR. 1993. Fine genetic mapping of the Batten disease locus (CLN3) by haplotype analysis and demonstration of allelic association with chromosome 16p microsatellite loci. Genomics 16:455–460.

Mohandas N, Chasis JA. 1993. Red blood cell deformability, membrane material properties and shape: regulation by transmembrane, skeletal and cytosolic proteins and lipids. Semin Hematol 30:171–192.

Mohler CW, Fine SL. 1981. Long-term evaluation of patients with Best's vitelliform dystrophy. Ophthalmology 88:688–692.

Mulberg AE, Tulk BM, Forgac M. 1991. Modulation of coated vesicle chloride channel activity and acidification by reversible protein kinase A-dependent phosphorylation. J Biol Chem 266:20590–20593.

Müller H, Schmidt U, Lutz HU. 1981. On the mechanism of red blood cell shape change and release of spectrin-free vesicles. Acta Biol Med Germ 40:413–417.

Noji T. 1980. Electron microscopic histochemical study of arylsulfatase of the rabbit ocular tissues. Jpn J Ophthalmol 24:396–406.

O'Gorman S, Flaherty WA, Fishman GA, Berson EL. 1988. Histopathologic findings in Best's vitelliform macular dystrophy. Arch Ophthalmol 106:1261–1268.

Ohkuma S, Poole B. 1978. Fluorescence probe measurement of the intralysosomal pH in living cells and the perturbation of pH by various agents. Proc Nat Acad Sci USA 75:3327–3331.

Okami T, Yamamoto A, Takada T, Omori K, Uyama M, Tashiro Y. 1990. Immunocytochemical localization of Na+,K+-ATPase, in rat retinal pigment epithelial cells. J Histochem Cytochem 38:1267–1275.

Okuzaki H, Osada Z. 1995. Ordered-aggregate formation by surfactant-charged gel interaction. Macromolecules 28:380–382.

Palczewski K, Jäger S, Buczylko J, Crouch RK, Bredberg DL, Hofmann KP, Asson-Batres MA, Saari JC. 1994. Rod outer segment retinol dehydrogenase: substrate specificity and role in phototransduction. Biochemistry 33:13741–13750.

Palek J, Jarolim P. 1993. Clinical expression and laboratory detection of red blood cell membrane protein mutations. Semin Hematol 30:249–283.

Palmer DN, Barns G, Husbands DR, Jolly RD. 1986. Ceroid lipofuscinosis in sheep. II. The major component of the lipopigments in liver, kidney, pancreas and brain is low molecular weight protein. J Biol Chem 261:1773–1777.

Palmer DN, Martinus RD, Cooper SM, Midwinter GG, Reid JC, Jolly RD. 1989. Ovine ceroid lipofuscinosis: the major lipopigment protein and the lipid-binding subunit of mitochrondrial ATP synthase have the same NH2-terminal sequence. J Biol Chem 264:5736–5740.

Palmer DN, Bayliss SL, Clifton PA, Grant VJ. 1993. Storage bodies in the ceroid lipofuscinoses (Batten disease): low molecular weight components, unusual amino acids and reconstitution of fluorescent bodies from nonfluorescent components. J Inherited Metab Dis 16:292–295.

Penn JS, Anderson RE. 1991. Effects of light history on the rat retina. Prog Retinal Res 11:75–98.

Philp NJ, Nachmias VT. 1987. Polarized distribution of integrin and fibronectin in retinal pigment epithelium. Invest Ophthalmol Vis Sci 28:1275–1280.

Pisano JM, Firestone RA. 1981. Lysosomotropic agents. III. Synthesis of N-retinyl morpholine. Synth Commun 11:375–378.

Raines MF, Bhargava SK, Rosen ES. 1989. The blood-retinal barrier in chloroquine retinopathy. Invest Ophthalmol Vis Sci 30:1726–1731.

Rakoczy PE, Kennedy C, Thompson-Wallis D, Mann K, Constable I. 1992. Changes in retinal pigment epithelial cell autofluorescence and protein expression associated with phagocytosis of rod outer segments in vitro. Biol Cell 76:49–54.

Rakoczy PE, Mann K, Cavaney DM, Robertson T, Papadimitreou J, Constable IJ. 1994. Detection and possible functions of cysteine protease involved in digestion of rod outer segments by retinal pigment epithelial cells. Invest Ophthalmol Vis Sci 35:4100–4108.

Ramsey MS, Fine BS. 1972. Chloroquine toxicity in the human eye: histopathologic observations by electron microscopy. Am J Ophthalmol 73:229–238.

Regan CM, de Grip WJ, Daemen FJM, Bonting SL. 1980. Degradation of rhodopsin by a lysosomal fraction of retinal pigment epithelium: biochemical aspects of the visual process. XLI. Exp Eye Res 30:183–191.

Remé CE. 1977. Autophagy in visual cells and pigment epithelium. Invest Ophthalmol Visual Sci 16:807–814.

Rideout D, Jaworski J, Dagnino R Jr. 1988. Environment-selective synergism using self-assembling cytotoxic and antimicrobial agents. Biochem Pharmacol 37:4505–4512.

Rizzolo LJ, Heiges M. 1991. The polarity of the retinal pigment epithelium is developmentally regulated. Exp Eye Res 53:549–553.

Rizzolo LJ, Zhou S, Li Z-Q. 1994. The neural retina maintains integrins in the apical membrane of the RPE early in development. Invest Ophthalmol Vis Sci 35:2567–2576.

Robert S, Tancrede P, Salesse C, LeBlanc RM. 1983. Interactions in mixed monolayers between distearoyl-L-phosphatidylethanolamine, rod outer segment phosphatidylethanolamine and all-trans-retinal. Biochim Biophys Acta 730:217–225.

Robison WG Jr, Kuwabara T, Bieri JG. 1979. Vitamin E deficiency and the retina: photoreceptor and pigment epithelial changes. Invest Ophthalmol Vis Sci 18:683–690.

Robison WG Jr, Kuwabara T, Bieri JG. 1980. Deficiencies of vitamins E and A in the rat: retinal damage and lipofuscin accumulation. Invest Ophthalmol Vis Sci 19:1030–1037.

Rosenthal AR, Kolb H, Bergsma D, Huxsoll D, Hopkins JL. 1978. Chloroquine retinopathy in the rhesus monkey. Invest Ophthalmol Vis Sci 17:1158–1175.

Rothman H, Feeney L, Berman ER. 1976. The retinal pigment epithelium: analytical subcellular fractionation with special reference to acid lipase. Exp Eye Res 22:519–532.

Rouslahti E, Reed JC. 1994. Anchorage dependence, integrins, and apoptosis. Cell 77:477–478.

Rózanowska M, Jarvis-Evans J, Korytowski W, Boulton ME, Burke JM, Sarna T. 1995. Blue light-induced reactivity of retinal age pigment: in vitro generation of oxygen-reactive species. J Biol Chem 270:18825–18830.

Rozet JM, Gerber S, Bonneau D, Souied E, Frézal J, Munnich A, Kaplan J. 1995. Exclusion of the cone-specific a-subunit of the

transducin gene in Stargardt's disease. Invest Ophthalmol Vis Sci 36(4): S919.

Sackmann E, Duwe H-P, Engelhardt H. 1986. Membrane bending elasticity and its role for shape fluctuations and shape transformations of cells and vesicles. Faraday Discuss Soc 81:281–290.

Sakai N, Decatur J, Nakanishi K, Eldred GE. 1996. Ocular age pigment A2-E: an unprecedented pyridinium bisretinoid. J Amer Chem Soc 118:1559–1560.

Sarks SH. 1976. Ageing and degeneration in the macular region: a clinico-pathological study. Br J Ophthalmol 60:324–341.

Sarks SH, Van Driel D, Maxwell L, Killingsworth M. 1980. Softening of drusen and subretinal neovascularization. Trans Ophthalmol Soc UK 100:414–422.

Schremser J-L, Williams TP. 1995a. Rod outer segment (ROS) renewal as a mechanism for adaptation to a new intensity environment. I. Rhodopsin levels and ROS length. Exp Eye Res 61:17–24.

Schremser J-L, Williams TP. 1995b. Rod outer segment (ROS) renewal as a mechanism for adaptation to a new intensity environment. II. Rhodopsin synthesis and packing density. Exp Eye Res 61:25–32.

Seglen PO. 1983. Inhibitors of lysosomal function. Meth Enzymol 96:737–764.

Shanthaveerappa TR, Bourne GH. 1964. Histochemical studies on the distribution of acid phosphatase in the eye. Acta Histochem 18:317–327.

Sheetz MP, Singer SJ. 1974. Biological membranes as bilayer couples: a molecular mechanism of drug-erythrocyte interactions. Proc Nat Acad Sci USA 71:4457–4471.

Siakotos AN, Koppang N. 1973. Procedures for the isolation of lipopigments from brain, heart and liver, and their properties: a review. Mech Ageing Devel 2:177–200.

Snyder LM, Lutz HU, Sauberman N, Jacobs J, Fortier NL. 1978. Fragmentation and myelin formation in hereditary xerocytosis and other hemolytic anemias. Blood 52:750–761.

Stark WS, Tan KEWP. 1982. Ultraviolet light: photosensitivity and other effects on the visual system. Photochem Photobiol 36:371–380.

Stark WS, Miller GV, Itoku KA. 1984. Calibration of microspectrophotometers as it applies to the detection of lipofuscin and the blue- and yellow-emitting fluorophores in situ. Meth Enzymol 105:341–347.

Staurenghi G, Delori FC, Goger DG, Weiter JJ. 1993. Lipofuscin in Stargardt's disease. Invest Ophthalmol Vis Sci 34(4):1167.

Stone EM, Nichols BE, Streb LM, Kimura AE, Sheffield VC. 1992. Genetic linkage of vitelliform macular degeneration (Best's disease) to chromosome 11q13. Nature Genetics 1:246–250.

Streeten BW. 1961. The sudanophilic granules of the human retinal pigment epithelium. Arch Ophthalmol 66:391–398.

Sugasawa K, Deguchi J, Okami T, Yamamoto A, Omori K, Uyama M, Tashiro Y. 1994. Immunocytochemical analyses of distributions of Na,K-ATPase and GLUT1, insulin and transferrin receptors in the developing retinal pigment epithelial cells. Cell Struc Func 19:21–28.

Swartz JG, Mitchell JE. 1973. Phospholipase activity of retina and pigment epithelium. Biochemistry 12:5273–5278.

Takahashi K, Kobayashi T, Yamada A, Tanaka Y, Inoue K, Nojima S. 1983. Release of vesicles containing acetylcholinesterase from erythrocyte membranes by treatment with dilauroylglycerophosphocholine. J Biochem 93:1691–1699.

Tapper H, Sundler R. 1995. Bafilomycin A1 inhibits lysosomal, phatosomal, and plasma membrane H+-ATPase and induces lysosomal enzyme secretion in macrophages. J Cell Physiol 163:137–144.

Taschner PEM, de Vos N, Thompson AD, Callen DF, Doggett N, Mole SE, Dooley TP, Barth PG, Breuning MH. 1995. Chromosome 16 microdeletion in a patient with juvenile neuronal ceroid lipofuscinosis (Batten disease). Am J Hum Genet 56:663–668.

Traboulsi EI, Green WR, Luckenbach MW, de la Cruz ZC. 1987. Neuronal ceroid lipofuscinosis: ocular histopathologic and electron microscopic studies in the late infantile, juvenile, and adult forms. Graefes Arch Clin Exp Ophthalmol 225:391–402.

Tyynelä J, Palmer DN, Baumann M, Haltia M. 1993. Storage of saposins A and D in infantile neuronal ceroid-lipofuscinosis. FEBS Lett 330:8–12.

Tyynelä J, Baumann M, Henseler M, Sandhoff K, Haltia M. 1995. Sphingolipid activator proteins in the neuronal ceroid-lipofuscinoses: an immunological study. Acta Neuropathol 89:391–398.

Van Dyke RW, Rost KV. 1993. Ethinyl estradiol decreases acidification of rat liver endocytotic vesicles. Hepatology 18:604–613.

Van Norren D, Vos JJ. 1974. Spectral transmission of the human ocular media. Vision Res 14:1237–1244.

von Rückmann A, Fitzke FW, Bird AC. 1995. Distribution of fundus autofluorescence with a scanning laser ophthalmoscope. Br J Ophthalmol 79:407–412.

Weingeist TA, Kobrin JL, Watzke RC. 1982. Histopathology of Bests's macular dystrophy. Arch Ophthalmol 100:1108–1114.

Weiter JJ, Delori FC, Wing GL, Fitch KA. 1986. Retinal pigment epithelial lipofuscin and melanin and choroidal melanin in human eyes. Invest Ophthalmol Vis Sci 27:145–152.

Weiter JJ, Delori F, Dorey CK. 1988. Central sparing in annular macular degeneration. Am J Ophthalmol 106:286–292.

Weitz M, Bjerrum OJ, Ott P, Brodbeck U. 1982. Quantitative composition and characterization of the proteins in membrane vesicles released from erythrocytes by dimyristoylphosphatidylcholine: a membrane system without cytoskeleton. J Cell Biochem 19:179–191.

Wilbers KH, Haest CWM, von Gentheim M, Deuticke B. 1979. Influence of enzymatic phospholipid cleavage on the permeability of the erythrocyte membrane. I. Transport of non-electrolytes via the lipid domain. Biochim Biophys Acta 554:388–399.

Wilcox DK. 1988. Vectorial accumulation of cathepsin D in retinal pigmented epithelium: effects of age. Invest Ophthalmol Vis Sci 29:1205–1212.

Wing GL, Blanchard GC, Weiter JJ. 1978. The topography and age relationship of lipofuscin concentration in the retinal pigment epithelium. Invest Ophthalmol Vis Sci 17:601–607.

Wrigstad A, Wihlmark U, Roberg K, Brunk UT, Nilsson SEG. 1995. Lipofuscin formation and photooxidative cell damage in RPE cell cultures: an in vitro model for age related macular degeneration. Invest Ophthalmol Vis Sci 36(4):S433.

Young RW. 1967. The renewal of photoreceptor cell outer segments. J Cell Biol 33:61–72.

Young RW, Bok D. 1969. Participation of the retinal pigment epithelium in the rod outer segment renewal process. J Cell Biol 42:392–403.

Yuan CC, Crabb JW, Fishman GA, Jacobson S, Musarella MA. 1994. Exclusion of cellular retinaldehyde binding protein (CRALBP) as a candidate gene for Stargardt's disease. Invest Ophthalmol Vis Sci 35(4):1788.

Zanotti G, Marcello M, Malpeli G, Folli C, Sartori G, Berni R. 1994. Crystallographic studies on complexes between retinoids and plasma retinol-binding protein. J Biol Chem 26:29613–29620.

Zimmerman WF, Lion F, Daemen FJM, Bonting SL. 1975. Biochemical aspects of the visual process. XXX. Distribution of stereospecific retinol dehydrogenase activities in subcellular fractions of bovine retina and pigment epithelium. Exp Eye Res 21:325–332.

Zimmerman WF, Godchaux W III, Belkin M. 1983. The relative proportions of lysosomal enzyme activities in bovine retinal pigment epithelium. Exp Eye Res 36:151–158.

34. Aging and Bruch's membrane

JOHN MARSHALL, ALI A. HUSSAIN, CARLA STARITA,
DAVID J. MOORE, AND ANN L. PATMORE

Bruch's membrane is an enigma that has long puzzled both clinicians and scientists. Throughout the literature both its origins and its nomenclature are subject to confusion and debate, with authorities making claim and counterclaim which vary with the passage of time. It is thus variously described as the innermost layer of the choroid, or the outermost layer of the retina. In reality its components are derived from both sources, and therefore both interpretations may be useful in any given set of circumstances. What is indisputable is that Bruch's membrane lies between the outer retina and its metabolic supply, and that changes on the inner surface of Bruch's are a common finding in age-related retinal diseases. For clarity this chapter will first describe the anatomy of the membrane, and then its age-related changes, before looking at the possible causes of the morphological changes and their functional significance.

ANATOMY

Although anatomists have actively discouraged the use of eponyms, and in many tissues such discouragement has resulted in their abandonment, in ocular tissues they still reign supreme. Bruch's membrane is named after the Zurich anatomist Carl Bruch, who first demonstrated a structureless membrane between the choroid and retina. In early reports he is said to have made his dissection using a fine brush and a flat knife. Any who have attempted the isolation of Bruch's membrane will be aware of the difficulties implicit in such a procedure and one can only admire the patience and dissecting skills of Bruch. Because of an apparent lack of substructure in early microscopic observations, this so-called structureless membrane was termed the *lamina vitrea* and, as such, was one of the three so-called glass membranes of the eye. Improved methodology led Wolfrum (1908) to note that Bruch's membrane was apparently composed of three layers, including what appeared to be an inner thin basal membrane adjacent to the pigment epithelium, a layer of loose fibrous tissue, and a layer of elastin. These observations led Wolfrum to remove Bruch's

membrane from the other glass membranes, such as Descemet's membrane of the cornea and the capsule of the lens. Further microscopic studies showed that unlike these other glass membranes, which had clearly defined borders, the extent of Bruch's membrane was in some ways difficult to define. Bruch's membrane lies adjacent to the pigment epithelium of the retina throughout the distribution of the former. It is pierced by the exit of the optic nerve posteriorly, while anteriorly it extends to the *ora serrata*. Beyond the *ora serrata* it becomes modified, but some structural resemblance is still seen extending beneath the pigmented epithelium of the ciliary body. Embryologically, the epithelial surface of Bruch's membrane is apparent by the seventh week of development and the choroidal aspect becomes apparent by the ninth week (Braekevelt and Hollenberg, 1970). At 12 weeks, collagen is deposited and the basic requirements of the adult structure are defined (O'Rahilly, 1975). The thickness of the system varies with both age and topography. It is, on average, at its thinnest in the central region of the young eye, being in the order of two μm in thickness. Empirically, the dimensions of the membrane are again difficult to determine in that, while its internal aspect is cleanly defined beneath the basal layer of the retinal pigment epithelium (RPE), its external aspect is multivariant, as its components lie adjacent to and between the capillaries of the choriocapillaris. It is the lack of definition of this external aspect that makes a clean anatomical isolation of Bruch's membrane virtually impossible.

ULTRASTRUCTURE

On light microscopic examination, even with high-performance objectives, Bruch's membrane can only be resolved into three sublayers—the basement membrane of the pigment epithelium, a layer of collagen, and a zone of elastin. The collagenous layer appears as the most external of these layers and is most easily seen where it extends outward between the lumen of the capillaries of the choriocapillaris. In this location, collagen fibers appear to have a brushlike arrangement, with their long

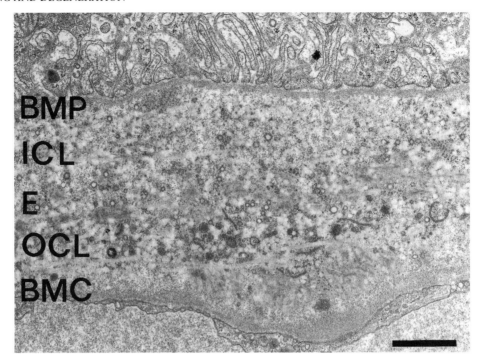

FIGURE 34-1. Transmission electron micrograph of Bruch's membrane in an 18-year-old human retina, showing the five layers of Bruch's membrane. From the outside in these are: (BMC)—basement membrane of the choriocapillaris; (OCL)—outer collagenous layer; (E)—elastin layer; (ICL)—inner collagenous layer; (BMP)—basement membrane of the pigment epithelium. The bar marker is 1 μm.

axes predominantly oriented from the choroid toward the retina. Using periodic acid-Schiff (PAS) staining, the basement membrane of the RPE can be clearly determined, and it appears as an uninterrupted layer throughout the distribution of Bruch's membrane. Since the advent of the electron microscope and studies undertaken on Bruch's membrane during the early 1960s, it has been almost universally accepted that Bruch's membrane can be defined as having a five-layered structure (Sumita, 1961; Lerche, 1963; Garron, 1963; Hogan, 1961). From outside to inside these layers are defined as (a) the basement membrane of the choriocapillaris; (b) the outer collagenous layer; (c) the elastin layer; (d) the inner collagenous layer, and (e) the basement membrane of the RPE. Although most authors use this format, a novel classification has been proposed by Gass (1987). In his definition Gass excludes the basement membranes from Bruch's membrane. He does this as he considers that, from a pathophysiological point of view, it is better to think of Bruch's membrane as being part of the choroidal stroma. Such a definition would avoid the confusion that could be created when defining the external limit of the outer collagenous layer within the intercapillary pillars of the choriocapillaris, where the basement membrane of the choroidal capillary en-

dothelium is not present. Currently, most textbooks still prefer the pentalaminar system and, as a consequence, it will be used throughout the current chapter (Hogan et al., 1971).

To demonstrate the pentalaminar structure, Bruch's membrane is usually illustrated in transverse section (Fig. 34-1). It should be remembered, however, that most of the fibers in the three fibrous layers are organized such that their long axes run parallel to the plane of the membrane (Fig. 34-2). As will be discussed, the fibers run at a variety of angles to each other and collectively present a complex, multilayered, gridlike structure. The functional significance of this stereospatial array will be discussed later. In transverse plane, the absolute dimensions of the five layers will vary according to age. However, their percentage contribution remains relatively stable. These are listed in Figure 34-3, together with the respective fibrous components and collagen types.

The Basement Membrane of the Choriocapillaris

This is the only discontinuous layer of Bruch's membrane, being absent where Bruch's membrane projects outward between the capillaries of the choriocapillaris,

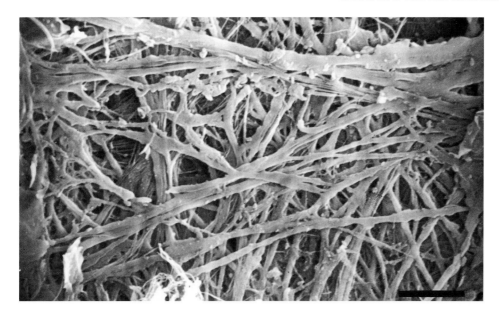

FIGURE 34-2. Scanning electron micrograph of the surface of the inner collagenous layer of Bruch's membrane of a 76-year-old, in which the basement membrane of the pigment epithelium had been removed. The multilayered gridlike structure is clearly illustrated, as is the primary orientation of the collagen fibers parallel to the surface of Bruch's membrane. The bar marker is 5 μm.

in the so-called intercapillary columns. Where the curvature of the capillary wall moves away from the backward projections of Bruch's, its basement membrane is laid down over choroidal elements. It is the continuity of this basement membrane structure around the vessels, but its discontinuity as a contribution to Bruch's membrane, that gives rise to its exclusion from the definition of Bruch's membrane proposed by Gass (1987). In the young eye, this basement membrane has an average thickness of 0.14 μm and, like all basement membranes, it appears to have two components. There is a pale, or electron-translucent layer adjacent to its germinal cell layer and a more remote, darker, or electron-dense layer. On high-power examination, the dense layer appears to be granular but with fine filaments which extend through into the adjacent collagen fibers. This layer is predominantly composed of collagens type IV and VI, together with laminin and heparin sulphate (Fig. 34-3). There is also some possibility of small amounts of collagen type V appearing in this layer. Some reports indicate that there may be focal differences in the distribution of these various components. Collagen type VI has been reported to be found only on the choroidal aspect of the basement membrane of the choriocapillaris and not on the side adjacent to Bruch's membrane. This collagen has been suggested to be involved in the anchorage of capillary endothelial cells, particularly in the region of pericytes (Marshall et al., 1993; Rittig et al., 1990).

The Outer Collagenous Layer

The outer collagenous layer consists of a network of collagen fibers which are predominantly oriented in the plane of the membrane and embedded in a mucopolysaccharide protein matrix. The outer portion of this layer extends between the capillaries of the choriocapillaris and the outer collagenous fibrils become continuous with those of the choroidal stroma and subcapillary tissue. At the inner aspect of this layer, some of the collagen fibers also protrude through the overlying elastin layer and into the inner collagenous layer. In the young, the thickness of the outer collagenous layer away from the intercapillary columns is approximately 0.7 μm and the individual collagen fibers have a diameter of 60 nm and a characteristic banding pattern with a periodicity of 64 nm. The components of this layer have been identified as collagen types I, III, and V; fibro-nectin; chondroitin sulphate; dermatan sulphate; and proteoglycans (Fig. 34-3).

The Elastin Layer

The elastin, elastic, or middle elastic layer has been termed the "backbone" of Bruch's membrane and again, in the young, is about 0.8 μm thick. Collectively, the fibers in this layer effectively form a continuous but perforated sheet extending from the edge of the optic nerve to the *pars plana* of the ciliary body. The layer consists of an array of linear elastin fibers, which form

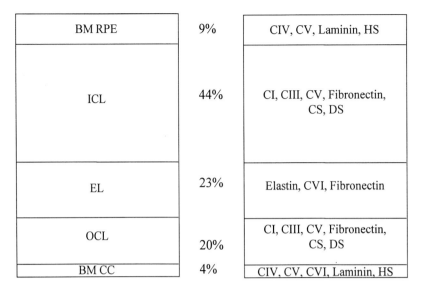

FIGURE 34-3. Diagram to show the pentalaminar structure of Bruch's membrane, together with relative percentage contribution to thickness and collagen and fibrous content. (BMRPE)—basement membrane of the retinal pigment epithelium; (ICL)—inner collagenous layer; (EL)—elastin layer; (OCL)—outer collagenous layer; (BMCC)— basement membrane of the choriocapillaris.

a grill-like structure several fibers thick. The fibers vary considerably in size and shape, but generally they are long and thin and predominantly their long axes run parallel to the surface of Bruch's membrane. Where the fibers intersect, they form dense nodes with few, if any, small porelike openings between them. However, away from these nodes there are less dense areas where interfibrillar spaces, or pores, are about 1 μm in diameter. It is through these pseudo-pores that collagen fibers may pass from both the outer and inner collagenous layers. Although elastin is the major component of this layer, it also contains collagen type VI, fibronectin, and possibly a sulphated proteoglycan (Fig. 34-3).

The Inner Collagenous Layer

In the young the inner collagenous layer is the largest single component of Bruch's membrane, having twice the dimensions of the outer collagenous layer. Given the discursion of collagen fibers through the layer of elastin, it is perhaps not surprising that the structure and composition of the two layers are identical. In transverse sections the greater dimensions of the inner collagenous layer often give the impression of a higher concentration of collagen fibers, or fibers of greater length than those in the outer collagenous layer, but this impression is erroneous.

The Basement Membrane of the Retinal Pigment Epithelium

This basement membrane is an uninterrupted layer extending over the entire surface of Bruch's membrane. In the young the bilaminar structure of this layer can be clearly seen, with an electron-translucent inner layer approximately 0.04–0.05 μm in thickness, and an outer, more electron-dense layer approximately 0.1 μm in thickness. Through the granular layer fine filaments are seen to extend, which pass into the collagen fibers of the inner collagenous layer. On its inner surface tonofilaments are seen to pass from the plasma membrane of the RPE in the region of hemidesmosomes. The basement membrane of the RPE does not appear to extend inward into the extracellular space presented by the basal infoldings of the basal membrane of the pigment epithelial cells, although it does slightly increase in thickness adjacent to some infoldings. The chemical components of this layer are similar to those of the basement membrane of the choriocapillaris, with the exception of collagen type VI. The basement membrane of the pigment epithelium is part of the continuum of basement membranes that extends from the margins of the optic nerve through to the pupillary edge of the iris.

The basic pentalaminar structure of Bruch's membrane, readily identified in childhood, is preserved throughout life, but undergoes a series of insidious changes with age.

MORPHOLOGY OF AGING BRUCH'S MEMBRANE

It is well documented that Bruch's membrane progressively increases in thickness throughout life, apparently doubling over a normal human lifespan (Hogan and Alvarado, 1979; Sarks, 1976; Newsome et al., 1987; van der Schaft, 1992; Ramrattan et al., 1994). Only one study has measured the relative dimensional changes in each of the substrata of the membrane; although only a limited sample size was employed, there was some indication that a greater alteration occurred within the inner layers of the membrane (Newsome et al., 1987). The increase in thickness of the membrane is due both to the remodeling of its fibrous structure and the deposition of the material within it. It is the latter mechanism that gives rise to an increasingly disorganized appearance within the pentalaminar substructure (Hogan and Alvarado, 1967; Sarks, 1976; Grindle and Marshall, 1979).

From histological examination the earliest alterations to the substructure are apparent during late childhood and early teens, although they become really prominent by the early twenties.

The first changes are the accumulation of granular, membranous, filamentous, and vesicular material between the basement membrane of the RPE and the inner collagenous layer (Hogan and Alvarado, 1967; Grindle and Marshall, 1975; Feeney-Burns and Elsick, 1985; Killingsworth, 1987). The membranous filaments may be long and extensive arrays, or predominantly vesicular (Fig. 34-4). The buildup of this material within the inner collagenous layer increases with age until it occupies a large proportion of the layer. There is also an increase in the collagen content of the membrane. This collagen is of two types. The first is similar to the 64 nm–periodicity collagen, which is an intrinsic component of the membrane throughout life. The second type appears in quantity after the age of 40 and is typified by the accumulation of clumps of collagen that possess a banding periodicity of 100–140 nm (Hogan and Alvarado, 1967; van der Schaft et al., 1991). This latter collagen, termed *wide-spaced collagen,* has also been found within other aging membrane systems in the eye, such as Descemet's membrane (van der Schaft et al., 1991).

Senescent changes are not limited to the collagenous layers; the elastin layer also shows a progressive accumulation of granular and fine fibrillar, electron-dense material (Hogan et al., 1971; Newsome et al., 1987). In some eyes calcification of the elastin layer has been

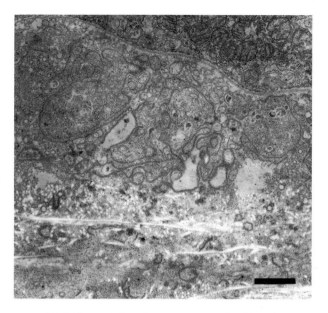

FIGURE 34-4. Transmission electron micrograph of Bruch's membrane in a 47-year-old human retina, showing the accumulation of membranous debris between the basement membrane of the pigment epithelium and the inner collagenous layer. Two sorts of debris can be identified, long membranous sheets and coated, membrane-bound bodies. The bar marker is 1 μm.

shown to be apparent, but usually not until the fourth decade of life (van der Schaft, 1992). It has been stated that degeneration of elastin introduces calcification (Kline, 1947), therefore it is not surprising that with increasing age the elastin layer has been ascribed as possessing an increasingly holey or moth-eaten appearance (Hogan et al., 1971).

From the age-related structural changes described it appears that there is considerable remodeling of the membrane. Evidence to support this concept is supplied by the work of Karwatowski et al. (1991), who demonstrated a 50% decrease in the solubility of Bruch's membrane collagen between birth and 90 years of age. Change in solubility may be due to the cross-linking of collagen components. Such a change could be brought about by the nonenzymic glycosylation of long-lived protein structures, giving rise to large, amorphous macromolecules known as *advanced glycosylated end products* (AGEs) (Vasan et al., 1990). Although AGEs are found in many parts of the body, as yet they have not been reported in Bruch's membrane.

A number of studies have demonstrated a senescent increase in the lipid content of Bruch's membrane (Pauleikhoff et al., 1990; Sheraidah et al., 1993; Holtz et al., 1994). Initial histochemical analysis demonstrated the absence of detectable phospholipid and neutral fats below the age of 30 years, with faint to moderate accumulation in middle life and higher levels of accumulation in the elderly (Pauleikhoff et al., 1990). Two subsequent studies using chromatographic methods to assess the quantity of extractable lipid in Bruch's membrane have since shown no detectable lipid within the first three decades of life, yet progressively accelerating accumulation thereafter (Sheraidah et al., 1993; Holtz et al., 1994). A further finding common to all three studies was that the ratio of phospholipids to neutral fats varied between individual eyes.

BASAL LINEAR, BASAL LAMINAR DEPOSIT

Perhaps the most prominent changes in aging Bruch's membrane occur on its innermost aspect, that is, between the basement membrane of the RPE and the basal membrane of the RPE cell. Unfortunately, reviewing the literature of this interface is confounded and confused by a nomenclature which individual authors have changed and different authors have used somewhat randomly. Key publications and their use of nomenclature

are summarized in Fig. 34-5 and an attempt at reinterpreting the morphological findings into a systematic pattern is shown in Fig. 34-6. From Fig. 34-5 it can be seen that the pentalaminar structure described by Hogan and Alvarado (1967) can be used as the key. In 1976 Sarks published a keynote clinical histopathological study following the aging changes in the outer retina in a captive population in an old peoples' home in Australia. Sarks described the accumulation of amorphous material between the pigment epithelium and its basement membrane. She termed this *basal linear deposit*. Subsequently, Feeney-Burns and Ellersieck (1985) published a morphological study in which the identical deposit was now termed *linear basal deposit*. Further confusion was contributed by Sarks et al. (1988), when they withdrew the term *basal linear deposit* and introduced a new term, *basal laminar deposit*, which they then further subdivided into late and early basal laminar deposit. More recently, even more confusion has been added by Green and Enger (1993), as in this publication basal laminar deposit was cited internal to the basement membrane of the RPE, whereas basal linear deposit was now placed in the inner collagenous layer.

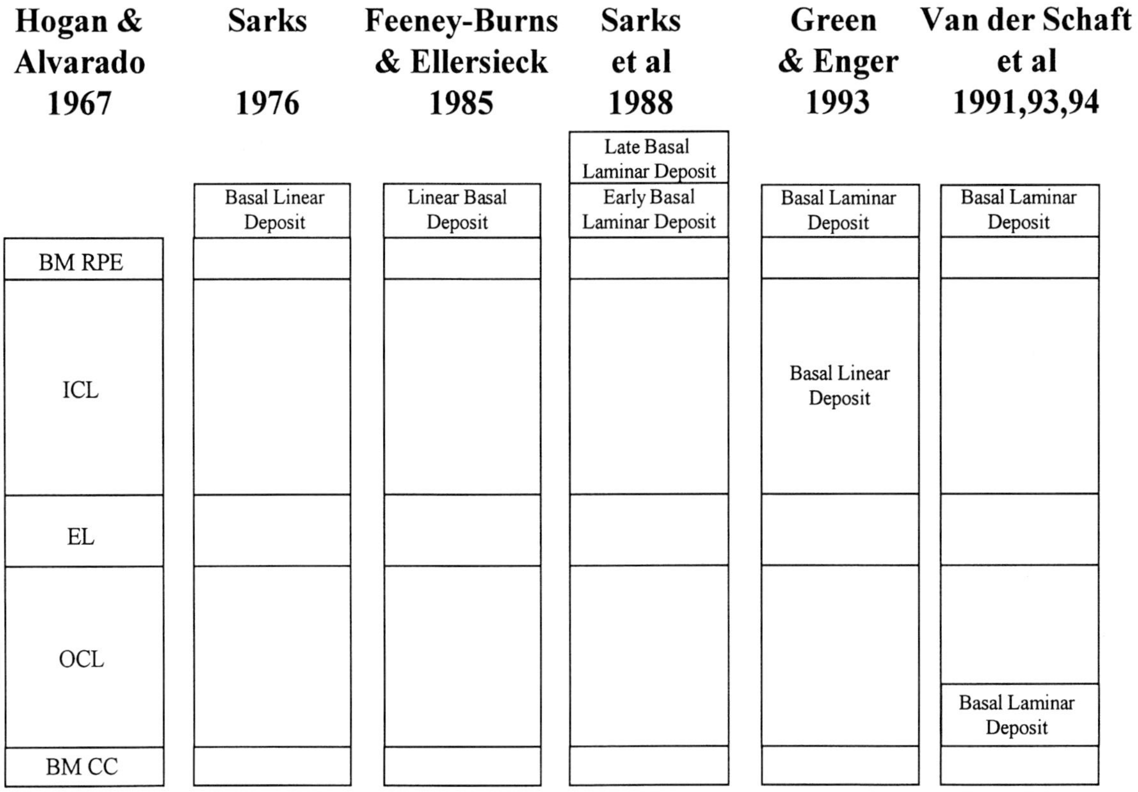

Hogan & Alvarado 1967	Sarks 1976	Feeney-Burns & Ellersieck 1985	Sarks et al 1988	Green & Enger 1993	Van der Schaft et al 1991,93,94
			Late Basal Laminar Deposit		
	Basal Linear Deposit	Linear Basal Deposit	Early Basal Laminar Deposit	Basal Laminar Deposit	Basal Laminar Deposit
BM RPE					
ICL				Basal Linear Deposit	
EL					
OCL					
					Basal Laminar Deposit
BM CC					

FIGURE 34-5. Summary diagram to illustrate the nomenclature and location of layers and deposits in key references.

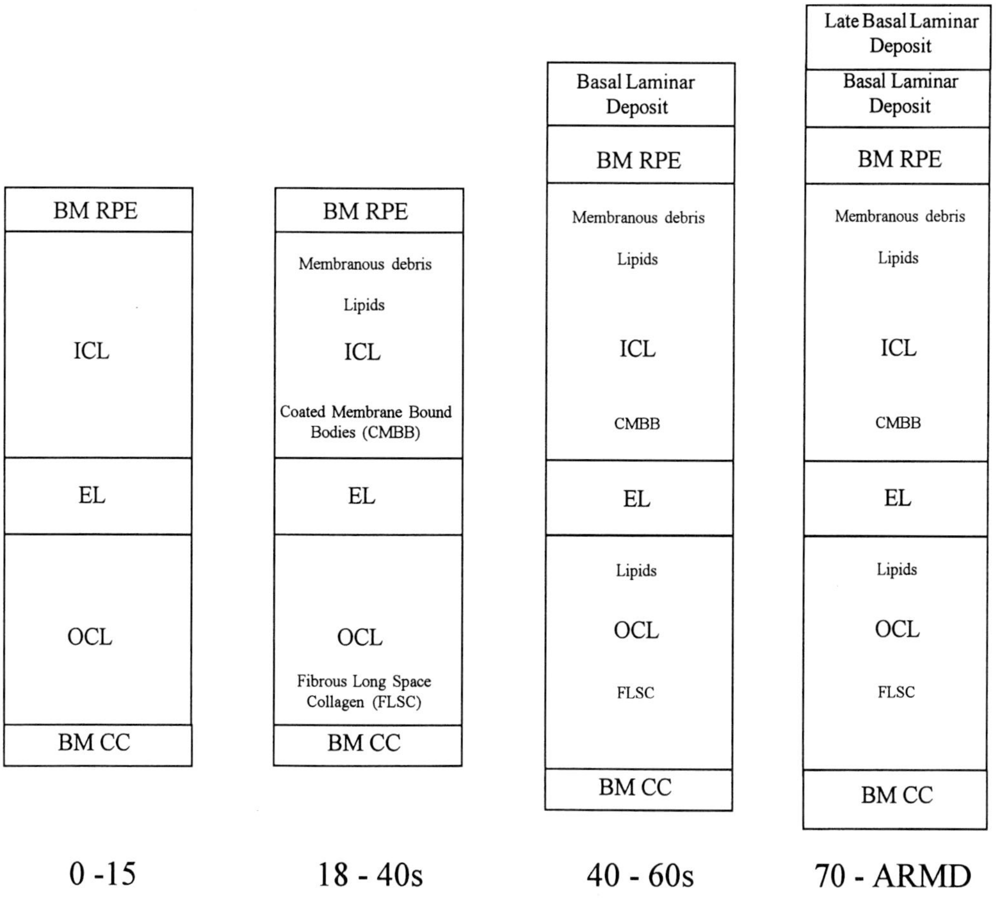

FIGURE 34-6. Summary diagram to indicate changes in the pentalaminar structure with increasing age and to clarify confusion implicit in Figure 34-5. For description see text.

Finally, in a series of papers by van der Schaft et al. (1991; 1993; 1994) basal laminar deposit was cited as occurring both internal to the basement membrane of the RPE and internal to the basement membrane of the choriocapillaris. Fig. 34-6 is an attempt to resolve the confusion in the literature. Starting from the pentalamina of Hogan et al. 1971, the first series of changes are seen in late adolescence and early adult life and occur predominantly within the two collagenous layers. This results in the increase in membranous debris and coated membrane-bound bodies predominantly in the inner collagenous layer and increase in fibrous wide-spaced collagen initially in the outer collagenous layer. In late middle age these changes are still apparent and increasing in magnitude together with the deposition of lipids. By the late fifties in many individuals some deposition of material is beginning to occur internal to the basement membrane of the RPE. Although, to maintain precedent, the term *basal linear deposit* should be used in this figure, the term *basal laminar deposit* is more anatomically correct and therefore will be adapted for

the present chapter (Sarks, 1988). From the late sixties the increase in deposition beneath the epithelium accelerates and two distinct layers of basal laminar deposit can be determined. The late basal laminar deposit is superimposed between the pigment epithelial cell and the initial basal laminar deposit. It is suggested that the displacement of the deposition described by Green and Enger derives from confusion with membranous debris and coated vesicles, while that of van der Schaft's group may be derived from a similar appearance of such debris in the outer collagenous layer.

The basal laminar deposit is eosinophilic, but also stains with Picro-Mallory and therefore must contain collagen. It has a striated appearance which is often palisading, or brushlike (Löffler and Lee, 1986). On electron microscopy, the striations resemble wide-spaced collagen and the spaces between the clumps often seem to contain membranous material. The late form of basal laminar deposit is a thick hyalinized layer which no longer stains with Picro-Mallory. On electron microscopy it appears to be an amorphous material but is laid down in a series of relatively thick layers. Its appearance and substructure is similar to that seen, but highly amplified, in Sorsby's pseudoinflammatory dystrophy (Capon et al., 1989). Throughout both early and late deposition of basal laminar deposits, membranous debris is also observed. It is this superimposition of two ultrastructural changes that may have given rise to some of the confusion summarized in Fig. 34-5 and 34-6.

DRUSEN

The deposits thus far described are often referred to as *diffuse deposits*. However, discrete focal aggregations also occur on the surface of Bruch's membrane. Clinically discrete spots, known as *drusen,* are often seen in the aging fundus (Weld, 1854). Drusen again suffer from a confusion between clinical and histopathological literature. Clinically, drusen may be characterized by the terms *hard* and *soft,* their size, and their behavior subsequent to injection of sodium fluorescein. Histologically, they may be classified as small, hard, round drusen and extensive, diffuse, soft drusen; or by their ultrastructural appearance, such as diffuse drusen, basal laminar drusen, or papillary drusen; or by their histochemical staining. As they vary in size, shape, elevation, distribution, and degree of pigmentation (Bressler et al., 1988) numerous classifications have been attempted (Bressler et al., 1989; Klein et al., 1992; Garner et al., 1994; Sarks et al., 1994; Bird et al., 1995).

Hard drusen occur in 80% of postmortem eyes, are normally small, being under 63 μm in diameter, but can become larger with their amorphous contents becoming less compact (Coffey and Brownstein, 1986; Bressler et al., 1989). On fluorescein angiography, hard drusen are hyperfluorescent (Bird and Marshall, 1986; Sarks et al., 1994), and it has been demonstrated that such drusen are rich in phospholipids (Pauleikhoff et al., 1992). Generally, hard drusen do not cause loss of vision, nor do they signify the onset of a pathological condition (Sarks et al., 1994).

Soft drusen are usually larger than hard drusen and have less well defined boundaries. They rarely occur before the age of 55 (Garner et al., 1994). Soft drusen also show a different behavior on fluorescein angiography in that they appear hypofluorescent. Their behavior is thought to be related to their high content of neutral fats which would inhibit the entry of any water-soluble dyes (Pauleikhoff et al., 1992). Soft drusen may contain vesicles, membranous debris, and wide-spaced collagen (Green et al., 1985; van der Schaft et al., 1992). Eyes with soft drusen are more likely to show visual loss (Eagle, 1984). It should be emphasized that drusen are not static, in that over time they may increase or decrease in size and may disappear completely. This natural process may also be accelerated by laser treatment, which has demonstrated that focal application may have widespread consequences for disappearance of drusen remote from the site of irradiation.

ORIGINS OF AGE-RELATED CHANGES

Given that Bruch's membrane may be considered either part of the choroid or the retina, it is perhaps not surprising that both tissues play a role in its aging. It sits between the outer blood–retinal barrier of the pigment epithelium and the major source of metabolic input to the retina, the choroidal vasculature. In the literature many roles have been assigned to it. Clearly, like all basement membrane systems, it provides support and an organized substructure for the cells attached to it. It has also been postulated that its elastic properties have special implications for the overlying photoreceptor cells. Leure de Pree (1968) suggested that as Bruch's membrane has no natural frequency it may act as a dampener to modulate the pulsations of the choroidal circulation and thus prevent the pulsations from disrupting the organization of the outer segments. Other authors have suggested that, given its key location, it may act to selectively filter molecular moeities traveling across it. In this respect, the demonstration of anionic sites and glycosaminoglycans, such as heparin sulphate, within Bruch's membrane may filter some macromolecules (Wislocki and Ladman, 1955; Pino et al., 1982; Call and Hollyfield, 1990). The presence of highly negatively charged entities, such as glycosaminoglycans, within the basement membrane system is thought to present an electrostatic barrier to the passage of large macromolecules, many of which possess a negative charge at physiological pH (Kanwar et al., 1980). The basement membrane of the choriocapillaris is rich in anionic sites and heparin sulphate proteoglycans, and trace studies have revealed that this is the site at which the large macromolecules are restricted in their passage from the capillary lumen (Wislocki and Ladman, 1955; Pino and Essner, 1980; Pino et al., 1982; Call and Hollyfield, 1990). This restriction acts to limit the passage of entities of 70,000 daltons, or larger (Pino and Essner, 1980). Entrapment or delay to any macromolecular systems passing across Bruch's membrane may contribute to changes within the system, and in turn may have secondary consequences. It may therefore be helpful to briefly review the components involved in movement of material across Bruch's membrane from the choroid to the retina and the retina to the choroid.

THE DELIVERY OF METABOLITES
BY THE CHOROIDAL CIRCULATION

The choroid supplies the major portion of the metabolic demands of the retina (Dollery et al., 1969; Alm and Bill, 1972a; Shabo and Maxwell, 1972; Alder et al., 1983; Ahmed et al., 1993). Unlike the intraretinal vessels, in which the blood–retinal barrier is in the endothelial cells, the endothelial cells of the choriocapillaris contain fenestrations and are therefore leaky (Berstein and Hollenberg, 1965; Hogan et al., 1971; Spitznas and Reale, 1975). Fenestrated vessels are usually found in organs where large movement of fluid occurs between lumen and ablumenal compartments, such as the renal glomerulus (Levick, 1991). In the choriocapillaris the fenestrations measure 80 nm in diameter and, unlike those of the kidney, they have been suggested to possess diaphragms (Burns et al., 1986). The majority of the fenestrations face Bruch's membrane and to this extent the endothelial cell bodies and nuclei are located on the lateral and posterior surface of the vessels (Hogan et al., 1971). This is presumably to minimize the distance over which metabolic exchange occurs. Due to the presence of the fenestrations the capillaries of the choroid, unlike those of the retina, leak most plasma components, even large proteins (Cunha-Vaz et al., 1966; Pino and Essner, 1981; Raviola and Butler, 1983; Burns et al., 1986). Animal studies have suggested that the choroidal fenestrations are permeable to proteins of up to 70,000 daltons in weight (Pino and Essner, 1981).

Although the vast majority of the transcapillary flux occurs through the fenestrations, like all capillaries other routes also exist. Some small flux of metabolites may occur through the intracellular junctions of the endothelial cells and larger molecular entities may cross the endothelium by pinocytosis (Bungaard, 1983; Levick, 1991).

Differences in the dimensions of the capillaries of the two retinal vascular supplies may also influence the input of metabolites. The vessels of the choriocapillaris possess a width of at least 20 μm (Hogan et al., 1971) and are much wider than those of the retinal capillaries, which measure only 6 μm (Leber, 1903). The resistance of the choroidal capillaries is therefore much lower than that of the retinal capillaries, as evidenced by a rate of blood flow which is two hundred times greater in the former (Alm et al., 1973). This high choroidal rate of flow no doubt aids metabolic exchange by maintaining high concentration gradients across the vessel walls. High rates of flow also exist in the kidney, where high transcapillary transport also occurs (Folkow and Neil, 1971). In animal studies these high flow rates ensure that only 5% of the oxygen carried by the choroidal circulation is extracted (Alm and Bill, 1970), as opposed to an arteriovenous oxygen difference of 38% in the retinal vessels (Hickam et al., 1963). The regulation of blood flow in both sources of supply is unclear. The intraretinal vessels experience some regulation as blood flow increases in the dark and decreases in the light (Bill and Sperber, 1990). In contrast, blood flow in the choroidal capillaries is thought not to be so heavily autoregulated, as it alters with changes in intraocular pressure and blood pressure (Alm and Bill, 1972a; 1973). A greater regulatory mechanism in the retinal vessels is thought to be required to maintain a constant oxygen tension within the inner retina (Pournaras et al., 1978). A decrease in blood flow within the retinal capillaries could be traumatic, due to the already high degree of oxygen extraction (Alm and Bill, 1972). Tight regulation of choroidal circulation does not appear to be necessary, as reduction in choroidal blood flow will not significantly reduce the supply of nutrients to the retina (Törnquist and Alm, 1979). High flow rates within the choroid have also been suggested to act as a heat sink to conserve heat and counteract heat losses as a result of evaporation from the surface of the cornea (Sliney, 1986). Conversely, it has been proposed that the high rate of blood flow could act as a cooling mechanism to dissipate heat and prevent temperature rise in the retina, due to excessive absorption of optical radiation (Parver et al., 1980). With increasing age there is a loss of choroidal vascular elements. Studies have demonstrated that there is a progressive decrease in the thickness of the choroid from 200 μm at birth to 80 μm by the age of 90 years (Ramrattan et al., 1994). Using histological and resin-casting techniques, numerous authors have demonstrated an age-related decrease in the density and lumen diameter of the vessels of the choriocapillaris (Sarks, 1976; Bird et al., 1990; Olver et al., 1990; Ramrattan et al., 1994). Similar changes have been observed in other capillary beds, such as that of the testes (Takizawa and Hatakeyama, 1978). A decrease in the density and dimensions of the choroidal capillary bed is likely to reduce the potential for metabolic support. However, it is not known if this has a significant effect on the actual metabolic flux required to sustain the photoreceptors.

As the dimensions of the choroidal capillaries decrease, the width of intercapillary columns of Bruch's membrane increase (Sarks, 1976; Olver et al., 1990). As the columns widen they also show an increase in fibrous content and deposition of membranous debris. Killingsworth (1996) has suggested that at least some of the debris within the columns and in the outer collagenous layer may be derived from the death of cells within the choroid and that the coated vesicles in this region may represent incompletely degraded components of cellular elements that have passed into the membrane structure.

PIGMENT EPITHELIAL-DERIVED MATERIAL

The most widely held view for the accumulation of membranous debris of vesicular material within Bruch's membrane with age is that such material originates from the retinal pigment epithelium (Feeney-Burns et al., 1990; Ishibashi et al., 1986a, 1986b). It is suggested that in the young the phagocytic degradation of photoreceptor discs results in almost complete catabolism, with breakdown products that can either be recirculated to the photoreceptor cells or voided by the basal surface of the pigment epithelium. The voided material then has an unimpeded passage across Bruch's membrane into the choriocapillaris. It is suggested that with increasing age, the effects of progressive photochemical damage and impaired lytic activity by components of the RPE result in the egestion of material from the RPE that is inappropriately digested and therefore in a less degraded form (Marshall, 1986; Boulton et al., 1989; Kennedy et al., 1995). There are two concepts for the way in which debris accumulates on the inner aspect of Bruch's membrane. These concepts can be broadly categorized as active processes, or passive ones. Active accumulation is said to occur through the egestion of packets of cytoplasm, which bud off from the basal membrane of the RPE (Feeney-Burns and Ellersieck, 1985; Ishibashi et al., 1986). This process (confusingly termed "apoptosis" in those studies) may account for the senescent decrease in the infolding of the basal membrane of the RPE. However, it is difficult to explain in what form the material is transported from the secondary lysosomes to the basal membrane and, further, it does not account for the large arrays of membranous material seen within aging Bruch's membrane (Killingsworth, 1987). Marshall (1984) has postulated an alternative hypothesis whereby macromolecules passively moving into Bruch's membrane undergo concentration and free-energy aggregation (Pauleikhoff et al., 1990). This process is analogous to that of a Langmuir trough experiment, whereby artificial membranes are created in the absence of an energy source. Marshall considers that membrane aggregation of this sort also accounts for the sheets of membranous material seen in the subretinal space in the Royal College of Surgeons rat (Ansell and Marshall, 1974). In this animal the discs are shed from the photoreceptor cells, but not taken up by the underlying pigment epithelium. As part of the extracellular breakdown process the discs begin to fuse one with another in a free-energy situation to form huge continuous sheets.

With increasing age, more and more debris is seen within Bruch's membrane and such debris will include secondary lysosomes and coated membrane-bound bodies (Killingsworth, 1987). Killingsworth has supported the suggestion of Feeney-Burns and Ellersieck (1985) that the coated membrane-bound bodies represent RPE-derived plasma membrane-bound systems and that they are released via pinching off the basal plasma membrane of the RPE. The contents of such systems, the so-called vesicle-like bodies, give the indication that these are degrading cellular organelles. It should be remembered, however, that such vesicles are typical products of cell extraction techniques and almost certainly require zero energy in their formation.

With increasing age, the deposition of material between the pigment epithelium and its basement membrane infers some change in the metabolic function of the RPE, or significant change in the transport characteristics of the Bruch's membrane complex. Sarks (1976) has suggested that the highly membranous early form of basal laminar deposit may derive from impeded transport of waste materials through Bruch's membrane and that this in turn may contribute to the rather more organized structure of the late phase of basal laminar deposition. Although, again, the layering or wavelike deposition of late basal laminar deposit may be interpreted as the endpoint of a discontinuous manufacturing or voiding process from the RPE. Some evidence exists that cross-correlates photoreceptor and RPE status with that of debris deposition. For example, in a study by Sidikkaro et al. (1988) the quantity of debris accumulating at the basal surface of the RPE in culture was increased when outer segments had been exposed to radiation. This would suggest that if the phagocytic capacity of the RPE was stretched by, for example, excessive light exposure or other insult to photoreceptors, such as a genetic disorder, then the deposition of debris within Bruch's membrane might increase and, as it were, artificial or accelerated aging might take place. By contrast, if photoreceptor cells were lost from an area, then with time debris-dependent changes in Bruch's membrane might clear.

TRANSPORT ACROSS BRUCH'S MEMBRANE AND PUTATIVE CHANGES WITH AGE

Given the location and age-related changes within Bruch's membrane, it is perhaps not unreasonable to expect senescence-related alteration in its transport properties. Bird and Marshall (1986) proposed a model in which solute and fluid flux are impaired, as a result of increasing deposition of debris within Bruch's membrane as a function of age. This model is illustrated in

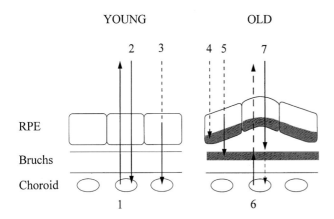

YOUNG   OLD

2   3   4 5   7

RPE

Bruchs

Choroid

1   6

FIGURE 34-7. Diagram to summarize key changes in vectorial transport mechanism between the retina and choroid as a function of age. For description see text.

Fig. 34-7 and described below. In the young eye, Bruch's membrane is free of deposits and presents a negligible barrier to the inward flux of metabolites from the choroid (1) and from the outward flux of both water (2) and waste material (3). In the older eye, the insidious effects of photochemical damage to the retina and the phagocytosis of photoreceptor discs give rise to the accumulation of lipofuscin in the RPE (4). The detrimental effect of lipofuscin on the RPE cell, even if only in occupying cell volume, results in incomplete catabolism of photoreceptor outer segments and the accumulation of debris within Bruch's membrane (5). The chemical nature of these deposits may determine their effects on the exchange capabilities of the membrane. Lipid-rich deposits, particularly those with a high content of neutral fats, may impose a significant hydrophobic barrier on the membrane. Such a barrier may inhibit the inward flux of water-soluble metabolites (6). Such a hydrophobic barrier would also restrict the net outflow of water from the retina (7). This model has been used to explain the formation of some pigment epithelial detachments (PEDs) in the elderly (Bird and Marshall, 1986). If a significant barrier to water movement could be generated, then fluid would collect between the pigment epithelium and Bruch's membrane. The continued active pumping of water and ions by the RPE outward would increase the volume of this fluid and ultimately detach the cells from their basement membrane. Originally, this mechanism of PED formation was proposed for those detachments which occurred in the absence of neovascularization of the subepithelial space. Therefore, in this original model, the concept was that water came from the retina and was trapped in its outward passage. In reality, most pigment epithelial detachments occur in the presence of a neovascular membrane; therefore, it could be argued that the subepithelial fluid orig-

inated from the choroid. However, in order for fluid to pool beneath the pigment epithelium, one must postulate some form of barrier that prevents it from entering the choroidal circulation and draining. Thus, regardless of whether a new vessel is present or absent, there is a requirement for some sort of hydrophobic barrier in Bruch's membrane in order to explain the observed clinical findings. Until relatively recently, few references confirmed a limited resistance to the movement of water across Bruch's membrane (Lyda et al., 1957; Fisher, 1987). The work of Pauleikhoff et al. (1990; 1992) seems to suggest that the lipid accumulation within Bruch's membrane with increasing age could be the site of a hydrophobic barrier and therefore could result in the entrapment of water. Within an inert extracellular system such as Bruch's membrane there is no active transport, and fluid movement is governed by passive processes. However, in vivo, active cellular processes, hydrostatic considerations, and osmotic gradients will all influence the flow across Bruch's membrane. It would be impossible to duplicate such a complex milieu in an in vitro investigation, and even if it was possible it would render analysis of the contribution of individual components extremely complex. In empirical studies, it is common to measure fluid movement either as a result of defined osmotic gradient, or due to a defined hydrostatic pressure. However, to measure water transport in response to an osmotic gradient, a knowledge of the membrane's permeability to the solute driving the gradient is required, as well as the stability of this relationship between samples. It is, therefore, more common to measure the fluid movement due to hydrostatic pressure (Fisher, 1982; 1987; Curry, 1984; Katz et al., 1992).

HYDRAULIC PERMEABILITY OR CONDUCTIVITY

The assessment of hydraulic permeability is, in essence, the measurement of bulk flow of fluid through a test membrane in response to an applied pressure. It is usually expressed as the hydraulic conductivity of the membrane. Experimentally, the conventional way to measure flux across a semipermeable membrane is to utilize an Ussing chamber and trap the subject membrane between the two compartments of the chamber (Ussing and Zerahn, 1950). Recently, two studies have been undertaken on the movement of water across Bruch's membrane–choroid samples using such chambers (Moore et al., 1995; Starita et al., 1996). Both of these studies evaluated the ability of water to move through Bruch's membrane in samples isolated from both peripheral retina and the macula. Both utilized samples in which a complex of Bruch's membrane and choroid were employed in the interface of the Ussing chamber. Complex samples of this kind were used because of the inability to systematically remove choroid from the external surface of Bruch's membrane. In pilot studies both authors demonstrated that reproducible results were obtained when hydraulic conductivity was measured retina to choroid. In the obverse direction, greater difficulties were experienced, presumably resulting from collapse of the choroidal vascular components under the applied pressure. In the system employed by Moore et al. (1995) hydraulic conductivity was measured in response to a changing pressure gradient. By contrast, the study of Starita et al. (1996) utilized a constant pressure head. Both studies showed a decrease in hydraulic conductivity in age, with that of the macular Bruch's membrane decreasing more rapidly than that of the periphery (Fig. 34-8). Both studies showed an exponential relationship, but the decay constants in the two studies varied. The Moore group found a halving of hydraulic conductivity for every 9.5 years of life, while the Starita group found the same decay over 15 years. The comparative data from these studies, together with that of Fisher (1987), is summarized in Table 34-1. It should be remembered that Fisher used an indirect method to obtain hydraulic conductivity, applying a known pressure to deform or bow an isolated disc of Bruch's membrane. The rate of decline of this membrane distortion as the tissue dome relaxed toward the flat plane was used to calculate the outflow through the membrane at the applied pressure and thus enabled calculation of hydraulic conductivity. In the studies of the Moore and Starita groups flow through the system

was measured directly. There are clear differences between Fisher's studies and those based on direct flow. This can be summarized as follows:

1. The age-related loss of hydraulic conductivity is minimal in Fisher's studies compared to the other two.
2. His values are lower at all age intervals. This is of interest in that Fisher claimed that his tissue preparation contained only Bruch's membrane. Thus, if the choroid was making a significant contribution to the restraint of water movement then his values should have been higher than those of the Moore and Starita groups.
3. There is a contradiction in the mode of decay of permeability between Fisher and the other two studies. Given the limited number of samples available to Fisher, he expressed his data as a linear decline in hydraulic conductivity (P < 0.02), with the value halving between the ages of 22 and 71 years. It is not possible to assess the fit of his data to an exponential equation, as he did not fully report the boundary conditions of his experiment.

Although Fisher and the other two studies show a similar trend in hydraulic conductivity, that is, decrease with increasing age, the discrepancy between the magnitude and time course of this decay warrants further discussion. It is perhaps pertinent to mention that Fisher also measured senescent variation in the hydraulic conductivity of the lens capsule (Fisher, 1987); he found that in the young eye the lens capsule was approximately six times less permeable to water than Bruch's membrane. Unlike Bruch's membrane, the hydraulic conductivity of the capsule increased by a factor of over 50% over an average lifetime. Fisher also suggested further differences between these two membrane systems, in that the young's modulus of elasticity of Bruch's membrane increases with age as the membrane becomes less flexible, while that of the lens decreases. Changes in the elasticity of Bruch's membrane with age are an important consideration in the disparity between the mode of senescent change in hydraulic conductivity reported in studies by the Moore and Starita groups and that reported by Fisher. Fisher postulated that with increasing pressure the various components of the membrane would be compressed and therefore resistance would increase. It could be argued that the greater elasticity of the young would allow greater compression and therefore measurements of fluid movement may be an underestimate. Further, in the elderly, it could be suggested that the senescent deposition of material within Bruch's membrane could either prevent membrane compression or increase its apparent effects. For example, debris within the membrane may provide additional resistance to compression, thereby maintaining a greater number of flow routes through the membrane, or com-

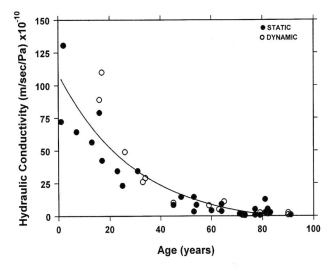

FIGURE 34-8. Age-related variation in hydraulic conductivity of Bruch's membrane as a function of age, from Moore et al., 1995 *(open circles)* and Starita et al., 1996 *(closed circles)*. Although the exponential relationships for these two sets of data differ, they do show good general agreement.

TABLE 34-1. *Summary of published data on measurements of hydraulic conductivity of Bruch's membrane*

Parameter	Findings, by reference		
	Fisher, 1987	Moore et al., 1995	Starita et al., 1996
Experimental method	Membrane relaxation	Dynamic method (continuous pressure changes)	Static method (fixed pressure)
Tissue preparation	Isolated Bruch's membrane	Bruch's–choroid complex	Bruch's–choroid complex
Number of eyes	6	13	23
Age range (years)	22–71	16–90	1–91
Tissue diameter	2.5 mm	4 mm	3.5 mm
Pressure	up to 2700 Pa	486.65–3406 Pa	583.98–2336 Pa
Hydraulic conductivity m·sec^{-1} Pa^{-1} × 10^{-10}	2.8–1.52	110.54–2.45	130.6–0.52
Age profile	linear	exponential $t_{1/2}$ = 9.5 years	exponential $t_{1/2}$ = 15 years

pression of a membrane containing debris may increase the percentage of internal space of the membrane taken up by debris and therefore reduce the number of available routes for flow. Fisher's concept is, however, dependent upon the fundamental requirement that increased pressure deforms the structure of the membrane and, in turn, decreases the rate of flow. The study of the Moore group demonstrated that flow as independent of the applied pressure over a physiological range of pressures. Further, although subtle differences exist between the data of the Moore and Starita groups, there is extremely good agreement when they are plotted together (Fig. 34-8).

The most surprising finding of the recent studies on water movement through Bruch's membrane is that the decay is exponential and that most of the loss of flow occurs in early life, long before significant buildup of debris within the membrane system. Many senescent changes in biological tissues follow a linear time course (Weale, 1993; 1995). In the limited number of studies where a sufficient number of samples of aging Bruch's membrane have been reported to be presented graphically, the overall thickness of the membrane also shows a linear relationship with age (Ramrattan et al., 1994). In the Ramrattan study, 120 eyes were studied and the authors demonstrated a linear relationship between increase in thickness and age, with membranes having overall dimensions that ranged from 2 μm in the first decade of life to 4.7 μm by the tenth decade. Unfortunately, this study did not measure the relative changes in the five sublayers within Bruch's membrane. In a more limited study, changes in thickness within the substrata of the membrane have been reported (Newsome et al., 1987). Although change appeared greater within

the inner layers of the membrane, no one layer seemed to dominate overall increase in thickness, and the age bands presented were too broad to enable direct comparison with the hydraulic conductivity data.

Many other studies of Bruch's membrane and its adjacent tissues show senescent changes to be most apparent after the age of 40, with some of these increasing in rate with progressive age (Severin et al., 1967; Sarks, 1976; Grindle and Marshall, 1978; Wing et al., 1978; Marshall et al., 1979; Gartner and Henkind, 1981; Feeney-Burns et al., 1984; van der Schaft, 1991; Curico et al., 1993; Ramrattan et al., 1994). It is difficult to reconcile the early rapid decline in hydraulic conductivity of Bruch's membrane with either the linear changes in thickness of the membrane, or those which become apparent from the age of forty. One could argue that the fit of the data of Moore et al. (1995) and Starita et al. (1996) to a monoexponential decay is fortuitous and aided by the small sample size. However, chance is an unlikely explanation for both the hydraulic conductivity of macular and peripheral samples adhering to the same mode of decay.

SITE OF MAXIMUM RESISTANCE WITHIN BRUCH'S MEMBRANE

Given the absence of significant morphological change in the overall membrane, or in any given substrata in the first four decades of life, a second series of experiments were undertaken by Starita et al. (1997). These experiments were an attempt to determine the layer in which change was occurring in early life that brought about the dramat-ic increase in resistance to flow (Starita et al.,

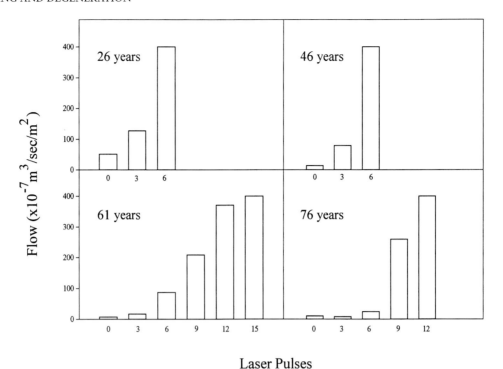

Laser Pulses

FIGURE 34-9. Histogram 😊 show the effect of laser ablation of Bruch's membrane on flow. Flow was determined in samples of Bruch's membrane obtained from four donors, age range 26 to 76 years. The bars for zero pulses corresponded to baseline flow prior to ablation. Total loss of barrier resulted in flow rates that could not be measured and these are represented as 400×10^{-7} m³/sec/m² in the bar charts. The data shows that a higher number of pulses is required to abolish membrane resistance with increasing age and that in young individuals the loss of resistance is progressive, while in the older individuals the first few pulses often have relatively little effect.

1997). In this series of experiments Bruch's membrane–choroid samples were again mounted in a modified Ussing chamber. However, in this chamber the innermost aspect of Bruch's membrane was irradiated in a controlled fashion with an argon fluoride excimer laser (193 nm). When argon fluoride excimer lasers are used to ablate the cornea, it has been shown that, depending on the hydration characteristics, at a radiant exposure of 180 mJ/cm², between 0.22 and 0.25 μm of tissue are removed per pulse (Krueger and Trokel, 1985). This ablation takes place over the entire area over which the beam falls, and typically such areas are in the order of millimeters in diameter. Starita et al. (1997) argued that if the ablation rate of Bruch's membrane was similar to that of the choroid it should be possible to progressively ablate the exposed subepithelial surface of Bruch's membrane while simultaneously measuring its hydraulic conductivity. The resistance to flow should drop to near zero immediately on ablation of the high-resistance barrier and thus locate the barrier to within 0.25 μm. Empirically, it was shown that, under the stated conditions, the ablation rate for Bruch's membrane was typically 0.11 μm per pulse. Findings of this study are summarized in Fig. 34-9, where two compo-

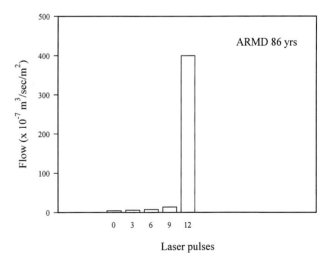

FIGURE 34-10. Histogram showing the effect of laser ablation on flow across Bruch's membrane of a donor affected with age-related macular degeneration. In this eye, where histology showed significant basal laminar deposit, the first nine pulses have virtually no effect on flow. This number of pulses would therefore again indicate high resistance in the inner collagenous layer.

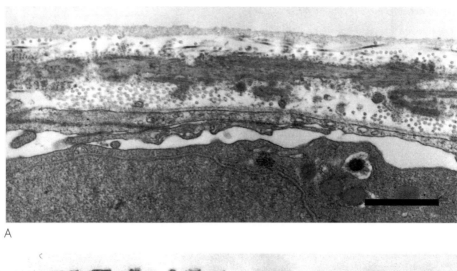

A

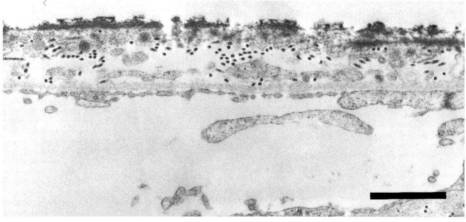

B

FIGURE 34-11. Transmission electron micrograph of isolated Bruch's membrane preparation from a 46-year-old donor. (A) unablated area showing all five layers of Bruch's membrane. (B) area of membrane retrieved from the Ussing chamber subsequent to ablation of sufficient material to remove high-resistance barrier. Note: all layers of the membrane internal to the layer of elastin have been removed. Bar marker is 1 μm.

nents are noted. First, more pulses are required to remove the high-resistance barrier with age; second, in younger eyes the effect of ablation is progressive, while in older eyes the first few pulses have a limited effect. The importance of this second finding is demonstrated in Fig. 34-10, the ablation characteristics and resistance drop recorded for an age-related macular degeneration (AMD) patient. In this patient the first nine pulses effected virtually no change in flow, while the final three pulses broke the barrier. On examining the specimens in electron microscopy subsequent to irradiation, the site of the barrier was seen to lie somewhere within the inner collagenous layer, as all samples had elastin and an intact outer collagenous layer and basement membrane complex of the choriocapillaris (Fig. 34-11). These findings suggest that throughout life a major barrier to flow

of water to Bruch's membrane lies within the inner collagenous layer. It further suggests that in later life an even denser barrier begins to be laid down internal to the inner collagenous layer. Simplistically, then, in the young, increase in resistance is due to some change within the inner collagenous layer that does not result in a morphologically detectable endpoint, while in the elderly this progressive change is further compounded by changes that give rise to either lipid entrapment or the basal laminar deposit. The work of Starita et al. (1997) in identifying the location of the high-resistance barrier has led to two further lines of investigation—first, a morphometric investigation of the various layers within Bruch's membrane and their changes with age, second, a biochemical study of the properties of aging collagen.

MORPHOMETRY OF THE FIBROUS LAYERS OF BRUCH'S MEMBRANE

In this study sections have been cut parallel to the plane of Bruch's membrane and examined in the electron microscope. By a grid analysis system, attempts have been made to estimate the space in the membrane not occupied by fibrous components. It could be argued that moving water molecules take the line of least resistance and therefore pass between, rather than through the fibrous elements. On this analysis the space between fibers is deemed to be "pore space," and the diameters of the "pores" vary within each of the three fibrous layers and with age. Typical illustrations of pore sizes in the various fibrous layers of a 75-year-old are seen in Fig. 34-12. By evaluating the number of sections between viewed samples, the lengths of the pores may also be estimated. Given the length, tortuosity, and pore size, modeling of movement of water and molecules through this system may be undertaken.

APPLICATION OF PORE THEORY TO TRANSPORT OF FLUIDS THROUGH BRUCH'S MEMBRANE

The porosity of individual layers of Bruch's membrane can be estimated by examining transmission electron microscopical (TEM) photomicrographs of sequential sections at various depths parallel to the surface. Within given limitations, classical pore theory formulations can then be applied to predict the transport characteristics of individual layers of the membrane. For Newtonian fluids in the absence of turbulent flow, the rate of transport through a capillary column is given by the Poiseuille equation:

$$F = \frac{P\Pi r^4}{8\eta l} \tag{34-1}$$

where

F = flow (m³/sec/m² surface area)

P = pressure diffential between the two surfaces of the membrane (Pa)

r = pore radius (m)

η = viscosity of fluid; saline, 0.97×10^{-3} (Pa sec)

l = pore length (m)

For a heterogeneous membrane with different pore sizes and distribution densities, the above equation is modified appropriately:

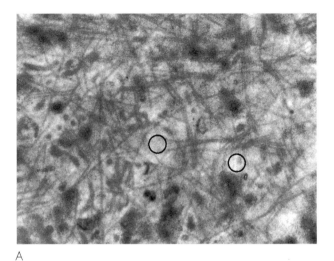

A

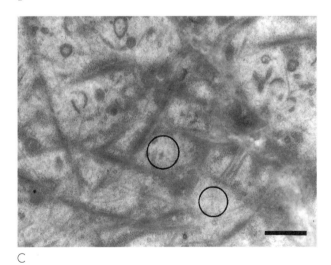

B

C

FIGURE 34-12. Transmission electron micrographs of Bruch's membrane sectioned tangentially to its surface, showing (A) the inner collagenous layer, (B) the layer of elastin, and (C) the outer collagenous layer. The dark circles give some indication as to the inter-fiber space, or pores. Analysis of material such as this has been utilized in the generation of results shown in Tables 34-2 and 34-3. The bar marker is 1 μm.

$$F = \sum_{1}^{i} \frac{P\Pi r_i^4}{8\eta l} \sigma_i \qquad (34\text{-}2)$$

where

$r_i = r_1, r_2, ...r_n$, radii of different pores

$\sigma_I = \sigma_1, \sigma_2, ...\sigma_n$, distribution density of individual pores

The TEM photomicrographs of individual layers of Bruch's membrane can be used to determine individual pore radii and their relative surface densities (see Fig. 34-12). Application of the pore theory model to biological membranes requires certain assumptions and modifications. First, the pores must be relatively large, so as to allow bulk flow and thereby permit the use of the Poiseuille equation. Second, the idealized pores must be cylinders of length equal to the thickness of an individual layer of Bruch's membrane. Minor considerations are that the pores are electrically neutral and that the membrane does not undergo pressure-induced compression.

As an example, the above simplified theory has been applied to Bruch's membrane from two elderly donors aged 75 and 81 years. Flow rates were calculated through individual layers at a unitary pressure differential of 1 Pa (Tables 34-2, 34-3).

The highest porosity, or largest pore size, was always observed in the elastin layer of the membrane, and computed flow rates were also considerably higher there. Flow in the outer collagenous zone was about 26%–52% of that in the elastin layer. The inner collagenous zone presented with the lowest porosity and in the two donors accounted for 5%–17% of the flow rate of the elastin layer. These rather simplistic calculations are in agreement with the excimer-based membrane sub-

fractionation techniques identifying the inner collagenous layer as the major site of the resistance barrier to fluid transport in Bruch's membrane.

BIOCHEMICAL STUDY OF COLLAGEN AGING

From Fig. 34-3 it can be seen that the inner collagenous layer contains collagens type I, III, and V; fibronectin; chondroitin sulphate; and dermatan sulphate. Each of the collagen types constitute an element for structural stabilization of extracellular matrices such as Bruch's membrane. The strength of the system emanates from the extensive intra- and interchain cross-linkage of collagen primarily involving disulphide and lysine-derived coupling (Siebold et al., 1988). With increasing age it has been shown in other collagenous tissues that increase in rigidity occurs and results from increased cross-linkage. Such cross-linkages are primarily S–S bonds. This dynamic remodeling of collagen could be an underlying mechanism contributing to the change in the stereospatial architecture of the collagen fibers with age and, again, contributing to a decline in hydraulic conductivity. This could also further promote deposition of lipidlike material and increase the likelihood of the formation of advanced glycosylation end products (AGEs). If Bruch's membrane behaves like any other similar tissues then an increase in S–S bonds should occur in the first four decades of life. While direct analysis of S–S bonds is not possible and indirect analysis of these entities subsequent to bond breaking is extremely difficult, -SH bonds are relatively easy to quantify. Any increase in S–S bonds as a function of age should be associated with a complementary decrease in -SH bonds. Starita et al. (1998) undertook both a histochemical and fluorometric analysis of thiol groups in Bruch's membrane, us-

TABLE 34-2. *Transport characteristics of individual layers of Bruch's membrane in a 75-year-old human donor*

Inner collagenous layer thickness 1.35×10^{-6} m			Elastin layer thickness 0.6×10^{-5} m			Outer collagenous layer thickness 0.75×10^{-6} m		
Pore radius $r_i \times 10^{-6}$ m	Pore density, $\sigma_i \times$ $10^{11}/m^2$	Flow $m^3/sec/m^2$ $\times 10^{-6}$	Pore radius, $r_i \times 10^{-6}$ m	Pore density, $\sigma_i \times$ $10^{11}/m^2$	Flow $m^3/sec/m^2$ $\times 10^{-6}$	Pore radius, $r_i \times 10^{-6}$ m	Pore density, $\sigma_i \times$ $10^{11}/m^2$	Flow $m^3/sec/m^2$ $\times 10^{-6}$
r_1 0.27	3.81	0.6072	r_1 0.465	2.858	9.02	r_1 0.405	1.905	2.767
r_2 0.21	3.81	0.2222	r_2 0.3	0.952	0.52	r_2 0.36	0.952	0.863
r_3 0.18	7.62	0.2399	r_3 0.27	0.952	0.341	r_3 0.33	0.952	0.6094
r_4 0.135	6.669	0.06643	r_4 0.24	0.952	0.2131	r_4 0.285	2.858	1.018
Total flow		1.136			10.09			5.257
Relative flow*		0.11			1.0			0.52

*Flow in the elastin layer is designated 1.0.

Pore size was determined from TEM micrographs of individual layers as follows: A grid template consisting of a descending gradient of fixed radii was placed on top of the micrographs, and the maximum pore size (r_1) together with frequency of occurrence was first obtained for each layer. This procedure was repeated for progressively smaller sizes, with r_4 being the smallest clearly discernible pore.

TABLE 34-3. *Transport characteristics of individual layers of Bruch's membrane in an 80-year-old human donor*

Inner collagenous layer thickness 1.35×10^{-6} m			Elastin layer thickness 0.6×10^{-6} m			Outer collagenous layer thickness 0.9×10^{-6} m		
Pore radius, $r_i \times 10^{-6}$ m	Pore density, $\sigma_i \times 10^{11}/m^2$	Flow $m^3/sec/m^2 \times 10^{-6}$	Pore radius, $r_i \times 10^{-6}$ m	Pore density, $\sigma_i \times 10^{11}/m^2$	Flow $m^3/sec/m^2 \times 10^{-6}$	Pore radius, $r_i \times 10^{-6}$ m	Pore density, $\sigma_i \times 10^{11}/m^2$	Flow $m^3/sec/m^2 \times 10^{-6}$
r_1 0.195	1.905	0.083	r_1 0.51	0.9527	4.35	r_1 0.3	0.9257	0.337
r_2 0.18	4.7635	0.15	r_2 0.39	0.9527	1.49	r_2 0.24	4.7635	0.711
r_3 0.15	4.7635	0.072	r_3 0.3	0.9527	0.52	r_3 0.21	2.858	0.25
r_4 0.135	1.905	0.019	r_4 0.24	1.905	0.43	r_4 0.18	9.529	0.45
Total flow		0.324			6.79			1.748
Relative flow*		0.05			1.0			0.26

*Flow in the elastin layer is designated as 1.0.

ing a modification of the method of Ogawa et al. (1979). This technique used homogenized discs of Bruch's membrane and choroid and quantified thiols fluorometrically after reaction with 7 diethylamino-3-(4-maleimidylphenyl)-4-methylcoumarin(cpm) (Ayers et al., 1986). The results are shown in Fig. 34-13 and, although few eyes in the younger age group were obtained, there is a clear decrease in thiol groups as a function of age, showing a 58% reduction in the macular region of Bruch's membrane and choroid between the ages of 37 and 86. Of concern to the authors was that while Bruch's membrane was increasing in thickness with age, the choroid

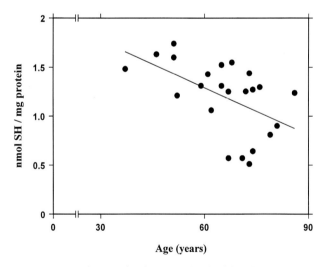

FIGURE 34-13. Showing the changes in levels of free thiols in macular samples expressed per milligram protein as a function of age. Data shows a significant loss of free thiols during the aging process with a 58% reduction between the ages of 37 and 86 years. Linear regression parameters were, nM SH/mg protein = $-0.016*$ Age $+2.25$, r = -0.524, p < 0.01.

was decreasing. Therefore, they also expressed their results in terms of unit protein in the sample and, again, there was a significant age-dependent decrease. In order to determine which proportion of the thiols was in the choroidal compartment and which was in Bruch's membrane, a second series of experiments was undertaken in which the excimer laser was used to ablate away either Bruch's membrane or an equivalent volume of tissue from the choroidal surface. These experiments showed that almost 50% of the thiols measured in the samples were derived from Bruch's membrane alone. This is strong indirect evidence that cross-linkages of collagen play a major role in the age-related changes in the permeability of Bruch's membrane in the young. It further supports the previous observations of Karwatowski et al. (1991) that also indirectly inferred greater cross-linkage of fibers, in that the solubility of extracted collagen from Bruch's membrane decreases linearly as a function of age. In a further study it was shown that the normal mature enzymically formed collagen cross-linkages, such as hydroxylysyl-pyridinoline, which stabilized the structure of collagen, did not change with age, but additional unidentified cross-links responsible for molecular aggregation and decrease in solubility were detected (Karwatowski et al., 1995). In addition to the lysinehydroxylysine-derived cross-linkage sites there are abundant cysteine residues. These have the potential for forming both intra- and intermolecular disulphide bonds—the former would be involved in monomer stabilization and the latter may result in disulphide stabilized networks (Siebold et al., 1988). As such, disulphide bridging accounts for nearly 88% of intramolecular bonds in type IV collagen with elastin also possessing a potential for cystein-based cross-linkage.

Any reduction in the level of free thiols has ramifications for the structural and functional integrity of

Bruch's membrane. If the increased disulphide bridging occurred between collagen chains, intermolecular, the result would be greater rigidity of the matrix at the expense of reduction of porosity of the membrane. Both inter- and intramolecular increases in nonphysiological disulphide bridging are likely to cause further conformational alterations in the polypeptide backbone, leading to exposure of other normally hidden and protected potential cross-linking sites. Exposed lysine and hydroxylysine residues, for example, can undergo nonenzymic glycosylation and, following molecular rearrangement and stabilization to Amadori products, can react with other protein molecules to form AGEs (Vasan et al., 1996). The combination of greater component cross-linkage, due to either lysine-derived or disulphide bridging with the entrapment of passing protein molecules, will certainly reduce porosity and result in further significant reduction in transport capacity.

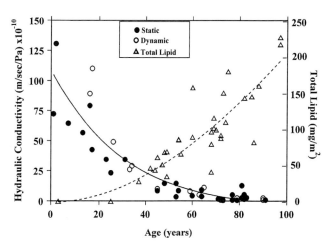

FIGURE 34-14. Hydraulic permeability and lipid content of Bruch's membrane–choroid complex comparing data from Moore et al., 1995, ("dynamic"; *open circles*), Starita et al., 1996, ("static"; *dark circles*), with lipid content data of Holz et al., 1994 *(triangles)*. Note the dramatic loss of hydraulic conductivity long before buildup of lipids.

LIPID ACCUMULATION

First analysis of the data would seem to indicate that because the major changes in hydraulic conductivity of Bruch's membrane occur within the first four decades of life (Moore et al., 1995; Starita et al., 1996) and because lipid accumulation only becomes of significance after the age of forty (Pauleikhoff et al., 1990; Holz et al., 1994), the original hypothesis of Bird and Marshall (1986) was in error. It should be remembered that the total lipid content of Bruch's membrane increases from O mg/m² during the first three decades to 220 mg/m² by the tenth. Since the studies of the Holz (1994), Moore (1995), and Starita (1996) groups contained eyes from roughly similar age groups, direct comparisons could be made between them. To aid analysis, data from all three studies were subdivided into four sample groups of comparable age. The age groups were 1–21, 22–44, 45–69, and 70–88. The number of donor eyes in each group varied for each study, but in almost all cases the Holz group had the most samples. For each group the mean values were calculated for total extractable lipids and resistance of Bruch's membrane. Fig. 34-14 and 34-15 show that the data gave rise to a nonlinear relationship between the level of lipid deposits and the resistance of the membrane to fluid transport. Both figures demonstrate that low-level accumulation of lipid, up to approximately 50 mg/m², does not appear to influence resistance to any appreciable extent. Such levels will be present during the first four decades of life and therefore would support the existence of an alternative mechanism for the rapid decline in hydraulic conductivity during this period. The figures are, however, a clear demon-

stration that in later life lipid accumulation leads to significant alteration in the resistance of the membrane. Thus, these results support the original hypothesis of Bird and Marshall (1986) that lipid deposition in the aging macula would be expected to impart hydrophobic properties to Bruch's membrane and thus interfere with local fluid dynamics.

THE IMPLICATIONS OF AGING IN BRUCH'S MEMBRANE FOR METABOLIC SUPPLY OF THE OUTER RETINA

From the data, the general pattern of age-related change may be illustrated in Fig. 34-16. In the young, each of the three fibrous layers has pore sizes which are maximal, but those of the inner collagenous layer are smallest. This would suggest that in the young diffusion is at its maximum and the rate-limiting layer is the inner collagenous layer. From late teens to late thirties, the fibrous content and membranous debris, coated membrane-bound bodies, and wide-spaced collagen begins to accumulate, causing a net reduction in effective pore size, which results in decreased flow. From forties to sixties, this process is exacerbated and results in a significant increase in the thickness of the various layers, increasing tortuosity and further decreasing pore size. Again, maximal resistance is in the inner collagenous layer and is further exacerbated by the presence of lipids. From late sixties to disease state, the system undergoes further degenerative change with now an in-

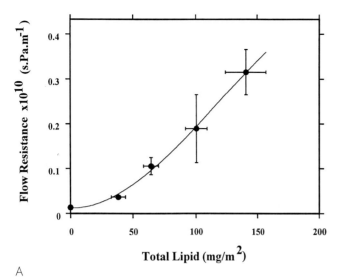

A

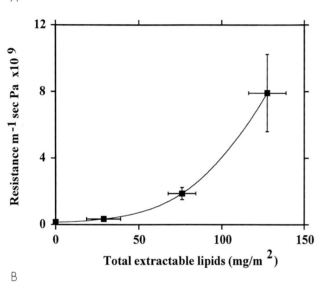

B

FIGURE 34-15. Graphs showing the relationship between resistance to flow (the reciprocal of hydraulic conductivity) and extractable lipid. For comparative purposes the data were grouped in 15-year age bands. The cross-plots refer to the mean (±SEM) for each age band. No point for the 0 to 15-year age band is shown, because of the lack of hydraulic conductivity values within this region. (a) Moore et al., 1995; (b) Starita et al., 1996.

creasing problem due to significant amounts of basal laminar deposit. From the limited studies using the excimer laser on age-related macula (Starita et al., 1997) this layer seems to be highly resistant to flow. This model, dependent upon specific changes within individual layers of Bruch's membrane, may explain why exponential changes in resistance are observed during early life, while changes in overall thickness of the membrane are linear (Fig. 34-17).

In order to obtain some estimate of the fluid exchange

capabilities in man and the impact of the above variations with age, a number of assumptions and simplifications must be made. First, no value for the flow rate through the RPE in man is currently available; for this analysis the rate must be assumed to be similar to those obtained for other species (Frambach and Marmor, 1982; Negi and Marmor, 1986; Hughes et al., 1984; Tsuboi and Pedersen, 1988; Tsuboi, 1987). Second, although osmosis must play a role in fluid movement, in the absence of data it will be assumed that the osmotic pull of the choroid is negligible. Third, in the absence of direct measurement, the hydrostatic pressure dissipated across Bruch's membrane is taken as 4 mm Hg (533 Pa) (Emi et al., 1989). With these assumptions and the measured values of hydraulic conductivity, some estimate of total fluid exchange can be made. The basic equation for hydraulic conductivity is as follows:

$$Lp = (J/S)/P \qquad (34\text{-}3)$$

where Lp is the hydraulic conductivity of the membrane, J is the flux/unit area, S is the area and P the applied pressure. By rearranging we can solve for J/S, the flow/unit area.

$$J/S = (Lp \cdot P) \qquad (34\text{-}4)$$

Substituting the hydraulic conductivities measured for a 17-year-old and 90-year-old of, respectively, 110.5 × 10^{-10} and 2.2 × 10^{-10} m/sec/Pa (Moore et al., 1995), it is determined that Bruch's membrane can pass 2000 μl/hour/cm² in the young, a figure dropped to 46 μl/hour/cm² in the 90-year-old.

From these simplistic calculations it would appear that the young Bruch's membrane has a potential to cope with flow rates far in excess of those produced by the pigment epithelium. This does not, however, hold for the aged Bruch's membrane. With a 4 mm Hg pressure differential the Bruch's membrane potential capacity for flow in the elderly is only marginally higher than the largest estimate of 32 μl/hour/cm² for the fluid movement through the RPE. Thus, in the young, Bruch's membrane does not constitute a rate-limiting resistance to flow; by contrast, in the elderly it may be a far more significant barrier and may impact upon the homeostasis of the overlying photoreceptor cells.

It would appear then that changes in the movement of fluid through Bruch's membrane as a function of age arise in response to at least three mechanisms. The first mechanism occurs in early life and may relate to changes in the effective "pore size" within fibrous layers of the membrane due to collagen cross-linkage and entrapment of other protein molecules. A second mechanism is apparent in midlife and relates to the progressive accumulation of lipids. Finally, in some individuals a com-

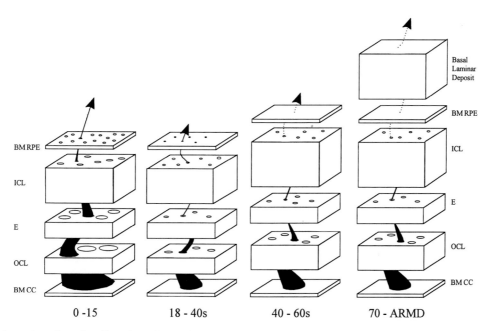

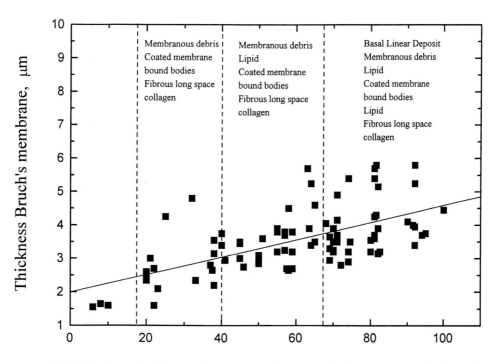

FIGURE 34-16. Schematic to show the effect of membrane changes as a function of age on fluid flow through the system. In early childhood pore sizes are such that little if any impedence occurs to the passage of molecular moeities through the system. By late teens to early forties changes in pore size and collagen cross-linkage may begin to effect overall transport capacity. In late forties to early sixties pore size changes are further exacerbated by accumulation of lipids and increase in membrane thickness. Depending on the class of lipid, fluid flow may be further compromised. In early seventies to later life these changes are further exacerbated by deposition of material at the interface between the pigment epithelium and the basement membrane of the RPE in the form of basal laminar deposits.

FIGURE 34-17. Graph showing the data of Ramrattan et al., 1994, with a linear increase in thickness of Bruch's membrane as a function of age. The age groups illustrated in Figure 34-16 and accompanying changes are superimposed.

689

bination of the effects of both of these systems may lead to a significant reduction in the transport capacity of the system, such that changes begin to occur at the interface between the pigment epithelium and Bruch's membrane and result in the deposition of basal laminar deposit. Whether the production of this basal laminar deposit is a sign of advanced senescence or an indication of disease has yet to be resolved.

REFERENCES

Ahmed J, Braun RD, Dunn R, Linsenmeier RA. 1993. Oxygen distribution in the Macaque retina. Invest Ophthalmol Vis Sci 34:516–521.

Alder VA, Cringle SJ, Constable IJ. 1983. The retinal oxygen profile in cats. Invest Ophthalmol Vis Sci 24:30.

Alm A, Bill A. 1972. The oxygen supply to the retina: II. Effects of high intraocular pressure and of increased arterial carbon dioxide tension on the uveal and retinal blood flow in cats: a study with labelled microspheres including flow determination in brain and some other tissues. Acta Physiol Scand 84:306–316.

Alm A, Bill A. 1973. Ocular and optic nerve blood flow at normal and increased intraocular pressure in monkeys (Macaca irus): a study with radioactively labelled microspheres including flow determinations in brain and some other tissues. Exp Eye Res 15:15.

Alm A, Bill A, Young F. 1973. The effects of pilocarpine and neostigmine on the blood flow through the anterior uvea in monkeys: a study with radioactively labelled microspheres. Exp Eye Res 15:31.

Ansell PL, Marshall J. 1974. The distribution of extracellular acid phosphatase in the retina of retinitis pigmentosa rats. Exp Eye Res 19:273–279.

Ayers SC, Warner GL, Smith KL, Lawrence DA. 1986. Fluorometric quantitation of cellular and non-protein thiols. Analytical Biochem 154:186–193.

Berstein MH, Hollenberg MJ. 1965. Fine structure of the choriocapillaris and the retinal capillaries. Invest Ophthalmol Vis Sci 4:1016.

Bill A, Sperber GO. 1990. Aspects of oxygen and glucose consumption in the retina: effects of high intraocular pressure and light. Graefes Arch Clin Exp Ophthalmol 228:124–127.

Bird AC, Bressler NM, Bressler SB, Chisholm IH, Coscas G, Davies MD, De Jong PTVM, Klaver CCW, Klein BEK, Klein R, Mitchell P, Sarks JP, Sarks SH, Soubrane G, Taylor HR, Vigerling JR. 1995. The International ARM Epidemiological Study Group. An international classification and grading system for age related maculopathy and age related macular degeneration. Surv Ophthalmol 39:367–374.

Bird AC, Marshall J. 1986. Retinal pigment epithelial detachments in the elderly. Trans Soc Ophthalmol UK 105:674–682.

Bird AC, Pauleikhoff D, Olver J, Maguire J, Sheraidah G, Marshall J. 1990. The correlation of choriocapillaris and Bruch's membrane changes in ageing. Invest Ophthalmol Vis Sci 31:228.

Boulton M, McKechnie NM, Breda J, Bayly M, Marshall J. 1989. The formation of autofluorescent granules in cultured human RPE. Invest Ophthalmol Vis Sci 30:82–89.

Braekevelt C, Hollandberg M. 1974. Development of the retinal pigment epithelium, choriocapillaris and Bruch's membrane in the albino rat. Exp Eye Res 9:124.

Bressler N, Bressler S, Fine S. 1988. Age related macular degeneration. Surv Ophthalmol 32:375–413.

Bressler N, Bressler S, West S, Fine S, Taylor HR. 1989. The grading and prevalence of macular degeneration in Chesapeake Bay waterman. Arch Ophthalmol 107:847–852.

Bungaard M. 1983. Vesicular transport in capillary endothelium: does it occur? Fedn Proc 42:2425–2430.

Burns MS, Bellhorn RW, Korte GE, Heriot WJ. 1986. Plasticity of the retinal vasculature. In: Osborne N, Chader G, eds, Progress in Retinal Research, Oxford: Pergamon Press, 253–308.

Call T, Hollyfield J. 1990. Sulphated proteoglycans in Bruch's membrane of the human eye: localisation and characterisation using cupromeronic blue. Exp Eye Res 51:451–462.

Capon MR, Marshall J, Krafft J, Alexander RA, Hiscott PS, Bird AC. 1989. Sorsby's fundus dystrophy: a light and electron microscopic study. Ophthalmology 96:1769–1777.

Coffey A, Brownstein S. 1986. The presence of macular drusen in post mortem eyes. Am J Ophthalmol 102:164–171.

Cunha-Vaz JG, Shakib M, Ashton N. 1966. Studies on the permeability of the blood ocular barrier. Br J Ophthalmol 50:441.

Curico CA, Millican CL, Allen KA, Kalina RE. 1993. Ageing of the human photoreceptor mosaic: evidence for selective vulnerability of rods in the central retina. Invest Ophthalmol Vis Sci 34:3278–3296.

Curry FE. 1984. Mechanics and thermodynamics of transcapillary exchange. In: Geiger SR, Renkin EM, Michel CC, eds, Handbook of Physiology Section 2; The Cardiovascular System. Bethesda: Amer Physiological Soc 4:309–374.

Dollery C, Bulpitt C, Kohner E. 1969. Oxygen supply to the retina from the retinal and choroidal circulations at normal and increased arterial oxygen tensions. Invest Ophthalmol Vis Sci 8:588.

Eagle RC. 1984. Mechanisms of maculopathy. Ophthalmology 91:613–625.

Emi K, Pederson JE, Toris CB. 1989. Hydrostatic pressure of the suprachoroidal space. Invest Ophthalmol Vis Sci 30:233–238.

Feeney-Burns L, Ellersieck MR. 1985. Age related changes in the ultrastructure of Bruch's membrane. Am J Ophthalmol 100:686–697.

Feeney-Burns L, Hilderbrand ES, Eldridge S. 1984. Ageing human RPE: morphometric analysis of macular, equatorial and peripheral cells. Invest Ophthalmol Vis Sci 25:195–200.

Feeney-Burns L, Burns RP, Gao C. 1990. Age-related macular changes in humans over ninety years old. Am J Ophthalmol 109:265–278.

Fisher RF. 1982. The water permeability of basement membrane under increasing pressure: evidence for a new theory of permeability. Proc Royal Soc B 216:475–496.

Fisher RH. 1987. The influence of age on some ocular basement membranes. Eye 1:184–189.

Folkow B, Neil E, eds. 1971. Circulation. New York: Oxford University Press.

Frambach DA, Marmor MF. 1982. The rate and route of fluid reabsorption from the subretinal space of the rabbit. Invest Ophthalmol Vis Sci 22:292–302.

Garner A, Sarks S, Sarks JP. 1994. Degenerative and related disorders of the retina and choroid. In: Garner A, Klintworth GK, eds, Pathobiology of Ocular Disease: A Dynamic Approach, 2nd ed., New York: Marcel Dekker 631–674.

Garron LK. 1963. The ultrastructure of the RPE with observations on the choriocapillaris and Bruch's membrane. Trans Am Ophthalmol Soc 61:545.

Gartner S, Henkind P. 1981. Ageing and degeneration of the human macula. I. Outer nuclear layer and photoreceptors. Br J Ophthalmol 65:23–28.

Gass JDM. 1987. Stereoscopic Atlas of Macular Diseases. Vol 1. Diagnosis and Treatment. 3rd ed. St Louis: Mosby.

Green WR, Enger C. 1993. The 1992 Lorenz E Zimmerman Lecture. Age related macular degeneration histopathologic studies. Ophthalmology 100:1519–1535.

Green WR, McDonnell PJ, Yeo JH. 1985. Pathologic features of senile macular degeneration. Ophthalmology 92:615–627.

Grindle CFJ, Marshall J. 1978. Ageing changes in Bruch's membrane and their functional implications. Trans Soc Ophthalmol UK 98: 172–175.

Hickam J, Frayser R, Ross J. 1963. A study of retinal venous blood oxygen saturation in human subjects by photographic means. Circulation 27:375.

Hogan MJ. 1961. Ultrastructure of the choroid: its role in the pathogenesis of choroidal diseases. Trans Pat Coast Oto Ophthalmol Soc 42:61.

Hogan MJ, Alvarado J. 1967. Studies on the human macula. IV Ageing changes in Bruch's membrane. Arch Ophthalmol 77:410–420.

Hogan MJ, Alvarado JA, Weddell JE. 1971. Histology of the Human Eye: An Atlas and Textbook. Philadelphia: Saunders.

Holz F, Sheraidah G, Pauleikhoff D, Bird AC. 1994. Analysis of lipid deposits extracted from human macular and peripheral Bruch's membrane. Arch Ophthalmol 112:402–406.

Hughes BA, Miller SS, Machen TE. 1984. Effects of cyclic AMP on the fluid absorption and the ion transport across the frog retinal pigment epithelium. J Gen Physiol 83:875.

Ishibashi T, Sorgente N, Patterson R, Ryan SJ. 1986a. Ageing changes in Bruch's membrane of monkeys: an electron microscopic study. Ophthalmologica 192:179–190.

Ishibashi T, Patterson R, Ohnishi Y, Inomata H, Ryan SJ. 1986b. Formation of drusen in the human eye. Am J Ophthalmol 101:342–353.

Kanwar YS, Linker A, Farquar MG. 1980. Increased permeability of the glomerular basement membrane to ferritin after removal of glycosaminoglycans (heparin sulphate) by enzyme digestion. J Cell Biol 86:688.

Karwatowski WSS, Jefferies TE, Duance VC, Albon J, Bailey AJ, Easty DL. 1991. Collagen and Ageing in Bruch's membrane. Biochem Soc Trans UK 19:349(S).

Karwatowski WSS, Jefferies TE, Duance VC, Albon J, Bailey AJ, Easty DL. 1995. Preparation of Bruch's membrane and analysis of age-related changes in the structural collagens. Br J Ophthalmol 79:944–952.

Katz MA, Barrette T, Krasovich M. 1992. Hydraulic conductivity of basement membrane with computed values for the fibre radius and void volume ratio. Am J Physiol (Heart Circ Physiol 32) 263: H1417–H1421.

Kennedy CJ, Rakoczy PE, Constable IJ. 1995. Lipofuscin of the retinal pigment epithelium: a review. Eye 9:763–771.

Killingsworth MC. 1987. Age related components of Bruch's membrane in the eye. Graefes Arch Clin Exp Ophthalmol 225:406–412.

Killingsworth MC. 1996. Choroidal cell death may contribute to the formation of age-related deposits in Bruch's membrane. (Unpublished work.)

Klein BA. 1947. Angioid streaks: a clinical and histopathological study. Am J Ophthalmol 30:955–968.

Klein R, Klein BEK, Linton KLP. 1992. Epidemiology of age related maculopathy: the beaver dam eye study. Ophthalmology 99:933–943.

Krueger RR, Trokel SL. 1985. Quantitation of corneal ablation by ultraviolet laser light. Arch Ophthalmol 103:1741–1742.

Leber T. 1903. Circulationsund Ernährungsverhältnisse des Auges. In: Graefe A, Sämisch T, eds, Handbuch der gesamten Augenheilkunde. Leipzig: Springer-Verlag.

Lerche W. 1963. Electron microscopic observations of Bruch's membrane in the human eye. Ber Dtsch Ophthalmol Ger 65:384.

Leure de Pree A. 1968. Ultrastructure of the retinal pigment epithelium in domestic sheep. Am J Ophthalmol 65:383–398.

Levick JR. 1991. Haemodynamics: pressure, flow and resistance. In: An Introduction to Cardiovascular Physiology. London: Butterworth 90:117.

Löffler KU, Lee WR. 1986. Basal linear deposit in the human macula. Graefes Arch Clin Exp Ophthalmol 224:493–501.

Lyda W, Eriksen N, Krishna N. 1957. Flow and permeability studies in a Bruch's membrane choroid preparation. Am J Ophthalmol 44:362–369.

Marshall GE, Kontas AGP, Lee WR. 1993. Collagens in ocular tissue. Br J Ophthalmol 77:515–524.

Marshall J. 1984. Radiation and the ageing eye. Ophthalmol Physiol Opt 4:1–23.

Marshall J. 1986. Light damage and ageing in the human macula. Res Clin Forums 7:27–43.

Marshall J, Grindle J, Ansell PL, Berwein B. 1979. Convolutions in human rods: an ageing process. Br J Ophthalmol 63:181–187.

Moore DJ, Hussain AA, Marshall J. 1995. Age-related variation in the hydraulic conductivity of Bruch's membrane. Invest Ophthalmol Vis Sci 36:1290–1297.

Negi A, Marmor MF. 1986. Quantitative estimation of the metabolic transport of subretinal fluid. Invest Ophthalmol Vis Sci 27:1564–1568.

Newsome DA, Huh W, Green WR. 1989. Bruch's membrane age-related changes vary by region. Curr Eye Res 6:1211–1221.

Ogawa H, Taneda A, Kanaoka Y, Sekine T. 1979. The histochemical distribution of protein-bound sulphedral groups in human epidermis by the new staining method. J Histochem Cytochem 27:942–946.

Olver J, Pauleikhoff D, Bird AC. 1990. Morphometric analysis of age changes in the choriocapillaris. Invest Ophthalmol Vis Sci 31:229.

O'Rahilly R. 1975. The prenatal development of the human eye. Exp Eye Res 21:23.

Parver L, Auker C, Carpenter D. 1980. Choroidal blood flow as a heat dissipating mechanism in the macula. Am J Ophthalmol 89:641.

Pauleikhoff D, Harper CA, Marshall J, Bird AC. 1990. Ageing changes in Bruch's membrane: a histochemical and morphological study. Ophthalmology 97:171–178.

Pauleikhoff D, Zuels S, Sheraidah GS, Marshall J, Wessing A, Bird AC. 1992. Correlation between biochemical composition and fluorescein binding of deposits in Bruch's membrane. Ophthalmology 99:1548–1553.

Pino RM, Essner E. 1980. Structure and permeability to ferritin of the choriocapillary endothelium in the rat. Cell and Tissue Res 208:21–27.

Pino RM, Essner E. 1981. Permeability of the rat choriocapillaris to haeme proteins: restriction of tracers by a fenestrated endothelium. J Histochem Cytochem 29:281–290.

Pino RM, Essner E, Pino LC. 1982. Localisation and chemical composition of anionic sites in Bruch's membrane of the rat. J Histochem Cytochem 30:245–252.

Pournaras C, Tsacopoulos M, Chapuis P. 1978. Studies on the role of prostaglandins in the regulation of retinal blood flow. Exp Eye Res 26:687–697.

Ramrattan RS, van der Schaft TL, Mooy CM, de Bruijn WC, Mulder PGH, de Jong PTVM. 1994. Morphometric analysis of Bruch's membrane, the choriocapillaris and the choroid in ageing. Invest Ophthalmol Vis Sci 35:2857–2864.

Raviola G, Butler JM. 1983. Unidirectional vesicular transport mechanisms in retinal vessels. Invest Ophthalmol Vis Sci 24:1465–1474.

Rittig M, Lutjein-Drecoll E, Rauterberg J, Jander R, Mollenhauer J. 1990. Type VI collagen in the human iris and ciliary body. Tissue and Cell Res 259:305–312.

Sarks SH. 1976. Ageing and degeneration in the macular region: a clinico-pathological study. Br J Ophthalmol 60:324–341.

Sarks SH, Sarks JP, Killingsworth MC. 1988. Basal laminar deposit, membranous debris and drusen. In: Zingirian M, Piccolino F, eds, Retinal Pigment Epithelium. Milan: Kugler and Ghedini 187–190.

Sarks J, Sarks S, Killingsworth MC. 1994. Evolution of soft drusen in age related macular degeneration. Eye 8:269–283.

Severin SL, Tour RL, Kershaw RH. 1967. Macular function and the photostress test 1. Arch Ophthalmol 77:2–7.

Shabo AL, Maxwell DS. 1972. The blood aqueous barrier to tracer protein: a light and electron microscopic study of the primate ciliary process. Microvac Res 4:142.

Sheraidah G, Steinmetz R, Maguire J, Pauleikhoff D, Marshall J, Bird AC. 1993. Correlation between lipids extracted from Bruch's membrane and age. Ophthalmology 100:47–51.

Sidikkaro Y, Trüb PR, Morse L. 1988. The formation of drusen-like nodules by cultured RPE enhanced by UV irradiated rod outer segments. Invest Ophthalmol Vis Sci 28:9.

Siebold B, Deutzmann R, Kuhn K. 1988. The arrangement of intra- and intermolecular disulphide bonds in the carboxyterminal, non-collagenous aggregation and cross-linking domain of basement membrane Type IV collagen. Eur J Biochem 176:617–624.

Sliney DH. 1986. Physiological factors in cataractogenesis: ambient ultraviolet radiation and temperature. Invest Ophthalmol Vis Sci 27:781–790.

Spitznas M, Reale E. 1975. Fracture forces of fenestrations and junctions of endothelial cells in human choroid vessels. Invest Ophthalmol Vis Sci 14:98–107.

Starita C, Hussain AA, Pagliarini S, Marshall J. 1996. Hydrodynamics of ageing Bruch's membrane: implications for macular disease. Exp Eye Res 62:565–572.

Starita C, Hussain AA, Patmore A, Marshall J. 1997. Localisation of the site of major resistance to fluid transport in Bruch's membrane. Invest Ophthalmol Vis Sci 38:762–767.

Starita C, Willmott N, Hussain AA, Marshall J. 1998. Fluorometric quantitation of thiol groups in Bruch's membrane and their importance in the ageing process. (In preparation.)

Sumita R. 1961. The fine structure of Bruch's membrane in the choroid. Acta Soc Ophthalmol Jpn 65:1188.

Takizawa T, Hatakeyama S. 1978. Age associated changes in the human adult testis. Acta Path Jpn 28:541–554.

Törnquist P, Alm A. 1979. Retinal and choroidal contribution to retinal metabolism in vivo: a study in pigs. Acta Physiol Scand 106:351.

Tsuboi S. 1987. Measurement of the volume flow and the hydraulic conductivity across the isolated dog retinal pigment epithelium. Invest Ophthalmol Vis Sci 28:1776–1782.

Tsuboi S, Pederson JE. 1988. Volume flow across the isolated RPE of cynomolgus monkey eyes. Invest Ophthalmol Vis Sci 29:1652–1655.

Ussing HU, Zerahn K. 1950. Active transport of sodium as the source of electric current in the short circuited isolated frog skin. Acta Phys Scand 23:111–127.

van der Schaft TL, de Bruijn WC, Mooy CM, Ketelaars DAM, de Jong PTVM. 1991. Is basal laminar deposit unique for AMD? Arch Ophthalmol 109:420–425.

van der Schaft TL, Mooy CM, Bruijn WC, Oron FG, Mulder PGH, de Jong PTVM. 1992. Histological features of the early stages of age-related macular degeneration: a statistical analysis. Ophthalmology 99:278–286.

van der Schaft TL, Mooy CM, de Bruijn WC, de Jong PT. 1994. Early stages of AMD: an immunofluorescence and electron microscopic study. Br J Ophthalmol 77:657–661.

Vasan S, Zhang X, Kapurniotu A, Bernhagen T, Teichberg S, Basgen J, Wagele D, Schih D, Terlecky I, Bucala R, et al. 1996. An agent cleaving glucose-derived protein cross-links in vitro and in vivo. Nature 382:275–278.

Weale RA. 1993. Have human biological functions evolved in support of a life span. Mech Age Dev 69:65–77.

Weale RA. 1995. The lifelong preservation of sight. In: Adaptations in Ageing. London: Academic Press, 93–119.

Weld C. 1854. Rudiments of Pathological History. London: George Busk, 282.

Wing GL, Blanchard GC, Weiter JL. 1978. The topography and age relationship of lipofuscin concentration in the retinal pigment epithelium. Invest Ophthalmol Vis Sci 17:601–607.

Wislocki GB, Ladman AJ. 1955. The demonstration of the blood ocular barrier in the albino rat by means of the intravitum deposition of silver. J Biophys Biochem Cytol 1:501–509.

Wolfrum M. 1908. Contribution to the anatomy and histology of the choroid in man and higher animals. Graefes Arch Clin Ophthalmol 67:307.

35. Bruch's membrane, drusen, and age-related macular degeneration

ROBYN GUYMER AND ALAN C. BIRD

With age there is accumulation of debris in Bruch's membrane. In some subjects this results in retinal pigment epithelial detachment (PED), choroidal neovascularization (CNV), or geographic atrophy with consequent visual loss (Fig. 35-1 and Plate 35-I). An international classification and grading system for age-related macular degeneration has recently been agreed upon, in which age-change at the level of Bruch's membrane is known as *age-related maculopathy* (ARM) and the resulting complications causing visual loss as *age-related macular degeneration* (AMD) (International ARM Epidemiological Study Group, 1995). The terms are restricted to subjects aged 50 years or more. The strategic location of Bruch's membrane between the retina and its primary source of nutrition, the choriocapillaris, makes diffusion through it essential for the health of the retina (Bok, 1985). Bruch's membrane normally forms a semipermeable filtration barrier through which nutrients pass from the choriocapillaris to the photoreceptors and cellular breakdown products travel in the opposite direction. Any interference with these processes could lead to disease.

AMD has long been recognized as the commonest cause of blindness and partial sight in Western societies (Leibowitz et al., 1984; Kahn and Moorhead, 1973). Moreover, a recent study on causes of blind and partially sighted registrations in England and Wales shows that AMD is now the leading cause of partially sighted registration among the working population (16–64 years), and contributes equally with glaucoma and diabetes to blind registration in this age group (Evans, 1985). AMD is also the only cause for registration that increased in prevalence over the last decade, with other common causes such as cataract, diabetes, and glaucoma all falling. This may only reflect an aging population and better treatment of other sight-threatening conditions, but evidence exists that the increase may be more than would be expected from these changes alone (Evans, 1995; Evans and Wormald, 1996). Other indications of a possible rise in prevalence of AMD is seen in Japan, where this disease, which was considered rare 20 years ago, has become a common cause of poor vi-

sion in urban communities (Kubo et al., 1989; 1990). Clearly AMD is a major health problem, and to date there is no effective treatment which has had a major impact on the rates of blindness caused by this disorder (Moorfields Macular Study Group, 1982; Chisholm, 1983; Macular Photocoagulation Study Group, 1991; 1993).

As a result of recent clinical observation and laboratory research, new pathogenetic concepts have been formulated concerning the origin of the material in Bruch's membrane, its chemical composition, its influence upon retinal function, and the reactions it evokes.

BRUCH'S MEMBRANE CHANGES

Focal Deposits: Drusen

The clinical hallmark of ARM is the presence of drusen, pale deposits seen ophthalmoscopically at the level of Bruch's membrane. Historically they have been divided into hard and soft drusen according to the nature of their margins. Hard drusen are defined as less than 63 μm, and are discrete with distinct margins. This arbitary size was decided upon for clinical classification of drusen as being equivalent to the width of a second-order tributary venule in the posterior pole. Hard drusen appear not to signify risk of visual loss, and therefore their presence does not form a criterion for the diagnosis of ARM. Soft drusen have indistinct edges, tend to be large, and may be confluent. Irregularity of pigmentation at the level of the RPE is commonly seen in subjects with drusen (Fig. 35-2).

Although drusen and disciform lesions were both recognized in the last century (Donders, 1855; Tay and Hutchinson, 1878), a causal relationship between the two conditions was not recognized until much more recently. In 1937 Verhoeff and Grossman noted an association of these "senile changes" with disciform lesions and in 1940 Gifford and Cushman proposed that drusen predisposed to disciform detachments of the macula (Verhoeff and Grossman, 1938; Gifford and

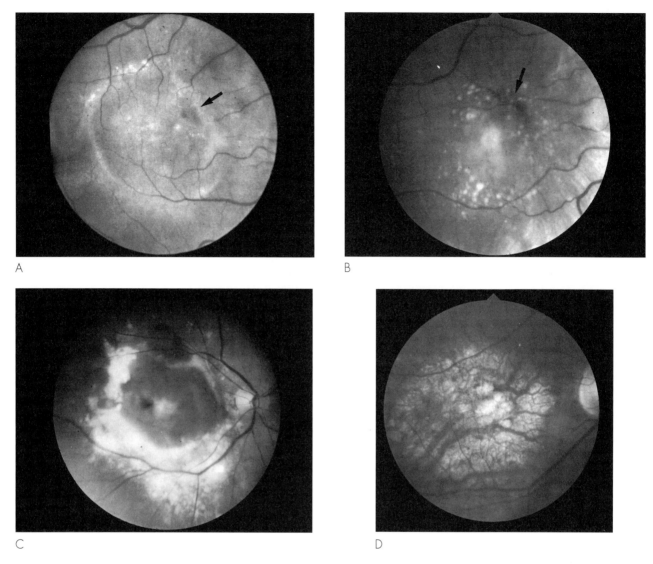

FIGURE 35-1. Fundus photographs. (a) Pigment epithelial detachment with neovascular notch *(arrow)*, (b) subretinal choroidal neovascular membrane *(arrow)* with associated retinal hemorrhage and exudate, (c) end-stage disciform lesion with massive subretinal exudate, (d) geographic atrophy. (See also Plate 35-I.)

Cushman, 1940). Gass, Teeters, and Bird were responsible for formulating the concept of the evolution of AMD when they confirmed the association of drusen with AMD, and proposed that choroidal neovascularization (CNV) was the initiating response leading to visual loss (Gass, 1967; 1972; Teeters and Bird, 1973).

The prevalence of all types of drusen within the elderly Western population has been estimated at between 10–80%, depending upon definitions and methods used to detect them (Leibowitz, 1984; Gibson et al., 1985; Coffrey and Brownstein, 1986). The risk of visual loss in subjects with drusen has been estimated. In a hospital population with bilateral drusen the overall risk of a

sight-threatening lesion was 8.6% over 1 year, 16.4% over 2 years and 23.5% over 3 years (Holz et al., 1994b). A much lower cumulative risk of 12.5% over 5 years was identified in another study (Smiddy and Fine, 1984). The disparity between the two studies is likely to be due to a higher prevalence of hard drusen in the latter. Several authors have noted that greater numbers and confluence of drusen, and focal hyperpigmentation at the level of the retinal pigment epithelium (RPE) were associated with greater-than-average risk of visual loss (Gass, 1973; Holz et al., 1994b; Strahlman, et al., 1983; Smiddy and Fine, 1984; Bressler et al., 1988; Bressler et al., 1990). Estimates of risk of visual loss also exist in

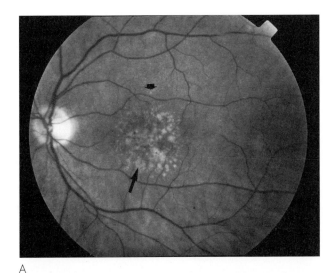

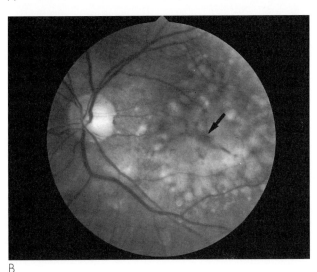

FIGURE 35-2. Fundus photographs. (a) hard *(small arrow)* and soft drusen *(large arrow)*, (b) confluent soft drusen with pigment figure *(arrow)*.

those already suffering unilateral visual loss from AMD. There is an overall risk of 12–15% per year of developing a disciform lesion in the other eye, but this risk is even higher if the better eye has high-risk drusen (Gass, 1973; Bressler et al., 1990). People with unilateral tears of the RPE have an 80% risk of a similar lesion in the other eye over three years (Schoeppner et al., 1989).

Diffuse Deposits

Diffuse thickening of Bruch's membrane is due to accumulation of material external to the basement membrane of the RPE (called by some basal linear deposits) and internal to the basement membrane of the RPE (called by

some basal laminar deposits). Although well documented histologically, diffuse deposits have received little attention by clinicians until recently, since no recognizable clinical correlate of their presence existed. However, diffuse rather than focal deposits would logically be expected to have the greater influence on the outcome of disease. Studies on Sorsby fundus dystrophy, a condition where a continuous layer of abnormal material of up to 30 microns in thickness is deposited between the inner collagenous layer of Bruch's membrane and the basement membrane of RPE (Capon et al., 1989), have provided evidence of a clinical sign that may correlate to a thickened Bruch's membrane. It has been suggested that the prolonged, patchy choroidal-filling phase on fluorescein angiography seen in Sorsby fundus dystrophy may indicate the presence of diffuse thickening of Bruch's membrane (Hoskin et al., 1981; Polkinghorne et al., 1989). This pattern of choroidal filling is also seen in patients with known choroidal hypoperfusion as part of general vascular disease (Foulds et al., 1971; Gaudric et al., 1982; Friedman et al., 1964). This angiographic sign has been identified in patients with AMD (Pauleik-hoff, 1990b), and it could represent the clinical correlate of the reduced cross-sectional area of choriocapillaris identified by light and electron microscopy in eyes with AMD (Sarks, 1978; Sarks et al., 1988; Tso, 1985; Olver et al., 1990; McLeod and Luddy, 1994). It is not possible to identify whether Bruch's membrane thickening precedes choriocapillaris changes in AMD, so the causal relationship between the two is in doubt. An initial abnormality in the choriocapillaris could lead to reduced diffusion of waste material from Bruch's membrane into the choroidal circulation, thus allowing it to accumulate in Bruch's membrane. Alternatively, the diffuse deposits in Bruch's membrane may induce secondary changes in the capillaries by acting as a barrier to diffusion between the RPE and choroid. There is good evidence that diffusible agents from the RPE regulate the choriocapillaris, and a reduction of the hydraulic conductivity of Bruch's membrane may alter the accessibility of these molecules to the capillaries, resulting in the vessels reverting to the more common tubular arrangement of capillary beds (Piguet et al., 1992; Korte et al., 1984; Henkind and Gartner, 1983). The potential significance of this clinical sign has been established by demonstrating discrete areas of scotopic threshold elevation of up to 3.4 log units and slow dark-adaptation corresponding closely to regions of choroidal perfusion abnormality (Chen et al., 1992; Steinmetz et al., 1993). These deficits correspond well with symptoms of poor vision in the dark, dark-adapted central scotomas, and fading vision in bright light, which are so commonly complained of by subjects with ARM (Steinmetz et al., 1993).

A unifying mechanism has been proposed to explain the functional loss and changes in Bruch's membrane and the choroid. Normal photoreceptor function is dependent on the free diffusion through Bruch's membrane of large molecule complexes as they pass from the choriocapillaris to the RPE. Predictably, such molecules would not pass freely through a hydrophobic layer of debris, and functional deficit would ensue. The magnitude of change would depend upon the thickness and chemical composition of the material within Bruch's membrane, and would be particularly marked in the presence of a large quantity of neutral lipids. Thus, loss of sensitivity, slow dark-adaptation, and changes in the choriocapillaris may indicate the presence of diffuse deposits that are sufficiently thick or hydrophobic to compromise metabolic exchange between the choroid and retina. Early scotopic dysfunction, implying poor rod function, may be explained by the lack of a vital nutrient such as vitamin A. Significantly, rods are more dependent on a constant supply of vitamin A than the cones, which have some ability to recycle vitamin A and so are less dependent upon its diffusion across Bruch's membrane. Recently it has been shown that the functional deficits in Sorby's fundus dystrophy can be reversed by vitamin A supplementation (Jacobson et al., 1995).

There is little information to date concerning the clinical implications of diffuse deposits because of the lack of clinical information as to their presence or absence. In one study it was recorded that geographic atrophy is much more likely to occur, and that loss of two lines or more of Snellen's visual acuity is three times greater in patients with abnormal choroidal perfusion than in one without this clinical sign (Piguet et al., 1992). Admittedly, the evidence for diffuse thickening is indirect and awaits verification.

PATHOGENESIS OF BRUCH'S MEMBRANE CHANGE

The first change to be identified by histopathology is the deposition of extracellular material including wide-spaced collagen and membrane-bound bodies external to the basement membrane of the RPE in the inner collagenous layer of Bruch's membrane. As the disorder progresses, these deposits may be found throughout Bruch's membrane, and in the intercapillary pillars in the inner choroid. This may give rise to diffuse thickening of Bruch's membrane (which is named by some authors *basal linear deposits*) or focal deposits. Focal collections of this material enlarge by the addition of amorphous material to form discrete drusen (Green and Enger, 1993) (Fig. 35-3). Hard drusen are formed of dense hya-

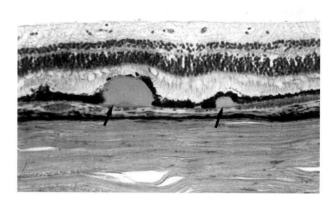

FIGURE 35-3. Light micrograph showing discrete hard drusen within Bruch's membrane *(arrows)*.

line material that is apparently continuous with the inner collagenous layer and is often densely opaque on electron microscopy. Soft drusen are formed by focal accentuations of the membranous debris within Bruch's membrane (soft membranous drusen) or may be derived from clusters of small hard drusen (soft clusters) (Sarks, 1976; 1980; Garner et al., 1994; Sarks et al., 1994). In late disease an additional deposit occurs as an even layer of collagenous material between the plasma membrane and basement membrane of the RPE, and it has been called *basal laminar deposits*.

The mechanisms which result in deposition of debris in Bruch's membrane with age are not well understood. It is believed that this material is derived from the RPE (Farkas et al., 1971; Marshall, 1987; Feeney-Burns and Ellersieck, 1985; Hogan, 1972; Grindle and Marshall, 1978; Burns and Feeney-Burns, 1980). There is good evidence that the RPE discharges cytoplasmic material throughout life into the inner portion of Bruch's membrane (Ishibashi et al., 1986; Rungger-Branche et al., 1988; Reme, 1977). By this means it is believed that the RPE achieves cytoplasmic renewal, a mechanism common to all metabolically active but nondividing cells.

The RPE is involved in the phagocytosis of photoreceptor cell outer segments, which are shed daily in vast quantities. The ingested outer segments material is contained within a phagosome, and a primary lysosome fuses with the vacuole in order to deliver degradative enzymes into the phagosome. Upon delivery of enzymes, degradation of the contents of the phagocytic vacuole occurs. Incompletely digested material forms residual bodies which contain the fluorescent pigmented granules of lipofuscin (Dorey et al., 1989; Feeney, 1978; Feeney-Burns and Eldred, 1984; Katz et al., 1986; Weiter et al., 1986; Boulton et al., 1989; 1990; Boulton, 1991;

Wyszynski et al., 1989; Deguchi et al., 1994; see also Chapter 33). Residual bodies may fuse with melanophores, forming melanolipofuscin (Feeney, 1978; Boulton et al., 1990; Weale, 1989—also see Chapter 4). The residual bodies are all acidified, indicating that lysosomal vesicles are constantly fusing with the long-term phagosomes, a conclusion supported by the observation by Feeney that all phagosomes showed degradative enzyme activity (Feeney, 1978). From this, residual bodies would be expected to have a finite half-life, a conclusion supported by the observation that lipofuscin slowly disappears with atrophy of the outer retina (von Rückmann et al., 1995). Vesicles may also form within the cytoplasm which contain waste products of metabolic activity, a process called *autophagy*. Some of the products resulting from degradation of the contents of these various intracytoplasmic vesicles are recycled, and it is assumed that the remainder is discharged into Bruch's membrane. It has not been proven that the photoreceptors represent the original source of abnormal material or that it is derived from phagosomes, since neither rhodopsin sequences nor phagosomal enzyme activity have been shown in Bruch's membrane deposits using monoclonal antibodies. However, the presence of docosohexanoic acid implies that material derived from the rod outer segment contributes to the debris (Reme, 1977). It is likely that the quantity of material discharged into Bruch's membrane reflects the metabolic activity of the RPE, which in turn is related to photoreceptor outer segment renewal (Reme, 1977; Ishibashi et al., 1986).

With age there is progressive accumulation of material in the RPE. In vitro studies report that there are very few fluorescent lipofuscin granules in young eyes but with increasing age the quantity of fluorescent granules increases. After increasing in the first two decades of life, lipofuscin remains stable until middle life, rising thereafter. At age 40, residual bodies occupy approximately 8% of cytoplasmic volume of the RPE, and by 80 this has increased to 19%. Only recently has a technique been available whereby in vivo imaging of autofluorescence of the fundus could be achieved using a scanning laser ophthalmoscope (Woon et al., 1990; Delori et al., 1995; von Rückmann et al., 1995; see Chapter 11). The optical characteristics and distribution imply that the fluorescence is derived from lipofuscin in the RPE. Early results show that there is little autofluorescence in the young but that it increases with age, although refinements of this technique are required before accurate quantification is achieved (personal observation).

The cause for the accumulation and its effect on cell function are unknown. Accumulation may be due to an absolute deficiency of lysosomal enzymes, such that there is defective degradation of phagosomal material. It has been demonstrated that in the presence of antisense cathepsin-D and cathepsin-S, RPE cells in culture rapidly accumulate cytoplasmic inclusions when fed rod outer segments (Rakoczy et al., 1994). This is presumed to be the result of reduced ability to degrade the contents of phagosomes due to lack of active cathepsin. The evidence concerning the level of enzyme activity is mixed (Boulton et al., 1991; Wyszynski et al., 1989), but most studies imply that total activity increases with age. In addition, there is experimental evidence that increasing phagosomal load in cultured RPE cells results in a rise in degradative enzyme activity (Boulton, 1991; Boulton et al., 1991). The finding that all residual bodies have enzyme activity suggests that there may be competition for newly produced lysosomes such that they may not be freely available to new phagosomes. Thus, even if there is increased total enzyme activity, there may still be a relative deficiency, with defective breakdown of newly ingested photoreceptor outer segment material within the RPE. It is also postulated that the substrate for degradation may be altered by peroxidation, resulting in compounds which cross-link biological molecules, causing them to be indigestible by lysosomes. The unsaturated fatty acids from the photoreceptor outer segments would be liable to free-radical damage, particularly in the high oxygen tension of RPE and outer segments, and in high light levels (Wing et al., 1978).

Accumulation of debris in Bruch's membrane may be visible microscopically by the age of ten years and is universal by 40 years. This is thought to result from failure to clear the debris deposited into this region. The mechanism of clearance is not clear but both the diffusion characteristics of Bruch's membrane and the nature of the material deposited by the RPE may contribute to incomplete clearance. The material to be cleared may be abnormal as a consequence of incomplete degradation, possibly due to failure of degradative enzymes, although there is little evidence to support or deny this possibility. Alternatively, there may be changes in Bruch's membrane which make clearance more difficult. As Bruch's membrane ages the collagen fibers cross-link, resulting in a decrease in the solubility of the collagen. It is also possible that nonenzymatic glycosylation of collagen, which occurs in other collagens throughout the body, may occur in Bruch's membrane (Karawatowski et al., 1991). The interfiber matrix of Bruch's membrane is composed largely of heparan sulfate and chondroitin/dermatan sulfate, and it has been suggested that the chondroitin sulfate side chains provide the initial filtration barrier for material from the choriocapillaris. Proteoglycans increase in Bruch's membrane with age, and changes in the negatively charged field may impede the passage of negatively charged macromolecules and affect normal filtration (Marshall, 1987; Hewitt and Newsome, 1985; Hewitt et al., 1989; Marshall et al., 1994).

An alternative mechanism for clearance of material from Bruch's membrane is suggested by the observation that drusen disappear as a consequence of laser photocoagulation (Haut et al., 1991; Figueroa et al., 1994; Weizig, 1988; Sigelman, 1991; Frennesson and Nilsson, 1995). It is evident that the effect is widespread, in that a few laser lesions cause clearance of drusen over a large area. Studies show that laser photocoagulation induces blood-borne macrophages and choroidal pericytes to engulf drusen material, leading to their regression (Duvall and Tso, 1985; Wallow and Tso, 1973; Tso, 1973; Gloor, 1974). As a consequence, it has been postulated that cells of the choriocapillaris may play a role in normal clearance of the debris from Bruch's membrane, and that this process is accelerated as a reaction to photocoagulation (Duvall and Tso, 1985). Similar observations have been made of intrusions from the endothelial cells of choriocapillaris into the outer portion of Bruch's membrane in rat, chick, and humans (Leeson and Leeson, 1967; Matsusaka, 1968; Yamamoto and Yamashita, 1989; 1990; 1994). If these intrusions represent a normal mechanism of clearance of Bruch's membrane debris, a defect in this process would represent a potential mechanism in the pathogenesis of age-related Bruch's membrane change. Furthermore, the possibility exists that choroidal neovascular membranes, rather than a novel process occurring in response to Bruch's membrane changes, may be a distortion of a normal phenomenon.

Despite the universal acceptance that the material in Bruch's membrane is derived from RPE, little information exists as to the exact relationship between the accumulation of debris in both structures. It is possible only to speculate on the factors which determine this relationship. If it were variation in activity of degradative enzyme activity, low activity would cause buildup of residual bodies in the RPE, and possible discharge into Bruch's membrane of large molecules which might clear slowly. Thus, a direct correlation would exist between RPE lipofuscin accumulation and Bruch's membrane thickness. A direct correlation would also exist if the ability to recycle the products of degradation was different from one person to another. By contrast, an inverse relationship could be expected if efficiency of RPE cytoplasmic renewal differed from one individual to another. High levels of renewal would result in low levels of accumulation in RPE but increase in the quantity of material deposited into Bruch's membrane, resulting in an inverse relationship between changes in the two structures. Elucidation of the association between accu-

mulation of debris in these two structures will help in the understanding of the sequence of events leading to AMD.

Drusen vary widely in their appearance and location from one patient to another, although there is remarkable symmetry between the two eyes of an individual with respect to drusen size, density, and particularly fluorescence on angiography (Coffrey and Brownstein, 1986; Hutchinson and Tay, 1875; Barondes et al., 1990). These observations imply that there is great variation in the precise mechanisms which determine the formation of drusen from one subject to another but not between the two eyes of a single individual.

CHEMICAL COMPOSITION OF BRUCH'S MEMBRANE DEPOSIT

It has been suggested that the chemical composition of the deposits in Bruch's membrane has a major influence on the subsequent outcome of disease (Bird and Marshall, 1986). Bruch's membrane stains with periodic acid-Schiff, and changes in staining characteristics have been considered to imply increase in lipid content (Sarks, 1976; Farkas et al., 1971; Hogan and Alvarado, 1967; Green, 1977; Feeney-Burns and Ellersieck, 1985). However, the commonly used method of dehydration of tissues with alcohol removes much of the lipid. Only recently have techniques been employed histologically to investigate lipid deposition. A study of frozen tissue was undertaken using histochemical staining techniques on thirty human eyes with an age range between 1 and 95 years. The composition and ultrastructure of Bruch's membrane were recorded by electron microscopy on the same specimens. The results were analyzed in three age groups, 0–30 years, 31–60 years, and older than 60 years, and showed progressive accumulation of lipids in Bruch's Membrane with age. Differences were found in the specific types of lipids present, but the composition of diffuse and discrete deposits within the individual appeared to be similar. Some eyes stained for neutral lipids alone, some stained predominantly for phospholipids, and others stained equally for both neutral lipids and phospholipids (Pauleikhoff et al., 1990c) (Fig. 35-4). To support these findings material extracted by lipid solvents from tissue of fresh eyes was analyzed by thin-layer and gas chromatography (Sheraidah et al., 1993). After separation, the chemical species were identified by mass spectroscopy. Little or no lipid was extracted from donors under 50 years old. Over 50 years old, the study confirmed the conclusion that the quantity of lipid in Bruch's membrane increases with age, and that the ratios of phospholipids to neutral fats varies from one subject to another (Fig. 35-5). It was also found that the

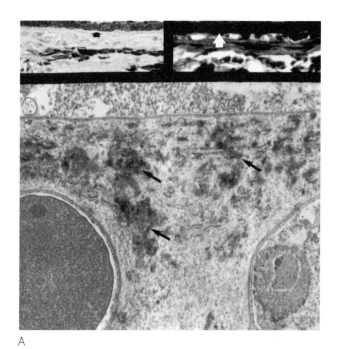

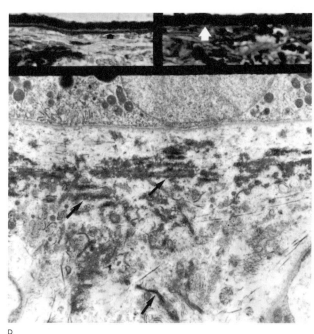

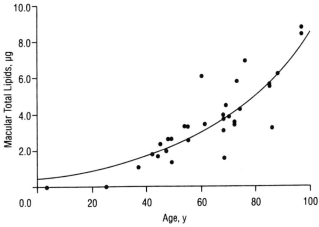

FIGURE 35-5. Relationship between total lipids extracted from macular Bruch's membrane and donor age. (Courtesy of Holz, Sheraidah, et al., 1994. Copyright 1994 American Medical Association.)

quantity of lipid extracted was higher from the macula than from the periphery. The lipids consisted of phospholipids, triglycerides, fatty acids, and free cholesterol (Holz et al., 1994a). Extracellular deposits of lipid thought to be derived from blood have cholesterol esters as the major fraction of the total lipids. Very little cholesterol ester was found in either the macula or the periphery of Bruch's membrane, and no more than 50% of the phospholipids was phosphotidylcholine, supporting the concept that the abnormal material is cellular in origin (Fig. 35-6) (Sheraidah et al., 1993; Holz et al., 1994a).

FIGURE 35-4. Light and electron micrographs of diffuse deposits in Bruch's membrane. (a) The staining of Bruch's membrane with bromine Sudan Black B *(large white arrow)* and lack of stain for oil red O *(small black arrow)* indicates that the lipids in this specimen are predominantly phospholipids rather than neutral fats. The electron micrograph shows an increase in electron-dense material within Bruch's membrane *(black arrows)*. (b) The staining of Bruch's membrane with oil red O *(small black arrow)* and lack of staining with bromine Sudan Black B *(large white arrow)* indicates that the lipids in this specimen are predominantly neutral fats rather than phospholipids. The electron micrograph shows an increase in electron-dense material within Bruch's membrane *(black arrows)*. Reproduced by permission of D. Pauleikhoff.

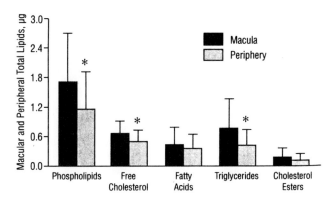

FIGURE 35-6. Composition of lipids extracted from the human macular and peripheral Bruch's membrane. Data represented as mean ± SD for 32 eyes. Asterisk indicates $P<.001$. (Courtesy of Holz, Sheraidah, et al., 1994. Copyright 1994 American Medical Association.)

PATHOGENESIS OF LESIONS CAUSING VISUAL LOSS

Some understanding of the potential mechanisms by which the nature of deposits in Bruch's membrane determine the particular manifestation of AMD comes from the reconstruction of the potential events that lead to PEDs (Bird and Marshall, 1986). In earlier discussion it was believed that the detachment was induced by passage of fluid through Bruch's membrane from the choriocapillaris, the physical attachment of pigment epithelium to Bruch's membrane having been disturbed by progressive accumulation of debris on the inner surface of Bruch's membrane (Gass, 1967). The assumption that fluid was derived from choroid was understandable, since the fluorescein which fills the sub-pigment-epithelial space during fluorescein angiography is derived from the choroid rather than the retina. This explanation, however, requires either higher hydrostatic pressure in the choroid than in the subretinal space or, alternatively, flow induced by an osmotic pressure gradient from the choroid into the sub-pigment-epithelial space. The little evidences that exists does not support this concept (Foulds, 1976). Another proposal was that choroidal blood vessels grow through Bruch's membrane and proliferate on the outer surface of flat pigment epithelium, and exudation from these new vessels may be an alternative source of sub-RPE fluid (Gass, 1984). However, neovascularization is not universal in PEDs (Barondes et al., 1992), implying that neovascularization is not always the initiating event in the pathogenesis of PEDs. An alternative concept was proposed in 1986, in which it was suggested that the sub-pigment-epithelial fluid is derived from the RPE rather than from the choroid (Bird and Marshall, 1986). It is widely accepted that fluid is pumped from the retina to Bruch's membrane due to active movement of ions by the pigment epithelial cells. If Bruch's membrane became hydrophobic, a significant resistance to water flow could be generated at this level, causing fluid to collect between the pigment epithelium and Bruch's membrane. This alternative explanation for the pathogenesis of PEDs had the advantage over previous concepts, in that it was compatible with the three observed behavioral characteristics of PEDs, which were unexplained at that time:

1. The flattening of a PED after scatter laser. This could be explained by the destruction of pigment epithelial cells, and therefore the destruction of some of the pump, by photocoagulation. This would cause reduction in the volume of fluid being moved into the sub-pigment-epithelial space and, predictably, would be followed by flattening of the pigment epithelium.

2. The observation that flattening of PEDs was accompanied by loss of vision. Tissue failure as manifest by visual loss might be associated with reduction of fluid pumped into the sub-pigment-epithelial space, which would itself be accompanied by flattening of the pigment epithelium onto Bruch's membrane. The alternative, that flattening itself may cause visual loss, is clearly not correct since therapeutic flattening by treating neighbororing new vessels complexes is not accompanied by visual loss (Maguire et al., 1991).

3. The occurrence of RPE tears. The pigment epithelial pump might be powerful enough to produce tangential stress in the detached tissues sufficient to cause tearing of the pigment epithelium (Bird, 1991). It has been shown that fluid movement across the RPE is not influenced by wide changes in pressure gradients across the cells so that hydrostatic pressure gradients generated across the RPE would not suppress the pump function (Tsuboi, 1987). If, however, the fluid were derived from choroid driven by hydrostatic pressure, fluid movement would cease as pressure within the detachment increased.

The observed entry of fluorescein from the choroid into the sub-pigment-epithelial space during fluorescein angiography could be explained by movement down a concentration gradient rather than the movement following fluid flow. The observed slow flow of fluorescein into the subpigment epithelial space in patients at risk of suffering a pigment epithelial tear would be in accord with the proposal that in these patients the hydrophobicity in Bruch's membrane would be high.

It is evident that decreased hydraulic conductivity of Bruch's membrane would be an essential prerequisite to the accumulation of fluid in the sub-pigment-epithelial space. Fisher had reported that the hydraulic conductivity of Bruch's membrane decreased with age, and he predicted from extrapolation of his data that by the age of 130 there would be no flow of water through Bruch's membrane (Fisher, 1987). More recently, Moore et al. (1995) have shown an exponential decrease in hydraulic conductivity with increasing age, with changes being more marked in the macula than in the periphery. The age-related profile of conductivity was compared with the corresponding profile of lipid extracted from Bruch's membrane by Holz et al., and an inverse association between the two parameters was found (Holz et al., 1994a; Moore et al., 1995—also see Chapter 34). Further support for the reduction in hydraulic conductivity may come from histopathological studies under electron microscopy where empty spaces were noted between the RPE basement membrane and the inner collagenous layer of Bruch's membrane in eyes with basal linear deposits. This was thought to suggest an impedance of fluid and solute movement across Bruch's membrane (Loffler and Lee, 1986).

The concept that hydrophobicity of Bruch's membrane may be important to disease is illustrated by observations on the relationship of the characteristics of drusen and the lesion subsequently causing visual loss. Drusen characteristics on fluorescein angiography provide insight into their chemical composition. It has been hypothesized that hyperfluorescent drusen may be hydrophilic, allowing free diffusion of water-soluble sodium fluorescein into the deposits where they may bind to polar molecules (Bird and Marshall, 1986), whereas hypofluoresent drusen would imply hydrophobic drusen. It is concluded that the former are rich in polar compounds, the latter rich in neutral fats. This hypothesis was recently supported by in vitro staining, in that the specimens with deposits containing few neutral lipids bound sodium fluorescein, while those with high levels did not (Pauleikhoff et al., 1992). It has been shown that eyes with hypofluorescent drusen are at risk of developing a PED, whereas those with hyperfluorescent drusen are at risk of CNV (Pauleikhoff et al., 1990a; Chuang and Bird, 1988; Schoeppner et al., 1989). These findings are compatible with PEDs resulting from impedence of outward flow of fluid by a hydrophobic Bruch's membrane.

Impedance of metabolic exchange between choroid and RPE may also compromise photoreceptor function and eventually lead to cell death, which is seen clinically as geographic atrophy.

At present, the determinants of Bruch's membrane change that predispose to neovascularization are less clear. The precise reason why hyperfluorescent drusen predispose to neovascularization has not been identified (Pauleikhoff et al., 1990a). Vessel growth is thought to occur when there is an imbalance between stimulating and inhibiting substances. It is likely that blood vessel growth is suppressed by the metabolic environment of Bruch's membrane and may be due to a diffusible agent produced by the RPE (Penfold et al., 1986; Killingsworth et al., 1990). Inhibitors of neovascularization are also believed to be released from the RPE, and any disruption to their diffusion through Bruch's membrane to the choroid could result in new vessel formation (Glaser et al., 1985). The presence of macrophages in Bruch's membrane have also been implicated, since activated macrophages have been long recognized as stimulating blood vessel growth (Killingsworth et al., 1990). Once geographic atrophy ensues, the risk of new vessels is minimal, most likely due to the disappearance of the RPE, choriocapillaris, and debris and along with them any angiogenic factor (Killingsworth et al., 1990).

RISK FACTORS IN AMD

Those factors that determine risk of developing age-related macular disease are not well defined but clinical studies imply that both genetic and environmental factors are involved. It has been shown that there is greater concordance between siblings than spouse in the prevalence and quality of change in Bruch's membrane, showing that genetic factors are important to the pathogenesis of disease (Piguet et al., 1993). Subsequent twin and sibling studies support this conclusion (Heiba et al., 1994; Silvestri et al., 1994; Klein et al., 1994). These findings also imply that either environment is not important or the variation in environment in the communities under study is insufficient for its effect to show. AMD has been shown to be rare in South African blacks, which could be explained on a genetic basis (Gregor and Joffe, 1978), but a similarly low rate was found in rural southern Italy (personal observation), implying that environmental factors may be important. The most persuasive evidence of environmental influence comes from Japan, where age-related macular disease was rare 20 years ago but purportedly is now common in urban communities (Kubo et al., 1989; 1990). The search for major environmental influences on AMD has led to a number of possible factors being proposed, and in some their possible relevance to the disease process is evident. Lack of antioxidant vitamins C, D, and E is proposed by those who believe AMD is related to generation of free radicals in the retina. Smoking and sun exposure, which would also contribute to free-radical production, have also been implicated. Zinc deficiency may play a role as it is a coenzyme in the lysosomal degradative processes within the RPE. It has also been shown that carotinoids may be protective to the macula. Various epidemiological studies have been undertaken to assess the possible role of these factors in AMD, but the evidence is mixed and no clear risk factors have emerged except possibly for smoking. While there may be an association between these factors and AMD, none have been shown to sufficiently alter the odds ratio to influence the risk of disease sufficiently to account for observed changes in prevalence (Seddon et al., 1994; Newsome et al., 1988; Eye Disease Case Control Study Group, 1993; Sperduto et al., 1990; West et al., 1989).

The genes responsible for transmitting risk of AMD are unknown, but candidate genes may become evident as mutations responsible for dominantly inherited disorders with some homology to AMD become known. It has been identified that mutations in TIMP3 gene are responsible for Sorsby fundus dystrophy (Weber et al., 1994), and the locus of the gene for both Doyne honeycomb dystrophy and malattia levantinese is on chromosome 2p (Gregory et al., 1996; Héon et al., 1996). It is possible that mutations may influence the risk of AMD by either altering turnover rates of outer segments or influencing rates of lysosomal degradation, RPE efficiency in discharging material, or Bruch's membrane diffusional characteristics. The disorder may be polygenic, such that many processes may be altered, giving a graded risk dependent upon the presence of one or several mutant genes.

CONCLUSION

Bruch's membrane lies in a critical position, separating a rich nutrient source, the choriocapillaris, from the RPE and photoreceptors, which are metabolically very active cells. Alterations in the structure or composition of Bruch's membrane that interfere with its function could potentially have repercussions on both sides of the membrane. This is most obvious in AMD where the precise nature of the changes in Bruch's membrane may ultimately determine the outcome of this disease.

There is increasing circumstantial evidence that age-related macular disease represents a spectrum of disease in which patients behave differently one from another. Many clinically identifiable clues exist that allow the variants of disease to be defined and that provide a basis upon which the determinants of disease may be defined. Both laboratory and clinical observations lend circumstantial support to the concept that reduced hydraulic conductivity of Bruch's membrane gives rise to retinal PEDs. In addition, the functional deficits so common in the elderly can be explained by alternation of the diffusion characteristics of Bruch's membrane. The corollary is that subretinal neovascularization occurs as a result of changes that are different from those which give risk to PEDs. The factors which determine the nature of Bruch's membrane change and the relative importance of genetic and environmental influences in dictating these changes are unknown but are amenable to investigation.

REFERENCES

Barondes M, Pauleikhoff D, Chisholm IH, Minassian D, Bird AC. 1990. Bilaterality of drusen. Br J Ophthalmol 74:180–182.

Barondes MJ, Pagliarini S, Chisholm IH, Hamilton AM, Bird AC. 1992. Controlled trial of laser photocoagulation of pigment epithelial detachments in the elderly: a four year review. Br J Ophthalmol 76:5–7.

Bird AC. 1991. Doyne lecture: pathogenesis of retinal pigment epithelial detachment in the elderly: the relevance of Bruch's membrane change. Eye 5:1–12.

Bird AC, Marshall J. 1986. Retinal pigment epithelial detachments in the elderly. Trans Ophthalmol Soc UK 105:674–682.

Bok D. 1985. Retinal photoreceptor-pigment epithelium interactions. Invest Ophthalmol Vis Sci 26:1659–1694.

Boulton ME. 1991. Aging of the retinal pigment epithelium. In: Osborne NN, Chader GJ, Progress in Retinal Research, vol. 11. Oxford: Pergamon Press, 125–152.

Boulton ME, McKechnie NM, Breda J, Bayly M, Marshall J. 1989. The formation of autofluorescent granules in cultured human RPE. Invest Ophthalmol Vis Sci 30:83–89.

Boulton ME, Docchio F, Dayhaw-Braker P, Ramponi R, Cubeddu R. 1990. Age related changes in the morphology, absorption and fluorescence of melanosomes and lipofuscin granules of the retinal pigment epithelium. Vis Res 30:1291–1303.

Boulton M, Moriarty P, Unger W, Bishop P. 1991. Modulation of lysosomal enzyme content in cultured human RPE. Invest Ophthalmol Vis Sci 32(suppl):1056.

Bressler NM, Bressler SB, Seddon TM, Gragoudas ES, Jacobson LP. 1988. Drusen characteristics in patients with exudative versus non-exudative age-related macular degeneration. Retina 8:109–114.

Bressler SB, Maguire MG, Bressler NM, Fine SL. 1990. Relationship of drusen and abnormalities of the retinal pigment epithelium to the prognosis of neovascular macular degeneration. Arch Ophthalmol 108:1442–1447.

Burns RP, Feeney-Burns L. 1980. Clinico-morphological correlations of drusen and Bruch's membrane. Trans Amer Ophthalmol Soc 78:206–225.

Capon MRC, Marshall J, Kraft JI, Alexander RA, Hiscott PS, Bird AC. 1989. Sorsby's fundus dystrophy: a light and electron microscopic study. Ophthalmology 96:1769–1777.

Chandra SR, et al. 1974. Natural history of disciform degeneration of the macula. Amer J Ophthalmol 78:579–582.

Chen JC, Fitzke FW, Pauleikhoff D, Bird AC. 1992. Functional loss in age-related Bruch's membrane change with choroidal perfusion defect. Invest Ophthalmol Vis Sci 33:334–340.

Chisholm IH. 1983. The recurrence of neovascularisation and late failure in senile disciform lesions. Trans Ophthalmol Soc UK 103:354–359.

Chuang EL, Bird AC. 1988. The pathogenesis of tears of the retinal pigment epithelium. Amer J Ophthalmol 105:285–290.

Coffrey AJH, Brownstein S. 1986. The prevalence of macular drusen in postmortem eyes. Am J Ophthalmol 102:164–171.

Deguchi Y, et al. 1994. Acidification of phagosomes and degradation of rod outer segments in rat retinal pigment epithelium. Invest Ophthalmol Vis Sci 35:568–569.

Delori FC, Arend O, Staurenghi G, Goger D, Dorey CK, Weiter JJ. 1995. Lipofuscin and drusen fluorescencein aging and age related macular degeneration. Invest Ophthalmol Vis Sci 36:718–729.

Donders FC. 1855. Beitrage zur pathologischen Anatomie des Aüges. Albrecht von Graefes Archiv fur Opthalmologie 1, abs 2:106–118.

Dorey CK, Wu G, Ebenstein D, Garsd A, Weiter JJ. 1989. Cell loss in the ageing retina: relationship to lipofuscin accumulation and macular degeneration. Invest Ophthalmol Vis Sci 30:1691–1699.

Duvall J, Tso MOM. 1985. Cellular mechanisms of resolution of drusen after laser coagulation: an experimental study. Arch Ophthalmol 103:694–703.

Evans J. 1995. Causes of blindness and partial sight in England and Wales 1990–1991. Studies on medical and population subjects No. 57. London: Her Majesty's Stationary Office.

Evans J, Wormald R. 1996. Is the incidence of registrable age-related macular degeneration increasing? Br J Ophthalmol 80:2–3.

Eye Disease Case Control Study Group. 1993. Antioxidant status and neovascular age related macular degeneration. Arch Ophthalmol 111:104–109.

Farkas T, Sylvester V, Archer D, Altona M. 1971. The histochemistry of drusen. Am J Ophthalmol 71:1206–1215.

Feeney L. 1978. Lipofuscin and melanin of human retinal pigment epithelium: fluorescence, enzyme cytochemical and ultrastructural studies. Invest Ophthalmol Vis Sci 17:583–600.

Feeney-Burns L, Eldred GE. 1984. The fate of the phagosome: conversion to "age-pigment" and impact in human retinal pigment epithelium. Trans Ophthalmol Soc UK 103:416–421.

Feeney-Burns L, Ellersieck M. 1985. Age-related changes in the ultrastructure of Bruch's membrane. Am J Ophthalmol 100:686–697.

Figueroa MS, Regueras A, Bertrand J. 1994. Laser photocoagulation to treat macular soft drusen in age-related macular degeneration. Retina 14:391–396.

Fisher RF. 1987. The influence of age on some ocular basement membranes. Eye 1:184–189.

Foulds WS. 1976. Clinical significance of trans-scleral fluid transfer. Trans Ophthalmol Soc UK 96:290–308.

Foulds WS, Lee WR, Taylor WOG. 1971. Clinical and pathological aspects of choroidal ischaemia. Trans Ophthalmol Soc UK 91:325–341.

Frennesson IC, Nilsson SEG. 1995. Effects of argon (green) laser treatment of soft drusen in early age-related maculopathy: a 6 months prospective study. Br J Ophthalmol 79:905–909.

Friedman E, Smith TR, Kuwabara T, Beyer CK. 1964. Choroidal vascular patterns in hypertension. Arch Ophthalmol 71:842.

Garner A, Sarks S, Sarks JP. 1994. Degenerative and related disorders of the retina and choroid. In: Garner A, Klintworth GK, eds, Pathobiology of Ocular Disease, 2nd ed. New York: Marcell Dekker, 631–674.

Gass JDM. 1967. Pathogenesis of disciform detachment of the neuroepithelium. 3. Senile disciform macular degeneration. Am J Ophthalmol 63:617–644.

Gass JDM. 1972. Drusen and disciform macular detachment and degeneration. Trans Am Ophthalmol Soc 70:409–436.

Gass JD. 1973. Drusen and disciform macular detachment and degeneration. Arch Ophthalmol 90:206–217.

Gass JD. 1984. Pathogenesis of tears of the retinal pigment epithelium. Br J Ophthalmol 68:513–519.

Gaudric A, Coscas G, Bird AC. 1982. Choroidal ischemia. Am J Ophthalmol 94:489–498.

Gibson JM, Rosenthal AR, Lavery J. 1985. A study of prevalence of eye disease in the elderly in an English community. Trans Ophthalmol Soc UK 104:196–203.

Gifford SR, Cushman B. 1940. Certain retinopathies due to changes in the lamina vitrea. Arch Ophthalmol 23:60–75.

Glaser BM, Campochiaro PA, Davis JL Jr, Sato M. 1985. Retinal pigment epithelial cells release an inhibitor to neovascularization. Arch Ophthalmol 103:1870–1875.

Gloor BP. 1974. On the question of the origin of macrophages in the retina and vitreous following photocoagulation. Graefes Arch Clin Exp Ophthalmol 190:183–194.

Gragoudas ES, et al. 1976. Disciform degeneration in the macula. II. Pathogenesis. Arch Ophthalmol 94:755–757.

Green WR, Enger C. 1993. Age related macular degeneration histopathological studies. Ophthalmol 100:1519–1535.

Green WR, Key SN. 1977. Senile macular degeneration: a histopathological study. Trans Am Ophthalmol Soc 75:180–250.

Gregor Z, Bird AC, Chisholm IH. 1977. Senile disciform macular degeneration in the second eye. Br J Ophthalmol 61:141–147.

Gregor Z, Joffe L. 1978. Senile macular changes in the black African. Br J Ophthalmol 62:547–550.

Gregory CY, Evans K, Wijesurya SD, Kermani S, Jay MR, Plant C, Cox N, Bird AC, Bhattacharya SS. In press. The gene responsible for autosomal dominant Doyne's honeycomb retinal dystrophy maps to chromosome 2p16. Hum Genet.

Grindle CFJ, Marshall J. 1978. Aging changes in Bruch's membrane and their functional implications. Trans Ophthalmol Soc UK 98:172–175.

Haut J, Renard Y, Kraiem S, Bensoussan C, Moulin F. 1991. Preventive treatment using laser of age-related macular degeneration of the contralateral eye after age-related macular degeneration in the first eye. J Fr Ophthalmol 14:473–476.

Heiba IM, Elston RC, Klein BEK, Klein R. 1994. Sibling correlations and segration analysis of age-related maculopathy: the beaver dam eye study. Genet Epidemiol 11:51–67.

Héon E, Piguet B, Munier F, Sneed SR, Morgan CM, Forni S, Pescia G, Schorderet D, Taylor CM, Streb LM, et al. 1996. Linkage of autosomal dominant radial drusen (Malattia leventinese) to chromosome 2p 16-21. Arch Ophthalmol 114:193–198.

Henkind P, Gartner S. 1983. The relationship between retinal pigment epithelium and the choriocapillaris. Trans Ophthalmol Soc UK 103:444.

Hewitt TA, Newsome DA. 1985. Altered synthesis of Bruch's membrane proteoglycans associated with dominant retinitis pigmentosa. Curr Eye Res 4:169–174.

Hewitt TA, Nakazawa K, and Newsome DA. 1989. Analysis of newly synthesized Bruch's membrane proteoglycans. Invest Ophthalmol Vis Sci 30:478–486.

Hogan MJ. 1972. Role of the retinal pigment epithelium in macular disease. Trans Am Acad Otolaryngol Ophthalmol 76:64–80.

Hogan MJ, Alvarado J. 1967. Studies on the human macula. IV: Aging changes in Bruch's membrane. Arch Ophthalmol 44:410–420.

Holz FG, Sheraidah G, Pauleikhoff D, Bird AC. 1994a. Analysis of lipid deposits extracted from human macular and peripheral Bruch's membrane. Arch Ophthalmol 112:402–406.

Holz FG, Wolfensberger TJ, Piguet B, Gross-Jendroska M, Wells JA, Minassian DC, Chisholm IH, Bird AC. 1994b. Bilateral macular drusen in age-related macular degeneration: prognosis and risk factors. Ophthalmology 101:1522–1528.

Hoskin A, Sehmi K, Bird AC. 1981. Sorby's pseudo-inflammatory macular dystrophy. Br J Ophthalmol 65:859–865.

Hutchinson J, Tay W. 1875. Symmetrical central chorio-retinal disease occurring in senile persons. Royal Lond Ophthalmol Hosp Rep 83:275–285.

International ARM Epidemiological Study Group. 1995. An international classification and grading system for age related macular maculopathy and age related macular degeneration. Surv Ophthalmol 39:367–374.

Ishibashi T, Sorgente N, Patterson R, Ryan SJ. 1986. Pathogenesis of drusen in the primate. Invest Ophthalmol Vis Sci 27:184–193.

Jacobson SG, Cideciyan AV, Regunath G, Rodriguez FJ, Vandenburgh K, Sheffield VC, Stone EM. 1995. Night blindness in a TIMP3-associated Sorsby's fundus dystrophy is reversed by vitamin A. Nature Genet 11:27–32.

Kahn HA, Moorhead HB. 1973. Statistics on Blindness in the Model Reporting Areas 1969-70. United Status Department of Health, Education and Welfare Publication No. (NIH) 73-427. Washington, DC:US Government Printing Office.

Karawatowski WSS, Jeffries TE, Duance VC, Albon J, Easty DL. 1991. Collagen and ageing in Bruch's membrane. Invest Ophthalmol Vis Sci 32(suppl):687.

Katz ML, Drea C, Robinson WG. 1986. Relationship between retinol and lipofuscin in the retinal pigment epithelium. Mech Ageing Dev 35:291–305.

Killingsworth MC, Sarks JP, Sarks SH. 1990. Macrophages related to Bruch's membrane in age related macular degeneration. Eye 4:613–621.

Klein ML, Mauldin WM, Stoumbos VD. 1994. Heredity and age-related macular degeneration: observations in monozygotic twins. Arch Ophthalmol 112:932–937.

Korte GE, Repucci V, Henkind P. 1984. RPE destruction causes choriocapilary atrophy. Invest Ophthalmol Vis Sci 25:1135–1145.

Kubo N, Ohno Y, Yanagawa H, Yuzawa M, Matsui M, Uyama M. 1989. Annual Estimated Number of Patients with Senile Disciform Macular Degeneration in Japan. Research Committee on Chorioretinal Degenerations: Ministry of Health and Welfare of Japan, Tokyo 136–139.

Kubo N, Ohno Y, Yuzawa M, Matsui M, Uyama M, Yanagawa H. Murase T. 1990. Report on Nationwide Clinico-Epidemiological Survey of Senile Disciform Macular Degeneration in Japan. Research Committee on Chorioretinal Degenerations: Ministry of Health and Welfare of Japan, Tokyo 121–124.

Leeson TS, Leeson CR. 1967. Choriocapillaris and lamina elastica (vitrea) of the rat eye. Br J Ophthalmol 51:599–616.

Leibowitz H, et al. 1984. The Framingham Eye Study monograph: an ophthalmological and epidemiological study of cataract, glaucoma, diabetic retinopathy, macular degeneration and visual acuity in a general population of 2631 adults, 1973–75. Surv Ophthalmol 25(suppl):335–610.

Loffler KU, Lee WR. 1986. Basal linear deposit in the human macula. Graefes Arch Clin Exp Ophthalmol 224:493–501.

Macular Photocoagulation Study Group. 1991. Argon laser photocoagulation for neovascular maculopathy: five year results from randomized clinical trials. Arch Ophthalmol 109:1109–1114.

Macular Photocoagulation Study Group. 1993. Five year follow-up of fellow eyes of patients with age related macular degeneration and unilateral extrafoveal choroidal neovascularization. Arch Ophthalmol 111:1189–1199.

Maguire JI, Benson WE, Brown GC. 1991. Treatment of foveal pigment epithelial detachments with contiguous extrafoveal choroidal neovascular membranes. Am J Ophthalmol 109:523–529.

Marshall GE, Konstas AGP, Reid GG, Edwards JG, Lee WR. 1994. Collagens in the aged macula. Graefes Arch Clin Exp Ophthalmol 232:133–140.

Marshall J. 1987. The ageing retina: physiology or pathology. Eye 1:282–1295.

Matsusaka T. 1968. Undescribed endothelial processes of the choriocapillaris extending to the retinal pigment epithelium in chick. Br J Ophthalmol 52:887–892.

McLeod DS, Lutty GA. 1994. High-resolution histologic analysis of the human choroidal vasculature. Invest Ophthalmol Vis Sci 35(11):3799–3811.

Moore DJ, Hussain AA, Marshall J. 1995. Age related variation in the hydraulic conductivity of Bruch's membrane. Invest Ophthal Vis Sci 36:1290–1297.

Moorfields Macular Study Group. 1982. Retinal pigment epithelial detachments in the elderly: a controlled trial of argon laser photocoagulation. Br J Ophthalmol 66:1–16.

Newsome DA, et al. 1988. Oral zinc in macular degeneration. Arch Ophthalmol 106:192–198.

Olver J, Pauleikhoff D, Bird A. 1990. Morphometric analysis of age changes in the choriocapillaris. Invest Ophthalmol Vis Sci 31(suppl):47.

Pauleikhoff D, Barondes MJ, Minassian D, Chisholm IH, Bird AC. 1990a. Drusen as a risk factor in age related macular disease. Am J Ophthalmol 109:38–43.

Pauleikhoff D, Chen JC, Chisholm IH, Bird AC. 1990b. Choroidal perfusion abnormalities in age related macular disease. Am J Ophthalmol 109:211–217.

Pauleikhoff D, Harper CA, Marshall J, Bird AC. 1990c. Aging changes in Bruch's membrane: a histochemical and morphological study. Ophthalmology 97:171–178.

Pauleikhoff D, Zuels S, Sheraidah G, Marshall J, Wessing A, Bird AC. 1992. Correlation between biochemical composition and fluorescein binding of deposits in Bruch's membrane. Ophthalmology 99:1548–1553.

Penfold PL, Killingsworth MC, Sarks SH. 1986. Senile macular degeneration: The involvement of giant cells in atrophy of the retinal pigment epithelium. Invest Ophthalmol Vis Sci 27:364–371.

Piguet BP, Palmvang IP. Chisholm IH, Bird AC. 1992. Evolution of age-related macular disease with choroidal perfusion abnormality. Am J Ophthalmol 113:657–663.

Piguet B, Wells JA, Palmvang IB, Wormald R, Chisholm IH, Bird AC. 1993. Age-related Bruch's membrane change: a clinical study of the relative role of heredity and environment. Br J Ophthalmol 77:400–403.

Polkinghorne PJ, Capon MR, Berninger TA, Lyness AL, Sehmi K, Bird AC. 1989. Sorsby's fundus dystrophy: a clinical study. Ophthalmology 96:1763–1768.

Rakoczy PE, Mann K, Cavaney DM, Robertson T, Papadimitreou J, Constable IJ. 1994. Detection and possible functions of a custeine protease involved in digestion of rod outer segments by retonal pigment epithelial cells. Invest Ophthalmol Vis Sci 35:4100–4108.

Reme C. 1977. Autophagy in visual cells and pigment epithelium. Invest Ophthalmol Vis Sci 16:807–814.

Rungger-Branche E, Englert U, Leuenberger PM. 1988. Exocytic clearing of degraded membrane material from pigment epithelial cells in frog retina. Invest Ophthalmol Vis Sci 28:2026–2037.

Sarks JP, Sarks SH, Killingsworth MC. 1994. Evolution of soft drusen in age related macular degeneration. Eye 8:269–283.

Sarks SH. 1976. Ageing and degeneration in the macular region: a clinico-pathological study. Brit J Ophthalmol 60:324–341.

Sarks SH. 1978. Changes in the Region of the Choriocapillaris in Aging and Degeneration. Kyoto: 23rd Concilium Ophthalmol, 228–238.

Sarks SH. 1980. Drusen and their relationship to senile macular degeneration. Aust J Ophthalmol 8:117–130.

Sarks SH, Sarks J, Killingsworth C. 1988. Evolution of geographic atrophy of the retinal pigment epithelium. 2:552–577.

Schoeppner G, Chuang EL, Bird AC. 1989. The risk of fellow eye visual loss with unilateral retinal pigment epithelial tears. Am J Ophthalmol 108:683–685.

Seddon JM, et al. 1994. Dietary carotenoids, vitamins A, C and E and advanced age related macular degeneration. JAMA 272:1413–1420.

Sheraidah G, Steinmetz R, Maguire J, Pauleikhoff D, Marshall J, Bird AC. 1993. Correlation between lipids extracted from Bruch's membrane and age. Ophthalmology 100:47–51.

Sigelman J. 1991. Foveal drusen resorption one year after perifoveal laser photocoagulation. Ophthalmol 98:1379–1383.

Silvestri G, Johnston PB, Hughes AE. 1994. Is genetic predisposition an important risk factor in age-related macular disease? Eye 8:564–568.

Smiddy WE, Fine SL. 1984. Prognosis of patients with bilateral macular drusen. Ophthalmology 91:271–277.

Sperduto R, et al. 1990. Do we have a nutritional treatment for age related cataract or macular degeneration? Arch Ophthalmol 108:1403–1405.

Steinmetz RL, Haimovici R, Jubb C, Fitzke FW, Bird AC. 1993. Symptomatic abnormalities of dark adaptation in patients with age-related Bruch's membrane change. Br J Ophthalmol 77:549–554.

Strahlman ER, Fine SL, Hillis A. 1983. The second eye of patients with senile macular degeneration. Arch Ophthalmology 101:1191–1193.

Teeters VW, Bird AC. 1973. The development of neovascularization of senile disciform macular degeneration. Amer J Ophthalmol 76:1–18.

Tso MOM. 1973. Photic maculopathy in rhesus monkey: a light and electron microscopic study. Invest Ophthalmol Vis Sci 12:17–34.

Tso MOM. 1985. Pathogenetic factors of aging macular degeneration. Ophthalmology 92:628–635.

Tsuboi S. 1987. Measurement of the volume flow and hydraulic conductivity across the isolated dog retinal pigment epithelium. Invest Ophthalmol Vis Sci 28:1776–1782.

Verhoeff FH, Grossman HP. 1938. Pathogenesis of disciform degeneration of the macula. Arch Ophthalmol 19:561–585.

Von Rückmann A, Fitzke FW, Bird AC. 1995. Distribution of fundus autofluorescence with a scanning laser ophthalmoscope. Br J Ophthalmol 119:543–562.

Wallow IHL, Tso MOM. 1973. Repair after xenon arc photocoagulation: an electron microscopic study of the evolution of retinal lesions in rhesus monkeys. Am J Ophthalmol 75:957–972.

Weale RA. 1989. Do years or quanta age the retina? Photochem Photobiol 50:429–438.

Weber BH, Vogt G, Pruett RC, Stohr H, Felbor U. 1994. Mutations in the tissue inhibitor of metalloproteinases-3 (TIMP 3) in patients with Sorsby's fundus dystrophy. Nature Genetics 8:352–356.

Weiter JJ, Delori FC, Wiung GL, Fitch KA. 1986. Retinal pigment epithelial lipofuscin and melanin and choroidal melanin in human eyes: absorption profiles show increased optical density with age. Invest Ophthalmol Vis Sci 27:145–152.

Weizig PC. 1988. Treatment of drusen-related ageing macular degeneration by photocoagulation. Trans Am Ophthalmol Soc 86:276–290.

West S, et al. 1989. Exposure to sunlight and other risk factors for age related macular degeneration. Arch Ophthalmol 107:875–879.

Wing GL, Blanchard GC, Weiter JL. 1978. The topographical and age relationship of lipofuscin concentration in the retinal pigment epithelium. Invest Ophthalmol Vis Sci 17:601–607.

Woon WH, Fitzke FW, Chester GH, Greenwood DG, Marshall J. 1990. The scanning laser ophthalmoscope: basic principles and applications. J Ophthalmol Photog 12:17–23.

Wyszynski RE, Brunar WE, Cano DB, Morgan KM, Davis CB, Sternberg P. 1989. A donor age-dependent change in the activity of alpha-mannosidase in human cultured RPE cells. Invest Ophthalmol Vis Sci 30:2341–2347.

Yamamoto T, Yamashita H. 1989. Pseudopodia of choriocapillary endothelium. Jpn J Ophthalmol 33:327–336.

Yamamoto T, Yamashita H. 1990. Pseudopodia of choriocapillary endothelium in ocular tissues. Jpn J Ophthalmol 34:181–187.

Yamamoto T, Yamashita H. 1994. Electron microscopic observation of pseudopodia from choriocapillary endothelium. Jpn J Ophthalmol 38:129–138.

36. Age-related retinal pigment epithelial detachments

STEPHEN G. SCHWARTZ, DAVID R. GUYER,
AND LAWRENCE A. YANNUZZI

Detachment of the retinal pigment epithelium (RPE) is a prominent feature of many diseases, which can be broadly categorized into four etiologies. Three of these, idiopathic (exemplified by central serous chorioretino-pathy [CSC], inflammatory (typified by the Vogt-Koyanagi-Harada [VKH] syndrome), and ischemic, are discussed more fully in Chapter 22. The fourth (and most prevalent) etiology is degenerative, the archetype of which, age-related macular degeneration (AMD), will be discussed here. Within the exudative form of the disease, vascularized PEDs are more common than purely serous detachments. Two published series of patients with exudative AMD, imaged by intravenous fluorescein angiography (FA), report that 3–5% of eyes present with purely serous detachments, 21–29% present with vascularized detachments, and 15–21% present with both serous and vascularized PEDs (Yannuzzi et al., 1992; Freund et al., 1993). The identification of choroidal neovascularization (CNV) associated with RPE detachment has sight-threatening implications because 90% of patients with exudative AMD lose vision to the level of 20/200 or worse (Yannuzzi, 1989).

THE PATHOPHYSIOLOGIC BASIS OF RPE DETACHMENT

The cell monolayer of the RPE is bounded on its apical surface by the photoreceptors of the neurosensory retina and on its basal surface by the collagenous fibers of Bruch's membrane. The forces maintaining adhesion between the neurosensory retina and the RPE are well described (Frambach and Marmor, 1982; Negi and Marmor, 1983; 1984; 1986). The high oncotic pressure within the choriocapillaris, in combination with the high hydrostatic pressure on the retina, creates a net flow of fluid from vitreous to choroid. However, the tight junctions interconnecting the RPE cells within the monolayer resist this fluid vector; therefore, the RPE cells use active ion transport mechanisms to pump fluid out of the eye, which may help maintain retinal adhesion. The RPE cells are theoretically capable of trans-

porting more than half of the vitreous volume per day (Chihara and Nao-i, 1985).

In contrast, less is known about the forces maintaining normal adhesion between the RPE and Bruch's membrane, as well as the processes by which this adhesion may be disrupted. In vitro, the RPE–Bruch's membrane interface is disrupted by the toxins hemicholinium-3 and sodium iodate, which implies a complex anatomic and/or physiologic bond (Yoon and Marmor, 1993).

Bruch's membrane contains five layers; from innermost to outermost, they are the basal lamina of the RPE cell monolayer; the inner collagenous zone; an elastic layer; the outer collagenous zone; and the basal lamina of the choriocapillaris. Therefore, what is described clinically as a "pigment epithelial detachment" is actually, in histologic terms, a separation of the RPE cell monolayer with its basal lamina from the inner collagenous zone, or, more precisely, an intra-Bruch's membrane detachment. This area, between the basal lamina and the inner collagenous zone, is also the site at which drusen develop. The confluence of multiple soft drusen may be confused with a small serous PED, as the distinction between these two structures, on clinical, angiographic, and histopathologic grounds, may be difficult (Green et al., 1985). Generally, however, a lesion greater than 300 microns in diameter is classified as a PED (Elman and Fine, 1989).

Bruch's membrane undergoes many histochemical and ultrastructural changes with age, several of which are important factors in the pathogenesis of vascularized RPE detachment. One theory, summarized by Pauleikhoff et al. (1990), relates to lipid metabolism within the RPE. Normally, waste products generated by the RPE cell monolayer are transported through Bruch's membrane into the choroid. However, in the aging eye, waste products such as lipofuscin progressively accumulate within the RPE cells and eventually in Bruch's membrane, which manifests histochemically as an increase in the lipid content of Bruch's membrane. Theoretically, then, Bruch's membrane becomes more hydrophobic in character, impeding the normal membrane hydraulic conductivity and promoting fluid accumulation in the sub-RPE space. This becomes magnified in the macula, where in vitro studies (Moore et al., 1995) suggest that the normal vitreous-to-choroid fluid vector declines with aging at a faster rate than in the peripheral retina.

CNV is the pathognomonic feature which differentiates vascularized PEDs from purely serous detachments. However, the precise pathogenesis of vascularized RPE detachment is currently unknown; whether the CNV is the cause or the effect of the PED has never been conclusively determined. Gass (1984) proposed that an invasive choroidal neovascular membrane first penetrates Bruch's membrane into the sub-RPE space with what may be undetectable anatomic and physiologic consequences ("occult" CNV), and that only later does this membrane exude fluid and/or blood, leading to serous or hemorrhagic detachment of the RPE. This more classical explanation, that the CNV causes the PED, is supported by the common clinical finding that successful laser photocoagulation of the neovascularization may cause flattening of the detachment with stabilization or improvement of visual acuity (see below).

Alternatively, there is a growing body of evidence that suggests that the converse of this theory can also be correct, and that the subretinal neovascularization is actually a secondary complication of a preexisting serous PED. Green et al. (1985), for example, proposed that thickening of the inner aspect of Bruch's membrane, drusen formation, and serous RPE detachment represent a progression of disease that only later leads to invasion of CNV. This theory is supported by the observation that many eyes with purely serous RPE detachments later develop neovascularized disease; in fact, approximately 30% of these eyes will develop CNV by 1 year (Poliner et al., 1986; Elman et al., 1986). However, this finding may be an artifact of the relatively low sensitivity of FA in the detection of CNV. For example, it is now generally accepted that digital indocyanine green videoangiography (ICG-V) may, under certain circumstances, localize areas of CNV that were undetectable by FA (see below). Therefore, many PEDs that by clinical and FA criteria appear avascular may actually be associated with CNV.

Chuang and Bird (1988) have suggested that the PED comes first, and have supported this proposal with data indicating that cultured human RPE cells can inhibit in vitro vascular endothelial cell proliferation (Glaser et al., 1985). The implication, therefore, is that detachment of the RPE would interfere with its normal antiangiogenic function and allow the ingrowth of CNV. Further evidence for this idea comes from studies of hu-

man macular collagens. The age-dependent thickening of Bruch's membrane (Ramrattan et al., 1994) is due at least in part to the deposition of type IV collagen in the basal lamina of the choriocapillaris, while the inner and outer collagenous zones contain types I, III, and V (Marshall et al., 1994). In vitro evidence (Roberts and Forrester, 1990) suggests that type I collagen stimulates endothelial cell differentiation and migration, while type IV collagen has an inhibitory effect. Thus, Marshall et al. (1994) have proposed that the type IV collagen normally found in the outermost layer of Bruch's membrane prevents the ingrowth of CNV, and that disruption of this type IV collagen (for example, by detaching the RPE) would allow migrating endothelial cells access to the type I collagen of the outer and inner collagenous zones, thus promoting further invasion of the neovascular membrane.

Further insight into the mechanism of vascularized RPE detachment comes from the study of retinal–choroidal anastomoses (RCAs), which may be found in a majority of eyes with CNV and PEDs (Kuhn et al., 1995). Eyes with vascularized PEDs and RCAs may represent the same phenomenon as eyes with what were identified by Hartnett et al. (1992) as a "retinal vascular abnormality" (see below); in the same paper, these authors cited animal studies (Bellhorn et al., 1980) indicating that experimental damage to photoreceptor cells induces retinal neovascular complexes to invade the RPE and become anatomically more like choroidal vessels. Therefore, it is possible that, in at least some eyes, retinal neovascularization may be the first step in the pathogenesis of vascularized RPE detachment, and that separation of the RPE and ingrowth of CNV are both secondary complications of the disruption of the RPE and/or Bruch's membrane by these invading retinal-derived angiomatous lesions (Slakter et al., 1998).

CLINICAL CONSIDERATIONS

PEDs (Fig. 36-1 and Plates 36-I, 36-II) are discrete dome-shaped elevations of the RPE, with sharply delineated margins caused by the firm adherence of the RPE to Bruch's membrane, and may be associated with turbid subretinal fluid, hemorrhage, lipid exudate, areas of pigment epithelial proliferation and/or atrophy, and overlying neurosensory retinal detachment (Yannuzzi et al., 1979). Other characteristic features include an encircling orange ring and a pigment band on the dome of the elevation that may form linear figures. This pigment, composed of both lipofuscin and melanin, usually indicates a chronic detachment (Yannuzzi, 1989).

The vascularized RPE detachments found in exuda-

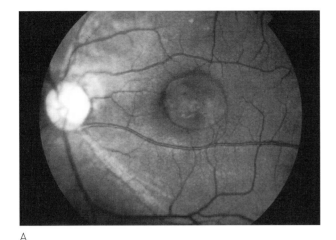

A

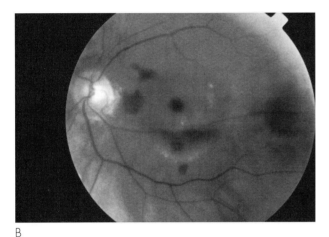

B

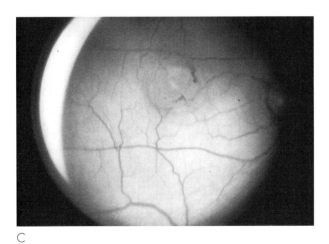

C

FIGURE 36-1. Variations of pigment epithelial detachment (PED). (A) PED in a darkly pigmented individual. (B) Hemorrhagic PED. (C) PED associated with atrophic changes. (see Plates 36-I, 36-II.)

tive AMD differ from those found in other conditions (see above and Chapter 22). For example, idiopathic polypoidal choroidal vasculopathy (IPCV) is a rare macular disorder characterized by nodular, polypoidal subretinal excrescences with interconnecting vascular channels, usually located in the peripapillary region and associated with serosanguineous detachments of both the RPE and the neurosensory retina. IPCV can be distinguished from exudative AMD on clinical, angiographic, demographic, and prognostic grounds. On biomicroscopic examination, IPCV is characterized by a conspicuous lack of drusen. Angiographically, the lesions of IPCV lack the significant fluorescein leakage characteristic of CNV (see below). The majority of reported patients with IPCV are black, and generally younger than patients with exudative AMD. And perhaps most important, the natural course of IPCV is considerably more benign than that of exudative AMD (see below); many patients maintain good visual acuity even without laser photocoagulation treatment (Yannuzzi et al., 1990).

Angiographic Characteristics

In the early phase of FA, a PED will hyperfluoresce evenly and diffusely beneath the entire detachment. The intensity, but not the size, of this hyperfluorescence will increase throughout the middle phase. In the late phase, homogeneous pooling of dye into the subretinal space completely fills the PED, often with sharp, well-demarcated margins (Yannuzzi, 1989). Such substances as subretinal hemorrhage and macular xanthophyll may cause areas of relative hypofluorescence within the PED (Yannuzzi et al., 1979). In contrast, CNV is characterized by a lacy subretinal hyperfluorescence in the early phase, which increases in both size and intensity during the late phase (Schatz et al., 1979).

Certain angiographic features may differentiate a vascularized PED from a purely serous detachment; one widely reported indicator is a flattened or notched border of the detachment (Gass, 1984). Other clues to the presence of CNV include a hot spot, or focal area of increased hyperfluorescence (more readily visible through an atrophic overlying RPE) and a gravity-dependent meniscus, or fluid level, of hemorrhage (Schatz et al., 1979).

Failure to visualize CNV by FA is often secondary to signal blockage by blood and/or serosanguineous material (Weiter et al., 1988). Visualizing CNV within a PED is additionally complicated by the leakage of fluorescein dye into the detachment itself, thus obscuring the localization of a neovascular complex. Such limitations have led to the investigation of an alternative angiographic dye, indocyanine green (ICG), which has two biophysical properties which result in enhanced imaging of the choroidal circulation and its pathology as compared with FA (Flower, 1972; Flower and Hochheimer, 1972; Hayashi and de Laey, 1985; Bischoff and Flower, 1985; Destro and Puliafito, 1989). First, ICG absorbs and emits energy in the near-infrared range, enhancing penetration through subretinal hemorrhage, turbid serosanguineous exudation (as in a PED), and other substances which may block transmission of sodium fluorescein. Second, ICG has a higher protein-binding capacity than fluorescein, which makes it relatively less likely to leak out of the intravascular compartment. The combination of digital imaging systems or scanning laser ophthalmoscopes with ICG cameras has resulted in high-resolution digital ICG videoangiography (ICG-V) (Guyer et al., 1992; Yannuzzi et al., 1992).

ICG-V may, in some patients, precisely localize areas of CNV that could not be localized by FA in eyes with occult CNV both with and without PEDs (Yannuzzi et al., 1994; Guyer et al., 1994; Lim et al., 1995; Guyer et al., 1996), and recent evidence indicates that ICG-V may be superior to FA in detecting CNV in eyes with PEDs (Yuzawa et al., 1995). Various examples of PEDs, as well as their corresponding angiograms (both FA and ICG-V), are illustrated in Figures 36-2 to 36-4 and Plate 36-III.

Natural History

As mentioned above, both Poliner et al. (1986) and Elman et al. (1986) found that approximately 30% of eyes with serous PED will develop CNV by one year. Risk factors for neovascularization cited by both of these studies were advanced patient age and large PED size. Other risk factors for CNV and/or loss of central vision noted by these studies and others (Lewis and Pautler, 1988) include the notch sign, neurosensory retinal detachment, subretinal fluid in the same eye, disciform scarring in the fellow eye, and the following findings on FA: hot spots, late filling, and irregular filling.

Singerman and Stockfish (1989) were among the first authors to demonstrate the grim prognosis associated with vascularized RPE detachments. They studied 55 eyes with PED associated with CNV that was either subfoveal or unidentifiable in location; 82% of these eyes lost two or more lines of vision at one year, and 62% lost six or more lines. The presence of both hemorrhage and exudate on initial presentation correlated significantly with poor initial visual acuity, and advancing patient age was a significant risk factor for reduction in

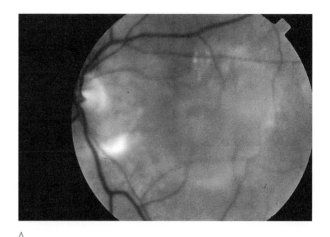

A

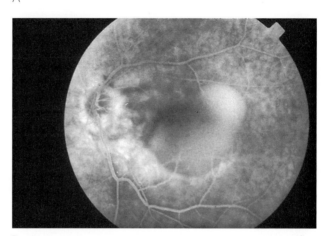

B

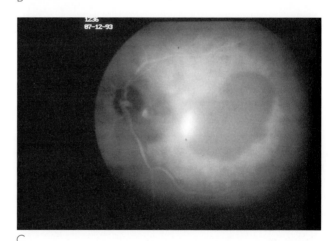

C

FIGURE 36-2. Angiographic findings in pigment epithelial detachment (PED). (A) Fundus appearance. (B) Fluorescein angiography reveals no obvious signs of choroidal neovascularization. (C) Digital indocyanine green videoangiography better delineates the hyperfluorescent vascularized component of the PED from the hypofluorescent serous portion.

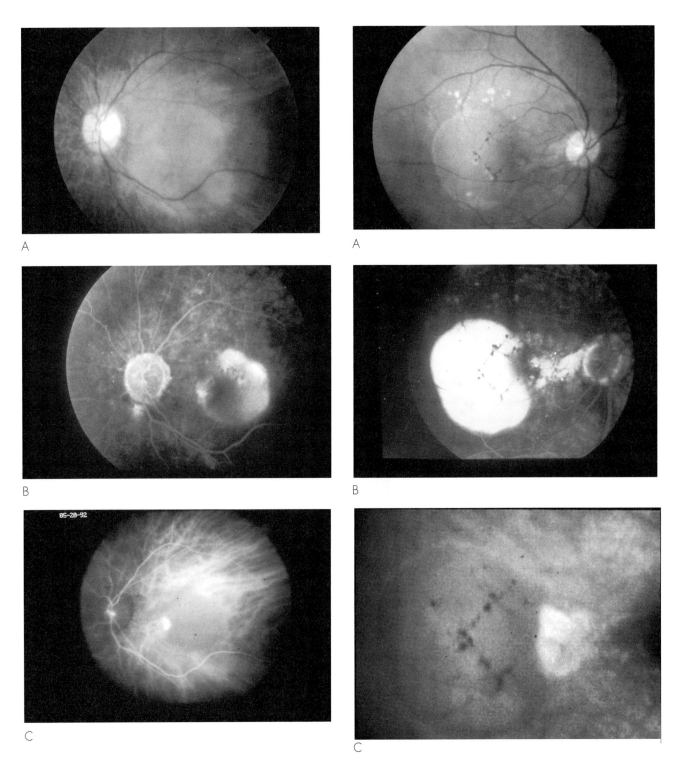

FIGURE 36-3. Further angiographic findings in pigment epithelial detachment (PED). (A) Fundus appearance. (B) Fluorescein angiography reveals classic hyperfluorescence. (C) Digital indocyanine green videoangiography better delineates the hyperfluorescent vascularized portion of the PED from the hypofluorescent serous component.

FIGURE 36-4. Pigment epithelial detachment associated with atrophic changes. (A) Fundus appearance (see Plate 36-III). (B) Fluorescein angiography reveals a notch nasally. (C) Digital indocyanine green videoangiography reveals a hyperfluorescent vascularized area nasally with an adjacent hypofluorescent serous portion.

both initial and final visual acuity. The initial size of the PED, however, was not a significant risk factor.

In an attempt to predict the natural history of PEDs on angiographic grounds, Casswell et al. (1985) categorized PEDs by FA criteria into four groups: early fluorescence, late fluorescence, shallow detachment with limited fluorescence, and irregular fluorescence. The PEDs associated with shallow detachment and limited fluorescence ("drusen" type) appeared to be at the lowest risk for subsequent development of CNV, while those with irregular fluorescence were at highest risk. The late fluorescence group carried the highest risk for RPE rips.

Similarly, Hartnett et al. (1992) described six types of PED: pseudovitelliform (a yellow subretinal lesion surrounded by small drusen), confluent drusen, serous PED, vascular PED, hemorrhagic PED, and retinal vascular abnormality. The pseudovitelliform and confluent drusen forms were associated with the best prognosis, while the serous PEDs, vascular PEDs, hemorrhagic PEDs, and retinal vascular abnormality subtypes, which were associated with CNV, carried the poorest prognosis.

Therapeutic Options

Laser photocoagulation is the only form of therapy proven effective against CNV. The Macular Photocoagulation Study Group (MPSG) has demonstrated the efficacy of laser photocoagulation of classic CNV secondary to AMD and has established guidelines for treatment of these lesions (MPSG 1982; 1990; 1991a; 1991b). However, there is less convincing evidence in the literature regarding laser photocoagulation of PEDs associated with CNV. The MPSG, for example, specifically excluded eyes with PED from its original study (MPSG, 1982).

The Moorfields study (1982), the first prospective controlled clinical trial to study the efficacy of laser photocoagulation of serous PEDs, reported successful flattening of these lesions but recruitment for the study was terminated prematurely when treated eyes were found to have greater visual loss than the control eyes. However, a retrospective review of the Moorfields data indicates that many of these presumed avascular PEDs were actually associated with underlying CNV (Pagliarini et al., 1992) and were thus treated inappropriately with a scatter pattern of laser photocoagulation instead of a confluent, intense treatment. In contrast, later studies (Singerman, 1988; Weiter et al., 1988) of FA-guided laser photocoagulation of vascularized PEDs reported anatomic obliteration and/or visual stabilization or improvement in approximately half of treated eyes. The standard of care now practiced by many authorities, is

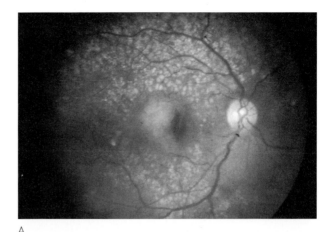

A

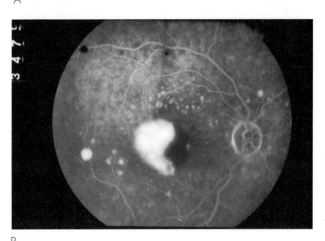

B

FIGURE 36-5. Retinal pigment epithelial (RPE) rip. (A) Fundus appearance. Note the exposed choroid temporally and the heaped-up RPE nasal to this area. (B) Fluorescein angiography reveals a hyperfluorescent area, representing exposed choroid, and hypofluorescent blockage, representing heaped-up RPE.

to photocoagulate vascularized PEDs when possible, but not to treat purely serous detachments.

RPE rips (Fig. 36-5) may complicate PEDs in both treated and untreated eyes. A small RPE rip may resemble a focal area of CNV at the margin of a PED. However, by clinical examination and on FA, the rip is usually flat and atrophic at its base (as compared to a thickened or elevated area of CNV), often with a sharp edge with a convexity toward the center of the PED. The distinction between CNV and an RPE rip is important, because laser photocoagulation of an RPE rip may induce thermal contraction, tissue shrinkage, and hemorrhage without resolving the PED (Yannuzzi, 1989).

RPE rips are probably associated with tractional forces exerted by contracture of sub-RPE fibrovascular tissue and typically occur on the side of the PED opposite the CNV (Weiter et al., 1988). Rips can occur as a

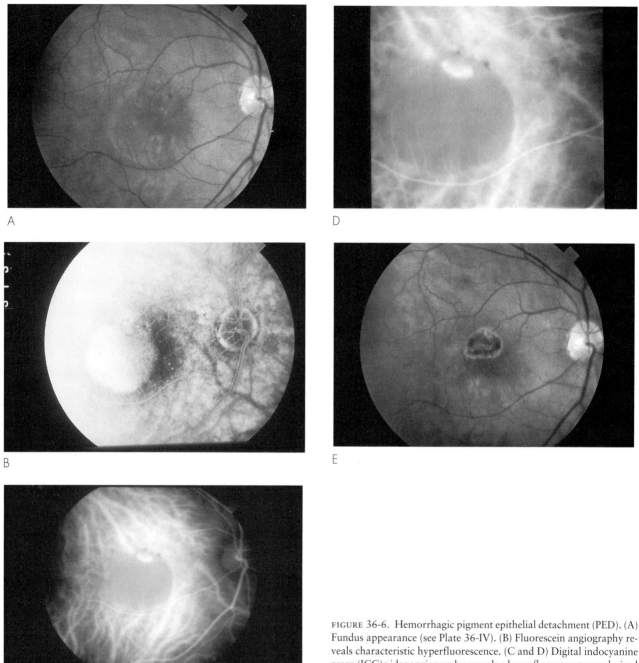

FIGURE 36-6. Hemorrhagic pigment epithelial detachment (PED). (A) Fundus appearance (see Plate 36-IV). (B) Fluorescein angiography reveals characteristic hyperfluorescence. (C and D) Digital indocyanine green (ICG) videoangiography reveals a hyperfluorescent vascularized portion superior to the hypofluorescent serous component. (E) ICG-guided laser photocoagulation was applied, with subsequent resolution of the PED.

consequence of laser therapy, but many occur spontaneously; Lewis and Pautler (1988) found an approximately equal incidence of RPE rips regardless of treatment. The Moorfields study originally reported that RPE rips occurred earlier in treated than in untreated eyes; however, it appears that treatment may merely precipitate a rip in a PED which is already predisposed to such an event (Barondes et al., 1992).

Because of its relatively enhanced imaging of the choroidal circulation (see above), ICG-V may be used to guide laser photocoagulation in some eyes that are ineligible for FA-guided treatment under MPSG criteria. Two representative cases are illustrated in Figures 36-6 and 36-7 and Plate 36-IV. However, ICG-guided laser photocoagulation is less successful in obliterating occult CNV in eyes with associated PED than in eyes without

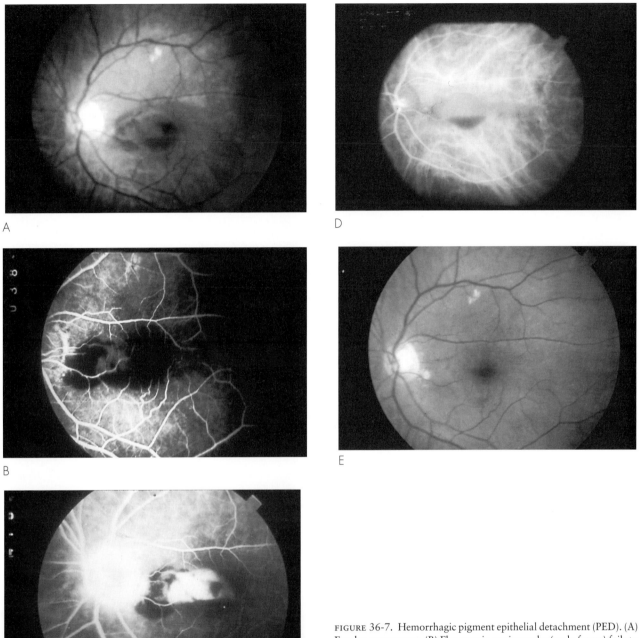

FIGURE 36-7. Hemorrhagic pigment epithelial detachment (PED). (A) Fundus appearance. (B) Fluorescein angiography (early frame) fails to reveal well-defined choroidal neovascularization (CNV). (C) Fluorescein angiogram, late frame. (D) Digital indocyanine green (ICG) videoangiography reveals a focal area of CNV nasally. (E) ICG-guided laser photocoagulation was applied, with subsequent resolution of the PED.

PED (Slakter et al., 1994; Schwartz et al., 1995). There are several possible explanations for this observation, but there is new evidence implicating the role of RCA (which, again, may be present in a majority of eyes with CNV and PED) in preventing adequate treatment of occult CNV associated with PED. Eyes with occult CNV and PED with RCA appear to have a relatively poorer response to laser photocoagulation treatment than eyes

with occult CNV and PED without RCA. The anastomotic vessels, therefore, are thought to be more resistant to direct laser photocoagulation, which may lead to higher rates of laser failure (Slakter et al., 1998).

Only about 13% of all eyes with exudative AMD meet MPSG guidelines for FA-guided laser photocoagulation (Freund et al., 1993) and about half of these eyes experience untreatable persistence or recurrence of

CNV within 12 months of treatment, yielding an over-all treatment rate of approximately 6.5% at one year. Of the 87% of eyes with occult CNV that are ineligible for FA-guided laser photocoagulation, as many as 29% of these (Guyer et al., 1996), or 25% of all eyes with ex-udative AMD, will be eligible for ICG-guided laser pho-tocoagulation. We have found (Schwartz et al., 1998) obliteration of occult CNV in 48% of eyes without PED and 23% of eyes with PED, for an overall anatomic suc-cess rate of 36% at one year. Thus, 25% of eyes with exudative AMD are eligible for ICG-guided laser pho-tocoagulation, and CNV is obliterated in 36% of these eyes, yielding an additional 9% treatment rate at one year.

Therefore, ICG-guided laser photocoagulation can potentially double the number of eyes with exudative AMD, both with and without vascularized PED, that can be successfully treated at 12 months. However, it is humbling to note that even with the combined benefits of both FA- and ICG-guided laser photocoagulation, only about 16% of all patients with newly diagnosed ex-udative AMD can be successfully treated at one year. The overwhelming majority of these patients remain un-treatable.

In spite of the apparently promising success of ICG-guided laser photocoagulation treatment in the man-agement of patients with occult CNV, exudative AMD, particularly when associated with vascularized PED, re-mains an extremely difficult and complex disease with a generally unfavorable prognosis. Thus, attention must remain focused on developing new imaging techniques above and beyond ICG-V, as well as alternative thera-peutic strategies, such as pharmacologic agents and sur-gical intervention, for this very challenging condition.

REFERENCES

Barondes MJ, Pagliarini S, Chisholm IH, Hamilton AM, Bird AC. 1992. Controlled trial of laser photocoagulation of pigment ep-ithelial detachments in the elderly: 4 year review. Br J Ophthalmol 76:5–7.

Bellhorn RW, Burns MS, Benjamin JV. 1980. Retinal vessel abnor-malities of phototoxic retinopathy in rats. Invest Ophthalmol Vis Sci 19:584–595.

Bird AC, Marshall J. 1986. Retinal pigment epithelial detachments in the elderly. Trans Ophthalmol Soc UK 105:674–682.

Bischoff PM, Flower RW. 1985. Ten year experience with choroidal angiography using indocyanine green dye: a new routine examina-tion or an epilogue? Doc Ophthalmol 60:235–291.

Caswell AG, Kohen D, Bird AC. 1985. Retinal pigment epithelial de-tachments in the elderly: classification and outcome. Br J Ophthal-mol 69:397–403.

Chihara E, Nao-I N. 1985. Resorption of subretinal fluid by transepi-thelial flow of the retinal pigment epithelium. Graefe's Arch Clin Exp Ophthalmol 223:202–204.

Chuang EL, Bird AC. 1988. The pathogenesis of tears of the retinal pigment epithelium. Am J Ophthalmol 105:285–290.

Destro M, Puliafito CA. 1989. Indocyanine green videoangiography of choroidal neovascularization. Ophthalmology 96:846–853.

Elman MJ, Fine SL. 1989. Exudative age-related macular degenera-tion. In: Ryan SJ, ed, Retina. St Louis: Mosby, 1103–1141.

Elman MJ, Fine SL, Murphy RP, Patz A, Auer C. 1986. The natural history of serous retinal pigment epithelium detachment in patients with age-related macular degeneration. Ophthalmology 93:224–230.

Flower RW. 1972. Infrared absorption angiography of the choroid and some observations on the effects of high intraocular pressures. Am J Ophthalmol 74:600–614.

Flower RW, Hochheimer BF. 1972. Clinical infrared absorption an-giography of the choroid [letter]. Am J Ophthalmol 73:458–459.

Frambach DA, Marmor MF. 1982. The rate and route of fluid re-sorption from the subretinal space of the rabbit. Invest Ophthalmol Vis Sci 22:292–302.

Freund KB, Yannuzzi LA, Sorenson JA. 1993. Age-related macular de-generation and choroidal neovascularization. Am J Ophthalmol 115:786–791.

Gass JDM. 1984. Serous retinal pigment epithelial detachment with a notch: a sign of occult choroidal neovascularization. Retina 4:205–220.

Glaser BM, Campochiaro PA, Davis JL Jr, Sato M. 1985. Retinal pig-ment epithelial cells release an inhibitor of neovascularization. Arch Ophthalmol 103:1870–1875.

Green WR, McDonnell PJ, Yeo JH. 1985. Pathologic features of se-nile macular degeneration. Ophthalmol 92:615–627.

Guyer DR, Puliafito CA, Mones JM, Friedman E, Chang W, Ver-dooner SR. 1992. Digital indocyanine-green angiography in chorio-retinal disorders. Ophthalmology 99:287–291.

Guyer DR, Yannuzzi LA, Slakter JS, Sorenson JA, Hope-Ross M, Or-lock DA. 1994. Digital indocyanine-green videoangiography of oc-cult choroidal neovascularization. Ophthalmology 101:1727–1737.

Guyer DR, Yannuzzi LA, Slakter JS, Sorenson JA, Hanutsaha P, Spaide RF, Schwartz SG, Hirschfeld JM, Orlock DA. 1996. Classi-fication of choroidal neovascularization by digital indocyanine green videoangiography. Ophthalmology 103:2054–2060.

Hartnett ME, Weiter JJ, Garsd A, Jalkh AE. 1992. Classification of retinal pigment epithelial detachments associated with drusen. Graefes Arch Clin Exp Ophthalmol 230:11–19.

Hayashi K, de Laey JJ. 1985. Indocyanine green videoangiography of choroidal neovascular membranes. Ophthalmologica 190:30–39.

Kuhn D, Meunier I, Soubrane G, Coscas G. 1995. Imaging of chorio-retinal anastomoses in vascularized retinal pigment epithelial de-tachments. Arch Ophthalmol 113:1392–1398.

Lewis MM, Pautler SE. 1988. Retinal pigment epithelial detachments with choroidal neovascular membranes in age-related macular de-generation: natural history versus laser photocoagulation. In: Git-ter KA, Schatz H, Yannuzzi LA, McDonald HR ed, Laser Photoco-agulation of Retinal Disease: From the International Laser Symposium of the Macula. San Francisco: Pacific Medical Press, 207–215.

Lim JI, Sternberg P Jr, Capone A Jr, Aaberg TM Sr, Gilman JP. 1995. Selective use of indocyanine green angiography for occult choroidal neovascularization. Am J Ophthalmol 120:75–82.

Marshall GE, Konstas AGP, Reid GG, Edwards JG, Lee WR. 1994. Collagens in the aged human macula. Graefe's Arch Clin Exp Oph-thalmol 232:133–140.

[MPSG] Macular Photocoagulation Study Group. 1982. Argon laser photocoagulation for senile macular degeneration: results of a ran-domized clinical trial. Arch Ophthalmol 100:912–918.

[MPSG] Macular Photocoagulation Study Group. 1990. Krypton

laser photocoagulation for neovascularized lesions of age-related macular degeneration. Arch Ophthalmol 108:816–824.

[MPSG] Macular Photocoagulation Study Group. 1991a. Argon laser photocoagulation of neovascular maculopathy. Arch Ophthalmol 109:1109–1114.

[MPSG] Macular Photocoagulation Study Group. 1991b. Subfoveal neovascular lesions in age-related macular degeneration: Guidelines for evaluation and treatment. Arch Ophthalmol 109:1242–1258.

[MMSG] Moorfields Macular Study Group. 1982. Retinal pigment epithelial detachments in the elderly: a controlled trial of argon laser photocoagulation. Br J Ophthalmol 66:1–16.

Moore DJ, Hussain AA, Marshall J. 1995. Age-related variation in the hydraulic conductivity of Bruch's membrane. Invest Ophthalmol Vis Sci 36:1290–1297.

Negi A, Marmor MF. 1983. The resorption of subretinal fluid after diffuse damage to the retinal pigment epithelium. Invest Ophthalmol Vis Sci 24:1475–1479.

Negi A, Marmor MF. 1984. Experimental serous retinal detachment and focal pigment epithelial damage. Arch Ophthalmol 102:445–449.

Negi A, Marmor MF. 1986. Quantitative estimation of metabolic transport of subretinal fluid. Invest Ophthalmol Vis Sci 27:1564–1568.

Pagliarini S, Barondes MJ, Chisholm IH, Hamilton AM, Bird AC. 1992. Detection of subpigment epithelial neovascularization in cases of retinal pigment epithelial detachments: a review of the Moorfields treatment trial. Br J Ophthalmol 76:8–10.

Pauleikhoff D, Harper CA, Marshall J, Bird AC. 1990. Aging changes in Bruch's membrane: a histochemical and morphologic study. Ophthalmol 97:171–178.

Poliner LS, Olk RJ, Burgess D, Gordon ME. 1986. Natural history of retinal pigment epithelial detachments in age-related macular degeneration. Ophthalmology 93:543–551.

Ramrattan RS, van der Schaft TL, Mooy CM, de Bruijn WC, Mulder PGH, de Jong PTVM. 1994. Morphometric analysis of Bruch's membrane, the choriocapillaris, and the choroid in aging. Invest Ophthalmol Vis Sci 35:2857–2864.

Regillo CD, Benson WE, Maguire JI, Annesley WH Jr. 1994. Indocyanine green angiography and occult choroidal neovascularization. Ophthalmology 101:280–288.

Roberts JM, Forrester JV. 1990. Factors affecting the migration and growth of endothelial cells from microvessels of bovine retina. Exp Eye Res 50:165–172.

Schatz H, Yannuzzi LA, Gitter KA. 1979. Subretinal neovascularization. In: Yannuzzi LA, Gitter KA, Schatz H, eds, The Macula: A Comprehensive Text and Atlas. Baltimore: Williams & Wilkins, 180–201.

Schwartz SG, Guyer DR, Yannuzzi LA, Slakter JS, Sorenson JA, Valentini EP, Orlock DA. 1995. Indocyanine-green videoangiography-guided laser photocoagulation of primary occult choroidal neovascularization in age-related macular degeneration. Invest Ophthalmol Vis Sci 36(suppl):186.

Schwartz SG, Guyer DR, Yannuzzi LA, Slakter JS, Sorenson JA, Valentini EP, Spaide RF, Orlock DA. 1998. Indocyanine-green-guided laser photocoagulation of primary occult choroidal neovascularization secondary to age-related macular degeneration. (In preparation.)

Slakter JS, Yannuzzi LA, Sorenson JA, Guyer DR, Ho AC, Orlock DA. 1994. A pilot study of indocyanine green videoangiography-guided laser photocoagulation of occult choroidal neovascularization in age-related macular degeneration. Arch Ophthalmol 112:465–472.

Slakter JS, Yannuzzi LA, Schneider U, Guyer DR, Sorenson JA, Spaide RF, Fisher YL, Orlock DA. 1998. Retinal choroidal anastomoses and occult choroidal neovascularization. (In preparation.)

Singerman LJ. 1988. Laser photocoagulation for choroidal neovascularization associated with pigment epithelial detachment. In: Gitter KA, Schatz H, Yannuzzi LA, McDonald HR, ed, Laser Photocoagulation of Retinal Disease: From the International Laser Symposium of the Macula. San Francisco: Pacific Medical Press, 201–205.

Singerman LJ, Stockfish JH. 1989. Natural history of subfoveal pigment epithelial detachments associated with subfoveal or unidentifiable choroidal neovascularization complicating age related macular degeneration. Graefes Arch Clin Exp Ophthalmol 227:501–507.

Weiter JJ, Jalkh AE, Smets E. 1988. Classification of retinal pigment epithelial detachments in age-related macular degeneration. In: Gitter KA, Schatz H, Yannuzzi LA, McDonald HR, ed, Laser Photocoagulation of Retinal Disease: From the International Laser Symposium of the Macula. San Francisco: Pacific Medical Press. 193–199.

Yannuzzi LA, Gitter KA, Schatz H. 1979. Detachment of the retinal pigment epithelium. In: Yannuzzi LA, Gitter KA, Schatz H, eds, The Macula: A Comprehensive Text and Atlas. Baltimore: Williams & Wilkins, 166–179.

Yannuzzi LA. 1989. Retinal pigment epithelial detachment. In: Yannuzzi LA, ed, Laser Photocoagulation of the Macula. Philadelphia: Lippincott, 49–63.

Yannuzzi LA, Sorenson J, Spaide RF, Lipson B. 1990. Idiopathic polypoidal choroidal vasculopathy. Retina 10:1–8.

Yannuzzi LA, Slakter JS, Sorenson JA, Guyer DR, Orlock DA. 1992. Digital indocyanine green videoangiography and choroidal neovascularization. Retina 12:191–223.

Yannuzzi LA, Hope-Ross M, Slakter JS, Guyer DR, Sorenson JA, Ho AC, Sperber DE, Freund KB, Orlock DA. 1994. Analysis of vascularized pigment epithelial detachments using indocyanine green videoangiography. Retina 14:99–113.

Yoon YH, Marmor MF. 1993. Retinal pigment epithelium adhesion to Bruch's membrane is weakened by hemicholinium-3 and sodium iodate. Ophthalmic Res 25:386–392.

Yuzawa M, Kawamura A, Yamaguchi C, Shouda M, Shimoji M, Matsui M. 1995. Indocyanine green videoangiographic findings in detachment of the retinal pigment epithelium. Ophthalmology 102:622–629.

37. Epidemiology of age-related retinal pigment epithelial disease

ANAT LOEWENSTEIN, NEIL M. BRESSLER, AND SUSAN B. BRESSLER

The retinal pigment epithelium (RPE) is involved in many diseases including age-related macular degeneration (AMD), the most common abnormality affecting the RPE in older people, and less common macular dystrophies that may affect younger individuals. While epidemiological data on AMD continues to accumulate each year, there is virtually no epidemiological data on other abnormalities of the RPE. Thus, the aim of this chapter is to summarize the known epidemiological data on AMD and to emphasize some epidemiological considerations on some macular dystrophies.

AGE-RELATED MACULAR DEGENERATON

AMD can be divided into two main categories: *non-neo-vascular* (also termed atrophic or dry) and *neovascular* (also termed exudative or wet). The condition also can be divided into an *early stage* (drusen, hyperpigmentation, and mottled depigmentation of the RPE), usually not associated with significant visual loss, and a *late stage* (geographic atrophy or abnormalities associated with choroidal neovascularization) usually associated with visual loss (Ferris et al., 1984). The purpose of this chapter is to describe the epidemiological features of AMD, including the definition of the disease, its prevalence and incidence, risk factors, and possible areas for future research. This epidemiological data can be useful for planning future eye services, as well as for planning intervention trials designed to evaluate preventive and treatment strategies (Mitchell et al.,1995).

AMD usually is defined as any non-neovascular abnormalities which could progress to atrophy or choroidal neovascularization (CNV), or CNV associated with these non-neovascular abnormalities (Bressler et al., 1988). This definition considers non-neovascular AMD to include certain features of drusen and pigmentary alterations of the RPE. Drusen are yellow deposits seen in the outer retina predominantly in the central macula on ophthalmoscopic examination. On histopathologic examination, drusen correspond to deposits external to the RPE and usually within Bruch's membrane. When

they are small clinically (in which the greatest linear dimension is less than 64 μm), they usually have distinct boundaries and, therefore, often are termed hard drusen. When they are larger clinically (in some studies greater than 63 μm and in other studies greater than 125 μm) they usually have indistinct borders and, therefore, often are termed *soft drusen*. Since the terms *hard drusen* and *soft drusen* have different definitions when used to describe histopathologic features, since there is a high correlation between small and hard drusen as well as between large and soft drusen, and since measuring the size of drusen may be easier than determining if the borders of drusen are distinct or indistinct, many studies only use the size of drusen but not *hard* or *soft* to describe drusen clinically.

Pigmentary abnormalities include focal areas of hyperpigmentation and depigmentation (Green and Key, 1985). Focal hyperpigmentation is caused by RPE hypertrophy and hyperplasia, while depigmentation is caused by atrophy of the RPE and choriocapillaries. When the atrophic borders are well delineated and the larger choroidal vessels are seen, the term *geographic atrophy* (GA) is applied. When the depigmentation of the RPE is mottled and its boundaries are poorly defined, then the term *nongeographic atrophy* (NGA) or *RPE degeneration* is used (Klein et al., 1992).

The neovascular form of AMD involves the ingrowth of choroidal new vessels or CNV into the sub-RPE space. Clinically, a gray to green subretinal lesion may be apparent, which might be accompanied by detachment of the RPE, subretinal fluid, subretinal hemorrhage, lipids, or cystic retinal edema. Based on the fluorescein angiographic appearance, CNV is termed *classic CNV* or *occult CNV* (MPS, 1991a). Classic CNV is an area of bright, well-demarcated hyperfluorescence first detected during the early phase of the angiogram, with leakage of dye at the boundary of the classic CNV in the mid and late phases of the angiogram (MPS, 1991b). Features of occult CNV may include (1) fibrovascular pigment epithelial detachment (PED), an irregular elevation of the RPE with well or poorly demarcated boundaries and with persistent staining or leakage of

716

fluorescein by 10 minutes; and (2) late leakage of unde-termined source, leakage in the late phase of the an-giogram, usually accompanied by stippled dots of hy-perfluorescence that do not correspond to an area of either classic CNV or a fibrovascular PED in the early or mid phase of the angiogram (MPS, 1991b). CNV is accompanied by fibrous proliferation histologically; when the fibrosis is visible clinically, the lesion often is termed a *disciform scar.*

PREVALENCE

Prevalence of AMD Based on Morphological Findings

A number of studies performed throughout the world have reported on the prevalence of AMD in different populations (Leibowitz et al., 1980; Klein and Klein, 1982; Martinez et al., 1982; Gibson et al., 1985; Wu, 1987; Jonasson and Thordason, 1987; Vinding, 1989; Bressler, 1987; Klein et al., 1992; Mitchell, 1993; Scha-chat et al., 1995; Vingerling et al., 1995; Mitchell et al., 1995). These studies have used a variety of definitions of AMD as well as different methods of clinical exami-nation and documentation. These important differences make comparisons difficult among the studies. For ex-ample, several studies have identified cases of AMD based solely on clinical examination without documen-tation or evaluation of stereoscopic photographs of the macula obtained with a standardized protocol. Clinical examination may have poor sensitivity for detecting ear-ly macular abnormalities of AMD which can be docu-mented by fundus photography (Leibowitz et al., 1980). The most reliable information on the prevalence of AMD probably can be obtained from studies which used stereoscopic color fundus photographs of the mac-ula obtained with a standardized protocol and an ob-jective, reliable system for grading those photographs for maculopathy. These studies are summarized in Table 37-1. In each of the studies listed in the table, the preva-lence of AMD is stratified into "early AMD" (drusen and abnormalities of RPE that are not expected to be as-sociated with marked central visual loss) and two fea-tures, geographic atrophy (GA) of the RPE and CNV, that usually are associated with marked central visual loss. Although all three features (early AMD, GA, and CNV) are considered to be part of the spectrum of AMD, the prevalence is listed separately because these features have a different impact on vision (GA and CNV often are associated with visual acuity of 20/200 or worse, while cases of early AMD may or may not go on to visual loss depending on whether atrophy or CNV de-velops in the remaining lifetime of these cases).

For early AMD, defined fairly similarly in all five studies listed in Table 37-1, the prevalence was strong-ly age related in four of the studies. The prevalence of any large drusen (>63 μm in size) was not age related by decade in the Rotterdam Study (Vingerling et al., 1995), although the prevalence of ten or more large drusen was age-related. Thus, despite slightly different methods of grading, and slightly different definitions used to identify early AMD, features that comprise ear-ly AMD do appear to be age related in these different populations. As discussed below, people with early AMD likely are at a higher risk of developing severe cen-tral visual loss because of the development of GA or CNV than people without early AMD (Klein et al., 1997).

The prevalence of "late AMD" (GA or CNV) is avail-able from three of the studies listed in Table 37-1. Both of the features of late AMD were age related in all three studies, and involved approximately 1% of the popula-tion in their sixties to early seventies and approximate-ly 5% to 10% of the population in their seventies and older. In general, in each decade the prevalence of CNV was higher than the prevalence of GA. In the United States, where the number of people over age 65 (ap-proximately 35 million in 1995) or over age 75 is ex-pected to at least double over the next 35 years (as the baby boomers reach these ages), the absolute number of people with GA or CNV will represent an even greater public health problem than is seen with AMD today.

Prevalence of AMD as a Cause of Visual Loss

The prevalence of visual loss associated with features of AMD in a variety of epidemiological studies indicates that AMD is the leading cause of severe, irreversible cen-tral visual loss among adults aged 65 years and older in Western countries (Hyman, 1992; Ghafour et al., 1983; Klein et al., 1991a; Sommer et al., 1991; Cooper, 1990; NAEC, 1983). In the Beaver Dam Eye Study, 57% of the participants who were legally blind (20/200 or worse in the better seeing eye) had AMD. More specifically, of the 77 eyes with CNV, 37 (48%) had a visual acuity of 20/200 or worse, and of 34 eyes with GA, 14 eyes (42%) had such a reduced visual acuity (Klein et al., 1991b; 1995). Thus, of all participants who had a visual acuity of 20/200 or worse in an eye from AMD, the decrease was associated with CNV in approximately 75% of the cases and with GA in approximately 25%. The Beaver Dam Eye Study also confirmed that participants who had features of early AMD (drusen or abnormalities of the RPE) but not GA or CNV did not have a significant decrease in visual acuity.

In the Baltimore Eye Survey (Sommer et al., 1991),

TABLE 37-1. *Prevalence of AMD from studies based on fundus photograph grading*

Study	Number	"Early AMD" * (%)	Geographic atrophy** (%)	Choroidal neovascularization/ scar (%)	Reference
Chesapeake Bay Watermen Study					
60–69 years old	163	15	0	0	Bressler, 1987
70–79 years old	94	28	3	2	
Beaver Dam Eye Study (BDES)					
65–74 years old	1249	18.0	0.2	1	Klein et al., 1992
≥75 years old	717	29.7	3.2	5.3	
Rotterdam Study					
65–74 years old	3247	51.4	0.4	0.4	Vingerling et al., 1995
75–84 years old	2301	56.0	1.3	2.4	
≥85 years old	1006	52.6	3.7	7.4	
Blue Mountains Eye Study					
55–64 years old	1142	2.6	—	—	Mitchell et al., 1995
65–74 years old	1160	8.5	—	—	
75–84 years old	569	15.5	—	—	
≥85 years old	82	28.0	—	—	
Barbados Eye Study					
60–69 years old	565	32.7	—	—	Schachat et al., 1995
70–79 years old	197	40.6	—	—	
≥80 years old	16	50.0	—	—	

*"Early AMD" was defined in the Chesapeake Bay Waterman Study and the Barbados Eye Study as the presence of large drusen (>63 μm), confluent drusen, or focal hyperpigmentation of the RPE; in the BDES as the presence of soft indistinct drusen or reticular drusen, or the presence of any drusen type (except hard indistinct) with RPE degeneration or increased retinal pigment in the macular area; in the Rotterdam Study as the presence of any intermediate size drusen; in the Blue Mountains Eye Study as either soft indistinct drusen or soft distinct drusen in the presence of any retinal pigment abnormality, or drusen between 64 and 250 μm in size.

**Data estimated from data in published figures from the studies and calculations made from figures.

the late stage of AMD was the leading cause of blindness in white participants 65 years of age and older, accounting for 16 (38%) of the 42 eyes with 20/200 or worse vision. An additional 4 (10%) of these 42 eyes had AMD in combination with cataract or primary open-angle glaucoma contributing to vision of 20/200 or worse. The prevalence of 20/200 or worse vision from AMD was age dependent, increasing to 29.1 per 1,000 participants 80 years of age or older. However, AMD was not a cause of 20/200 or worse vision among all of the black participants.

INCIDENCE

Drusen and RPE Abnormalities

The Chesapeake Bay Watermen Study was the first published report on the incidence and disappearance of drusen and RPE abnormalities, although a larger epidemiological study (the Beaver Dam Eye Study) recently confirmed this information (Klein et al., 1997). In the Chesapeake Bay Watermen Study, the appearance of large drusen, focal hyperpigmentation, or the early stage of AMD (defined as either large drusen, focal hyperpigmentation, or NGA) over a five-year follow-up period in all age groups combined was 8%, 3%, and 9%, respectively. The incidence of all of these features was found to be age-related, occurring in 5%, 1%, and 7%, respectively, of participants aged 50–59 years; 17%, 3%, and 14%, respectively, of participants aged 60–69 years; and 17%, 9%, and 26%, respectively, of participants aged 70 years or more. During this follow-up period, disappearance of large drusen, focal hyperpigmentation, and the early stage of AMD occurred in 34%, 58%, and 28%, respectively, of participants who had these features at the baseline examination. Such disappearance had been reported in non-population-based studies previously (Javornik et al., 1992; Sebag et al., 1992; Sarks, 1980; Green and Enger, 1993; Dastgheib and Green, 1994) and may be related to removal of the drusen material by macrophages or multinucleated giant cells (Dastgheib and Green, 1994). Among participants with no large drusen at baseline, those participants with numerous small drusen (<64 μm in diameter) at the baseline examination were more likely to develop new large drusen by the five-year follow-up examination. Since all of the participants were men, no data exist concerning the incidence of AMD in women. A follow-up study from the BDES recently confirmed that the incidence of age-related maculopathy significantly increased with age (Klein et al., 1997). The incidence of large drusen, soft indistinct drusen, and RPE abnormalities being 2.1%, 1.8%, 0.9%, respectively for patients 43–54 years old; and 17.6%, 16.3%, 12.9%, respectively, for participants aged 75 years or older. Both the Beaver Dam Eye Study and the Chesapeake Bay Watermen follow-up study showed that large areas of small drusen were associated with an increased risk of developing large drusen.

Geographic Atrophy or Choroidal Neovascularization

Participants with no GA or CNV in either eye. The incidence of late GA or CNV in people with the early stage of AMD in both eyes is not precisely known. Of the 483 participants in the Chesapeake Bay Watermen Study, GA did not develop in any patient; CNV developed in one participant by the five-year follow-up examination (Bressler et al., 1995). In a report from follow-up examinations of the BDES (Klein, 1995; 1977), the incidence of late ARM varied from 0% in persons 43 to 55 years old to 3.5% in those 75 years old or older at baseline. Late ARM was more likely to develop in eyes with soft indistinct drusen (6.5% vs. 0.1%) at baseline than eyes without these features. In a prospective study from a retina clinic population on 126 individuals with bilateral drusen, the incidence of CNV development over a two-year follow-up period in patients 65 years of age or older was 21.45%; that of PED 4.63%; and that of GA 7.67% (Holtz et al., 1994).

Fellow eye of individuals who have neovascular AMD in the first eye. Patients affected with CNV in one eye are at high risk of developing CNV in the other (fellow) eye. Studies investigating the incidence of CNV in these fellow eyes are summarized in Table 37-2. Many of these studies (Gass, 1973; Chandra et al., 1974; Gregor et al., 1977; Bressler et al., 1990; Yuzawa et al., 1991) were limited because they were retrospective, involved very few participants, or did not incorporate standardized protocols for annual evaluations incorporating fluorescein angiograms. These studies estimated the yearly incidence of developing neovascular AMD in the fellow eye to range from 3% to 15%. This relatively wide range of values may be explained by the differing presentations of CNV in the first eye (disciform scarring, well-demarcated CNV, poorly demarcated CNV), as well as differing proportions of patients lost to follow-up.

Some of most reliable information on the incidence of CNV in the fellow eye of someone who has CNV in the first eye can be derived from the Macular Photocoagulation Study (MPS) reports. These studies included a larger number of participants, of whom relatively few were lost to follow-up, and on whom data was collected prospectively with detailed information collected by utilizing biannual fundus photographs and annual fluorescein angiography. In one MPS report, during a five-year follow-up period, CNV developed in 28% of fellow eyes that originally had been free of any sign of CNV at baseline. This cumulative incidence rate yielded an estimated annual incidence rate of 6% per year, on average. The incidence of severe visual loss was dependent on whether the fellow eye developed CNV. By the five-year examination, eyes still free of neovascular maculopathy had lost a mean of 0.2 lines (1 letter) of visual acuity from baseline level; eyes with neovascular maculopathy at baseline had lost a mean of 1.8 lines of visual acuity by the five-year follow-up visit; eyes free of

TABLE 37-2. *Incidence of CNV in the fellow eye to an eye with CNV*

Study	Number of eyes	Incidence	Reference
Gass et al.	91	34%/48 months	Gass, 1973
Chandra et al.	36	36%/22 months	Chandra et al., 1974
Gregor et al.	104	12%/12 months	Gregor, 1973
Strahlman et al.	84	11%/27 months	Strahlman et al., 1983
Bressler et al.	127	13%/12 months	Bressler et al., 1990
		22%/24 months	
		29%/36 months	
Yuzawa et al.	183	10.4%/52 months	Yuzawa et al., 1991
MPS, 1993	228	26%/60 months	MPS Group, 1993
MPS, 1997	670	35%/60 months	MPS Group, 1997

neovascular maculopathy at baseline in which neovascular maculopathy developed during follow-up had lost a mean of 9.1 lines of visual acuity (MPS, 1995).

RISK FACTORS

Numerous potential risk factors for the development of AMD have been studied, including environmental factors, nutritional factors, gender, ocular features (refractive error, iris color, cataract, macular abnormalities), and others. From population-based studies (Klein, 1991b; 1992; Goldberg et al., 1988; Taylor et al., 1992; West et al., 1989), case control studies (Blumenkranz et al., 1986; EDCCSG, 1992; 1993), and interventional trials (Bressler et al., 1990; MPS, 1997), the risk factors can be divided into those which suggest (Table 37-3) and those which do not readily suggest (Table 37-4) the possibility of intervention.

Features that Suggest an Intervention

Light exposure. It has been theorized that light may lead to the generation of activated forms of oxygen in the outer retina and choroid, which in turn might cause lipid peroxidation of the photoreceptor outer segment membranes (Young, 1988). Short-term exposures to UV and blue visible light can cause retinal damage in animals, comparable with those seen in humans following

sun gazing (Ham, et al., 1982; Tso, 1989; Ewald and Ritchey, 1970). The long-term changes induced in laboratory animals by exposure to visible light have limited similarities to changes seen in AMD. For example, the animal studies may show basal *laminar* deposits (long-spaced collagen-like fibrils between the basal lamina of the RPE cells and the inner aspect of the basement membrane of the RPE [Gottsch et al., 1993]), but not changes believed to be specific for AMD, namely basal *linear* deposits (phospholipid vesicles and electron-dense granules within the inner aspect of Bruch's membrane) (Bressler et al., 1994). In addition, the intense, short degree of light exposure used in many of these experimental studies may be different from the chronic light exposure that typically occurs in a person's lifetime. Initial data collected from the Chesapeake Bay Watermen Study found no association between carefully ascertained individual ocular exposure to UVB or two bands of UVA and AMD (West et al., 1989). This study did report significantly higher exposures to blue or visible light over the preceding twenty years among the eight individuals in the study group who had GA or neovascular AMD (Taylor et al., 1992), supporting an association between ocular exposure to visible light and an increased risk of vision-impairing AMD in a phakic population, seen only in later life. However, this latter data should be regarded with caution, given the relatively few number of eyes that had CNV or GA in this specific population at the baseline examination, the in-

TABLE 37-3. *Risk factors for AMD for which an intervention might be possible*

Risk factor	For	Reference
Left ventricular hypertrophy	AMD*	Leibowitz et al., 1980
Reduced vital capacity, history of lung infection	AMD*	Leibowitz er al., 1980
Cerebrovascular disease	AMD*	Hyman et al., 1983
Atherosclerosis	AMD*	Hyman et al., 1983
Low vitamin A and C in diet	AMD*	Klein et al., 1992
Current smoking	Non-neovascular and neovascular	Hyman, 1992; Christen et al., 1996; Seddon et al., 1996
High plasma vitamin A levels	Non-neovascular and neovascular	Hyman, 1992
Greater caloric intake	Non-neovascular and neovascular	Hyman, 1992
Exposure to blue and visible light	Non-neovascular and neovascular	Taylor, 1992
Low serum antioxidant index	Neovascular AMD	Eye Disease Case-Control Study, 1993
Diastolic blood pressure >95	Neovascular AMD	Hyman, 1992
Antihypertensive medications	Neovascular AMD	Hyman, 1992
Low serum carotenoids	Neovascular AMD	Eye Disease Case-Control Study, 1993
High serum cholesterol	Neovascular AMD	Eye Disease Case-Control Study, 1993
No vitamin C supplementation	Early and late age-related maculopathy	Mares-Perlman et al., 1995
Lycopene (carotenoid)	Early and late age-related maculopathy	Mares-Perlman et al., 1995

*AMD: not specified as to whether risk factor was for non-neovascular, neovascular, or both forms of AMD.

TABLE 37-4. *Risk factors for AMD for which an intervention might not be possible*

Risk factors	For	Reference
Age	AMD*	Maltzman, 1979; Leibowitz et al., 1980; Klein, 1992
Decreased hand grip strength	AMD*	Leibowitz et al., 1980
Hyperopia	AMD*	Leibowitz et al., 1980
Lesser education	AMD*	Leibowitz et al., 1980
Short stature	AMD*	Leibowitz et al., 1980
Greater elastotic degeneration	Neovascular AMD	Blumenkranz et al., 1986
Positive family history	Non-neovascular and neovascular	Hyman, 1992
Light iris color	Non-neovascular and neovascular	Hyman, 1992

*AMD: not specified as to whether risk factor was for non-neovascular, neovascular, or both forms of AMD.

direct methods used for calculating visible light exposure, and the lack of consistent data from other studies to support this. For example, the Beaver Dam Eye Study found a limited association between lifetime sunlight exposure and neovascular form of AMD among male participants only (Klein, 1992). The Eye Disease Case-Control Study did not show a positive association between lifetime sunlight exposure and the neovascular form of macular degeneration (EDCCS Group, 1992). Thus, there is limited and inconsistent experimental and clinical data that evaluates the theory that light exposure leads to macular degeneration. Recommending that patients reduce the exposure to reduce the development or progression of AMD may not be warranted until further investigation provides more data in this regard (Bressler and Bressler, 1995).

Antioxidants. The theory that light exposure might cause AMD led to the hypothesis that oxygen-free radicals, liberated by light exposure, could be causing the damage that results in AMD and may be inhibited from causing AMD by manipulating levels of antioxidants, such as vitamin C and E or beta-carotene in the outer retina (Young, 1988; Goodman, 1984). According to this theory, oral ingestion of megadoses of micronutrients and minerals might deliver increased tissue levels of substances with antioxidant capabilities at the level of the outer retina, preventing peroxidation of the photoreceptor membrane lipids. Animal studies have shown that altered levels of dietary vitamin A or E can lead to retinal degeneration (Hayes, 1972). Rats that receive dietary supplementation of vitamin C are less vulnerable to experimentally induced retinal phototoxicity (Organisciak et al., 1985). However, the level of deficiency of various antioxidants produced in these experiments is much more profound than that ever attained clinically, and the histopathological picture in the deficient animals differed from the histopathology of AMD. This

also was investigated clinically in a variety of epidemiological studies. The Baltimore Longitudinal Study on Aging performed at a geriatrics center in Baltimore (West et al., 1994) found that participants with the highest plasma levels of vitamins E and C and beta-carotene were less likely to have any evidence of AMD than participants with the lowest blood levels of these substances. Dietary intake was not evaluated in this study. Only vitamin E and the index composed of the three antioxidants showed statistical significance; furthermore, there was no evidence that micronutrient supplements were protective.

The Eye Disease Case-Control Study evaluated the relationship between antioxidants and AMD in patients with neovascular AMD, both by biochemical analysis of serum levels and detailed history of dietary consumption (EDCCS Group, 1992; Seddon et al., 1994). Both measures were taken, since each has strengths and weaknesses as an indicator of antioxidant status. Serum levels can add to an understanding of the relationship between AMD and the availability of antioxidants for two reasons. First, estimates of levels of antioxidants in the serum are based on direct measurement and, as such, are not influenced by the limited amount of information available on the levels of these compounds in foods. Second, levels of nutrients in serum better reflect the actual level of nutrients absorbed, which is quite variable for carotenoids for example, reflecting the actual amount of these substances available to the tissue (Nierenberg et al., 1991). However, serum levels tend to reflect recent nutritional intake within a few days preceding the test, and therefore may not reflect the tissue level of long-term exposure. Dietary consumption, as measured by a food-frequency questionnaire, summarizes behavior over a prolonged period of time, and therefore is less subject to transient fluctuations. In the Eye Disease Case-Control Study, it was found that individuals with higher serum levels of various carotenoids or with greater dietary consumption of carotenoid-containing food sources were significantly less likely to have neovascular AMD (EDCCS Group, 1993; Seddon, 1994). High vitamin C consumption also was associated with a marginal reduction in disease risk. Serum levels of vitamin E and C, and dietary intake of vitamin E were not associated with the presence or absence of neovascular AMD (Seddon et al., 1994).

In a recently published nested case-control study within the population-based cohort of the 4926 participants of the Beaver Dam Eye Study (Mares-Perlman et al., 1995), the average levels of individual carotenoids were similar in cases and controls. Patients with either soft drusen or GA or CNV were less likely than controls to use supplements containing vitamin C, vitamin E, or zinc, although this finding was statistically significant only for vitamin C. Average levels of vitamin E (alphatocopherol) were significantly lower in cases than in controls. However, the difference was not statistically significant after controlling for levels of cholesterol in serum. Persons with levels of lycopene (the most abundant carotenoid in the serum) in the lowest quintile were twice as likely to have AMD. Levels of carotenoids that compose macular pigment (lutein and zeaxanthin) in the serum were unrelated to AMD. The investigators concluded that very low levels of only lycopene and not other dietary carotenoids or tocopherols were associated with AMD. Lower levels of vitamin E in subjects with GA or CNV than in controls might be explained by lower levels of serum lipids. These data, although suggestive of an association between increased dietary or serum levels of certain antioxidants and a decreased risk for AMD, do not necessarily translate into a causal relation. For example, people taking vitamin supplementation also might be those individuals who follow regular exercise programs and have better access to health care. Furthermore, even though the theory that antioxidants may play a protective role against the development or progression of AMD might be supported by these case-control studies, the findings have been inconsistent and conflicting with respect to specific micronutrients.

With respect to zinc, one prospective clinical trial evaluated oral zinc for the prevention of AMD progression, and found that less vision loss occurred in the patients treated with zinc than in those given a placebo. These differences diminished among subjects followed for up to 24 months. No long follow-up or details for the cause of visual loss exists in this study (Newsome, 1988). Furthermore, the Eye Disease Case Control Study found higher serum zinc levels in their patients with neovascular AMD compared with their control subjects, although the difference was not sta-

tistically significant (EDCCS Group, 1993). Thus, until results of randomized clinical trials prove that micronutrients are beneficial and clarify the risk of any long-term potential toxicity, physicians probably should be reluctant to recommend that micronutrients be used as a preventive measure for the development or progression of AMD.

Association with risk factors for cardiovascular disease. Several studies have found a positive association between risk factors for cardiovascular disease and AMD (Hyman et al., 1983; Goldberg et al., 1988; Blumenkranz et al., 1985; Delaney et al., 1982) and others have not (EDCCS Group, 1992; Malzman et al., 1979; Kahn et al., 1977; Klein et al., 1993). As mentioned below, definite systemic hypertension increased the estimated five-year incidence rate to develop CNV in the fellow eye of a patient who had CNV in one eye (MPS, 1997). Regardless of the inconsistencies, interventions aimed at lessening these risk factors might be appropriate; AMD might be just an additional health reason to treat high blood pressure and other cardiovascular disease or risk factors associated with this condition.

Smoking. Several studies have found a positive association between cigarette smoking and AMD (Hyman et al., 1983; Goldberg et al., 1988; Blumenkranz et al., 1986; EDCCSG, 1992; Malzman et al., 1979; Delaney et al., 1982, Kahn et al., 1977; Klein et al., 1993). This risk factor recently was confirmed by two prospective cohort studies that found cigarette smoking increased the relative risk of AMD by 2.4 and 2.46 for 25 cigarettes per day for women and men, respectively (Seddon et al., 1996; Christen et al., 1996). Past heavy smokers had a relative risk of 2.0 and 2.45 for women and men, respectively. Current smokers of less than 25 cigarettes per day did not have a significant increase in risk for AMD. Again, AMD might be an additional health reason to refrain from smoking.

Features That Do Not Readily Suggest an Intervention

Non-ocular features. Age and other risk factors not readily suggesting an intervention are listed in Table 37-4. Of note, the neovascular stage of AMD may be less prevalent among blacks than among whites. For example, in the MPS, only 0.8% of the patients were black. The percentage of blacks in other reports studying CNV due to ocular histoplasmosis or idiopathic causes also was low, reaching only 0.9% (Jampol, 1992). In the Baltimore Eye Survey, blacks had more than twice the overall age-adjusted rate of legal blindness (1.75%) as did whites (0.76%) (Tielsch, 1990). A later report presenting data on the causes of blindness and their distribution according to age showed that all AMD-related blindness was found in whites. The leading cause of blindness among blacks was cataract, followed by open-angle glaucoma (Sommer, 1991). In a retrospective review at a tertiary retinal referral center, only 1.4% of 1725 patients identified as having CNV were black, even though black patients comprised 15% of all patients seen at this center (Pieramici et al., 1994). The prevalence of neovascular AMD in blacks also was reported by Schachat and colleagues from data from a large population of persons primarily of African descent (Schachat et al., 1995). Although the early stage of AMD occurred quite frequently (28.7%) in older individuals of this population, CNV occurred in only 0.1%. Thus, although both the non-neovascular (Klein and Klein, 1982; Schachat et al., 1995; Sommer et al., 1991) and neovascular (Schachat, 1995, Pieramici, 1994) forms of AMD occur in black patients, the non-neovascular features may be similarly prevalent in blacks and whites, while the neovascular form of AMD may be rarer in blacks than whites.

Another risk factor which does not readily suggest an intervention is gender. In one population-based study there was no difference between men and women in the prevalence of the early stages of AMD (Mitchell et al., 1995). Another population based study reported that the prevalence of the early stages of AMD was higher in men (Vingerling et al., 1995). In the Beaver Dam Eye Study, there was no statistically significant difference in the prevalence of drusen between sexes in all age groups studied. RPE hyperpigmentation or hypopigmentation was more common in men than in women under 65 years old, but the reverse was true for men and women aged 75 years and older. In subjects aged 75 years and older, women had a significantly higher prevalence of neovascular AMD than men (6.7% vs. 2.6%) (Klein et al., 1992).

Ocular features that identify risk of fellow eye to develop CNV. Several retrospective studies found that large drusen, confluence of drusen, and focal hyperpigmentation were associated with an increased risk of developing CNV (Smiddy and Fine, 1984; Bressler et al., 1988b; Gragoudas et al., 1976). These findings were confirmed by a prospective study of participants in the Macular Photocoagulation Study (Bressler et al., 1990), in whom one eye had an extrafoveal CNV and the fellow eye had no CNV at the time of enrollment. Twenty-eight percent developed CNV within five years. Only 10% of fellow eyes with no large drusen or focal hyperpigmentation developed CNV during follow-up, whereas 58% of fellow eyes with both large drusen and RPE hyperpigmen-

tation developed CNV. Only 18 eyes had GA in the fellow eye at baseline; however, 8 of these eyes developed CNV within five years. A follow-up study of fellow eyes of eyes enrolled in the MPS trial for juxtafoveal or subfoveal CNV recently confirmed these results. In this study, 35% developed CNV within five years. The presence of five or more drusen, focal hyperpigmentation, one or more large drusen in these fellow eyes, or definite hypertension increased the risk to develop CNV in five years from 7% to 87% (MPS, 1997).

Future Research

Clarification of the role of dietary supplementation with antioxidant micronutrients or zinc for preventing the development or progression of AMD awaits further investigation through well-designed randomized clinical trials of representative populations in individuals with and without AMD. The National Institutes of Health–sponsored multicentered randomized clinical trial, the Age-Related-Eye Disease Study (AREDS), had been designed to evaluate the therapeutic risks and benefits of these agents on the rate of development and progression of AMD and age-related cataract. Besides providing us with the answer to these important questions, additional data from the BDES, AREDS, and other studies hopefully will further our understanding of the natural evolution and progression of macular degeneration.

OTHER DISEASES OF THE RETINAL PIGMENT EPITHELIUM

Other diseases of the RPE include pattern dystrophies (a group of hereditary macular dystrophies in which slowly progressive granular or reticular pigment abnormalities appear at the level of the pigment epithelium, usually in midlife), Best's disease (an autosomal dominantly inherited disease with a typical vitelliform lesion in the macula), fundus flavimaculatus (a hereditary disease in which an array of irregular ill-defined yellowish flecks at the level of the RPE is associated with macular atrophy) and a variety of other relatively rare disorders. The prevalence of these disorders is unknown; the risk factors that might be associated with variable expressivity of these dystrophies also are unknown. However, any epidemiological studies on AMD need to take into account that other RPE pathologies may masquerade for drusen and pigmentary abnormalities of AMD and may need to be excluded. Furthermore, these relatively rare RPE diseases may predispose to choroidal neovascularization, again masquerading for advanced AMD in epidemiological studies on AMD.

REFERENCES

Blumenkranz M, Russell SR, Robey MG. 1986. Risk factors in age-related maculopathy complicated by choroidal neovascularization. Ophthalmology 96:552–558.

Bressler NM, Bressler SB. 1995. Preventative ophthalmology: age-related macular degeneration. Ophthalmology. 102:1206–1211.

Bressler NM, Bressler SB, West SK, Fine SL, Taylor HR. 1987. The grading and prevalence of macular degeneration in Chesapeake watermen. Arch Ophthalmol 107:847–852.

Bressler NM, Bressler SB, Fine SL. 1988a. Age-related macular degeneration. Surv Ophthalmol 32:375–413.

Bressler NM, Bressler SB, Jacobson L. 1988b. Clinical characteristics of drusen in patients with exudative versus non-exudative age-related macular degeneration. Retina 8:109–114.

Bressler NM, Silva JC, Bressler SB. 1994. Clinicopathologic correlation of drusen and retinal pigment epithelial abnormalities in age-related macular degeneration. Retina 14:130–142.

Bressler NM, Munoz B, Maguire MG, Vitale SE, Schein OD, Taylor, HR, West, SK. 1995. Five-year incidence and disappearance of drusen and retinal pigment epithelial abnormalities. Arch Ophthalmol 113:301–308.

Bressler SB, Maguire MG, Bressler NM, Fine SL. 1990. Macular Photocoagulation Study Group. Relationship of drusen and abnormalities of the retinal pigment epithelium to the prognosis of neovascular macular degeneration. Arch Ophthalmol 110:1442–1447.

Chandra SR, Gragoudas ES, Friedman E, Van Burskirk EM, Klein ML. 1974. Natural history of disciform degeneration of the macula. Am J Ophthalmol 78:579–582.

Christen WG, Glynn RJ, Manson JE, Ajani UA, Buring JE. 1996. A prospective study of cigarette smoking and risk of age-related macular degeneration in men. JAMA 276:1147–1151.

Cooper R. 1990. Blind registrations in Western Australia: a five year study. Aust NZ J Ophthalmol 18:421–426.

Dastgheib K, Green WR. 1994. Granulomatous reaction in Bruch's membrane in age-related macular degeneration. Arch Ophthalmol 112:813–818.

Delaney WV Jr, Oates RP. 1982. Senile macular degeneration: a preliminary study. Ann Ophthalmol 14:21–24.

[EDCCS Group] Eye Disease Case-Control Study Group. 1992. Risk factors for neovascular age-related macular degeneration. Arch Ophthalmol 111:1701–1708.

[EDCCS Group] Eye Disease Case-Control Study Group. 1993. Antioxidant status and neovascular age-related macular degeneration. Arch Ophthalmol 111:104–109.

Ewald R, Ritchey CL. 1970. Sun gazing as the cause of foveo-macular retinitis. Am J Ophthalmol 70:491–497.

Ferris F, Fine S, Hyman L. 1984. Age-related macular degeneration and blindness due to neovascular maculopathy. Arch Ophthalmol 102:1640–1642.

Gass JDM. 1973. Drusen and disciform macular detachment and degeneration. Arch Ophthalmol 90:206–217.

Gass JDM. 1974. A clinicopathologic study of a peculiar foveomacular dystrophy. Trans Am Ophthalmol Soc 72:139–156.

Ghafour I, Allan D, Foulds W. 1983. Common causes of blindness and visual handicap in the west of Scotland. Br J Ophthalmol 67:209–213.

Gibson J, Rosenthal AR, Lavery JA. 1985. Study of the prevalence of eye disease in the elderly in an English community. Trans Ophthalmol Soc UK 104:196–203.

Goldberg J, Flowerdew G, Smith E. 1988. Factors associated with age-related macular degeneration: an analysis of data from the first National Health and Nutrition Examination Survey. Am J Epidemiol 128:700–710.

Goodman D. 1984. Vitamin A and retinoids in health and disease. N Eng J Med 310:1023–1031.

Gottsch J, Bynoe LA, Harlan JB. 1993. Light-induced deposits in Bruch's membrane of protoporphyric mice. Arch Ophthalmol 111:126–129.

Gragoudas E, Chandra SR, Friedman E, Klein ML. 1976. Disciform degeneration of the macula. Arch Ophthalmol 94:755–757.

Green W, Enger C. 1993. Age-related macular degeneration in histopathologic studies: the 1992 Lorenz E. Zimmerman Lecture. Ophthalmology 100:1519–1535.

Green W, Key SN. 1985. Pathologic features of senile macular degeneration. Ophthalmology 92:615–627.

Gregor Z, Bird AC, Chisholm LH. 1977. Senile disciform macular degeneration in the second eye. Br J Ophthalmol 61:141–147.

Ham WT Jr, Mueller HA, Ruffolo JJ Jr, Guerry D 3rd, Guerry RK. 1982. Action spectrum for retinal injury from near-ultraviolet radiation in the aphakic monkey. Am J Ophthalmol 93:299–306.

Hayes K. 1972. Retinal degeneration in monkeys induced by deficiencies of vitamin E or A. Invest Ophthalmol Vis Sci 13:499–510.

Holtz GG, Wolfensberger TJ, Bertrandt P, Bross-Jendroska M, Wells FA, Minassian DC, Chisholm IH, Bird AC. 1994. Bilateral macular drusen in age-related macular degeneration: prognosis and risk factors. Ophthalmology 101:1522–1528.

Hyman L. 1992. Epidemiology of AMD. In: Hampton G, Nelsen PT, eds. Age-Related Macular Degenerations: Principles and Practices. New York: Raven Press 1–35.

Hyman L, Lilienfeld AM, Ferris FL. 1983. Senile macular degeneration: a case-control study. Am J Epidemiol 118:213–227.

Jampol LM, Tielsch J. 1992. Race, macular degeneration, and the Macular Photocoagulation Study. Arch Ophthalmol 110:1699–1700.

Javornik N, Hiner CJ, Marsh MJ. 1992. Changes in drusen and RPE abnormalities in age-related macular degeneration. Invest Ophthalmol Vis Sci 33:1230.

Jonasson K, Thordason K. 1987. Prevalence of ocular disease and blindness in a rural area in the eastern region of Iceland during 1980 through 1984. Acta Ophthalmol 65:40–43.

Kahn H, Leibowitz HM, Ganley JP. 1977. The Framingham Eye Study. II. Association of ophthalmic pathology with single variables previously measured in the Framingham Heart Study. Am J Epidemiol 106:33–41.

Klein BEK, Klein R. 1982. Cataracts and macular degeneration in older Americans. Arch Ophthalmol 100:571–573.

Klein R, Klein BEK, Linton KLP. 1991a. The Wisconsin age-related maculopathy grading system. Ophthalmology 98:1128–1134.

Klein R, Klein BEK, Linton KLP, DeMets DL. 1991b. The Beaver Dam Eye Study: visual acuity. Ophthalmology 98:1310–1315.

Klein R, Klein BEK, Linton KLP. 1992. Prevalence of age-related maculopathy: the Beaver Dam Eye Study. Ophthalmology 99:933–943.

Klein R, Klein BEK, Frank T. 1993. The relationship of cardiovascular disease and its risk factors to age-related maculopathy: the Beaver Dam Eye Study. Ophthalmology 100:406–414.

Klein R, Wang Q, Klein BEK, Moss SE, Meuer SM. 1995. The relationship of age-related maculopathy, cataract, and glaucoma to visual acuity. Invest Ophthalmol Vis Sci 36:182–191.

Klein R, Klein BEK, Jensen SC, Meuer SM. 1997. The 5-year incidence and progression of age-related maculopathy: the Beaver Dam Eye Study. Ophthalmology 104:7–21.

Leibowitz H, Krueger DE, Maunder LR. 1980. The Framingham Eye Study Monograph: An ophthalmologic and epidemiological study of cataract, glaucoma, diabetic retinopathy, macular degeneration, and visual acuity in a general population of 2631 adults, 1973–1975. Surv Ophthalmol 24(s):335–457.

Liu I, White L, LaCroix AZ. 1989. The association of age-related macular degeneration and lens opacities in the aged. Am J Public Health 79:765–769.

Malzman V, Mulvihill MN, Greenbaum, A. 1978. Senile macular degeneration and risk factors: a case-control study. Ann Ophthalmol 88:1197–1201.

Mares-Perlman J, Bride WE, Klein R, Klein BEK, Bowem P, Stacewicz-Sapuntzkis M, Palta M. 1995. Serum antioxidants and age-related macular degeneration in a population-based case-control study. Arch Ophthalmol 113:1518–1523.

Martinez G, Cambvell AJ, Rinken J, Allan BC. 1982. Prevalence of ocular disease in a population study of subjects 65 years old and older. Am J Ophthalmol 94:181–189.

Mitchell P, Smith W, Attebo K, Want JJ. 1995. Prevalence of age-related maculopathy in Australia: the Blue Mountains Eye Study. Ophthalmology 102:1450–1460.

Mitchell R. 1993. Prevalence of age-related macular degeneration in persons aged 50 years and over resident in Australia. J Epidemiol Commun Health 47:42–45.

[MPS Group] Macular Photocoagulation Study Group. 1991a. Laser photocoagulation of subfoveal neovascular lesions in age-related macular degeneration: results of a randomized clinical trial. Arch Ophthalmol 109:1220–1231.

[MPS Group] Macular Photocoagulation Study Group. 1991b. Subfoveal neovascular lesions in age-related macular degeneration: guidelines for evaluation and treatment in the Macular Photocoagulation Study. Arch Ophthalmol 109:1242.

[MPS Group] Macular Photocoagulation Study Group. 1995. Five year follow-up of fellow eyes of patients with age-related macular degeneration and unilateral extrafoveal choroidal neovascularization. Arch Ophthalmol 111:1189–1199.

[MPS Group] Macular Photocoagulation Study Group. 1997. Risk factors for choroidal neovascularization in the second eye of patients with juxtafoveal or subfoveal choroidal neovascularization secondary to age-related macular degeneration. Arch Ophthalmol 115:741–745.

[NAEC] National Advisory Eye Council. 1983. Vision Research: A National Plan: Bethesda: Department of Health and Human Services, 198312-4 (NIH publication no 83-2469).

Newsome DA, Swarts M, Leone LC, Elston RC, Miller E. 1988. Oral zinc in macular degeneration. Arch Ophthalmol 106:192–198.

Nierenberg D, Stukel TA, Baron JA, Dain BJ, Greenberg ER. 1991. Determinants of increase in plasma concentration of beta-carotene after chronic oral supplementation. Am J Clin Nutr 53:1443–1449.

Organisciak D, Wang H, Li W, Tso MOM. 1985. The protective effect of ascorbate in retinal light damage of rats. Invest Ophthalmol Vis Sci 26:1580–1588.

Pieramici D, Bressler NM, Bressler SB, Schachat AP. 1994. Choroidal neovascularization in black patients. Arch Ophthalmol 112:1043–1046.

Rosenberg T, Faurchou S, Nielsen N. 1977. The clinical classification of maculopathies in adults. A survey. Acta Ophthalmol 55(s):3–23.

Sarks S. 1980. Drusen and their relationship to senile macular degeneration. Aust NZ J Ophthalmol 8:117–130.

Sarks S, Sarks JP. 1994. Age-related macular degeneration: atrophic form. In: Ryan SJ, Schachat AP, Murphy RB, Patz A, eds, Retina, vol 2. St Louis: Mosby 1071–1102.

Schachat A, Hyman L, Leske C, Connell AMS, Yu SY, and the Bar-

bados Eye Study Group. 1995. Features of age-related macular degeneration in a black population. Arch Ophthalmol 113:728–735.

Schatz H, McDonald HR. 1989. Atrophic macular degeneration: rate of spread of geographic atrophy and visual loss. Ophthalmology 96:1541–1544.

Sebag M, Peli E, Lahay M. 1992. Image analysis of changes in drusen area. Acta Ophthalmol 69:603–610.

Seddon JJ, Ajani UA, Sperduto RD, Hiller R, Blair N, Burton TC, Farber MD, Gragoudas ES, Haller J, Miller DT. 1994. Dietary carotenoids, vitamins A, C, and E, and advanced age-related macular degeneration. JAMA 272:1413–1420.

Seddon JM, Willett WC, Speizer FE, Hankinson SE. 1996. A prospective study of cigarette smoking in age-related macular degeneration in women. JAMA 276:1141–1146.

Smiddy W, Fine SL. 1984. Prognosis of patients with bilateral macular drusen. Ophthalmology 91:271–277.

Sommer A, Tielsch JM, Katz J. 1991. Racial differences in the cause-specific prevalence of blindness in East Baltimore. N Eng J Med 325:1412–1417.

Strahlman ER, Fine SL, Hillis A. 1983. The second eye involvement with senile macular degeneration. Arch Ophthalmol 101:1191–1193.

Taylor H, West S, Munoz B. 1992. The long term effects of visible light on the eye. Arch Ophthalmol 110:99–104.

Teeters V, Bird AC. 1973. The development of neovascularization of senile disciform macular degeneration. Am J Ophthalmol 76:1–18.

Tielsch JM, Sommer A, Witt K, Katz J, Royal RM. 1990. Blindness and visual impairment in an American urban population: the Baltimore Eye Survey. Arch Ophthalmol 108:286–290.

Tso M. 1995. Experiments on visual cells by nature and man: in search of treatment for photoreceptor degeneration. Invest Ophthalmol Vis Sci 30:2430–2454.

Vinding T. 1989. Age-related macular degeneration. Macular changes, prevalence and six ratio: an epidemiological study of 1,000 aged individuals. Acta Ophthalmol 67:60–616.

Vinding T. 1990. Visual impairment of age-related macular degeneration: an epidemiological study of 1,000 aged individuals. Acta Ophthalmol 68:162–167.

Vingerling J, Dielmans I, Hofman A. 1995. The prevalence of age-related maculopathy in the Rotterdam Study. Ophthalmology 102:205–210.

Werner J, Steele VG, Pfoff DS. 1989. Loss of human photoreceptor sensitivity associated with chronic exposure to ultraviolet radiation. Ophthalmology 96:1552–1558.

West SK, Rosenthal FS, Bressler NM. 1989. Exposure to sunlight and other risk factors for age-related macular degeneration. Arch Ophthalmol 107:875–879.

West SK, Vitale S, Hallfrisch J. 1994. Are antioxidants of supplements protective for age-related macular degeneration. Arch Ophthalmol 112:222–227.

Wu L. 1987. Study of aging macular degeneration in China. Jpn J Ophthalmol 31:349–367.

Young R. 1988. Solar radiation of age-related macular degeneration. Surv Ophthalmol 23:2525–269.

Yuzawa M, Hagita K, Egawa T. 1991. Macular lesions predisposing to senile disciform macular degeneration. Jpn J Ophthalmol 35:87–95.

Index

Page references followed by the letter *f* are for figures.
Page references followed by the letter *t* are for tables.